C0-ALU-567

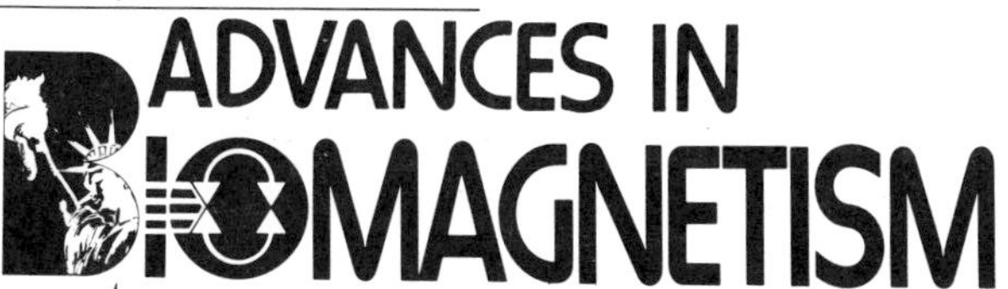
ADVANCES IN
BIOMAGNETISM

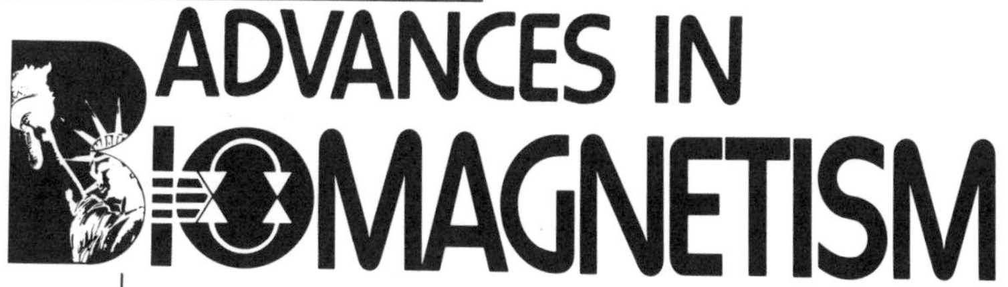

Edited by

Samuel J. Williamson
New York University
New York, New York

Manfried Hoke
Westfälische Wilhelms-Universität Münster
Münster, Federal Republic of Germany

Gerhard Stroink
Dalhousie University
Halifax, Nova Scotia, Canada

and

Makoto Kotani
Tokyo Denki University
Tokyo, Japan

PLENUM PRESS • NEW YORK AND LONDON

Library of Congress Cataloging-in-Publication Data

International Conference on Biomagnetism (7th : 1989 : New York, N.Y.)
Advances in biomagnetism / edited by Samuel J. Williamson ... [et al.].
p. cm.
"Proceedings of the Seventh International Conference on Biomagnetism, held August 1989, in New York, New York"--T.p. verso.
Includes bibliographical references.
ISBN 0-306-43483-0
1. Biomagnetism--Congresses. I. Williamson, Samuel J. II. Title.
QP82.2.M3I54 1989
612'.0142--dc20 89-49359
CIP

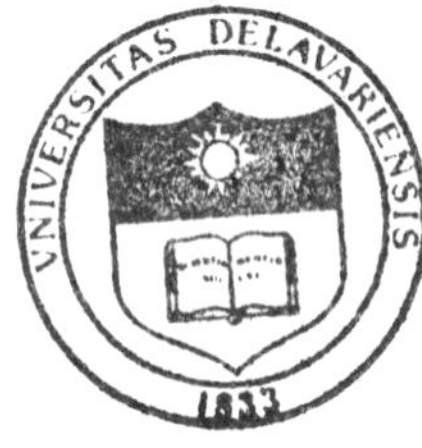

Proceedings of the Seventh International Conference on Biomagnetism, held August 13–18, 1989, in New York, New York

A Division of Plenum Publishing Corporation
233 Spring Street, New York, N.Y. 10013

Printed in the United States of America

CONFERENCE ORGANIZATION

Co-Chairmen

Lloyd Kaufman
Department of Psychology
New York University
New York City, USA

Samuel J. Williamson
Department of Physics
New York University
New York City, USA

Local Committee

Douglas Brenner
Sarah Curtis
Yael Cycowicz
Jinchu Huang
Gladys Klemic
Yoshio Okada
Urs Ribari
Carlo Salustri
Barry Schwartz
Juna Suk
Jia-Zhu Wang

Program Committee

AMERICAN SECTION

Chairman:
Prof. Gerhard Stroink
Department of Physics
Dalhousie University
Halifax, Canada

Prof. Daniel Barth
Department of Neurology
UCLA School of Medicine
Los Angeles, USA

Prof. Paulo Costa Ribeiro
Departamento da Fisica
Pontifica Universidade Catolica
Rio de Janeiro, Brazil

ASIAN SECTION

Chairman:
Prof. Makoto Kotani
Department of Electronics
Tokyo Denki University
Tokyo, Japan

Dr. Hisashi Kado
Acoustics Section
Natl. Electrotechnical Laboratory
Tsukuba, Japan

Prof. Hiroyoshi Mori
School of Medicine
The University of Tokushima
Tokushima, Japan

EUROPEAN SECTION

Chairman:
Univ.-Prof. Dr. med. Manfried Hoke
Inst. für Experimentelle Audiologie
Westfälische Wilhelms-Universität
Münster, FRG

Prof. Riccardo Fenici
1st Di Clin. Medica Generale
Università Cattolica del Sacro Cuore
Rome, Italy

Dr. Maria J. Peters
Department of Applied Physics
University of Twente
Enschede, The Netherlands

Dr. Victor Vvedensky
Kurchatov Institute of Atomic Energy
Moscow, USSR

Advisory Committee

Sponsors

Air Force Office of Scientific Research (USA)

Biomagnetic Technologies, Inc.

Office of Naval Research (USA)

Siemens AG

Yokogawa Medical Systems/GE

New York University

A Topical Conference of the American Physical Society

PREFACE

This volume celebrates the 20th anniversary of the first application of superconducting magnetic field sensors to biomagnetism by providing a comprehensive survey of advances in biomagnetic research worldwide. "Biomagnetism" is the investigation of biological processes as reflected by accompanying magnetic fields. It embraces basic and clinical research, as well as applications in medicine and occupational health. The contents of this book are the proceedings of the 7th International Conference on Biomagnetism, held from August 13 through 18, 1989, at New York University – in the heart of the Greenwich Village area of Manhattan. Topics include studies of the brain, heart, liver, lungs, muscle, tissue *in vitro*, advances in instrumentation, development of theory, and related topics.

Interdisciplinary in emphasis, this presentation begins with a set of tutorials by five outstanding professors: John Wikswo, Toivo Katila, Gian Luca Romani, Gerhard Stroink, and Stephen Swithenby. These tutorials were especially prepared to serve as an introduction for readers who are relatively new to the subject. They are followed by three presentations that mark the 20th anniversary of the first application of a SQUID sensor to biomagnetism (the acronyn SQUID is shorthand for *s*uperconducting *qu*antum *i*nterference *d*evice). Articles by James Zimmerman and Edgar Edelsack look back to the catalytic process that affected a marriage between Zimmerman's SQUID and David Cohen's magnetically shielded room. The accomplishment of these three pioneers in recording the extremely weak magnetic field of the heart with great clarity stimulated international interest in biomagnetic phenomena. Roger Koch follows this retrospective with his own prospective by describing recent dramatic advances in the development of SQUIDs that work at much higher temperatures than conventional ones. With a "high T_c SQUID" liquid helium can be replaced as a coolant by a small-scale refrigerator that cycles gaseous nitrogen. Some benefits are small size, simplicity in refrigeration, versatile configurations for sensor arrays, and reduced cost. Recent technological achievements provide substance to the prediction that the next 20 years will yield manifold advances in biomagnetic applications, perhaps even the introduction of a "personal SQUID" whose versatility would be analogous to the personal computer's.

The major emphasis of this volume are 11 invited and 172 contributed articles, which are grouped according to specialized topics. Three major advances are revealed. Most dramatic is the unveiling of newly developed large arrays of magnetic sensors – some commercial and others in research laboratories – which can sample simultaneously a field pattern from many more positions than was previously possible. They substantially speed data acquisition and provide greatly enhanced recording quality. The second advance is in techniques for deducing information about the distributed nature of underlying current patterns. To date, interest has been nearly exclusively directed toward a single localized patch of activity, for example in the heart or brain. Going hand in hand with these developments is the third advancement: graphics that begin to portray the time evolution of widespread patterns of electrical current. Thus the interplay is revealed of distributed biological activity, as in several separate regions of the brain. Emphasis in biomagnetism is advancing from the study of single, isolated events to an appreciation for the ensemble of activity.

A conference for four hundred participants can be a success only by virtue of dedicated contributions from many individuals. Selection of invited presentations and supervision of referees for all of the presentations was the responsibility of the Program Committee. Marc Hoke, Makoto Kotani, and Gerhard Stroink were Chairmen of the European, Asian, and American Sections, respectively, and are Co-Editors of this volume. They and members of the Program Committee ensured that contributions were scrutinized by at least two peer reviewers, thus setting a high standard for acceptance. Members of the Program Committee, Advisory Committee, and Organizing Committee are listed after this preface. Jia-Zhu Wang deserves special acknowledgement for helping with the editorial preparation of this volume. We wish to thank as well our many colleagues at New York University, in particular Robert Kivetz and Michelle Gaillard for invaluable administrative help and the assistance of their staffs with local arrangements; Sek Lien for his talented contributions to design and graphics of conference publications and John Yadrick for overall guidance; and especially the Neuromagnetism Group at NYU, which put heart and soul into a great effort to make this conference the acknowledged success it was.

We as Co-Chairmen wish to thank especially the six Sponsors of the conference, whose contributions were essential for attaining the highest quality for all the presentations that are set forth in this book.

Samuel J. Williamson
Lloyd Kaufman

Co-Chairmen

CONTENTS

Tutorials

Biomagnetic Sources and Their Models (*invited*) 1
J.P. Wikswo, Jr.

Principles and Applications of SQUID Sensors (*invited*) 19
T.E. Katila

Fundamentals of Neuromagnetism (*invited*) 33
G.L. Romani

Principles of Cardiomagnetism (*invited*) 47
G. Stroink

Biomagnetic Studies of Organs other than the Heart and Brain (*invited*) 57
S.J. Swithenby

20th Anniversary of the SQUID's Introduction

Evaluation of the SQUID and its Use in Biomagnetic Research (*invited*) 67
J.E. Zimmerman

A Vicennial View of SQUID Magnetocardiography (*invited*) 73
E. Edelsack

Present Status and Future of DC SQUIDs made from High T_c Superconductors (*invited*) 81
R.H. Koch, W.J. Gallagher, V. Foglietti, B. Oh, R.B. Laibowitz, G. Koren A. Gupta, and W.Y. Lee

Neuromagnetism: Auditory Evoked Responses

Activation of the Human Auditory Cortex by Various Sound Sequences: Neuromagnetic Studies (*invited*) 87
R. Hari

Selective Averaging in Auditory Evoked Magnetic Field Experiments 93
K.B. Mikkelsen, K. Saermark, J. Lebech, C.K. Bak, and E. Basar

Frequency-Specific Sources of the Auditory N19-P30-P50 Response Detected by a Multiple Source Analysis of Evoked Magnetic Fields and Potentials 97
M. Scherg, R. Hari, and M. Hämäläinen

Replicability for Localization of the P1, N1, and P2 Components of the Auditory Evoked Response in an Unselected Group of Subjects 101
S. Baumann, R. Rogers and A. Papanicolaou, and C. Saydjari

Nonstationary Dynamics of Sequential Magnetic Dipole Source Changes Associated with N100 Auditory Evoked Responses 105
R.L. Rogers, A.C. Papanicolaou, S. Baumann, C. Saydjari, and H.M. Eisenberg

Event Related Potentials and Fields Evoked by Auditory Stimuli: Effects of Interstimulus Interval and Selective Attention 109
S. Kuriki, F. Takeuchi, and M. Murase

Neural Mechanisms of Selective Auditory Attention 113
D. Arthur, S. Hillyard, E. Flynn, and A. Schmidt

Neuromagnetic Responses to Infrequent Changes in Periodicity Pitch 117
S.T. Lu, R. Hari, and M. Sams

Paired Tone Presentation Enhances Responses of Human Auditory Cortex to Rare Frequency Changes 121
J. Rif, R. Hari, and J. Tiihonen

Neuromagnetic Responses of the Human Auditory Cortex to Different Types of Deviant Stimuli 125
M. Sams, E. Kaukoranta, M. Hämäläinen, and R. Näätänen

Specificity of Neuromagnetic Responses in the Human Auditory Cortex to Consonants of Monosyllable Speech Sounds 129
S. Kuriki, M. Murase, and F. Takeuchi

Neuromagnetism: Somatomotor and Nerve Activity

Short-Latency Somatosensory Evoked Magnetic Fields Recorded over the Brachial Plexus and Cervical Spine in Man 133
G. Curio, S.N. Erné, J. Sandforth, J. Scheer, R. Stehr, and L. Trahms

Intraoperative Recording of the Magnetic Field of a Human Nerve 137
J.P. Wikswo, W.P. Henry, R.N. Friedman, A.W. Kilroy, R.S. Wijesinghe, J.M. van Egeraat, and M.A. Milek

A Comparative Study of Compound Action Potentials and Currents 141
K.W. Kim, D.J. Engle, and R.J. Sclabassi

Estimation of Both Conduction Velocities and the Number of Firing Nerve Fibers from Magnetic Fields Outside a Volume Conductor 145
S. Ueno and S. Suzuki

Source Localisation from Somatosensory Neuromagnetic Data 149
R.J-M. Grognard and A.D. Seagar

Short Latency Median Nerve Somatosensory Evoked Magnetic Fields and Electrical Potentials 153
C.L. Lim, C. Rennie, C. Yiannikas, E. Gordon, G.J. Sloggett, R.J-M. Grognard, and A.D. Seagar

On the Frontal Components of Somatosensory Scalp Responses to Median Nerve Stimulation: Neuromagnetic Demonstration of an Anterior, Midline Generator 157
P.M. Rossini, L. Narici, V. Pizzella, G.L. Romani, and R. Traversa

Spatiotemporal Modeling of Somatosensory Evoked Magnetic Fields 161
C. Baumgartner, D.S. Barth, and W.W. Sutherling

Magnetic Localization of Somatically Evoked Responses in the Human Brain 165
J. Suk, J. Cappell, U. Ribary, T. Yamamoto, and R.R. Llinás

Evoked and Spontaneous Magnetic Activity of the Human Somatosensory Cortex 169
J. Tiihonen, R. Hari, M. Kajola, and M. Hämäläinen

ECD Tracing for Middle Latencies of Neuromagnetic Responses to Right Tibial Nerve Stimulation 173
Y. Uchikawa, T. Hasegawa, M. Kotani, K. Kida, H. Yamamoto, and H. Hosaka

Neuromagnetic Localization of Sensorimotor Cortex Sources Associated with Voluntary Movements in Humans 177
D. Cheyne, R. Kristeva, W. Lang, G. Lindinger, and L. Deecke

Measurement of Neuromagnetic Fields Preceding Triggered and Self-Paced Finger Movements 181
Y. Mizutani, K. Okano, and S. Kuriki

Neuromagnetic Localization of Late Pain-Related Fields 185
R. Wakai, J. Joseph, E. Howland, M. Backonja, F. Potenti, O. Baffa, and C. Cleeland

Multi-Dimensional Vector Analysis of Evoked Responses 189
J. Suk and D. Brenner

Neuromagnetism: Visually Evoked Responses

Identification of Multiple Sources in Transient Evoked Neuromagnetic Responses 193
C.J. Aine, J.S. George, P.A. Medvick, S. Supek, E.R. Flynn, and I. Bodis-Wollner

Spatial / Temporal Resolution of Multiple Sources: Path of Activation in Human Visual Cortex 197
J.S. George, C.J. Aine, P.A. Medvick, and E.R. Flynn

A Frequency Domain Technique for Using Evoked Magnetic Fields to Test Multi-Stage Models of Sensory Processing 201
M.P. Regan and D. Regan

Ultra-High Resolution Analysis of Auditory and Visual Brain Responses Using Zoom-FFT 205
D. Regan and M.P. Regan

Neuromagnetic Measurements of Visual Responses to Chromaticity and Luminance 209
J. Krauskopf, G. Klemic, O.V. Lounasmaa, D. Travis, L. Kaufman, and S.J. Williamson

Brain Activity Related to Spatial Visual Attention 213
B. Luber, L. Kaufman, and S.J. Williamson

Temporal Variability of the Neuromagnetic Evoked Field: Implications for Human Performance Assessment 217
G.W. Lewis, L.J. Trejo, P. Naitoh, M.H. Blankenship, and M. Inlow

Crossmodal Interactions of Auditory Stimulus Presentation on the Visual Evoked Magnetic Response 221
C. Busch, G. Wilson, C. Orr, and A. Papanicolaou

Scalp Distribution of Magnetic Fields Generated by Horizontal Eye Movements and Eye Blinks 225
M.T. Oakley, G. Sullivan, S.B.W. Roeder, and E.R. Flynn

Neuromagnetism: Spontaneous Activity and Higher Functions

A Modality-Specific Neuromagnetic P3 229
J.D. Lewine, S.B.W. Roeder, M.T. Oakley, D.L. Arthur, C.J. Aine, J.S. George, and E.R. Flynn

Cortical Resource Allocation During Mental Rotation Determined by Magneto- and Electro- Encephalography 233
G.F. Wilson, C. Busch, A. Papanicolaou, C. Oliver, and C. Orr

Alpha Suppression Related to a Cognitive Task 237
B.J. Schwartz, C. Salustri, L. Kaufman, and S.J. Williamson

Visualizing and Rhyming Cause Differences in Alpha Suppression 241
L. Kaufman, M. Glanzer, Y.M, Cycowicz, and S.J. Williamson

Phase Relationships in Synchronous Magnetic and Electric Alpha Activity in the Parieto-Occipital Area of the Human Brain 245
V.L. Vvedensky, K.G. Gurtovoy, A.P. Grebenkin, S.P. Naurzakov, V.I. Ozhogin, and S.Yu. Shabanov

Distribution of Phase for Alpha Rhythm Measured by Multichannel Magnetometer over Occipital Head 249
K.G. Gurtovoy, M.J. Kajola, and V.L. Vvedensky

Coherence Analysis of Alpha Rhythm MEG Measured Simultaneously at Two Positions 253
N. Kasai, H. Kado, M. Higuchi, M. Nakanishi, K. Chinone, and M. Koyanagi

Method for Locating Sources of Human Alpha Activity 257
S.J. Williamson, J.-Z. Wang, and R.J. Ilmoniemi

Neuromagnetic Imaging of Synchronized Mu Activity 261
L. Narici, G. Iori, I. Modena, G.L. Romani, G. Torrioli, R. Traversa, and P.M. Rossini

Sleep Spindles in Magnetoencephalography and Electroencephalography 265
N. Nakasato, K. Hatanaka, K. Seki, T. Yoshimoto, and H. Kado

Neuromagnetism: Clinical Applications and Physiology

Magnetoencephalography in Epilepsy Research and Its Perspectives (*invited*) 269
M. Balish and S. Sato

Recent Developments on the Physiological Basis of Magnetoencephalography (MEG) (*invited*) 273
Y.C. Okada

Application of a Multichannel MEG-System in Temporal Lobe Epilepsy 279
H. Stefan, S. Schneider, K. Abraham-Fuchs, J. Bauer, H. Feistel, U. Neubauer, and W.J. Huk

Mapping of MEG and EEG in Normals and Epileptic Patients 283
Yu.A. Kholodov, A.M. Gorbach, V.M. Verkhlutov, R.A. Maragey, and V.A. Konyshev

Template Analysis on Interictal Neuromagnetic Data from Cases of Focal and Generalized Epilepsy 287
G.B. Ricci, S.N. Erné, C. Del Gratta, M. Peresson, V. Pizzella, G.L. Romani, and G. Torrioli

Comparison of Dynamic Spatiotemporal Field Structures of Dorsolateral Fronto-Central Seizures and Hand Sensorimotor Cortex 291
W.W. Sutherling, C. Baumgartner, T.M. Darcey, and D.S. Barth

Pre- and Postoperative Magnetoencephalography in Partial Epilepsy. A Case Story 295
A. Sabers, J. Roenager, and the Hvidovre Epilepsy Surgery Group K. Saermark, C.K. Bak, J. Lebech, and K.B. Mikkelsen

Multiple Source Modeling of the Human Epileptic Spike Complex in the Magnetoencephalogram 299
C. Baumgartner, W.W. Sutherling, S. Di, and D.S. Barth

A Method to Separate Contributions of Different Foci in Interictal Epileptic Activity 303
R. Stehr, Ch. Lefèbre, D. Janz, W. Scheuler, S.N. Erné, L. Trahms, and J. Wedemeyer

Ischemic and Epileptic Lesions Measured by AC- and DC-MEG 307
J. Vieth, G. Sack, P. Schueler, P. Grummich, and S. Schneider

Neuropathological Dynamics of Magnetic, Auditory Steady-State Responses in Alzheimer's Disease 311
U. Ribary, R.R. Llinás, A. Kluger, J. Suk, and S.H. Ferris

The Use of Flash and Pattern Evoked Fields in the Diagnosis of Alzheimer's Disease 315
R.A. Armstrong, B. Janday, A. Slaven, and G.F.A. Harding

Objective Evidence of Tinnitus in Auditory Evoked Magnetic Fields 319
M. Hoke, H. Feldman, C. Pantev, B. Lütkenhöner, K. Lehnertz, and W. Kumpf

Magnetic Observation of Spreading Cortical Depression in Anaesthetized Rabbits 323
A.R. Gardner-Medwin, N. Tepley, G.L. Barkley, J. Moran, S. Nagel-Leiby, R.T. Simkins, and K.M.A. Welch

Observation of Spreading Cortical Depression in Migraine Patients 327
N. Tepley, G.L. Barklay, J.E. Moran, R.T. Simkins, and K.M.A. Welch

Comparative Study of Transmembrane Potential and Magnetic Evoked Field Due to Applied Electric Field in the Turtle Cerebellum 331
L. Lopez, Y.C. Okada, C.Y. Chan, and C. Nicholson

Conductivity Boundaries May Produce Stronger Magnetic Fields than the Primary Source: Comparison of Three Analytical Methods 335
J.-C. Huang, Y.C. Okada, and C. Nicholson

In Vivo Neuromagnetic Study of Normal and Pathological Intracellular Current in Rat Cortex 339
S. Di, C. Baumgartner, W.W. Sutherling, and D.S. Barth

Cardiomagnetism: Cardiac Conduction and Physiology

Contribution Maps in Magnetocardiography (*invited*) 343
A. van Oosterom, T.F. Oostendorp, and G. Huiskamp

High Resolution Magnetocardiography, Source Localization and Multichannel Magnetometry 349
G. Albrecht, M. Burghoff, F. Gieβler, W. Haberkorn, and H. Nowak

Dynamic Magnetic Study of the Heart Conduction System 353
Yu. Zhuravlev, A. Lipovich, A. Matlashov, E. Godik, and Yu. Gulyaev

Evaluation of Techniques Used to Extract His-Purkinje System Spatial Distributions 357
R. Lamothe, G. Stroink, and C.J. Kafer

Magnetocardiographic Localization of a Pacing Catheter 361
R.R. Fenici, G. Melillo, A. Cappelli, C. De Luca, and M. Masselli

Magnetocardiographic Localization of Kent Bundles 365
R.R. Fenici, G. Melillo, A. Cappelli, C. De Luca, and M. Messelli

Application of a Biomagnetic Multichannel System to the Comparative Localization of Accessory Conduction Pathways in Patients with WPW Syndrome 369
K. Abraham-Fuchs, A. Weikl, S. Schneider, W. Moshage, G. Röhrlein, A. Wirth, K. Bachmann, and R. Schittenhelm

Detection of Accessory Pathway in Patients with WPW Syndrome by Means of the Isomagnetic Map and MRI 373
M. Nomura, Y. Nakaya, K. Watanebe, M. Katayama, A. Takeuchi, K. Fujino, and H. Mori

ECG and MCG Studies on the HIS-Purkinje Activity in a Case of Congenital Heart Block 377
M. Leiniö, J. Montonen, M. Mäkijärvi, K. Mäkiniemi, J. Nenonen, T. Katila, and P. Siltanen

High-Resolution Magnetocardiographic Mapping of the Pre-Excitation in Wolff-Parkinson-White Syndrome 381
M. Mäkijärvi, J. Nenonen, M. Leiniö, J. Montonen, K. Mäkiniemi, T. Schulman, T. Katila, and P. Siltanen

Analysis of High Resolution MCG Recordings of Patients with Ventricular Tachycardia 385
J. Montonen, M. Leiniö, K. Mäkiniemi, M. Mäkijärvi, J. Nenonen, T. Katila, and P. Siltanen

Detection of Magnetic Atrial Flutter Waves in Isolated Rabbit Hearts 389
P. Costa Ribeiro, A.C. Bruno, E. Parente Ribeiro, S.J. do Carmo, E. Costa Monteiro and A. Fonseca Costa

The Magnetic Field of Isolated Rabbit Heart 393
R.S. Gonnelli, G.F. Durin, A. Sanmartino, and E. Rosettani

Cardiomagnetism: Other Clinical Applications

What Does an Electrocardiologist Expect of a Magnetocardiogram? (*invited*) 397
K. Harumi, S. Mashima, H. Tsunakawa, T. Hashimoto, K. Shimizu, and G. Nishiyama

Clinical Value of Magnetoencephalographic Mapping (*invited*) 403
Y. Nakaya, H. Mori, and M. Nomura

Biomagnetic Imaging in the Cardiac Catheterization Laboratory (*invited*) 409
R.R. Fenici and G. Melillo

Detection of the Abnormal Repolarization Vector in Diabetes Mellitus by Means of the Isomagnetic Map 417
M. Nomura, K. Watanabe, M. Katayama, A. Takeuchi, K. Fujino, Y. Nakaya, and H. Mori

Magnetocardiography in Patients with the Long QT-Syndrome 421
K. Brockmeier, L. Schmitz, L. Trahms, and S.N. Erné

Measurement of Cardiac Magnetic Field Vector 425
Y. Sakauchi, H. Kado, N. Awano, N. Kasai, M. Higuchi, K. Chinone, M. Nakanishi, K. Ohwada, and S. Kariyone

Classification of Infarcts Using Electric and Magnetic Inverse Solutions 429
C. Purcell, G. Stroink, and T.J. Montague

Descrimination Between Patients with Myocardial Infarction and Those with Ventricular Tachycardia Using Magnetic and Potential Map Extrema and Trajectory Plots 433
J. Lant, G. Stroink, D. Vardy, and M.J. Gardner

Magnetocardiographic and Electrocardiographic Recordings of Patients with Ventricular Tachycardia 437
G. Stroink, D. Vardy, R. Lamothe, and M. Gardner

Atrial and Ventricular Tachycardias: Invasive Validation and Reproducibility of Magnetocardiographic Imaging 441
R.R. Fenici, G. Melillo, A. Cappelli, C. De Luca, and M. Masselli

The Influence of Heart Motion on Magnetic Fields 445
U. Tachinardi, S.S. Furuie, S. Sirota and C.P. Melo

Effect of Constitutional Variables on Magnetocardiogram 449
J. Nousiainen, O.S. Oja, and J. Malmivuo

Magnetocardiography in Patients with Cardiomyopathy and Operated Congenital Heart Disease 453
L. Schmitz, K. Brochmeier, L. Trahms, S.N. Erné

The Magnetocardiogram in Patients with Systolic and Diastolic Overload of the Right Ventricle ... 457
M. Katayama, M. Nomura, K. Watanabe, A. Takeuchi, K. Fujino, Y. Nakaya, and H. Mori

Pneumomagnetism

Magnetic Microparticles can Measure Whole-Body Clearance, Cell Organelle Motions, and Protein Polymer Viscoelasticity (*invited*) ... 461
P.A. Valberg and K.S. Zaner

Estimation of Energy of Intracellular Movement and Apparent Viscosity by Magnetometry ... 469
I. Nemoto, K. Ogura, and H. Waki

Intracellular Motility of Pulmonary Macrophages from Smokers and Non-Smokers Estimated by Cytomagnetometry ... 473
P. Gehr, M. Klauser, and V. Im Hof

Welding Fume Retention in Lungs of Previously Unexposed Subjects ... 477
M. Forsman and P. Högstedt

In Vivo SQUID Measurements of the Magnetised Human Thorax ... 481
D. Rassi, B.H. Blott, H. Al-Sewaidan, S. Davies, and C. Ni

A Study of Magnetic Contaminants in Post Mortem Lung Samples from Asbestos Miners ... 485
D. Rassi, V. Timbrell, H. Al-Sewaidan, S. Davies, O. Taikina-aho, and P. Pääkkö

Effects of Latex and Different Doses of Silica on Behavior of Iron Particles in Rabbit Lungs ... 489
Y. Aizawa, T. Takata, K. Hashimoto, M. Tominaga, H. Tatsumi, M. Kotani, and K. Chiyotani

Research on Biomagnetic Technique Used for Tracing Pneumoconiosis of Metallurgical Workers ... 493
B. Yu, K. Xiang, P. Hu, L. Li

Tissue Susceptiblity

The Hamburg Biosusceptometer for Liver Iron Quantification ... 497
D.N. Paulson, R. Engelhardt, R. Fischer, and H.C. Heinrich

The Calibration Problem in Liver Iron Susceptometry ... 501
R. Fischer, E. Eich, R. Engelhardt, H.C. Heinrich, M. Kessler, and P. Nielsen

Magnetic Mapping of DC Fields Related to Tissue Susceptibility in the Human Body ... 505
S. Di Luzio, G. Obletter, S. Comani, C. Del Gratta, and G.L. Romani

Diverse Applications

Ionic Currents Within Developing Chick Eggs ... 509
S.M. Freake, B.S. Janday, S.J. Swithenby, and I.M. Thomas

Magnetic Field Measurements of the Electric Organ of Gymnotus Carapó 513
O. Baffa, S. Lopes Côrrea, C.A. Pelá, and A. Tannus

Measurement of Magnetic Field Near An Acute Surgical Injury on the Rabbit's Thigh 517
Z. Trontelj, J. Pirnat, J. Lužnik, V. Jazbinšek, V. Valenčič, D. Križaj, L. Vodovnik, and A. Jerčinović

Biochemical Magnetite Formation and Its Application 521
T. Hamaya and K. Horikoshi

Immunosensor Using Bacterial Magnetites 525
N. Nakamura and T. Matsunaga

Localized Stimulation of the Human Cortex by Opposing Magnetic Fields 529
S. Ueno, T. Matsuda, and M. Fujiki

Modeling, Theory, and Data Processing

Volume Current Effects on MEG and Modeling (*invited*) 533
E. Ducla-Soares

Impact of Different Noise Sources on Dipole Localization in the Spherical Model: A Simulation 539
D.S. Buchanan

Monte Carlo Analysis of Localization Errors in Magnetoencephalography 543
P.A. Medvick, P.S. Lewis, C. Aine, and E.R. Flynn

A Variation Principle for the Return Current in Encephalography 547
L. Heller

Magnetoencephalographic Localization of Simulated Evoked Response Sources Affirms the Importance of Adequate Modeling 551
P.J. DeRego and A.F. Badeau

Improved Methods for MEG Inverse Dipole Estimation 555
L. Goldstein, P. Teale, and M. Reite

Influence of the Finite Pickup Coil Size on the Location of Current Sources with Quadrupolar Components 559
V. Jazbinšek, Z. Trontelj, S.N. Erné, and L. Trahms

Considerations on a Spatio-Temporal Two-Dipole Model 563
K. Lehnertz, B. Lütkenhöner, M. Hoke, and C. Pantev

Rule-Based Location of Multiple Current-Dipole Sources from Biomagnetic Data 567
N.M. Palfreyman, K.D. Singh, and S.J. Swithenby

A Linear Estimation Approach to Biomagnetic Imaging 571
W.H. Kullmann, K.D. Jandt, K. Rehm, H.A. Schlitt, W.J. Dallas, and W.E. Smith

Discussion of Biomagnetic Imaging System and Reconstruction Algorithm 575
H. Haneishi, N. Ohyama, and K. Sekihara

Direct Approach to an Inverse Problem: A Trial to Describe Signal Sources by Current Elements Distribution 579
H. Kado, S. Kashiwaya, M. Higuchi, and H. Miura

Magnetic Fields of Current Monopoles 583
A.S. Ferguson and D. Durand

Localised and Distributed Source Solutions for the Biomagnetic Inverse Problem, I 587
C.J.S. Clarke, A.A. Ioannides, and J.P.R. Bolton

Localised and Distributed Source Solutions for the Biomagnetic Inverse Problem, II 591
A.A. Ioannides, J.P.R. Bolton, R. Hasson, and C.J.S. Clarke

Random Dipoles as a Model for Spontaneous EEG and MEG Activity 595
J.C. De Munck, P.C.M. Vijn, and H. Spekreijse

Theory and Properties of Lead Field Synthesis Analysis 599
S.E. Robinson

Minimum Norm Estimation of Current Distributions in Realistic Geometries 603
C.W. Crowley, R.E. Greenblatt and I. Khalil

Localizing Abnormalities in Mapping 607
S.S. Furuie, U. Tachinardi, S. Sirota, and C.P. Melo

Preliminary Tests of MEG and EEG Localization in a Homogeneous Saline Head 611
R. Maniewski, D. Cohen, B.N. Cuffin, K. Yunokuchi, and C. Purcell

Projective Methods for the Magnetic Direct Problem 615
S.L. Gonzalez, R. Grave de Peralta, R. Biscay, J.C. Jimenez, R.D. Pascual, J. Lemagne, and P.A. Valdes

Mechanism of Flux Reversal Phenomena in Spatial Distributions of the Magnetoencephalograms 619
K. Iramina and S. Ueno

Constructing a Realistically Shaped Model of the Human Head 623
V.A. Konyshev, R.A. Maragey, Yu.A. Kholodov, V.M. Verkhlutov, and A.M. Gorbach

Compression of Biomagnetic Data by Combining Linear Predictive and Variable-Length Coding 627
B. Lütkenhöner, C. Pantev, M. Hoke, and K. Lehnertz

Interactive Control and Data Processing in Multichannel SQUID Instrumentation Systems 631
J.H. Voskamp, R. Niessen, A.J. van der Wal

Channel Capacity of Multichnnel Magnetometers 635
P.K. Kemppainen and R.J. Ilmoniemi

Instrumentation

A 24-Channel Planar Gradiometer: System Design and Analysis of Neuromagnetic Data (*invited*) 639
M.S. Hämäläinen

Improved SQUID Magnetometer with an External Feedback Circuit 645
Y. Igarashi, T. Goto, T. Hayashi, N. Fujimaki, K. Kawabe, T. Shimura, and H. Hayashi"

Designing Planar Gradiometer Arrays: Preliminary Considerations 649
A.C. Bruno and P. Costa Ribeiro

Pb-In Wire Bonding for Superconducting Connection between Thin Film DC-SQUID and Pickup Coil 653
S. Kiryu, T. Ogashiwa, K. Chinone, N. Kasai, H. Kado, N. Ishikawa, M. Nakanishi, and M. Koyanagi

A Single-Chip SQUID 657
N. Fujimaki, H. Tamura, H. Suzuki, T. Imamura, S. Hasuo, and A. Shibatomi

A Multi-Channel Biomagnetometer 661
C.N. Guy, A. Cayless, S. Walker, and K. Leedham-Green

A Nine Channel DC SQUID System for Biomagnetism 665
P. Carreli, C. Del Gratta, V. Foglietti, I. Modena, A. Pasquarelli, V. Pizzella, M. Pullano, G.L. Romani, and G. Torrioli

Development and Performance of a Multichannel System for Studies of Biomagnetic Signals of Brain and Heart 669
S. Schneider, K. Abraham-Fuchs, G. Daalmans, W. Folberth, H.E. Hoenig, H. Reichenberger, G. Röhrlein, H. Seifert, and A. Wirth

A 24-Channel Magnetometer for Brain Research 673
M. Kajola, S. Ahlfors, G.J. Ehnholm, J. Hällström, M.S. Hämäläinen, R.J. Ilmoniemi, M. Kiviranta, J. Knuutila, O.V. Lounasmaa, C.D. Tesche, and V. Vilkman

MicroSQUID: A Close-Spaced Four Channel Magnetometer 677
D.S. Buchanan, D.B. Crum, D. Cox, and J.P. Wikswo

Preliminary Measurements with MicroSQUID 681
J.P. Wikswo, R.N. Friedman, A.W. Kilroy, J.M. van Egeraat, and D.S. Buchanan

Sequential Spatially Distributed Activity of the Human Brain Detected Magnetically by CryoSQUIDs 685
G.A. Klemic, D.S. Buchanan, Y.M. Cycowicz, and S.J. Williamson

Techniques and Methodology

The LANL Gradiometer Orientation Device 689
D.B. van Hulsteyn, L. McGavran, L. Heller, J. George, P. Medvick, and E. Flynn

Magnetometer Position Indicator for Multichannel MEG 693
S. Ahlfors and R.J. Ilmoniemi

Subject and Gradiometer Positioning for MEG Recording: A Preliminary Report 697
P. Teale, J.E. Zimmerman, J. Edrich, S. Linnville, and M. Reite

The Positioning of Magnetometer Pickup Coil in Dewar by Artificial Signal Source 701
M. Higuchi, K. Chinone, N. Ishikawa, H. Kado, N. Kasai, M. Nakanishi, M. Koyanagi, and Y. Ishibashi

Neuromagnetometer® Calibration Using an Array of Small Coils 705
D.S. Buchanan and D.N. Paulson

Spatial Fourier Technique for Calibrating Gradiometers 709
A.C. Bruno, C.S. Dolce, S.D. Soares, amd P. Costa Ribeiro

On the Spatial Locating Accuracy of Multichannel Magnetometers 713
J. Knuutila and M.S. Hämäläinen

Experimental Accuracy of Localization of Current Dipoles in a Spherical Phantom 717
D.N. Paulson and D.S.Buchanan

Environmental Noise Cancellation for Biomagnetic Measurements 721
S.E. Robinson

Electronic Noise Suppression in Multichannel Neuromagnetic System 725
A. Matlashov, Yu. Zhuravlev, A. Lipovich, A. Alexandrov, E. Mazaev, V. Slobodchikov, and O. Wazhiewski

Thermal Noise of a Biomagnetic Measurement Dewar 729
J. Nenonen, T. Katila, and J. Montonen

Noise Cancellation in Biomagnetometers 733
J. Vrba, J. McCubbin, S. Lee, A.A. Fife, and M.B. Burbank

Three-Dimensional Volumetric Reconstruction for Neuromagnetic Source Localization 737
J.S. George, P.S. Jackson, D.M. Rankin, and E.R. Flynn

An Integrated Stimulus Generation and Data Acquisition System for the Investigation of Auditory Evoked Magnetic Fields 741
E. Ross, B. Lütkenhöner, M. Hoke, and C. Pantev

Study on a Design Method of a Magnetically Shielded Room by Using Models 745
K. Yamazaki, K. Unno, and K. Seino

Preparation of High-T_c Superconducting Magnetic Shields by a Low Pressure Plasma Spraying 749
K. Tachikawa, O. Tsukamoto, Y. Shimbo, K. Niki, M. Ono, M. Kabasawa, and S. Kosuge

Author Index 753

Subject Index 759

BIOMAGNETIC SOURCES AND THEIR MODELS

John P. Wikswo

Living State Physics Group
Department of Physics and Astronomy
Vanderbilt University
Nashville, TN 37235, U.S.A.

INTRODUCTION

Over the past twenty-five years, the study of biomagnetic phenomena has evolved into an interdisciplinary research effort involving individuals whose primary training has most often been in either biology, engineering, medicine, physics, or psychology. The goal of this tutorial is to present to a similarly eclectic audience the essential physics and electrophysiology required to describe the biological sources of magnetic fields, the spatial variation of these fields, and how the sources and their fields can be modeled mathematically. Introductory physics courses tend to concentrate on simple systems such as isolated electric charges in vacuum, currents flowing in circular coils, and circuits with discrete batteries, wires, and resistors. Introductory biology courses seldom address bioelectric phenomena in detail. As a result, many of us enter biomagnetism with an intuition that is ill-prepared to describe how biological cells produce currents that flow throughout an inhomogeneous body that has a complicated geometry. It is even harder to understand the spatial variation and information content of the magnetic fields associated with these currents. In complex systems such as the human heart or brain, the simple equations presented in an introductory physics course must be written in a more general form, usually involving vector or tensor calculus. Rigorous and quantitative treatment of this material can be found in several chapters in the volume edited by Williamson *et al.* (1983), in the text by Hobbie (1988), and in the review by Wikswo *et al.* (1979). Kuffler *et al.* (1984) and Macfarlane and Lawrie (1989) provide comprehensive treatments of neurophysiology and cardiac electrophysiology, respectively. In this tutorial, I will concentrate on presenting a more qualitative, pictorial approach to the subject than do any of these references. I hope that I will describe the concepts in a manner that will allow someone whose background does not span all of physics, mathematics, and biology to develop an appreciation for the interdisciplinary subtleties of the subject without the distraction of numerous equations or extensive physiological descriptions. Because of space limitations, I will not discuss how magnetic materials, either of biological origin or from contamination, can produce magnetic fields.

Since, out of necessity, this tutorial can provide only a cursory view of the subject, two messages should be emphasized at the outset: the physiological and bioelectric phenomena at play in biomagnetism are exquisitely complicated, and the physical laws that ultimately describe them are elegant in their simplicity and generality. We now will proceed to show how these physical laws can describe biomagnetic phenomena, and in doing so will attempt to develop our own intuitive grasp of the subject.

Advances in Biomagnetism
Edited by S.J. Williamson *et al.*
Plenum Press, New York

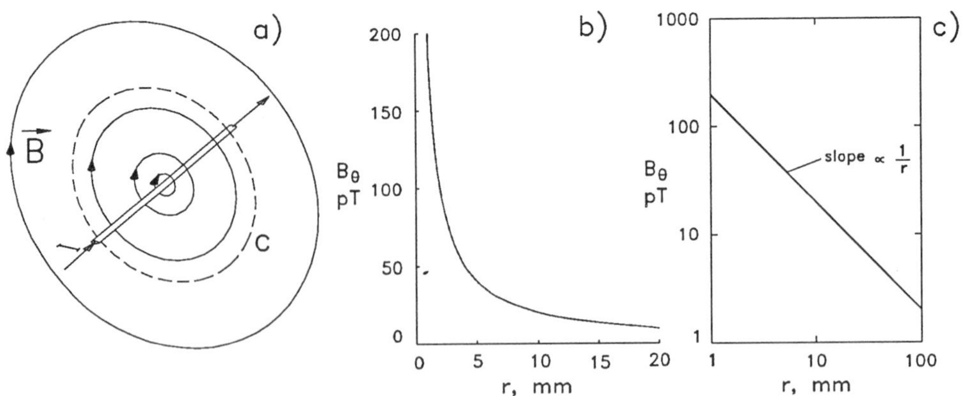

Figure 1. a) The magnetic field $\vec{B}$ produced by a current I flowing in a long, straight wire. b) Linear and c) log-log plots of the strength of the magnetic field (B_θ) encircling a wire that is carrying a 1 μA current.

SOURCES OF MAGNETIC FIELDS

As a first step toward understanding biomagnetic fields, it is useful to consider the magnetic field produced by a long wire carrying a current I. The magnetic field $\vec{B}$ from this current encircles the wire, as shown in Figure 1a. Since a magnetic field has both magnitude and direction, it is a vector quantity, which we so identify by placing an arrow above the symbol, as in $\vec{B}$. The direction (or sign) of the magnetic field encircling the wire must be chosen by mathematical convention, since the cylindrical symmetry of the problem does not provide a distinction between clockwise or counterclockwise field lines. By the right hand rule, if the extended thumb of the right hand is placed along the wire with the thumb pointing in the direction of the flow of current, the direction of the field is defined by the fingers as they wrap around the wire. The strength of the magnetic field is easily determined by Ampere's law, which, in the simple form that is applicable to our cylindrically-symmetric problem, states that the magnetic field along the closed curve c (shown in Fig. 1a by the broken circle) times the length of c is equal to a fundamental constant μ_o (the magnetic permeability of free space) times the net current threading c. Because c is threaded only by the wire, the net current is I. Ampere's law can be rearranged to yield an expression for the component of the magnetic field that is tangential to c, i.e. B_θ, at a distance r from the wire:

$$B_\theta(r) = \frac{\mu_o I}{2\pi r}, \tag{1}$$

where μ_o equals $4\pi \times 10^{-7}$ tesla-meter/ampere. In SI units, the magnetic field strength is measured in tesla. The proportionality of B_θ to $1/r$ is shown by the hyperbola in Fig. 1b and the line of slope -1 in the log-log plot in Fig. 1c. In these graphs, I is assumed to be a biologically-realistic current of 1 microampere (μA), which produces a 20 picotesla (10^{-12} T = 1 pT) magnetic field 10 mm from the wire. This field strength, less than one millionth of the 5×10^{-5} T magnetic field of the earth, would best be measured with a Superconducting QUantum Interference Device (SQUID) magnetometer.

If we take the wire in the previous example and bend it into the circle shown in Fig. 2a, the magnetic field is strengthened along the axis of the circle and is reduced outside the loop. As a result, the vertical component of the field at a distance z along the axis of a loop of radius a is given by a somewhat more complicated equation

$$B_z(z) = \frac{\mu_o I a^2}{2(a^2 + z^2)^{3/2}}. \tag{2}$$

If the loop is small in size, the field at the center of the loop is stronger than for a larger loop carrying equal current, but falls off more quickly close to the loop, as shown in Fig. 2b.

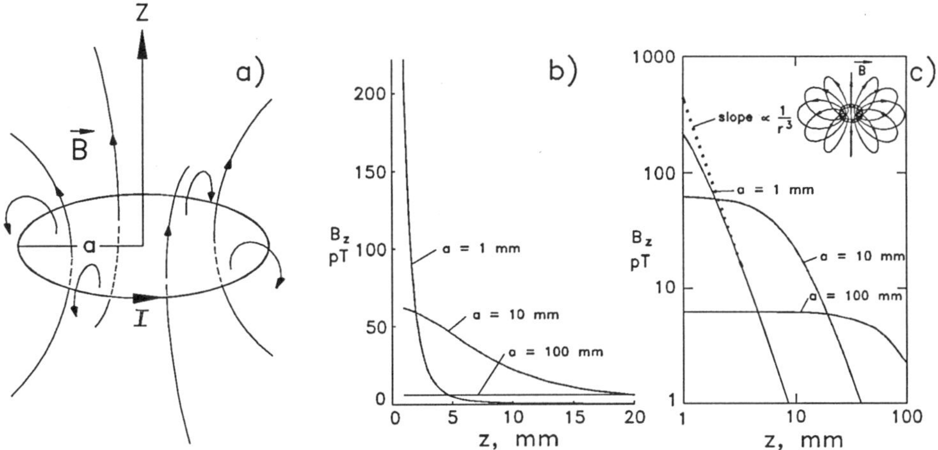

Figure 2. a) The magnetic field $\vec{B}$ produced by a current I flowing in a loop of wire of radius a. b) Linear and c) log-log plots of the strength of the magnetic field B_z along the axis of the loop, which is carrying a 1 μA current, for loops of three different radii. The inset in c) shows the dipolar magnetic field of a small current loop.

Figure 2c and Eq. (2) show that when the distance from the loop is much larger than the radius, the magnetic field falls off as $1/z^3$, independent of the size of the loop. In this far-field case, the spatial variation of the magnetic field has the pattern shown in the inset of Fig. 2c. The field is axisymmetric, comes out of the upper side of the loop, and reenters on the lower side, just as if the loop had a north pole immediately above it and a south pole immediately below. It is important to note that since isolated magnetic poles (monopoles) have not yet been found to exist, magnetic field lines must form closed curves that neither start nor stop, and hence the current loop does not really have two magnetic poles. Even so, it is useful to describe the current loop as if it were a magnetic "dipole," and hence its field pattern in Fig. 2c is "dipolar." The strength of the magnetic field is proportional to the product of the current I and the area of the loop πa^2, and this product is termed the "moment" (or strength) of the magnetic dipole.

We must now examine the sources of current that produce the magnetic field. In the simple circuit in Fig. 3a, the voltage, V, current, I, and resistance, R, obey Ohm's law, $V = IR$. If we write this as $I = V/R$, we see that for a fixed voltage, the current that flows in the circuit is inversely proportional to the resistance. As with the example in Fig. 3a, an introductory physics class is most likely to discuss magnetic fields that are produced by currents flowing in circular loops of wire. The batteries are usually kept far away from, rather than as an integral part of, the coil that produces the magnetic field. For biological systems, it would be more realistic to have both the battery, which serves as the voltage source, and the resistor, which limits the current, as integral parts of the coil, as in Fig. 3b. This figure also emphasizes the fact that the magnetic field is produced not only by the Ohmic (passive) current flowing through the wire and the resistor, but also by the electrochemically- or metabolically-driven (active) currents within the battery. Since discrete wires are seldom found in biological systems, the situation in Fig. 3c is an even better example, since the battery is placed on the surface of a container of electrically-conductive fluid such as saline, so that the current I flowing out of the positive electrode next to the resistor is dispersed into a current density $\vec{J}$ that flows throughout the saline and then returns to the negative electrode next to the battery. A current dipole is a mathematical idealization of a source for which the current flows out at one location and returns at another location that is an infinitesimal distance away. When viewed from far away, our current source looks like a current dipole whose moment q equals I times the electrode separation. If this current dipole were placed deep in a large volume of saline, its electric field would be proportional to q/r^3, where r is the distance between the dipole and the point where the field is measured. As

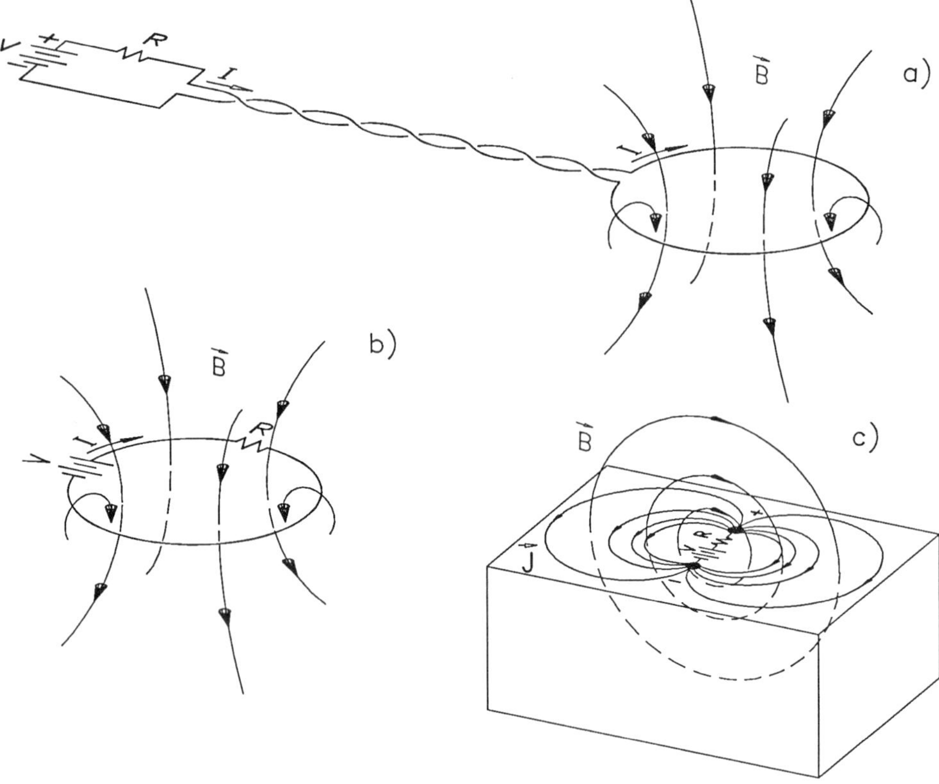

Figure 3. a) A loop of wire and its magnetic field $\vec{B}$, when the battery is far away. It follows from Ampere's law that the magnetic field from the leads connecting the battery to the loop is negligible because the leads are tightly twisted. b) A loop of wire that contains a voltage source and a current-limiting resistor. c) The current and magnetic field distributions from a current source located on the surface of a conducting bath of saline. The source can be thought of as a current dipole whose moment (i.e. strength) is the product of the spacing between the positive and negative electrodes times the current passing between them.

shown in the figure, a magnetic field encircles the *primary* current flowing within the current source. The magnetic field from this current dipole would be proportional to q/r^2. Note that for this simple source, the electric and magnetic fields are everywhere perpendicular to each other. As we will see, the current dipole is one of the most important concepts in biomagnetism, although magnetic dipoles are useful for interpreting the magnetic fields from magnetic materials in the body and also have been used to analyze the magnetocardiogram (MCG).

The calculation of the electric fields produced by current sources is a key problem in bioelectricity. By combining Ohm's law with the constraint that electric charge can neither be created nor destroyed, it is possible to show that the electric voltage V in the conductor obeys Laplace's equation, a general formula with analytical solutions for many situations. Since Laplace's equation has been well-studied by mathematicians, physicists, and engineers, there exists both an intuition and a mathematical tool kit that allows this equation and the voltage distribution it describes to be analyzed with comparative ease. A detailed knowledge of V can then be used to determine the electric current density $\vec{J}$ everywhere in the conductor.

Ampere's law, as we showed above, can be used to compute the magnetic field encircling the current source in Fig. 3c but, the net current enclosed by the imaginary curve c in Fig.

1a must now include the primary current I within the battery minus the return current $\vec{J}$ that would flow between the outside of the battery and c. This return current flows in a direction opposite to that of I and hence produces a magnetic field that partially cancels the field from the primary source I. There are several other ways to compute the magnetic field from the currents flowing in Fig. 3c. The law of Biot and Savart allows us to determine the magnetic field $\vec{B}(\vec{r})$ at the point $\vec{r}$. To do this, both the Ohmic current $\vec{J}$ returning through the saline and the primary current I within the battery and resistor are broken into small segments of current. The magnetic field produced by the entire current distribution is then computed by the vector addition of the contribution of each segment. Another approach uses a mathematical slight-of-hand to show that as long as the saline is homogeneous and has no boundaries, the summed contributions of $\vec{J}$ to $\vec{B}$ cancel themselves out, leaving only the magnetic field produced by I as it flows from the negative terminal, through the battery and resistor, and to the positive terminal. In this case, the current dipole alone appears to be the source of the magnetic field. While different mathematical operations are required in the three approaches, the results obtained are identical.

The problem of computing the magnetic field from electric current sources in conducting media is complicated by inhomogeneities. Suppose that the right-hand third of the saline bath in Fig. 3c has a conductivity that is substantially lower than that of the left-hand two-thirds. The lines of current density $\vec{J}$ would bend at the interface between these two regions, and this bending of current lines would alter the magnetic field, just as bending the wire in Fig. 1 into the loop in Fig. 2 changed the field. The actual calculation of how $\vec{J}$ is affected by the inhomogeneity can be a rather involved application of Laplace's equation, but this calculation is necessary before it is possible to determine $\vec{B}$. As always, the law of Biot and Savart can be used to compute the magnetic field $\vec{B}$ from the current density $\vec{J}$. Ampere's law is still valid, but because the symmetry of the original problem has been destroyed by the inhomogeneity, this law is of little practical value. A pedagogically-useful approach is to imagine that the saline bath remains homogeneous and extends to infinity in all directions, but that secondary current sources K are added to the bath at the locations that would correspond to the surfaces bounding the inhomogeneities. The strength of these secondary sources is adjusted to bend the current lines into the configuration that would exist in the inhomogeneous system. With this approach, the magnetic field is determined by the primary and secondary current sources and not by the Ohmic currents.

BIOLOGICAL CURRENT SOURCES

By now, we should have begun to develop an intuition regarding the relationship between electric currents and magnetic fields. In extending this discussion to examples that are more relevant to biology, we must address the problem of identifying a biological equivalent of Fig. 3b and 3c that does not utilize metal wires or electrodes or good, plastic insulators. We will first look at the current source and then turn to the necessary insulators and wires. Possibly one of the simplest sources of electric charge is a small glass sphere that is rubbed across a piece of silk so that the sphere has a net positive charge on its surface. When this sphere is in dry air (Fig. 4a), the electric field $\vec{E}$ points radially outward, just as does the hair on the head of a person who is touching the top of a high-voltage static electricity generator. This is consistent with Coulomb's law, which states that electric field lines start and stop on charges.

If we were to drop our glass sphere into a jar of electrically-conductive saline solution, the electric charge would no longer be trapped on the surface of the sphere, but could move away along the radial electric field lines, as shown in Fig. 4b. When viewed from far away, our charged sphere looks like a current monopole, i.e. a point source of current. If we modify Ohm's law to apply to continuous media rather than discrete circuit components, we find that the electric current density $\vec{J}$ equals the electric field $\vec{E}$ times the saline conductivity σ. Thus, we have radial lines of $\vec{J}$. Because of $\vec{J}$, the charge on the sphere decreases exponentially in time, so that 63% of the charge has left the sphere in an interval known as the "relaxation time." The relaxation time depends strongly upon whether the substance into

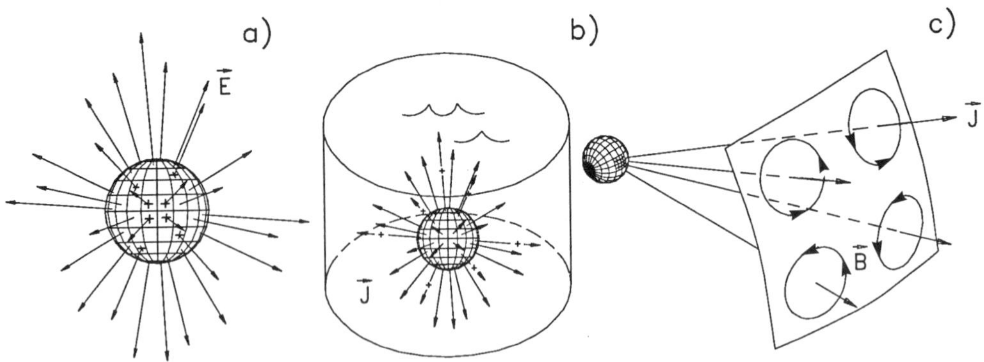

Figure 4. a) The electric field $\vec{E}$ produced by a positively-charged sphere in air. b) The electric current density $\vec{J}$ produced when the sphere in a) is immersed in saline to form a point current source. c) An illustration of how the magnetic fields $\vec{B}$ from the lines of current in b) cancel each other so that a point current source produces no magnetic field.

which the charge is placed is a conductor or an insulator. In quartz, an excellent insulator, the relaxation time is 9×10^5 s, while in copper, it is 1.5×10^{-19} s. Since the relaxation time for sea water is 2×10^{-10} s, the radial electric current produced when our charged sphere is dropped into saline will be significant for less than a billionth of a second. Because of this short time-scale, a charged object dropped into saline is not a good biological battery!

We can learn two other important points from the example in Fig. 4. First, if an object is made of saline or another reasonable conductor, free charges in such a system will distribute themselves throughout the system virtually instantaneously, at least on the time scale of the bioelectric signals we will consider. This type of argument provides the basis for the quasi-static approximation that is usually used in biomagnetic calculations. In this approximation, the bioelectric and biomagnetic fields at any instant in time can be viewed as being produced by the electric charges and currents extant at that same instant in time. Phase shifts, propagation delays, and the electric field induced by the time dependence of the biomagnetic field can all be safely ignored as long as the events considered are slow in comparison to the relaxation time. This in turn greatly simplifies the mathematics required to describe the electric and magnetic fields and their sources. As we will see later, the only significant exception to the quasi-static approximation that we need worry about relates to the electric fields across a nerve membrane, and this exception arises from the poor conductivity of nerve membrane and the ability of a nerve membrane to store electric charge. This should not be surprising when we consider that the duration of the nerve action potential and the relaxation time of nerve membrane are both about one millisecond.

Since the diffusion of electric charge through a conductor may be hard to envision, it is worthwhile to develop a simple analogy. Suppose that we pour a liter of water into a large, shallow tank. If we ignore any waves, we find that the water spreads out uniformly over the tank in a reasonably short time. Returning to our earlier definition of the quasi-static limit, we see that ignoring the waves is valid as long as we are interested in slow phenomena, such as the overall level of water in the tank. However, if we filled the tank with a dense plastic sponge, it would take much longer for the water to move to the far edges of the tank. Because the sponge has a capacity to hold water and the pores of the sponge delay the spread of the water, initially most of the water would remain close to the point where it was poured onto the sponge. Only with time would the water level in the tank reach equilibrium everywhere. Hence, external stimuli that disturb the water level in the tank might occur slowly enough to be treated as being quasi-static in a water-filled tank, but not in a water- and sponge-filled one. In most cases of interest to biomagnetism, the electrical properties of the human body are those of an oddly-shaped, saline-filled tank.

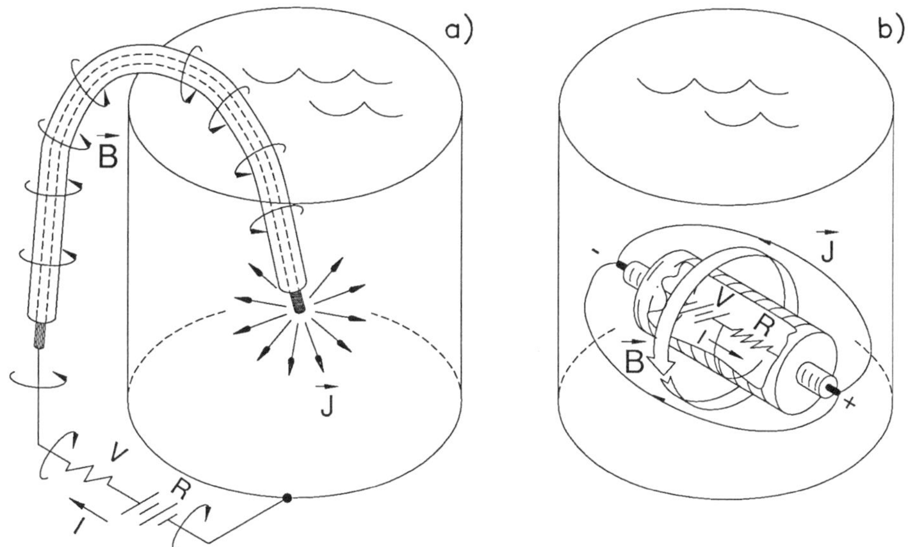

Figure 5. a) A point current source formed by the end of a wire immersed in a saline-filled metal bucket and connected to a battery. b) A self-contained current source consisting of two electrodes connected to a battery and a resistor, which are surrounded by a layer of insulation. The magnetic field, indicated by the broad arrow, encircles the source.

Our example of the charged sphere immersed in saline can also be used to demonstrate that a point source of current produces no magnetic field. Because of the spherical symmetry of the example in Fig. 4b, the current must flow radially away from our charged sphere, with the same current density in all directions. If we think of the current as flowing along the discrete lines shown in Fig. 4c, we realize that at a given distance from the source, each line of current must produce an equal magnetic field encircling the line, just as we saw in Fig. 1a. However, because each line of current has an identical line of current as a neighbor, the magnetic fields in the space between the two lines will be oppositely directed and will cancel each other out. It follows that everywhere outside the point current source the magnetic field is zero.

Our first attempt to create a biological battery was unsuccessful, so we will try another. Suppose we take an insulated wire, connect it to a battery and a resistor, and place one end in a metal bucket filled with saline, as shown in Fig. 5a. A wire connected to the bucket completes the electrical circuit, so that a steady current flows from the battery, through the resistor, along the wire, across the saline, and back to the battery. From the point of view of the electric fields in the bucket, the point current source formed by the end of the wire is almost identical to the spherical source of charge in Fig. 4. In this case, however, as charge flows away from the end of the wire and into the saline, this "lost" charge is immediately replaced by more charge provided by the battery, so that the electric field and current in the bucket do not decay quickly, but instead are steady. It is important to recognize that the spherically-symmetric current distribution outside the end of the wire produces no magnetic field, but the current flowing along the wire does. As we indicated before, when computing biomagnetic fields, it is important to include all of the electric currents that are flowing in the system. In the isolated sphere example, the stored charge had potential energy, which was dissipated as the charge flowed out into the saline. In the example in Fig. 5, electrical energy originating from the electrochemical processes within the battery is dissipated as the charge moves through both the resistor and the saline. As long as the battery is capable of providing this energy, the currents will flow. In our water analogy, in the steady state the surface of the water can be sloped only while water is being poured into the tank at one location and

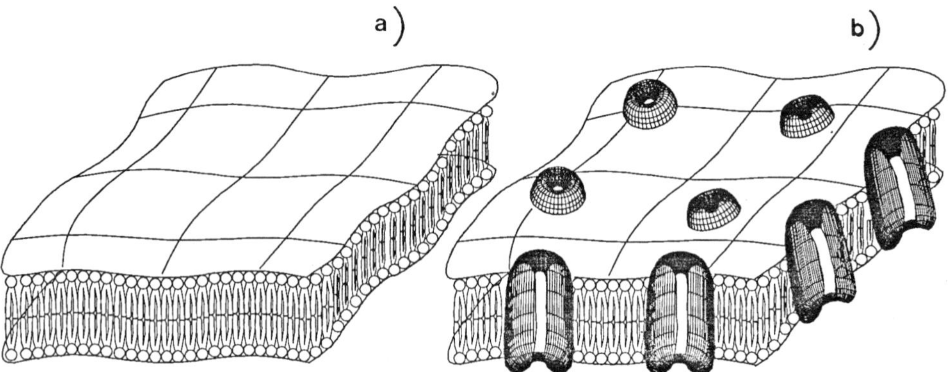

Figure 6. a) A schematic diagram of a segment of phospholipid membrane. Charged, hydrophilic head groups that are in contact with the water inside and outside the cell form the two surfaces of the membrane. Hydrophobic tails on the phospholipid molecules form the middle of the membrane and are responsible for the high electrical resistance of the membrane. b) The same membrane as a), but with ion-selective channel proteins spanning the membrane.

is drained out at another. The quasi-static limit is still valid as long as the current flow is either steady or changes slowly in comparison to the relaxation time.

The wire immersed in a bucket is not biologically realistic, but it suggests the key components for a biological battery: a source of electrical energy, and some form of an insulated conductor that allows the current to flow over a macroscopic distance without shorting itself out. Without insulation, positive and negative charges would cancel each other in the short relaxation time of less than a nanosecond. Figure 5b shows a simple system that is a reasonable approximation of many biological current sources: a voltage source, a current-limiting resistor, a layer of insulation, and a region from which current leaves the source and another at which it returns to the source. Just as in Fig. 3c, this current source looks like a current dipole whose field falls off as $1/r^3$ and has an encircling magnetic field that falls off as $1/r^2$.

In everyday life, insulating materials are made of plastic, ceramic, or glass, but none of these materials are available for constructing biological insulation. Figure 6 shows a phospholipid membrane that serves as the layer of insulation separating the inside and the outside of biological cells. The membrane is remarkably thin, less than one thousandth of the diameter of a typical nerve cell. While phospholipid is not a very good insulator in comparison to glass or quartz, it is sufficiently good that the membrane of a 1 mm long segment of 100 μm diameter nerve axon will have a resistance of 300 kilohms (kΩ), in which case a 70 mV potential difference across the membrane would result in a 0.2 μA current crossing that segment of membrane. As we will see later, the time-dependent voltages and currents in nerve and muscle cells arise not from the simple phospholipid membrane in Fig. 6a, but from the more complicated one in Fig. 6b in which the membrane is spanned by gating proteins that have time- and voltage-dependent conductances to specific ions.

THE RESTING MEMBRANE POTENTIAL

The cell membrane is a truly important component of a biological battery, since the relatively high electrical resistance of the membrane allows the inside of the cell to remain at a potential that is negative with respect to the outside. This can be observed experimentally, as illustrated in Fig. 7a. A microelectrode, made from a micropipette filled with a concentrated salt solution, can penetrate a cell membrane with minimal damage to the cell and thus can be used to measure the transmembrane potential, V_m. In typical nerve and muscle cells, V_m

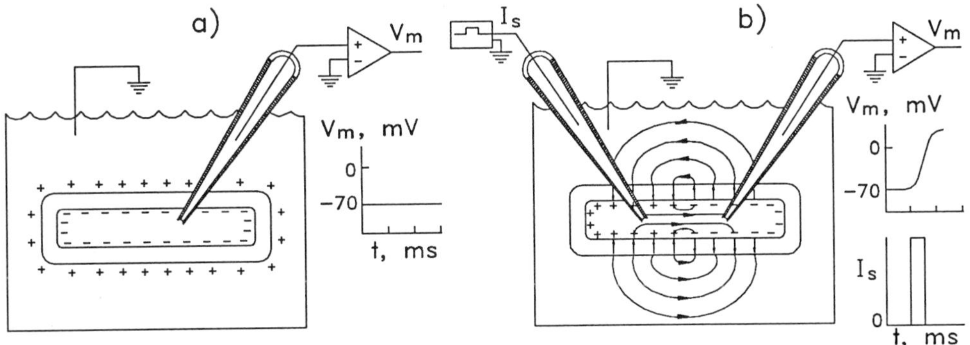

Figure 7. a) A measurement of the transmembrane resting potential using a glass microelectrode and a high-impedance amplifier. b) A measurement of an action potential initiated by an electrical stimulus I_s applied by a second microelectrode.

ranges from -70 to -90 mV. This potential difference means that there must be an excess of negative charge on the inside of the cell membrane, and an excess of positive charge on the outside. The positive and negative charges are dispersed uniformly over the outer and inner surfaces of the membrane, respectively, because like charges repel and opposite charges attract, and because charge is free to move through the relatively-good conductors formed by the intracellular and extracellular fluids, but not through the poorly-conducting membrane. Outside the resting cell, the electric fields from the two layers of charge cancel perfectly, as they do inside the cell, so that there is no electric field in either region. Within the membrane, however, the electric fields from the negative charge on the inner surface and the positive charge on the outer surface have the same magnitude and direction and hence add, producing an electric field of approximately 10^6 volts/meter inside the phospholipid. The capacity of the membrane to store electric charge arises from the fact that the opposite charges on the two surfaces of the membrane are held in place by this electric field.

A number of different mechanisms contribute to the resting transmembrane potential. Inside the cell, there is a high concentration of negatively-charged proteins that are too large to cross the membrane, but the corresponding positive counter-ions are free to cross the membrane and hence can exit the cell, leaving the inside of the cell slightly negative. Furthermore, the inside of a typical nerve or muscle cell has a high concentration of K^+ ions and a low concentration of Na^+ ions. The reverse is true for the extracellular fluid. As a result, there is a small but steady flux of Na^+ ions into the cell and of K^+ ions out. The cell must expend metabolic energy to operate a "sodium-potassium pump" that balances these ionic fluxes and maintains the cell in an electrochemical steady state. This pump in general moves 3 Na^+ ions out of the cell for every 2 K^+ that it moves into the cell, and as a result produces an electric current across the membrane that contributes to the negative transmembrane resting potential. The most important mechanism for producing V_m is the fact that the resting membrane is more permeable to some ions than to others. Each species of ion moves across the membrane at a rate that is determined both by the permeability of the membrane to the ion and by the net force on that ion. This force is the result of both the chemical concentration difference for that ion and the electric potential difference across the membrane. The steady state membrane potential occurs when all of the inward ionic currents are balanced by the outward currents. In the resting cell, the resistance of the membrane to K^+ ions (which tend to move outward) is typically 30 times smaller than to Na^+ ions (which tend to move inward). However, when V_m is at -70 mV, the net force on K^+ ions is one-thirtieth of the net force on Na^+, and as a result, the two ionic currents cancel and the cell potential remains constant in time. While there is a higher concentration of Cl^- outside of the nerve than inside, the electric potential difference across the membrane of the resting cell almost exactly balances this concentration difference, so that the chloride current is negligible at rest.

The resting membrane potential is stable against small disturbances. If a small amount of positive charge is added to the inside of a nerve cell, it will locally make the potential less negative. But this added charge will quickly diffuse away, so that in a millisecond or so, the originally-applied charge will move back across the membrane, thus allowing the membrane to return to its original potential everywhere. As a result of this, the small disturbance will be significant only within a few millimeters of the point where the charge is applied. While this passive response can be of the utmost importance in the short dendrites of the brain, it is not an acceptable method for moving information over the long distances of the peripheral nervous system. In our analogy, a drop of water applied to the surface of our sponge will not be felt very far away.

THE NERVE ACTION POTENTIAL

Although V_m is stable against small stimuli, larger ones produce a drastically-different effect. If an appropriate mechanical, chemical or electrical stimulus is applied to a nerve or muscle cell, it will induce a conformational change in the gating proteins that span the membrane, as in Fig. 6b. These proteins have an axial channel that will allow certain ions to pass through the protein (and hence across the membrane) when the protein is in one configuration but not when it is in another configuration. Earlier, we showed that the electric field in a resting membrane can be very strong; changes in this strong electric field can produce a conformational change in a gating protein. As shown in Fig. 7b, a second microelectrode can be connected to an electric pulse generator (i.e. a stimulator) so as to inject positive charge into the cell. For this example cell, when the stimulus raises V_m to –50 mV, which is above the stimulation threshold, the reduction in the membrane electric field triggers a conformational change in the sodium-channel protein, causing the permeability of the membrane to Na^+ to suddenly increase by two orders of magnitude. This results in a large influx of Na^+ ions, and V_m rises to +40 mV. That region of the cell is then termed "depolarized." In Fig. 7b, the inside of the cell is depolarized (positive) near the stimulating electrode, but is still negative at the opposite end. Because of the potential gradient along the axis of the cell, intracellular positive charge moves to the right, the transmembrane potential in the middle of the cell increases to –50 mV, and as a result the membrane in the middle of the cell becomes more permeable to Na^+. The right-ward flowing intracellular current continues, the region of high-sodium permeability also moves to the right, and eventually the right-most regions of the cell become positive. But here we see the fundamental aspects of the biological battery we have been searching for: when viewed from the outside, the outer surface of the cell is positive at the right end and negative on the left end. Inside the cell, electric current flows from left to right, and outside the cell, the current returns in the opposite direction. The inside and outside of the current source are separated by a layer of insulation. The similarity with Fig. 5b is perfect, except that for peripheral nerves, the current source moves along the nerve.

After a nerve cell has been stimulated, it is necessary to reset the transmembrane potential in preparation for a second stimulus, unless the animal you are constructing needs to "take only a single step." The cell is reset in two ways. First, the sudden increase in sodium permeability, which lasts for only a millisecond, is immediately followed by a decrease in sodium permeability. However, the inside of the depolarized cell still has an excess of positive charge, and decreasing the sodium permeability does little to reduce this. A transient increase in potassium permeability allows sufficient K^+ to leave the cell to return V_m to its resting value, or even to a slightly more negative value. The net effect of the depolarizing, inward Na^+ current and the repolarizing, outward K^+ current is to return the cell to its resting potential, but with a small chemical imbalance, which is subsequently corrected by the sodium-potassium pump.

THE PROPAGATING ACTION POTENTIAL

Figure 8 shows a rather simplified motor neuron as well as circuits that explain how the action potential propagates along the axon. The axon in Fig. 8a is a tube of phospholipid membrane filled with a saline medium, and thus serves as our insulated conductor. As we

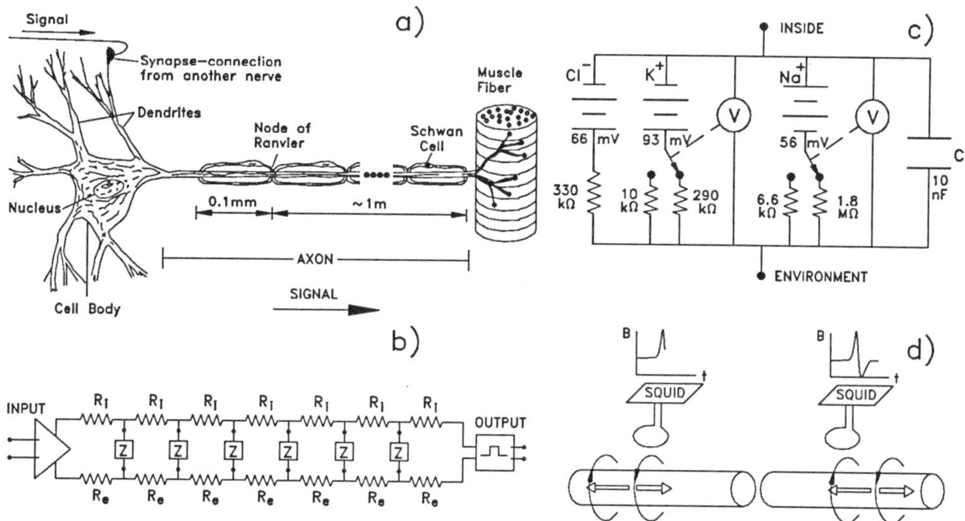

Figure 8. a) A motor neuron that connects a neuron from the brain to a muscle fiber. b) A schematic representation of a motor neuron, with the input amplifier connected to the output stimulator by an electrical cable consisting of an intracellular resistance R_i, an extracellular resistance R_e, and a membrane element Z. c) An overly-simplified circuit for Z that exhibits the voltage-dependent changes in sodium and potassium conductance associated with a nerve action potential. The values of the components correspond to a 1 mm by 1 mm patch of membrane. A more realistic model would replace each voltmeter, switch, and pair of resistors with a continuously-variable, time- and voltage-dependent resistor. d) The action current and magnetic field distributions that move along a nerve with a propagating nerve action potential. The magnetic field is measured with a Superconducting QUantum Interference Device (SQUID) magnetometer.

discussed earlier, because the resting membrane is leaky to potassium and chloride ions, a passive voltage would be conducted only a millimeter or two before being shorted out by the leakage pathway across the membrane provided by the membrane elements Z in Fig. 8b (shown in more detail in Fig. 8c). Hence, the propagation of signals over long nerves is dependent on the large sodium and potassium currents that are triggered by a stimulus, for example from another nerve. The voltage-controlled switches and resistors in Fig. 8c represent the variable ionic permeabilities discussed above; the batteries represent the chemical concentration gradients, and C represents the capacity of a segment of the membrane for storing electric charge. Extending our water analogy, the batteries correspond to the pressures in three different supply pipes that fill the tank from the bottom, and the resistance in series with each battery corresponds to a valve that limits the flow of water in each pipe. The capacitance corresponds to the size of the tank and thus its ability to store water. Depending upon the difference between the pressure at the bottom of the tank and the pressure in a particular pipe, water can flow through the valve in either direction, either raising or lowering the water level in the tank. When this level rises, so does the pressure at the bottom of the tank, and at some point the tank pressure will exceed the pressure in one or more of the pipes and the filling will slow and eventually stop. Opening one of the valves further will change the balance of flows between the pipes and the tank, until a new water level is reached. While it might not seem practical, it would be possible to propagate a water wave down a long tank by locally adding and then removing water from the tank by means of the successive opening and closing of valves distributed along the bottom of the tank. A nerve does just this by having ion channels distributed along its length, as shown by the boxes labeled Z in Fig. 8b.

Figure 8d shows how the depolarized region moves along the nerve, at a velocity of up to 120 m/s. It is important to recognize that the propagation velocity of a nerve is very

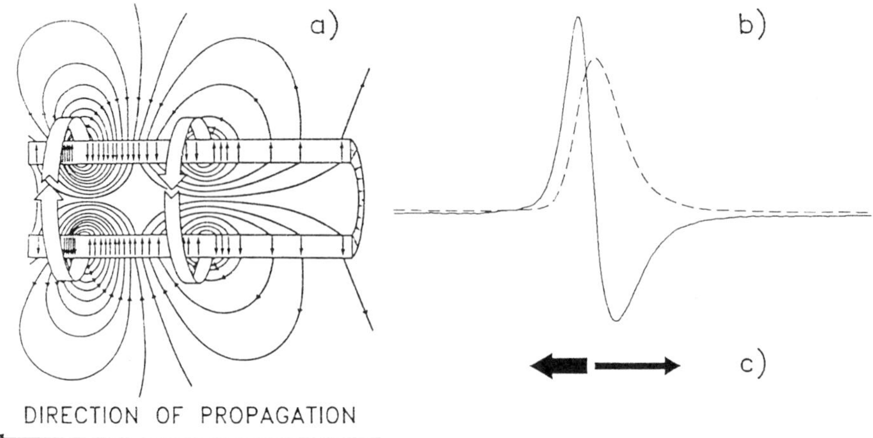

Figure 9. a) The electric current (thin arrows) and magnetic field (wide arrows) associated with a propagating nerve action potential. The thickness of the membrane is greatly exaggerated. b) The corresponding transmembrane potential (dashed) and the axial, intracellular action currents (solid). c) The depolarization (D) and repolarization (R) current dipoles consistent with a) and b).

much less than what one might expect from our earlier discussions of the quasi-static limit. In our discussion of Fig. 4b, we assumed that the conductivities were high and the capacitance (the ability of the material to store charge) was low. In situations involving cell membranes, neither of these conditions are met, and as a result, the quasi-static approximation does not apply within the membrane. This problem can be avoided, however, by treating the entire nerve as a time-dependent voltage source, just like the idealized source in Fig. 5b, in which case all electric and magnetic fields *outside of the source* are consistent with the quasi-static approximation. We already saw what adding the sponge did to our tank analogy; now try to imagine what would happen if we took a cylindrical sponge, wrapped it with a layer of plastic with small holes and many valves, and then immersed it in the tank!

BIOMAGNETIC FIELDS FROM NERVE AND MUSCLE

Now that we have described our biological battery, we need to show how this concept applies to the magnetic signals produced by various biological tissues. The electric and magnetic fields associated with the propagating nerve action potential are shown in Fig. 9a. Close to the nerve, Ampere's law indicates that the magnetic field is proportional to the intracellular action current. As a general rule, the waveform describing the axial, intracellular current closely resembles the time-derivative (i.e. the slope) of the transmembrane action potential waveform. Hence a monophasic (i.e. single polarity) action potential will produce a biphasic action current which can be detected by its biphasic magnetic field, as shown in Fig. 10a. The pair of opposing current dipoles in Fig. 9c is a good model for the source of the nerve action currents and fields. Since the magnetic field from a single current dipole decreases as $1/r^2$, it follows that the magnetic field from the opposing pair falls off as $1/r^3$. The transition from a $1/r$ fall-off close to the nerve to a $1/r^3$ fall-off far away is shown in Fig. 10b. The magnetoneurogram (MNG) from human peripheral nerves is difficult to detect from outside the body because of this rapid fall-off, even though such nerves are bundles of thousands of individual nerve fibers and carry total currents on the order of 1 μA.

Skeletal muscle fibers have electric and magnetic fields that are quite similar to those of peripheral nerve; but, since a single, small nerve fiber might activate 50 or more larger muscle fibers, muscle signals are much stronger. However, skeletal muscles have a graded response to stimuli that involves the recruitment and repeated firing of groups of fibers. While this generally results in good muscle control, it produces complicated time- and spatial-

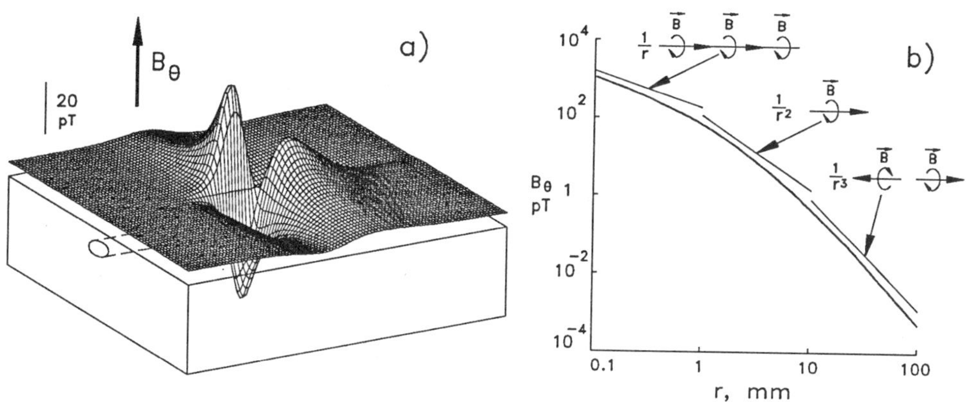

Figure 10. a) A theoretical prediction of the output of a magnetometer as it is scanned above an active nerve immersed in a conducting bath. b) A plot of the fall-off of the neuromagnetic field with distance from the nerve. Close to the surface of the nerve, the field falls off as $1/r$, as if it were produced by current in a long wire. Further away, the finite length of the depolarization or repolarization current causes the peak depolarization or repolarization field to fall off as $1/r^2$, as if the field were produced by a single current dipole. Even further away, both the depolarization and repolarization dipoles contribute to the field at the measurement point, and the field falls off as $1/r^3$, consistent with it being produced by an opposing pair of current dipoles.

dependences of the fields, which are recorded as the magnetomyogram (MMG).

The electric and magnetic fields produced by cardiac muscle are in some ways easier to understand than the fields from nerves and skeletal muscle. Unlike peripheral nerves, which are single cells of up to a meter in length, cardiac muscle is made up of a large number of individual cells, each on the order of 15 μm in diameter and 100 μm long. The intracellular spaces of adjacent cardiac cells are interconnected by a structure termed an "intercalated disk", which contains proteins that provide channels for the movement of ions between cells. Because of the electrical interconnections provided by these intercalated disks, cardiac tissue functions as if it was a syncytium, i.e. a single large cell. This is in contrast to skeletal muscle cells, which are not interconnected and can be stimulated individually. The electrical resistance of the intercalated disks results in the axial resistance of a strand of cardiac tissue being higher than that of a corresponding strand of peripheral nerve, and the propagation velocity is lower. As shown in Fig. 11a, the current and magnetic field distributions are similar to those of our original current source in Fig. 5b. However, the shape of the cardiac action potential in Fig. 11b is quite different from the nerve action potential in Fig. 9b, primarily because of a secondary inward current that brings Ca^{++} ions into the cell and maintains a long, depolarized plateau. Because the repolarization phase of the cardiac action potential is a hundred times longer than the depolarization phase, the repolarization currents are one-hundredth of the depolarization currents. As a result, the depolarization dipole is much more prominent than the repolarization one. For this reason and because of the large temporal and spatial separation of depolarization and repolarization, Fig. 11a shows only depolarization dipoles and a single loop of magnetic field. The single field maximum and the mirror-image minimum in Fig. 11c are characteristic of a single dipole current source, in contrast to the pair of current dipoles for peripheral nerve that result in the two maxima and two minima in Fig. 10a.

Our discussion of cardiac muscle has so far been limited to one-dimensional strands of tissue, such as the Purkinje fibers in the cardiac conduction system and the papillary muscle bundles within the ventricles. The vast majority of cardiac muscle, however, is a

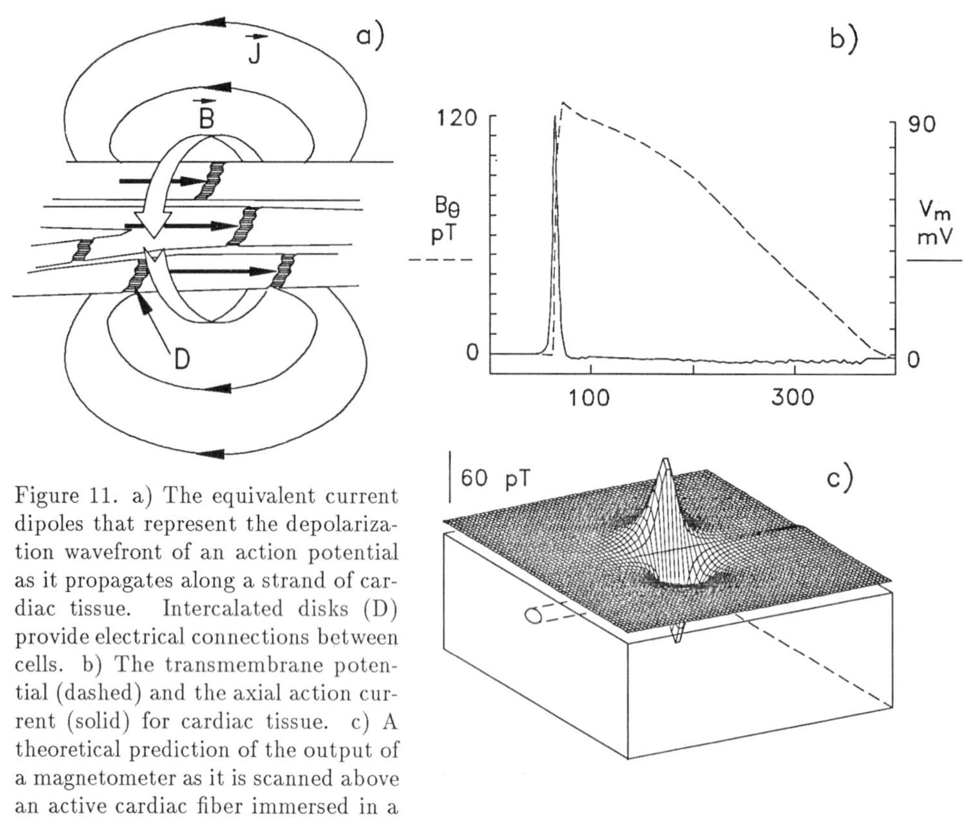

Figure 11. a) The equivalent current dipoles that represent the depolarization wavefront of an action potential as it propagates along a strand of cardiac tissue. Intercalated disks (D) provide electrical connections between cells. b) The transmembrane potential (dashed) and the axial action current (solid) for cardiac tissue. c) A theoretical prediction of the output of a magnetometer as it is scanned above an active cardiac fiber immersed in a conducting bath.

three-dimensional structure in which adjacent cells in all directions are interconnected. As a result, the depolarization wavefront in cardiac muscle is an extended surface, shown in Fig. 12a, that moves through the heart with a velocity of 1 m/s. The isolated current dipoles that we have used so far to describe our current sources are not appropriate in this case. It is better to divide the depolarization wavefront into many small segments, each of which has its own dipole. The magnetocardiogram (MCG) is determined by the sum of the magnetic fields of each segment of the wavefront. If we make the segments small enough, it is appropriate to think of the current dipole associated with each segment in terms of a current dipole density, termed the "impressed current" density $\vec{J}^i$, that is dispersed uniformly over the wavefront as is illustrated in Fig. 12b. It is worthwhile to note that it is theoretically possible for $\vec{J}^i$ to have an electrically-silent yet magnetically-detectable component that is tangential to the depolarization wavefront, but there have yet to be any conclusive experimental demonstrations that such sources exist in nature. If these sources occur, their anomalous fields may be most obvious close to the surface of the heart.

Calculations of the magnetic field from the distributed sources in the heart proceed with the same techniques we described before. We can use the law of Biot and Savart if we include the magnetic fields from both the primary, impressed current $\vec{J}^i$, and from the Ohmic return current $\vec{J}$. In cases of high symmetry, we can use Ampere's law. If the medium surrounding the heart is homogeneous, isotropic (the electrical properties are the same in all directions), and extends to infinity, then the contribution from $\vec{J}$ cancels out and only the magnetic field from $\vec{J}^i$ need be considered. In the inhomogeneous case, we can include secondary current sources $\vec{K}$ to account for the inhomogeneities.

The concepts we have presented so far can provide a rudimentary explanation of the magnetic fields of the brain, which are recorded as the magnetoencephalogram (MEG).

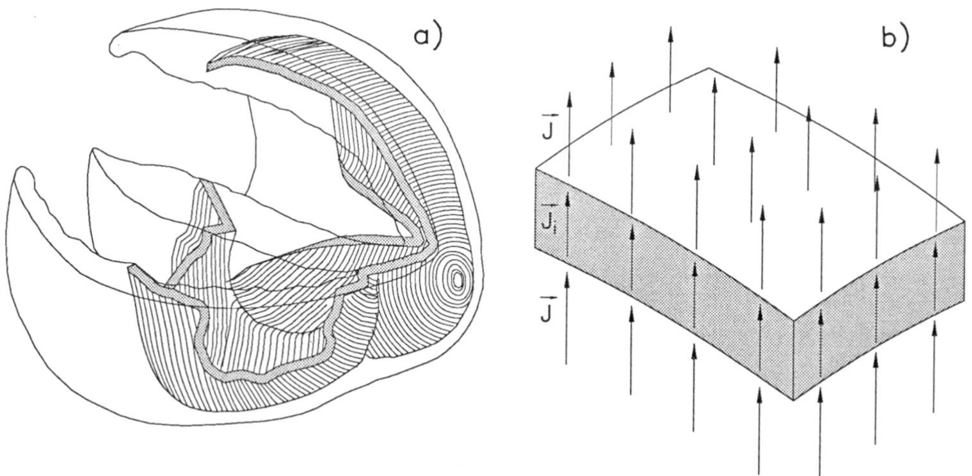

Figure 12. a) The depolarization wavefront propagating through the heart. The near chamber is the right ventricle and the far one is the left ventricle. (Adapted from a drawing by Ronald Selvester, personal communication). b) A representation of the current sources within a small segment of the wavefront in terms of an impressed current density $\vec{J^i}$, and the Ohmic current $\vec{J}$ that it produces.

Figure 13a shows a rather simplified view of the evoked field (EF) that is produced by the localized cortical response that immediately follows a sensory stimulus such as a pure tone applied to one ear, a flashing light seen by one eye, or an electrical stimulus applied to a finger. The magnetic field at an instant in time leaves the head at one location and reenters at another, with the actual locations depending on the specific stimulus used. If the field strength were plotted as a map, there would be a single, localized maximum, and a corresponding, symmetric minimum. Referring to our two-dipole source of a propagating nerve action potential (Figs. 9a and 10a) and the single-dipole source of a propagating cardiac action potential (Figs. 11a and 11d), we see that Fig. 13a suggests that the EF is produced by a single dipole. Observations so far of the time-evolution of MEG maps do not in general suggest propagation, but instead the data are consistent with the turning-on and turning-off of a stationary dipole, possibly followed by the energizing of another dipole. Electrical measurements suggest that the principal electrical activity arises from graded, post-synaptic potentials occurring in the dendrites of cortical neurons. While in the past it was believed that these dendrites behaved as simple, passive electrical cables, there is mounting evidence that dendrites too have ion-selective channels that control their electrical response to stimuli from connecting neurons. Of the different types of cortical neurons, those with dendritic networks that are spherically-symmetric about the cell body produce electric currents along the dendrites that have little or no external magnetic field, just as occurred in our example of the spherical current source. Only those neurons with dendrites that are centered about a point that is displaced from the cell body, such as in Fig. 13b, can result in a measurable current dipole moment with its characteristic field. If the synapses that are active in an evoked response are excitatory, the intradendritic space will become positive, and hence the cell body will be a source of positive current flowing into the adjacent tissue. If the synaptic input is inhibitory, the cell body will appear to be a current sink. Hence the sign of the dipole moment will depend upon the nature of the input, and could change during a response. Unfortunately, the magnetic field from a single cortical neuron is too weak to be detected outside the skull, and the evoked magnetic fields observed so far arise from the combined activity of 10^4 to 10^5 neurons, which are often in close proximity and appear to be functioning as a single unit.

So far, we have ignored the effects of the boundary of the conductor that contains the

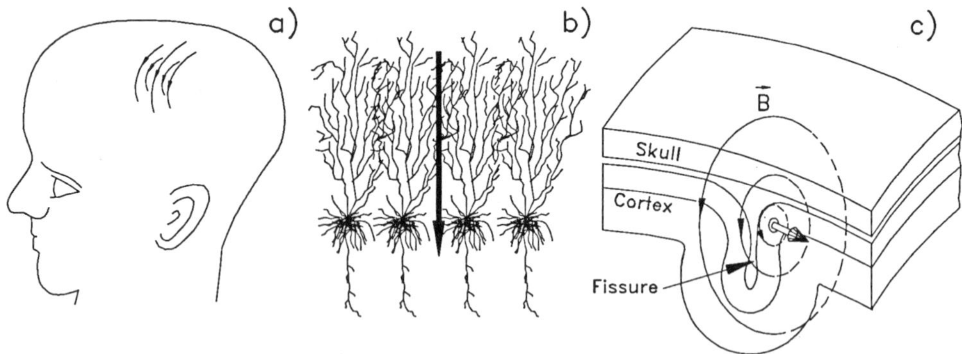

Figure 13. a) The magnetic field outside the skull from an evoked cortical response. b) The effective current dipole that describes the summed contributions of the dendritic activity of a population of simultaneously-activated cortical neurons. c) The relationship between the cortical dipole, the cortical fissures, and the evoked magnetic field.

current sources. For the MEG, the boundary formed by the skull has a profound effect, in that a radially-oriented current dipole will produce no external magnetic field. Hence the dipole that we detect with the MEG must be oriented tangential to the skull, and as a result the MEG arises primarily from cortical neurons located in the fissures, as shown in Fig. 13c.

Obviously most biological current sources are much more complex than the simple ones we have just described; but, the principles that govern their electric and magnetic fields are the same as those we have outlined. We can now shift our attention to the harder problem of obtaining a description of the biological sources given measurements of their fields.

THE INVERSE PROBLEM AND MODELLING

Early in our discussion, we described how to calculate a magnetic field from a knowledge of the currents that produced it. We start with a detailed description of both the geometry and the electrical conductivity of the region that has current flowing in it. Given the source distribution $\vec{J}^i(\vec{r}\,')$, where $\vec{r}\,'$ specifies the locus of points that spans the conducting region, we can use Laplace's equation and Ohm's law to calculate $V(\vec{r}\,')$ and $\vec{J}(\vec{r}\,')$ everywhere in the conductor. We then use the law of Biot and Savart to calculate $\vec{B}(\vec{r})$, where $\vec{r}$ corresponds to the location where we want to know the fields. Such calculations constitute solutions to the "forward problem." Ideally, it would be as straightforward to solve the "inverse problem" of determining exactly what sources, i.e. what $\vec{J}^i(\vec{r}\,')$, produced a measured magnetic field $\vec{B}(\vec{r})$ or electric potential $V(\vec{r})$, but in fact it is not.

There are many different techniques that can be used in solving the inverse problem. The most common is the least-squares approach that starts with an initial guess as to the source distribution, computes the field that this source would produce, compares the mean-squared error between the observed and calculated fields, and then adjusts the source to minimize this error. This process is repeated until the solution converges on a single set of source parameters, or until the investigator gives up. Unfortunately, it is an undisputable consequence of Laplace's equation that, in general, the three-dimensional inverse problem has no unique solution. Many, or even an infinite number of solutions, could produce the same external fields. While mathematical, physical, physiological, and/or metabolic constraints may eliminate certain solutions and guarantee a stable, repeatable calculation, there is always the justifiable concern that the sources that are estimated to have produced the observed fields may have little resemblance to the actual physiology.

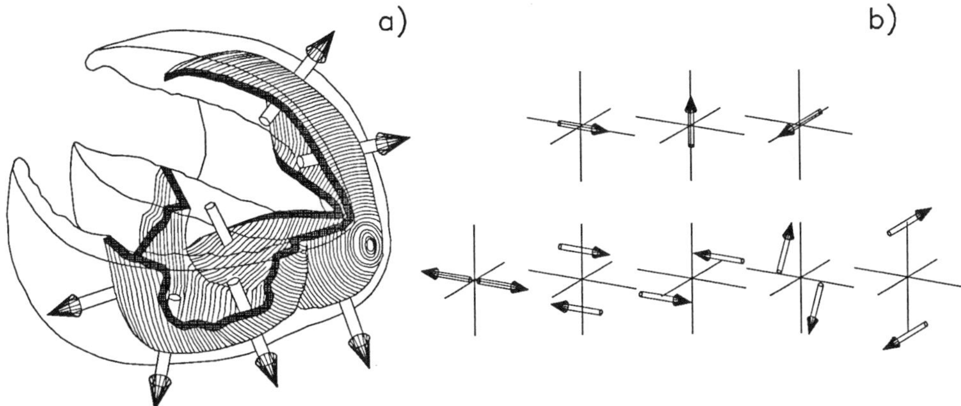

Figure 14. a) A multiple-dipole model for a cardiac activation wavefront. b) A pictorial representation of the first 8 terms of a multipolar current source model.

Based upon this caveat regarding the lack of a unique solution to the inverse problem, it is reasonable to ask what can be learned from either electric or magnetic measurements. If the exact nature of the current source is well known, for example a simple current dipole, then the time-dependent location, strength, and orientation of the dipole can be determined. If the source is more complex, it is necessary to use a more complex model. Fields from action potentials propagating along a nerve require a pair of dipoles. Since the cardiac wavefront in Fig. 12a resembles a sheet of current sources, one might model it as a large number of current dipoles, each of which accounts for the contribution of a portion of the wavefront, as shown in Fig. 14a. However at this level of complexity, problems of stability, uniqueness and noise often set in. While such a model may produce valid results when used for a forward calculation, it may not produce the expected result when used in an inverse one. The modeler is often tempted to use a mathematically-elegant but physiologically-unrealistic solution that consists of a multipole series such as that in Fig. 14b. The first three terms of the multipole series are simply three current dipoles with perpendicular orientations. The next five terms are the quadrupoles, which can be thought of as being constructed from pairs of dipoles. Octapoles and hexadecapoles follow. Mathematically, each of these sources would be superimposed at a single point and their strengths would be adjusted to best fit the observed field. This approach is productive if the primary goal is to obtain a compact mathematical description of the fields, but may provide little insight into the physiology or pathology of the biological sources. Overall, the safest approach to modeling is to first master the forward calculation that provides the desired level of physiological detail without becoming mathematically intractable, and then to use this model as the starting point for an inverse calculation. The modeler must recognize the possibility that constraints may have to be added to the inverse model, for example to prevent the individual cardiac dipoles in Fig. 14a from pointing in the wrong direction.

THE FUTURE

The lack of a unique solution to the inverse problem plagues bioelectric and biomagnetic measurements alike, and thus biomagnetism should not be thought of as the panacea for the limitations of bioelectric techniques. Instead, the enthusiasm for biomagnetism arises from a number of situations where fundamental or practical differences between the two techniques can be exploited. For example, a radial cortical current dipole will have a simple electric pattern but no external magnetic field, while a tangential dipole will have a clear magnetic signature. Thus the MEG is good for studying activity located in a cortical fissure.

Biomagnetic fields are influenced less strongly by intervening tissue, such as the skull, than are bioelectric fields and for this reason magnetic localization of bioelectric current sources may prove to be mathematically easier, more accurate, and/or more convenient than electrical localization. The MEG does not require a reference electrode, as does the EEG. As the number of magnetometers in multichannel SQUID systems is increased, it will become easier to map the MEG than to prepare and apply a large number of scalp electrodes. Biomagnetic fields are more closely related to intracellular currents than are extracellular potentials and thus, magnetic measurements on single nerve or muscle fibers readily allow determination of the transmembrane action potential without penetration of the cell membrane. It is easier to detect steady electric currents flowing within a person or animal by detecting the associated magnetic field than by recording surface electric potentials at the skin.

Fundamental differences between electric and magnetic fields may also exist. For example, we should now recognize that magnetic fields provide information about currents while electric measurements provide information about voltage. But current and voltage are related by Ohm's law to the resistance. In systems such as the heart, the complexity and importance of the electrical resistance of anisotropic tissue is acknowledged but poorly understood. There is reason to believe that biomagnetic recordings may help explain several confusing aspects of the propagation of cardiac activity. There may even exist physiological current sources that are magnetically-detectable yet electrically-silent, but these have yet to be found.

Thus, for either practical or fundamental reasons, biomagnetic measurements may provide solutions to problems in clinical medicine or basic science. Perhaps even more exciting applications of this new technology are awaiting discovery. In any case, the critical evaluation of emerging biomagnetic techniques will require a balanced and thoughtful comparison of both the measurement of electric and magnetic fields and the modeling of their sources.

ACKNOWLEDGEMENTS

The preparation of this manuscript has been supported by National Institutes of Health Grants NS 19794 and NS 24751 and by the College of Arts and Science of Vanderbilt University. I am indebted to Licheng Li for the skill and care with which she prepared illustrations. I thank John Barach, Richard Friedman, Nestor Sepulveda, Carlos Trenary, Ranjith Wijesinghe, and Leonora Wikswo for their comments on the manuscript, and Sam Williamson for his encouragement and patience.

REFERENCES

Hobbie, R.K., 1988, "Intermediate Physics for Medicine and Biology," Wiley, New York.

Kuffler, S.W., Nichols, J.G., and Martin, A.R., 1984, "From Neuron to Brain," Sinauer, Sunderland, Massachusetts.

Macfarlane, P.W., and Lawrie, T.D.V, (Editors), 1989, "Comprehensive Electrocardiology: Theory and Practice in Health and Disease," Pergamon Press, New York.

Wikswo, J.P., Jr., Malmivuo, J. A. V., Barry, W.H., Leifer, M.C., and Fairbank, W.M., 1979, Theory and Application of Magnetocardiography, in: "Cardiovascular Physics", D.N. Ghista, E. Van Vollenhoven and W. Yang, Eds., Karger, Basil, pp.1-67.

Williamson, S. J., Romani, G.-L., Kaufman, L., and Modena, I., (Editors), 1983, "Biomagnetism, An Interdisciplinary Approach," Plenum, New York.

PRINCIPLES AND APPLICATIONS OF SQUID SENSORS

T. Katila

Laboratory of Biomedical Engineering
Faculty of Information Technology
Helsinki University of Technology
02150 Espoo, FINLAND

INTRODUCTION

Since the discovery of superconductivity by Kamerlingh Onnes in 1911 this physical phenomenon has found several important applications. The application described here is the use of superconductive magnetometers for measuring weak biomagnetic fields. Superconductive devices work only at low temperatures; such a temperature is usually maintained with the aid of liquid helium. Storage and use of liquid helium requires special thermally isolated dewars.

Since 1970, Superconducting Quantum Interference Device (SQUID) magnetometers have been used for biomagnetic studies (Cohen et al 1970). In the 70's most SQUID magnetometers were single channel devices and they were used at magnetically unshielded measurement sites. Cohen reported in 1979 a two-channel "2-D" planar gradiometer and Seppänen et al. in 1983 a 3-channel first-order vector gradiometer. In 1984, the 3+1 channel system (Ilmoniemi et al. 1984) and finally 1985 the BTi 5-channel system (Williamson et al. 1985) were reported. These were systems finally designed for studies in a magnetically shielded room (MSR), and working at sensitivities adequate for biomagnetic studies $\leq 50 fT/\sqrt{Hz}$. During the last few years, the number of channels has first grown to seven and thereafter to 24 and 37. The sensitivity of 7-channel devices has increased to 5-7 $fT/\sqrt{Hz}$ and one-channel device to 3 $fT/\sqrt{Hz}$ (Nenonen et al., these proceedings).

The discovery by Bednorz and Müller in 1986 of a new class of superconductors with higher transition temperatures than known before initiated a search for superconductivity at liquid nitrogen temperature and higher. Superconductivity at 90 K was observed in the perovskite type Y-Ba-Cu-0-system in 1987. In the Bi-Sr-Ca-Cu-O-system, a phase with a superconducting transition temperature of 110 K, and in the Tl-Ca-Ba-Cu-O-system 125 K have been reported. However, it is not yet clear how well the new materials will be suited for magnetometric applications. Systems have also been constructed, where the cryogenic temperatures needed for the use of SQUIDs are reached without the use of liquified helium.

QUANTIZATION OF MAGNETIC FLUX

To understand the functioning of superconducting flux transformers and SQUIDs we will have to discuss briefly the principles of the Ginzburg-Landau theory of superconductivity. In this theory, a wave function type presentation is used for superelectrons:

Advances in Biomagnetism
Edited by S.J. Williamson *et al.*
Plenum Press, New York

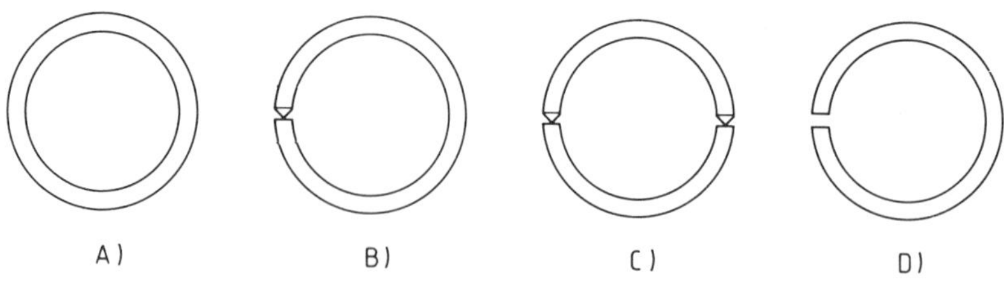

Fig. 1. *Rings made of superconducting material: A) a closed ring made of s.c. material, B) an s.c. ring with a weak link in it, C) an s.c. ring with two weak links, and D) an open ring.*

$$\psi(\vec{r}) = \sqrt{n_s(\vec{r})}e^{i\Theta(\vec{r})}, \tag{1}$$

where ψ is the Ginzburg-Landau *order parameter,* with a close resemblance to the quantum mechanical wave function. The order parameter is a complex number, describing the behaviour of the superelectrons with a density of n_s and a quantum phase Θ. It is assumed that superconducting electrons are bound as Cooper pairs, consisting of two electrons. The order parameter describes the collective behaviour of a number of Cooper pairs.

The name *superconductivity* refers to a specific physical property, namely that the electrical resistance of a material is identically zero below the critical temperature, T_c. This perfect electric conductivity is true, however, only below a critical frequency, a critical electric current density and a critical external magnetic field. Another remarkable physical property of the superconducting material is the perfect diamagnetism, $\chi = -1$. The magnetic flux does not penetrate inside a superconductive region. This is called the *Meissner-effect.* The Meissner effect can be utilized to make extremely effective shields against magnetic fields.

A more detailed study would reveal that the magnetic flux through any loop made of superconducting material is not necessarily zero, but it is quantized. According to the Ginzburg-Landau theory, the phase along a closed path l inside the superconductor must fullfill the condition:

$$\oint_l \nabla\Theta \cdot d\vec{l} = n\ 2\pi, \qquad (n = 0, \pm 1, \pm 2, ...) \tag{2}$$

A very similar condition is faced in quantum mechanics in the quantization of electronic orbits in an atom.
In the presence of a magnetic field with a vector potential $\vec{A}$, the quantum mechanical generalized momentum operator $\vec{\hat{p}} = -i\hbar\nabla$ can be expressed as a sum of a kinetic contribution and a contribution due to the magnetic field. The supercurrent flows close to the surface of the superconductor only. Therefore one can write Eq. (2) for Cooper pairs of superelectrons as,

$$\oint_l \vec{A} \cdot d\vec{l} = \int_S \vec{B} \cdot d\vec{S} = n\frac{h}{2e} = n\Phi_0. \tag{3}$$

Thus the magnetic flux through an area S surrounded by the path l inside a superconducting material is quantized in units of the natural *magnetic flux quantum* , whose value is $\Phi_0 \cong 2.07 \cdot 10^{-15}$ Wb.

The quantization of the magnetic flux is illustrated in Figs. 1 and 2. In Fig. 1A), a closed ring made of superconducting material, 1B) one weak link in an otherwise s.c. ring, 1C) two weak links in an s.c. ring, and 1D) an open s.c. ring, are depicted.

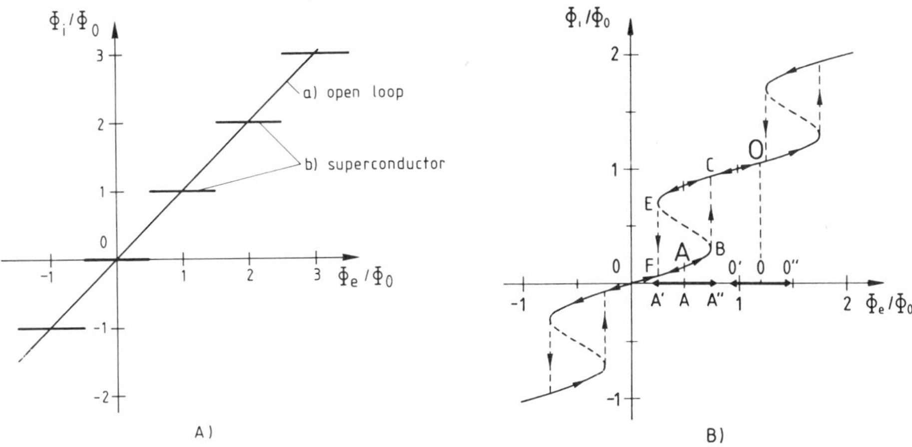

Fig. 2. *The magnetic flux inside superconducting loops* (Φ_i) *as a function of the extenally applied flux* Φ_e*, the fluxes are normalized by the flux quantum* Φ_0*.*
(A) a) An open loop, made of a superconductor or normal metal (cf. Fig. 1D), b) a closed superconducting loop (cf. Fig. 1A).
(B) A SQUID-ring with one weak link in the ring, (Fig. 1B, for details see text).

Fig. 2 shows the internal magnetic flux Φ_i penetrating the superconducting ring when an external magnetic flux Φ_e is applied on it. Both magnetic fluxes are given in units of the magnetic flux quantum Φ_0. For an open s.c. ring or a ring at normal metallic state $\Phi_i \simeq \Phi_e$, shown by curve a) in Fig. 2A. In the superconducting state, for the solid s.c. ring of Fig. 1A), the flux quantization of Eq. (3) is valid, and the magnetic flux can appear only as multiplets of the flux quantum Φ_0. This is demonstrated by the integer steps (curve b) in Fig. 2A. Fig. 2B shows the relationships of external and internal magnetic fluxes, when the superconducting rings contain one weak link (rf-SQUID). This case will be discussed in detail later.

FLUX TRANSFORMER

As long as a loop of wire stays superconducting, the loop not only encloses an integer number of magnetic flux quanta, $n\Phi_0$, but it also will resist any attempt to change the internal magnetic flux Φ_i:

$$\delta\Phi_i = 0. \tag{4}$$

Eq. (4) shows the principle of flux transformers of superconducting magnetometers and gradiometers.

A magnetic flux transformer may contain two or more coils, usually coupled in series, as shown in Fig. 3. A change of the magnetic flux through one of the coils causes a change in the magnetic flux in the other coils. E.g. the two-coil system of Fig. 3a) depicts the conventional magnetometric coil configuration. The coil L_1 is called the main sensing coil; any external magnetic field to be measured should act on it. The signal coil L_{sg} is coupled to the sensor of the magnetic flux, the SQUID in this case. Application of Eq. (4) gives:

$$\Delta\Phi_1 + \Delta\Phi_{sg} = 0. \tag{5}$$

Thus, the change of the magnetic flux is transferred from the sensing coil L_1 to the signal coil L_{sg}. If the influence of the sensing element (SQUID) is neglected, optimum

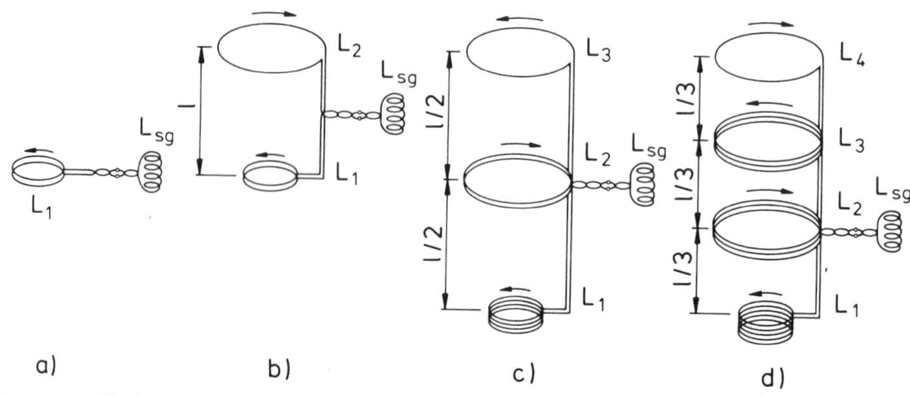

Fig. 3. *Coil configurations of superconducting magnetometers and gradiometers: a) a magnetometer, b) a first order, c) a second order, and d) a third order axial, asymmetric gradiometer.*

flux transfer is obtained, if $L_1 = L_{sg}$.

Physically, the flux transfer is caused by a shielding supercurrent I_{sg}, maintaining the magnetic flux constant inside the superconducting loop. The loop consists here of the coils L_1 and L_{sg} and of interconnecting wires; the inductance of the latter is neglected in the following. Any external magnetic flux $\Delta\Phi_e$ introduced at the sensing coil is compensated for by the change of the shielding current:

$$\Delta\Phi_e = (L_1 + L_{sg})\Delta I_{sg}. \tag{6}$$

When $L_1 \simeq L_{sg}$, about half of the magnetic flux introduced into the sensing coil is transferred to the sensing element connected to the coil L_{sg}. Differential magnetometers, usually called gradiometers, are preferred to simple magnetometers, since they offer more effective rejection of external magnetic noise.

The first-order gradiometer, shown in Fig. 3b), has two sensing coils, L_1 and L_2; the second order gradiometer (Fig. 3c) has three and the third order gradiometer (Fig. 3d) four sensing coils. All the gradiometers shown are axial, i.e. all sensing coils are uniaxial. These gradiometers are also asymmetric, the diameter of the main sensing coil, L_1, is smaller than that of the compensating coils $(L_2, L_3, ...)$ If the areas of the main sensing coil and the compensating coils are the same, and the coils are wound in opposition, as depicted in Fig. 3, all gradiometers are insensitive to external uniform magnetic fields. It is easily seen that the second order gradiometer is insensitive also to the uniform (first) gradient of the external magnetic field. The third order gradiometer is, in addition to the homogeneous fields and to the first gradient, insensitive also to the second gradient of the external magnetic field.

Typical diameters of the main sensing coils are between 1 and 3 cm. The distance between coils usually varies from 3 to 15 cm.

JOSEPHSON EFFECT

The Josephson junction is the basic component of the SQUID. In the early 1960's Josephson derived the currently famous relation for a supercurrent through a weak link in a superconductor (Josephson 1962). In Fig. 4 A) a sandwich type weak link, a thin oxide layer between two superconductors, is shown schematically. This part also presents the symbols used in the following. Parts B) and C) of Fig. 4 depict two

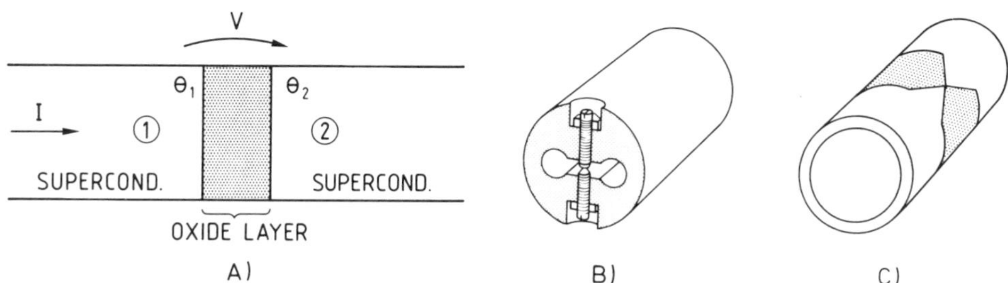

Fig. 4. *A) An oxide weak link; B) a point contact, and C) a constriction type weak link in an rf-SQUID.*

constructions of rf-SQUIDs both having one weak link in the superconducting ring, a point contact screw type weak link (B) or a constriction type weak link (C).

Josephson predicted that the supercurrent I_s through the weak link is a periodic function of the G-L phase difference $\Delta\theta = \theta_2 - \theta_1$:

$$I_s = I_c sin(\Delta\theta) \tag{7}$$

where I_c is the critical current of the weak link. The critical current is the maximum supercurrent through the weak link. For a typical weak link with a normal resistance of around 1Ω, I_c is 1 mA or less, in practical devides between 1μA and 1 mA. According to Eq. (7), a supercurrent will flow through the weak link even in the absence of a voltage difference across it. This is called the DC Josephson effect.

On the other hand, a nonzero voltage V across the weak link in Fig. 4A causes a new effect. In the presence of this voltage a pair of electrons would gain energy by an amount of 2 eV by crossing the Josephson junction. Since superconducting electrons cannot, due to the energy gap, receive this energy it is radiated out as a photon: $hf = 2eV$. In other words,

$$V = \Phi_o f = \frac{1}{2\pi}\Phi_o \frac{d(\Delta\theta)}{dt}, \tag{8}$$

where f is the frequency of the radiation. The phenomenon that a voltage across the Josephson junction produces current oscillations, is called the AC Josephson effect.

SQUIDS

Although the first biomagnetic measurements by Baule and McFee (1963) were done using coil magnetometers, conventional magnetometers are usually not sensitive enough for biomagnetic measurements. The SQUID is the most sensitive magnetic flux detector at low frequencies, known today. We first discuss the characteristics of the rf-SQUID. The rf-SQUID is essentially a superconducting ring with one weak link in it, such as shown in Fig. 1B). Two early practical constructions were presented in Figs. 4B) and C).

RF-SQUID. In the superconducting state, the current I_s contributes a shielding term to the flux inside the ring:

$$\Phi_i = \Phi_e + L_s I_s, \tag{9}$$

where L_s is the inductance of the ring. The corresponding dependence of Φ_i on Φ_e at low frequencies is shown in Fig. 2B.

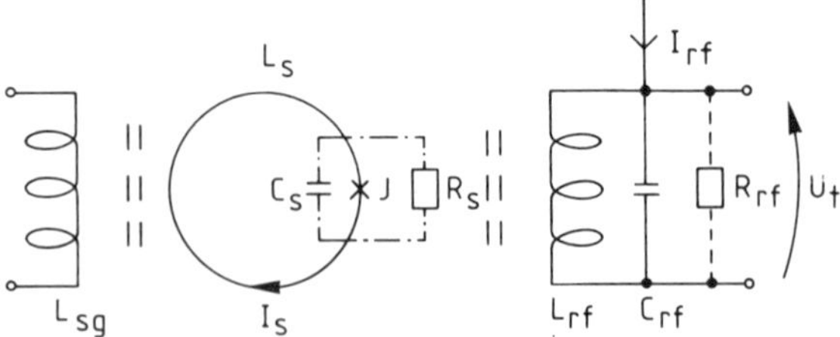

Fig. 5. *Coupling of an rf-SQUID to the signal coil L_{sg} and to the tank circuit (L_{rf}, C_{rf}, R_{rf}). The voltage of the tank circuit U_t is usually amplified by a room temperature amplifier.*

The rf-SQUID is coupled inductively to the signal coil L_{sg} and to the inductance L_{rf} of the rf-resonance circuit, as shown in Fig. 5. The flux transformer transforms part of the slowly varying external magnetic flux, affecting the main sensing coil L_1, through the signal coil L_{sg} to the SQUID. This shifts the working point (e.g. A on Fig. 2B). The rf-circuit introduces an alternating magnetic flux Φ_e, shifting the working point back and forth around A (A'⇔ A"). In reaching point B with increasing external flux Φ_e, the internal flux Φ_i jumps from the value at B to C. Correspondingly, with decreasing flux from C to E, a flux jump E → F occurs. The hysteretic path BCEFB causes hysterisis-losses in the tank circuit of the rf-SQUID. A similar rf-amplitude around the working point "O", with rf-oscillations O'⇔ O" would not yet cause any hysterisis at all. Around "O", flux jumps and hysteresis would start at considerably higher rf-amplitudes only. Thus the hysteresis enclosed depends on the rf-amplitude and the working point.

A more accurate analysis requires the inclusion of the normal resistance R_s and capacitance C_s of the junction. The total current through the weak link now becomes:

$$I_s = I_c \sin(\Delta\Theta) + \frac{\hbar}{2eR_s}\frac{d(\Delta\theta)}{dt} + \frac{\hbar}{2e}C_s\frac{d^2(\Delta\theta)}{dt^2}. \tag{10}$$

Application of Eq. (2) along a path inside the superconductor, but across the weak link gives,

$$2\pi\frac{\Phi_i}{\Phi_o} + \Delta\theta = n\ 2\pi, \qquad \text{with n} = 0, \pm1, \pm2, ... \tag{11}$$

Equations (9), (10), and (11) cover the functioning of the rf-SQUID.

Since the characteristic curve of the rf-SQUIDs (Fig 2B) is periodic, the period being the flux quantum Φ_0, the output voltage U_t of the rf-circuit of the rf-SQUID must also be periodic in Φ_0, (see Fig. 6).

The average value of the output voltage $< \hat{U}_t >$ has in practice an approximately

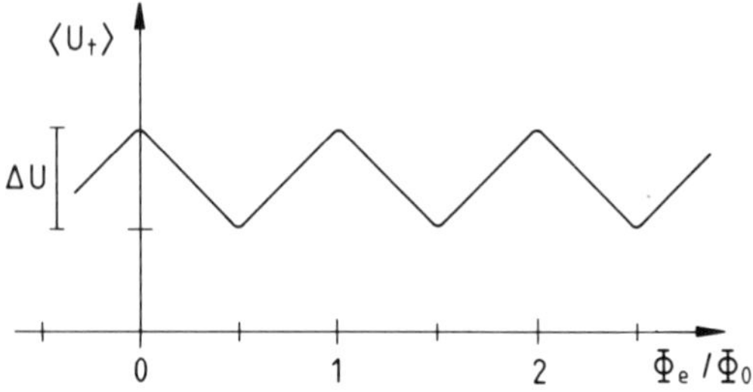

Fig. 6. *The average output voltage $< \hat{U}_t >$ of an rf-SQUID amplifier as a function of the externally applied magnetic flux Φ_e.*

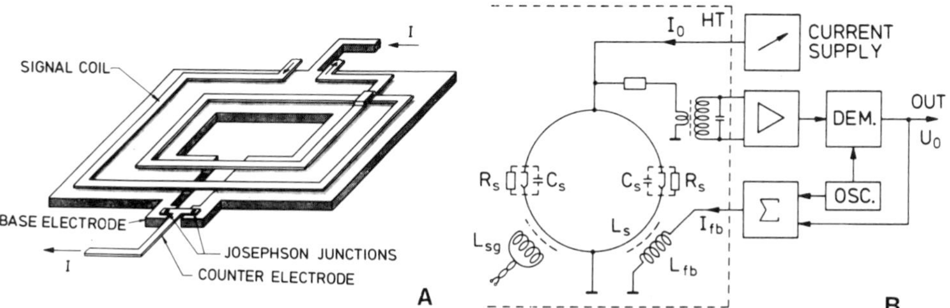

Fig. 7. (A) *The dc-SQUID shown schematically. The superconducting ring contains two Josephson junctions. View from Ryhänen et al. (1989).*
(B) The coupling of the dc-SQUID as a magnetometer. A constant current I is driven through the device and the average output voltage is detected. For details, see text

triangular shape. The sensitivity G_s of the magnetometer, i.e. the ratio between the averaged output voltage and the external magnetic flux is as follows,

$$G_s = \frac{d < \hat{U}_t >}{d\Phi_e} \simeq \frac{\omega_0}{k}\sqrt{\frac{L_{rf}}{L_s}}, \tag{12}$$

where k is the coupling coefficient between the rf-coil and the one hole SQUID-loop, with inductances L_{rf} and L_s, correspondingly. However, to determine the sensitivity of the system in magnetic measurements, we have also to consider the noise.

DC-SQUID. In the dc-SQUID, there are two weak links in a superconducting ring (Fig. 7A). In the RSJ-model, both weak links are replaced by a Josephson-element (J), normal resistance across the link (R_s) and the junction capacitance (C_s), as shown in Fig. 7B. A constant current I from an external supply is driven through the dc-SQUID. The average of the voltage $< V >$ across the SQUID is measured. We next calculate $< V >$ as a function of the external magnetic flux introduced into the dc-SQUID through the signal coil L_{sg} of the flux transformer.

A more thorough study would require both weak links to be described separately using equations similar to Eq. (10). However, we make the assumptions that both junctions (a and b) are similar and that a resistive model can be used, neglecting the junction capacitances. The current I through the device is given as (see Eqs. (8) and (10)),

$$I = I_c(\sin\Delta\theta_a + \sin\Delta\theta_b) + 2\frac{V}{R_s}. \tag{13}$$

From this, the voltage V can be deduced,

$$V = \frac{R_s}{2}(I - 2I_c\sin\delta_o\cos\pi\frac{\Phi_i}{\Phi_o})). \tag{14}$$

In Eq. (14), the symbol $\delta_o = \frac{1}{2}(\Delta\theta_a + \Delta\theta_b)$ and Eq. (11), modified for two weak links, has been applied. The average output voltage can now be obtained by calculating the period of the AC-Josephson effect and then by using Eq. (8), one obtains

$$< V >= \Phi_o f = \frac{R_s I}{2}\sqrt{1 - 4\frac{I_c^2}{I^2}\cos^2(\pi\Phi_e/\Phi_o)}, \tag{15}$$

by further making the simplifying approximation that the shielding effect is small and thus $\Phi_i \simeq \Phi_e$. The result of Eq. (15) is shown in Fig. 8B. The average voltage

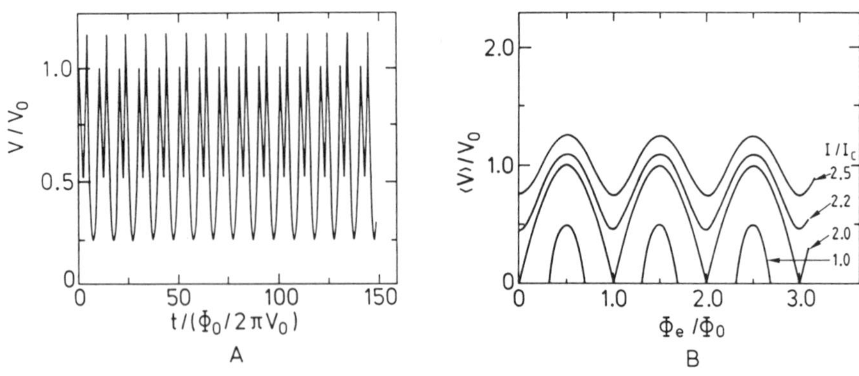

Fig. 8. *(A) Josephson oscillations in the output voltage of a dc-SQUID. (B) The average output voltage $< V >$ as a function of externally applied magnetic flux Φ_e, the constant current I as a parameter.*

$< V >$ is nonzero, if $I > 2I_c \cos(\pi\Phi_e/\Phi_o)$.

At nonzero $< V >$ the time dependence of V shows an oscillating behaviour. A computer simulation of such oscillations in the output voltage of the dc-SQUID is shown in Fig. 8A. A value $I = 2I_c$ and an externally applied magnetic flux $\Phi_e = \Phi_o/4$ are assumed. The unit of the vertical (voltage) scale is $V_o = R_s I_c$. With figures typical of a practical Josephson junction $V_o = 1...10\ \mu V$. The (horizontal) time unit $t_o = \Phi_o/(2\pi V_o)$ would be of the order of 0.1 ns for those parameter values. Thus the basic frequency of oscillations in Fig. 8A is of the order of 1 GHz. This frequency, however, varies as a function of the externally applied field, even though the current I is kept constant.

In practical devices, the oscillatory behaviour of V is not measured, but only the time average voltage $< V >$ after amplification. A somewhat simplified dependence of $< V >$ on Φ_e is presented in Fig. 8B. The value of the bias current I is used as a parameter. The strongest signal is obtained for $I = 2I_c$. The output is periodic much the same way as the output of the rf-SQUID shown in Fig. 6. Even the typical peak-to-peak output is of the same order of magnitude (10μV) for both types of SQUIDs. Thus the sensitivities G_s (Eq. 12) are also quite comparable. However, the dc-SQUIDs can possess a lower noise level than the rf-SQUIDs.

SQUID-MAGNETOMETERS

Since the output voltages of both rf- and dc-SQUIDs are highly nonlinear, feedback is used in practical measurements to linearize the response. We explain here the linearization of the dc-SQUID response with the aid of Fig. 7B. The SQUID and various coils surrounding it are at helium temperature (HT) inside the helium dewar. The constant current I is fed from a current source at room temperature. The working point is stabilized by phase sensitive detection and feedback. For this purpose, a signal at an intermediate frequency is added. The frequency chosen must be above the highest signal frequency, which usually is between 100 Hz and 10 kHz in biomagnetic measurements. Typical phase detection frequencies of rf-SQUID systems are between 10 and 100 kHz, somewhat higher for dc-SQUIDs. The signal for phase detection is produced by a separate oscillator and it is fed into the SQUID through the feedback coil (L_{fb}) and into the reference input of the demodulation detector.

The changes in the output voltage V of the dc-SQUID are fed via a transformer and an amplifier to the demodulation detector. The fast oscillation visible in Fig 8A is

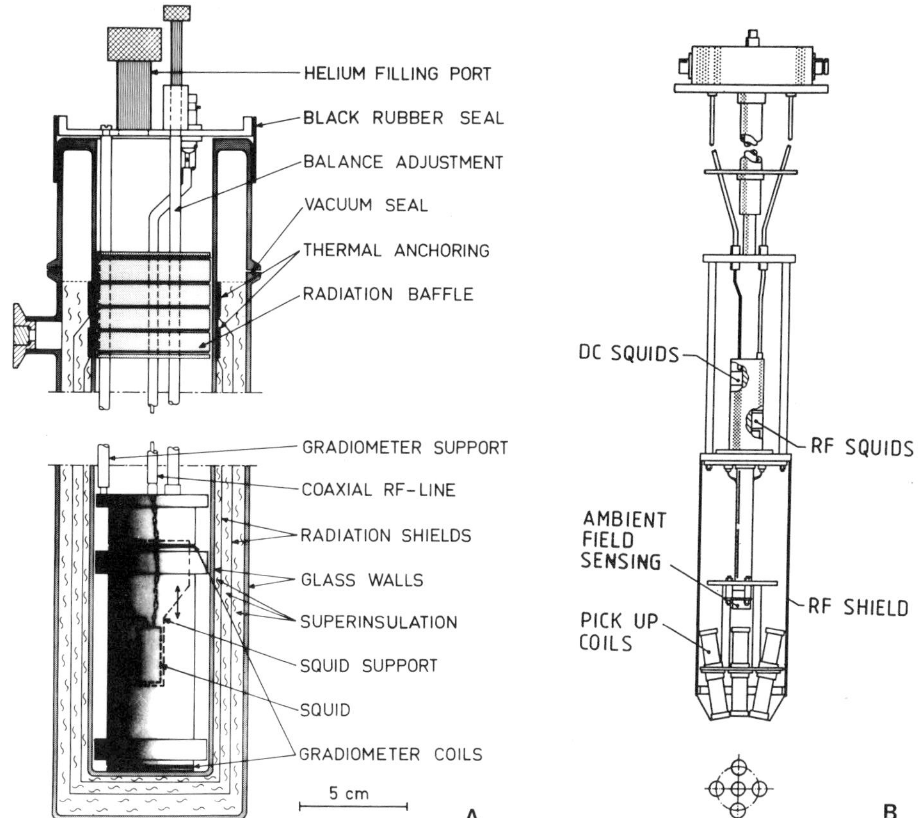

Fig. 9. *(A) A small size, laboratory made, first-order SQUID gradiometer. This one-channel instrument was built in 1972 (Saarinen et al. 1974).*
(B) The insert of a 5-channel second-order gradiometer. The instrument was installed in 1984 (Williamson et al. 1985).

not used in detection, only the average value $< V >$. The output is proportional to the on-phase and on-frequency component of V. A signal proportional to the output of the device is sent back to the feedback coil, to compensate for any magnetic flux introduced into the SQUID by the signal coil L_{sg}. Thus the dc-SQUID is effectively working as zero point detector. Any low frequency flux change due to the signal coil is compensated for by the corresponding feedback signal. This method assures excellent linearity, high sensitivity and a wide dynamic range. However, one drawback of the phase sensitive detection is that the zero point is arbitrary.

Two practical constructions of SQUID gradiometers are shown in Fig. 9. The rf-SQUID based instrument of Fig. 9A is a laboratory made first-order gradient magnetometer (Saarinen 1974). The dewar is superinsulated and it uses liquid helium for cooling. The two radiation shields are made of copper wires. Liquid helium is filled up to the radiation baffle. Thus the gradiometer coils and the SQUID are immersed in liquid helium. The SQUID was a laboratory made, point contact rf-SQUID of the two-hole type, popular in the 70's (Zimmerman 1972). The small size dewar remains cold throughout one normal working day. In a remote nonmagnetic measurement site, as well as in the MSR, the best sensitivity obtained was about $20fT/\sqrt{Hz}$.

The BTi 5-channel second-order gradiometer, the insert of which is shown in Fig. 9B, was the first commercial multichannel magnetometer. The positioning of the five main sensing coils is depicted below the main figure. The diameter of the coils is 15 mm, the base length 40 mm and the separation between channels 20 mm. The white noise level is given as $20fT/\sqrt{Hz}$ when the measurements are made in a double-wall mu-metal MSR. The axes of the gradiometers are tipped so that the coils are actually tangential to a spherical surface, which together with the concave bottom of the dewar makes the instrument suitable for brain studies. Signals produced by the second-order gradiometers are detected by the dc-SQUIDs.

The third instrument described here is a 7-channel first-order gradiometer, drawn schematically in Fig. 10 A (Knuutila et al. 1987). The first-order gradiometers are connected to dc-SQUIDs (manufactured by IBM) inside superconducting Nb-shields, also containing the impedance matching transformers. The imbalance of the gradiometers is below 1 %, considered to sufficient for studies in an MSR. The preamplifiers are mounted at the top of the dewar (manufactured by CTF Systems Inc.) which has a curved, tilted bottom. The inner diameter of the tail of the dewar is 140 mm and the radius of the curvature of the concave cap is 125 mm. The diameter of the sensing coils is 20 mm and the coil separation 37 mm. Thus the 7 coils cover a relatively wide area in brain studies. The sensitivity of the system is 5 - 6 $fT/\sqrt{Hz}$, comparable to the 7-channel system of BTi, when using first-order gradiometers.

MAGNETICALLY SHIELDED ROOMS AND GANTRIES

The first order gradiometer is useful at a remote measurement site without a magnetic shielding. However, its rejection of external magnetic disturbancies is not high enough in an unshielded laboratory. Strong environmental magnetic noise is always present in laboratories and hospitals. Especially strong sources of magnetic noise are

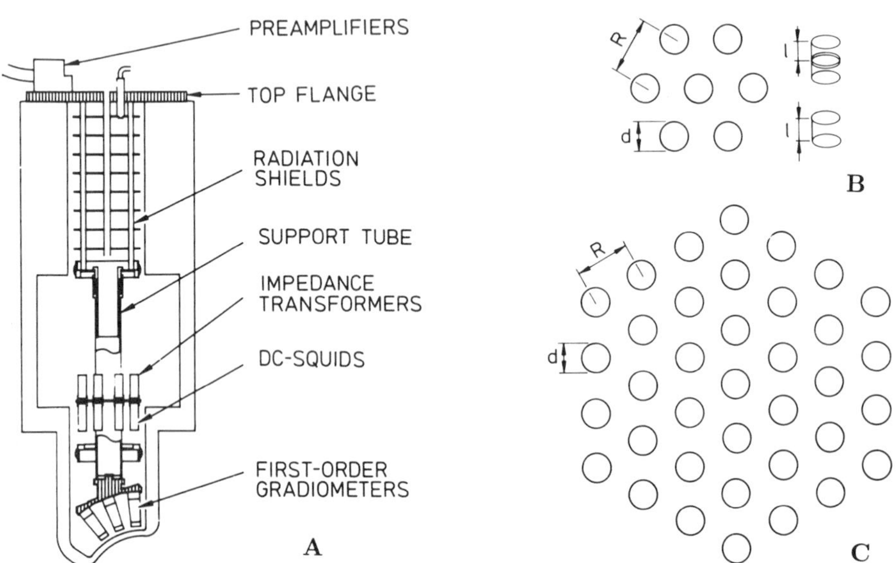

Fig. 10. *(A) A 7-channel dc-SQUID first-order gradiometer (Knuutila et al. 1987) (B) A popular hexagonal arrangement of the pick-up coils of the 7-channel magnetometers. (C) A hexagonal extension to 37 channels.*

various electronic equipment, moving large ferromagnetic objects close to the measurement site and building vibrations. Under favourable conditions, the rejection of second or third order gradiometers can be sufficient for biomagnetic studies in a laboratory. Usually high resolution magnetic measurements in laboratories or hospitals are possible only inside a magnetically shielded room. An MSR provides both low and radiofrequency electric and magnetic shielding. Inside a high quality MSR, usually with at least three mu-metal layers on the walls, a first-order gradiometer is a very sensitive measuring instrument (Mager 1981, Erne et al. 1981, Kelhä 1982). A two-wall structure is less expensive, nevertheless, high sensitivity has been obtained using, in two-wall rooms, both first- and second-order gradiometers. Recently, a wall construction with two layers of mu-metal and at least one layer of aluminum has become popular. Typically, the inner dimensions of an MSR vary from 2.25 x 2.25 x 2.25 m^3 (Mager 1981) to 3 x 4 x 2.4 m^3 (BTi/Vacuumschmelze MSR). For effective magnetic shielding and ease of use, proper door design is essential. Typical attenuation figures are between 40 dB and 60 dB for very low frequency magnetic fields, 50 dB-90 dB at 1 Hz and $\geq$ 80 dB at $>>$10Hz.
The dewar, together with the sensors, must be mounted on a gantry system, which provides the necessary freedom to locate and orientate the sensors relative to the subject. In addition, it is often possible to move the subject bed or the chair horizontally. In constructing the gantries for mangetically unshielded measurement sites, large metal parts and especially magnetic materials have to be avoided, since they would turn external magnetic fields into gradient noise. In addition, such a gantry must be extremely free of mechanical vibrations.

The old gantry designs often had 3 translational degrees or freedom, or 2 rotational angles, alternatively. Nowadays, the gantries of commercial instrumentations, used in an MSR, may even offer both the three translational and the three rotational degrees of freedom. This makes the positioning of the system relatively easy. Usually tilting of the dewar by approximately 45° is possible. Manual positioning can be locked by an automatic braking system. The mounting of the gantry can be done on the ceiling, the walls or the floor.

A sensor positioning indicator may be used to record the subsequent positions and orientations of the sensor system. E.g. in biomagnetic studies of the human head, reference points are usually fixed on the head, and the positioning is given relative to these points. Inductive position detection systems work at an accuracy of the order of one millimeter. A more advanced system would use data collected on the actual geometry of the head (or the torso). Such data is obtained from the CT- and MRI-pictures of the subject.

NOISE AND SENSITIVITY

External magnetic noise is in general much stronger than the biomagnetic fields to be measured. Since the gradient noise is also high in laboratories and hospitals, a magnetically shielded room is a preferred measurement site in most cases. In Fig. 11, we see the field noise in various measurement sites in a laboratory or hospital (curves 1 - 7) and a remote nonmagnetic measurement site (curve 8). Although the magnetic shielding of the MSR facilitates biomagnetic measurements, the MSR itself is made of electrically conducting material and it is also a source of magnetic noise (Nenonen et al. 1988). By taking the noise consideration carefully into account in designing the MSR and the experiments, this contribution can be minimized.

Currently, the limiting factor in high-sensitivity biomagnetic studies is either the noise of the SQUID-magnetometer or the thermal noise of the dewar (Nenonen et al., these proceedings). Fig. 11 also depicts the sensitivity of a 7-channel first-order gradiometer in an MSR (Knuutila et al. 1987) and the sensitivity of a single-channel system in the same MSR (Nenonen et al., these proceedings). Finally, the shadowed broad line indicates a future goal of the noise in biomagnetic studies. This value has been obtained by extrapolation of the trends in the past and by making comparisons between the signal-to-noise ratios in bioelectric and biomagnetic studies.

Finally, we present in Table I some representative parameters of selected biomagnetic instrumentations. The Rome IEES and the Shimadzu instruments are designed to work in a magnetically unshielded measurement site. The other instruments require an MSR for proper functioning. Presently, the 7-channel systems can reach sensitivities between 5 and 7 $fT/\sqrt{H}$ and prototypes of commercial instruments with up to 37 channels have recently been made public. Several other multichannel systems are introduced in these proceedings. In the future, the number of channels will continue to increase and the sensitivity improve.

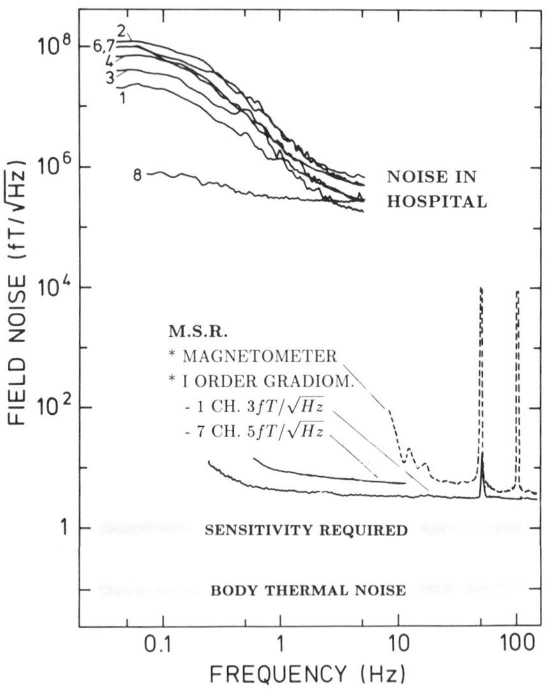

Fig. 11. *External magnetic field noise in unshielded laboratory and hospital measurement sites and in a remote nonmagnetic cottage. In addition, instrument noise curves are given, measured in a magnetically shielded room.*

Table I. (below) *Characteristics of some multichannel biomagnetometers. In these proceedings, several new multichannel systems are introduced, e.g. a miniature 4-channel system (Buchanan et al.), a 9-channel system (Carelli et al.) and a 12 position, 24- channel planargradiometer-system (Hämäläinen). For references to the various instruments and for further studies see the review articles listed at the end of this paper.*

Table I

INSTRUMENT	NO OF CHANN.	ORDER	d mm	l mm	R mm	NOISE $fT/\sqrt{Hz}$
BTi/NYU-New York	5	II	15	40	20	20
ISSE-Rome	4	II	15	70	21	50
BTi 607	7	II	15	40	20	20
BTi/PTB-Berlin	7	I	15	78	20	7
Shimadzu	7	II	25	35	38	<100
HUT/LT-Helsinki	7	I	20	60	37	5
Siemens Krenikon	37	I	27	70	27	12
BTi 6000	37	I	20	50	20	10

REFERENCES

Baule, G. and McFee, R. (1963). Detection of the magnetic field of the heart, Am. Heart J. 66, pp. 95-96.

Bednorz, J.G. and Müller, K.A. (1986). Possible High T_c Superconductivity in the Ba-La-Cu-O System, Z. Phys. B64, pp. 189-193.

Cohen, D., Edelsack, E.A., and Zimmerman, J.E. (1970). Magnetocardiograms taken inside a shielded room with a superconducting point-contact magnetometer. Appl. Phys. Letters 16, pp. 278-280.

Cohen, D. (1979). Magnetic Measurement and Display of Current Generators in the Brain. Part I: The 2-D Detector, in Proceedings of the 12th International Conference on Medical and Biological Engineering, Jerusalem, pp. 15-16.

Erné, S.N., Hahlbohm, H.-D., Scheer, H., and Trontelj, Z. (1981). The Berlin Magnetically Shielded Room (BMSR), Section B: Performances, in Erné, S.N., Hahlbohm, H.-D., and Lübbig, H., Eds., in Biomagnetism, Walter de Gruyter, Berlin, pp. 79-87.

Ilmoniemi, R.J., Hari, R., and Reinikainen, K. (1984) A four-channel SQUID magnetometer for brain research, Electroenceph. Clin. Neurophysiol. 58, pp. 467-473.

Josephson, B.D. (1962) Possible new effects in superconductive tunneling, Phys. Letters 1, pp. 251-253.

Kelhä, V.O., Pukki, J.M., Peltonen, R.S., Penttinen, A.J., Ilmoniemi, R.J., and Heino, J.J. (1982). Design, Construction and Performance of a Large-Volume Magnetic Shield, IEEE Trans. Magn., Mag-18, pp. 260-270.

Knuutila, J., Ahlfors, S., Ahonen, A., Hällström, J., Kajola, M., Lounasmaa, O.V., Vilkman, V., and Tesche, C. (1987). Large-area low-noise seven-channel dc SQUID magnetometer for brain research. Rev. Sci. Instrum. 58, pp. 2145-2156.

Mager, A. (1981). The Berlin Magnetically Shielded Room (BMSR), Section A: Design and Construction, in Erné, S.N., Hahlbohm, H.-D., and Lübbig, H., Eds., in Biomagnetism, Walter de Gruyter, Berlin, pp. 51-78.

Nenonen, J. and Katila, T. (1988). Thermal Noise in a Magnetically Shielded Room, in Biomagnetism '87, Atsumi, K., Kotani, M., Ueno, S., Katila, T., and Williamson, S.J., Eds., Tokyo Denki University Press, Tokyo, pp. 426-429.

Saarinen, M., Karp, P.J., Katila, T.E, and Siltanen, P. (1974). The magnetocardiogram in cardiac disorders, Cardiovasc. Res. 8, pp. 820-834.

Seppänen, M., Katila, T., Tuomisto, T., Varpula, T., Duret, D., and Karp, P. (1983). Measurement of Biomagnetic Fields Using Multichannel Superconducting-Magnetometer Techniques, Il Nuovo Cimento 2D, pp. 166-174.

Williamson, S.J., Pelizzone, M., Okada, Y., Kaufman, L., Crum, D.B., and Marsden, J.R. (1985). Five channel SQUID installation for unshielded neuromagnetic measurements, in Weinberg, H., Stroink, G., and Katila, T., Eds., Biomagnetism : Applications and Theory, Pergamon Press, New York, pp. 46-51.

Zimmerman, J.E. (1972). Josephson effect devices and low-frequency field sensing. Cryogenics 12, pp. 19-31.

RECENT REVIEW ARTICLES
for further references

Hoke, M. (1988). SQUID-Based Measuring Techniques- A Challange for the Functional Diagnostics in Medicine, in The Art of Measurement, Kramer, B., Ed., VCH Verlagsgesellschaft mbH, Weinheim, pp. 287-335.

Ryhänen, T., Seppä, H., Ilmoniemi, R., and Knuutila, J. (1989). SQUID Magnetometers for Low Frequency Applications, J. Low Temp. Physics, 76, pp. 287-386.

Weinberg, H., Stroink, G., and Katila, T. (1988). Biomagnetism, in Encyclopedia of Medical Devices and Instrumentation, John G. Webster, Ed., John Wiley and Sons, New York, pp. 303-322.

Williamson, S.J., Robinson, S.E., and Kaufman, L. (1988). Methods and Instrumentation for Biomagnetism, in Biomagnetism '87, Atsumi, K., Kotani, M., Ueno, S., Katila, T., and Williamson, S.J., Eds., Tokyo Denki University Press, Tokyo, pp. 18-25.

FUNDAMENTALS ON NEUROMAGNETISM

Gian Luca Romani

Istituto di Fisica Medica, Universita' *"G. D'Annunzio"*, Via dei Vestini, 66100 Chieti, and
Istituto Elettronica Stato Solido - CNR. Via Cineto Romano 42, 00156 Roma, ITALY

INTRODUCTION

Although the first attempt to detect a magnetic signal associated with bioelectric activity in the human brain traces back to the late sixties, and was performed by means of a non-superconducting sensor (Cohen, 1968), it was only four years later than a SQUID was successfully used to record a human magnetic alpha rhythm with a satisfactory signal-to-noise ratio (Cohen, 1972). Some years later (Brenner et al., 1975), magnetic signals associated with brain activity evoked by peripheral sensory stimulation were also detected. Hughes and co-workers (1977) examined some cases of generalized epilepsy, but the identification of the most promising application of the neuromagnetic method in the clinical field, namely the study of focal epilepsy, was achieved by the independent work of two groups at the beginning of the nineteeneighties (Barth et al., 1982; Barth et al., 1984; and Modena et al., 1982; Chapman et al., 1983). During the last decade impressive progress have been achieved in the field of neuromagnetism. Fundamental understanding on the structural organization of primary areas in the human brain (Romani et al., 1982a; Pantev et al., 1988; Hari and Kaukoranta, 1985) has been accompanied by important findings on higher levels of brain functions, such as different sounds processing (Hari and Lounasmaa, 1989), or the effect of memory (Lounasmaa et al., 1989). The generators of some of the natural rhythms, like alpha and mu, have been found to be partly localized in specific cortical areas (Chapman et al., 1984) and, even more fascinating, they are likely to be synchronized in an impressive "resonant", macroscopic response (Narici et al., 1987). The noninvasive investigation of focal epilepsy has proved to be a new, powerful tool for pre-operative diagnosis in a widespread disease (Ricci et al., 1985; Rose et al., 1987). But also in more complex pathologies, such the photoconvulsive response in generalized epilepsy, the neuromagnetic investigation has provided significant new information (Ricci et al., 1989). Finally, at least other two major results have been obtained, which have remarkable value for future clinical use: the preoperative evaluation for appropriateness to implant a cochlear prosthesis in deaf patients, and the detection of pathological neural activity associated with tinnitus (Hoke, 1988).

It would be too long to describe in detail all the significant results which have been achieved in the last ten years, and it would go beyond the purposes of the present article, that has been conceived with a *tutorial* structure. After a brief overview of the used nomenclature and of the methodology of magnetic measurements, we will dwell on the genesis of neuromagnetic fields from neural bioelectric activity, with the aim to demonstrate why and when the magnetic approach may really be advantageous, and the kind of information we can learn magnetically. Then, a brief description of the procedure commonly used for source localization will serve as an introduction to a rapid survey of some of the most important results so far obtained in the study of evoked fields, spontaneous activity, and in the clinical field. The reader interested in a complete description of neuromagnetic studies is addressed to recent review articles (Hari and Ilmoniemi, 1986; Hoke, 1988; Romani and Rossini, 1988; Hari and Lounasmaa, 1989).

EXPERIMENTAL NOMENCLATURE AND MEASUREMENT METHODOLOGY

Movements of electrically charged particles, namely ions, inside, across, and outside cellular membranes are responsible for potential differences across the scalp. They also produce magnetic fields

Advances in Biomagnetism
Edited by S.J. Williamson *et al.*
Plenum Press, New York

measurable outside the head: however, as we will see in a following section, the contribution to the generated field from intracellular, transmembrane and extracellular currents respectively is significantly different. By suitably placing a pair of electrodes at appropriate locations on the scalp, it is possible to measure an electroencephalogram (EEG) which, in general, reflect the evolution of electric signals associated with spontaneous activity. When the measurement is related to potential variations produced by sensory stimulation the recorded signal is commonly referred to as evoked potential (EP) or event-related potential (ERP). Similarly, we will call *magnetoencephalogram* (MEG), *evoked field* (EF), and *event-related field* (ERF) the recording of magnetic signals respectively associated with the cerebral activities mentioned above.

Recording of magnetic fields over the scalp is performed by means of SQUID based sensors: these have been described elsewhere in this volume. It is worth reminding, however, that the state of the art nowadays permits to detect the field simultaneously at several sites of the head. The component of the magnetic field perpendicular to the scalp, $\mathbf{B}_n$, is typically measured by means of detection coils featuring an interferometric geometry, namely that of a *first-order-*, or of a *second-order axial gradiometer*. Alternatively, new instruments are being setup (Kajola et al., this volume), which use *first-order planar gradiometers*. In this case the transverse derivative of $\mathbf{B}_n$ is measured, thus providing different kind of information on the cerebral field. We will come back to this point, since it turns to have fundamental importance for the problem of source localization.

MODELING NEURAL BIOELECTRIC ACTIVITY

It has been already said that ionic currents in the cerebral cells produce magnetic fields. This phenomenon is due to a general physical behavior, predicted by the Ampere's law and summarized by the Biot-Savart law: whenever an electric current flows, a magnetic field is generated in the surrounding space. Its intensity strongly diminishes with distance whereas its direction and orientation are given the right-hand rule: if the current flows along the thumb, the field lines follow a circular pattern identified by the other fingers. This statement is valid for any conductor along which a current flows, and holds also for neural cells, where the role of "moving electric charges" is basically played by Na^+ and K^+ ions. Figure 1 schematically illustrates the pattern of ionic currents which flow inside, across, and outside the membrane of a neuron, and specifically in a portion of it, like an axon or a dendritic tree. A detailed description of the ionic exchange on both sides of the membrane, as well as of the time evolution of this phenomenon would not fit the limits of the present article: the interested reader is therefore addressed to a recent review (Williamson and Kaufman, 1989). We want to stress here only some basic aspects of this neural process, which turn to have a fundamental importance for the structure of the generated magnetic fields.

Current pattern produced by neural excitations

The first point we want to remark regards the distribution of ionic currents: the *intracellular current* is basically a concentrated ionic flow inside the membrane, and along it in a very small portion of the total dendritic or axonal length. This is represented by an arrow in Fig. 1, and is what is accounted for by the simplest and most used model source, namely a *current dipole*. The *transmembrane current* follows a radial pattern, in that it isotropically flows through a cross section of the "cylindrically" shaped neural membrane. The *extracellular current* flows backward in the surrounding medium in order to close the loop and satisfy the current continuity requirement. Differently from what happens to the intracellular current, the pattern is now widespread in the surrounding medium, but again an axial symmetry is mantained, at least as far as the medium has homogeneous conductivity.

Action potentials and postsynaptic activity

The second point concerns the time evolution of this bioelectric event. The pattern illustrated in Fig. 1 actually represents a *depolarization* process, with respect to the " unperturbed " resting state of the membrane. This phenomenon, that, for example, may be initiated by a perturbation provided by an excitatory synapse, is followed by a *repolarization* process, during which the membrane returns to its initial state, thanks to the Na-K pump. In this second event the overall current pattern is reversed, with the intracellular current pointing backward and the extracellular current pointing in a forward direction. At this point a fundamental distinction between two neural mechanisms needs to be made: either the depolarization and repolarization *fronts* rapidly move along the axon, as a propagating excitation, linked together and separated by less than few milliseconds in time, and less than few millimeters in space for a cortical unmyelinated axon, or the depolarization process is relatively localized, typically at a cortical level, is "mediated" by synaptic activity and is followed by a much slower repolarization process, in an overall time scale that can reach even hundreds of milliseconds, and usually may involve several thousands of adjacent dendrites. The two phenomenona are commonly referred to as *action potential currents* and *postsynaptic currents*, respectively.

The substantial difference in the time scale supports the idea that action potential currents, beside their evident role in the peripheral nervous system, are also responsible for measured brain-stem activity (Erne' et al., 1987) and, possibly, for early components of cortical response (Rossini et al., 1989). On the other hand, postsynaptic currents, such as those involving apical dendrites of pyramidal neurons which feature a preferential alignement perpendicularly to the cortical surface, are commonly supposed to generate stimulus-related and event-related responses.

The equivalent current dipole

The current dipole model, briefly described above, may account for both bioelectric phenomena. The current patterns of a travelling action potential are indeed well represented by two oppositely directed current dipoles moving along the axon. A single dipole may account for postsynaptic activity of an apical dendrite. However, as will be discussed below, it is more likely that an equivalent current dipole (ECD) represents a large number of neurons simultaneously and synchronously active.

We will not describe in detail the current dipole (CD) source, in that it has been already explained in a different article of this volume. It is useful, however, to recall here that a CD is a vector defined by the relation **Q** = I**L**, the intensity of which, namely Q = IL is expressed in ampere-meter, and decreases as the square of the distance from the site where the current flow is concentrated. The current pattern associated with this source, when immersed in a homogeneously conducting medium, well reproduces the one illustrated in Fig. 1.

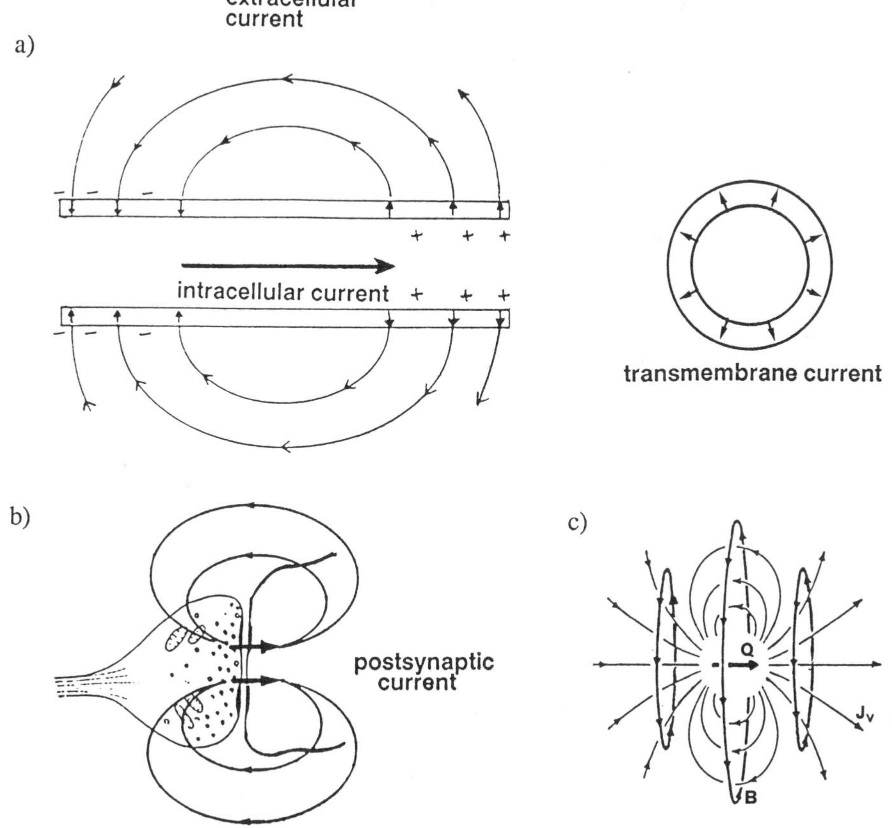

Fig.1. a) Current pattern associated with the depolarization front of an axon potential (top), (b) and with a postsynaptic potential. c) A current dipole model source.

The field generated by such a source in an infinite medium with homogeneous conductivity may be calculated by integrating the Biot-Savart law. An interesting property is that if we divide the current pattern in two parts, the primary current and the volume currents (see Fig. 1), it happens that the *net* contribution to the field at any point in space from volume currents is zero. This occurs because of the symmetry of the paths of volume currents in the medium, the contribution from one region of space being cancelled by contribution from another region.

A reasonable question at this point would regard transmembrane currents, which are not accounted for by the model. Indeed, also their contribution to the field is negligible: this was mathematically calculated by Swinney and Wikswo (1980), but can also be qualitatively demonstrated, as made by Williamson and Kaufman (1989). These authors pointed out that the contribution of the transmembrane current must be basically smaller than that of intracellular (primary) currents because of the radial symmetry of the pattern (see Fig. 1) which produces substantial cancellation of the field from inversely directed currents on opposite sides of the membrane. Additionally, due to the thinness of the neural membrane, the volume containing the transmembranic current flow is much smaller than the intracellular volume where the primary current flows. On the basis of these two arguments Willliamson and Kaufman (1989) conclude that 'it is ironic that the transmembrane current, which gives rise to the cellular excitation in the first place, plays no appreciable direct role in producing the detected magnetic field'.

Estimation of neural population size from the detected field

It is instructive to use the Biot-Savart law to evaluate the magnetic field generated by a current dipole accounting for postsynaptic activity in a single neuron. The expression for Q has been obtained in various way by different authors (Hari and Ilmoniemi, 1986; Williamson and Kaufman, 1989). We will use a very simple approximation which leads, however, to the same result. We assume that a dendritic tree having a diameter d and a length L behaves like a conductor featuring a conductivity σ. The total resistance is given by the Ohm's law ($I = V / R$): $R = 4 L / (\pi d^2 \sigma)$, and the dipole moment is:

$$Q = \pi d^2 \sigma V / 4$$

by substituting the following typical values (Williamson and Kaufman, 1989), $d \approx 4\ \mu m$, $\sigma \approx 0.25\ \Omega^{-1} m^{-1}$, and $V \approx 10$ mV, we obtain $Q \approx 3 \times 10^{-14}$ Am. The resulting magnetic field may be derived by the Biot-Savart law:

$$\mathbf{B} = (\mu_0 / 4\pi)\, \mathbf{Q} \times \mathbf{r} / r^3$$

where μ_0 is the permeability of free space and has a value of $4\pi \cdot 10^{-7}$ newton/ampere^2 in the SI units. The permeability of biological tissues may be considered equal to that of free space, as long as there are no ferromagnetic particles within the tissue. The magnetic induction B can be easily calculated at a point, say, 4 cm away from the neuron in a transverse direction. This assumption is reasonably realistic if we consider, for instance, a pyramidal neuron in the somatosensory or the auditory cortex. The resulting value, $B \approx 0.002$ fT, is evidently too weak to be detected by any magnetic sensor. As a field of 100 fT (or more) is typically measured outside the scalp in response to somatosensory or auditory stimulation, the implication is that a large number of neurons, 50,000 or more, coherently act to generate that field, adding their individual responses to form the macroscopic signal. This also explains why post-synaptic activities give a larger field than action potentials: to build up a detectable field many action potentials must occur in adjacent axons within 1 ms, since the signal is only 1 ms long. On the other hand, post-synaptic activities last for 10 ms or more, so that there is much more time to add up all single fields. Furthermore, in the case of an action potential, the generated field is the sum of the two fields coming from two opposite dipoles, namely a magnetic quadrupole, so that its amplitude is more rapidly decreasing with the distance between the source and the sensor.

We want to stress once more that the hypothesis that postsynaptic activity is responsible for the macroscopic fields measured in response to stimulation of sensory systems is not physiologically unrealistic. Actually, in most primary areas several cortical layers contain a population of neurons, namely *pyramidal cells*, which present a preferential allignement in a direction orthogonal to the cortex surface. It is therefore not unlikely that postsynaptic currents flowing along the apical dendrites, and simultaneously involving a large group of cells, may produce fields large enough to be detected at a scalp level. On the contrary, it is much harder to reveal magnetic signals related to action potential currents, such as, for instance, those flowing along a myelinated axon of the peripheral sensory system. An experimental *in vitro* verification of the quadrupolar aspect of these last type of phenomena was given by Roth and coworkers (1985) . More recently, the travelling magnetic signal produced by stimulation of the median nerve at the wrist was measured in vivo at several positions along the nerve path (Erne' et al., 1988). The distribution of the field over the biceps was used to localize the equivalent generator and the agreement with the actual location of the nerve in the arm, as inferred by MRI pictures, was definitively good. An interesting finding was the absence of a clearcut repolarization front in the measured signals. This might be in contrast with the theory of two oppositely travelling dipoles (or a magnetic quadrupole). The authors, however, suggested that, while the depolarization front is triggered by the electric stimulation, the repolarization process might be somewhat spread in time: as the overall duration of the phenomenon is of the order of 1 ms, a small desynchronization of the same order of magnitude may produce a significant reduction of the "macroscopic" field, and eventually its immersion in the noise.

Spherical medium

The independence of magnetic field of volume currents holds in case of an infinite medium with homogeneous conductivity. A convenient approximation for the head is a spherical medium, with homogeneous conductivity. The modelling medium requires further complexity when interpreting electric potential data. In this case a three, concentric, sphere model is preferred, each shell endowed with a homogeneous conductivity and accounting for a specific "component" of the head: cerebral tissue and fluid, skull (with a conductivity about 80 times smaller than the others), and the scalp. This higher complexity is needed since volume currents are affected by the conductivity of the tissues surrounding the primary source. In case of magnetic measurements, however, the component of the field perpendicular to the sphere surface is still independent of volume currents. This means that the three sphere model and the single sphere one are completely identical, as far as the normal component of the field is measured.

By measuring only $\mathbf{B}_n$, however, an important limitation comes out: only tangential dipoles contribute to it. This means that we are somewhat "blind" with respect to radially oriented current flows, namely all those involving apical dendrites in areas located in convolutions of the cortex. A second implication is that a dipole located in the center of the sphere is magnetically "silent".

Toward a realistic medium

It should be remarked that the homogeneously conducting sphere model is only a first approximation and, indeed, it acceptable only if the perpendicularity to the sphere surface is saved. On the other hand only some portions of the head are satisfactorily reproducible by means of a sphere, in particular the occipital area. The temporal zone, extremely important for many measurements of focal epilepsy, is poorly represented by a sphere with a unique radius. Furthermore, the development of multichannel systems has, ironically, worsened the situation! The gradiometers are indeed positioned according to a fixed radius of curvature (typically chosen between 12 and 16 cm), and the relatively careful orienting with respect to the head of a single channel system is definitively lost. This means that it is illusory to pretend to measure the normal component of the field with a large multichannel system: rather, a certain portion of the normal component and another of the tangential component will be detected by the gradiometers, and the relative percentage will be in general different for each of them.

A first progress consists in fitting the sphere to the inner surface of the skull, i.e. to the brain surface and in evaluating the contribution to the field from volume currents flowing in the sphere. Hamalainen and Sarvas (1987) have indeed demonstrated that the greatest part of volume currents indeed flow inside the skull, due to the small value of the bone conductivity. Only a few percent of volume currents actually reaches the scalp surface, and consequently, the total magnetic induction **B** may be calculated by considering the model source as immersed in a "smaller" sphere with a homogeneous conductivity equal to that of the cerebral tissue.

A second improvement consists in expressing in a mathematical form (by triangulation) the actual surface of the brain, as derived from MRI data. The forward problem is then solved by assuming that this surface enclose a medium with homogeneous conductivity, and the potential over the surface and the field outside it is evaluated. Hamalainen and Sarvas (1987) have demonstrated the feasibility of this procedure, whereas Ducla-Soares and co-workers (Ducla-Soares, this volume) experimentally verified the goodness of the approach.

The final step consists in considering a realistic multi-layer medium, and in solving the forward problem therein. As it has recently pointed out (Hamalainen and Sarvas, 1989), this sophisticated procedure is important to evaluate the electric potential over the scalp, but it is not necessary when calculating the magnetic field, a brain-shaped homogeneous conductor being indeed more than sufficient to get all the relevant information on the field. The obvious penalty we pay in going toward a realistic head model is that the procedure for calculating the field is increasingly time-consuming. This might not fit the requirement of a rapid data analysis when handling a wide scale clinical screening.

Information contained in $\mathbf{B}_n$

Before concluding this section we want to stress that the amount of information contained in a measurement of $\mathbf{B}_n$ may indeed completely characterize the field. As Hari and Ilmoniemi pointed out (1986), the two tangential component of the field may be calculated by measuring the transverse derivatives of $\mathbf{B}_n$. The Maxwell's equations require that outside the body, where there are no biological sources, *curl* $\mathbf{B} = 0$. Using for simplicity a cartesian coordinate system, where $\mathbf{B}_n = \mathbf{B}_z$, the vectorial relation written above gives:

$$\partial \mathbf{B}_x / \partial z = \partial \mathbf{B}_z / \partial x$$

$$\partial \mathbf{B}_y / \partial z = \partial \mathbf{B}_z / \partial y$$

The components $\mathbf{B}_x$ and $\mathbf{B}_y$ may be evaluated by integrating the above expressions. The physical meaning of this fact is that, although the radial component of the magnetic field is produced by the primary current alone, the way $\mathbf{B}_n$ changes in space is determined by both primary and volume currents.

The transverse derivatives of $\mathbf{B}_n$ may be easily detected using planar gradiometers. A "hybrid" multichannel system using both axial gradiometers, thus measuring $\mathbf{B}_z$, and planar gradiometers, to detect $\partial \mathbf{B}_Z / \partial x$ and $\partial \mathbf{B}_Z / \partial y$, would permit to adequately reconstruct the total magnetic field.

PROCEDURE FOR SOURCE LOCALIZATION

In this section we will briefly describe the steps which may be followed to achieve source localization on the basis of a magnetic field map recorded over the scalp. Then we will try to point out some parameters of the experimental procedure which may significantly affect the quality of results.

Localization procedure

The first *inevitable* assumption, intrinsically linked to the non-uniqueness of the inverse problem, is whether or not the experimental map may be interpreted by the simple dipole model. This is still an experimenter's decision, and turns to have a fundamental importance for the final result. Other choices may alternatively be made, like complex-many-dipole configurations, etc.; however, we will consider only the simplest case. The process to find the dipole location (three parameters) and strength (two parameters, for the tangential component of the dipole only!) has a recursive structure (Romani and Leoni, 1985):

1) A first guess of the dipole position and strength in the sphere is made. The choice of a good first guess may significantly speed-up the process.
2) The magnetic field generated by such a source is calculated (forward problem), and
3) The difference between the theoretical and the experimental field distribution is evaluated, typically adopting the χ^2 as a figure of merit to be optimized.
4) A new dipole location and strength is generated, and the χ^2 is then evaluated and compared with the previous value. A smaller χ^2 value means a better approximation to the real source. By means of such an iterative procedure, a new set of parameters is obtained at each iteration. A progressive reduction of the figure of merit implies that the rate of reduction becomes smaller and smaller. The fit is truncated when the variation reaches a pre-defined threshold. The final set of parameters provides the best approximation for the equivalent source accounting for the measured field distribution. It is clear that, again, the choice of the threshold is crucial, and depends exclusively on the experimenter's skill.
5) Finally, the 95% confidence interval may be calculated. This is performed by simple statistical tests that produce little variation in the parameter space starting from the fitted values, with the aim to check the stability of the fit itself. A small 95% confidence interval means a reliable fit and viceversa.

Experimental accuracy and reproducibility

It is worth stressing that the "final" result of a neuromagnetic measurement is, in general, the identification of a specific source responsible for a certain cerebral activity. The procedure illustrated above provides the "best location and strength" of an equivalent source accounting for the measured pattern: However, the reliability and the accuracy of these values are affected by several factors which must be carefully considered.

System noise, for instance, directly influences the signal-to-noise ratio, and dramatically depends on whether or not the meaurement is performed in a shielded environment. Brain noise, that is uncontrolled signals from activity other than the one under investigation, constitutes a disturbing background (Hari, personal communication). More in general, noise from other sources in the body, such as the heart, may also produce fastidious artifacts, particularly if the measurement is performed with magnetometer coils or with long-baseline first-order gradiometers (Erne, personal communication).

Large effects are definitively introduced by errors in positioning the dewar with respect to the subject's head. This task can be performed in several ways. One method consists in taping around the subject's head three small rf transmitters, and in monitoring their signal by means of an appropriate receiver, fixed to the dewar, to identify their relative position. Another method uses the superconducting array to record an ac, low-frequency signal fed to three tiny copper coils, i.e. magnetic dipoles, fixed at specific, anatomically significant location of the subject's head. A source localization procedure with a six-(times three) parameter fit is carried out immediately before and after each measurement to check possible variations in system positioning. This method was independently proposed by Knuutila and Ilmoniemi (1985) and by Erne' and co-workers (1987). The second group performed a detailed analysis on the performance of the procedure using simulations and including the effect of noise, and demonstrated a pretty good accuracy in the assessment of relative positioning, provided the number of detection coils was high enough (19 or more), and the copper coils were at least three. These two requirements are linked to the need for having enough simultaneous information from the array, and to avoid ambiguities in the minimization process.

We have already discussed the problem of a realistic head model, and therefore it is needless to say how profoundly the choice of the medium may affect the localization accuracy. Before concluding, however, it is worth mentioning a last factor which, probably, has not been sufficiently recognized. The assumption that a biological signal is basically reproducible is commonly made whenever more than a single cerebral response is needed to improve the signal-to-noise ratio, i.e. in all evoked response measurements. This assumption, equivalent to the idea that the brain response is stationary, is wrong. Indeed, recent analyses performed by several groups on evoked potential responses by means of sophisticated selection criteria (Gevins, 1984; Cerutti et al., 1987), and first results obtained with the same approach in case of evoked field measurements (Liberati, personal communication), have shown that the cerebral response is significantly varying across repetitive stimulation, ranging from what is currently referred to as an actual evoked signal, to weaker, or even completely missing responses. This effect has a fundamental importance, in that the final morphology of the averaged signal may be profoundly affected by the "non-valid" responses, and the subsequent "topographic" analysis may be misleading or even definitely wrong. Therefore, great care should be taken to ensure as much as possible a reproducible cerebral response, by controlling all the psychological parameters that may influence subject's concentration and motivation. Additionally, the power (and the risks) of advanced response selection criteria - such as those based on auto-regressive moving averages (ARMA), or any other which may provide a statistical significance to the chosen response - should be adequately exploited.

EXAMPLES OF NEUROMAGNETIC STUDIES

Tonotopic and amplitopic organization of the auditory cortex

The investigation of the human auditory cortex by neuromagnetic measurements gave the first non-invasive confirmation that human neurons, similarly to what happens in animals, are tuned to different tonal frequencies and serially located along the floor and roof of the Sylvian fissure. Such a logarithmic progression, namely a *tonotopic* organization, strictly reproduces that of the acoustic epithelium within the cochlea. Equivalent dipoles feature progressively deeper localization with respect to the delivery of acoustic stimuli containing more acute frequencies. This regular functional structure was previously demonstrated using pure tones, sinusoidally modulated at low frequency, as acoustic stimuli (Romani et al., 1982a; Romani et al., 1982b). More recently, a similar result was obtained using tone bursts with different frequency: the logarithmic behavior with frequency was observed for the component of the evoked response with 100 msec delay, namely *latency*, from the stimulus onset (Pantev et al., 1988). The results are

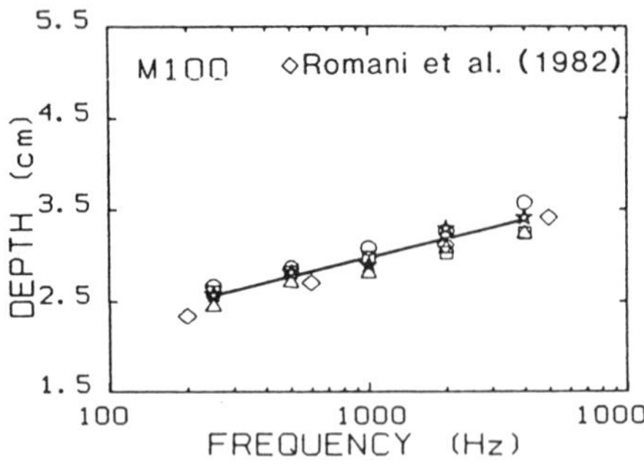

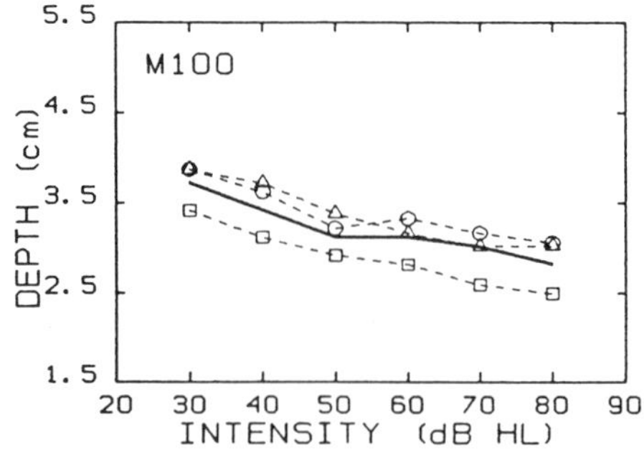

Fig. 2. Tonotopic and amplitopic organization of the auditory cortex (modified from Hoke, 1988, and including data from Romani et al., 1982a)

illustrated in Fig. 2. It should be remarked that the two experiments used significantly different stimulation paradigms. However, the agreement of the results reported in Fig. 2 is impressively good, and provides a concrete argument for the long-lasting debate on whether or not the steady-state and the transient modalities may provide consistent and coherent information on the cortex functional organization.

But the auditory cortex seems to have an even more intriguing characteristic: a regular progression of cortical sites also exists with respect to the intensity of the acoustic stimulation. This spatial representation of stimulus intensity, namely *amplitopic* organization, locates sources elicited by more intense sounds at more superficial sites, whereas the depth increases with increasing stimulus frequency (see Fig. 2). Moreover, a slight anterior shift of the dipole location with increasing intensity antiparallels the one observed with increasing frequency. This fact has an important consequence (Hoke, 1988): the way intensity is coded at a cochlear level is the same as for frequency. Both higher intensity and frequency elicit areas toward the beginning of the cochlear partition. By contrast, the cortical representation of intensity and frequency is "bidimensional", in that for each intensity an isofrequency line exists, and an isointensity exists for each frequency as well. These two sets of parallel isolines are crossing each other.

Spontaneous- and synchronized spontaneous activity

The neuromagnetic approach to the study of spontaneous activity, although fundamentally limited by the lack of simultaneity in the analysis of MEG distribution, has provided evidence that the sources of the predominant alpha rhythm might be located within a relatively discrete area of a few square centimeters on both sides of a cross formed by the calcarine and interhemispheric fissures and at an average depth of 5 cm (Chapman et al., 1984). These authors proposed and used for these measurement a new analytical approach, namely the *relative covariance* method (RCM), in which the covariance between magnetic and electric signals is calculated, after appropriate filtering in the bandwidth of interest (i.e. around 10 Hz). The covariance coefficient is divided by the variance of the electric signal similarly filtered, to compensate for possible variations of source intensity during sequential recordings. In this way the relative covariance coefficient is obtained. A similar procedure is carried out for all successive measurements, obviously maintaining unchanged the electric lead used for calculating the reference variance. Finally, a scalp distribution for the relative covariance coefficient is achieved, which reflects that of the magnetic field over the scalp. In-phase MEG and EEG signals give positive RC values, whereas out-of-phase signals produce negative RC values. Chapman and co-workers (1984) stressed that a great limitation of the RCM is the fundamental hypothesis that EEG and MEG signals reflect the activity of the same sources, and that the information on the time evolution of the rhythmic activity is completely lost. Nevertheless, the RCM has permitted a significant advance in the study of rhythmic- and quasi-rhythmic activity, with important benefit in the clinical field (see below).

The neuromagnetic investigation of spontaneous activity has provided recently other significant new information on the process that links natural rhythms to evoked responses. It had been known since mid nineteenfifties that the cerebral response to flash stimulation was structured in several components at specific latencies, but might be "concluded" by an oscillation, namely *after discharge*, peaked at the alpha frequency (about 10 Hz) (Regan, 1972). Narici and co-workers (1987) observed a similar phenomenon with a completely different stimulation paradigm: a sequence of brief stimuli were delivered to the subjects with a specific repetition rate and for a period lasting 1 to 2 s. Each sequence of stimuli was separated by the following one by a non-stimulating period of equal duration. In this way the brain was supposed to have time enough to recover its initial unperturbed state before the successive stimulation. A surprising observation was that the cerebral response, elicited and increasingly enhanced during the "train" of stimuli, lasted well beyond the end of the last stimulus, with a typical oscillating behavior thus resembling that of an after discharge. A second observation was that the response was sharply *tuned* at a "resonant" frequency: by varying the repetition rate of the train of stimuli in a relatively wide range, Narici and co-workers observed a *resonant* response in the non-stimulated period only at a precise rate, and practically no response at all for all other rates. The third significant finding was that this resonant response, which might have been expectable in the visual modality, was observed also in the somatosensory modality. Visual stimulation elicited responses tuned at about 10 Hz, whereas somatosensory resonant response was peaked around 6-8 Hz, with often a contribution at the second harmonic. Figure 3 shows some of these responses obtained from various subjects in the two modalities. In the same figure also the frequency behavior of the responses is reported: it is worth stressing the impressive similarity between the frequency response in the visual modality and the measured spectral density for the alpha rhythm of the same subjects.

A successive series of experiments (Narici et al., 1988; Narici and Romani, 1989) provided further information on the possible genesis of this phenomenon. Detailed field mapping performed in both modalities showed that the distribution of the tuned response over the occipital and parietal scalp, respectively, actually featured a dipolar distribution, that permitted to carry out source localization. In brief, these authors found that the observed phenomenon was likely to be an effect of *synchronization* of at least part of the generators responsible for spontaneous activity, in particular the alpha- and mu-rhythms.

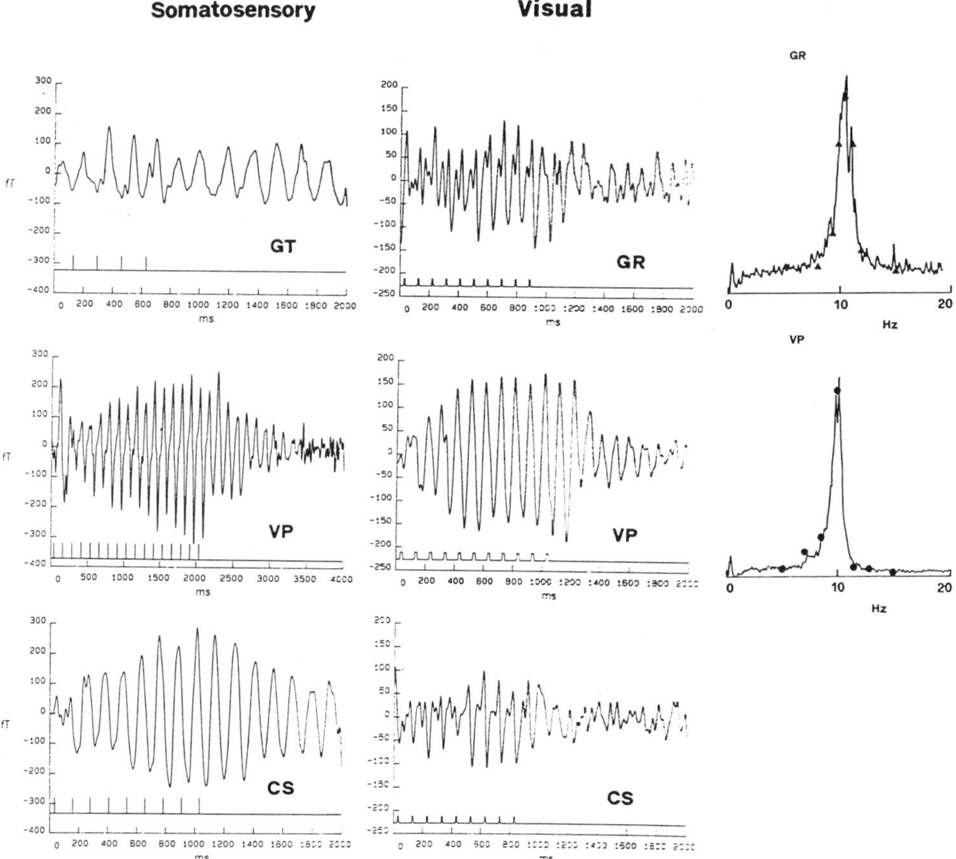

Fig. 3. Synchronized spontaneous responses obtained for different subjects in the somatosensory and visual modality. The frequency behavior of the visual responses and the spectral densities of the alpha rhythm for two subjects are shown together on the right.

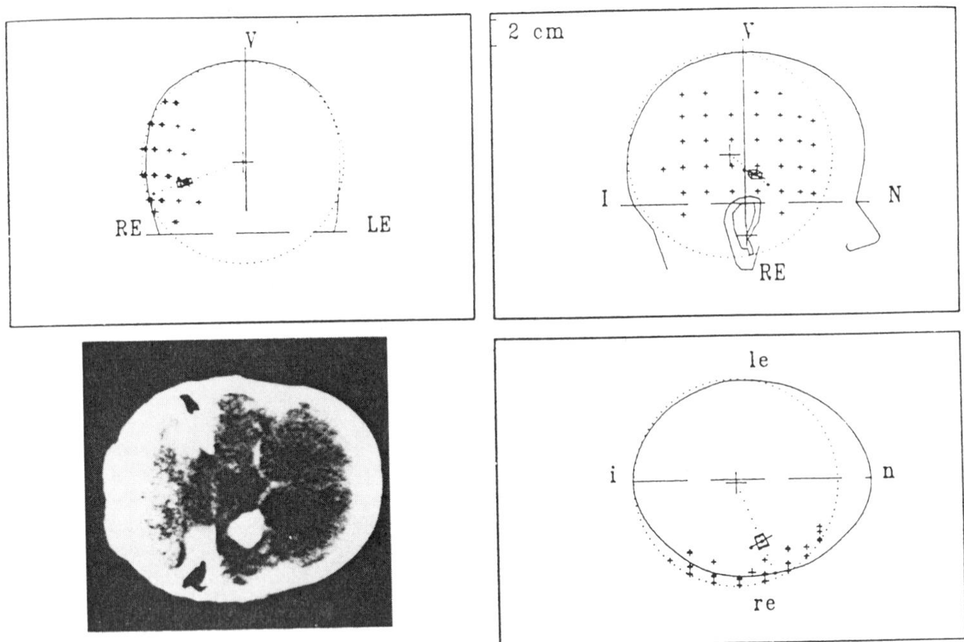

Fig. 4. Neuromagnetic localization of the ECD accounting for the measured activity in a patient affected by a calcification in the right uncus area. The result was obtained using the relative covariance method.

The cortical location of the generators of the resonant visual response was basically coincident with the area where previous studies had observed generation of alpha rhythm (Chapman et al., 1984), whereas the generators of the mu-rhythm were likely to be localized in the somatosensory cortex, close to the area where the first cortical components of the somatosensory evoked response are generated. Finally, these authors pointed out significant implications that these findings might have for the understanding of the generation of the "traditional" evoked responses, which indeed might share part of the population of generators for natural rhythms to build up a reinforced response at specific frequencies (Regan, 1972).

Clinical applications

The analysis of "spike" activity during interictal period in focal epilepsy undoubtedly represents one of the most promising applications of the neuromagnetic method in the clinical field. Selection of EEG spikes with a large amplitude, and consequently with a good signal-to-noise ratio, and subsequent averaging of the corresponding MEG signals, has permitted to obtain quite often clearcut dipolar field maps and to carry out a source localization procedure to identify the location of the active focus (Barth et al., 1982; Barth et al., 1984). The quasi-rhythmic polymorphic activity often accompanying spike activity was shown to be much more powerfully investigable using the relative covariance method, illustrated above

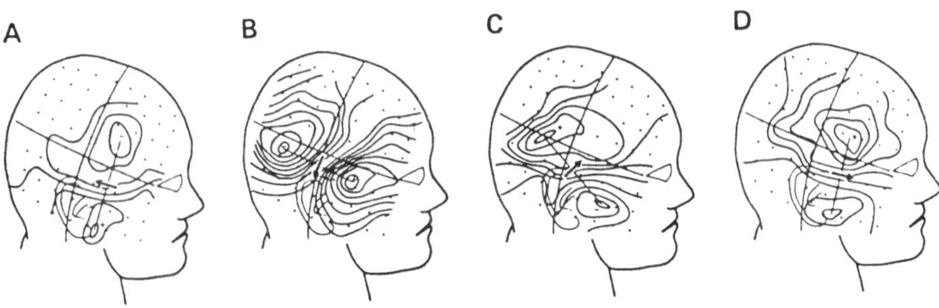

Fig. 5. Magnetic field maps revealing a discharge sequence between two sources underlying an interictal complex in the right temporal lobe (After Barth et al., 1984).

(Chapman et al., 1983; Ricci et al., 1985). Fig. 4 shows and example of neuromagnetic localization obtained with the RCM, whereas Fig. 5 illustrates the successive activation of two cortical sources underlying an interictal spike complex in the temporal lobe. The results obtained by the neuromagnetic study have been also compared with direct measurements perfomed on the exposed cortex during surgery, with a quite satisfactory agreement (Ricci et al., 1985; Rose et al., 1987). There are still several problems that should be clarified before a widespreading of the technique in everyday practice. In particular, i) the brain area generating a single epileptic discharge may be not invariant, ii) there may be different neuronal populations contributing to a single epileptic patterns, iii) there is little support to the idea that intercritical activity and activity during seizures should come from the same generators. All these questions must be adequately answered in order to assess the neuromagnetic method as a valid pre-operative diagnostic means. A parallel solution of the inverse problem in the realistic head will fasten the achievement of this goal.

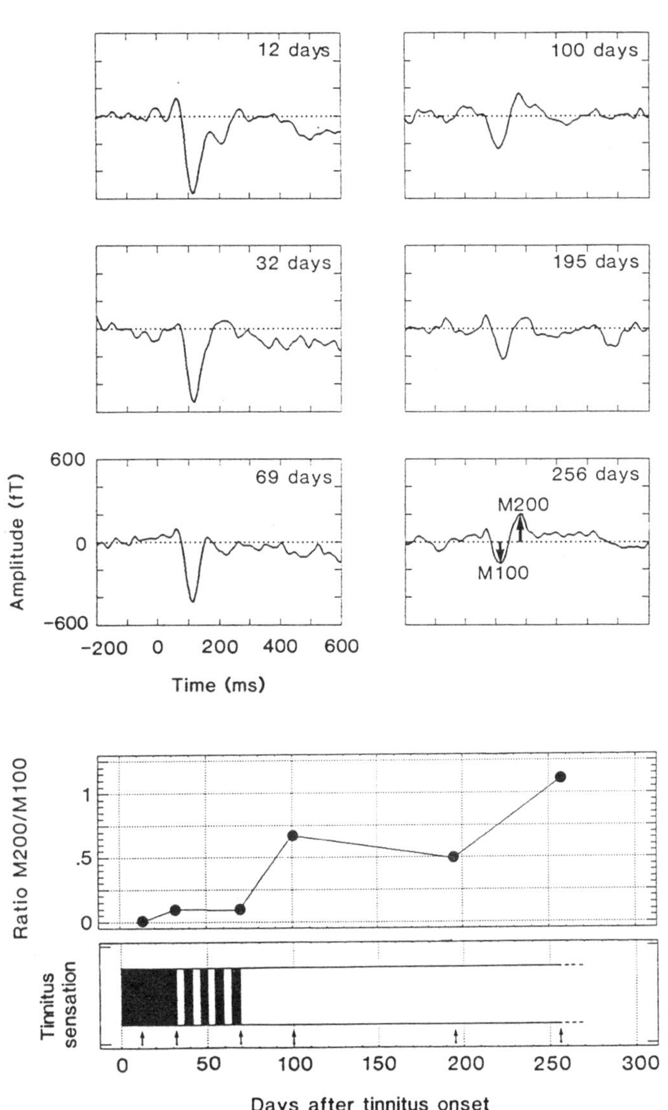

Fig. 6. (Top) Observed variation with time of the morphology of the magnetic 100 and 200 components in the evoked auditory response from one subject suffering for a noise trauma. The time evolution of the M200/M100 ratio is compared with the "subjective" sensation of tinnitus (bottom; black field: permanent tinnitus; bars: intermittent tinnitus; blank field: no tinnitus).

Before concluding this section we want to mention two other promising clinical applications of the neuromagnetic method. We have already seen that at the end of a localization procedure not only the coordinates but also the strength of the ECD are evaluated. This fact may have fundamental importance if an estimate of the active neural population is needed as, for instance, in cases of hearing loss. The decision whether or not the implantation of a cochlear prostesis is appropriate, strongly depends on the knowledge of the residual number of excitable neurons in the auditory cortex. Moreover, direct stimulation of the acoustic nerve in cases of total cochlear deafness may be performed by means of an electrode or by an electrode array surgically implanted in the inner ear. Investigation of brain-stem evoked potentials permits only to conclude that some responsive nerve fibers still exist, but no information is gathered on the number of surviving active neurons in the cortex, information on which depends the choice of implanting a single-channel electrode or, rather, a much more expensive but effective twenty-channel system (Hoke, 1988).

Finally, it is worth mentioning that the neuromagnetic method has been successfully applied to the study of patients affected by ringing in the ear, namely *tinnitus*. This disease, associated with various hearing defects, has been supposed to be linked to abnormal spontaneous activity, and has an impressively high incidence in industrialized countries (14-15% of the population), (Hoke, 1988). A systematic study recently performed on a relatively large population of patients affected by tinnitus, as compared with a normal group, clearly showed objective evidence that in the auditory evoked magnetic response the component with 200 msec latency is delayed and dramatically depressed. whereas the amplitude of the 100 msec component is significantly increased (Hoke et al., 1989). These authors conclude that the ratio between the amplitude of the 200 msec component and that of the 100 msec component may well serve as a figure of merit to objectively diagnose tinnitus below the age of 50. Very recently, Pantev and co-workers (1989) could verify the goodness of this hypothesis by studying tinnitus remission for a period of 256 days in one case where tinnitus had been provoked by a noise trauma (see Fig. 6).

CONCLUSIONS

The purpose of the present *tutorial* was not at all to provide a complete review of neuromagnetic studies: rather, we tried to point out the basic principles of a simple modeling of neural activity, with specific emphasis on cortical activity, since it has been at this level that so far the most interesting results have been obtained. Some practical considerations regarding the measuring procedure and the data analysis procedure have been illustrated, in that they might turn to be advantageous for the experimenter who would like to initiate research activity in this field. Evident limitations in space have forced to describe only very few examples of what has been achieved by the neuromagnetic method: our hope, however, is that they may serve of encouragement for much more impressive progress in a very near future.

ACKNOWLEDGEMENTS

The author is indebted to all members of the biomagnetic group in Roma. Special thanks are due to G. Torrioli for help during the preparation of the article, and to V. Pizzella for a critical revision of the manuscript.

REFERENCES

Barth, D.S., Sutherling, W., Engel Jr., J., and Beatty, J. (1982). Neuromagnetic localization of epileptiform spike activity in the human brain. Science, 218:891-894.

Barth, D.S., Sutherling, W., Engel Jr., J., and Beatty, J. (1984). Neuromagnetic evidence of spatially distributed sources underlying epileptiform spikes in the human brain. Science, 223:293-296.

Brenner, D., Williamson, S.J., and Kaufman, L. (1975). Visually evoked magnetic fields of the human brain. Science, 190:480-482.

Cerutti, S., Baselli, D., Liberati, D., and Pavesi, G. (1987). Single sweep analysis of visual evoked potentials through a model of parametric identification. Biol. Cybern., 56:111-120.

Chapman, R.M., Romani, G.L., Barbanera, S., Leoni, R., Modena, I., Ricci, G.B., and Campitelli, F. (1983). SQUID instrumentation and the relative covariance method for magnetic 3-D localization of pathological cerebral sources. Nuovo Cimento Lett., 38:549-554.

Chapman, R.M., Ilmoniemi, R., Barbanera, S., and Romani, G.L. (1984). Selective localization of alpha brain activity with neuromagnetic measurements. Electroenceph. clin. Neurophysiol., 58:569-572.

Cohen, D. (1968). Magnetoencephalography: Evidence of magnetic fields produced by alpha-rhythm currents. Science, 161:784-786.

Cohen, D. (1972). Magnetoencephalography: Detection of the brain's electrical activity with a superconducting magnetometer. Science, 175:664-666.

Erne', S.N., Scheer, J.H., Hoke, M., Pantev, C., and Lütkenhöner, B. (1987). Brain stem auditory evoked magnetic fields in response to stimulation with brief tone pulses. Intern. J. Neurosci., 37:115-125.

Erne', S.N., Narici, L., Pizzella, V., and Romani, G.L. (1987). The positioning problem in biomagnetic measurements: a solution for arrays of superconducting sensors. IEEE Trans. Magn. MAG-23: 1319-1322.

Erne', S.N., Curio, G., Trahms, L., Trontelj, Z., and Aust, P. (1988). Magnetic activity of a single peripheral nerve in man. In: Atsumi, K., Kotani, M., Ueno, S., Katila, T., and Williamson, S.J. (Eds), Biomagnetism '87, Tokyo Denki University Press, 166-169.

Gevins, A.S. (1984). Analysis of the electromagnetic signals of the human brain: milestones, obstacles, and goals. IEEE Trans. BME-31:833-850.

Hämäläinen, M.S., and Sarvas, J. (1987). Feasibility of the homogeneous head model in the interpretation of neuromagnetic fields. Phys. Med. Biol., 32:91-97.

Hämäläinen, M.S., and Sarvas, J. (1989). Realistic conductivity geometry model of the human head for interpretation of neuromagnetic data. IEEE Trans. BME-36:165-171.

Hari, R., and Kaukoranta, E. (1985). Neuromagnetic study of somatosensory system: Principles and examples. Prog. Neurobiol. 24:233-256.

Hari, R., and Ilmoniemi, R.J. (1986). Cerebral magnetic fields. CRC Critical Reviews in Biomed. Engineer., 14:93-126.

Hari, R., and Lounasmaa, O.V. (1989). Recording and interpretation of cerebral magnetic fields. Science, 244:432-436.

Hoke, M. (1988). SQUID-based measuring techniques - A challenge for the functional diagnostics in medicine. In: The art of measurement, Kramer, B. (Ed.), VCH Verlagsgesellschaft mbH, Weinheim, 287-335.

Hoke, M., Feldmann, H., Pantev, C., Lütkenhöner, B., and Lehnertz, K. (1989). Objective evidence of tinnitus in auditory evoked magnetic fields. Hearing Res., 37:281-286.

Hughes, J.R., Cohen, J., Mayman, C.I., Scholl, M.L., and Hendrix, D.E. (1977). Relationships of the magnetoencephalogram to abnormal activity in the electroencephalogram. J. Neurol., 217:79-93.

Knuutila, J., Ahonen, A.I., Hämäläinen, M.S., Ilmoniemi, R.J., and Kajola, M.J. (1985). Design considerations for multichannel SQUID magnetometers. In: Hahlbohm, H.D., and Lübbig, H. (Eds), SQUID85: Superconducting Quantum Interference Devices and their applications. Walter de Gruyter, Berlin-New York, 939-944.

Lounasmaa, O.V., Hari, R., Joutsiniemi, S.-L., and Hämäläinen, M. (1989). Multi-SQUID recordings of human cerebral magnetic fields may give information about memory processes. Europhys. Lett., 9:603-608.

Modena, I., Ricci, G.B., Barbanera, S., Leoni, R., Romani, G.L., and Carelli, P. (1982). Biomagnetic measurements of spontaneous brain activity in epileptic patients. Electroenceph. clin. Neurophysiol., 54:622-628.

Narici, L., Romani, G.L., Salustri, C., Pizzella, V., Modena, I., and Papanicolaou, A.C. (1987). Neuromagnetic evidence of synchronized spontaneous activity in the brain following repetitive sensory stimulation. Intern. J. Neurosci., 32:831-836.

Narici, L., Modena, I., Peresson, M., Pizzella V., Romani, G.L., and Torrioli, G. (1988). Time, spatial, and frequency analysis of evoked field and synchronized spontaneous activity under repetitive visual stimulation. In: Atsumi, K., Kotani, M., Ueno, S., Katila, T., and Williamson, S.J. (Eds), Biomagnetism '87, Tokyo Denki University Press, 134-137.

Narici, L., and Romani, G.L. (1989). Neuromagnetic investigation of synchronized spontaneous activity. Brain Topography, in press.

Pantev, C., Hoke, M., Lenhertz, K., Lütkenhöner, B., Anogianakis, G., and Wittkowski, W. (1988). Tonotopic organization of the human auditory cortex revealed by transient auditory evoked magnetic fields. Electroenceph. clin. Neurophysiol., 69:160-170.

Pantev, C., Hoke, M., Lütkenhöner, B., Lenhertz, K., and Kumpf, W. (1989). Tinnitus remission objectified by neuromagnetic measurements. Hearing Res., 40:261-264.

Regan, D. (1972). Evoked potentials in psychology, sensory physiology and clinical medicine. London, Chapman & Hall; New York, Wiley.

Ricci, G.B., Leoni, R., Romani, G.L., Campitelli, F., Buonomo, S., and Modena, I. (1985). 3-D neuromagnetic localization of sources of interictal activity in cases of focal epilepsy. In:

Weinberg, H., Stroink, G., and Katila, T. (Eds), Biomagnetism: Applications and Theory, Pergamon Press, New York-Toronto, 304-310.

Ricci, G.B., Chapman, R.M., Erne', S.N., Narici, L., Peresson, M., Pizzella, V., Romani, G.L., Torrioli, G., and Cilli, M. (1989). Neuromagnetic topography of photoconvulsive response in man. Electroenceph. clin. Neurophysiol., in press.

Romani, G.L., Williamson, S.J., and Kaufman, L. (1982a). Tonotopic organnization of the human auditory cortex. Science, 216:1339-1340.

Romani, G.L., Williamson, S.J., Kaufman, L., and Brenner, D. (1982b). Characterization of the human auditory cortex by the neuromagnetic method. Exp. Brain Res., 47:381-393.

Romani, G.L., and Leoni, R. (1985). Localization of cerebral sources with neuromagnetic measurements. In: Weinberg, H., Stroink, G., and Katila, T. (Eds), Biomagnetism: Applications and Theory, Pergamon Press, New York-Toronto, 205-220.

Romani, G.L., and Rossini, P. (1988). Neuromagnetic functional localization: Principles, state of the art, and perspectives. Brain Topography, 1:5-22.

Rose, D.F., Smith, P.D., and Sato, S. (1987). Magnetoencephalography and epilepsy research. Science, 238:329-335.

Rossini, P.M., Narici, L., Romani, G.L., Traversa, R., Cecchi, L., Cilli, M., and Urbano, A. (1989). Short latency somatosensory evoked responses to median nerve stimulation in healthy humans: electric and magnetic recordings. Intern. J. Neurosci. 46:67-76.

Roth, B.J., Woosley, J.K., and Wikswo, J.P. Jr. (1985). An experimental and theoretical analysis of the magnetic field of a single axon. In: Weinberg, H., Stroink, G., and Katila, T. (Eds), Biomagnetism: Applications and Theory, Pergamon Press, New York-Toronto, 78-82.

Swinney, K.R., and Wikswo, J.P. Jr.(1980). A calculation of the magnetic field of a nerve action potential. Biophys. J., 32:719-731.

Williamson, S.J., and Kaufman, L. (1989). Theory of neuroelectric and neuromagnetic fields. In: Grandori, F., Hoke, M., and Romani, G.L. (Eds.), Auditory electric and magnetic fields, Karger, in press.

PRINCIPLES OF CARDIOMAGNETISM

G. Stroink

Departments of Physics and Physiology & Biophysics
Dalhousie University.
Halifax, N.S., Canada, B3H-3J5

INTRODUCTION

Cellular currents that initiate the periodic muscle contractions of the heart will also generate volume currents in the ionic, conductive medium of the body. These volume currents create potential differences at the body surface which can be displayed as the electrocardiogram (ECG). Both cellular and volume currents produce small magnetic fields near the body surface. A recording of these periodic magnetic field changes constitute a magnetocardiogram (MCG).

While it is now over a hundred years ago that the first ECG was measured, the first MCG was recorded just over 25 years ago by Baule and McFee (1963). They used large coils, with two million turns each, in a gradiometer arrangement. The development of the SQUID and the use of a shielded room made high quality (low noise) MCG's possible (Cohen, Edelsack and Zimmerman, 1970). Improvements in gradiometer designs enabled several groups to operate in an unshielded or moderately shielded environment. These developments made MCG technology accessible to many researchers.

Fig. 1 shows a typical MCG with similar features as a ECG. Fig. 1 also shows the potential distributions and the magnetic field distribution at the body surface during the peak of the R -wave. The figures demonstrate the similarities and differences that can be expected when measuring magnetic fields and potentials. The amount of new information contained in the MCG has been debated extensively (e.g. Plonsey, 1972). There are several theoretical arguments that demonstrate that the MCG contains unique information not obtainable from ECG recording and several experimental studies support this. To investigate this further more studies are needed, however the number of MCG research projects is still relatively small; they comprise only a minute fraction of the vast ECG research effort.

Lately the development and use of multiprobe sensors makes mass screening not only simple an safe, but also a quick procedure that would be acceptable to the medical community. In addition new high resolution MCG probes provide us with a signal to noise ratio that is essentially the same as that in high resolution ECG. These new developments will stimulate research to explore further the unique capabilities of the MCG. Reviews on MCG have recently written by Siltanen (1989), as well as by Weinberg, Stroink and Katila (1988). A tutorial article has been written by Fenici (1983).

Advances in Biomagnetism
Edited by S.J. Williamson *et al.*
Plenum Press, New York

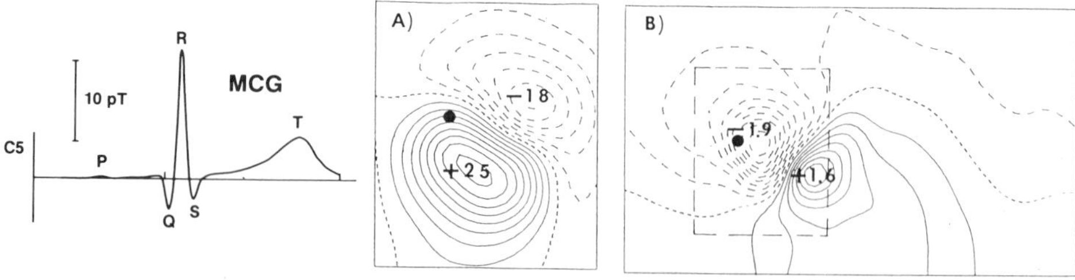

Fig.1. A typical MCG (left) at one of the locations of a 56 lead Magnetic Field Map -MFM (A) at R- wave maximum. For comparison we also show a 120 lead Body Surface Potential Map -BSPM (B) at the same time instance. The dashed box (24 cm x 28 cm) on the BSPM represents the area on the body where the MFM is obtained. The dot in both maps reflects the location where the midline of the anterior torso and the level of the 4th intercostal space intersects.

THE HEART

As a cardiac muscle cell prepares to contract, a wave of depolarization sweeps the length of the cell starting a selective diffusion of ions to and from the extracellular medium. The ion concentration gradients across the cell membrane generate a primary current density $\mathbf{j_p}$ in each cell, pointing in the direction of propagation of the depolarization. One can group many such current dipole elements, in many cells, together and integrate them over a small volume to form a current dipole moment **p** (units A.m). A wavefront of dipoles, with a width of about 0.5 mm, will propagate with a velocity of about 0.5 mm/s, through the muscle mass to depolarize the heart chambers.

Cardiac activity starts in the right atrium at the sino-atrial (S-A) node. From the S-A node this wavefront spreads throughout the atria, but cannot cross the non-conductive boundary between atria and ventricles. The atrioventricular (A-V) node, located at this boundary, provides the only conductive path between the atria and the ventricles. From here, the conduction follows the bundle of His, which divides itself into the left and right bundle branches and finally splits into a network of Purkinje fibers reaching into the inner and outer sides of the ventricular wall, the endo- and epicardium respectively. Depolarization of the ventricular muscle cells starts at the septum, continues towards the apex and then reaches the remainder of the left and right ventricular mass (Fig. 2). Generally, it spreads from the endocardium towards the epicardium. After the muscle cells have depolarized, repolarization follows.

To calculate the magnetic field and potential at a point **r**, due to the dipoles **p** at the wave front, we have to sum the contribution at **r** of each individual current dipole. However, we can, as a approximation, sum these current dipole elements to obtain an resultant current dipole, **J**(t). This current dipole, which for convenience we locate near the center of the heart, changes, according to Fig.2 in direction and magnitude during the depolarization process. This total dipole moment is often referred to as "heart vector", "electric force vector" or "activity" by cardiologists. This vector can be used to interpret the different deflections observed in the MCG or ECG leads.

The strength of the signal measured, electrically or magnetically, will reflect the strength of **J**(t) at the different times during the heart cycle. It is therefore not surprising that the ECG and MCG shows similarities in the overall waveform. Similar nomenclature to describe different aspects of the heart cycle is used in the MCG as in the ECG. In Fig. 1 (left) the P wave reflects the atrial repolarization, the R- wave the ventricular depolarization and the T-wave the ventricular repolarization. The atrial repolarization starts during the PR-segment and extends into the R- wave but is, during this interval, swamped by this much larger signal.

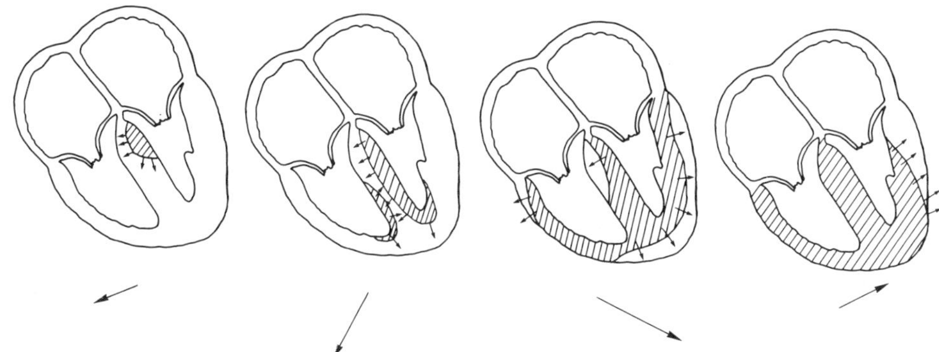

Fig. 2. A wavefront of depolarization, represented by current dipoles **p**, sweeping over the ventricals. The total dipole moment **J**(t) is shown at the bottom of each figure.

CALCULATING CARDIAC FIELD AND POTENTIALS

The Forward problem

Infinite homogeneous medium If one knows all the cardiac sources and the properties of the medium in which these sources are active one can calculate V(**r**,t) and **B**(**r**,t) on the surface of the torso. Such calculations are known as forward solutions. The simplest model of cardiac activity is that of the resultant current dipole source **J**(t), as defined above, inside an infinite, homogeneous and isotropic conducting medium. The mathematical expression for the potential, V, and magnetic field, **B**, due to such a current dipole are well known. It is interesting to note that the ohmic volume currents generated by this current dipole in such an infinite medium can be ignored in the calculations of V (Hobbie, 1973) and **B** (Cohen et al., 1976), each for different reasons.

Magnetic field maps (MFM) of cardiac activity are normally obtained in a plane near the anterior surface. It is instructive to plot the magnetic field ($\mathbf{B}_Z$) and potential (V) contour lines created by this simple model, in such a xy-plane at a distance z=d from the origin of **J**(t) for different values of α, the angle between the dipole and the perpendicular distance between the dipole and the plane. From such plots one finds that:

- with **J**(t) perpendicular to the measuring plane (α=0), $\mathbf{B}_Z$ in that plane is zero, whereas V shows a single maximum.
- for any value of α>0 the potential map and the magnetic map show two extrema. For the magnetic map the location of these extrema is independent of α The distance, d, between the dipole and the plane is always given by the simple equation: $d=\delta/\surd 2$, where δ is the separation of the extrema of the magnetic field. Such a simple relation between d and δ does not exist for the separation of the extrema of the potentials. In fact for a given d, δ goes gradually from $d.\surd 2$ for α=90 to infinity for α=0 degrees.
-the x,y coordinates of the dipole is determined by the midpoint of the separation of the extrema of the magnetic field. This information is not readily available from the potential maps.

These observations suggest, that under these ideal model assumption, the MFM is particularly valuable in sensing and characterizing tangential dipoles (α=90°) in the myocardium, whereas potential measurements will be sensitive to transmural dipole components perpendicular (α=0°) to the observation plane.

A piecewise homogeneous torso. One can approximate the human torso by introducing compartments resembling the major organs, each with its separate uniform conductivity. The presence of a boundary influences the current distributions in the conductive medium. This influence can be represented by secondary current sources located at the boundary and perpendicular to it. For simple geometries (e.g. an infinite plane) one can show that these secondary current dipoles influence the potentials at this boundary, but not $\mathbf{B}_Z$. This insensitivity of $\mathbf{B}_Z$ and the sensitivity of V to boundary layers of simple geometry suggests that the MCG can have a distinct advantage over the ECG in localizing cardiac sources. Several studies (e.g. Horacek, 1973) used different source models and elaborate heart and torso models to calculate the relative contribution of the boundaries to the *magnitude* of the MCG and ECG signals. The general conclusion after evaluating the results of such forward calculations (Hosaka et al., 1976) is that, when averaged over many different sources, located in different regions of the heart, the effect of the boundaries on the *magnitude* of the calculated signal is as large for the MCG as for the ECG.

Because the overall magnitude of the MCG or ECG is normally not a primary factor in analyzing *contour maps*, as measured in most research labs, Purcell et al. (1988) investigated the effects of the torso boundaries on the body surface potential maps (BSPM's) and magnetic field maps (MFM's), produced by single dipoles located at different locations near the cardiac blood mass. As can be expected the effect of the torso boundaries on the topology of the MFM due to sources perpendicular to the anterior surface is large. For other dipole directions the boundaries influence the magnetic and potential maps, on average, about equally, although for particular dipole locations and/or direction either the BSPM or MFM is influenced the least by the boundaries. In general the potential and magnetic maps complement each other. E.g. it is advantageous to make MCG measurements to study sources parallel to the anterior plane in the presence of larger sources perpendicular to this plane, which would dominate a potential measurement.

As an illustration we show in Fig. 3 contour maps of B_Z at the anterior surface plane due to a single current dipole in the septum of the heart pointing parallel (Fig. 3a&b) and perpendicular (Fig. 3c) to this surface. Torso boundaries can have unexpected results on the magnetic field patterns (Purcell et al., 1988), as is also demonstrated in Fig. 3 c&d. The study shows that dipoles located assymmetrically relatively to the different body compartments, in particular, can create field patterns that deviate substantially from the symmetric patterns expected in an infinite homogeneous medium (see Fig. 3d).

To computate the potentials and magnetic fields due to a realistic excitation wavefront in a realistic healthy or diseased heart requires extensive computer power. Steps towards such a complete model, which should include anisotropic conduction properties of the heart muscle fibers, have been taken by several researchers. It is expected that the MCG will be particularly sensitive to such an anisotropic conduction and that, consequently, with such realistic models more definite conclusions can be drawn about the independence of information content in the ECG and MCG (Roth et al., 1988).

The inverse solution

The most challenging aspect in MCG studies is to use the measured magnetic fields or potentials, or both, to determine the cardiac sources. Because there is no unique solution to this problem, assumptions have to be made as to the nature of these sources. When the cardiac activity is confined to a small volume, one chooses, usually, a current dipole in an infinite, isotropic, homogeneous medium as the source. The inverse solution will attempt to fit the observed field values to such an equivalent current dipole (ECD), to which one then tries to give a physiological meaning. This procedure is suprisingly successful, perhaps because of the compact and often dipolar nature of the measured MFM's. However it is clear that such a fit to model data shown in Fig. 3 c&d, will give erroneous answers.

Lately bounded conductors with piecewise homogeneous conductivity for the realistically shaped lung, heart and torso have been used as part of an inverse solutions

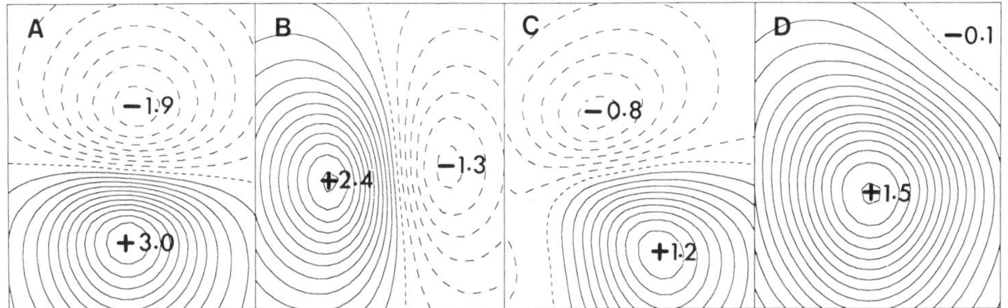

Fig.3. Contour maps of $\mathbf{B}_z$ generated by current dipoles p_x (3a), p_y (3b), and p_z (3c) located at the septum, where ventricular activity starts. Also is shown B_z due to p_y at a location on the far left side of the left ventricle (3d). The area shown is the same as that in Fig. 1. Each dipole has a strength of 1 A-m. The extrema of each map are given in pT.

of BSPM's and MFM's (Purcell et al., 1988). Because of the complex geometries involved special techniques are required to make such solutions run fast. Even so, such programs are presently limited to considering a single current dipole as source, using a fixed torso geometry for different subjects and they do not take into account anisotropic conductivities in the heart, known to influence the magnetic field maps. In addition such inverse solutions have to be validated with implanted current sources (Fenici et al., 1989) or computer simulations (Purcell, 1988).

INSTRUMENTATION AND METHODS.

Almost all MCG research is done with SQUID based magnetometers with a typical noise level of 25 fT/√Hz. Different gradiometer systems are used in the several MCG research laboratories. Second or higher order gradiometer systems with the short baseline (4 cm), are generally used in an unshielded or moderate shielded environment; first order systems, with a relatively long baseline (10-16 cm), in a shielded room. Most gradiometers have a coil diameter of approximately 2.5 cm.

Although several attempts have been made to introduce standard MCG methodologies, several measuring techniques are in use. The standard (Finnish) grid, introduced during Biomagnetism Conferences in Grenoble and Rome, is based on a 36 point flexible grid, which, on average, for adults results in measuring point separations of approximately 5 cm in the y-direction (head to toe) and 3.5 cm in the x-direction (right to left arm). The sign of the magnetic flux is positive when the flux is directed towards the subject. In our clinical studies, which aim at measuring patients within one hour, we use a 56 point fixed grid with a 4 cm spacing. This spans a grid that is larger than the standard grid and larger than necessary for accurate inverse solutions to a current dipole in a homogeneous medium (Abraham-Fuchs et al., 1988). However recent studies of infarct patients have shown that the outer measuring points of the larger grid have clinical significance (Lant et al., 1989a).

In vectormagnetocardiography (VMCG) the aim is to measure the magnetic dipole moment **m**, the largest component in a multipole expansion of the magnetic field of the heart. Theoretically this moment is closely linked to the current dipole source **J**(t) and is perpendicular to it. **m** is derived from a measurement, usually at a single location, of all three orthogonal vector components of **B**. The results can then be compared, on an equal footing, with the conventional vector electrocardiographic (VECG) measurements obtained by using e.g. the Frank lead system. VMCG measurements are, in principle, easy and quick to perform, making it attractive as a mass screening method.

THE NORMAL MAGNETOCARDIOGRAM

Several studies have attempted to characterize the normal MCG. From a study of 31 men and 10 women (Saarinen et al., 1978) the median, upper and lower quartile MCG's were calculated for each gridpoint of the standard grid. Murakami et al., (1988) also published the incidence of characteristic normal MCG's at each gridpoint. Average values for the amplitude of the QRS complex of 60 normal subjects have been published by Fujino et al. (1984).

Another means of characterizing a relatively large amount of data is by calculating time integral maps over specific time segments during the heart cycle. This method, borrowed from BSPM techniques, leads to a single value for each measuring point, which can then be averaged over the group, mapped and compared with other subject groups. In Fig.4 we have plotted the average time integral MFM over the commonly used time segments of 22 normals and compared them with a patient group (inferior MI). The method maintains the dominant heart vector (ECD) direction during the time segment as can be seen by comparing Fig.4 with Fig.2 during initial (Q-zone) and late (LATQRS) ventricular depolarisation. As we will see later such maps are sensitive indicators of cardiac abnormalities.

Recently Nousiainen et al. (1986) presented results on the VMCG of normals and compared their data with VECG data of the same persons. The VMCG is more sensitive than the electrical vector in the terminal phase of the QRS, when the activation in the heart appears in a more tangential direction. A similar conclusion can be drawn from the time integral maps (Lant et al., 1989a) and theoretical calculations (Hosaka et al., 1976).

THE ABNORMAL MAGNETOCARDIOGRAM

Because of space limitations, we discuss here only those clinical studies that has recently drawn a large amount of interest in the magnetocardiographic community. Siltanen (1989) as well as Mori and Naskaya (1988) recently published a survey of clinical MCG studies for a large number of cardiac abnormalities.

Ventricular Hypertrophy This increase of the left or right ventricular muscle mass, leading to stronger electric activity in that region, has been studied by a number of researchers. When a ventricle hyperthrophies, the ECD, during depolarization, shifts towards the direction of the hypertrophied area. In general it is found that for this condition the MCG amplitude divided by the normal MCG is larger in the MCG recordings than the same ratio in ECG recordings, which suggests advantages of the MCG over the ECG. In fact in a MCG study of 95 patients with left ventricular hypertrophy (LVH) Fujino et al. (1984) introduced criteria for the diagnosis of LVH in MCG with a sensitivity, specificity and predictive value at least as good or better than that for the established criteria for LVH using the standard 12 lead ECG. A study of 37 cases with right ventricular hypertrophy (RVH) shows that the sensitivity of the MCG for RVH is substantially higher (73 vs 31%) than that of the ECG (Mori and Nakaya, 1989). This is presumably due to the fact that the right ventricular wall is located close, and the increased "electromotive force" is generally parallel to the anterior chest wall. Both factors are favorable for MCG measurements.

Myocardial infarction Although, as yet, no MCG's have been recorded during the acute phase of myocardial infarction in man, some work has been reported on the MCG changes during coronary occlusion in dogs. Of particular importance is the fact that MCG can measure DC shifts relative to a previous established baseline and consequently can determine the absolute value of the DC shifts during different segments of the MCG of the injured heart; such ECG measurements are not possible (Cohen et al. 1983).

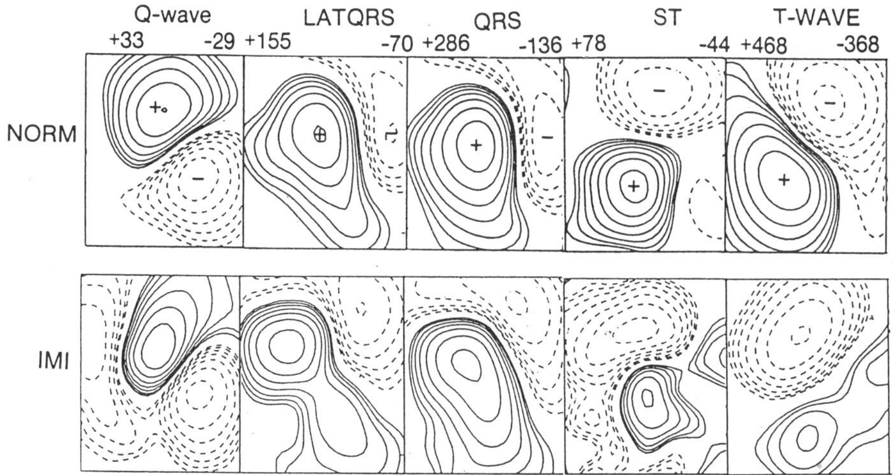

Fig. 4. Average integral maps during several time intervals of a group of 22 normals and a group of 7 patients with inferior myocardial infarction (IMI). Units are in pT.s.

Several studies, both experimental and theoretical, have documented the MCG changes due to previous myocardial infarction. Characteristic MCG's of MI patients have been published by Murakami et al., (1988). In general the MFM's, after infarction, can be understood in terms of the infarction dipole. This can be defined as the difference of the current dipoles forming the excitation wavefront just before and after the infarction. This difference can be approximated by subtracting the MFM of a normal subject, from that of the infarction patient. Mathematical methods like the singular value decomposition or KL-expansion can be used to characterize the MCG of normals. The first eigenfunctions of this expansion can then be applied to the measured maps of MI-patients (Stroink et al., 1985) to obtain the required difference map. This method allows one to obtain spatial maps, assumed to be due to the infarction dipole, that can then be used for localization and evaluation purposes.

A recently published study (Lant et al, 1989b) provides a qualitative and quantitative analysis of MFM and BSPM time integrals over the different time segments of non-Q wave, inferior and anterior infarct patients (see Fig. 4). The analysis, borrowed from BSPM studies (Montague et al., 1986), suggests that significant differences between different subject groups occur for the BSPM's during the Q-wave and Q-zone interval; for the MFM's during late QRS and S-T interval. Using a statistical analysis this study showed that the BSPM is most discriminatory in classifying MI's during depolarization, MCG techniques more so during the repolarization.

HIGH RESOLUTION MAGNETOCARDIOGRAPHY

High resolution MGC generally relates to the measurements of the very small signals (smaller than 1 pT) associated with the conduction system or with arrhythmias. The aim of such studies is to detect such signals noninvasely for diagnostic purposes and to make use of the localization capabilities of the MCG to assist in a clinical diagnosis. The results are often compared with high resolution electrocardiography.

His-Purkinje System. The large volume of work on the electrical activity of the His- Purkinje system (HPS) have been reviewed by Berbari (1989) and Siltanen (1989) from the ECG and MCG point of view respectively. Non-invasive ECG recordings of the bundle of His were first reported around 1975. They are characterized by a ramp like pattern starting about 40-50 ms before the onset of the QRS. Different recording and analysis techniques have attempted to separate the His bundle signals and that of the proximal bundle branches from the underlying atrial repolarization.

Around 1980 the first MCG measurements of a ramp pattern attributed to the HPS-MCG were reported (Farrell et al., 1980). The measurement showed good agreement with theoretical predictions. However some questions about the origin of the ramp patterns remain unresolved. Animal experiments suggested that atrial repolarization alone can explain the ramp patterns. This is supported by MCG measurements on subjects with 1st degree block (Lorenzana et al., 1985). However based on a simultaneous recording of atrial monophasic action potentials, HPS electrograms and HPS-MCG it was concluded that the atrial contribution to the ramp pattern is small (Fenici et al., 1985).

Recent theoretical calculations demonstrate that the MCG of the bundle of His is probably too small to observe on the body surface and that the ramp patterns are due both to the left bundle branch and the atrial repolarization (Kafer, 1988). The model was used (Lamothe et al., 1989) to test the variety of methods to extract the atrial repolarization pattern from the measured MCG maps to reveal the HPS pattern. These simulations demonstrate the sensitivity of these methods to the assumption made concerning the stability of the AR pattern during the PR segment. It suggests that the dipolar patterns in both the BSPM and MFM's may not necessarily be due to the HPS.

Kent-Bundle. The extra conduction pathway, at the A-V ring, is known as the Kent-bundle. If associated with tachycardia it is called the Wolff- Parkinson-White (WPW) syndrome. In both the MCG and ECG it manifests itself by a short PR-interval, an anomalous broad QRS complex that includes a "delta wave" and ST-segment alterations. Because of the often dipolar patterns associated with the delta wave, the non- invasive MCG has been used to localize the Kent bundle in three dimensions, which can then be compared with the results of invasive measurements using catheters and fluoroscopy. Results on 5 patients investigated invasively (Oeff and Erne, 1989) show that the MCG can localize the Kent bundle to within 2 cm, sufficiently close to use the MCG as a non-invasive tool prior to surgery to remove, if necessary, this extra pathway. These clinical MCG measurements (Fenici et al., 1988), combined with the catheter studies, provide an almost ideal testing ground to validate the different inverse solutions (Katila et al., 1988).

Late potentials. Evidence obtained from epicardial and endocardial potential mapping has verified that myocardium with delayed ventricular activity is a source for reentry, a mechanism presumed to be involved with many life-threatening arrhythmias like ventricular tachycardia (VT). Such delayed activity can be recorded non-invasively with HR-ECG as small potentials (25 μV) during the last 40 ms of the high pass filtered QRS.

Late fields (LF) of the same structure as the late potentials have been observed by several groups. However the S/N ratio of such signals is small and it is not yet clear if this is due to a higher noise level in HR-MCG systems as compared to the HR- ECG system or to a lower sensitivity of the MCG for this type of signals (Stroink et al., 1989). Comparing MFM and BSPM of normals, patients with MI and patients with MI and VT, reveals, however, that a plot of the MFM extrema as a function of time during the QRS and ST-T intervals shows promise to identify, with a relatively high sensitivity, patients with VT.

Several studies have attempted to localize the origin of ventricular arrhythmias by using mapping techniques with the ECD as the source model. In one study the arrhythmogenic area was reproducibly localized in the area of the right ventricle which appeared the most severely damaged at echocardiography (Fenici et al., 1989). In another (Schmitz et al., 1988), 3D localization of the earliest ventricular depolarization, pacemaker induced, suggests that a localization accuracy of 5 mm can be obtained, as verified by MRI and invasive endocardial potential mapping. Because HR-ECG has achieved poor results in the localization of arrhythmogenic foci it is important to explore the MCG techniques further in the hope of providing the clinician with a non invasive technique to determine where ablation of the affected cardiac tissue should occur.

ACKNOWLEDGEMENTS

This work is supported by the Nova Scotia Heart Foundation, the Medical Research Council (MRC) and the Narural Science and Engineering Council (NSERC) of Canada. Special thanks are extended to R. Lamothe, G. A. Tan and P. B. Charlebois.

REFERENCES

Abraham-Fuchs, K., Schneider, S., and Reichenberger, H., 1988, MCG inverse solution: influence of coil size, grid size, number of coils and SNR., IEEE Trans. Biomed. Eng., 35(8):573.

Baule, G., and McFee, R., 1963, Detection of the magnetic field of the heart, Am. Heart J., 66:95.

Berbari, E. J., 1988, High resolution electrocardiography, CRC critical reviews in Biomed. Eng., 16(1):67.

Cohen, D. and Hosaka, H., 1976, Magnetic field produced by a current dipole. J. Electrocard., 9:409.

Cohen, D., Edelsack, E. A., and Zimmerman, J. E., 1970, Magnetocardiograms taken inside a shielded room with a superconducting point-contact magnetometer, Appl. Phys. Lett., 16:278.

Cohen, P., Savard, P., Rifkin, R. D., Lepeschkin, E., and Strauss, W. E., 1983, Magnetic measurement of S-T and T-Q Segment Shifts in Humans, Circ. Res., 53:274.

Farrel, D. E., Tripp, J. H., and Norgren, R., 1980, Magnetic study of the His-Purkinje conduction system in man, IEEE Trans. Biomed. Eng., 27:345.

Fenici, R. R., 1983, Clinical assessment of the magnetocardiogram, in "Biomagnetism, an interdisciplinary approach", S. J. Williamson, G. L. Romani, L. Kaufman and I. Modena, eds., NATO ASI Series, Plenum Press, New York.

Fenici, R. R., Masselli, M., Lopez, L., and Melillo, G., 1989, Clinical magnetocardiography localization of arrhytmogenic structures, in: "Advances in Biomagnetism; functional localization," S. N. Erne and G. L. Romani, eds., World Scientific, Singapore, p. 102.

Fujino, K., Sumi, M., Saito, K., Murakami, M., Higuchi, T., Nakaya, Y., and Mori, H., 1984, Magnetocardiograms of patients with left ventricular overloading recorded with a second-derivative SQUID gradiometer, J. Electrocardiol., 17:219.

Hobbie, R. K., 1973, The electrocardiogram as an example of electrostatics, Am. J. Phys., 41:824.

Horacek, B. M., 1973, Digital model for studies in magnetocardiography, IEEE Trans. Magn., 9:440.

Hosaka, H., Cohen, D., Cuffin, B. N., and Horacek, B. M. 1976, The effect of the torso boundaries on the magnetocardiogram, J. Electrocardiol., 9:418.

Katila, T., Montonen, J., Makijarvi, M., Nenonen, J., Raivio, M., and Siltanen, P., 1988, Localization of the accessory cardiac conduction pathology, in: "Biomagnetism 87," K. Atsumi, M. Kotani, S. Ueno, T. Katila, and S. J. Williamson, eds., Tokyo Denki Univ. Press, Tokyo, p. 274.

Lamothe, R. M., Stroink, G. and Kafer, C. J., 1989, Evaluation of techniques to extract HPS- Purkinje system spatial distributions. These proceedings.

Lant, J., Stroink, G., Rautaharaja, P., and Montague, T. J., 1989a, Identification of best magnetocardiographic leads for diagnosing myocardial infarction, To be published.

Lant, J., Stroink, G., ten Voorde, B., Horacek, B. M., and Montague, T. J., 1989b, Complementary nature of electrocardiographic and magnetocardiographic data in patients with ischemic heart disease, To be published in J. Electrocard.

Lorenzana, H. E., Pipes, P. B., Zaitlin, M. P., and James, D. A., 1985, A study of the P-R segment in the human magnetocardiogram, In: "Biomagnetism: Aplications and Theory," H. Weinberg, G, Stroink, and T. Katila, eds., Pergamon, New York, p. 142.

Montague, T. J., Johnstone D. E., Spencer, A., Lalonde L.D., Gardner M. J., O'Reilly, M. G. and Horacek, B. M., 1986, Non-Q-Wave acute myocardial infarction: Body surface potential map and ventriculographic patterns, Am J Cardiol., 58: 1173-1180.

Mori, H., and Nakaya, Y., 1988, Clinical value of the magnetocardiogram, in, "Biomagnetism 87," K. Atsumi, M. Kotani, S. Ueno, T. Katila and S. J. Williamson, eds., Tokyo Denhi Univ. Press, Tokyo, p. 82.

Murakami, M., Watanabe, K., Takeuchi, A., Katayama, M., Nomura, M., Fukuda, Y., Sumi, M., Nakaya, Y., and Mori, H., 1988, The QRS wave of the magnetocardiogram in myocardial infarction, in: "Biomagnetism 87", K. Atsumi, M. Kotani, S. Ueno, T. Katila and S. J. Williamson, eds., Tokyo Denki Univ. Press, Tokyo, p. 354.

Nousiainen, J. J. O., Lekkala, J. O. and Malmivuo, J. P. V., 1986, Comparative study of the normal vector magnetocardiogram and vector electrocardiogram, J. Electrocardiology, 19(3):275.

Plonsey, R., 1972, Comparative capabilities of electrography and magnetocardiography. Am. J. Cardiol., 29: 735-6.

Oef, M. and Erne S.N., 1989, Invasive measurements to validate magnetic localization of ventricular preexcitation in Wolff- Parkinson- White Syndrome. in: "Advances in Biomagnetism, functional localization", S. N. Erne and G. L. Romani, eds., World Scientific, Singapore.

Purcell, C. J., Stroink, G. and Horacek, B. M., 1988, Effect of torso boundaries on electric potential and magnetic field of a dipole, IEEE Trans. Biomed. Eng., BME, 35:671.

Purcell, C. J., 1988, A comparison of electric and magnetic body surface mapping using single moving dipole inverse solutions. Ph. D. Thesis, Dalhousie University.

Saarinen, M., Siltanen, P., Karp, P. J., and Katila, T. E., 1978, The normal magnetocardiogram: I. Morphology, Ann. Clin. Res., 10 (Suppl. 21):1.

Schmitz, L., Jeff, M., and Erne, S. N., 1988, Localization of arrhythmogenic areas in the human heart, 1988, in: "Biomagnetism 87," K. Atsumi, M. Kotani, S. Ueno, T. Katila and S. J. Williamson, eds., Tokyo Denki Univ. Press, Tokyo, p. 286.

Siltanen, P., 1989, Magnetocardiography, in: "Comprehensive Electrocardiology", P. W. MacFarlane and T. D. Veitch Lawrie, eds., Pergamon Press, New York.

Roth, B.J., Guo, W. and Wikswo, J.P., 1988, The effects of spiral anisotropy on the electric potential and magnetic field at the apex of the heart, Math. Biosc., 88: 191.

Stroink, G., MacAulay, C., Montague, T. J., and Horacek, B. M., 1985, Normal and abnormal components in magnetocardiographic maps of a subject with a myocardial infarction, Med. Biol. Eng. Comput., 23 (Suppl.):61.

Weinberg, H., Stroink, G., and Katila, T., 1988, Biomagnetism, in: "Encyclopedia of medical devices and instrumentation", J. G. Webster, ed., John Wiley & Sons, Inc., New York.

BIOMAGNETIC STUDIES OF ORGANS OTHER THAN THE HEART AND BRAIN

S.J.Swithenby

Physics Department, Open University, Milton Keynes MK7 6AA, U.K.

INTRODUCTION - THE DIVERSITY OF FIELD SOURCES

In the heart and brain coherent ionic currents flow across appreciable volumes producing detectable magnetic fields. In this paper I will survey other organs and processes which give rise to measurable fields. These are too diverse and numerous for the survey to be encyclopaedic: instead I will concentrate on those that have either attracted most attention or, in my view, seem most promising. They are:

- **Contaminant magnetic material in the body** The body may contain, as contaminants, ferromagnetic or ferrimagnetic material. Magnetite Fe_30_4 is commonly found in dust and is easily inhaled. It is a strong ferrimagnet and as little as a fraction of a gram of magnetite in the lungs is easily detectable. By measuring the field outside the chest it is possible to both monitor the dust burden of the lungs and assess lung function. The measurements are entirely non-invasive.
- **Intrinsic magnetic material in the body** Overall, biological tissue is diamagnetic (with a susceptibility of order $10^{-5}m^{-3}$) though, significantly, it does contain some paramagnetic material. In the Earth's field; the presence of a biological organism changes the local magnetic induction by about 500 pT. SQUID magnetometers have sufficient sensitivity to map the local susceptibility variations of tissues as a way of probing their composition. This idea underlies a method of measuring stored iron levels in the liver.
- **Quasi dc ionic currents** Because of the difficulty of making reliable dc electrode measurements on biological systems, many potentially significant electrophysiological processes are unexplored. 'Injury current' is an example. This may be a simple epiphenomenon, but it has been suggested that the currents have a significant role in the repair process. A linked suggestion is that the ionic currents that accompany development help to 'shape' the organism. DC magnetic field studies of such phenomena may allow monitoring of hidden injuries and help to elucidate fundamental biological processes.

In biomagnetic terms the sources I will be discussing produce 'strong' magnetic fields. Detection with SQUIDs and, in some cases, with fluxgate magnetometers, is straightforward. However, there is a complication. In each case the magnetic field is essentially constant over periods of less than say 10 seconds. To put it another way the signal power spectrum is concentrated in the bandwidth between dc and about 0.1 Hz. Because of both low frequency noise and, more fundamentally, the inability of SQUIDs to measure *absolute* magnetic fields, we cannot just position a subject with respect to a detection system and passively observe the signal evolve in time. Instead, the essentially dc signal is converted into an ac signal by

Advances in Biomagnetism
Edited by S.J. Williamson *et al.*
Plenum Press, New York

movement of the subject with respect to the magnetometer(s). This is a little inconvenient but does have an important advantage. During the scanning process each detector gives information about the field at all the positions it occupies. So, it is possible to assemble a complete field map with just one detector. The cost implications are obvious.

MAGNETOPNEUMOGRAPHY

Magnetopneumography is the study of the remanent magnetisation of contaminant particles in the thorax (Stroink 1985, Legros et al. 1989, Kalliomaki et al. 1983). It offers a non invasive means of measuring the lung dust load and of studying the viscomechanical properties of the local environment of the magnetised particles.

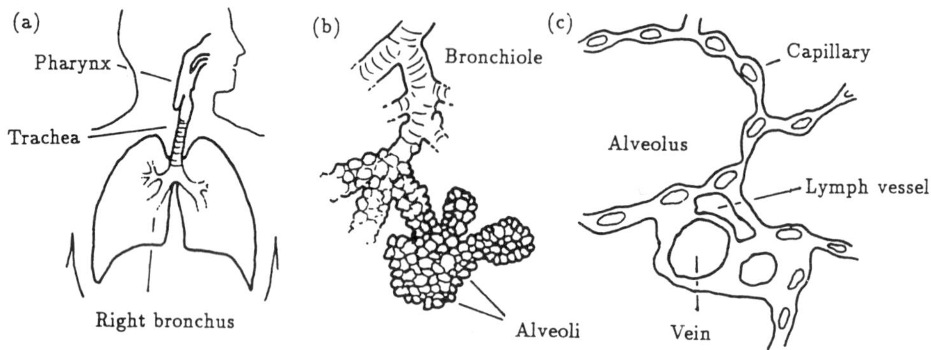

Fig. 1. The airways of the respiratory system; (a) a macroscopic view, (b) the tracheo-bronchiolar tree, and (c) alveoli showing blood and lymph vessels.

As a background to magnetopneumography it is essential to have a basic understanding of the anatomy of the lung. The airways of the lung subdivide progressively and terminate in a honeycomb like structure of chambers known as alveoli (Figure 1). Typically there are about 300 million alveoli in the two lungs with an average diameter of about 250 microns, giving a total alveolar wall area of about 60 square metres. These walls are very thin, consisting essentially of structural membranes and capillaries. Gaseous exchange through the walls between the blood and alveolar volume is rapid.

The efficient functioning of the lungs can be disrupted by any process that impedes the gas-exchange process. This may occur because of; inadequate ventilation of the alveoli (e.g. in asthma, emphysema, tubercolosis, silicosis, and pulmonary edema), reduced diffusion through the alveolar wall (e.g. in emphysema, tubercolosis, silicosis, edema and fibrotic conditions), and decreased oxygen transport from the lungs.

We are particularly concerned with lung conditions that are linked with exposure to dust. Although the nose acts as an efficient filter, particles with a diameter of less than about 5 microns are drawn into the lungs. The larger particles within this group settle in the bronchioles. These are cleared by the action of cilia that move the mucus coating of the bronchioles towards the pharynx. Particles with a diameter of about 1 micron become trapped on the alveolar surfaces. There they are engulfed by macrophages and carried up towards the moving carpet of mucus. However, an excess of dust causes the deposition of fibrous tissue and a reduction in both ventilation and diffusion. The overall efficiency of the lungs depends on the interplay between the rate of and duration of dust inhalation and the effectiveness of the lung clearance mechanisms.

Techniques for magnetopneumography The wide variety of instruments and of protocols used in lung magnetisation measurements are all variants on the basic theme of first magnetising the chest with a field of 30–100 mT and then presenting the now magnetised chest to a sensitive field detector. The timing of this sequence varies but, typically, the magnetising field is applied for a few seconds with measurements subsequently occupying minutes to hours.

A common system consists of Helmholtz coils which generate a uniform magnetic field

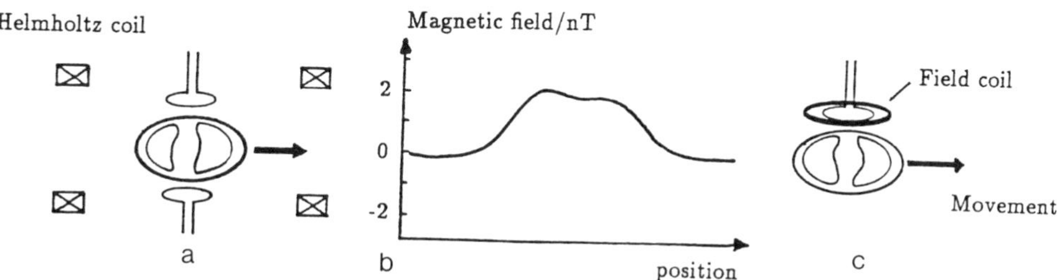

Fig. 2. (a) A uniform field lung-measurement system. (b) The signal as a function of position for a scan across the anterior surface of the chest of a contaminated subject. (c) A localised field lung-measurement system

and one or two small detectors (Figure 2a). The patient is moved on a horizontal bed. Placing detectors above and below the chest (Aittoniemi 1981) increases the information available about the magnetisation distribution. In this arrangement fluxgate magnetometers are used as it is difficult to place cryogenic instrumentation below the patient. Of course, with only one detector above the patient, more sensitive SQUID systems can be used. Figure 2b shows schematically the result of a simple uniform magnetising field measurement.

The main variant on the above arrangement (Figure 2c) was developed by Freedman and his colleagues (1984). They used a small coil to magnetise only a small region of tissue. This offers advantages in terms of mapping the distribution of magnetic material.

There are many factors that complicate the interpretation of magnetopneumography data. As an example, I will go through the calculation of a parameter of perceived clinical importance, the total dust load. The first step is to estimate from the data the total magnetic moment M_t of the dust in the lungs. Unfortunately, the observed fields depend on geometric factors such as the shapes of the lungs and the magnetising coils, the distribution of the dust, the position and geometry of the detector etc. In principle, lung models can be used to calibrate a given detection system, but uncertainties remain. A more elegant approach is to use a mutipole analysis of the measured field to calculate a value for M_t without making any assumptions about geometric factors.

The second more problematic step is to decide on a value for the specific remanent magnetic moment M_{rs} of the dust. This quantity –the magnetic moment per unit mass – depends on the applied magnetising field; for magnetite a saturation value $M_{rs}(\max)$ is reached for applied fields above about 10^5 Am^{-1}. $M_{rs}(\max)$ depends markedly on the nature of the magnetic particles, the particle size, and the fraction of the dust that is magnetic. Even for pure (magnetic) dusts the range is from of order 0.1 Am^2kg^{-1} to 50 Am^2kg^{-1}. It seems clear that the amount of dust in the lungs can only be calculated if the dust can be examined! This can't be done in the lungs but it is feasible to sample the dust in the working environment of the subject group and measure its magnetic properties. The empirical value of $M_{rs}(\max)$ is then assumed to be valid for the material deposited in the lungs. This *in-vitro* to *in-vivo* extrapolation is of questionable validity and it remains a major problem in magnetopneumography. However, with this caveat, we now have all that is needed to calculate the dust load; assuming that the saturation value of M_t has been found, the mass of dust is simply the measured $M_t(\max)$ divided by the assumed value of $M_{rs}(\max)$.

Some information can be gained about the contaminant particles *in vivo* by coercivity measurements. After magnetisation it is possible to demagnetise either partially or totally by applying a short oppositely oriented-field pulse; it is found (Kalliomaki et al 1983) that the ratio of the pre and post demagnetisation signals depends on the dust involved. Such techniques are very promising; they can serve to fingerprint the lung dust and reduce the uncertainties both in comparing subjects with uncertain dust exposure histories and in calculating the mass of dust present.

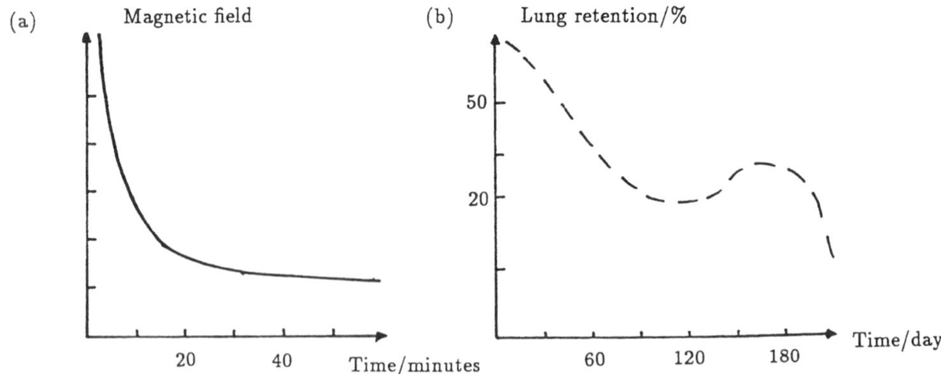

Fig. 3. (a) Relaxation in a normal human subject following inhalation of magnetite dust (Cohen 1978) (b) Clearance of magnetite in a dwarf donkey (adapted from Halperin et al. 1981). The anomalous increase in signal is attributed to migration of the dust to positions of increased detector sensitivity.

Following magnetisation the remanent field, if measured repeatedly, is seen to fall with time – to 'relax' (Figure 3a). Relaxation will be discussed later. For the moment, it is worth noting that it is quite straightforward to extrapolate the results to estimate a t=0 signal. Relaxation should not be confused with 'clearance' (Figure 3b) – the process of elimination of dust from the lungs. It can be observed magnetically following an inhalation of magnetic dust by periodically remagnetising the subject and observing the induced moment.

In this discussion I have emphasised the considerable problems that arise in magnetopneumography, both in measurement and in interpretation. On a more optimistic note, the technique is highly sensitive – as little as 1–20 mg of deposited dust (depending on the fraction that is magnetic) can be detected. In contrast, at least 1 gram of uniformly deposited welding dust is the minimum visible using X-rays.

Applications of magnetopneumography Since 1973, magnetopneumography has been used to study dust loads and clearance rates in many groups of workers. I will briefly review this work, emphasising the correlations between these quantities, as measured magnetically, and (i) the incidence and severity of respiratory illnesses, and (ii) the the results of other clinical tests. However, a word of caution is necessary. Because of variations in both the protocols used and the subjects studied, it is in many cases difficult to compare results of different groups. In addition, we should not expect precise correlations as there is known to be extreme variability in tolerance of exposure to dust.

Welders Mild steel welders in shipyards who use the manual metal arc technique have been studied extensively (see Legros et al. 1989 for references). On average welders with ten years exposure are found to be carrying about 1 gram of dust in their lungs but the inter subject variability extends over a factor of ten. The average deposition rate is 100 mg per year with 20 per cent of the dust cleared each year after exposure ceases. High lung dust loads are associated with radiologically visible abnormalities but there is no observed correlation with the results of standard spirometric tests. Reports vary on the extent of the correlation with incidence of chronic bronchitis. In most studies no difference has been found between the average dust loads of smokers and non smokers, although there is separate evidence that smoking affects clearance rates.

Welders of stainless steel have much higher dust loads than their mild steel counterparts because of a much lower rate of clearance from the alveoli. In the subjects studied there was no radiologically observable damage in spite of this increased contamination.

Iron and steel workers are found to have dust loads that depend markedly on the exact process in which the worker is involved. However, as with mild steel welders, there is a link between high dust load and radiologically visible damage.

Foundry workers are a difficult group to study because the amount of magnetic material in the dust varies greatly with working location. However, many studies have taken place and, within well defined groups, good correlations are observed between magnetically determined dust loads and radiologically observed changes associated with silicosis.

Coal miners carry appreciable dust loads but only a very small fraction of the dust is ferrimagnetic. Although magnetic measurements have been able to distinguish the dust loads of miners from those of control groups and the computed dust loads agree with autopsy data, there has been no observation of correlations with radiological findings.

Asbestos miners inhale fibres to which magnetite particles adhere; typically 4 per cent of the fibre mass is magnetite. A weak correlation has been found between the magnetic signal and both duration of exposure and radiological evidence of damage, but the method has proved a poor predictor of quality of lung function. Smokers appeared to have a *reduced* fibre burden, possibly because of constriction of the airways.

It is clear that magnetopneumography has potential in the early diagnosis of occupation related lung disease. However, in most cases, further work is needed to clarify the physiological processes involved in the cycle of dust deposition and clearance.

Several groups have studied clearance with magnetic methods. Their findings are in general agreement with radioactive tracer results. The advantage of the magnetic method is that it carries no known risk and can be used in human studies. One interesting and perhaps important observation is that clearance is significantly slower in smokers.

Relaxation – Cytomagnetometry Clearance from the alveoli takes place over months or years. In contrast, relaxation – the reduction in the observed signal on repeated measurement without remagnetising – takes place in minutes to hours. It occurs because of the physical reorientation of the magnetised particles (Figure 3a).

For a few hours after the first deposition of magnetic particles, when they are in an extracellular environment, relaxation is slow. However the particles are quickly ingested by macrophages and, once engulfed, relaxation is enhanced by the actin driven motion within the cell (Legros et al. 1989, Brain et al. 1985 and 1989).

The rate of phagocytosis can be monitored non-invasively by measurement of the changing relaxation rate as particles are engulfed, but it is the subsequent study of the phagocytosed particles that has become of increasing interest. This type of investigation has been termed *cytomagnetometry*. It is not limited to the lungs, but can be used wherever there are accessible macrophages – in humans, animals and in cell cultures. It allows the investigation of the internal dynamics of cells using probes (i.e. the particles) that are of a well characterised size similar to that of organelles. Mentioning just two studies will serve to indicate the potential of cytomagnetometry. Of immediate clinical relevance was a study of the effects of perfluorochemical emulsions, which are possible blood substitutes, on macrophage function (see Brain et al. 1985 for references). The second more fundamental study (Nemoto et al. 1989) was of the dependence of cytoplasmic movement on temperature and ATP concentration.

At a more phenomenological level, relaxation in the lungs is found to be independent of the exact nature of the occupational exposure but, overall, it is much more rapid in smokers than in non smokers. This suggests some enhancement in macrophage activity in smokers.

IRON STORAGE MEASUREMENTS

Magnetic susceptibility measurements can be used to quantify human iron storage levels, particularly in the liver (Farrell 1983, Brittenham et al. 1983, Paulson et al. 1989). The technique, which was first developed around 1980, is non-invasive and is of particular interest for serial monitoring of patients who are at risk of clinically significant overload.

In an adult man there are typically 3 grams of iron actively involved in the storage and transport of oxygen and 1 gram held in storage. The main storage compound, ferritin, is a protein containing varying amounts of iron. It is mainly found in the liver (about 60 per cent).

Major changes in iron levels are clinically important. Reduction in stored iron may indicate chronic blood loss caused by, for example, malignancy, parisitic infection, gastrointestinal lesions etc. High stored iron levels are associated with high oral iron intake, hemachromatosis, chronic transfusion and, linked with this last factor, thalassemia. Hemachromatosis is a syndrome involving excessive iron uptake; it can lead to cirrhosis of the liver, diabetes, hepatic carcinoma and gonadal atrophy, but treatment by phlobotomy is successful if the condition is diagnosed promptly. Thalassemia is a genetically transmitted form of anaemia prevalent over much of the Middle and Far East (Figure 4). Sufferers are unable to synthesise hemoglobin adequately. The condition can be treated by regular transfusions but this leads to an excess of stored iron. In turn, this can be eliminated by the use of an iron chelating drug (Desferal), but the treatment regime is expensive and grossly disruptive.

In both hemachromatosis and thalassemia there is an obvious need for serial monitoring of stored iron. This cannot be achieved by the preferred technique, liver biopsy, because of the discomfort and risk involved. Magnetic biopsy is now a viable alternative.

The magetic susceptibility of the liver depends linearly on the iron concentration (Figure 5), but the contribution to the overall susceptibility of the iron, which is only present in small quantities, is small; for normal subjects it is only about 5%. Moreover, any *in vivo* susceptibility measurement is sensitive to both the liver and to surrounding tissue. It follows that, to find the iron related signal, substantial corrections to the measured signal are necessary.

Figure 6 shows a recently reported instrument (Paulson et al 1989). The measurement sequence is straightforward. The patient is raised on a motor controlled bed until there is the minimum convenient distance between skin and magnetometer. A superconducting magnet in the persistent mode applies a highly constant field of 20 mT to the liver and overlying tissue.

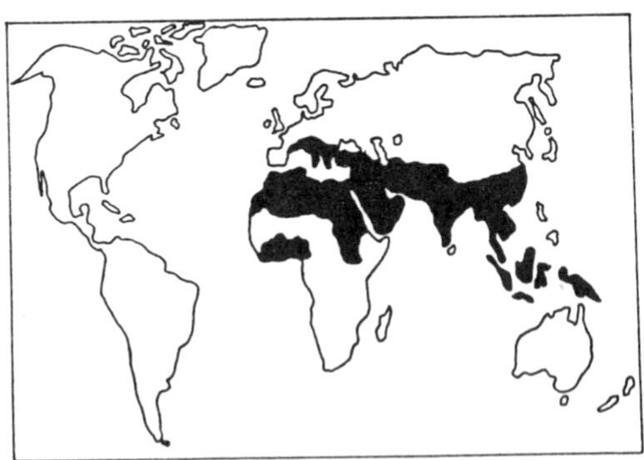

Fig. 4. Thalassemia is mainly found in the shaded regions.

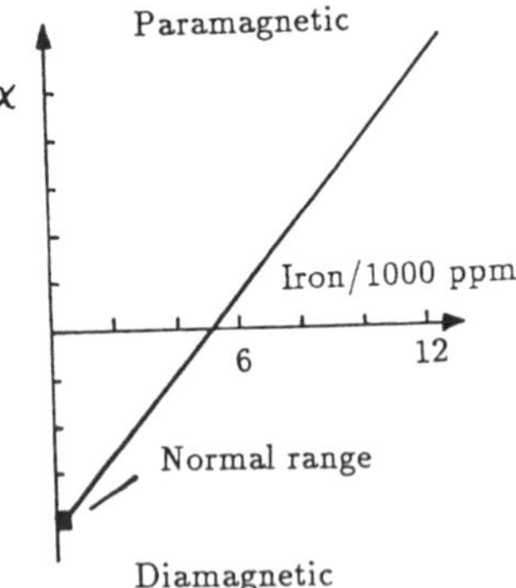

Fig. 5. The dependence of liver susceptibility on the the stored iron concentration. Note that, in normal subjects, the iron contribution is small.

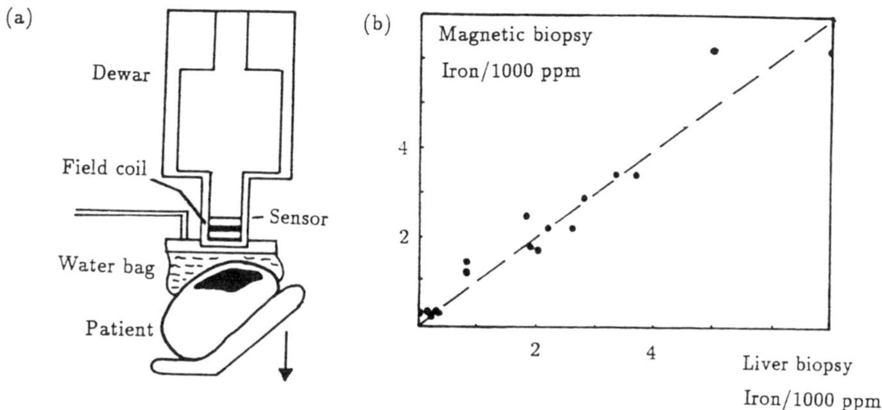

Fig. 6. (a) A liver susceptometer (Paulson et al. 1989). (b) A comparison of magnetic data recorded using (a) with the results of conventional invasive biopsy.

Then, while the outputs of two separate second order SQUID gradiometers are recorded, the bed is lowered by about 6 cm. Small coils fixed on the skin of the patient are used to define the initial position and to measure height during the lowering operation.

The use of a small field coil and gradiometers limits the sensitive volume to a region of a few centimetres depth directly below the instrument. Typically, with such an arrangement, the signal from the liver (all contributions) is 25% of the signal from the overlying tissue, but the exact ratio depends on both the detector-skin distance and the diameter of the detector coil. By using two detectors of different diameter and recording as a function of separation, it is possible to disentangle the two contributions, to eliminate certain instrumental artefacts, and to calculate χ_{liver}. Using a calibration graph such as Figure 5b the value of χ_{liver} can be converted into an iron concentration.

The water bag in Figure 6a simplifies the analysis. It is fed by a constant head device so that, as the torso is lowered, it is displaced by water. χ_{water} is very similar to χ_{tissue}, and therefore the presence of the bag reduces the dependence of the modelling on the details of the torso surface.

In the instruments reported to date random noise (ambient fields, vibrations etc.) has been reduced to a level equivalent to much less than 100 ppm of iron in the liver. Other instrumental related signals (attributable to magnetic materials in the system) may cause larger effects but they can easily be corrected for. Subject related uncertainties, as discussed above, are difficult to quantify from fundamental calculation, but are probably about 200 ppm stored iron. Empirically, excellent correlations are found between the results of invasive liver biopsies and magnetic data (Figure 6b). By comparison, the concentration of stored iron in normal livers is about 100–500 ppm and in subjects with overload is 1000-30000 ppm. It is clear that the magnetic technique is viable as a monitor of overload.

It is interesting to speculate on the technique's potential in monitoring iron deficiency. An accuracy corresponding to a stored iron level of about 50 ppm would be barely acceptable. Instrumental noise can probably be reduced to meet this target, but subject noise and uncertainties present major problems. For example, it has been calculated that a mere 1% change in assumed non-iron liver suceptibility, which may well be within the natural variation, corresponds to a 50 ppm change in the prediction of stored iron concentration. As there appears to be no obvious way of separately measuring this quantity *in vivo*, it may represent a fundamental uncertainty in absolute measurements.

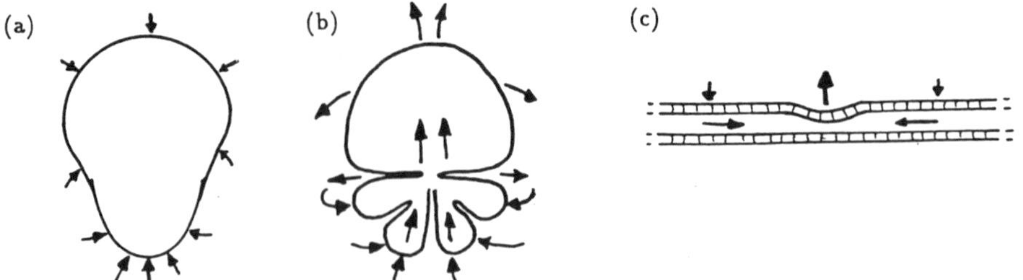

Fig. 7. Three examples of developing organisms in which continuous ionic currents have been detected (using vibrating probe electrometers). (a) Fucoid egg. (b) Silkworm (*Cecropia*) follicle. (c) Invaginating primitive streak of the chick.

QUASI DC IONIC CURRENTS

There are many electrophysiological processes which involve currents that are essentially constant over periods from a few seconds upwards. Typically current densities of order 1-10 μAcm^{-2} are involved. Often, though not always, the currents are associated with some departure from a previously established homeostatic equilibrium. Perhaps, the most obvious example is the injury current that flows when the electrical impedances and perhaps geometry of some region of tissue are disrupted. For the considerable period (perhaps days) it takes to establish a new equilibrium, ionic currents flow. There is some evidence that these currents or the electrical fields with which they are associated play an essential role in the repair process. An equally controversial suggestion is that the currents that are observed during the development of biological organisms (Figure 7) are a significant part of a complex electrical/chemical/mechanical system by which microscopic genetic information is converted into macroscopic physical shape changes.

We can also speculate on the relevance of dc processes in the brain. Clearly we might expect dc currents to be associated with 'injury' but might there also be detectable long term currents associated with more subtle processes, e.g. mood, memory formation etc.

SQUID magnetometry may help us to answer such questions and to better understand the systematics of dc electrophysiology. A suitable dc magnetometer system (Freake 1988) is shown schematically in Figure 8a. As mentioned previously, the dc signal is converted into an

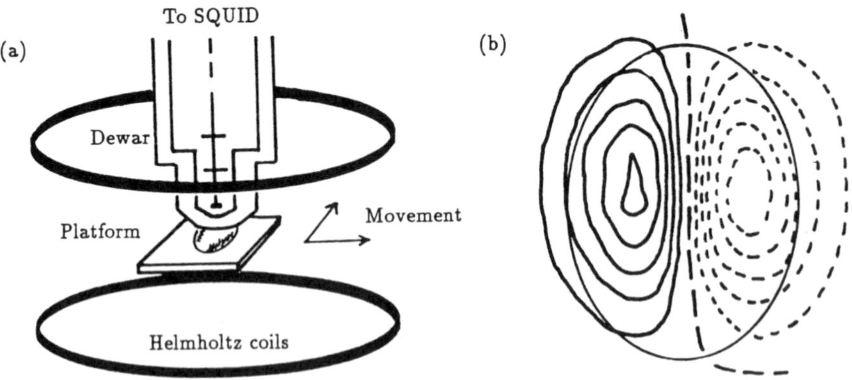

Fig. 8. (a) A magnetometer suitable for dc ionic current measurements. (b) The vertical dc magnetic field observed in a horizontal plane above a chick egg *in ovo* at 56 hours incubation time. The contour lines are spaced at 1 pT intervals with solid lines indicating positive B_z.

ac signal by moving the organism, in this case an egg, under the detector. The position of the platform supporting the organism is continuously recorded. The Helmholtz coils are used to reduce the ambient field to less than about 10^{-7} T thereby eliminating signals associated with the organism's diamagnetism. A single channel system of this type can provide a detailed map of the organism related magnetic field in a plane in of order minutes.

Partly because of the interest in making dc measurements on *small* organisms, considerable effort has been expended in making miniaturised magnetometers. The system in Figure 8a incorporates an asymmetric gradiometer in which the lowest coil is of diameter 4 mm and is 5.5 mm from the 300 K region. A spectacular recent achievement is the construction of a 4-channel system in which the sensing coils are of 3 mm diameter and are a mere 1.4 mm from the outside environment (Buchanan et al. 1989). In both these systems the miniaturisation exacts a price in terms of field sensitivity (in each case of order 100 $\mathrm{fTHz}^{-1/2}$) but this is more than compensated for by the reduction in source detector distance.

The first biomagnetic measurements using SQUIDs were reported by Cohen and colleagues (1975, 1980). In the second of these papers they catalogued a number of field sources including the scalp, abdomen and limbs. Typically the signals were equivalent to field values of order 1-10 pT. Since then extensive measurements of the dc fields associated with skeletal muscle have been made showing the existence of slowly changing microamp currents of characteristic form in normal subjects (see Swithenby 1988 for references). It is believed that the currents are associated with the inhomogeneity of muscle fibre membranes.

Though there are few dc studies to date there are hints of the possible clinical relevance of such measurements. Cohen and Kaufman (1975) have observed a dc shift in the magnetocardiogram associated with damage to the heart muscle. Barth et al. (1984) have identified a dc component in the fields generated in the rat brain during ictal episodes. Both these sudies suggest that localisation based on dc studies might identify sites of clinically significant electrophysiological disturbance. More work is needed to assess the accuracy and level of applicability of the methods and to identify problems of protocol etc.

An intriguing observation (Okada and Nicholson 1989) is of a dc field associated with the phenomenon of spreading depression in an *in vitro* preparation of the turtle cerebellum. This work indicates the feasibility of investigating magnetically whether the underlying mechanism of migraine is a similar macroscopic inhibition of cortical activity. The eventual clinical relevance is unclear.

Developmentally related currents have been detected in the chick egg *in ovo* (Swithenby 1988). Fields are detected from about 18 hours incubation and are present throughout subsequent stages. In the early period they are associated with the electrophysiologically very active extra-embryonic membranes, which compartmentalise the egg and create the appropriate conditions to both sustain the embryo and allow its subsequent development. (There is strong evidence that electrical parameters (ion concentrations, pH etc.) exert subtle controls over morphogenesis.) This work is at present beïng extended to allow more precise mapping of the currents both in the chick embryo and in other organisms.

The studies I have mentioned in the last few paragraphs are, in the main, preliminary in nature and the potential of dc measurements needs much more systematic exploration. In particular, I believe that there is great scope for investigation of the quasi dc behaviour of the brain. However, two words of warning. First, phenomenon gathering will not be enough; we must ask defined questions about carefully assembled subject groups in controlled conditions. Secondly, anyone venturing into such measurements must beware of topical ferromagnetic contamination and other sources of artefact. These have posed serious (sometimes intractable) problems to all those who have attempted detailed dc studies.

Concluding Remarks I have already indicated that my survey would be incomplete. There are many other biomagnetic field sources, including the potential difference across the retina, the action potentials in skeletal muscle, and skin potential differences. No doubt, with the improvements in instrumentation that have recently taken place, other sources will be reported in this conference.

REFERENCES

Aittoniemi K., Kalliomaki K., Katila T. and Varpula T. 1981, Practical magnetopneumography using fluxgate magnetometers. *in* "Biomagnetism" Walter de Gruyter, 476-484.

Barth D.S., Sutherling W. and Beatty J. 1984 Fast and slow magnetic phenomena in focal epileptic seizures. *Science* 226, 855-857

Brain J.D., Bloom S.B. and Valberg P.A. 1988, Magnetometry –a tool for studying the cell biology of macrophages. *in* "Biomagnetism '87" Tokyo Denki Univ. Press, Tokyo, 10-17

Brain J.D., Gehr P., Valberg P.A., Bloom S.B. and Nemoto I. 1985, Biomagnetism in the study of lung function. *in* "Biomagnetism: Applications and Theory", Pergamon Press, 378-387

Brittenham G.M., Farrell D.E., Harris J.W., Feldman E.S., Danish E.H., Muir W.A., Tripp J.H., Brennan J.N. and Bellon E.M. 1983, Diagnostic assessment of human iron stores by measurement of hepatic magnetic susceptibility. *Il Nuovo Cimento*, 2D, No. 2, 567-581

Buchanan D.S., Crum D.B., Cox D., and Wikswo Jr. J.P. 1989, *This volume*

Cohen D. and Kaufman L.A. 1975 Magnetic determination of the the relationship between the ST segment shift and the injury current produced by coronary artery occlusion. *Circ. Res.*. 36, 414-424

Cohen D. 1978, Report of the low field group: the magnetic field of the lung. *MIT/Francis Bitter Nat. Mag. Lab. Publication*, 78/1

Cohen D., Palti Y., Cuffin B.N. and Schmid S.J. 1980, *Proc. Natl. Acad. Sci. USA*. 77, 1447-1451

Freake S.M., Swithenby S.J. and Thomas I.M. 1988, A miniature SQUID magnetometer for the detection of quasi dc ionic current flow in developing organisms. *in* "Biomagnetism '87" Tokyo Denki Univ. Press, Tokyo, 434-437

Farrell D.E. 1983, The magnetic biopsy. *in* "Biomagnetism An Interdisciplinary Approach" Plenum Press, 483-499

Freedman A.P., Robinson S.E., Street M.C. and Camplone D. 1984, Effect of cigarette smoking on alveolar clearance of particles. *in* Proc. of 5th. World Conference on Biomagnetism, Vancouver, Canada. Pergamon, New York. 43-45

Halperin M., Williamson S.J. Spektor D.M., Schlesinger R.B. and Lippman M. (1981), Remanent magnetic fields for measuring particle retention and distribution in the lungs. *Exptl. Lung. Res.* 2, 27-35

Kalliomaki K., Kalliomaki P.L., Korhonen O., Pasanen J., Aittoniemi K. and Moilanen M. 1983, Magnetopneumography, *in* "Biomagnetism An Interdisciplinary Approach" Plenum Press, 533-568.

Le Gros V., Lemaigre D., Suon C., Pozzi J.P. and Liot F. 1989, Magnetopneumography: a general review. *Eur. Respir. J.*, 2, 149-159.

Nemoto I., Ogura K. and Toyotama H. 1989, Estimation of the energy of cytoplasmic movements by magnetometry: effects of temperature and intracellular concentration of ATP. *IEEE Trans. Biomed. Eng.*, BME–36, No. 6, 598-607

Okada Y.C. and Nicholson C. 1988, DC-coupled single trial measurements of the magnetic field during spreading depression in the cerebellum. *in* "Biomagnetism '87" Tokyo Denki Univ. Press, Tokyo, 202-205

Paulson D.N., Engelhardt R., Fischer R. and Heinrich H.C. 1989, The Hamburg biosusceptometer for liver iron quantification. *This volume*

Stroink G. 1985, Magnetic measurements to determine dust loads and clearance rates in industrial workers and miners. *Med. Biol. Eng. Computing.* 23, 44-49.

Swithenby S.J. 1988, Non invasive monitoring of ionic current flow during development by SQUID magnetometry. *Experientia*, 44, 673-678

EVOLUTION OF THE *SQUID* AND ITS USE IN BIOMAGNETIC RESEARCH

James E. Zimmerman

National Bureau of Standards Fellow (retired)
751 Gapter Road, Boulder CO, 80303, USA

INTRODUCTION

With benefit of several decades of hindsight, I think London's hypothesis, that superconductivity is a state characterized by long-range phase coherence, must have required great intellectual courage. He suggested that the theory of wave-particle duality known as quantum theory, hitherto applied only to submicroscopic systems such as individual atoms and molecules, should now be applied to vastly larger systems, such as a one-kilometer loop of superconducting wire. He proposed this startling hypothesis as a trivially simple way of understanding the Meissner effect, the exclusion of magnetic field from a bulk material when it is cooled through the superconducting transition temperature. A consequence of the hypothesis was that if magnetic field is trapped inside a hole or imperfection in a piece of bulk superconductor, the total flux contained within the hole must be quantized. The flux within the hole must be an integral multiple of a basic value, denoted Φ_o. He suggested $\Phi_o = h/e$ (Planck's constant divided by the electronic charge) as an obvious possibility for the magnitude of the quantum of flux. The quantity h/e had long been known as a factor in the magnetic effect in atomic spectra known as Zeeman splitting. In 1961, several years after London's death, it was shown experimentally (and immediately confirmed theoretically, as Prof. Bill Little once put it) that the flux quantum is $\Phi_o = h/2e$ (or 2.07×10^{-15} Wb), rather than h/e (Doll and Nabauer, 1961; Deaver and Fairbank, 1961). It was already known that the superconducting state involved electron pairing (with charge $2e$), but it seems no one had thought to relate this to flux quantization.

Figure 1 shows how quantum principles determine the electronic configuration in a superconducting ring and, for comparison, in an over-simplified concept of a single electron in an orbit around a proton, i.e., the hydrogen atom. The wavelength of the electron (or of electron pairs in the ring) is $\lambda = h/[(2)mv + (2)eA]$. Here m is the electron mass, v is the electron velocity, and the vector potential A is a quantity so defined that its line integral around any closed loop, such as an electron orbit or a superconducting ring, is equal to the magnetic flux Φ through the loop. This is written as: $\oint A \cdot ds = \Phi$. The requirement in quantum mechanics for a stable configuration of either of these two systems is that there be an integral number of wavelengths around the loop, i.e., $\oint (1/\lambda)\, ds = 0, \pm 1, \pm 2, \ldots$ (the sign being determined by whether the vector A points in the same direction, or opposite direction, to the path along which the integral is taken). For the hydrogen atom the eA term is nearly negligible, and the result is a set of discrete orbits. In Fig. 1 the electron is indicated in the sixth orbit. For the superconducting ring, the mv term is essentially negligible compared to eA, and the result is the set of discrete magnetic flux states, represented in Fig. 2a by evenly-spaced values on the vertical axis. If the external field is changed by bringing a magnet near, the flux within the ring remains unchanged, so lines representing the value of the flux within the loop are horizontal.

Advances in Biomagnetism
Edited by S.J. Williamson *et al.*
Plenum Press, New York

Fig. 1. (a) Simplified picture of the possible orbits for the electron in a hydrogen atom. (b) A superconducting ring of metal. Note the difference in scale.

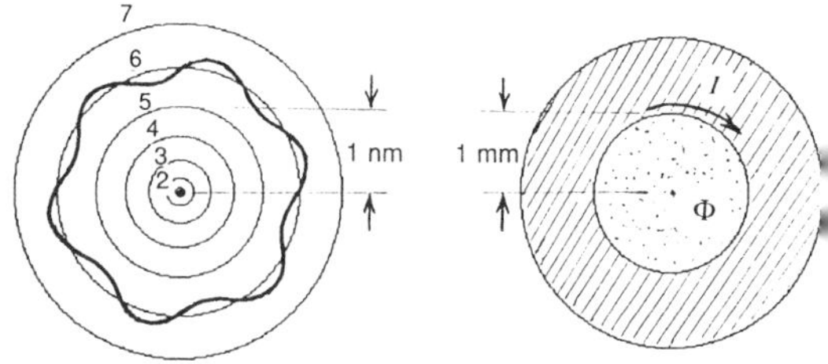

In 1962, Brian Josephson, then a graduate student, predicted superconducting tunnelling (the Josephson Effect) (Josephson, 1962). A tunnel junction is simply two metals separated by an insulating barrier sufficiently thin that electrons can "tunnel" through the barrier. The quantum mechanical wave function describing an electron in the metal cannot be abruptly terminated at the boundary, but weakly extends into the insulator. In effect, the insulator becomes a conductor, but with vastly attenuated current density. In a superconducting tunnel junction, or "Josephson junction," the amplitudes of the superconducting wave functions in each metal are similarly reduced within the insulator, but nevertheless their overlap couples one superconductor to the other. In addition to a tunnel current passing through the insulating barrier even where there is zero voltage across it, the Josephson effect includes magnetic quantum diffraction and interference effects, and an ac supercurrent of frequency $2eV/h$ when a potential difference V is impressed across a tunnel junction. Note that the ratio of the frequency of this oscillating current to the DC voltage is $2e/h$ = 486 megahertz/microvolt, just the inverse of the flux quantum. Experimental observation of the Josephson effect was reported a few months after Josephson's prediction (Rowell, 1963).

In 1963, in an experiment quite unrelated to the above, John Lambe and his colleagues at the Ford Scientific Laboratory discovered the rf-biased SQUID. In an experiment on nuclear magnetic resonance, they happened to observe that the X-band (X-band refers to a band of radio frequencies

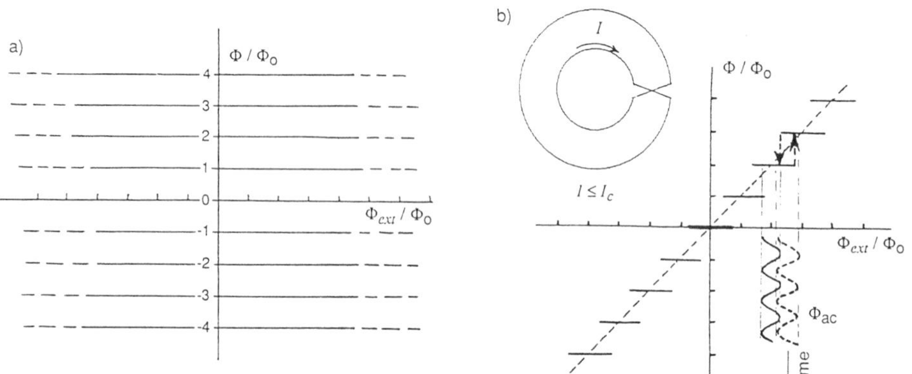

Fig. 2. (a) Value of the quantized magnetic flux Φ within a superconducting ring when the externally applied flux Φ_{ext} has the strength indicated on the horizontal axis, both expressed in units of the flux quantum Φ_0. (b) Flux in a ring with a weak connection *versus* applied flux, assuming only that the current circling the ring $I = (\Phi - \Phi_{ext})/L \leq I_c$. For this illustration, the critical current of the connection I_c is chosen to be slightly larger than $\Phi_0/2L$. The lower right quadrant illustrates two situations, described later in the text, where an *ac* field is applied in addition to the DC field, with time axis running downward. The solid sinusoidal line is for a DC field that is nearly an integral multiple of Φ_0 so that the ring current never reaches the critical value. The dashed sinusoidal line is for a DC field whose ring current is sufficiently close to the critical value that the AC field causes hysteretic response between the 3rd and 4th flux states on each cycle. Arrows depict the abrupt transitions when the AC field causes the critical current for each state to be exceeded.

centered around 10 GHz, or a wavelength of 3 cm) impedance of a bit of superconducting thin film varied periodically as a function of the dc magnetic field in the neighborhood. The periodicity of the variation was in the neighborhood of one or two nanotesla – it must have been obvious that they had a magnetic field sensor of unparalleled sensitivity. This exciting observation was so puzzling that at one time I was consulted for suggestions as to the fundamental nature of the phenomenon and how to investigate it experimentally. I was able to shed not the faintest glimmer of light on the subject.

There must have been a strong hint, however, that this effect in the X-band impedance of the thin film might be related to flux quantization or the Josephson effect or both. With this inspirational background, the group then embarked on their classic experiments on quantum interference between the DC tunnel currents of two junctions in parallel – the DC SQUID configuration. The results were reported in 1964 (Jaklevic et al. 1963a,b). Meanwhile, they continued the X-band experiments on thin films, and their first publication, later in 1964, reveals the influence of the double-junction experiments on their thinking. The paper shows a superconducting loop with two microbridges oriented parallel to the microwave electric field, with no mention of the microwave magnetic field (Lambe et al., 1964).

At the same time, early 1964, I suggested the use of small area metallic point contacts as a simple mechanism for demonstrating quantum effects in superconductors. I was able to do this because at the time I was working on a resistive control mechanism for electric power steering for automobiles. The mechanism was a pressure-sensitive resistive contact between two plates of poorly conducting material. I therefore knew something about electrical contacts, such as that the contact resistance between two semi-infinite pieces of metal is $R = \rho/D$, where ρ is the resistivity of the metal and D is diameter of the contact. The initial experiments by Arnold Silver and me on superconducting contacts between crossed wires showed convincingly their utility for demonstrating and studying quantum interference effects in superconductors (Zimmerman and Silver, 1964). These experiments, which took no more than two or three days, were the beginning of a five-year collaboration.

Silver and I completed a more extensive study of double-point-contact DC SQUIDs of various sizes and materials (Zimmerman and Silver, 1966). One of these had an inside diameter of nearly 10 mm, approaching the limit at which thermal fluctuations should wipe out the interference pattern. The wipeout occurs when the inductance L of the SQUID is large enough that $\Phi_0^2/2L$, the energy of one flux quantum in the SQUID ring, is comparable to the characteristic scale of thermal energy of current fluctuations $kT/2$, Boltzmann's constant times the absolute temperature. At the same time, Silver began a study of the 30 MHz impedance of small thin-film rings, in an attempt to understand the earlier X-band observations. Figure 3 is the 30 MHz version of John Lambe's X-band circuit. These experiments were not immediately successful, and we subsequently joined forces and used bulk superconducting rings with a single point contact as a "weak link" to permit easy modulation of flux in and out of the ring under the influence of a radio frequency (RF) field (Silver and Zimmerman, 1967).

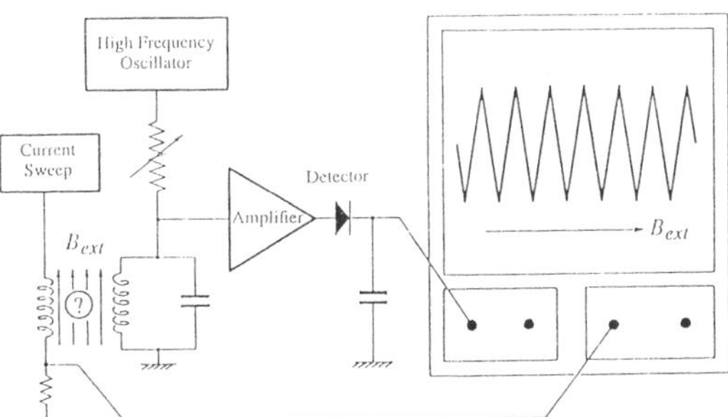

Fig. 3. A simple circuit for measuring high-frequency impedance, useful for observing magnetic resonance, or for displaying quantum effects in superconductors. A typical SQUID pattern is shown at the right, with output voltage varying periodically with increasing applied field B_{ext}.

The model that we used at that time, around 1965, was that the weak link should have a maximum supercurrent I_c of the order of Φ_o/L, so that the quantized flux states are truncated as shown in Fig. 2b (indicating that only one flux quantum enters when the ring current exceeds the critical current). If the externally applied field Φ_{ext} has both a slowly varying DC component and a rapidly varying *ac* component such as provided by a radio frequency (RF) source, the supercurrent maintains the flux in the ring unchanged unless the sum produces a total ring current that is less than I_c. If either is changed so that the ring current exceeds I_c, the ring switches to the next adjacent flux state (meaning simply that the number of flux quanta within the ring increases or decreases by one). With this "linear" model, it was qualitatively obvious that there would be quantum periodic discontinuities in the electrical impedance, as functions of both the DC and the RF field amplitudes applied to the ring. For example, with a very small RF field applied, the DC field can be set so that the ring remains always in the same quantum state (Fig. 2b, solid sinusoidal curve representing the RF field), with no energy loss. Or it can be set so the ring current $I = (\Phi - \Phi_{ext})/L$ is nearly I_c, so that the ring switches to the adjacent state and back with each RF cycle (Fig. 2b, dashed sinusoidal curve representing the RF field), with a specific energy dissipation per cycle. The onset of dissipation as the DC field is varied should be manifested as a discontinuity in both the real and the imaginary parts of the complex impedance of the ring.

Up to a point, the model was quite successful in interpreting our experimental results. It corrected the earlier misconceptions in showing that only one weak link is required rather than two, and in clarifying the coupling mechanism by showing that the plane of the ring should be perpendicular to the magnetic field and that the orientation of the weak link relative to the RF electric field is irrelevant. We developed a practical RF coupling circuit, and demonstrated the use of a phase-locked loop for SQUID magnetometers and other applications. Our 1967 paper interpreted the results both in terms of the linear model, and also in terms of the sinusoidal Josephson current-phase relation. Both models served our rather limited purposes equally well, except that the linear model was simpler to analyze.

Both models predicted periodic discontinuties in the RF impedance with increasing magnetic field. What we commonly observed, under conditions of good signal-to-noise ratio, was a triangular wave pattern, that is, discontinuities in the derivative rather that in the impedance itself. The observed pattern is a consequence of the rather complicated interaction between the SQUID and the resonant circuit to which it is coupled. This was shown analytically and, independently, by computer simulation, in 1970 (Zimmerman, Thiene and Harding, 1970; Simmonds and Parker, 1971). At around the same time, we developed mechanical analogs of simple electrical circiuts including Josephson junctions. By this mechanism we finally gained an elementary intuitive understanding of the full beauty and complexity of the operation of single and double-junction SQUIDs, including the dynamics of the transitions between flux states (Sullivan and Zimmerman, 1971). In our earlier work, we had simply assumed these transitions to be instantaneous, which was a workable assumption as long as the RF bias frequency was small compared to the frequency of self-resonance of the SQUID itself. Meanwhile, other significant developments were under way.

During 1968 and 1969, my colleagues and I worked at making stable point-contact SQUIDs, the most successful of which was the two-hole version with the contact bridging a narrow slot cut between the holes (Fig. 4). We also built a compact, production-prototype, RF electronic unit to be used in conjunction with a SQUID and phase-locked loop for use as highly sensitive laboratory magnetometer. The "phase-locked loop" is an electronic circuit which "feeds back" a current to apply a magnetic field to the SQUID exactly equal and opposite to the external field change being measured. The feed-back current is then a precisely linear measure of the external field change. This circuit was the prototype for practically all subsequent SQUID instruments.

In 1969 I was approached by John Wheatley to join him and others in forming a private company to manufacture and market SQUID magnetometers. And, at the end of 1969, Edgar Edelsack catalyzed a collaboration with David Cohen by which the three of us demonstrated the superior performance of the SQUID magnetometer for biomagnetic measurements. This was done in the last three days (and nights) of the decade, in the magnetically shielded room which Cohen had just finished building at the National Magnet Laboratory. It was the first time that an acceptable magnetocardiogram had been produced without time averaging (Cohen, Edelsack and Zimmerman, 1970), as illustrated in Fig. 5. The SHE Corporation was formally established in early 1970 to pro-

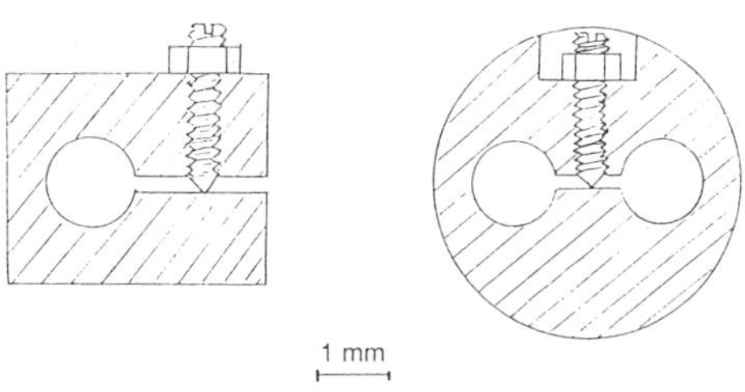

Fig. 4. Cross sections of two early types of stable point-contact SQUIDs. The two-hole version was the first to be used for biomagnetic measurements and was commercially produced for several years.

duce SQUIDs and related cryogenic instrumentation based on the two-hole RF SQUID.

Since 1970, research in biomagnetism has spread to many laboratories and, although SQUIDs are used routinely for many purposes, their primary application is for biomagnetic measurements. For several years after 1970, most research was carried out using single-channel instruments in a first or second-order gradiometer configuration to discriminate against magnetic interference. As interest and funding for biomagnetic measurement increased, we have seen in this decade increasing use of multi-channel instruments. And, in a rather expensive development, we now have major investments in multi-channel instruments and high-quality magnetically shielded enclosures for the ultimate in signal-to-noise ratio and in speed of data acquisition. Perhaps this conference will decide if the investment is justified.

It should be apparent that this paper is largely a narrative of my personal involvement with the development and applications of single and double-junction SQUID's, and does not do justice to the contributions of many others. The long-term dedication of John Clarke to the DC SQUID cannot be over-emphasized. The present wide-spread use and understanding of this device is owing largely the work of him and his students, many of whom are now pre-eminent in the field. Martin Nisenoff and John Goodkind (independently) made important contributions to the early development and application of the thin-film RF SQUID. Bill Goree and his colleagues established the first commercial firm to make and sell SQUID magnetometers and related instruments. Stable SQUIDs using

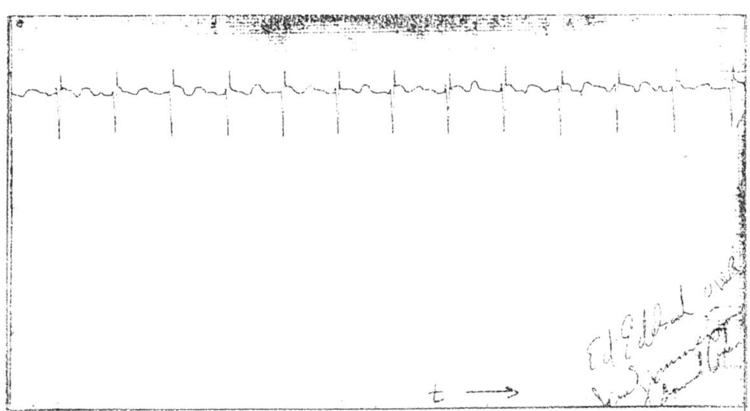

Fig. 5 First measurement of the magnetic field of the human heart using a SQUID sensor, obtained within the MIT magnetically shielded room. The signatures of the participants are shown on this data sheet at the lower right.

lightly oxidized point contacts were reported by Buhrman et. al. and by de Waele and de Bruyn Ouboter. SQUIDs of this type are still used in some laboratories, and are reported to be reliabl over long periods of time. In recent years, an enormous amount of work has gone into making reli able and highly sensitive DC SQUIDs and other Josephson devices by thin-film microcircuit tech niques.

As a final note, I must emphasize how much my own work was inspired and guided by others Acknowledgement is especially due to Jack Goldman, who coerced me into dropping my work o thermodynamic properties of paramagnetic alloys below 1 kelvin in favor of making superconduct ing devices after Jaklevic, et al. had had all the fun. And to Arnold Silver, who greatly simplifie early developments by introducing me to the linear model of the single-junction device, and wh also served as surrogate father in throwing cold water on my every idea and suggestion. And to John Wheatley who prodded me into figuring out how the SQUID coupling circuit worked, and wh also conned me into joining him in moonlighting and financing the founding of the SHE Corpora tion. And of course to Edgar Edelsack, who opened up the field of biomagnetism by getting me an David Cohen together to demonstrate the superiority of the SQUID in biomagnetic instrumentation and whose long-term interest in neurobiology and support through the Office of Naval Researcl made the whole development possible.

REFERENCES

Cohen, D., Edelsack, E.A., and Zimmerman, J.E., 1970, Magnetocardiograms taken inside a shielded room with a superconducting point-contact magnetometer. *Appl. Phys. Letters.* 16 278-280.

Deaver, B.S., and Fairbank, W.M., 1961. Experimental evidence for quantized flux in superconducting cylinders. *Phys. Rev. Lett.* 7, 43-46.

Doll, R., and Nabauer, M. 1961, Experimental proof of magnetic flux quantization in a superconducting ring. *Phys. Rev. Lett.* 7, 51-52.

Jaklevic, R., Lambe, J., Silver, A., and Mercereau, J.E., 1963a, Quantum interference effects in Josephson tunnelling. *Phys. Rev. Lett.* 12, 159-160.

Jaklevic, R., Lambe, J., Silver, A., and Mercereau, J.E., 1963b, Interference from a static vector potential in a field-free region. *Phys. Rev. Lett.* 12, 274-275.

Josephson, B.D., 1962, Possible new effects in superconductive tunnelling. *Phys. Letters* 1, 251-253.

Lambe, J., Jaklevic, R., Mercereau, J.E., and Silver, A.H., 1964, Microwave observation of quantum interference effects in superconductors. *Phys. Letters* 11, 16-17.

Rowell, J.B., 1963, Magnetic field dependence of the Josephson tunnel current. *Phys. Rev. Lett.* 11, 200-202.

Silver, A.H., and Zimmerman, J.E., 1967, Quantum states and transitions in weakly connected superconducting rings. *Phys. Rev.* 157, 317-341.

Simmonds, M.B., and Parker, W.H., 1971, Analog computer simulation of weakly connected superconducting rings. *J. Appl. Phys.* 42, 38-45.

Sullivan, D.B., and Zimmerman, J.E., 1971, Mechanical analogs of time-dependent Josephson phenomena. *Amer. J. Phys.* 39, 1504-1517.

Zimmerman, J.E., and Silver, A.H., 1964, Quantum effects in type II superconductors. *Phys. Letters* 10, 47-48.

Zimmerman, J.E., and Silver, A.H., 1966, Macroscopic quantum interference effects through superconducting point contacts. *Phys. Rev.* 141, 367-375.

Zimmerman, J.E., Thiene, P., and Harding, J.T., 1970, Design and operation of stable RF-biased superconducting point-contact devices and a note on the operation of perfectly clean metal contacts. *J. Appl. Phys.* 41, 1572-1580.

A VICENNIAL VIEW OF SQUID MAGNETOCARDIOGRAPHY

Edgar A. Edelsack

Senior Fellow, Institute for Technology and Strategic Research
School of Engineering and Applied Science
The George Washington University, Washington, D.C. 20037

INTRODUCTION

I am no historian and what follows is by no means an accurate narrative of the first attempt at SQUID magnetocardiography. The main protagonists in this tale are of course David Cohen and Jim Zimmerman. Their collaboration came about from quite different paths. I was an observer and an *amicus curiae* to this collaboration. The forces that shape science and technology today often have their origins in the immediate past. I will look back some twenty years to events that preceded the use of SQUIDS in biomagnetism and also try to look forward some twenty years to what could be in the future. I will recount some recollections of how this marriage between SQUIDS and biomagnetism was consummated.

EARLY DEVELOPMENTS

Somehow history never feels like history when you're living through it. It is often a confusing and sometimes contradictory set of events. In trying to recall the details surrounding the first SQUID biomagnetic measurements, I am reminded of Jean Cocteau's remark that history is facts which become lies in the end and legends are lies which become history in the end. For the field of biomagnetism, the past is little more than twenty-five years ago, beginning in 1963 with the pioneering work of Gerhart Baule and Richard McFee (1963). They used a coil of two million turns of wire with a ferrite core placed near the chest. They were able to detect a voltage across the coil induced by the time-rate of change of the cardiac field.

The year 1969 was exciting for both science and technology. It bears striking similarities to events of the present year. I will highlight a few similarities of past and present in the hope that it may be possible to learn from past failures how to do better in the future and also to learn from past successes how not to do worse in future. On July 20, 1969 the imagination of scientists, engineers and the general public were captured when Neil Armstrong landed on the moon. It was an unforgettable sight on that hot Sunday afternoon to see on television a man descending the steps of a lunar space craft. The history of the Apollo program is well documented. What is sometimes overlooked is that this monumental research and development program to explore outer space had its origin in 1961 with President Kennedy's announcement to start a program to land a man on the moon within a decade. It is an excellent example of where sustained government funding supporting competent scientists and engineers for a well-defined goal achieved a remarkable success. I will come back to this point at the end of my talk.

In 1967, I joined the Office of Naval Research in Washington and was given the opportunity of starting two small research programs. One program was in the field of superconductivity. The other was in biophysics. Why were these two programs chosen? I don't recall any special reason except that at that time, my boss Frank Isakson and I were both interested in these two topics.

Advances in Biomagnetism
Edited by S.J. Williamson *et al.*
Plenum Press, New York

Today, this reason would not be considered an adequate justification for starting a new research program. I did not have any specific idea of what research would be supported in the superconductivity program so I called it "Superconducting Elements". With this title it appeared possible to justify support of almost any good unsolicited research proposal in superconductivity. ONR operates its physics and electronics programs without the use of peer review. ONR staff are not permitted to solicit proposals from the research community. It only funds unsolicited proposals. I believe this may in part account for its continued vitality. It is able to fund small, high-risk research projects. This is often not possible for those U.S. funding agencies which use peer review. I believe such systems tend toward conservatism.

There was a competitive spirit among many ONR program managers to try to fund great science as opposed to simply good science. For science to be great, it must in part involve some surprises. It must bring discoveries of things few expected or even imagined. As a program manager, I became aware that those who had funds to dispense often attracted a following who sung their praises, assuring them they were correct in their scientific judgments. It was always delightful to hear songs of praise. The human brain appears designed to amplify such signals and attenuate those which contain criticism suggesting one is doing a miserable job.

The name of the biophysics program was chosen so as not to appear to be poaching on the turf of my biology and physiology colleagues. I called the program "Macromolecular Physics". Fortunately, no one ever asked me to define its meaning. Each research program had to have an objective. I dreamed up the one for the superconductivity program (Fig. 1). I don't recall the justification for the macromolecular physics program. An additional hurdle which had to be overcome before starting a new program was to provide our military and high-level civilian bosses with a list of potential applications (Fig. 2). The 1968 list of potential applications of superconductivity contains many of the same items being touted today in the U.S. as justifications for research programs in high temperature ceramic superconductors. I don't recall the list of potential applications for the biophysics program.

Research fortunately moves forward in new and exciting directions but the same old justifications seem to live on and on. There appears to be a strong emphasis in the United States today to justify support of research largely on its potential applications, and, often, this is synonymous with military applications. Some real dangers exist in overexploiting this approach. It is not always possible to provide breakthroughs or even significant new accomplishments at the beginning of each new fiscal year. SQUID magnetocardiography is an example of a serendipitous winner. No one in ONR in 1969, least of all I, expected SQUID magnetocardiography to be the main payoff from the superconductivity and biophysics programs. Support of science is often based on a large amount of blind faith. Today in Washington, research has to compete with many other requests for federal funding. There is strong pressure on Government science program managers to provide showcase applications for new research programs in order to make them attractive to Congress and to the heads of their agencies. You have to dangle a highly visible carrot to capture

Discovery, description, and exploitation of the unique properties of superconducting materials for the development of advanced instrumentation devices and measuring techniques of use to the Navy.

Fig. 1. Objectives of the superconducting elements program of ONR in 1967.

APPLICATIONS OF SUPERCONDUCTIVITY IN MILITARY ELECTRONIC SYSTEMS

High-Q Resonant Structures
Stabilized Oscillators
Magnetic Field Sensors
Receivers (μ wave and above)
Tunable Sources
Digital Logic Devices
Analog-to-Digital Converters

Fig. 2. Potential applications envisaged for the superconducting elements program.

new funding. In the future, I believe, it will be of the mutual benefit for researchers to collaborate closely with science program managers in the government to provide realistic and convincing reasons for sustained support of basic research. The oversell can be fatal. Witness cold fusion.

SQUID SENSORS

The first research contract under the new ONR superconducting elements program was to Jim Zimmerman who was then at Philco Ford Corporation. His task was to study the properties of SQUID magnetometers. The reason Jim's proposal was chosen above others was that it was relatively easy to justify it to my military bosses. At weekly ONR program council meetings new proposals were discussed and final decisions made. The justification I gave at one of these council meetings for support of Jim's project was that ultrasensitive superconducting magnetic sensors would one day replace the optically pumped magnetometers then used in the Navy to detect submarines. I claimed that they would revolutionize antisubmarine warfare, making magnetic detection of enemy submarines a relatively easy task. I was a little less exuberant in my written justification of Jim's project. I wrote "Dr. Zimmerman will study the properties of superconducting magnetic sensors in terms of practical, optimum and reliable operation. Magnetic signals of various kinds will be measured with these devices." This first contract was for some $82,000 (Fig. 3). It was the largest contract granted that year in superconductivity. Jim did a very fine job. In the second year (Fig. 4) his support went up slightly to $100,000, close to one sixth of the total funds of the 1968 ONR superconductivity program.

By 1969 Jim was at the National Bureau of Standards in Colorado working on improving the design of SQUID magnetometers and reducing their size and complexity so they were portable or at least transportable. The U.S. Navy still uses optically pumped magnetometers. Some 20 years after Jim's research, SQUID gradiometers that can be routinely used in the Navy do not exist. It is in large part due to the difficulties of taking a device that operates well in a laboratory and developing it into a rugged system with reliable refrigeration capable of being flown from an airplane traveling above the ocean. From laboratory to practical military application is not an easy road, I learned.

SUPERCONDUCTIVITY RR 011-11-01 – FY67

RESEARCH AREA	CONTRACTOR	INVESTIGATOR	FUNDING ($K)
MAGNETIC SENSORS			
NR 319-001	Philco-Ford	Zimmerman	82
NR 319-003S	Stanford	Fairbank	26
NR 319-007	Stanford	Little	20
NR 319-002	Stanford	Res. Inst. Chilton	39
			167
ELECTROMAGNETIC SENSORS			
NR 319-009	NRDL	Alger	10
NR 319-005	U. of Maryland	Ferrell	10
			20
MATERIALS			
NR 319-006	U. of Calif. Santa Cruz	Rosenblum	10
NR 319-004	Stanford	Little	20
			30
			207

Fig. 3. Level of funding support for participants in the ONR superconductivity program for 1967.

ONR Superconducting Elements Program 1968

NR No.	Contractor	Investigator	Current Annual Level (thousands)
319-001	Aeronutronic Division-Philco Ford (D)	J. Zimmerman	99.5
319-002	Stanford Res Inst (D,C)	F. Chilton	31.9
319-003	Stanford University (D)	W.M. Fairbank	20.0
319-004	Stanford University (M,C)	W.A. Little	30.0
319-005	University of Maryland (T)	R.A. Ferrell	20.0
319-006	University of Calif/Santa Cruz (M)	B. Rosenblum	38.5
319-007	Stanford University (D)	W.A. Little	23.0
319-009	Naval Radiological Defense Lab (D)	R. Alger	20.0
319-011	University of Minnesota (T)	A. van der Ziel	30.0
319-012	University of Rochester (D)	S. Shapiro	23.0
319-014	Naval Research Laboratory (C)	R. Hein	6.5
319-015	Arizona University (T)	R.H. Parmenter	24.7
319-017	Stanford Research Institute (D)	W. Goree	157.9
319-018	Massachusetts Institute of Tech	B. Lax	17.7
319-020	University of Southern California (D)	T. Smith	22.9
319-021	California Institute of Tech (D)	J. Mercereau	24.4
319-022	University of Calif/San Diego (M)	S. Schultz	13.0
319-028	Stanford University (D)	T. Geballe	14.8
		Total	617.8

10 - Devices (D) 3 - Materials (M) 3 - Theory (T) 3 - Conferences (C)

Fig. 4. Level of support for 1968 showed an increase.

I recall once when the superconductivity program was undergoing its annual review – an event which I dreaded – I was asked to justify its continued existence. At the end of my presentation, an admiral turned to me and said in exasperation "Edelsack, you give new meaning to the initials ONR - Office of No Results". In the eyes of that admiral the program was a failure. And he was correct, since the Navy to this day does not have an operational superconducting magnetometer. However, the fact that it is now possible to purchase multichannel SQUID biomedical systems from venders in several countries is testimony to the perseverance of those who followed in Jim Zimmerman's footsteps.

The year 1969, like the present year, saw its share of reported sighting of room temperature superconductors. In those days the materials were organic superconductors and copper chloride, as opposed to the present ceramic materials. However, all room temperature superconductor sightings, past and present, still remain in the Loch Ness Monster category – awaiting confirmation. The possibility of a room temperature superconductor looks a lot more promising today however, than it did then. In September 1969, the ONR Superconductivity Program sponsored the First International Symposium on the Physical and Chemical Problems of Possible Organic Superconductors. It was held in Hawaii. At that time a stage had been reached where many of the fundamental physical problems of achieving superconductivity at high temperatures which had blocked any real progress earlier were now fairly well understood. The great barrier appeared to be the interdisciplinary nature of the problem. No organic superconductors existed at that time. To sponsor an international meeting on a nonexistent material was to say the least, controversial. To hold it in Hawaii turned out to be a major administrative faux pas. The cry of dismay raised by several members of the superconductivity research community to this meeting almost rivaled the present-day storm over cold fusion. One well known researcher wrote to the then Chief of Naval Research stating that sponsoring this meeting was absurd because organic superconductors did not exist. He added the comment that one did have to go to Hawaii to discuss the properties of fictitious materials. Following his letter, there was pressure to cancel the meeting. It finally did take place. My travel request to attend was not approved.

Today, there are several organic superconductors, some with transition temperatures as high as 11 kelvin and ceramic superconductors with transition temperatures of 125 kelvin. There are research groups in Japan, the Soviet Union and elsewhere actively exploring the properties of organic superconductors. Next year, some 20 years after the first meeting, there will be a second conference on organic superconductors co-sponsored by the ONR Chemistry Program and the Department of Energy. This time it will be in California. Recently I was invited to join the organizing committee of this meeting by the same person who had the courage and foresight to organize the first meeting. I have every intention of attending this time.

MAGNETIC SHIELDING

Now to turn to the biophysics program. I had doubts if there would be sufficient interest in the program to make it viable. A few well known biophysicists were queried for ideas as to possible program content and technical direction. Responses ranged from suggested studies of extrasensory perception to exploring olfactory phenomena. Fears of lack of interest in the program proved unfounded when a number of persons approached ONR for support. Among those was David Cohen. He requested partial support to build a magnetically shielded enclosure at the Francis Bitter National Magnet Laboratory at MIT. He wished to continue his studies of the magnetic fields of the human heart (Cohen, 1975) and brain (Cohen, 1968) using techniques similar to that of Baule and McFee. He proposed to build a spherical shaped walk-in size room with sheets of high permeability material forming the surfaces of the room to intercept external magnetic fields and leave the interior relatively field-free (Fig. 5). My colleagues and I were enthusiastic about Cohen's idea. We recommended funding the construction of the room. However, there were others who greeted Cohen's proposal with skepticism. The National Magnet Laboratory was dedicated to producing very high magnetic fields. At this site we were suggesting the building of a room for the purpose of detecting extremely weak fields. I recall one critic remarking to me that if Cohen wanted to measure the weak magnetic fields from the human heart and brain he should build his enclosure in the remote desert and not at the one place in the United States dedicated to producing intense magnetic fields. I remember wanting to reply that perhaps Cohen didn't want to live in the desert. We pleaded our

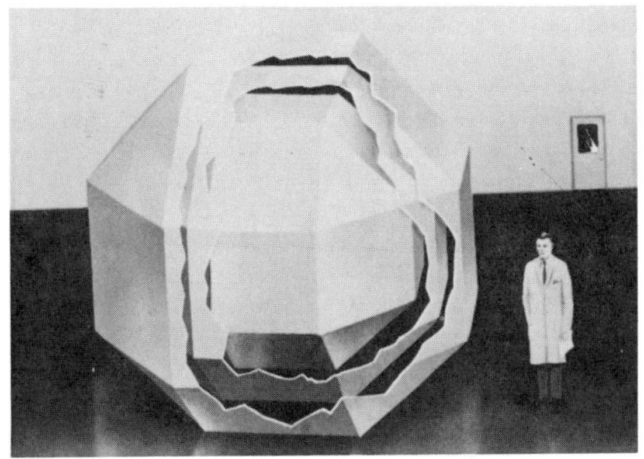

Fig. 5. Cohen's conception of a magnetically shielded room.

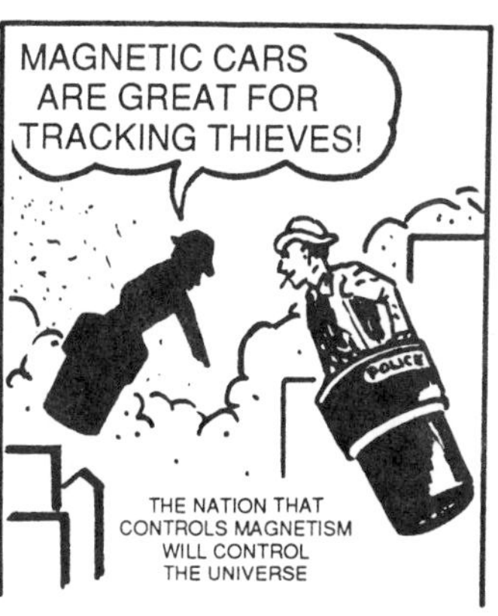
MAGNETIC CARS ARE GREAT FOR TRACKING THIEVES!
POLICE
THE NATION THAT CONTROLS MAGNETISM WILL CONTROL THE UNIVERSE

Fig. 6. During the late 1960's, magnetism attracted some public support.

case citing the military importance of understanding how the human brain and heart work. I stressed that in time of military conflict it was essential to know that both organs are functioning optimally. About that time a few cartoons appeared about magnetism (Figure 6 shows a modified version of one). Over the years I've wondered if a Dick Tracy cartoon in this spirit may have convinced some of the skeptics. Eventually, modest funds were made available.

A MARRIAGE OF TECHNIQUES

In retrospect, it did not require much insight to see that Jim's device might be useful in David's research. At the time it was not at all obvious to me. David and Jim were unaware of each other's effort. I approached them about collaboration. They were both interested. There was the problem of transporting Jim's SQUID system, dewar and electronics from Boulder to Boston. Jim solved that problem by agreeing to carry it all on the plane with him. No special authorizations were obtained to transport government-owned equipment or to perform research on humans. I hate to think what paper work would be required if the same exercise were attempted today. Jim arrived at the National Magnet Laboratory during the last week of December 1969. He and David quickly went about setting up his equipment in the shielded room. There was little I could do but wait around like an expectant father. The time finally arrived to make the first measurements. Jim agreed to be the subject. He undressed down to his shorts and sat in the shielded room, chest close to the helium dewar wall. Initial trials showed that, even within the shielded room, variations in external magnetic fields were a problem during normal working hours. During evening hours conditions improved (Fig. 7). This magnetocardiograph was taken on New Year's Eve, December 31, 1969. We realized that this was something of a special event and appended our signatures to this first SQUID magnetocardiograph. The director of the National Magnet Laboratory, Ben Lax, was present and added his signature.

David and Jim then decided to see if they could obtain a magnetoencephalogram. David had in 1968 discovered the magnetic field generated by spontaneous activity of the brain using an induction coil and signal averaging technique (Cohen, 1968). Being the least useful member of the trio I was drafted as the volunteer. Like Jim I undressed down to my shorts, entered the room and with some trepidation placed my head close to the tip of the dewar. The door closed and there I was alone. I wondered what would happen if the dewar broke and helium spilled all over me. Time seems infinitely long when you are trying to hold your head steady near the tip of a helium dewar. Finally, I asked "How are you fellows doing?" A faint reply came back: "Keep quiet and don't move". After some time I heard the request "Ed, please try to concentrate on something. We're not getting any signal". Finally the door opened. David and Jim told me that the experiment was over.

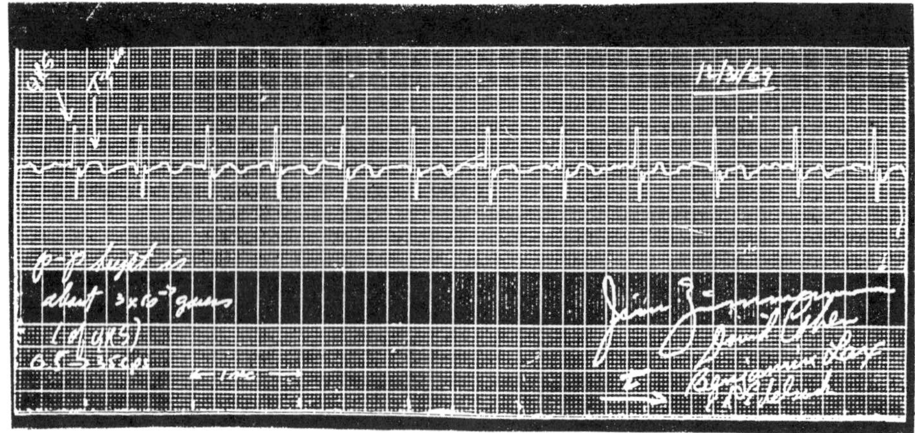

Fig. 7. First magnetocardiogram ever taken with a superconducting magnetometer.

The results were negative. From the look in their faces, I got their message. They didn't think that there was anything wrong with Jim's SQUID detector. The trouble they believed was that there was no signal emanating from the source, namely my head. Some two years later using a more sensitive detector and better source, Cohen was able to obtain a magnetoencephalogram (Cohen, 1972). In Figure 8, David, Jim and I are standing in front of the shielded room. Figure 9 is a photograph of David Cohen's charming secretary holding Zimmerman's SQUID magnetometer.

David and Jim wrote up their preliminary results and submitted a paper (Fig. 10) to *Applied Physics Letters* on February 2, 1970 (Cohen et al., 1970). Knowing that some of my bosses did not

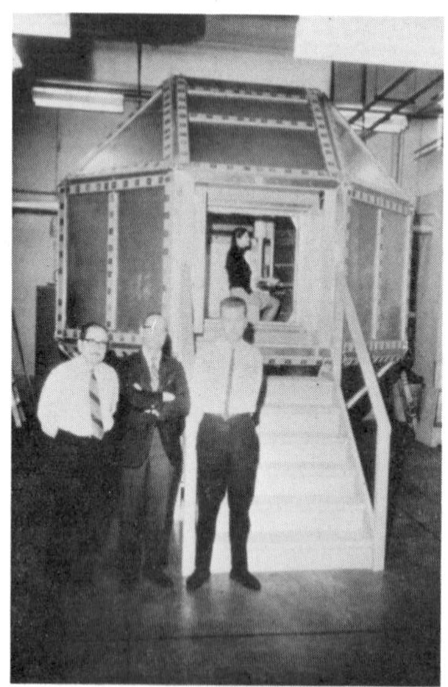

Fig. 8. Edelsack, Cohen, and Zimmerman before the magnetically shielded room at the Francis Bitter National Magnet Laboratory at M.I.T. For measurements, the doors for the room's magnetic shells are closed.

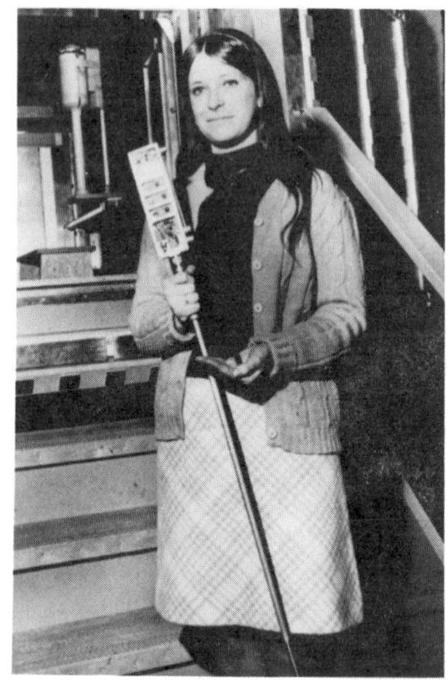

Fig. 9. The first SQUID system used to detect the magnetocardiogram. The long tube was inserted into a dewar filled with liquid helium, so that the SQUID mounted in the bottom of the tube becomes superconducting.

VOLUME 16, NUMBER 7 APPLIED PHYSICS LETTERS 1 APRIL 1970

MAGNETOCARDIOGRAMS TAKEN INSIDE A SHIELDED ROOM
WITH A SUPERCONDUCTING POINT-CONTACT MAGNETOMETER

David Cohen*
Francis Bitter National Magnet Laboratory,† *Massachusetts Institute of Technology, Cambridge, Massachusetts* 02139

Edgar A. Edelsack
Office of Naval Research, Washington, D. C. 20360

and

James E. Zimmerman‡
Aeronutronic Division,§ *Philco-Ford Corporation, Newport Beach, California* 92660

(Received 2 February 1970)

A point-contact (SQUID) magnetometer was used inside a shielded room to record the magnetic field of the human heart, without noise-averaging. The resulting magnetocardiograms, with the peak signal at about 3×10^{-7} G had a noise level of about 1×10^{-9} G (rms, per root cycle). They approach good medical electrocardiograms in clarity, and are an order-of-magnitude improvement in sensitivity over previous magnetic detectors of the heart. These results suggest new medical uses for this magnetometer.

Fig. 10. Article in *Applied Physics Letters* reporting the first use of a SQUID for magnetocardiography (with permission).

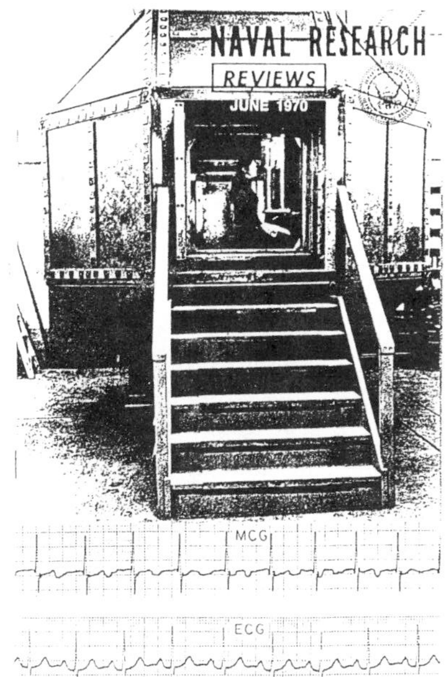

Fig. 11. Issue of *Naval Research Reviews* featuring an article on superconducting devices, with magnetocardiography illustrated on the cover.

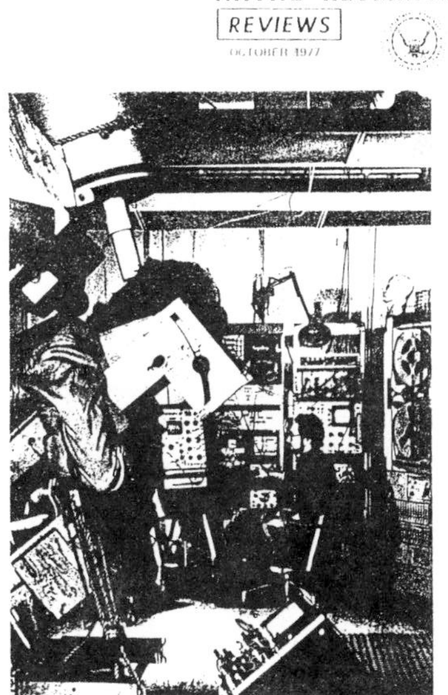

Fig. 12. Cover of *Naval Research Reviews* showing the unshielded arrangement in 1977 for recording visually evoked responses at New York University.

read *Applied Physics Letters*, but did read the ONR publication *Naval Research Reviews*, I arranged to have on the cover of the June 1970 issue a picture of the shielded room and a magnetocardiogram and an electrocardiogram (Fig. 11). Very soon, colleagues in the physiology and psychology group became interested in this research as a means of studying brain function. They were particularly interested in the technique of measuring evoked response using a variety of stimuli, including visual, tactile and auditory. Some years later I tried to measure evoked response from olfactory stimuli with little success. I don't know if anyone has successfully measured the evoked magnetic field from olfactory stimuli.

By the mid-1970s the ONR physiology and psychology program managers were supporting a few research groups in the United States working in biomagnetism. Among them was the N.Y.U Neuromagnetism Laboratory of our hosts, Professors Sam Williamson and Lloyd Kaufman. The cover of the October 1977 issue of *Naval Research Reviews* had a photograph of their laboratory (Fig. 12). The entire October 1985 issue of *Naval Research Reviews* was devoted to the topic of naval applications of superconductivity. It had on the inside cover a picture of the MIT shielded room, and, of course, the well-used picture of the first magnetocardiogram. ONR program managers quickly learned that a little publicity never hurts when pleading for additional funding.

WHAT'S AHEAD

I come from a family whose male members tend to live into their mid-90's, so I hope to attend the International Conference on Biomagnetism in the year 2009 and observe the 40th Anniversary of SQUID magnetocardiography. At that meeting perhaps there will be a celebration of another anniversary – the anniversary of a cooperative international program in space exploration which began during the last decade of the 20th century. Here I am not talking about another Apollo program, but rather a program to explorer "inner space" – the brain. This program would have been launched as a collaborative effort of researchers working at laboratories in many countries. They had successfully convinced their political leaders that participation in this international program to study the brain could truly benefit people in their own country, as well as all mankind. This program funded by science program managers from national and international funding agencies would have helped create an international center for biomagnetic research, where young researchers received further training and performed research using the most sophisticated techniques and advanced instrumentation available.

Exploring the "inner space" of the human brain and how it functions is among the ultimate challenges to which mankind can aspire. A technique that can non-invasively provide objective information about brain function must certainly have a very bright and a very exciting future in the 21st century.

REFERENCES

G.M. Baule, G.M., and McFee, R. (1963). Detection of the Magnetic Field of the Heart. *Am. Heart J.* 66, 95-96.

Cohen, D. (1968). Magnetoencephalography: evidence of magnetic fields produced by alpha-rhythm currents. *Science* 161, 784-786.

Cohen, D., Edelsack, E.A., and Zimmerman, J.E. (1970). Magnetocardiograms taken inside a shielded room with a superconducting point-contact magnetometer. *Appl. Phys. Lett.* 16, 278-280.

Cohen, D. (1972). Magnetoencephalography: detection of the brain's electrical activity with a superconducting magnetometer. *Science* 175, 664-666.

Cohen, D. (1975). Magnetic fields of the human body. *Physics Today* 28, 34-43.

PRESENT STATUS AND FUTURE OF DC SQUIDS MADE FROM HIGH T_c SUPERCONDUCTORS

R. H. Koch, W. J. Gallagher, V. Foglietti, B. Oh, R. B. Laibowitz, G. Koren, A. Gupta, and W. Y. Lee

IBM Research Division, Thomas J. Watson Research Center, Yorktown Heights, NY 10598.

INTRODUCTION

Superconducting QUantum Interference Devices (SQUIDs) have now been fabricated by a number of groups from high temperature (highT_C) superconductors [1-4]. Many reported devices operate at 77 K and noise measurements have been made on a small number of these highT_C SQUIDs. This paper will present a brief summary of the development of highT_C SQUIDs, review the performance of highT_C SQUIDs, including the issues of the periodicity and hysteresis of the response, the magnitude of the noise in the SQUIDs, and the manufacturability of the devices. The nature of the junctions forming the SQUIDs, which have been naturally occurring grain boundaries in all but a few of the reported devices, and the physical mechanisms responsible for the noise sources are discussed. We report our progress in attaching input coils to highT_C SQUIDs and our progress in fabricating "artificial barrier" junctions. Finally, the possible biomedical applications of these and future highT_C SQUIDs will be examined. This paper will focus thin film dc SQUIDs developed at IBM and not discuss progress in fabricating rf SQUIDs or important work in other laboratories throughout the world. While IBM is a leader in highT_C SQUID development, a more complete review would include much more than discussed in this paper.

A BRIEF HISTORY OF HIGH T_C SQUIDS

The first highT_C SQUIDs were made at IBM using thin films of $YBa_2Cu_3O_y$ soon after the discovery of high temperature superconductivity [1]. These devices, dc SQUIDs as shown in Fig. 1(a), consisted of a thin film of polycrystalline YBaCuO that was patterned into a loop typically 40 × 40 μm in size. The loop had many grain boundaries crossing it and these boundaries we found functioned as Josephson junctions of some unknown sort. This is a very easy way to make a SQUID, although the number of grain boundaries is usually many more than the required two around the loop. One has in effect "a SQUID of many junctions". At essentially the same time, J. E. Zimmermann and his colleagues at the NBS (now NIST) [2] followed a similar approach starting with a bulk sample of polycrystalline $YBa_2Cu_3O_y$ and a mechanical method of forming a constriction to make an rf SQUID. These two techniques have become the standard way of making highT_C SQUIDs today. While these types of SQUIDs are useful for demonstration and study, the yield and control of the junction characteristics for devices made in this way has always been poor.

Advances in Biomagnetism
Edited by S.J. Williamson *et al.*
Plenum Press, New York

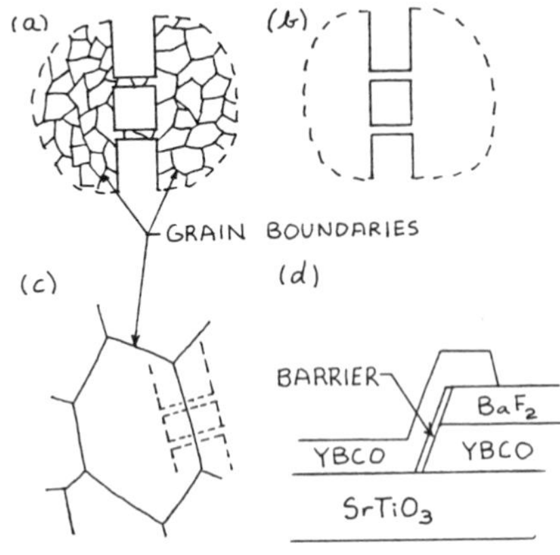

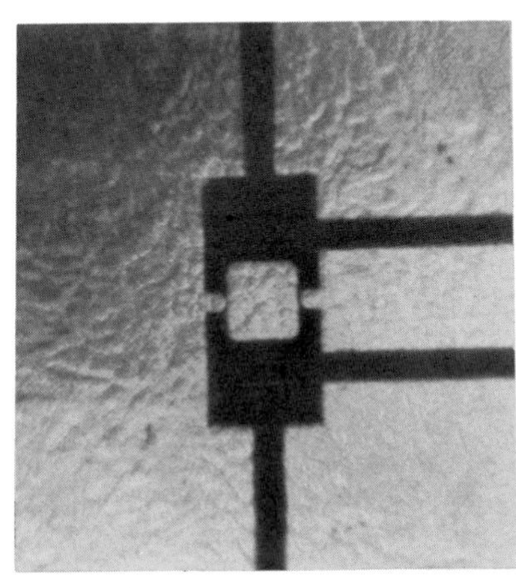

Fig 1. Four ways to make highT_C SQUIDs. Fig 2. A natural grain boundary TBCCO SQUID

As thin film technology improved, it became possible to grow a film with few, if any, grai boundaries around the loop forming the SQUID. A superconducting loop, as shown if Fig 1(b), without grain boundaries or junctions does not work as a SQUID. Many methods hav been tried by various groups throughout the world to make such a superconducting loop int a SQUID by attempting to make a weak link locally after the film has been fabricated. Thes ideas have included applying local heat to the links, using an e-beam, ion-beam, or current puls to locally damage the links, applying a local chemical contamination to "poison" the loop lo cally, etc. These approaches have not succeeded very well. The basic problem, of course, is tha a Josephson junction or weak link has to be similar in size to the coherence length of th superconductor in the tunneling direction. These methods, even though they can produce dam age over sub-micron dimensions, are still not able to alter the film on the scale of the coherenc length of YBCO which is about 20 Å or less.

A novel approach, developed at IBM [5], was to start with a substrate that had single o multiple grain boundaries across it and grow an epitaxial film on this substrate. The epitaxia film will reflect the substrate and hence there will be grain boundaries in the resulting film whic replicate the grain boundaries in the substrate. This is shown in Fig. 1(c). One has large grain with well defined grain boundaries and SQUIDs can be patterned such that a single grai boundary crosses each link. The method is probably the most controlled of all the natural grai boundary techniques that have been developed, but would be difficult to use in more highl integrated structures.

THE PRESENT STATUS OF NATURAL GRAIN BOUNDARY HIGH T_c SQUIDS

Fig. 2 indicates our present design for TlBaCaCuO-based highT_C SQUIDs [6, 7]. We hav found that making a natural grain boundary SQUID from $Tl_2Ba_2Ca_2Cu_3O_y$ instead o $YBa_2Cu_3O_y$ reduces the flux noise of the SQUID appreciably. The TlBaCaCuO material has superconducting transition temperature near 125 K whereas the YBCO compounds supercor duct at 93 K or so. This makes the TlBaCaCuO devices much better suited for operation at 7 K. The second major change from our earlier SQUID design, shown in Fig. 1(a), was a re duction in the amount of superconducting material forming the device to just a simple loop a can be seen. The four leads forming the voltage and current leads for the SQUID are made o gold. In general, SQUIDs of this design also have less magnetic hysteresis. In this contex hysteresis is defined as the difference in the indicated flux for the same actual applied flux be tween when the field is increasing or decreasing. The grain boundaries in our TBCCO films a fairly large, say an average of 5 microns in diameter. With this large grain size combined wit a small loop and pad area, the SQUID will often be working around a single grain bounda across the links and the number of excess grain boundaries in the pads will be minimized. Bot features reduce hysteresis and improve the periodicity of the response in a magnetic field as ca be seen in Fig. 3.

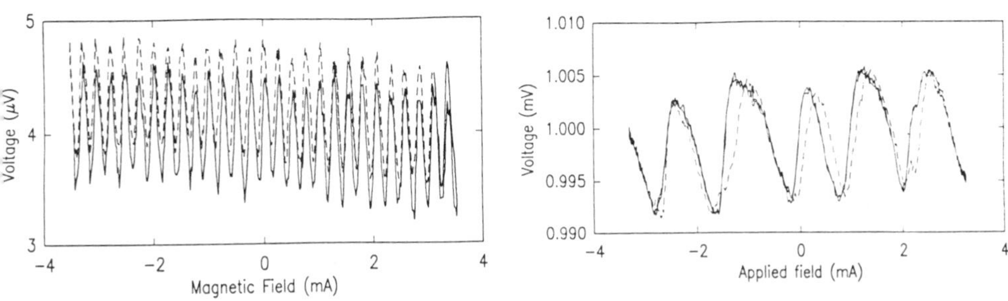

Fig 3. Voltage vs. flux curves for two TBCCO SQUIDs operating at 77 K.

The performance of these TBCCO SQUIDs at 77 K is better than we were ever able to achieve with any of our YBCO SQUIDs at any temperature. Figure 4 plots the temperature dependence of the noise of highT_C SQUIDs made from YBCO, BSCCO [8], and TBCCO. The hysteresis in the flux to voltage curve or the difference in the output voltage between increasing magnetic field (as shown in solid on Fig. 3) and decreasing field (shown in dashed) is fairly small. The fractional change h ≡ (difference)/(peak-to-peak value) is about 10^{-3} which is better than any of the YBCO SQUIDs. Figure 5 compares the energy resolution $\varepsilon \equiv S_\Phi/2L$ of these TBCCO SQUIDs with commercially available BTI rf and dc SQUIDs. The TBCCO SQUIDs have similar noise levels with these commercial SQUIDs and this noise level is adequate for most applications of SQUIDs, including all but the most demanding biomedical applications. The best 4.2 K niobium-based SQUIDs have noise levels of 10^{-32} J/Hz or less, which is much lower than any of the highT_C SQUIDs. Independent of the 1/f noise levels of the two types of SQUIDs, the white noise power levels for the highT_C SQUIDs will always be about 20 × higher than similarly designed lowT_C SQUIDs because of the higher operating temperature.

Up until mid-1988 it seemed that one would never be able to achieve these levels of performance with highT_C SQUIDs. The question to ask is what is better about the $Tl_2Ba_2Ca_2Cu_3O_y$ devices compared to SQUIDs made from $YBa_2Cu_3O_y$. The performance of any sensor is given by the amount of noise the sensor produces in the absence of a signal (in this case the voltage noise of the SQUID) normalized by the response of the sensor to a given amount of input signal (in this case the transfer function $\partial V/\partial\Phi$ of the SQUID). We have found that the difference between the TBCCO and YBCO SQUIDs is not the voltage noise of the device but the fact that the natural TBCCO grain boundary for reasons that we do not fully understand produces a larger responsivity to flux than the natural YBCO grain boundary.

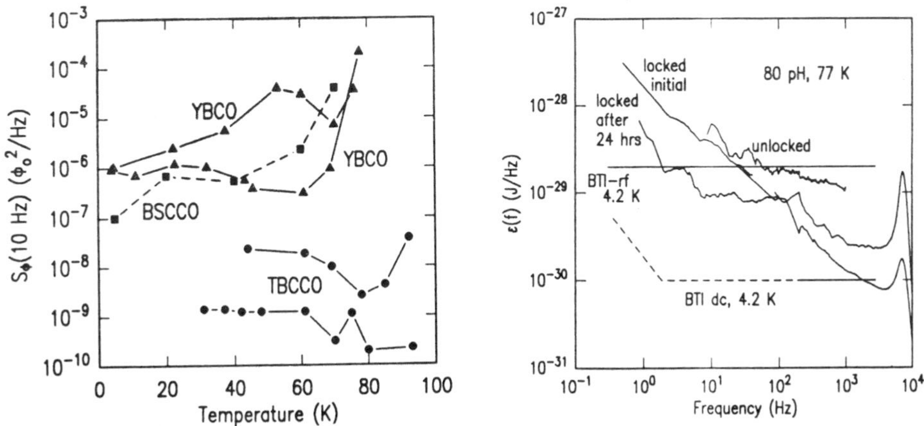

Fig 4. Noise vs. T for five highT_C SQUIDs. Fig 5. ε vs. f for highT_C and lowT_C SQUIDs.

Indicated in dashed lines are some measurements made on a BaSrCaCuO natural grain boun ary SQUID which shows performance levels similar to the YBCO SQUIDs. It is difficult make a definitive statement about the performance of BSCCO SQUIDs based on the measu ments from one device.

An important question to ask is what is the source of the 1/f noise in the SQUIDs. Ea expectations by us and others argued that the SQUID would be measuring its own magne field noise. The SQUID would sense the magnetic field of magnetic flux lines that were trapp in the superconducting body of the SQUID. The equilibrium motions of these flux lines wou result in low frequency flux noise in the SQUID. It turns out that nature is not that simp If one measures very carefully the dependence of the magnetic flux noise as the transfer functi of the SQUID is increased, one finds that there is no minimum flux noise which is independe of the size of the transfer function. In other words, as the SQUID becomes increasingly sen tive to magnetic flux, the magnetic flux noise it measures decreases. This is inconsistent w the aforementioned model. The noise mechanism is not one that is common in the low SQUIDs.

The noise performance of the TBCCO SQUIDs is clearly good enough for applications, b the hysteresis of the bare SQUID is too large to be useful. We found that by electronica locking up the SQUID in the normal feedback mode, the hysteresis goes away. We knew th this would happen, but we were delightfully surprised by the fact that when we did this the no did not increase. That was something good, but we are still not there yet.

THE NEXT CHALLENGES

Most applications, including biomedical applications, will need an input coil to concentra magnetic field into the loop of the SQUID. One approach to making an input coil is to ma a highT_C SQUID on one substrate and a highT_C input coil on a second substrate and flap the together like a sandwich to couple the input coil to the SQUID loop. B. Oh, of our group IBM Research, has made several single level input coils this way and coupled them to both l and highT_C SQUIDs [9]. He has found a coupling coefficient $\alpha \equiv M^2/L_S L_I$ of up to 0.1 and large increase in noise from the input coil. A single level input coil does not result in a lar improvement in the magnetic field sensitivity of the SQUID, perhaps a factor of four improv ment. The long term goal is to make a multiple level spiral input coil, and couple that to t SQUID. Our experiments with the single level coils strongly suggest that there should be fundamental obstacle in obtaining this goal.

The other major hurdle that needs to be resolved before highT_C SQUIDs are practical is develop a truly reliable technology for making Josephson junctions from highT_C supercondu tors. Today most highT_C SQUIDs use natural grain boundaries to provide the Josephson effe Natural grain boundaries can be engineered to some extent, but a junction that is made whe you want it, when you want it, and with good control over the critical current and resistance needed. There is a world-wide effort to fabricate such junctions for scientific and digital a plications. This is a difficult task because these applications usually require a high quality u shunted junction, whereas the naturally occurring shunting resistance usually found whe attempting to make an all highT_C junction is acceptable for SQUID operation.

In this spirit we have started to make edge junctions [10]. We call them "edge junctions" base on the method used to fabricate the devices. Fig. 1(d) shows a cross section of the fabricatic method and Fig. 6 is a picture of a edge junction SQUID. The rationale behind fabrication edge junctions is the realization that the c-axis of the superconducting crystal structure is "u (perpendicular to the plane of the substrate) in most highT_C films available today. The standa way of making a junction, a multiple layer junction, given the usual direction of the c-axi would mean tunneling parallel to the c-axis direction which is unlikely to work. The superco ducting coherence length is much longer perpendicular to the c-axis than parallel to the c-axi The optimal direction to tunnel is perpendicular to the c-axis and an edge junction does thi

Figure 7 demonstrates the operation of an artificial barrier SQUIDs at 6 K. The critical current of these devices vanished above 30 K which limited the maximum temperature of operation of the SQUIDs to about 28 K. The results are not very reproducible and we do not know the true nature of the weak link providing the Josephson effect, whether it is a SIS, a SNS, or a depression of the order parameter type of weak link. The important point here is that an artificial barrier Josephson junction has been fabricated. The YBCO edge junction SQUIDs could have lower noise than the natural grain boundary YBCO SQUIDs.

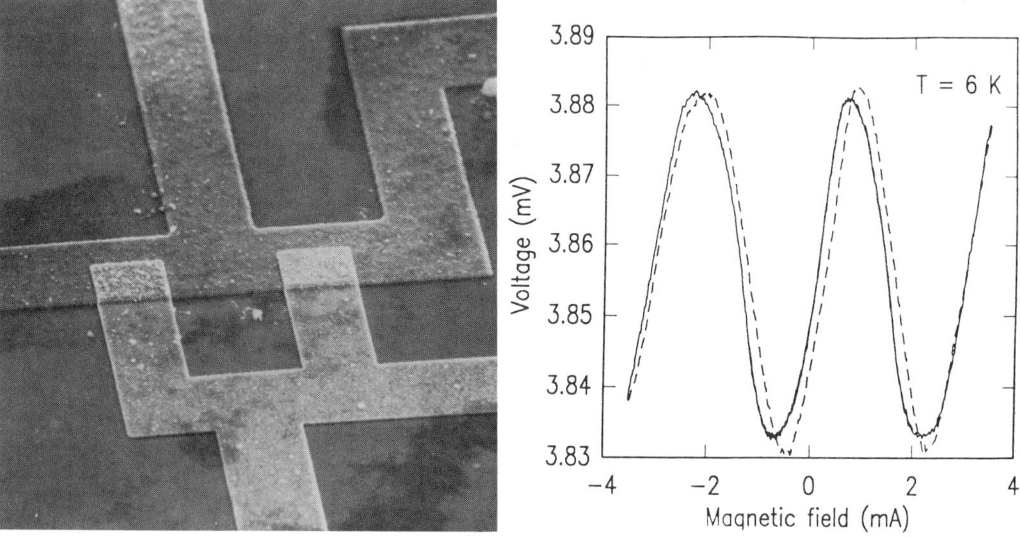

Fig 6. An YBCO edge junction highT_C SQUID.

Fig 7. The V vs. Φ curve for this SQUID.

SOME FUTURE TRENDS

Currently high T_c SQUIDs are in an unusual situation in terms of potential applications of highT_C superconductivity. Most future applications of highT_C superconductivity are in the dilemma that the material is not presently capable of satisfying the needs of the application. For instance, the present day critical current densities in a magnetic field for any highT_C superconducting wire is not high enough to be generally useful. Acceptable performance levels have been demonstrated for highT_C SQUIDs, although reductions in the flux noise levels would be advantageous. However, we should make it clear that good performance when the SQUID is coupled to an input coil or the ability to reproducibly make devices has not been achieved yet. We have learned enough about these two problems to believe that no fundamental reasons exist why this can't be done in a laboratory environment in the next few years.

The future of biomagnetometers will be strongly influenced by high temperature superconductivity. One dominate direction in biomagnetism is the emergence of 100+ channel systems. Such a system using lowT_C SQUIDs requires complex (and high risk) Josephson circuits in the cold space to read each channel or hundreds of readout circuits at room temperature with many hundreds of wires traversing from the warm to the cold space of the dewar. Both options are complicated and expensive. High T_C SQUIDs, on the other hand, could be used to make much simpler systems when combined with 77 K CMOS readout circuits. Most present day CMOS circuits work at 77 K and a single integrated CMOS chip could be used to read out and digitize the SQUID output at 77 K only millimeters away from the SQUID.

A drawback of present day biomagnetometers is their large size, primarily a result of the use of liquid helium cooling. High T_C cooling methods are much simpler and smaller. One can imagine Joule-Thompson cyrocoolers for biomedical applications about the size of a microscope slide. Room temperature nitrogen gas is injected in at one end and the other end cools to 77 K. Such devices are presently commercially available. One could build many highT_C SQUIDs and CMOS readout circuits on the cold end of the Joule-Thompson cyrocooler resulting in a multi-channel system about the size of a matchbox. The "matchbox" would be connected to a workstation with a simple digital link. This system could be placed very close to a person's heart or brain because of the thin wall "dewar" design available when operating at 77 K. Larger channel-number systems could be constructed from a number of the multi-channel "matchbox" systems that could closely adapt to the exact shape of each persons body, again improving performance over the rigid liquid helium dewar designs under development today.

The size of existing lowT_C systems is not only limited by the dewar size but also the need for operation of the system in a magnetically shielded room. The potential leverage obtainable from the size reduction of a highT_C system will need to be coupled to an improvement in noise cancellation techniques to make operation without the use of a shielded room possible. This should be possible using more sophisticated mathematical techniques for noise and interference cancellation, higher order gradiometers with more local reference magnetometers, and larger bandwidth feedback electronics.

One can envision a pocket size highT_C biomagnetometer (actually a gradiometer) that can be moved to the patient, instead of having to move the patient to a room size lowT_C biomagnetic system. The potential of such a small biomagnetometer could be enormous. Perhaps such a biomagnetometer would be useful in an operating environment or in the field at the scene of a medical emergency. The economy of operation might also allow such a system to be used in a patent monitoring system over extended periods of time. A useful analogy is to compare a lowT_C biomagnetometer with a highT_C biomagnetometer and to compare a mainframe computer with a personal computer. There is little doubt that a lowT_C biomagnetometer and a mainframe computer will always outperform the highT_C biomagnetometer or personal computer when measured in terms of field sensitivity or computing power. But as a lot of personal computer users have found, there are many applications where the ultimate in computing power is not needed, and the utility of a user-friendly system sitting on your desk is a overwhelming advantage. The flexibility, economy, and ease of use of a personal computer exceeds the mainframe and we expect this will also be the case with highT_C biomagnetic systems compared to their lowT_C predecessors. At the biomagnetism conference twenty years from now we believe that both lowT_C and highT_C biomagnetometers will present, but the highT_C systems will be the technology of choice for most clinical applications.

ACKNOWLEDGEMENT

This work was partially supported by the U.S. Office of Naval Research contract number N00014-88-C-0439.

REFERENCES

1 R. H. Koch, C. P. Umbach, G. J. Clark, P. Chaudhari, and R. B. Laibowitz, Appl. Phys. Lett. **51**, 200 (1987).
2 J.E.Zimmermann, J.A.Beall, M.W.Cromar, and R.H.Ono, Appl.Phys.Lett. **51**, 617 (1987).
3 B. Häuser, M. Diegel, and H. Rogalla, Appl. Phys. Lett. **52**, 844 (1988).
4 I.Takeuchi, J.S.Tsai, H.Tsuge, and N.Matsukura, Jpn.J.Appl.Phys. **27**, 2265 (1988).
5 P. Chaudhari, J. Mannhart, D. Dimos, C. Tsuei, C. C. Chi, M. M. Oprysko, and M. Scheuermann, Phys. Rev. Lett. **60**, 1653 (1988).
6 R. H. Koch, W. J. Gallagher, B. Bumble, and W. Lee, Appl. Phys. Lett. **53**, 951 (1989).
7 V.Foglietti, R.H.Koch, W.J.Gallagher, B.Oh, B.Bumble, and W.Y.Lee, Appl. Phys. Lett. **54**, 2259 (1989).
8 D. W. Face, J. T. Kucera, D. G. Steel, J. M. Graybeal, T. P. Orlando, and D. A. Rudman, Physica C **xx**, xxx (1990).
9 B.Oh, R.H.Koch, W.J.Gallagher, V.Foglietti, and W.Y.Lee, unpublished
10 R. B. Laibowitz, R.H.Koch, G. Koran, A Gupta, W.J.Gallagher, and V. Foglietti, unpublished

ACTIVATION OF THE HUMAN AUDITORY CORTEX BY VARIOUS SOUND SEQUENCES: NEUROMAGNETIC STUDIES

Riitta Hari

Low Temperature Laboratory
Helsinki University of Technology
02150 Espoo, Finland

INTRODUCTION

The neuromagnetic techique is rapidly establishing its role as a noninvasive tool to explore human auditory function (for recent reviews, see Hari, 1989; Hari and Lounasmaa, 1989). The supratemporal auditory cortex, embedded within the Sylvian fissure, is optimally situated for magnetoencephalographic (MEG) recordings: the subject can lie comfortably while magnetic field is measured over the lateral aspect of the head.

The usefulness of MEG is often compared with that of electric scalp potential recordings. Some auditory evoked potentials, like those originating in the brainstem, are widely applied in clinical assessment of peripheral auditory pathways. However, studies of long-latency evoked potentials have not contributed significantly to neurological diagnostics nor to our understanding about information processing along the auditory pathways. One important reason is the poor localization accuracy of the electric method, which has prevented interpretation of the recordings in terms of the underlying neural substrate. When sources cannot be separated it is not possible to study, for example, effects of different acoustic parameters or tasks on neural activity in specific brain areas. Consequently, too much emphasis has been paid on the peaks and bumps of the electric responses at descriptive level.

Many of these problems can be overcome with magnetic recordings which often allow accurate localization of the underlying neural sources. Having started from comparisons of the electric and magnetic response waveforms and distributions, the neuromagnetism community is now increasingly aiming at more functional approaches to probe neurophysiological properties of cortical networks.

Any abrupt sound evokes prominent changes in the cerebral magnetic field and the basic response waveform has now been documented in several laboratories. The first cortical deflection of the evoked response complex can be detected already 19 ms after the stimulus onset (Scherg et al., 1989), and the activity may continue for a few hundred milliseconds, depending on the stimulation parameters and the state of the subject. During this time the equivalent sources vary within an area of several square centimeters at the supratemporal auditory cortex (Hari et al., 1987). Some information already exists about the dependence of the response waveform and source configuration on physical parameters (frequency, intensity, rise time, etc.) of the sounds as well as on temporal aspects of the stimulation sequence; the latter will be discussed in this paper.

TIMING OF STIMULI AND AUDITORY RESPONSES

Interstimulus interval. It is well established that the shorter the interstimulus interval (ISI), the smaller is the amplitude of the auditory 100-ms response, N100m; usually an asymptotic level is reached at an ISI of about 500 ms (for a review, see Hari 1989). One explanation for the decrease of response amplitudes, when the ISI is shortened, is the limitation of contributing neural networks by active inhibition. Pure refractory phenomena, associated with neuronal fatigue, are improbable at these ISIs.

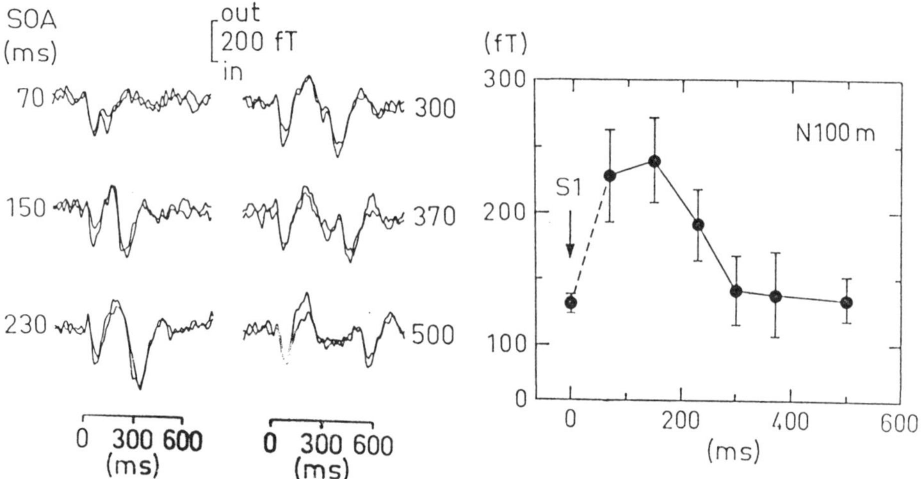

Fig. 1. *Left:* Responses of one subject to pairs of noise bursts with different sound onset asynchronies (SOAs) from the posterior field extremum. Two 50-ms noise bursts were presented in pairs (interpair interval 1.2 - 1.4 s) with 6 different SOAs (70, 150, 230, 300, 370, and 500 ms) randomly intermixed within the same stimulus train. The two superimposed curves illustrate repetitions of identical measurements. The responses have been digitally low-pass filtered at 45 Hz. N100m is directed downwards in the figure. *Right:* Mean (± S.E.M) amplitudes of N100m for 9 subjects as a function of SOA. The values at time 0 refer to responses to the first stimuli (S1) of the pairs. Adapted from Loveless et al. (1989).

Paired sound presentation. When short sounds are presented in pairs, the amplitude of N100m can be significantly larger to the second than to the first stimulus of the pair at sound onset intervals less than 300 ms (Loveless et al., 1989; Fig. 1). This phenomenon cannot be predicted from the recovery cycle of responses to single stimuli. The amplitude enhancement seems to be due to a central mechanism, since it can also be produced by presenting the two sounds to different ears. The underlying cellular mechanisms are unknown, and no animal data exist to make the interpretation easier.

Steady-state responses. When the stimulus repetition rate is increased above a few Hz, sinusoidal 'steady-state responses', phase-locked to the stimuli, can be recorded. This approach was favored in the early days of neuromagnetism: due to the fast stimulus repetition rate, averaged responses with sufficient signal-to-noise ratio could be recorded in rather short time even with noisy instruments, using narrow bandpass filtering centered at the stimulation frequency. We have observed that the responses to clicks, presented at rates between 10 and 70 Hz, are highest in amplitude around 40 Hz (Hari et al., 1989a; Fig. 2); the field maps suggest activation of the auditory cortex at all these frequencies. The amplitude enhancement around 40 Hz can be satisfactorily modeled by summation of 'middle-latency' responses, evoked by single clicks at 10 Hz, provided that a wide recording passband is used (see Fig. 2). Therefore, no 'resonance' mechanisms, hypothetized in the evoked potential literature for similar amplitude enhancement, need to be assumed.

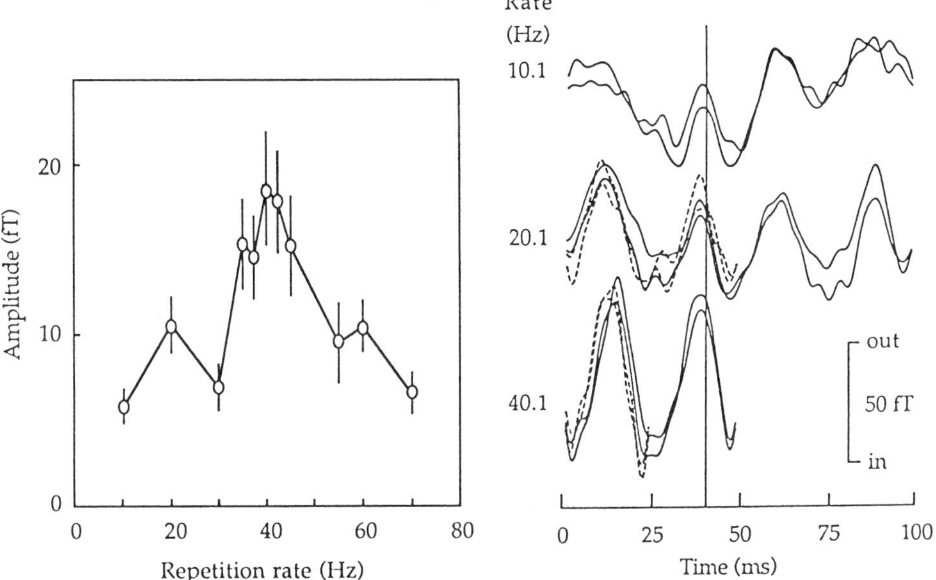

Fig. 2. *Left:* Mean (± S.E.M.; 10 subjects) amplitudes of the steady-state response to clicks as a function of stimulus repetition rate. *Right:* Responses of one subject to clicks presented at 10.1, 20.1, and 40.1 Hz (1, 2, and 2 cycles averaged, respectively). The recordings are from the posterior field extremum over the right hemisphere. The passband is 0.05 - 250 Hz, and about 1500 responses were averaged for each curve. The dotted lines illustrate the 'synthetic' curves calculated from the 10.1-Hz responses by multiplying the repetition rate by 2 and 4, respectively. The vertical line is at 40 ms. From Hari et al. (1989a).

Regularity of stimulation. The regularity of stimulus presentation also influences the response waveform. For example, a too-early stimulus, in a series of identical tone pips, evokes a large and delayed response at the auditory cortex, pointing to the importance of stimulus timing for the reactivity of cortical neurons (Hari et al., 1989b). The source area of the response to 'early' stimuli differs slightly from that of N100m to standard tones. An interesting question is whether this change of activity is triggered by neural mechanisms which code time, or whether it is due to changes in the frequency content of the stimulus sequence; long-term spectral changes are inevitable when timing or duration of tonal stimuli is varied.

Sound omission. If a tone is omitted in a regular sequence, a response can be detected 90 - 250 ms after the omission (Joutsiniemi and Hari, 1989; Fig. 3); the response depends strongly on the state of the subject and can even be missing if he does not pay attention to the tones. The equivalent source of this 'omission response' is anterior and superior to that of N100m to tones (Fig. 3). We have, therefore, suggested that the response gets contribution from the posterolateral frontal cortex, possibly from the frontal eye field. Animal experiments indicate the involvement of these areas in coding of stimulus timing. In addition, cerebral blood flow studies of humans have shown a local activation around the frontal eye field when the subjects were attentively listening to rhythmic patterns of sounds (Roland et al., 1981). It therefore seems possible to detect neuromagnetic activity from brain areas outside modality-specific cortices, which is encouraging for the future of MEG.

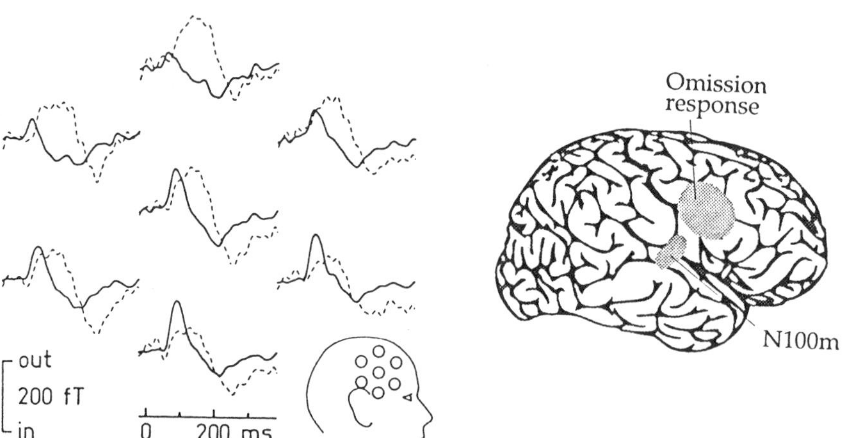

Fig. 3. *Left:* Magnetic responses of one subject to regularly occurring tones (continuous lines) and to stimulus omissions (dashed lines) at the anterior end of the right Sylvian fissure. 580 responses to tones and 80 to omissions were averaged. Passband is 0.05 - 40 Hz. Adapted from Joutsiniemi and Hari (1989). *Right:* Schematic illustration of average locations of the equivalent sources of responses to tones (N100m) and omissions in five subjects.

Infrequent stimulus deviance. Application of the 'oddball paradigm' further emphasizes the structure of the stimulus sequence for the evoked responses. In this approach infrequent 'deviants' are randomly interspersed among monotonously repeated 'standard' sounds. Different types of deviations have been observed to evoke strong magnetic responses, 'mismatch fields' (MMFs; for description of the electric counterpart of this response, see Näätänen and Picton, 1987), which are not present in responses to standard stimuli nor in those to deviants delivered in the absence of standards. In other words, MMF not only depends on the physical quality of the sound but also on the position of the stimulus in the sequence. MMF seems to reflect an automatic cerebral process since it can be elicited equally well when the subject ignores the stimuli or pays attention to them.

Using the oddball paradigm, we have tried to unravel reactions of the human brain to different variations in the auditory environment, like changes in tone frequency, duration, and intensity (Hari et al., 1984; Kaukoranta et al., 1989; Lounasmaa et al., 1989; Sams and Kaukoranta, 1989). The source areas of MMFs are usually anterior to those of N100m. Thus the change or novelty detectors, which possibly underlie MMF, are not located within the same cortical area as the generators of N100m.

CONCLUSIONS

These examples show that AEFs reflect the coding of complex sounds at the human auditory cortex. The temporal fine structure of stimulation sequences seems to have a very important role in determining cortical reactivity. Similar neural mechanisms may be involved in perception of other time-varying acoustic signals like speech sounds, and neuromagnetic studies might give information about the neurophysiological basis of these typically human functions.

ACKNOWLEDGMENTS

This work has been supported by the Academy of Finland and by the Körber Foundation (Hamburg). I acknowledge the collective effort of our interdisciplinary neuromagnetism group in producing the data reviewed in this paper.

REFERENCES

Hari, R., 1989, The neuromagnetic method in the study of the human auditory cortex. In "Auditory Evoked Magnetic Fields and Potentials," M. Hoke, F. Grandori, and G.-L. Romani, G.L., eds., Adv. in Audiol., Vol. 6, Karger, Basel, in press.

Hari, R., and Lounasmaa, O.V., 1989, Recording and interpretation of cerebral magnetic field, Science, 244:432.

Hari, R., Hämäläinen, M., Ilmoniemi, R., Kaukoranta, E., Reinikainen, K., Salminen, J., Alho, K., Näätänen, R., and Sams, M., 1984, Responses of the primary auditory cortex to pitch changes in a sequence of tone pips: neuromagnetic recordings in man, Neurosci. Lett., 50:127.

Hari, R., Pelizzone, M., Mäkelä, J.P., Hällström, J., Leinonen, L., and Lounasmaa, O.V., 1987, Neuromagnetic responses of the human auditory cortex to on- and off-sets of noise bursts, Audiology, 26:31.

Hari, R., Hämäläinen, M., and Joutsiniemi, S.-L., 1989a, Neuromagnetic steady-state responses to auditory stimuli, J. Acoust. Soc. Am., in press.

Hari, R., Joutsiniemi, S.-L., Hämäläinen, M., and Vilkman, V., 1989b, Neuromagnetic responses of human auditory cortex to interruptions in a steady rhythm, Neurosci. Lett., in press.

Joutsiniemi, S-.L., and Hari, R., 1989, Omissions of auditory stimuli may activate frontal cortex, Eur. J. Neurosci., in press.

Kaukoranta, E., Sams, M., Hari, R., Hämäläinen, M., and Näätänen, R., 1989, Reactions of human auditory cortex to changes in tone duration, Hearing Res., in press.

Lounasmaa, O.V., Hari, R., Joutsiniemi, S.-L., and Hämäläinen, M., 1989, Multi-SQUID recordings of human cerebral magnetic fields may give information about memory processes, Europhysics Lett., in press.

Loveless, N., Hari, R., Hämäläinen, M., and Tiihonen, J., 1989, Evoked responses of human auditory cortex may be enhanced by preceding stimuli, Electroenceph. Clin. Neurophysiol., in press.

Näätänen, R. and Picton, T., 1987, The N1 wave of the human electric and magnetic response to sound: A review and an analysis of the component structure. Psychophysiol., 24:375.

Roland, O.E., Skinhøj, E., and Lassen, N.A., 1981, Focal activation of human cerebral cortex during auditory discrimination, J. Neurophysiol., 45:1139.

Sams, M. and Kaukoranta, E., 1989, Neuromagnetic responses of the human auditory cortex to different types of deviant stimuli, this volume.

Scherg, M., Hari, R., and Hämäläinen, M., 1989, Frequency-specific sources of the auditory N19-P30-P50 detected by a multiple source analysis of evoked magnetic field and potentials, this volume.

SELECTIVE AVERAGING IN AUDITORY EVOKED MAGNETIC FIELD EXPERIMENTS

K.B.Mikkelsen, K.Saermark, J. Lebech, C.K.Bak, and E.Basar*

Technical University of Denmark, DK-2800 Lyngby, Denmark
*Medical University Lubeck, D-2400 Lubeck 1, FRG

INTRODUCTION

Since the first observation by Reite et al. (1978) of auditory evoked magnetic fields (AEF) from the human cortex several research groups have studied especially the late response occurring around 100 ms after application of the auditory stimulus. There appears by now to exist a general consensus that the 100-ms signal can be accounted for in terms of a model consisting of an equivalent current dipole (ECD) located in or close to the primary auditory cortex. The method normally used in analyzing experimental data (magnetic fields or electrical potentials) on evoked responses has been to collect a - large - number of single epochs followed by a simple averaging procedure, possibly after artifact rejection (see one of several reviews, e.g. Hari (1986)). The formation of a simple average is based on the assumption that the evoked response is superimposed on a noise background consisting of alpha-waves, theta-waves, instrumental noise etc. and that this noise averages out for a sufficiently large number of recorded epochs. Thus, in particular the evoked response and the spontaneous brain waves are considered as independent signals. This, however, need not be strictly true, and we give two remarks to elucidate this point. Firstly, earlier non published recordings of auditory evoked responses, (toneburst,1 kHz,random ISI) showed small oscillations, which appears to be time-locked to the stimulus. These oscillations may be, and probably are, brain waves trigged by the stimulus. Secondly, in a series of papers, e.g. (Basar 1980), Basar introduced a selective averaging and, further, the concept of an enhancement factor relating the prestimulus spontaneous activity to the poststimulus evoked activity. Basar also suggested that the analysis of the brain's responses should be performed as an analysis of a dynamical system so that the analysis of evoked responses should be extended by including the single epochs in the analysis. We note in this connection that Woody (1967) made use of a latency corrected average based on cross-correlation methods. The aim of the present paper is to contribute to a discussion of whether a simple averaging procedure, as normally used, can be considered as an adequate way of analyzing auditory evoked magnetic fields. In pursuing this aim we use the methods mentioned in the next section.

Advances in Biomagnetism
Edited by S.J. Williamson *et al.*
Plenum Press, New York

METHODS

In the present experiments we used a seven channel BTI-squid system, (second order gradiometer), equipped with a Probe Position Indicator system. The system was located at a magnetically quiet location, but not in a magnetically shielded room. The sensitivity is estimated to be between 15 to 20 fT/rHz. As stimuli we generally used tone-bursts (TB), and in all cases a prestimulus interval of 1 s was used, while a frequency of 1 kHz and a duration of 500 ms were chosen. Both randomly varying and constant inter-stimulus-intervals (ISI) were used. In all cases the post-stimulus time was 1 s and the total time epoch of 2 s was sampled with a frequency of 500 Hz. The number of epochs recorded at each measuring position was 100. Seven subjects (age 20-25 years) were examined for left hemisphere responses at 5 different cryostat positions, yielding 35 measuring positions for each subject, the cryostat positions being chosen so that both extrema in the dipole-like field distributions were covered. In a number of cases additional examinations were performed for right hemisphere responses, but here we essentially consider only left hemisphere results.
In analyzing the experimental data we used several different approaches:
1) Simple averaging. After rejection of sweeps containing obvious artefacts, the normal procedure for averaging across sweeps was used.
2) Rms selective averaging. Here we first evaluated the rms-value of the spontaneous activity in a prestimulus period both for raw and band-passed filtered data; several values of the length of the prestimulus period were tried. On the basis of the rms-value the sweeps were then grouped in three groups L,M,U. L consists of the sweeps with the 20% lowest rms-values, M consists of the sweeps with the 55% of the center rms-values while U contains sweeps with the 20% highest rms-values. The final 5% of the sweeps were discarded.
3) Correlation coefficient selective averaging. Here we first evaluated the correlation coefficient (cc) between each single sweep and the simple average over sweeps for a poststimulus period of 300 ms immediately after the trigger stimulus. On the basis of the cc-value the sweeps were then grouped in three groups L,M,U in a way similar to the one used in the rms-case above.
4) Latency corrected selective averaging. Here we first choose a reference recording, either the simple average or a single sweep. We then choose a small time window (less than 100 ms and centered at the latency value) from this reference recording and next for each sweep calculate the correlation coefficient between the window - used as a running window - and the sweep. In this way the latency difference relative to the reference recording can be determined and an average corrected for latency shifts can be found. This, essentially, is the method used by (Woody 1967).
5) Finally, a spectral density analysis was performed for each sweep by means of a maximum entropy method. For each measuring position the average of the spectral density can be found both for pre- and poststimulus periods.

RESULTS

We begin by showing, in Fig.1, a plot for a single sweep as simultaneously recorded by the seven squid channels. One notes that the various channels may show a different behavior although the interchannel distance is 2 cm only. In fact, in a time window immediately following the stimulus there may be a tendency for some channels to show a 'blocking' effect while others do not. This behavior, which was observed for many sweeps and individuals, is here seen in a much clearer way than in the similar EEG-observations by Basar (1980).

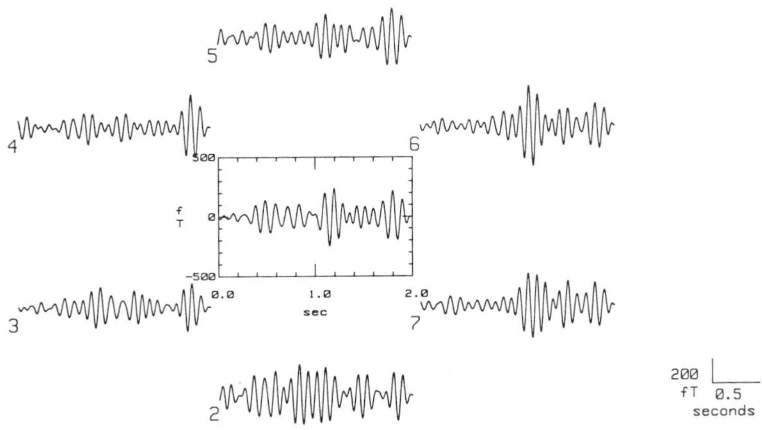

Fig. 1. A multiplot of a single sweep, recorded by seven squid channels (tone-burst, 1 kHz, random ISI), bandpass filtered in the frequency range 8 Hz to 13 Hz. The squid is located at T3. Stimulus occurs at time 1.03 sec.

Next we note that a spectral density analysis for (all of) the individual epochs shows almost the same behavior for the prestimulus period and for the poststimulus period. In fact one observes, Fig.2, a pronounced peak at alpha frequencies and only minor 'bumps' at lower frequencies.

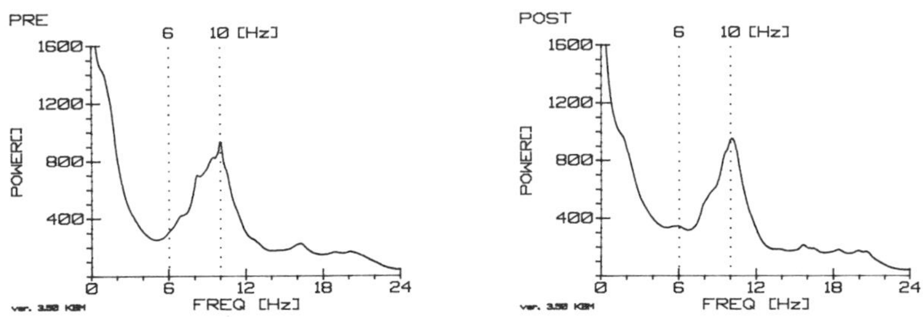

Fig. 2. Average of spectral density for all sweeps. Both pre- and poststimulus results are shown. The squid is located a few centimeters posterior to T3.

In contrast to this, a spectral density analysis of the simple average recording shows a pronounced peak at a frequency around 6 Hz and only a small or no response at alpha frequencies. This indicates that the poststimulus periods of the individual sweeps show inter-sweep phase differences or, equivalently, inter-sweep latency differences. This fact is also known from electrical evoked responses noted first, we believe, by (Woody 1967). In our opinion this fact is of importance in evaluating the nature of the source giving rise to the evoked response as it may indicate that the concept of a single equivalent dipole is only a first (rough) approximation.

We next consider the rms-selective averaging procedure and perform an average of the sweeps contained in each of the three groups L,M,U. We here find that these averages are almost equal to each other and to the average found by the simple averaging procedure. If, however, we instead use the correlation coefficient selective averaging the results are quite different. One now finds that group L gives practically no 100 ms response, that the M group gives a 100 ms signal very similar to the one observed for the simple average while group U, with the highest cc-values, gives a 100 ms peak response almost twice as large as for the simple average. The various cases are illustrated in Fig. 3, for lowpass (25 Hz) filtered data.

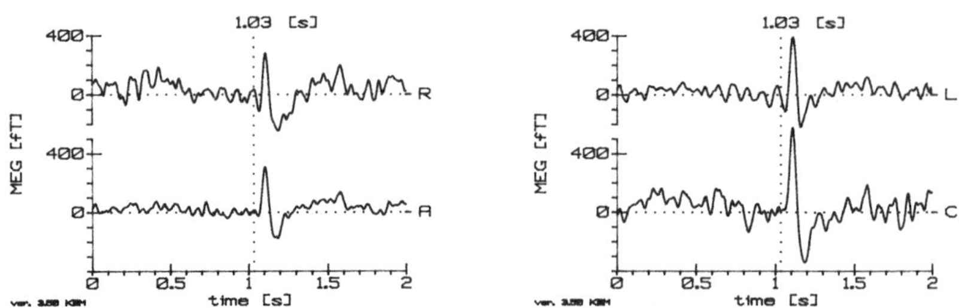

Fig. 3. A: Simple average, R: rms selective average (group L), C: cc selective average (group U), and L: latency corrected average. The squid is located a few centimeters posterior to T3.

Finally,if we apply a latency corrected selective averaging one first notes that the latencies of the individual epochs show a standard deviation of 35 ms. One further observes, relative to the simple averaging results, a considerable increase in the amplitude of the 100 ms signal, see Fig.3, and some minor modifications in the line shape. It should, however, be emphasized that for some measuring positions and for some individuals immediately after the stimulus a type of evoked alpha and/or theta rhythmicities were observed, which can be also recorded without filtering of MEF. (Evoked alpha rhythmicities are illustrated in Fig.1).

CONCLUDING REMARKS

Although the present analysis has not yet been carried to its end, we feel justified in stating that a simple averaging procedure is not the best possible form of analyzing magnetic field evoked responses unless a very large number of sweeps per measuring sessions and a relatively large number of measuring session are used so that the averaging, in effect, is over a large number of 'brain states'. In this case, however, one looses information about single 'brain states'. By selective averaging one can possibly get at least some information about 'brain states'.

REFERENCES

Reite M., Edric J., Zimmerman J. T. and Zimmerman J. E., 1978, Human magnetic auditory fields. Electroenceph. clin. Neurophysiol., 45: 114-117.

Hari, R. and Ilmoniemi, R.J., 1986, Cerebral magnetic fields. CRC Crit. Rev. Biomed. Eng., 14: 93-126.

Basar, E., 1980, EEG-BRAIN Dynamics. Relation between EEG and brain evoked potentials. Elsevier/North - Holland, Amsterdam.

Woody, C. D., 1967, Characteristics of an adaptive filter for the analysis of variable latency neuroelectric signals. Med. Biol. Engng., 5: 539-553.

FREQUENCY-SPECIFIC SOURCES OF THE AUDITORY N19-P30-P50 RESPONSE DETECTED BY A MULTIPLE SOURCE ANALYSIS OF EVOKED MAGNETIC FIELDS AND POTENTIALS

M. Scherg*, R. Hari and M. Hämäläinen

*Max Planck Institute for Psychiatry, Munich, FRG
and Low Temperature Laboratory,
Helsinki University of Technology, Espoo, Finland

INTRODUCTION

The first component of the middle latency auditory evoked fields (MAEFs) observed so far has been a peak at 30 ms (Pelizzone et al. 1987) corresponding to the P30 or P_a deflection of the middle latency auditory evoked potentials (MAEPs). The earlier part of the N19-P30 transient in the MAEP, a negative deflection around 19 ms, has been attributed to subcortical sources on the basis of scalp potential maps (Deiber et al., 1987). However, Scherg and von Cramon (1986) showed that N19 could also be explained by bilateral temporal lobe dipoles. Unilateral lesions of the auditory cortex or of the acoustic radiation resulted in a reduction of the strength of the tangential N19-P30 dipole up to a complete abolition in the lesioned hemisphere (Scherg and von Cramon, 1986; 1989). The aim of this study was to further clarify the origin of N19 by combining MAEF and MAEP measurements in the same subject. The spatio-temporal dipole model by Scherg and von Cramon (1986) was used to analyze the source structure of MAEPs and MAEFs. To study frequency specificity of N19-P30, the derived response technique by Don and Eggermont (1978) was applied to the MAEF.

METHODS

A 41-year-old male with normal peripheral hearing was studied. MEG was recorded with a 7-channel first order SQUID gradiometer (noise 5-6 fT/√Hz; Knuutila et al., 1987) from 4 positions over the right Sylvian fissure. Signals were analyzed from 24 of the 28 measurement locations. MAEPs were recorded around a coronal chain of 12 electrodes (cf. Scherg and von Cramon, 1986). Clicks (1 ms, 60 dB HL) were delivered to the left ear with an ISI of 285 ms, through a plastic tube transmitting frequencies up to 5 kHz for MAEFs and similarly low-pass filtered through earphones for MAEPs. Two replications with about 1600 averaged epochs were obtained for MAEFs in two conditions: clicks either alone or in the presence of high-pass filtered (2 kHz, 96 dB/oct) broadband masking noise (85 dB HL) on the same (left) ear. Thus, three responses were analyzed: wide-band, low-frequency response from cochlear input below 2 kHz and high-frequency derived response (wide-band response minus low frequency response). For the MAEP 10000 epochs were averaged during 5 runs in the wide-band condition only. A time frame of 6 ms pre- and 60 ms post-stimulus (MAEP: -5 to 55 ms) was analyzed after digital filtering (5 - 250 Hz). The brain electric source analysis (BESA) program by Scherg (1989), modified to account for MEG as well as EEG signals, was used to find the multiple sources underlying the MAEP and MAEF. In addition to locating dipole sources, the direct approach was used to reduce and separate the multi-channel signals into the temporal courses of the dipole moments, i.e. the waveforms associated with the local compound activities.

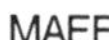

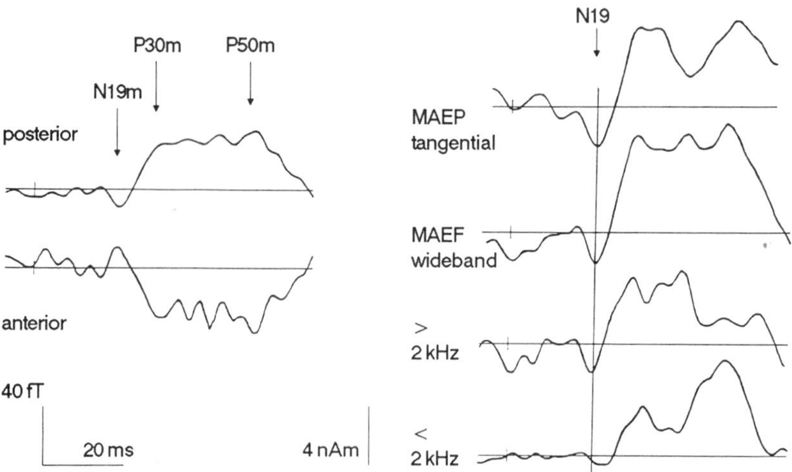

Fig. 1. Left: MAEF signals measured at the posterior and anterior end of the right Sylvian fissure. Right: Dipole moment waveforms, single source model. The tangential MAEP dipole in the right hemisphere behaves like the wide-band MAEF dipole. Note the latency shift and decrease of N19m with decreasing stimulus frequency.

RESULTS

The magnetic counterpart of the N19-P30 transient of the MAEP, the N19m-P30m, was clearly evident in the MAEF, with a polarity reversal between posterior and anterior coil locations (Fig. 1). The equivalent dipole for this transient had a depth of 38 mm. When fitting the peaks N19m and P30m separately, the source was about 5-8 mm deeper for the 19- than for the 30-ms response, both for MAEFs and MAEPs. The temporal courses of MAEF and tangential MAEP dipole moments in the right hemisphere were very similar (Fig. 1). For the MAEF this waveform was equal to the principal component of the 24 sensor signals, and it showed the N19m deflection more clearly than any individual sensor. Although N19 seemed to be preceded by a small positive deflection (P15) in both MAEP and MAEF, the signal-to-noise ratio was insufficient to determine this peak with certainty. In intracranial recordings P15 has been shown to be the first activity recordable from the surface of the primary auditory cortex (Celesia 1976). The derived responses (Fig. 1) revealed that the wide-band MAEF was composed of a N19m-P30m complex, which occurred about 3 ms later in the low-frequency than in the high-frequency band. The later activity P50m following the N19-P30 transient was also separable into an earlier high-frequency response, peaking at 38 ms, and into a later low-frequency response, peaking at 47 ms. Using a model with 2 simultaneously active sources the N19m-P30m complex could be clearly separated from P50m (Fig. 2). The sources of the latter activity were about 9 mm more anterior and 7 mm more superficial, and their dipole vectors pointed more anteriorly by 14° degrees. Both high-frequency sources were located about 11 mm posterior to the respective low-frequency sources and were oriented more posteriorly by 7 degrees. This frequency-specific organization and the separation of the equivalent dipole sources underlying the N19m-P30m-transient and P50m is depicted in Fig. 3. The tonotopy is most conspicuous in the x/depth-plane, which corresponds to a view of the right superior temporal plane from below.

DISCUSSION

The present results are the first demonstration of an auditory evoked magnetic deflection at 19 ms after click stimulation. Consistent with MAEP dipole source analysis, the MAEF sources suggest an origin of N19 and P30 in the primary auditory cortex. N19 seems to be the earliest activity from the auditory cortex which can be reliably recorded over the human scalp both electrically and magnetically. N19 appears to be generated predominantly by neurons specific to high frequencies, as

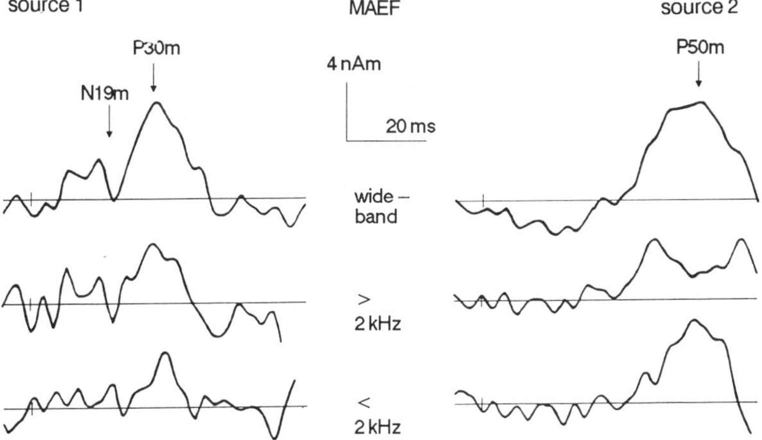

Fig. 2. MAEF dipole moment waveforms, two-source model. Note the clear separation of the N19m-P30m transient from the P50m waveform. For all components the earliest contributions stem from activation of neurons specific to the higher frequencies (> 2 kHz).

already proposed by Scherg and von Cramon (1989). In addition, the two-source model revealed distinct sources of the N19m-P30m complex and of the later P50m. As compared with N19m-P30m, the equivalent dipole of P50m exhibited a more anterior and lateral location. This suggests an origin of P50m in the paraconiocortical structures surrounding the primary auditory cortex. Evidence for this comes also from a source analysis of the late AEP (Scherg et al., 1989) showing that the P50

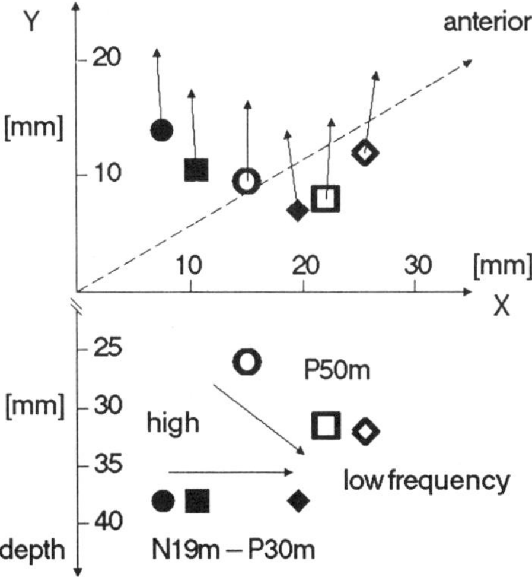

Fig. 3. Dipole locations and orientations of the two-source model as viewed from lateral (X/Y, top) and from below the superior plane (X/depth, bottom). Closed symbols: source 1, N19m-P30m, open symbols: source 2, P50m. Dipole location in the wide-band stimulus condition (squares) is closer to the high-frequency location (circles) for N19m-P30m and closer to the low-frequency location (diamonds) for P50m, indicating different frequency specificity (cf. Fig. 2). Depth was kept constant for N19m-P30m at the wide-band value of 38 mm when fitting high- and low-frequency responses separately. The x-axis forms a 45° angle with a line connecting the right ear canal and eye corner. The eye corner is located on the x-axis at x = 105 mm.

deflection was associated more with the dipole sources underlying the sustained potential (SP) than with the N100 dipoles. Similarly to P50m, the SP dipoles had the more anterior location and orientation. Further, the present study shows a frequency specificity not only for the N19m-P30m transient, i.e. for the primary auditory cortex, but also for the P50m. These results seem to reflect a tonotopic organization not only of the primary auditory cortex but also for the surrounding belt of association cortex in man. The observed anterior shift in dipole location towards lower frequencies is consistent with the changes in equivalent dipole location reported for N100m by Elberling et al. (1982). However, a similar anterior shift for N100m could not be found by Pantev et al. (1988), and for steady state auditory evoked fields (Romani et al. 1982) this shift was towards more posterior and more superficial locations. According to our findings (Fig. 2 & 3), a more superficial location may be due in part to a predominance of P50m activity in the steady state response with low frequency stimulation, compared to a predominance of P30m after high frequency stimulation (cf. Figs. 2 & 3). In conclusion, simultaneous activities in multiple areas of the auditory cortex may exert unknown effects on the location of a single equivalent dipole. Such effects as well as individual differences in location and tonotopy of these areas need to be studied in more detail, before the tonotopical organization of the human auditory cortex can be better understood. Our results have shown the usefulness of the derived response technique in measuring tonotopy and underline the need for multiple source models and simultaneous recordings in all channels.

ACKNOWLEDGEMENT

This work has been financially supported by the Körber Foundation, Hamburg. We are grateful to Patrick Berg for proof-reading the manuscript.

REFERENCES

Celesia, G. G., 1976, Organization of auditory cortical areas in man, Brain, 99:403.

Deiber, M. P., Ibanez, V., Fischer, C., Perrin, F., and Mauguière, F., 1988, Sequential mapping favours the hypothesis of distinct generators for Na and Pa middle latency auditory evoked potentials, Electroenceph. clin. Neurophysiol., 71:187.

Don, M., and Eggermont, J. J., 1978, Analysis of the click-evoked brainstem potentials in man using high-pass noise masking, J. Acoust. Soc. Am. 63:1084.

Elberling, C., Bak, C., Kofoed, B., Lebeck, J., and Saermark, K., 1982, Auditory magnetic fields. Source location and 'tonotopical organization' in the right hemisphere of the human brain, Scand. Audiol., 11:59.

Knuutila, J., Ahlfors, S., Ahonen, A., Hällström, J., Kajola, M., Lounasmaa, O. V., Vilkman, V., and Tesche, C., 1987, Large-area low-noise seven-channel dc SQUID magnetometer for brain research, Rev. Sci. Instrum., 58:2145.

Pantev, C., Hoke, M., Lehnertz, K, Lütkenhöner, B., Anogianakis, G., and Wittkowski, W., 1988, Tonotopic organization of the human auditory cortex revealed by transient auditory evoked magnetic fields. Electroenceph. clin. Neurophysiol., 69, 160.

Pelizzone, M., Hari, R., Mäkelä, J. P., Huttunen, J., Ahlfors, S., and Hämäläinen, M., 1987, Cortical origin of middle-latency auditory evoked responses in man, Neurosci. Lett., 82:303.

Romani, G. L., Williamson, S. J., Kaufman, L., and Brenner, D., 1982, Characterization of the auditory cortex by the neuromagnetic method. Exp. Brain Res., 47:381.

Scherg, M., 1989, Fundamentals of dipole source potential analysis, in: "Auditory Evoked Magnetic Fields and Potentials," M. Hoke, F. Grandori, and G. L. Romani, eds., Adv. Audiol., Vol. 6, Karger, Basel, in press.

Scherg, M., and von Cramon, D., 1986, Evoked dipole source potentials of the human auditory cortex, Electroenceph. clin. Neurophysiol., 65:344.

Scherg, M., and von Cramon, D., 1989, Dipole source potentials of the auditory cortex in normal subjects and in patients with temporal lobe lesions, in: "Auditory Evoked Magnetic Fields and Potentials," M. Hoke, F. Grandori, and G. L. Romani, eds., Adv. Audiol., Vol. 6, Karger, Basel, in press.

Scherg, M., Vajsar, J., and Picton, T. W., 1989, A source analysis of the human auditory evoked potentials, J. Cogn. Neurosci., submitted.

REPLICABILITY FOR LOCALIZATION OF THE P1, N1, AND P2 COMPONENTS OF THE AUDITORY EVOKED RESPONSE IN AN UNSELECTED GROUP OF SUBJECTS

S. Baumann, R. Rogers, A. Papanicolaou and C. Saydjari

Magnetoencephalography Laboratory, Division of Neurosurgery, University of Texas Medical Branch, and the Transitional Learning Community, Galveston, TX 77550, USA

INTRODUCTION

With few exceptions (Yamamoto et al, 1988) intrasubject replications have not been performed to test the reliability of dipole localization. Furthermore, although several studies have examined either the P1, N1 or P2 components of the auditory evoked magnetic field (EMF), most studies have localized one component in only a few subjects. Consequently, it is difficult to determine whether separate sources are responsible for these components. Also, only a few studies (Reite et al, 1988; Yamamoto et al, 1988) have included magnetic resonance images (MRIs) of each subject's brain onto which the location of the computed dipoles can be superimposed. We have begun a systematic effort to address these issues by testing a series of subjects at least twice and by superimposing dipole locations onto individual MRIs.

METHODS

Twelve subjects ranging in age from 21-54 years were each tested twice several days apart. Auditory stimuli were presented to the left ear and recorded contralaterally using a seven-channel, second-order gradiometer, dc SQUID system (BTi model 607) inside a magnetically shielded chamber. Tone bursts of 1 kHz sine waves with a 10 msec rise/fall time and a 30 msec plateau were delivered randomly every 2-3 seconds at a sound intensity of 95 dB with 50 dB white noise delivered to the right ear. Bandpass filters were set at 0.3 Hz - 50 Hz and the sampling rate was 200 Hz for a one second epoch including a 0.5 second pre-stimulus baseline. One hundred epochs were recorded and averaged at each of eight dewar locations for a total of 56 averaged EMF waveforms.

The data were fit to a model assuming a dipolar source in a homogeneous spherical conductor. A circular area of the scalp 10 cm in diameter and centered 7 cm above the right ear canal was digitized to provide a best-fitting sphere for that portion of each subjects' head. Dipole localization was performed using commercial software (BTi) that employs an iterative solution to find the best fit (expressed as the correlation coefficient r) between a forward solution and the obtained data. The results are listed in terms of five parameters - the three spatial coordinates of the dipole, (x, y, z), its orientation (psi) and

Advances in Biomagnetism
Edited by S.J. Williamson *et al.*
Plenum Press, New York

TABLE 1. Means (and Standard Deviations) of each peak during each testing session.

SESSIONS		DIPOLE	PARAMETERS			
	Latency (msec)	x (cm)	y (cm)	z (cm)	Psi (degrees)	Q (nA-m)
P1						
1st	49.86	.08	-4.80	5.61	-28.03	3.67
n=7	(2.67)	(1.08)	(1.0)	(.62)	(14.29)	(1.43)
2nd	49.86	.11	-5.09	5.69	-21.99	3.97
	(2.67)	(1.14)	(.96)	(1.13)	(15.45)	(1.79)
N1						
1st	91.58	-.03	-4.95	5.39	138.55	7.92
n=12	(10.33)	(1.07)	(.04)	(.61)	(21.78)	(3.68)
2nd	91.58	-.05	-4.89	5.44	134.03	9.40
	(10.33)	(.85)	(.90)	(.87)	(21.11)	(3.63)
P2						
1st	155.57	.18	-4.81	5.12	-43.92	5.84
n=7	(23.09)	(1.23)	(.49)	(1.08)	(21.13)	(2.17)
2nd	155.57	-.03	-4.98	5.22	-47.71	7.93
	(23.04)	(.87)	(.43)	(.62)	(18.79)	(3.14)

strength (Q). Dipoles were localized for several latencies at 5 msec intervals around each peak of interest.

To compare measurements between sessions for each peak a common latency was chosen by picking, within the range of latencies at which EMFs at the two extrema reached the highest amplitudes in both sessions, the latency with the highest mean correlation coefficient for both sessions. Correlation coefficients had to be above 0.9 for the N1 and the P2 and above 0.84 for the P1 for the data to be included for analysis.

To assess the replicability of measurements, parameter values for the second testing sessions were subtracted from those of the first session. A series of paired t-tests was performed on the mean difference values for each parameter to determine if there were any significant differences in the dipole parameters between sessions.

Magnetic resonance (MR) images were obtained from all subjects for purposes of comparing the calculated dipole locations with individual anatomy. Oil containing capsules were taped to the MEG fiduciary points (the nasion and both preauricular points) to align the MRI and MEG coordinate systems. The x axis extended from the inion to the nasion, the y axis from the right to the left preauricular point and the z axis was perpendicular to the x-y plane and through the intersection of the x and y axes. Serial coronal MRI sections 0.5 cm thick were taken at right angles to the x-y plane to show the supratemporal cortex.

RESULTS

Table 1 summarizes the data for all subjects. Table 2 summarizes the data on mean differences between the testing sessions for each of the components. Two types of difference scores are reported: the sign difference is the mean of the first session minus the mean of the second session; the absolute difference is the mean of the absolute values of the difference scores between sessions.

TABLE 2. Mean Differences (Standard Deviations) Between Sessions

PEAKS	DIFF.	x (cm)	y (cm)	z (cm)	Psi (degrees)	Q (nA-m)
P1	Sign	-.03	.29	-.07	-6.04	-.30
		(.55)	(.95)	(1.1)	(11.10)	(1.46)
(n=7)	Absolute	.46	.71	.86	10.58	1.07
		(.25)	(.64)	(.58)	(5.93)	(.96)
N1	Sign	.02	-.06	-.05	4.52*	-1.48
		(.45)	(.72)	(.63)	(4.47)	(2.81)
(n=12)	Absolute	.35	.55	.49	5.48	2.23
		(.26)	(.44)	(.38)	(3.08)	(2.20)
P2	Sign	.21	.17	-.10	3.79	-2.09
		(.84)	(.45)	(.70)	(8.29)	(2.38)
(n=7)	Absolute	.60	.32	.57	6.83	2.59
		(.58)	(.34)	(.34)	(5.58)	(1.71)

*p<.05

Paired t-tests on the sign differences in Table 2 did not reveal significant differences between sessions for any of the parameters except the N1 dipole orientation. In light of the fact that all the other parameters were not significantly different, this one finding may be a statistical aberration. Additionally, the absolute differences for location were all below 1 cm, but well above the 2-3 mm error seen on our system when measuring from a calibrated sphere. The mean differences computed using absolute values are a more realistic reflection of the amount of error inherent in making these measurements and tend to show a larger, but still nonsignificant, difference.

MR images in Figure 1 show scatterplots for the locations of the N1 dipoles for all subjects in each testing session. Except for one subject in the second session, all dipoles were located within approximately 1 cm of the center of the Sylvian fissure (marked by a cross). Distances from the center of the fisure were determined by viewing individual MR images.

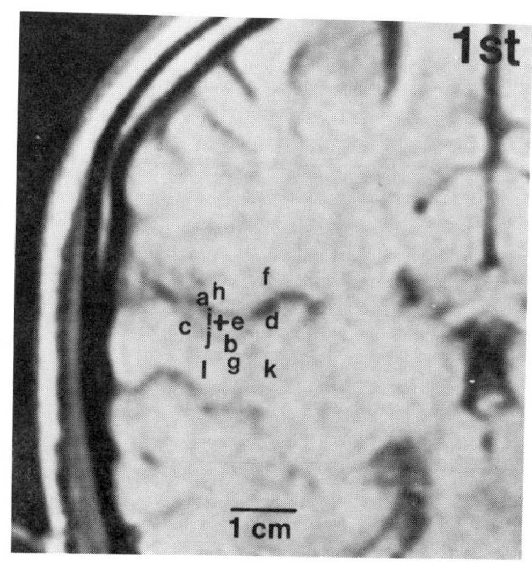

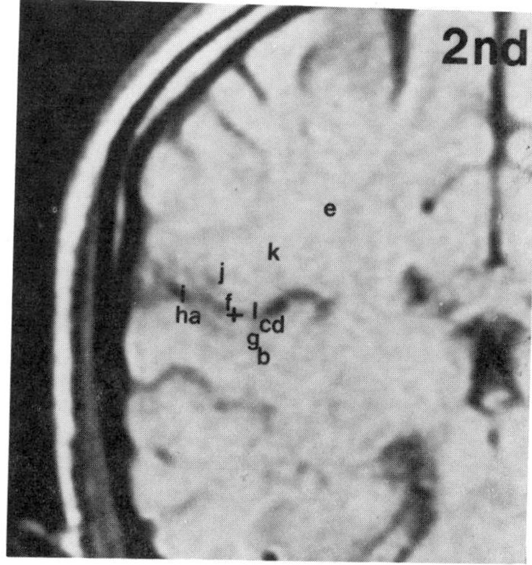

Figure 1. Scatterplots of N1 dipole locations around the center of the Sylvian fissure for all subjects (a-l) for each testing session.

Testing between components, significant differences were found in dipole orientation (Psi) and strength (Q) between N1 and P1 and between N1 and P2. Although no significant differences were found for dipole location, there is a trend suggestive of inferior movement along the z axis (see Table 1) going from P1 to N1 to P2. Also, five of the seven subjects showed anterior movement along the x axis for the P2. These data are suggestive of spatially distinct sources for the N1 versus the P1 and P2 components.

DISCUSSION

The main finding of this study is that localization of the P1, N1 and P2 components of the auditory evoked response replicate fairly well between sessions. A number of sources of error are present during the measurements that may account for the absolute difference values for dipole location being several mm larger than what can be obtained in recordings from a calibrated sphere. Foremost amongst these may be changes in attention during recording sessions. It is well known that the N1 and P2 are both affected by variations in attention. Despite efforts to motivate subjects to attend to the tones, changes in attention between sessions were quite noticeable for several of the subjects. Secondly, the bottom of the dewar has a radius of curvature that does not fit well to the flat side of the head. Unless the dewar is placed precisely in the same location and orientation for each testing session, distortions in the field measurements will not be the same.

The second finding of this study is that there are clear differences in dipole orientation and strength between the components and a noticeable, but nonsignificant, trend for the dipole location to move in the inferior-anterior direction from the P1 to N1 to P2. These results indicate that there are probably separate sources for each component. Some studies have reported that the P2 source is located anterior to the N1 source (Hari, 1988; Pelizzone et al, 1985). While we observed the same anterior movement in five subjects, two subjects displayed posterior movement of the P2 source, rendering the trend statistically non-significant.

Similarities in dipole orientation for both the P1 and P2 components, which are nearly 180° from the N1 dipole orientation, indicate that, if separate neuronal populations are responsible for producing each component, then the orientation of the dendritic fields may be similar for the P1 and P2 sources and quite different for the N1 source. On the other hand, if the same neuronal populations are responsible, reversal of current flow might be explained by summed responses to primarily excitatory and inhibitory sypatic potentials that may account for the N1 and P1/P2 components respectively.

REFERENCES

Hari, R. (1988). Neuromagnetic studies of the human auditory cortex. In Biomagnetism '87, ed. by K. Atsumi, M. Kotani, S. Ueno, T. Katila, S. Williamson, Tokyo Denki University Press, Tokyo, pp. 34-41.

Pelizzone, M., Williamson, S.J. and Kaufman, L. (1985). Evidence for multiple areas in the human auditory cortex. In Biomagnetism: Applications and Theory, ed. by H. Weinberg, G. Stroink and T. Katila, Pergamon Press, New York, pp. 326-330.

Reite, M., Teale, P., Zimmerman, J., Davis, K., and Whalen, J. (1988). Source location of a 50 msec latency auditory evoked field component. Electroencephalogr. Clin. Neurophysiol. 70:490-498.

Yamamoto, T., Williamson, S.J., and Kaufman, L. (1988). Magnetic localization of neuronal activity in the human brain. Proc. Natl. Acad. Sci., 85:8732-8736.

NONSTATIONARY DYNAMICS OF SEQUENTIAL MAGNETIC DIPOLE SOURCE CHANGES ASSOCIATED WITH N100 AUDITORY EVOKED RESPONSES

R.L. Rogers, A.C. Papanicolaou, S. Baumann,
C. Saydjari, H.M. Eisenberg

Magnetoencephalography Laboratory
Division of Neurosurgery
The University of Texas Medical Branch &
Transitional Learning Community
Galveston, Texas 77550, USA

INTRODUCTION

The source of the N100 component of auditory evoked magnetic fields (EMFs) has been localized in the auditory cortex in a number of MEG studies (see Hari, 1987 or Naatanen & Picton, 1987 for review). In those studies, equivalent dipole parameters were calculated for the magnetic field at a particular single latency during the time course of the N100 component (i.e. the latency at which the N100 reaches the highest amplitude at the two extrema or the one at which the isofield maps appear to have most distinct dipolar pattern). Yet, good dipolar patterns are often observed for a range of latencies reflecting the fact that not all EMFs recorded at the extrema reach maximal peak amplitude at precisely the same time. This suggested the possibility that the N100 may not be due to a stationary equivalent dipole but to a series of sources, a suggestion which has been supported by previous evoked potential studies (e.g. Wood and Wolpaw, 1982). In this experiment, we investigated that possibility as well as the question as to whether the N100 sources of EMFs resulting from ipsilateral and contralateral ear stimulation are distinct.

METHOD

Twelve normal adults were tested. EMFs were recorded over the right hemisphere to 1K tones (90db nHL, 50 msec duration) randomly delivered at a rate of between .33 to .5 sec to either the left (contralateral) or the right (ipsilateral) ear while white noise was delivered to the unstimulated ear. Measurements were made using a 7 channel BTi model 607 neuromagnetometer. One hundred EMFs were recorded and averaged at each of 56 locations over the right hemisphere during each stimulation condition, the order of which was randomized over the 12 subjects.

RESULTS

Clear EMF waveforms containing the N100 component were obtained from all subjects during both stimulation conditions. The peak of this component

Advances in Biomagnetism
Edited by S.J. Williamson *et al.*
Plenum Press, New York

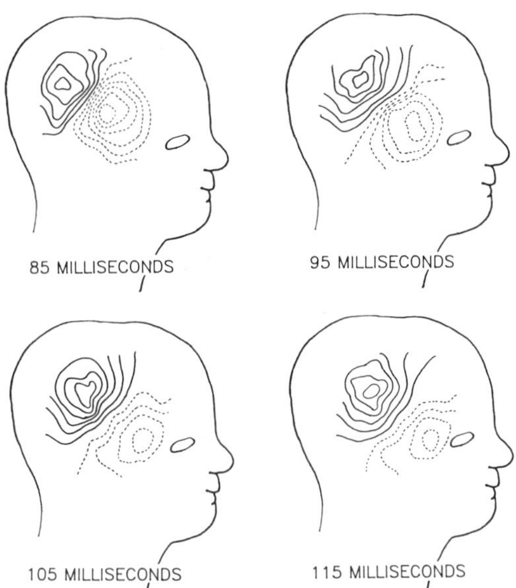

FIGURE 1. Isocontour maps of the N100 auditory evoked magnetic field in a single subject at successive 10 msec intervals during contralateral stimulation.

appeared within a latency range of approximately 30 msec starting at about 80 msec post-stimulus in all subjects. Isofield maps were constructed at 5 msec intervals from 80 to 110 msec. In most subjects all seven maps showed a clear dipolar pattern. In some, especially during the ipsilateral stimulation condition, only few of those maps, covering at least four consecutive latency points displayed a good pattern. We estimated the dipole parameters for those fields and retained for subsequent analysis only those for which good fits were obtained (correlation of the calculated and observed fields greater than .88).

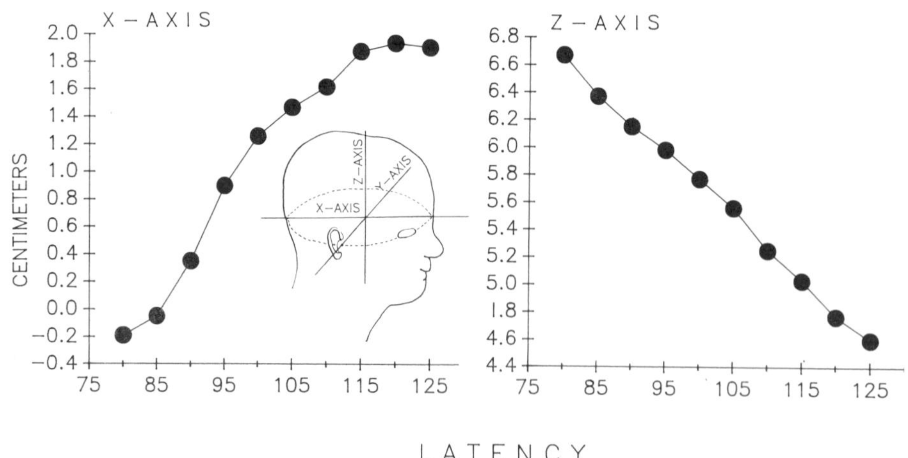

FIGURE 2. Demonstration of anterior-inferior movement of the N100 source.

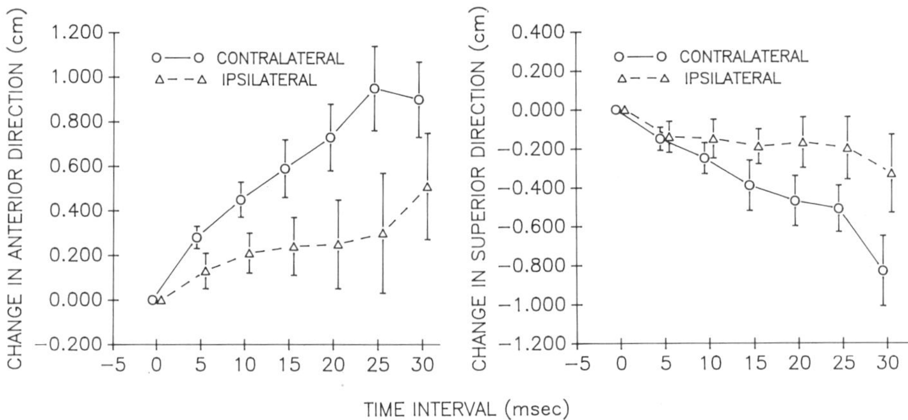

FIGURE 3. Relative movement of dipole location along the z- & x-axes averaged across 12 subjects indicating an anterior-inferior movement during successive 5 msec intervals around the N100 peak.

Inspection of sequential isofield maps (see Figure 1) suggests a progressive movement of the equivalent dipole in the anterior-inferior direction. This pattern was observed in 10 of the 12 subjects during both stimulation conditions, but most clearly during contralateral stimulation. The spatial parameters of the calculated equivalent dipoles at each successive latency confirmed this appearance of source movement, or of sequential progression of cortical excitation anteriorly (along the x axis) and inferiorly (along the z axis) as shown in Figure 2. This movement of the source appears to follow the slope of the temporal lobe. In fact, projection of the spatial parameters of the calculated dipoles onto sequential MR images of one subject confirmed this contention.

The reliability of this sequential progression of cortical excitation across subjects was statistically evaluated, through a series of linear regression analyses which revealed that during contralateral stimulation both the anterior and inferior progression of excitation (on the average 1 and .5 cm, respectively) was significant, whereas during ipsilateral ear stimulation the observed progression was not significant. Lateral movement of the source (along the y axis) was not reliable in either condition. Figure 3 shows the combined data from all 12 subjects.

DISCUSSION

The main finding in this study is that the magnetic N100 component appears to be generated by consecutive activation of adjacent sources extending anteriorly over the surface of the auditory cortex. This progression of excitation may well be mediated through cortico-cortical connections. As is well known (e.g. Braitenberg, 1978; Brugge and Reale, 1985), pyramidal cells send short axons down through superficial white matter layers that reemerge tangentially to synapse with adjacent pyramidal cells. Moreover, the primary auditory cortex in which the N100 sources appear to be located, contains an abundance of myelinated short cortical interconnections. The time constant for these pyramidal cells is approximately 8 msec and the propagation of excitation along these short cortico-cortical connections is in the order of 0.5 to 1.0 msec, which could well account for the observed temporal activation of adjacent sources.

The second finding of this study is that separate sources appear to account for responses to ipsilateral and contralateral stimulation. As Figure 3 illustrates, excitation due to ipsilateral stimulation does not progress as far as that of contralateral stimulation along the slope of the temporal lobe.

The present findings indicate the desirability of further studies to determine the type of stimulus information represented by the sequential excitation along the posterior-anterior dimension on the auditory cortex.

REFERENCES

Braitenberg, V., 1978, Cortical architectionics: General and areal, in: "Architectonics of the Cerebral Cortex", M.A.B. Brazier, H. Petsche, eds., Raven Press, New York.

Brugge, J.F., Reale, R.A., 1985, Auditory cortex, in: "Cerebral Cortex, Vol. 4", A. Peters, E.G. Jones, eds., Plenum Press, New York.

Hari, R., 1987, Neuromagnetic studies of the human auditory cortex: Recent results, in: "Biomagnetism 1987," K. Atsumi, M. Kotani, S. Ueno, T. Katila, S.J. Williamson, eds., Denki University Press, Tokyo.

Naatanen, R., Picton, T., 1987, The N1 wave for the human electric and magnetic response to sound: A review and analysis of the component structure, Psychophysiology, 24:375.

Wood, C.C., Wolpaw, J.R., 1982, Scalp distribution of human auditory evoked potentials. II. Evidence for overlapping sources and involvement of auditory cortex, Electroencephalogr. Clin. Neurophysiol., 54:25.

EVENT RELATED POTENTIALS AND FIELDS EVOKED BY AUDITORY STIMULI: EFFECTS OF INTERSTIMULUS INTERVAL AND SELECTIVE ATTENTION

Shinya KURIKI, Fumiya TAKEUCHI and Mitsunori MURASE

Research Institute of Applied Electricity
Hokkaido University
Sapporo 060, Japan

INTRODUCTION

Event related potentials (ERPs) evoked by auditory stimulation are sensitive to the interstimulus interval (ISI). When identical tone stimulus is given consecutively, the amplitude of the potential response is reduced, being smaller for shorter ISIs.[1] The ERPs are also modified by directing selective attention to the stimulus.[2] The response to the attended stimulus has an endogeneous negative wave, the latency and amplitude being dependent on the ISI.[3] Recent neuromagnetic studies[4,5] on event related fields (ERFs) indicate that neural activities in the auditory cortex are modified by the selective attention. In the present work we measured the ERPs and ERFs evoked by a pure tone and a short speech sound in the same paradigm. We studied how these responses are modified by short ISIs and by selective attention to either the tone or speech sound.

METHOD

We used a 1 kHz tone burst and a consonant-vowel speech sound /ka/ of 100 ms duration and 70 dB SPL as the standard stimuli. In the first measurement on the ISI dependence 1 kHz tone or /ka/ was delivered at a constant ISI binaurally to the subject. The subject was instructed to ignore the stimuli. The ISI was varied in different runs from 1400 ms down to 200 ms. In the second dichotic measurement 1 kHz tone and /ka/ were delivered in a random sequence to the left and right ear, respectively. The ISI was randomized between 200 and 300 ms. Besides the standard stimuli, target stimuli of a deviated tone of 1.02 or 1.05 kHz and a vowel /a/ were delivered to the left and right ear, respectively, at an occurrence probability of about 10% for each ear. The subject directed attention selectively to the stimuli at left or right ear by counting the number of the occurrence of the target stimulus. Only the responses to the standard stimuli were evaluated.

The ERPs were recorded at Cz on the scalp with Ag-AgCl electrodes referred to linked ears. The ERFs were recorded using a second order gradiometer at a location of the posterior surface of right and left hemispheres at which the response was maximum in each subject. A measurement run included 64 responses for each of the tone and speech sound, and several runs at a constant ISI in the first measurement or with a target stimulus in the second measurement were done for further data processing.

Advances in Biomagnetism
Edited by S.J. Williamson *et al.*
Plenum Press, New York

RESULTS

In the responses to the repeated tone or /ka/ in the first measurement, the peak-to-peak amplitude of N1(m)-P2(m) waves in the ERP and ERF decreased rapidly, in an exponential function of ISI, as it was shortened from 1400 to 500 ms. The peak latencies of the N1(m) and P2(m) waves were progressively delayed with the ISI decrease. Below 400 ms ISI, the ERF and ERP responses showed a much slower decrease of the amplitude. The waveform of the response to /ka/ at these ISIs differed from the response at longer ISIs in a way that the N1(m) wave was almost embedded in a newly developed wave with a longer latency. Figure 1 shows a comparison between the responses at a long ISI of 1400 ms and a short ISI of 200 ms. In the responses to 1kHz tone at the short ISI, N1(m) and P2(m) waves can be identified, though small and delayed, while in the responses to /ka/ at the short ISI the two waves are not clear.

The rapid decrease of the responses at short ISIs is due to the effect of habituation. The habituation is a function of acoustic resemblance of successive stimuli. The observations in the first measurement indicate that the amplitude of the response, and possibly the waveform, are affected by whether the preceding stimulus is identical or different when the ISI is very short. In the second measurement of selective attention, we therefore made separate averaging of the responses elicited by the stimulus which was preceded by a stimulus of the identical type (identical stimuli set) and the responses elicited by the stimulus which was preceded by a stimulus of different type (deviant stimuli set).

Figure 2 shows the grand averages across eight subjects of the ERF and ERP responses elicited by 1 kHz tone and /ka/, where the response when the relevant stimulus was attended and that when the irrelevant stimulus was attended are compared, and the difference response between them is shown in the lower trace. The measurement location of the ERFs is posterior side of the right hemisphere. The deflection of the N1m wave is taken upward as the deflection of the N1 wave in the ERPs. We made an analysis of variance to examine whether the attended and unattended responses have statistically significant differences. From those results, the waves in the difference response which differed significantly from zero ($P<0.05$) are indicated by an arrow.

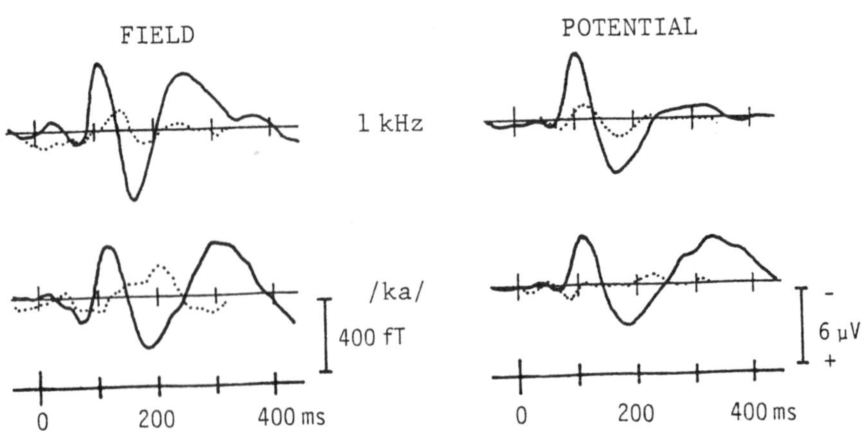

Fig.1. Examples of the ERF and ERP evoked by 1 kHz tone and /ka/ delivered at different ISIs of 1400 ms (solid line) and 200 ms (dotted line).

The difference responses of the potential to the identical stimuli set have a pronounced negative wave, which differs significantly from zero ($P<0.05$), at about the latency of N1 peak. The negative wave is evident for both 1 kHz and /ka/ stimuli. Contrary to this, the difference responses of the potential to the deviant stimuli set have less-pronounced and nonsignificant negative wave at about the N1 peak latency. An analysis of variance showed that there is a significant difference ($P<0.05$) of the negative wave between the responses to the identical and deviant stimuli sets. This difference indicates a dependence of the attention effect on the stimuli sequences in the potential responses.

On the other hand, in the difference responses of the field the negative wave, i.e., deflection toward the N1m peak, is not as large as that in the potential responses. No statistical significance of the negativity was found at about the N1m peak latency, though 20-30 % enhancement of the N1m wave was observed in the responses attended to the relevant stimuli. Moreover, there was no significant difference of the negativity between the responses to the identical and deviant stimuli sets. It is also noted that in both the potential and field responses to the deviant stimuli set a significantly positive wave ($P<0.05$) was observed at latencies above about 200 ms.

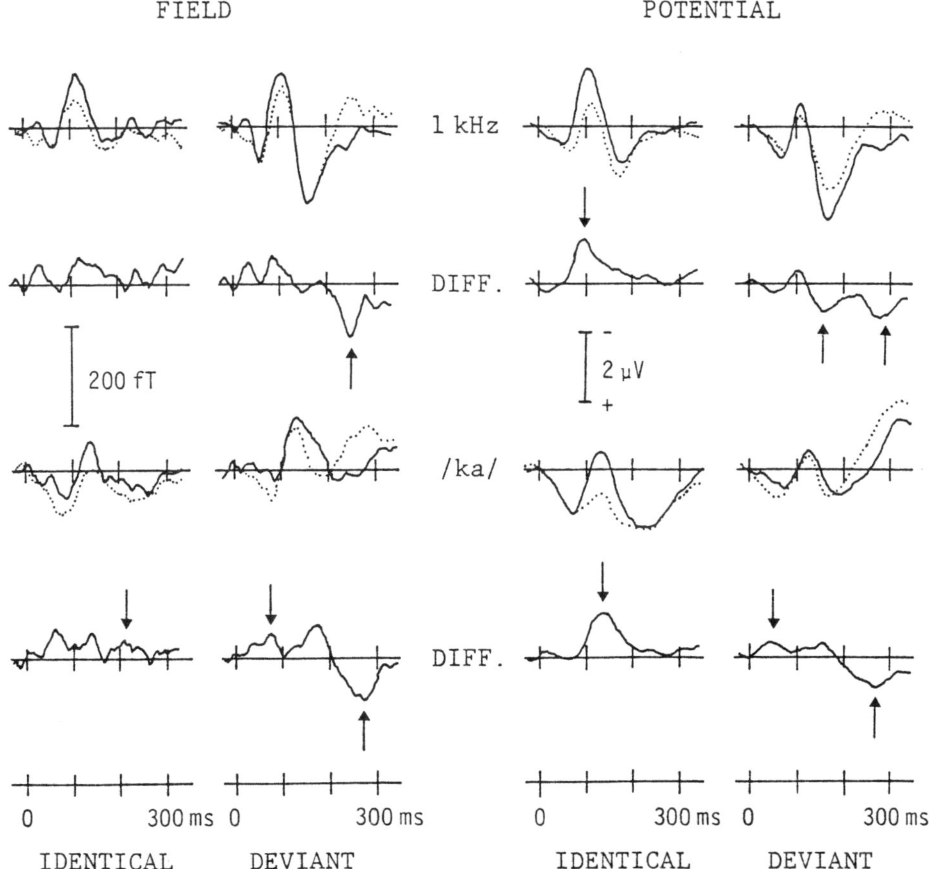

Fig.2. Grand averages of ERFs and ERPs when relevant stimulus was attended (solid line) and unattended (dotted line) and the difference response (lower trace). These responses are separately shown for identical and deviant stimuli sets. Waves in the difference response differing from zero at $P<0.05$ are indicated by solid arrows.

DISCUSSION

As can be seen in Fig.2, the responses to /ka/ delivered at 200-300 ms ISIs in the dichotic measurement have waveforms similar to the responses to 1 kHz tone. In contrast to this, the same responses have deformed waveforms (Fig.1) in the first measurement when /ka/ was delivered consecutively at similar short ISIs. This difference may be associated with the effect of short term habitation in which consecutive presentation of identical stimulus is crucial. The complex acoustic structure of /ka/ composed of a plosive consonant and a vowel is also an important factor to yield the deformed waveform of the responses.

The present dichotic measurement has shown that the selective attention manifests a component which enlarges the N1 wave in the ERPs evoked by the attended stimulus. This component appears as a negative wave in the difference response. The negative wave has a peak latency at about the N1 peak, in agreement with the early phase of the endogeneous negative component which appears in the ERPs measured at short ISIs.[6]

A new finding is that the negative component in the attended ERPs was significantly larger when they were evoked by the relevant stimuli which were preceded by the same stimulus in the random stimuli sequence. This fact seems to be related to the neural mechanisms underlying the selective attention in a way that the strength of the attention effect depends on the stimuli sequence. In addition, a positive component after 200 ms was observed in both the ERPs and ERFs evoked by the relevant stimuli which were preceded by a different stimulus, i.e., irrelevant stimulus. This component is a consequence of a positive shift of N2(m) wave, which should be also clarified in the relation to the stimuli sequence.

In the ERFs modulation of the waveform at about N1m peak in the attended responses was smaller in magnitude than that in the ERPs. The negative wave in the attended minus unattended response did not differ significantly from each other between the responses evoked by the same and different stimuli sequences. Comparing the responses measured over the right and left hemispheres, the difference wave in the attended minus unattended response was similar, indicating no significant hemispheric asymmetry, except for fluctuations of the waveform.

REFERENCES

1. H.Fruhstorfer, P.Soveri and T.Jarvilehto, Short-term habituation of the auditory evoked response in man, Electroenceph. clin. Neurophysiol., 28:153 (1970).
2. S.A.Hillyard, R.F.Schwent and T.W.Picton, Electrical signs of selective attention in human brain, Science, 182:172 (1973).
3. R.Näätänen, A.W.K.Gillard and C.A.Varey, Attention effects on auditory ERPs as a function of inter-stimulus interval, Biol. Psychol., 13:173 (1981).
4. S.Curtis, L.Kaufman and S.J.Williamson, Divided attention: selection based on location or pitch, in: Biomagnetism, K.Atsumi, M.Kotani, S.Ueno, K.Tatila and S.J.Williamson, eds., p.138, Tokyo Denki University Press, Tokyo (1988).
5. R.Hari, M.Hämäläinen, E.Kaukoranta, J.Mäkelä, S.L.Joutsiniemi and J.Tiihonen, Selective listening modifies activity of the human auditory cortex, Exp. Brain Res., 74:463 (1989).
6. J.C.Hansen and S.Hillyard, Endogeneous brain potentials associated with selective auditory attention, Electroenceph. clin. Neurophysiol., 49:277 (1980).

NEURAL MECHANISMS OF SELECTIVE AUDITORY ATTENTION

Deborah Arthur, Steven Hillyard[1], Edward Flynn and Al Schmidt[2]

Neuromagnetism Laboratory, MS M-715, Los Alamos National Laboratory, Los Alamos, NM 87545; [1]Neurosciences Dept., Univ. of California at San Diego; [2]Science & Technology Center, Westinghouse, Pittsburgh,PA.

Introduction

A fundamental goal of selective attention studies is to specify at which levels of sensory processing different kinds of information are selected or rejected. One key issue is whether stimulus selection occurs at early thalamic and primary cortical areas, or at levels of "higher" secondary and association cortex. In the auditory modality, selective attention to an attended stimulus elicits a large negative deflection, the "Nd" or "processing negativity" component. The physiological substrates of this selective attention effect remains controversial. Some authors have argued that the Nd wave represents (at least in part) an enhancement of the auditory evoked N1 wave, possibly by a mechanism of sensory gating (eg., Hillyard,1981), while others have suggested that the Nd arises from a wholly separate generator system (eg., Naatanen, 1982). Previous results from our laboratory suggest that the late Nd (Ndl) elicited under conditions of a long and constant inter-stimulus interval (ISI), stems from a region of auditory cortex distinct from that generating the evoked N1 component: possibly from auditory association areas (Arthur et al., 1989). Under conditions of a fast, variable ISI, selective attention elicits an additional component, the early Nd (Nde). We are using magnetoencephalography to assess the physiological substrates of both the early and late selective attention processes which occur at a fast, variable ISI.

Methods

The data were collected from 5 paid volunteers under conditions of a dichotic listening paradigm. Standard tone pips (1000 and 2500 Hz) with identical durations (60 msec) were dichotically presented with probabilities of 42.5% each at a random inter-stimulus interval of 200 to 400 msec. The subjects attended to tone bursts in one ear in order to respond to occasional target tone bursts (probability 7.5%) identical to standard tones in that ear except for duration. Four replications of each attention condition were recorded. Neuromagnetic responses were recorded over the left temporal cortex using a 7-channel neuromagnetometer and event-related potentials (ERPs) were recorded from Fz and Cz of the International 10-20 electrode system.

Both ERPs and event-related magnetic fields (ERFs) were quantified and analyzed under software control, with mean amplitudes of the N1 (latency range 110-160 msec), Nde (110-160 msec) and Ndl (230-500 msec) measured from the prestimulus baseline at either 10 msec intervals (70-170 msec) or 20 msec intervals (180-500 msec). Difference waves were obtained by subtracting ERPs and ERFs elicited by tones in non-attended ears from ERPs and ERFs elicited by identical tones when attended.

Isofield contour maps were constructed and a least squares procedure was applied to those neuromagnetic distributions which demonstrated two extrema of opposite polarity in order to estimate the location and orientation of the best fitting equivalent current dipole (ECD). The effect of measurement error on the fitted dipole model parameters was analyzed using 50-run Monte Carlo simulations (see Medvick et al., these proceedings, for details). If differences in Monte Carlo component source centroids exceeded 1.96 times the standard deviation of the mean for any one axis, the sources were taken to be different at a 95% confidence interval.

Results

Fig. 1 shows sample neuromagnetic responses of one subject over the posterior extremum to attended (dashed lines) and non-attended (solid) "standard" tones presented to the left ear. The event-related potentials recorded from Fz and Cz are also shown. Simultaneously recorded magnetic and electric responses were essentially identical in waveform. The first prominent magnetic deflection (N1m) peaks between 120-150 msec (across subjects) and corresponds to the electrical N1 component. In all subjects, the amplitude of the N1/N1m components was larger when subjects were attending targets in that ear compared to when their attention was directed to the opposite ear. The difference waves of the ERPs and ERFs contained a prominent Nd/Ndm, with distinct early and late phases. The early Nd/Ndm overlapped the N1/N1m component, while the late Nd/Ndm was a broader duration component with a latency range of approximately 200-500 msec.

Magnetic field patterns for N1m-attend (N1m-A), N1m-non-attend (N1m-NA), early Ndm and late Ndm resembled simple dipolar distributions so that ECD localization procedures were conducted. For each of these 4 components, 6 ECDs were calculated (left and right ears X 3 subjects). In 5 out of 6 observations, the ECD describing the N1m-A source could not be statistically distinguished from the ECD describing the N1m-NA source.

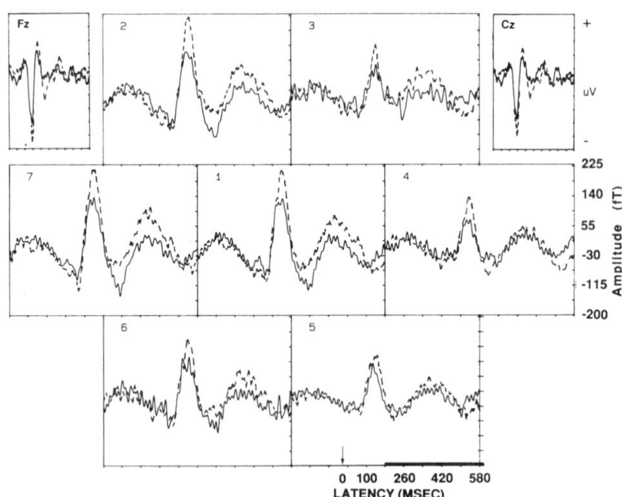

Figure 1 ERFs to left ear "standards" obtained over the posterior extremum of one subject are labeled 1-7. Simultaneously recorded ERPs from Fz and Cz are shown in the upper left and right boxes (negative amplitude down; same time scale as MEG). The dashed curves show responses when the left ear stimuli were attended, and the solid curves when the right ear was attended. The waveforms of a given type represent the average of approximately 400 responses.

Fig. 2 shows one subject's Monte Carlo results for (a) the N1m-NA source and the early Ndm (left panel) and (b) the N1m-NA source and the late Ndm (right panel). There is a clear separation in distribution of ECDs for the N1m-NA compared to the source distribution of the late Ndm (Fig. 2b). The Ndm activity is shifted about 2 cm anterior to the centroid of the N1m-NA. A similar anterior shift of ECDs describing the late Ndm was apparent in 3 of 6 observations; 1 out of 6 was posterior; 1 of 6 showed an Nd source that was dorsal to the N1m-NA source and 1 of 6 showed a late Nd source that was ventral to the N1m-NA. These shifts in sources were typically on the order of 15-20 mm across subjects.

There was more overlap between the source distributions of the early Ndm activity and the N1m-NA source (Fig. 2a). In 5 of 6 observations, there was significant overlap in the ECDs distribution for these two components. Although the sources could not be statistically distinguished in the Monte Carlo simulations, there was a tendency for the early Ndm centroid to be slightly shifted (1 cm or less) from the N1m centroid.

The orientation of ECDs suggests the N1m and Ndms may share common neural generators with the N1 and Nds of the ERP. In 4 of 6 observations, there was a shift in the dipole orientation line from central (N1m) to frontal (Ndm) regions. This pattern is consistent with ERP data reported in the literature.

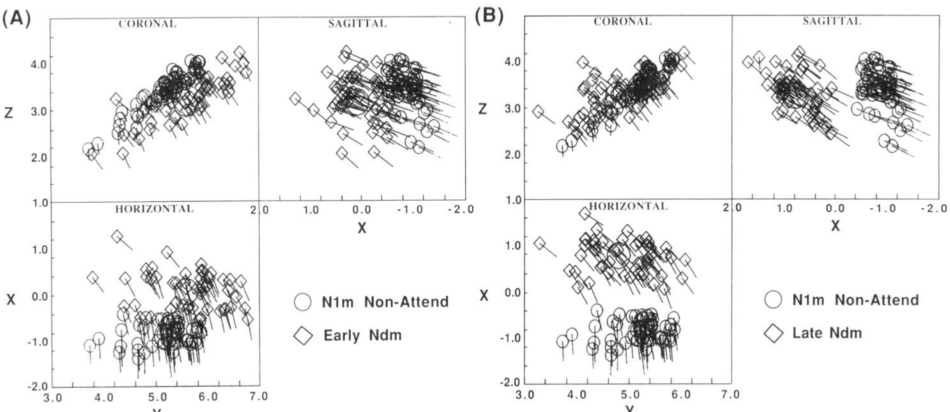

Figure 2 Monte Carlo generated ECD ensembles for event-related fields corresponding to (a) the N1m-NA and the early Ndm and (b) the N1m-NA and the late Ndm. Additive noise with a standard deviation of 15 fT was used for the N1m and 22 fT for the Ndms.

Discussion

The present results confirm earlier findings that the source of the late Ndm component has a somewhat different location in auditory cortex than the source of the N1m (Arthur et al. 1989). By contrast, the source of the early Ndm component could not generally be distinguished from the N1m source of activity. Curtis et al. (1987) reported similar results. These preliminary results suggest at least two functionally distinct mechanisms of selection: an early modulation of the N1 generator possibly due to increased "gating" of afferent input at or before the level of the auditory cortex (Hillyard, 1981) and a later "endogenous" process, perhaps reflecting an "attentional trace" in the sensory system (Naatanen, 1982).

It should be cautioned that comparisons of generator sources between different components such as the N1 and Nds are seldom straight forward. The problem is that the N1 component has been shown to arise from several distinct sources that overlap in time (Wood and Wolpaw, 1982). If the effect of attention were to modulate only one (or some subset) of these overlapping components, a dissociation may well be observed between the recorded field distributions of the entire unattended N1 component and the N1 subcomponent(s) that were enhanced by attention (ie., the early Nd). Despite this ambiguity in comparing component distributions, the close similarity in source localization between the N1m-NA and the early Ndm, taken together with the precise temporal correspondence between these two waveforms are supportive of the view that attention acts to gate the evoked sensory activity reflected in the N1 component. It cannot be determined from present evidence, however, whether the early gating of unattended-channel input is sustained throughout an entire train of stimuli or whether it develps progressively over successive stimuli in a train (Donald and Young,1982; Hansen and Hillyard, 1988).

Acknowledgements

This work was supported by the United States Army Research Institute, Alexandria VA and the United States Department of Energy contract W-7405-ENG-36 to D. Arthur and E. Flynn and by NIMH Grant MH-25594 and ONR Grant N00014-89-J-1806 to S. Hillyard. The authors wish to thank Dan Valdez for technical assistance and Wendy Tiee and Jeff Lewine for helping with data analysis. A special note of thanks to Marty Woldorff, without whose assistance this experiment would never have been completed.

References

Arthur, D. L., Lewis P. S. Medvick, P. A and Flynn, E. R., 1989, A neuromagnetic study of selective auditory attention. Submitted to Electroenceph. clin. Neurophysiol.

Curtis, S., Kaufman, L. and Williamson, S., 1987, Divided attention revisited: selection based on location or pitch, in: "Biomagnetism: 6th International Conference on Biomagnetism," K. Atsumi, M. Kotari, S. Vero, T. Katila and S. J. Williamson, eds., Tokyo Denki University Press, Tokyo.

Donald, M. W. and Young, M. J., 1982, A time-course analysis of attentional tuning of the auditory evoked response. Exp. Br. Res., 46:357.

Hansen, J. and Hillyard, S., 1988, Temporal dynamics of human auditory selective attention, Psychophysiology, 25:316.

Hillyard, S. A. 1981, Selective auditory attention: A rejoinder, Can. J. Psychol., 35:85.

Medvick, P. A., Lewis, P. S., Aine, C. and Flynn, E. R. Monte Carlo analysis of localization errors in magnetoencephalography, this volume.

Naatanen, R., 1982, Processing negativity: An evoked-potential reflection of selective attention. Psych. Bull., 92:605.

Wood, C. C. and Wolpaw, J. R., 1982, Scalp distribution of human auditory evoked potentials. II: Evidence for overlapping sources and involvement of auditory cortex. Electroenceph. clin. Neurophysiol., 54:25.

NEUROMAGNETIC RESPONSES TO INFREQUENT CHANGES IN PERIODICITY PITCH

Sing Teh Lu, Riitta Hari, and Mikko Sams

Low Temperature Laboratory, Helsinki University of Technology
02150 Espoo, Finland

INTRODUCTION

Periodic acoustic signals are perceived to have a pitch which does not depend on the spectral content of the sound. The existence of this kind of perception, usually called 'periodicity pitch', suggests that the temporal features of the sound, in addition to its spectral content, may form the basis for pitch detection (Langner, 1985; Warren and Bashford, 1988). Extraction of spectral information in the cochlea is explained by the 'place principle' (Pickles, 1988), and the tonotopic organization is retained also at the cortical level. There is no evidence of an analogous cortical place code for the temporal information involved in the periodicity pitch.

The auditory cortex is known to be necessary for the discrimination of periodicity pitch (Symmes, 1966). In the present work we studied whether neural correlates of the coding of the periodicity pitch might be found by neuromagnetic measurements in the auditory cortex of healthy humans.

METHODS

Magnetic responses were recorded with a 7-channel, first-order SQUID gradiometer in nine healthy adults. In four of them, the complete field pattern was measured from 35 - 49 locations over the right hemisphere; in the other five subjects the responses were recorded from one magnetometer position (7 channels) at the posterior field extremum. In addition to field mappings, some functional studies were carried out in three subjects (see Results). The recording passband was 0.05 - 100 Hz and the data were digitized at 1 kHz. The response to the first standard after each deviant was omitted from the analysis. Response amplitudes were measured in reference to a 40-ms prestimulus baseline.

Isocontour field maps were constructed during the peaks of the responses at 5 ms intervals, and the equivalent dipoles explaining the field patterns were found using a least-squares fit and by assuming that the head is a spherical conductor with a radius of 120 mm.

The stimuli were delivered through a plastic tube and an earpiece to the left ear. During the experiment, the subject was reading a book without paying any attention to the stimuli.

Advances in Biomagnetism
Edited by S.J. Williamson *et al.*
Plenum Press, New York

Two different stimuli were presented in an 'oddball paradigm' (90% standards, 10% deviants with an interstimulus interval (ISI) of 555 ms. The stimuli were 100-ms bursts of chopped noise (0 - 10 kHz), gated by either 80 or 240 Hz square waves. Since the sounds had identical (flat) frequency spectra but differed in their perceived pitch, no spectral cues were available for the detection of the pitch (Harris, 1963). Both stimuli served once as standards and once as deviants.

RESULTS

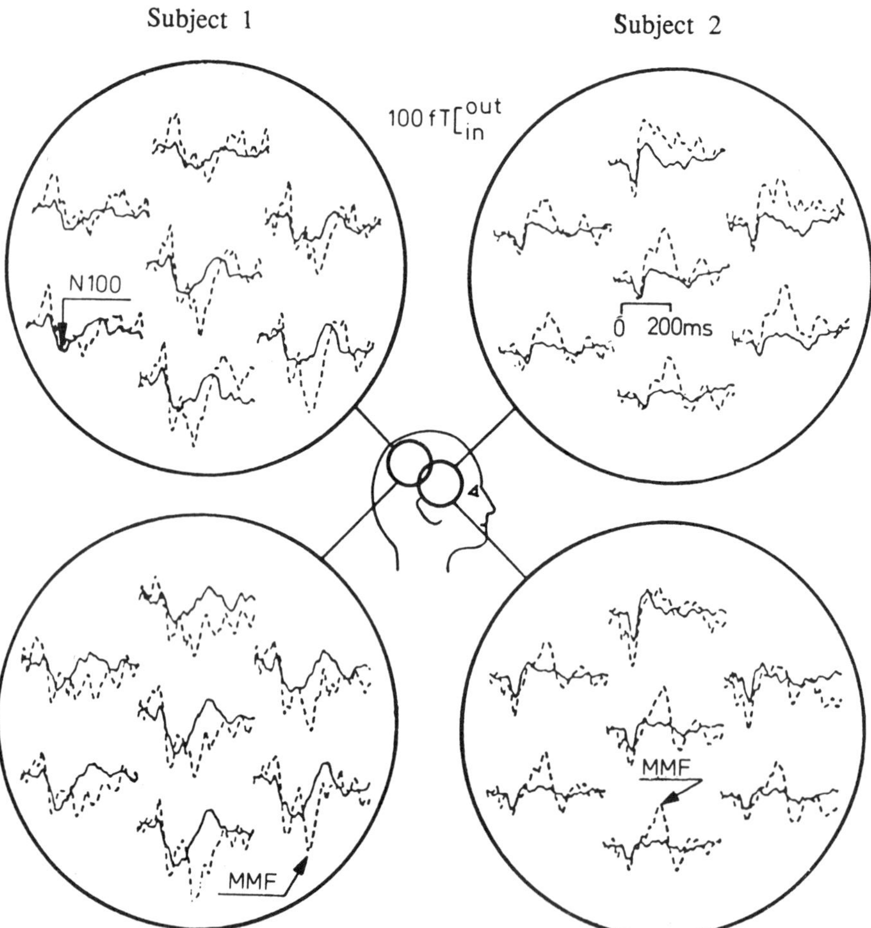

Fig. 1. 7-channel responses of Subject 1 over the posterior (left) and of Subject 2 over the anterior (right) end of the right Sylvian fissure to 80-Hz and 240-Hz standards (continuous lines, number of averaged responses N ≈ 450), and to 240-Hz and 80-Hz deviants (dashed lines in the upper and lower traces, respectively; N ≈ 50). The midpoints of the channels are separated by 36.5 mm. After averaging, the data were digitally low-pass filtered at 45 Hz.

Figure 1 shows responses of two subjects to standards and deviants. In Subject 1, the responses to standards consist of a deflection at 70 msec followed, at 125 msec, by N100m which is visible only in some channels. In Subject 2, a prominent deflection at 60 msec precedes N100m. In most subjects N100m was very small, evidently because of the short ISI and because noise was used as the stimulus. The responses to deviants have a distinct waveform, with a large deflection ('mismatch field', MMF) peaking at 200 msec in Subject 1 and at 210 msec in Subject 2.

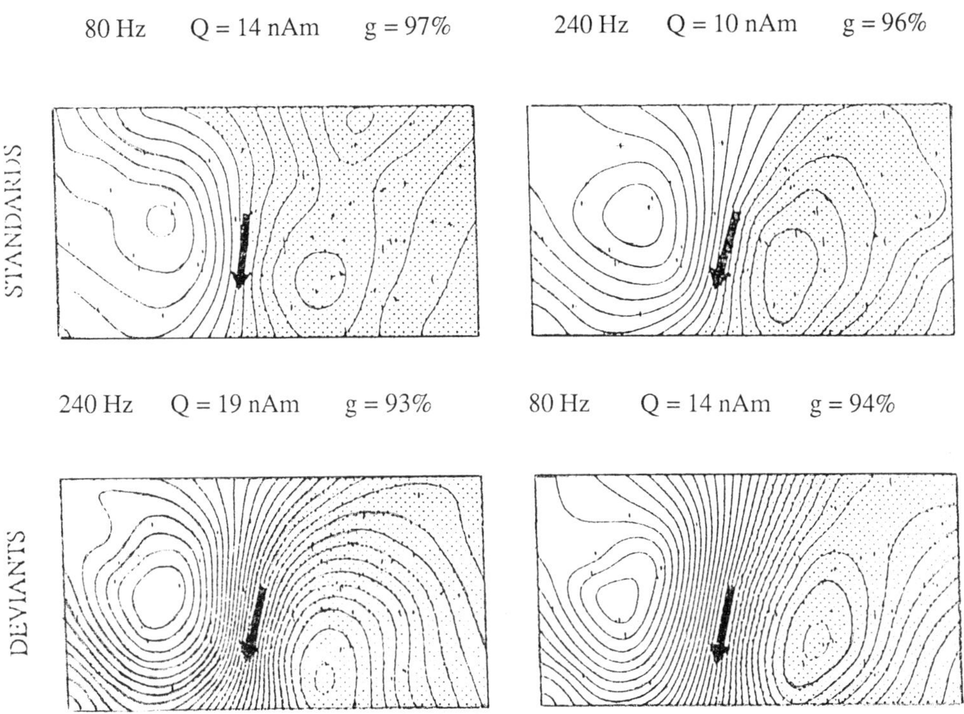

Fig. 2. Field maps of Subject 3 over the right hemisphere during N100m for both standards and deviants at frequencies of 80 and 240 Hz. The isocontours are separated by 10 fT and dashed areas indicate flux out of the skull. The arrows show the location of the equivalent current dipoles. Approximate measurement area is 8 cm x 16 cm.

Figure 2 illustrates isocontour maps of Subject 3 during N100m to standards (80 Hz and 240 Hz) and MMF to deviants (240 Hz and 80 Hz). The field patterns can be modelled by equivalent current dipoles, which explain 93 - 97% of the field variance. The locations of the sources agree with activation of the supratemporal auditory cortex.

The source locations for standards (N100) and deviants (MMF) differed in two subjects out of four at the 95%-confidence level; the variation was 11 - 12 mm in the plane parallel to the temporal skull surface. Sources for the two deviants differed in three subjects at the 95%-confidence level; the variation was 7 - 15 mm. No systematic features were seen in the source locations either between standards and deviants nor between different deviants.

In a control study with three subjects, MMF was larger in amplitude when the frequency difference between standards and deviants was bigger (standard 240 Hz and deviants 20, 80, or 120 Hz; or vice versa).

DISCUSSION

Because standards and deviants did not differ in their spectral content, the dissimilarities in responses must be due to differences in the temporal patterns of the sounds. MMF may, therefore, reflect activation of neural mechanisms involved in the coding of the periodicity pitch, which implies that MEG can be used to study its neural basis.

In the present paradigm, the representation of the standard stimulus must be stored, for example as a functional change in the neural network, up to the presentation of the deviant in order to generate the MMF. To our knowledge there are no animal data to indicate that such a memory trace would be coded by periodic temporal features of neural activity, even though the processing of a periodic sound is based on them. Therefore, our result might suggest that the time code of periodicity pitch is converted to a spatial code in cortex. Further studies are needed to find out whether this code is analogous to the tonotopic organization of the auditory cortex.

ACKNOWLEDGEMENTS

This work was financially supported by the Academy of Finland and by the Körber-Stiftung (Hamburg).

REFERENCES

Harris, G. G., 1963, Periodicity perception by using gated noise, J. Acoust. Soc. Am., 35:1229.

Langner, G., 1985, Time coding and periodicity pitch, in: "Time Resolution in Auditory System". A. Michelsen, ed., Springer Verlag, Berlin.

Pickles, J., O., 1988, An Introduction to the Physiology of Hearing. Academic Press, New York.

Symmes, D., 1966, Discrimination of intermittent noise by macaques following lesions of the temporal lobe. Exp. Neurol. 16: 201.

Warren, R. M., and Bashford, J. A., 1988, Spectral dominance or pitch averaging? J. Acoust. Soc. Am. 84: 2058.

PAIRED TONE PRESENTATION ENHANCES RESPONSES OF HUMAN AUDITORY CORTEX TO RARE FREQUENCY CHANGES

Josi Rif, Riitta Hari, and Jari Tiihonen

Low Temperature Laboratory
Helsinki University of Technology
SF-02150 Espoo, Finland

INTRODUCTION

An 'oddball paradigm', where monotonously repeated 'standard' sounds are randomly replaced by physically different 'deviants', has been recently used in several neuromagnetic studies. For example, a rare change in tone frequency evokes a special response, 'mismatch field' (MMF), with the source area close to that of the 100-ms response (N100m) to stimulus onset (Hari et al., 1984; Sams et al., 1985). The functional relation between the sources of N100m and MMF is still an unsolved question.

In a recent MEG-study, Loveless et al. (1989) observed, using a paired stimulus presentation, that N100m is larger to the second than to the first tone in the pair at onset intervals of less than 300 ms, in contrast to what would be predicted on the basis of the known recovery cycle of N100m. Previous stimuli evidently change the state of the neural network underlying the response, but the detailed mechanism is unknown. In the present work we used paired and single stimulus presentation to compare functional features of N100m and MMF. Different behavior of these responses would further support distinct generators.

METHODS

Eight healthy adults were studied in our shielded room. The magnetic field was measured over the right hemisphere with a 7-channel, first-order SQUID-gradiometer (field sensitivity 5 - 6 $fT/\sqrt{Hz}$; Knuutila et al., 1987). Stimulus trains, all presented to the left ear, consisted of two 50-ms tones: 'A' with a frequency of 1000 Hz and 'B' of 1200 Hz. An oddball paradigm was applied with 90% of stimuli as standards and 10% as deviants; the interstimulus interval was 745 ms. In the first condition, 'A' was the standard and 'B' the deviant. In the second condition paired stimuli were presented: the pair 'AA' as the standard and 'AB' as the deviant; tones of each pair were separated by 25 ms. During the measurements, the subject was reading, without paying attention to the stimuli.

The recording passband was 0.05 - 100 Hz and the data were digitized at 750 Hz. Responses coinciding with eye blinks or movements were rejected. Amplitudes of different deflections were analyzed in respect to a 50-ms prestimulus baseline. Isocontour field maps were constructed at 5 ms intervals during the peaks of the response and equivalent dipoles were searched using a least-squares fit and a spherical head model (radius 120 mm). For every stimulus condition and for each subject, the maps were based on measurements from 21 - 49 different locations, covering both field extrema over the right hemisphere.

Advances in Biomagnetism
Edited by S.J. Williamson *et al.*
Plenum Press, New York

RESULTS

Fig. 1 shows responses of one subject to standards and deviants in both conditions. The most prominent deflection N100m of the response to 'A' peaks at 92 ms. The response to the deviant 'B' peaks at 112 ms and is 55% higher in amplitude than N100m to 'A'. For paired stimulation N100m to 'AA' is smaller in amplitude than that to 'A' and no clear response is seen to the second tone of the pair. Responses to deviants 'AB' contain a N100m deflection similar to that to standards and a very strong deflection (MMF) at 208 ms, i.e., 127 ms after the onset of the second tone of the pair. The amplitude of MMF, measured from the subtraction curve, was 180% higher for 'AB' than 'B'.

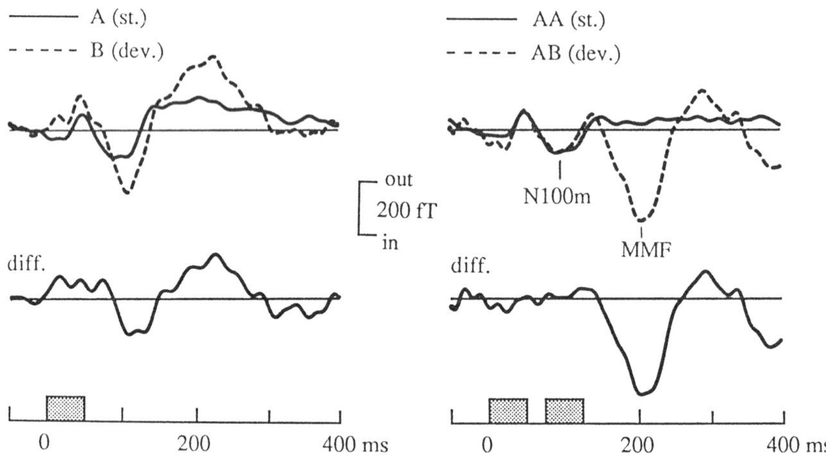

Fig. 1. Responses of one subject from the posterior end of the right Sylvian fissure during both conditions. The curves for standards are averages of about 300 responses and those for deviants of about 40 responses. The lowest traces illustrate subtraction curves (deviant minus standard). The stimulus durations are shown on the time scale. Passband is 0.05 - 40 Hz.

Fig. 2 shows a summary of the mean latencies and amplitudes of N100m and MMF during the two conditions in all subjects. The amplitude of MMF was 120 fT larger ($p < 0.001$), two-tailed t-test for pair differences) for 'AB' than 'B' and its latency was 13 ms longer (N.S.).

The field patterns were dipolar during the peaks of N100m and MMF during both conditions and could be satisfactorily explained by a single current dipole, the location of which agrees with activation of the supratemporal auditory cortex (Fig. 3). Isofield maps were also constructed on the basis of the subtraction curves (deviants minus standards). The location of the equivalent dipole, determined from these subtraction maps, was significantly ($p < 0.05$) more anterior than the source of N100m. The mean differences were 10 - 13 mm; this trend was seen in 6 subjects out of 8. The dipole moment, reflecting the strength of the cortical activation, was more than three times larger for MMFs to 'AB' than to 'B' ($p < 0.005$).

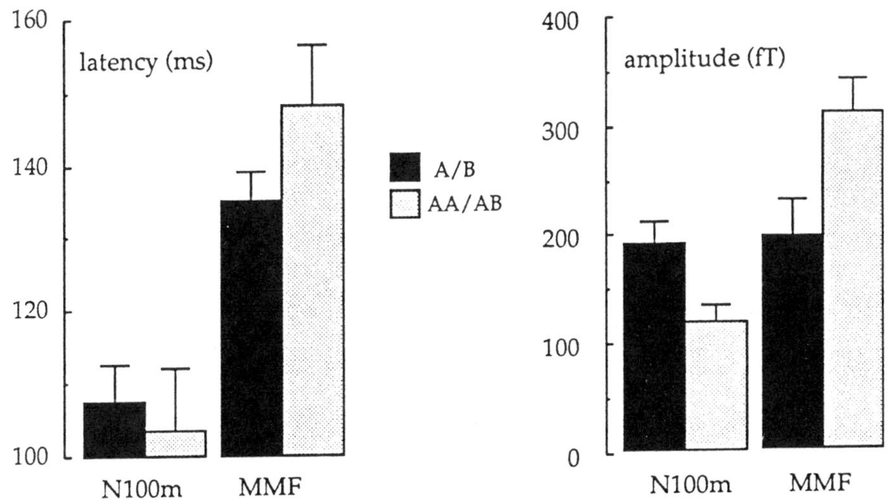

Fig. 2. Mean (± S.E.M.) latencies and amplitudes of N100m and MMF in both conditions in nine subjects ('A' vs. 'B' and 'AA' vs. 'AB').

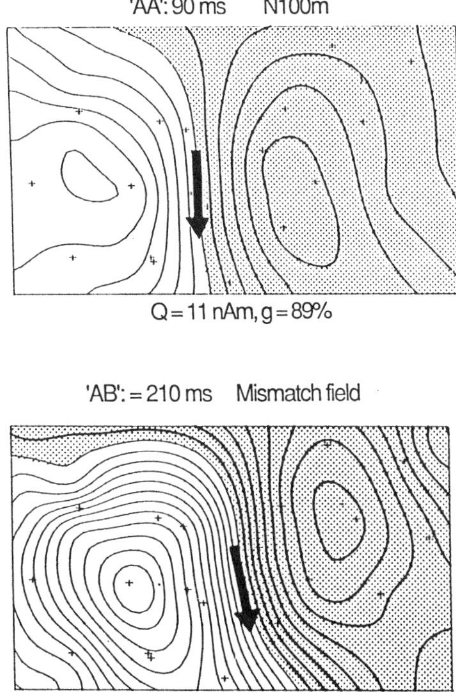

Fig. 3. Isocontour field maps of one subject during N100m to 'AA' and MMF to 'AB'. Measurements were carried out over the right auditory cortex from a 12 cm x 21 cm area.The dots show the measurement locations. Shaded areas indicate magnetic flux out of the skull; the isofield lines are separated by 20 fT. The arrows show the locations and orientation of the equivalent current dipoles.

DISCUSSION

MMF, like its electric counterpart 'mismatch negativity', has been suggested to be related to echoic sensory memory (Näätänen and Picton, 1987; Lounasmaa et al., 1989) but the neural generation mechanism has remained unclear. It has been suggested (for review and references, see Näätänen and Picton, 1987) that the deviants cause a 'mismatch' with a 'neural model', activated by the monotonously repeated standard stimuli. Unfortunately, it has not been possible to present any 'hard' neurophysiological correlates for this descriptive model. The present study shows significant and consistent differences between the source locations of MMF and N100m indicating that different cytoarchitectonic areas at the supratemporal auditory cortex are responsible for the generation of these two responses.

Further differences between N100m and MMF were evident in their different behavior during paired stimulation: N100m to the second tone of the pair was very small whereas MMF was about three times that to single stimulus presentation. This finding agrees with the neural model hypothesis: in the paired paradigm more 'A's were available to strengthen the model thereby enhancing the mismatch process. However, our further control studies cast doubt on the hypothesis that observed amplitude enhancement reflects some significant change in the storing of the memory trace. We rather believe it to be caused by the paired stimulus presentation.

The increase of MMF latency during the paired presentation might be associated with forward masking by the previous tone of the pair; similar latency delays were observed by Loveless et al. (1989) for N100m in paired stimulus presentation.

ACKNOWLEDGMENTS

This work has been finacially supported by the Academy of Finland and Körber Foundation (Hamburg).

REFERENCES

Hari, R., Hämäläinen, M., Ilmoniemi, R., Kaukoranta, E., Reinikainen, K., Salminen, J., Alho, K., Näätänen, R., and Sams, M., 1984, Responses of the primary auditory cortex to pitch changes in a sequence of tone pips: neuromagnetic recordings in man, Neurosci. Lett., 50:127.

Knuutila, J., Ahlfors, S., Ahonen, A., Hällström, J., Kajola, M., Lounasmaa, OV., Vilkman, V., and Tesche, C., 1987, A large-area low noise seven-channel DC SQUID magnetometer for brain research, Rev. Sci. Instr., 58:2145.

Lounasmaa, O.V., Hari, R., Joutsiniemi, S-l., and Hämäläinen, M.,1989, Multi-SQUID recordings of human cerebral magnetic fields may give information about memory processes, Europhys. Lett., 9:603.

Loveless, N., Hari, R., Hämäläinen, M., Tiihonen, J., 1989, Evoked responses of human auditory cortex may be enchanced by preceding stimuli, Electroenceph. Clin. Neurophysiol., 74:217.

Näätänen, R. and Picton, T., 1987, The N1 wave of the human electric and magnetic response to sound: a review and an analysis of the component structure, Psychophysiol., 24:375.

Sams, M., Hämäläinen, M., Anervo, A., Kaukoranta, E., Reinikainen, L., Hari, R., 1985, Cerebral neuromagnetic responses evoked by short auditory stimuli, Electroenceph. clin. Neurophysiol., 61:245.

NEUROMAGNETIC RESPONSES OF THE HUMAN AUDITORY CORTEX TO DIFFERENT TYPES OF INFREQUENT DEVIANT STIMULI

Mikko Sams*, Elina Kaukoranta*, Matti Hämäläinen, and Risto Näätänen*

*Department of Psychology, University of Helsinki, Ritarikatu 5, 00170 Helsinki, Finland; and Low Temperature Laboratory, Helsinki University of Technology, 02150 Espoo, Finland

INTRODUCTION

An infrequent "deviant" auditory stimulus presented among repetitive "standard" stimuli elicits a specific EEG signal termed the mismatch negativity (MMN; Näätänen et al., 1978) which is not seen in responses to standards. The MMN is elicited by practically any kind of auditory stimulus deviation, such as a change in frequency, intensity, duration, spatial locus of origin etc. (for a review, see Näätänen, 1989). We have also observed an analogous magnetic "mismatch field" (MMF) to a change in the frequency of a repetitive tone (Hari et al., 1984). On the basis of field mappings, MMF could be explained by activation of the supratemporal auditory cortex, close to the area where the N100m signal has its cortical origin. However, these earlier results did nor allow detailed comparisons of the sources of N100m and MMF.

In the present work, we report MMFs to different types of changes in simple physical features of an auditory stimulus (frequency, intensity, and duration). In addition, we show MMFs to changes in linear frequency modulations (glides) of short duration (see also Sams et al., 1989); such time-variant changes are important constituents of phonetic stimuli.

METHODS

We report here two experiments carried out in the magnetically shielded room of the Low Temperature Laboratory of the Helsinki University of Technology. In the first, the standard stimuli (100 ms, 1000 Hz, 80 dB SPL, probability (p) = 0.9) were presented to the subject's left ear once every 510 ms. Three different deviants (each with p = 0.033) were imbedded among the standard tones: frequency deviant (1500 Hz), intensity deviant (57 dB SPL), and duration deviant (50 ms). Seven subjects were run. In the second experiment, standard tones (33 ms, p = 0.9) were of linearly increasing or decreasing frequencies. One end of a stimulus was always 1000 Hz and the other either 1068, 1157, 1388, 1461 or 1540 Hz. The deviant stimulus (p = 0.1) was similar to a corresponding standard but presented backwards. Eight subjects were run. In both experiments, the subject was reading a book during the stimuli.

The magnetic field outside the head was measured with a 7-channel first-order SQUID-gradiometer (Knuutila et al., 1987). Magnetic signals elicited by the standard and deviant stimuli were recorded from 7 - 42 locations over the right hemisphere, digitized at 1100 Hz and averaged on-line. The isofield maps of MMFs for each deviant and of N100m for the standards were constructed by projecting the pickup coil locations onto a spherical surface whose radius was equal to the average distance of all pickup coils from the centre of the

Advances in Biomagnetism
Edited by S.J. Williamson *et al.*
Plenum Press, New York

sphere which was used to approximate the head. Least-squares fit was employed to determine the parameters of the equivalent dipoles that explained best the measured fields.

RESULTS

A conspicuous MMF at the latency of 120 - 180 ms was elicited by frequency, duration, and intensity deviants (Fig. 1). During MMF, the field maps showed two extrema of opposite polarities at the posterior and anterior measurement areas. Such patterns can be explained by equivalent current dipoles at the supratemporal auditory areas. The mean locations, on the xy-plane, of the three MMFs did not differ statistically significantly from each other.

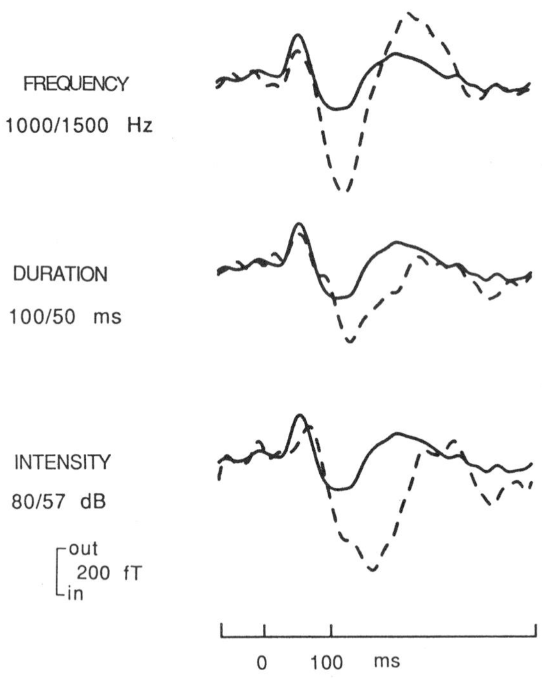

Fig. 1. MEG responses to standards (continuous lines) and frequency, duration, and intensity deviants (dashed lines). All the recordings were made from the same posterior temporal scalp location in one subject.

However, in two subjects, the source for the frequency MMF was significantly anterior to those for intensity and duration MMFs. In one subject, the sources for duration and intensity MMFs differed significantly. In another subject, the same was true for frequency and intensity MMFs. The mean locations of the sources for different MMFs were significantly more anterior, by approximately 10 mm, than the source for the N100m elicited by the standards.

The frequency glides presented as deviants also elicited a clear MMF which was of opposite polarities in the anterior and posterior ends of the Sylvian fissure. In addition, mappings in two subjects showed a dipolar field pattern confirming that even this MMF is generated at the supratemporal auditory cortex. The amplitude of the MMF was larger with larger glide magnitudes (Fig. 2).

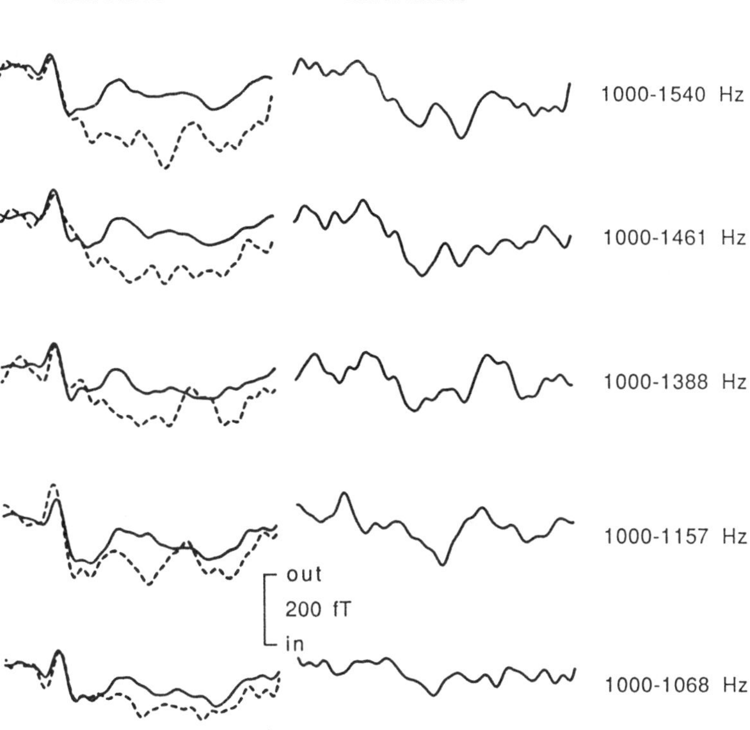

Fig. 2. *Left:* MEG responses to standards (continuous lines) and deviants (dashed lines) recorded from one location over the posterior temporal area in one subject. *Right:* Difference waveforms obtained by subtracting the responses to the standards from those to the deviants.

DISCUSSION

The present results show MMFs to deviations in frequency, intensity, and duration of an auditory stimulus. Each of these MMFs could be explained by neural activity in the supratemporal auditory cortex. The locations of the equivalent dipoles for these MMFs were anterior to that for N100m, suggesting that they result from activation of neuronal populations differing from that generating N100m. We propose that MMF reflects the activation of a pool of "novelty detectors" which respond to any change in the physical features of an auditory stimulus. The N100m signal could be more intimately related to the processing of the physical features of the stimulus. This is suggested by results of Näätänen et al. (1988), showing that the electric N100 is very sensitive to the frequency and to some extent also to the location of a tone. In a similar vein, the source location of N100m is dependent on the frequency (Pantev et al., 1988) and intensity (Pantev et al., 1989) of the tonal stimulus.

A neural network underlying such novelty detectors might include feature detectors, tuned to different physical characteristics of a stimulus, converging on novelty neurons. The repeated activation of feature detectors due to the presentation of the standard stimuli would gradually lead to habituation in the output of novelty neurons. However, when some parameter of the stimulus is changed a new set of feature detectors is activated sending a fresh input. Owing to this the novelty neurons respond again. Therefore, our results might also be regarded as providing indirect evidence for the existence of frequency, intensity, and duration detectors in the human auditory cortex (see also Kaukoranta et al., 1989).

The present results also demonstrate MMFs to a change in the direction of frequency changes within a brief tone. The standards and deviants consisted of exactly the same frequencies and, in comparison with the inter-stimulus interval, the stimulus duration was very short. It seems quite improbable that those detector elements underlying frequency MMFs could also explain the glide MMF. We suggest that underlying the present glide MMFs, there are detectors tuned to time-varying frequency changes, like those found in the auditory cortex of the cat (Whitfield and Evans, 1965). The present glides are of quite similar duration than the frequency transitions occurring at the beginning of such consonant-vowel syllables as [ba], [da], and [ga]. The magnitude and direction of the transition determines what phoneme is heard. Therefore, our results might indicate that the human auditory cortex contains neural mechanisms which can be automatically activated by stimulus features which are important constituents of speech sounds.

ACKNOWLEDGEMENTS

This study was supported by the Academy of Finland.

REFERENCES

Hari, R., Hämäläinen, M., Ilmoniemi, R., Kaukoranta, E., Reinikainen, K., Salminen, J., Alho, K., Näätänen, R., and Sams, M., 1984, Responses of the primary auditory cortex to pitch changes in a sequence of tone pips: neuromagnetic recordings in man, Neurosci. Lett., 50:127.

Kaukoranta, E., Sams, M., Hari, R., Hämäläinen, M., and Näätänen, R., 1989, Reactions of human auditory cortex to a change in tone duration, Hearing Res., in press.

Knuutila, J., Ahlfors, S., Ahonen, A., Hällström, J., Kajola, M., Lounasmaa, O.V., Vilkman, V., and Tesche, C., 1987, Large-area low-noise seven-channel de SQUID magnetometer for brain research, Rev. Sci. Instrum., 58:2145.

Näätänen, R., 1989, The role of attention in auditory information processing as revealed by event-related potentials and other brain measures of cognitive function. Behav. Brain Sciences, in press.

Näätänen, R., Gaillard, A. W. K., and Mäntysalo, S., 1978, Early selective attention effect reinterpreted. Acta Psychologica, 42: 313.

Näätänen, R., Sams, M., Alho, K., Paavilainen, P., Reinikainen, K., and Sokolov, E.N., 1988, Frequency and location specificity of human vertex N1 wave, Electroenceph. Clin. Neurophysiol., 69:523.

Pantev, C., Hoke, M., Lehnertz, K., Lütkenhöner, B., Anogianakis, G., and Wittkowski, W., 1988, Tonotopic organization of the human auditory cortex revealed by transient auditory evoked magnetic fields, Electroenceph. clin. Neurophysiol., 69:160.

Pantev, C., Hoke, K., Lehnertz, K., and Lütkenhöner, B., 1989, Neuromagnetic evidence of an amplitopic organization of the human auditory cortex, Electroenceph. clin. Neurophysiol., 72:225.

Sams, M., Kaukoranta, E., Hari, R., and Näätänen, R., 1989, Cerebral magnetic responses to changes in the direction of linear frequency transitions of a tone, XXXI International Congress of Physiological Sciences, Helsinki 1989, volume of abstracts.

Whitfield, I. C., and Evans, E. F., 1965, Responses of auditory cortical neurons to stimuli of changing frequency. J. Neurophysiol., 28:655.

SPECIFICITY OF NEUROMAGNETIC RESPONSES IN THE HUMAN AUDITORY CORTEX TO CONSONANTS OF MONOSYLLABLE SPEECH SOUNDS

Shinya KURIKI, Mitsunori MURASE and Fumiya TAKEUCHI

Research Institute of Applied Electricity
Hokkaido University
Sapporo 060, Japan

INTRODUCTION

Neuromagnetic method has high ability to localize a single current dipole of the neural source which is evoked by various sensory stimulations. In the auditory responses to tone bursts and short speech sounds differences were found in the location of dipole sources in the auditory cortex, depending on the frequency[1] and acoustic feature[2] of the stimuli. In this paper we report the location and its assessment of cortical dipole sources evoked by several monosyllable speech sounds. We found a statistically significant difference in the dipole locations between some speech sounds.

METHOD

The auditory stimuli of monosyllable speech sounds we used are consonant-vowels consisting of plosive consonants (/k/,/p/,/b/) or nasal consonant (/m/) and a vowel (/a/). Measurements are divided in two series, in which a stimuli set of /a/, /ka/, and pure tones with 200 ms duration or another set of /ba/, /pa/, and /ma/ with 80-90 ms duration were used. These sounds in each stimuli set were generated in random order at a repetition period of 1.5-1.7 s from a microcomputer and given binaurally to the subject. The intensity level of the sounds was 70-85 dB. The subject was reading a book without paying attention to the stimuli. Magnetic responses were measured using a second order gradiometer coupled with a SQUID at 35-45 locations over the lateral surface of two hemispheres. Averaging of 64 responses was done at each measurement location.

For the main components of N1m and P2m waves occurring at 100-140 and 160-200 ms after the stimulus onset in the responses, five parameters, i.e., three coordinates, the direction of current and the moment, of a best-fitting current dipole source were computed in a spherical conductor model. We developed a method to evaluate the confidence limit of the computed dipole parameters based on an empirically obtained statistic of the residual field, i.e., difference between the measured and theoretical fields.[3] The confidence limit of a parameter was determined by altering the relevant parameter until the variance of the residual field increased by a factor given by the statistic.

Advances in Biomagnetism
Edited by S.J. Williamson *et al.*
Plenum Press, New York

The locations of the N1m dipoles projected on a horizontal plane are shown in Fig.2, where the dipoles for /a/ and /ka/ measured in four subjects (ages 20-28 years) are shown in (a) and those for /ba/, /pa/, and /ma/ in two subjects (ages 24 years) are shown in (b). The 95% confidence region of the dipole location approximated by an ellipse is shown for pairs of the dipoles, connected with a solid line, between which the confidence region did not overlap each other. This separation of the confidence region indicates that the difference in the two dipole locations is statistically significant at a level of P<0.05. Figure 2(a) shows that three dipole pairs out of four pairs in the left hemisphere and one dipole pair in the right hemisphere have a significant separation that /ka/ dipoles are located laterally or lateral-posteriorly to /a/ dipoles. In Fig.2(b) a significant separation is found between /ba/ and /ma/ dipoles and /ba/ and /pa/ dipoles. The locations of the /ma/ (and /pa/) dipoles are lateral-posterior to the /ba/ dipoles in three all pairs (and two out of three pairs) across two hemispheres.

Locations of the N1m dipoles projected on the sagittal plane were also examined. In the superior-inferior direction significant separation was not found between any dipoles in the two stimuli sets. The relative locations of the dipoles along the anterior-posterior direction were as those found in the horizontal projections in Fig.2. For the P2m dipoles location differences between the specific monosyllables were not as clear as the N1m dipoles. Significant shift of /ka/ dipoles posteriorly or lateral-posteriorly to /a/ dipoles was found in three pairs out of seven across two hemispheres. Only a single dipole pair out of six across the hemispheres had a significant lateral-posterior shift of /ma/ dipole to /ba/ dipole.

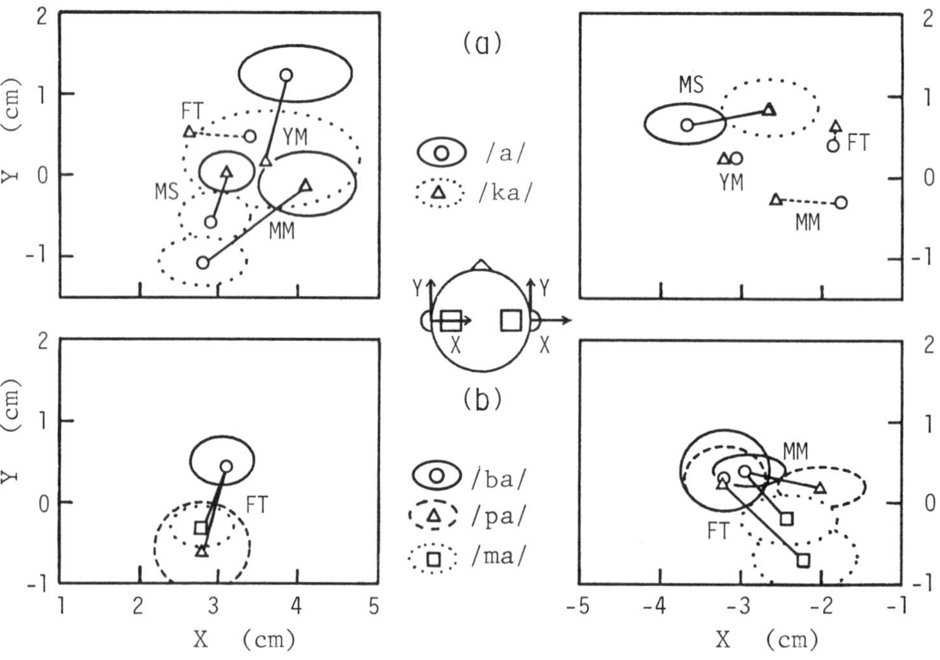

Fig.2. Location of N1m dipoles and 95% confidence region projected on a horizontal plane of two hemispheres, where origin (x=0, y=0) is the ear canal. Dipoles for /a/ and /ka/ syllables are shown in (a), and those for /ba/, /pa/, and /ma/ syllables are shown in (b).

RESULTS

From the responses in two subjects (ages 24 years), who were measured with all the stimuli of monosyllable sounds, peak latencies of the N1m and P2m components were evaluated. Figure 1 plots the averaged values of the peak latencies relative to the onset of the monosyllable sounds. Duration time of the consonant from its onset to the vowel onset determined visually from the waveform is also shown for comparison. The vowel /a/ and unvoiced plosives /ka/ and /pa/ have shorter peak latencies than voiced plosive /ba/ and nasal /ma/. The variation of the N1m and P2m latencies with different monosyllables does not follow the variation of the duration time of the consonant. This means that the N1m and P2m components are not evoked by the onset of the vowel. On the other hand, the shorter latencies of the vowel and unvoiced plosives than the voiced plosives and nasal indicate that the consonant onset solely does not evoke the N1m and P2m components. Acoustic structure of the consonant and the transition to the vowel may determine the evolution of the N1m and P2m components.

Parameters of a single current dipole of the N1m and P2m components were determined for all the monosyllables, except for a few cases where the responses had low signal-to-noise ratios due to small amplitudes. Locations of the computed dipoles were within an area 2-5 cm above and 1-4 cm posterior to the ear canal of both hemispheres. The depth of the dipoles from the scalp was 1.5-4 cm, indicating that they are located in the auditory cortex in the Sylvian fissure. 95% confidence limits were evaluated for these dipole locations along three coordinate axes fixed to each dipole. A part of the results on the dipole locations, including those of pure tones, will be published elsewhere.[4]

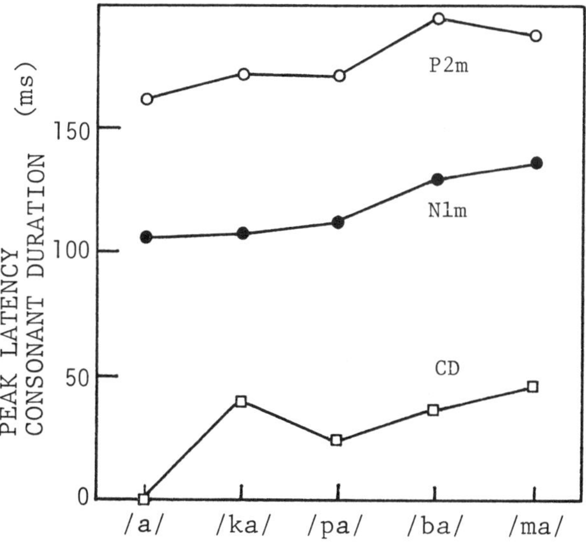

Fig.1. N1m and P2m latencies of the magnetic responses to different monosyllables and their consonant duration.

DISCUSSION

The variation of the N1m and P2m peak latencies in the magnetic responses to different consonants in Fig.1 is consistent with the results of previous study on the evoked potential.[5] Shorter latencies of N1 and P2 components are found in the potential responses to the consonant-vowels with unvoiced plosives than those with nasals and fricatives. These latency differences may be a consequence of differences in the energy, frequency, and their changes with time during a period between the consonant and the vowel. Therefore, the acoustic features are affecting the characteristics of the magnetic and potential responses.

We have measured spectrographs of the monosyllable sounds used in this work. The frequency spectrum and its change during the consonant-vowel transition, having a formant structure of vowel /a/, were similar between /pa/ and /ba/, but /pa/ was differentiated from /ba/ by a few sharp peaks at the consonant onset. Quite different spectrum was observed in /ma/. It had a component at a frequency of the second formant at the consonant onset and a subsequent long transition to the vowel. This component is probably associated with vibration of the vocal cords. On the other hand, /ka/ was characterized by a noise burst at the onset extending in wide frequencies.

The computed location of the dipole source of the auditory responses may represent a center of a population of neurons which are in active state. Then, the difference in dipole locations beyond the confidence region indicates that different areas are activated in the auditory cortex. In agreement with the clear difference in the spectrograph of the stimulus sounds, statistically significant difference was found in the horizontal dipole locations between /a/ and /ka/, and between /ma/ and /ba/. The significant location difference was also found between dipoles of /pa/ and /ba/, whose spectrographs differed slightly from each other. This sensitivity of the dipole location to the monosyllables having different acoustic characteristics implies that the neuromagnetic responses have a component specific to the consonant of speech sounds, and that the auditory cortex is involved in the neural process of speech sounds. In the superior-inferior direction no significant difference was found between these dipoles. This may be a consequence that the dipoles are located in the auditory cortex at the upper surface of the temporal lobe. The direction of the dipole current is nearly vertical, being downward for the N1m component and upward for the P2m component.[4]

REFERENCES

1. C.Pantev, M.Hoke, K.Lehnertz, B.Lütkenhöner, G.Anogianakis and W.Wittkowski, Tonotopic organization of the human auditory cortex revealed by transient auditory evoked magnetic fields, Electroenceph. clin. Neurophysiol.,69:160 (1988).
2. E.Kaukoranta, R.Hari and O.V.Lounasmaa, Responses of the human auditory cortex to vowel onset after fricative consonants, Exp. Brain Res.,69:19 (1987).
3. S.Kuriki, M.Murase and F.Takeuchi, Locating accuracy of a current source of neuromagnetic responses: simulation study for a single current dipole in a spherical conductor, Electroenceph. clin. Neurophysiol., to be published.
4. S.Kuriki and M.Murase, Neuromagnetic study of auditory responses in right and left hemispheres of the human brain evoked by pure tones and speech sounds, Exp. Brain Res., in press.
5. E.A.Lawson and A.W.K.Gaillard, Evoked potentials to consonant-vowel syllables, Acta Psychol., 49:17 (1981).

SHORT-LATENCY SOMATOSENSORY EVOKED MAGNETIC FIELDS RECORDED OVER THE BRACHIAL PLEXUS AND CERVICAL SPINE IN MAN

G. Curio, S.N.Erné*, J. Sandforth,
J. Scheer*, R. Stehr, and L. Trahms*

Depts. of Neurology
Universitätsklinika Steglitz/ R.Virchow, Berlin
*Physikalisch-Technische Bundesanstalt (PTB)
Institut Berlin

INTRODUCTION

Recently, non-invasive magnetic field measurements of evoked peripheral nerve activity in man have been reported (1,2,3). In this paper, recordings from the centripetal conduction path of this activity will be presented, with a focus on the spinal segmental dorsal horn generator ("P13") postulated by Desmedt (4) having a peak latency inter-individually varying between 12.6 and 15.0 ms (5). Concerning magnetic recordings from the dorsal neck, mainly late magnetic cervical somatosensory activity has been reported so far (6,7,8). Recently, a possible recording of early magnetic responses at the dorsal neck has been mentioned (2). In this study, considering the assumed dorsoventral orientation of the P13-generator, we scanned above the lateral neck in order to detect magnetic activity correlated to the P13-component of the spinal SEP.

EXPERIMENTAL PROCEDURE

The measurements were obtained upon conventional repetitive median nerve stimulation at the wrist (cathode proximal) with a rectangular constant current pulse of 0.1 ms duration (intensity just above the motor threshold) and 11/s repetition rate. Each run consisted of at least 4000 stimuli with up to 4 replications. The measurements were performed in the Berlin magnetically shielded room with the subject lying either on his left (right) side for recordings over the right (left) lateral neck, or in a prone (supine) position for recordings with the coil coplanar to the dorsal neck (Erb's point). The magnetic sensor was a single channel rf SQUID magnetometer having a 5 turn, 38 mm diameter pick-up coil and a white noise level of less than 8 $fT/\sqrt{Hz}$. Analog filtering was performed between 5 Hz (-3db, RC first order filters) and 1500 Hz (-3db, Bessel-filters 8th order). The sampling rate was 10 kHz. Electrical recordings of brachial plexus activity were obtained using conventional cup electrodes filled with electrode jelly, placed over Erb's point and referenced to the contralateral hand; for spinal recordings, an anterior to posterior neck derivation (larynx to spinous process of C6) was used. Impedances were below 5 kOhm; the ground electrode was located at the ipsilateral forearm.

Advances in Biomagnetism
Edited by S.J. Williamson *et al.*
Plenum Press, New York

RESULTS

a) Evoked Fields from Plexus Brachialis

Electrical SEP recordings from Erb's point show that in the investigated subject plexus activity occurs at about 11 ms (Fig. 1a). The magnetic field of 50 fT amplitude due to this activity was recorded near Erb's point (Fig. 1b). Similar to the peripheral nerve measurements of this subject (not shown), it exhibits a biphasic waveform with a small second lobe around 13 ms. In most of the magnetic recordings taken near the lower neck, this activity was picked up: in fig. 1c the magnetic field recorded at the dorsal lower neck is shown. Its amplitude depends critically on the geometric relation between coil and neck axis: Even slight re-adjustments of coil position could induce large changes in the amplitude of plexus-related fields.

b) Spinal Activity

Based on the hypothesis of a segmental dorsal horn SEP generator (4) with a dorsoventral direction of the intracellular current, the extremum of the corresponding magnetic field is expected at the upper lateral neck. The measurements of figs. 1e and 1f were taken with a mirror-like geometric arrangement of the set-up: 1e (1f) was recorded at the right (left) upper neck upon stimulation at the right (left) wrist. Fig. 1g shows the recording at the left upper neck upon right median nerve stimulation. In all of these cases, the temporal evolution of the magnetic field closely resembles the wave form of the spinal SEP, peaking around 15 ms for this subject (Fig. 1d). In addition, some later magnetic activity was found which in part coincides in time with the primary cortical response; its topography differed from spinal activity in that it could be measured also at the dorsal upper neck (not shown). Recordings from dorsal lower neck did not show any magnetic activity above the noise level at the latency of the early spinal response (Fig. 1c).

DISCUSSION

After median nerve stimulation, early somatosensory evoked magnetic activity can be recorded around the lower and upper neck.

a) Activity at plexus latency was observed around the lower neck. As for the peripheral nerve, the time evolution of the magnetic compound action field at the proximal plexus can be mono- or biphasic, depending on the investigated subject. Since the second lobe (at "spinal" latencies) of plexus related magnetic activity could be superimposed on true spinal activity, plexus activity has to be differentiated against intrinsic spinal fields, for example, by mapping over the ipsi- and contralateral neck.

b) For median nerve stimulation, the equivalent current dipole of P13 is assumed to be located at about the medullary segments C5/6 less than 1 cm lateral of the center of the neck and to point from posterior to anterior with a slight component in the contralateral direction (4,5,9). Accordingly, the corresponding magnetic field should be directed inward at the left upper neck and outward at the right one. This prediction is confirmed by the polarity reversal evident in figs. 1e and 1f/g. Due to the slight asymmetries of the generator location and direction, the corresponding magnetic field cannot be expected to be symmetric with respect to the symmetry plane of the neck. In order to demonstrate a polarity reversal without distortions due to this asymmetry, we have selected recordings with mirror-like arrangements of both sensor and stimulator for figs. 1e and 1f.

Notably, brainstem generators (e.g. cuneate nucleus, medial lemniscus (10)) and possible subcortical generators (thalamus, thalamocortical radiation (11)) may in addition be active during the activation of the spinal P13-generator. Two arguments in favor of a spinal origin of the magnetic field are the similar temporal evolution of early magnetic and spinal electric signals, and the onset latency of the first magnetic peak, which closely fits the sum of proximal plexus latency and one synaptic delay. Activity

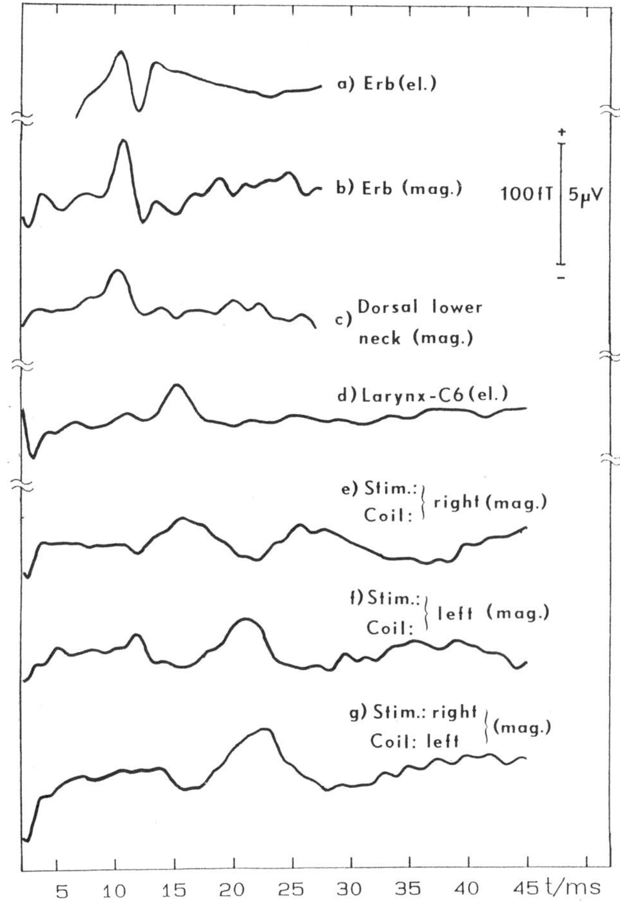

Fig. 1 Upon median nerve stimulation, electric (a) and magnetic (b) recordings near Erb's point show distinct plexus related activity, which is also picked up at the dorsal lower neck (c). SEP from an anterior to posterior neck derivation (d) identifies the spinal P13 component with a peak latency of 15 ms. Evoked magnetic fields recorded over the right (e) and left (f,g) upper neck show the corresponding activity with a characteristic polarity reversal. All recordings are digitally filtered between 20 and 500 Hz.

later than P13 might also be due to spinal generators (9), but at this latency some cerebral activity (even from the contralateral hemisphere) could be picked up by the magnetometer.

CONCLUSIONS

Upon median nerve stimulation, early evoked magnetic fields can be recorded near the cervical spine in man: (a) Plexus-related magnetic activity can be detected near the lower neck and needs to be taken into account when interpreting signals considered to be of spinal origin; (b) For the first time, the magnetic field generated by the segmental dorsal horn generator postulated by Desmedt (4) was detected, showing a polarity reversal across the upper lateral neck in agreement with the assumed dorsoventral direction of the intracellular current.

REFERENCES

1. S.N. Erné, G. Curio, L. Trahms, Z. Trontelj and P. Aust: Magnetic activity of a single peripheral nerve in man, in: "Biomagnetism 87", K. Atsumi, M. Kotani, S. Ueno, T. Katila and S.J. Willamson, eds., Tokyo Denki University Press, Tokyo (1988).
2. R. Hari, J. Hällström, J.Tiihonen and S.-L. Joutsiniemi: Multichannel detection of magnetic compound action fields of median and ulnar nerves, Electroenceph. clin. Neurophysiol. **72**; 277 (1989).
3. L. Trahms, S.N. Erné, Z. Trontelj, G. Curio and P. Aust: Biomagnetic functional localization of a peripheral nerve in man, Biophys. J. **55**; 1145 (1989).
4. J.E. Desmedt: Topographic mapping of generators of somatosensory evoked potentials, in: "Topographic Brain Mapping of EEG and Evoked Potentials", K. Maurer, ed., Springer Verlag , Berlin (1989).
5. Y.T. Hallström, U. Lindblom, B.A.Meyerson and T.S. Prevec: Epidurally recorded cervical spinal activity evoked by electrical and mechanical stimulation in pain patients, Electroenceph. clin. Neurophysiol. **74**, 177 (1989).
6. Y. Mizutani and S. Kuriki: Somatically evoked magnetic fields in the vicinity of the neck, IEEE-BME **33**; 510 (1986).
7. S. Kuriki and Y. Mizutani: Magnetic responses evoked in cervical cord and brain by somatic stimulation, in: cf. 1 (1988).
8. Y. Mizutani and S. Kuriki: Spinal evoked fields at neck by mixed and sensory nerve stimulations of various frequencies, in: cf. 1 (1988).
9. D. Jeanmonod, M. Sindou and F. Mauguière: Three transverse dipolar generators in the human cervical and lumbo-sacral dorsal horn: evidence from direct recordings on the spinal cord surface, Electroenceph. clin. Neurophsiol. **74**, 236 (1989).
10. I. Suzuki and Y. Mayanagi: Intracranial recording of short latency somatosensory evoked potentials in man: identification of origin of each component. Electroenceph. clin. Neurophsiol. **59**, 286 (1984)
11. P.M. Rossini, M. Cilli, L. Narici, M. Peresson, V. Pizzella, G.L. Romani, C. Salustri, R. Traversa and S.D. Luzio: Short-latency somatosensory evoked responses to median nerve stimulation: differences between electric and magnetic scalp recordings, in: cf. 1 (1988)

INTRAOPERATIVE RECORDING OF THE MAGNETIC FIELD OF A HUMAN NERVE

John P. Wikswo[1], W. Patrick Henry[1], Richard N. Friedman[1], Anthony W. Kilroy[2], Ranjith S. Wijesinghe[1], Jan M. van Egeraat[1] and Michael A. Milek[3]

[1]Department of Physics and Astronomy, Vanderbilt University Nashville, TN 37235, U.S.A.
[2]Department of Neurology, and [3]Department of Orthopedics and Rehabilitation, Vanderbilt University School of Medicine

INTRODUCTION

Accurate, quantitative assessment of nerve function during surgical procedures has been impeded by inherent limitations of extracellular electrophysiological recording techniques. Extracellular recordings are hampered by critical constraints on electrode placement, uncertainty in the conductivity of the moist layer on the outside of the nerve, and the risks involved in the essential elevation of the nerve in the air for recording. Our laboratory has developed a neuromagnetic current probe system that affords room- or body-temperature recording of magnetic signals as small as one millionth of the earth's magnetic field strength. In addition, we have designed and constructed an 'openable,' toroidal magnetic probe that can be placed around a nerve to assess the magnetic field arising from the electrical current flow within the active axons and across their membranes. A mathematical deconvolution model allows determination of the types and number of axons contributing to a compound nerve signal. Wikswo (1989) lists key references.

METHODS

The above developments made it possible to record the magnetic field from patients undergoing surgical section of the flexor retinaculum for decompression of the carpal tunnel. The median nerve was exposed proximal to the flexor retinaculum and followed distally to demonstrate the lateral and medial branches. Only a short segment (approximately 2 cm) of the nerve proximal to the flexor retinaculum was elevated into the air for stimulus application. The remainder of the nerve was immersed in physiological saline for the duration of the recording procedure. The nerve was stimulated at the elevated section with a 2.0 mA, 100 μs pulse applied by an electrophysiological stimulator (Grass) via stainless steel needle electrodes. The magnetic signal was recorded digitally (Acurex MDAS-7000) using an openable toroid positioned in the palm 6.0 cm distal to the stimulus electrodes. The measuring bandwidth was 1 Hz to 10 KHz. The recorded waveform (see Figure 1a.) is the average of 64 consecutive recordings made during a 22 second interval of 3 Hz stimulation. To suppress line frequency artifacts, each waveform to be averaged was triggered an odd number of 60 Hz half-cycles after the preceding trigger. A 2 μA, 1 ms calibration pulse preceded each

Advances in Biomagnetism
Edited by S.J. Williamson *et al.*
Plenum Press, New York

recording. In the reported case, the surgical procedure was accomplished with hemostasis assisted by a tourniquet inflated to 250 mmHg pressure around the upper arm. Recordings were made prior to and after section of the flexor retinaculum and deflation of the tourniquet. The conductivity of the saline bathing the nerve was assessed (YSI Model 35 conductivity meter) and corrected for the 31°C recording temperature.

The averaged waveform was analyzed using a mathematical deconvolution model developed in our laboratory (Wijesinghe, et al., 1989). In this model, the compound action current (CAC) is a sum of single fiber action currents (SFACs):

$$CAC(t_k,\ell) = \sum_{i=1}^{M} a_i \; SFAC_i\{t_k-\tau_i,\ell/(\tau_i-T_i)\} . \qquad (1)$$

t_k is the kth equally-spaced discrete time point in the CAC; ℓ is the propagation distance; M is the number of bins in the arrival time distribution (ATD); a_i is the number of fibers in the ith bin of the ATD; τ_i is the delay of the ith bin of the ATD; and T_i is the delay of the ith bin due to the virtual cathode effect (Wiederholt, 1970) and activation time. This equation can be used to determine a conduction velocity distribution histogram that provides an index of the number and type of viable axons in the nerve. Table 1 shows the parameters used in the deconvolution model as best available estimates for analysis of the magnetically-recorded nerve action current data obtained in this study.

RESULTS

Figure 1a shows the results of a representative experimental trial under the conditions described in the figure legend. The peak-to-peak amplitude of the CAC is 0.65 μA. The conduction velocity calculated from the stimulus artifact to the onset of the compound action current is 55 m/s. Pre-operative electrophysiological assessment in the clinic indicated a normal conduction velocity. Figure 1b shows the nerve CAC extracted from the trace in Fig. 1a by using appropriate scaling and offset corrections. The data of this trace were analyzed by applying the deconvolution model to determine the fiber composition of the nerve bundle. The histogram (Figure 2) generated by this calculation indicates the distribution of the number of fibers as a function of the conduction velocity of the fiber class. The total number of fibers was 8,652.

Table 1. Values of Deconvolution Model Parameters

Parameter	Value
Volume Fraction	0.63
Toroid Outer Radius	6.33 mm
Toroid Inner Radius	3.78 mm
Toroid Thickness	6.5 mm
Nerve Bundle Radius	2.0 mm
Nerve Sheath Thickness	0.4 mm
Propagation Distance	60 mm
Intercellular Conductivity	0.25 $\Omega^{-1}m^{-1}$
Extracellular Conductivity	1.25 $\Omega^{-1}m^{-1}$
Sheath Conductivity	8.37 $\Omega^{-1}m^{-1}$
Membrane Effective Resistance x Unit Area	4.80 Ωm^2
Membrane Effective Capacitance / Unit Area	2.7×10^{-5} Fm^{-2}
Temperature	31°C

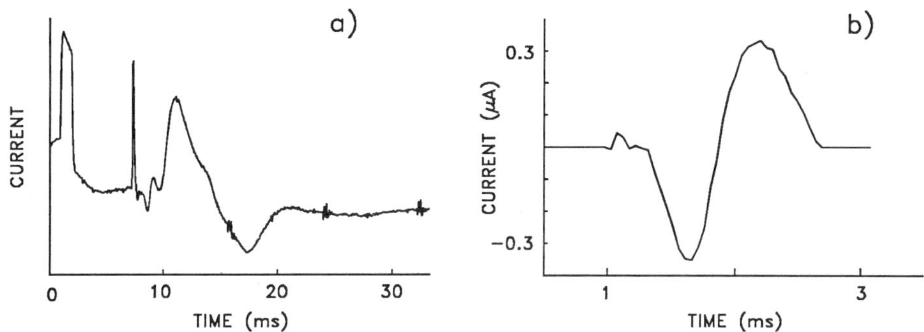

Fig. 1. The first intraoperative recording of the magnetic field of a human median nerve. a) A 2 μA, 1 ms calibration pulse precedes a sharp stimulus artifact followed by a biphasic nerve signal and finally by a large, biphasic muscle signal. Several line frequency artifacts are evident. (64 averages; 3 Hz stimulus rate). b) Nerve action current isolated from 1a with appropriate offset and scaling.

DISCUSSION

The 55.0 m/s conduction velocity indicated by the data falls at the lower end of the 55 - 73 m/s velocity range expected for the sensory (fastest) fibers of the 31-year-old patient (Hammer, 1982). At least four factors may account for a depressed conduction velocity, including age, temperature, interrupted circulation, and disease processes. Optimally, all of these parameters except the last should be known and used in applying the model. Age-related changes in conduction velocity have been well-established by EMG studies on humans (Kimura, 1978). The more quantitative, physical effects of temperature on nerve conduction properties are also well understood (Kimura, 1984). The clinical interest in avoiding ischemic damage to tissue during surgical procedures requiring tourniquet use for hemostasis has generated several papers on alterations in nerve function and structure resulting from prolonged interruption of the circulation (Rorabeck, 1980). Future magnetic studies may contribute to understanding of the mechanism(s) of progressive ischemic changes and may be helpful in establishing tourniquet application pressure/time safety limits, which are not well understood. The relative stability and ease of use of the present neuromagnetic current probe system should provide surgeons a means of monitoring the 'well-being' of the nerve during prolonged tourniquet application.

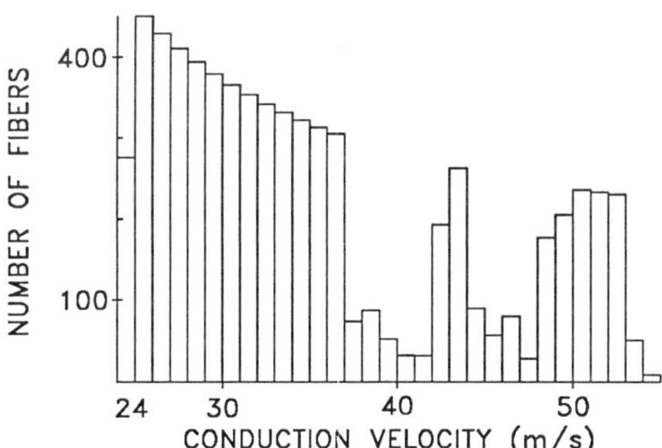

Figure 2. Conduction velocity distribution of human median nerve fibers in the palm, immediately distal to the nerve's exit from the carpal tunnel. This distribution was derived from the intraoperatively-recorded magnetic signal shown in Fig. 1.

By applying our deconvolution model to analyze the waveform shown in Fig 1a, we obtained an estimate of 8,652 fibers in the branch of the median nerve encircled by the magnetic probe. Unfortunately, we have been unable to locate histological information available on the number of fibers in the branch we studied. However, based on a fiber count of approximately 6,500 (between 5,500 and 7,500) for the median nerve just proximal to the flexor retinaculum (Rosenfalk, 1966), and considering that the median nerve divides into at least three branches proximal to the recording site, our model may be overestimating the number of viable fibers by a factor of ~4. This discrepancy is most likely due to systematic errors in our calculation due to improper assumptions about the parameters listed in Table 1, or to inaccuracies in the available information on these parameters.

Because the inaccuracies in the parameters have an even greater negative impact on conventional electrical measurements used in clinical determinations, the problem of quantitative description of the number of fibers could not be addressed previously. This problem had to be avoided by normalizing the histogram to a unit area and making decisions about the status of nerves based on the relative shapes of the distributions. When the parameters are corrected, the magnetic technique will provide a more quantitative approach and should afford accurate descriptions of the actual number of functional fibers present. To examine the source of the error(s) in the parameters, we are performing histological analyses on cadaver specimens of the studied nerve branch to gain quantitative information on the fiber number and diameter distributions as well as the fiber radii, sheath thickness and intercellular spaces. Also, combining electric measurements of voltage and magnetic measurements of current may allow us to achieve a more accurate estimate of the intracellular conductivity, the most influential parameter with the largest uncertainty (Wijesinghe, 1989).

The presented results demonstrate the effectiveness of the neuromagnetic probe system for intraoperative nerve recording in humans. Magnetic field recording should increase the accuracy and safety of intraoperative recording and encourage surgeons to take advantage of this information in making decisions for selecting nerve repair strategies. The neuromagnetic probe makes practical the intraoperative assessment of nerve damage resulting from a variety of accidents and/or pathologies and should be a valuable contribution to the surgeons' armamentarium for relieving many of these disorders.

ACKNOWLEDGEMENT

This work was supported in part by NIH Grant NS 19794.

REFERENCES

Buchthal, F. and Rosenfalk, A., 1966, Sensory potentials and conduction velocity in human sensory nerves, Brain Res., 3:1-122.

Hammer, C., 1982, "Nerve Conduction Studies," C.C.Thomas, Springfield, IL

Kimura, J., 1978, Method for determining median nerve conduction velocity across the carpal tunnel, J. Neurol. Sci., 38:1-10.

Kimura, J., 1984, Nerve conduction studies and electromyography, in: "Peripheral Neuropathy," P. J. Dyck, P. K. Thomas, E.H. Lambert, and R. Bunge, eds., W. B. Saunders, Philadelphia.

Rorabeck, C. H., 1980, Tourniquet-induced nerve ischemia: an experimental investigation, J. Trauma, 20:280-286.

Wiederholt, W. C., 1970, Threshold and conduction velocity in isolated mixed mammalian nerves, Neurology (Minneap.), 20:347-352.

Wijesinghe, R.S., Gielen, F.L.H. and Wikswo, J.P., Jr., 1989, (submitted).

Wikswo, J.P., Jr., 1988, Magnetic techniques for evaluating peripheral nerve function, in: "Proceedings of a Special Symposium on Maturing Technologies and Emerging Horizons in Biomedical Engineering," J. B. Myklebust, and G. F. Harris, eds., IEEE, Pistcataway, NJ.

A COMPARATIVE STUDY OF COMPOUND ACTION POTENTIALS AND CURRENTS

K.W. Kim, D.J. Engle, and R.J. Sclabassi

Departments of Neurological Surgery and Electrical Engineering
University of Pittsburgh, Pittsburgh PA 15260

INTRODUCTION

The recording of compound action potentials (CAPs) from peripheral nerves is a routine clinical investigative procedure in the operating room. Parameters such as amplitude, area, conduction velocity, and latency are used as measures for the functional integrety of the nerve. Pathology produces reduction in conduction velocities, desynchronization of compound nerve action potentials and, in severe disease, complete conduction block, leading to observable changes in these measurements. A number of technical difficulties exist which produce distortions in this data. For example, reliable and repeatable measurements of these parameters require careful electrodes placement. Also, changes in nerve moistness produces conductivity changes. These factors affect the amplitudes of the CAPs producing errors in the measured data (Wikswo et al, 1985).

Recently, a new technology for measuring compound action currents (CACs), using a toriod and a low input impedance amplifier, has been developed (Wikswo et al, 1983). This technology has been applied to the median nerve of the macaca fasicularis primate (Wikswo et al, 1985), *in vitro* bull frog sciatic nerves and earthworm nerve cords (Wijesinghe, 1988), and a lobster and a crayfish axon (Roth and Wikswo, 1985).

This study was designed to systematically measure and compare the properties of CAPs and CACs recorded from the *in vivo* sciatic nerve of a dog. The CAC data were obtained in preparation for applying the magnetic technique to human nerves in the operating room.

METHODS

Sixteen, 20 kilogram, adult mongrel dogs were studied. Both CAPs and CACs were measured for a variety of stimulating and recording parameters. The animals were anesthetized using a balanced narcotic technique. The sciatic nerve located on top of the semimembranous muscle, and approximately twelve centimeters in length was isolated. A deep tissue pocket was created overlying the exposed portion of the nerve.

The stimulation procedures were identical for recording both the CAPs and the CACs. Bipolar stimulating electrodes were positioned at the proximal or the distal end of the nerve, with recordings obtained for both conditions. The stimulus was applied from a constant voltage device with a constant width of 0.01 *ms*, and the stimulus frequency was maintained at 50 *Hz*. The data were acquired under computer control, with a sampling rate of 25 *kHz*.

Advances in Biomagnetism
Edited by S.J. Williamson *et al.*
Plenum Press, New York

For CAP recordings, a bipolar pair of wire electrodes, each 200 microns in diameter, were utilized. The bipolar electrodes were positioned under the nerve and used to lift the nerve away from the surrounding tissue during CAP recording. The signals were amplified with the gain adjusted between 200 and 1000 and the bandwidth was 10 to 10,000 *Hz*. The system readout was calibrated in *uVolts*. For CAC recordings, a toroid was positioned around the nerve, and the induced voltage was passed through the low impedance amplifier and processed in the same fashion as the CAPs. Signal strength was calibrated in *uAmps*.

For CAP recordings, the tissue pocket surrounding the exposed nerve was clear of excessive fluid; however, the nerve was maintained in a moist state. For CAC recordings, the pocket was filled with fluid at room temperature, with saline solution covering the nerve at a depth sufficient to completely submerge the nerve in the region where the recording toroid was located. The stimulating electrodes were not submerged in the fluid bath.

Descriptive parameters measured included polarity of the initial wave, area under the negative wave, area under the positive wave, width of the negative wave, width of the positive wave, peak negative amplitude, peak positive amplitude, latency to the peak negative wave, latency to the peak positive wave, and nerve diameter midway between the recording and the stimulating sites.

The data were statistically analyzed using the BMDP-6D package. Linear regressions were obtained between various descriptive parameters for both the PD and the DP conditions. A significance level of 0.05 was used in all cases to reject the null hypothesis that correlation coefficients were zero.

RESULTS

100 CAPs and 250 CACs were recorded. Of these, 50 CAPs and 183 CACs were analyzed. The remainder were discarded for technical reasons. For example, some of the measured CAC data drifted at one end, making it difficult to measure the parameters; some CAP data were embedded in stimulus artifact. The distance from the stimulating to the recording site was varied systematically between 2.5 cm and 8.0 cm. Data were obtained with both the stimulating electrodes distal and the recording device proximal (DP), and the stimulating electrodes proximal and the recording device distal (PD). Nerve diameters ranged from 0.30 *cm* to 0.60 *cm*. The averaged nerve diameter for all animals was 0.46 *cm*. CAP and CAC data appeared to be independent of nerve diameter if the proportional distribution of individual nerve fibers with different diameters is maintained across total nerve diameter.

Analysis of Compound Action Currents

For the PD condition, both the positive and the negative peak amplitudes decreased as distance increased. The slopes of the regression lines were -0.12 and -0.14 *uAmps/cm* respectively. While for the DP condition, only the peak positive amplitude decreased significantly as distance increased (slope=-0.44 *uAmps/cm*). The width of the positive wave increased significantly with distance for both conditions, with a slope of 0.07 and 0.09 *ms/cm* respectively in the regression line. All other conditions demonstrated insignificant regression coefficients.

Peak amplitude was analyzed as a function of changes in width. For the PD condition, the negative peak amplitude decreased significantly with the width of the negative wave (slope=-2.10 *uAmps/ms*). While for the DP condition, the peak positive amplitude decreased significantly with the width of the positive wave (slope=-5.20 *uAmps/ms*). No significant correlations were noted for all other conditions.

The positive area decreased as a function of distance for the DP condition, with a linear regression slope of -3.55 *uAmps.ms/cm*. No significant correlations were noted for all other conditions.

Both latencies of the positive and the negative peak amplitudes increased significantly as distance increased for both test conditions. The slopes for the PD condition were 0.14 and 0.09 *ms/cm* respectively, while the slopes for the DP condition were 0.15 and 0.21 *ms/cm* respectively.

Analysis of Compound Action Potentials

For the DP condition, the negative peak amplitude significantly decreased as a function of distance with the slope of the regression line being -61.40 *uVolts/cm*. None of the remaining peak positive amplitudes varied significantly as a function of distance. This appeared to be due to the high level of variability in the data. For the PD condition, the width of the positive wave increased significantly as a function of distance with slope being 0.33 *ms/cm*. For the DP condition, the width of the positive wave increased significantly as a function of distance (slope=0.11 *ms/cm*), while the width of the negative wave decreased significantly as distance increased (slope = -0.49 *ms/cm*).

The area of the positive wave increased signficantly with distance for the PD condition having a slope of 1.10 *uVolts.ms/cm*. However, the area of the negative wave did not change significantly with distance. The negative area for the DP condition significantly decreased as a function of distance (slope=-3.46 *uVolts.ms/cm*), while the positive area did not vary significantly with distance.

No significant differences were noted for peak ampitudes as a function of width, nor for latency as a function of distance for either test condition. Again, this finding appeared to depend on the high variability in the data.

Descriptive Parameters

Complete descriptive parameters for CACs and CAPs are listed in tabular form. The data shown were for the PD (CACs) and the DP (CAPs) conditions after averaging with same polarity.

Table 1

Compound Action Current (PD)

Dist (*cm*)	-Area (*uAmps.ms*)	+Area (*uAmps.ms*)	-Wdt (*ms*)	+Wdt (*ms*)	-Amp (*uAmps*)	+Amp (*uAmps*)	-Lat (*ms*)	+Lat (*ms*)
2.0	2.90	4.70	0.55	0.80	1.44	1.31	4.63	5.03
2.5	9.38	12.36	0.48	0.93	1.99	0.91	4.79	4.85
3.0	9.96	12.70	0.52	0.99	1.84	0.81	4.76	5.07
3.5	8.29	11.62	0.49	1.00	2.09	0.98	4.76	5.23
4.0	8.93	17.20	0.50	0.91	1.79	1.03	4.92	5.10
4.5	13.01	5.33	0.63	0.72	2.02	0.68	4.80	5.27
5.0	8.49	9.18	0.72	0.78	1.23	0.67	5.04	5.41
5.5	5.75	6.33	0.73	0.93	1.13	0.57	5.05	5.53
6.0	5.26	8.96	0.75	0.95	1.18	0.77	5.11	5.61
6.5	6.48	4.85	0.70	1.00	1.10	0.40	5.40	6.00
7.0	15.10	10.18	0.88	1.20	1.21	0.40	5.36	6.00
7.5	3.61	11.75	0.60	1.05	1.06	0.60	5.10	5.60
8.0	4.74	10.88	0.50	1.57	1.42	0.39	4.87	5.37

Table 2

Compound Action Potential (DP)

Dist. (cm)	-Area ($mVolts.ms$)	+Area ($mVolts.ms$)	-Wdt (ms)	+Wdt (ms)	-Amp ($uVolts$)	+Amp ($uVolts$)	-Lat (ms)	+Lat (ms)
3.5	3.60	0.06	0.70	0.50	371.10	39.11	5.20	5.90
5.0	1.95	0.62	0.40	0.60	681.80	146.60	4.80	5.20
6.0	1.34	3.63	0.49	1.10	413.00	206.40	5.04	5.50
6.5	1.70	4.20	0.60	1.90	236.70	153.70	5.20	5.90
7.0	2.00	3.55	0.75	1.45	644.20	142.70	5.20	5.90
7.5	4.00	3.70	0.80	1.60	559.10	224.10	5.20	5.80

DISCUSSION

CAPs have been routinely measured clinically to determine the degree of pathology in human peripheral nerve. Measurements of this type are used during surgery to decide if a damaged perpipheral nerve should undergo lysis or have a graft placed. Technical difficulties make this data difficult to interpret, thus the need for more robust measurement techniques. This study was undertaken to define the comparative properties of CAPs and CACs in an animal model prior to the utilization of the CAC technique in the operating room on human peripheral nerve.

From the above analysis of the PD condition, six parameter relationships are correlated significantly for CAC: amplitudes and latencies with distance, positive width with distance, and negative amplitude with width. But for CAP, only two parameter relationships are correlated significantly: positive width with distance and positive area with distance. For the analysis of the DP condition, CAC has six parameter relationships which correlate significantly: positive amplitude with distance, positive width with distance, positive area with distance, positive amplitude with width, and latencies of peak amplitudes with distance. Whereas for CAP, four parameter relationships are correlated significantly: negative amplitude, negative width, negative area, and positive width with distance. Totally, twelve CAC and six CAP parameter relationships are linearly correlated significantly. Therefore, the magnetic technique appears to provide more stable data than the electric technique.

ACKNOWLEDGEMENTS

This research was supported by NIH Grants NS 19794 to Dachling Pang, Department of Neurosurgery, University of Pittsburgh, and NS 23110 to John P. Wikswo, Living States Physics Laboratory, Department of Physics and Astronomy, Vanderbilt University, Children's Hospital of Pittsburgh, and the Copeland Fund of the Department of Neurological Surgery, University of Pittsburgh.

REFERENCES

B.J. Roth, and J.P. Wikswo, Jr., "Magnetic field of a single nerve axon: a comparison of theory and experiment," Biophysical Journal, 48:43-109(1985).

Wijesinghe, R.S., "Comparison of electric and magnetic techniques for the determination of conduction velocity distributions of nerve bundles," Ph.D. dissertation, Department of Physics and Astronomy, Vanberbilt University, Nashville TN (1988).

Wikswo, Jr., J.P., PC. Samson, and R.P. Giffard, "A low-noise low input impedance amplifier for magnetic measurements of nerve action currents," IEEE. Trans. Biomed. Eng., BME-30:215-221 (1983)

Wikswo, Jr., J.P., G.S. Abraham, and V.R. Hentz, "Magnetic assessment of regeneration across a nerve graft," in Biomagnetism Theory and Applications, H. Weinberg, G. Stroink, and K. Katila (Eds), Pergamon Press, pp 88-92 (1985).

ESTIMATION OF BOTH CONDUCTION VELOCITIES AND THE NUMBER OF FIRING NERVE FIBERS FROM MAGNETIC FIELDS OUTSIDE A VOLUME CONDUCTOR

Shoogo Ueno and Shuntaro Suzuki

Department of Electronics
Kyushu University
Fukuoka, 812, Japan

INTRODUCTION

In neuromagnetism study, it is important to know the relationship between magnetic fields produced by firing nerve fibers and the sources of action currents. Wikswo et al.(1980,1986) succeeded in estimating equivalent dipole sources of action currents by a transformer technique in which a ferrite toroidal core was introduced. In Wikswo's method, however, nerve bundle and the ferrite toroid should be interlinked to detect signals related to action currents. In the present report, we propose a method for estimating both conduction velocities and the number of firing nerve fibers from data of magnetic fields observed outside the body. Apart from neuromagnetism study, Barker et al. (1979a,1979b) reported a method for determining the distributions of conduction velocities within the alpha fiber group in human peripheral nerve trunks based on the analysis of the shape of compound action potentials recorded from surface electrodes. The method in the present report is useful for estimating both conduction velocities and the number of sources of which velocities distribute in a wide range.

METHOD

The inverse problem discussed here is shown in Fig. 1. A nerve bundle is located in a semi-infinite volume conductor with a uniform conductivity, and runs along the direction in parallel to the surface of the boundary. When action potentials propagate along fibers, magnetic fields can be produced outside the conductor. The magnetic field component normal to surface of the boundaly has no contribution from the volume current (Cohen and Hosaka, 1976). The waveforms of normal component of magnetic fields are due only to the current sources modeled by twin-dipole. We assume that the propagation of nerve excitation occurs independently in each fiber without any interaction among fibers.

Let us estimate both conduction velocities and the number of firing fibers from given waveforms at points a and b.

We introduce a "model waveform" which is a temporal change of magnetic fields produced by a traveling source of which conduction velocity is known.

As a simple case, we can estimate both conduction velocity and the number of sources of which velocities are the same. The number of sources, i.e., the number of firing fibers are estimated from the amplitude of the waveforms, adjusting the peak value of the model waveform. The conduction

Advances in Biomagnetism
Edited by S.J. Williamson *et al.*
Plenum Press, New York

velocity is determined from the time lag between the measured points. Once the conduction velocity and the number of sources are determined, the correct shape of waveform is obtained, adjusting both amplitude and duration of the model waveform. The amplitude increases in proportion to the number of sources, whereas the wave width i.e. duration, decreases in proportion to the velocity as shown in Fig. 2.

We apply this method to estimation of both conduction velocities and the number of sources. The procedure is shown in Fig.3. Decomposing the waveforms into each wave, sources of each group can be estimated. The procedure is given below.

(i) Estimate conduction velocities and the number of sources of the fastest group.

(ii) Obtain the shape of the fastest waveform.

(iii) Subtract the fastest wave component from the whole waveform.

(iv) As a result, the waveform excluding the fastest wave component is obtained.

(v) Repeat the procedure (i)-(iv) for estimation of the second and third components.

In subtracting process, it is essential to determine phase of wave components exactly.

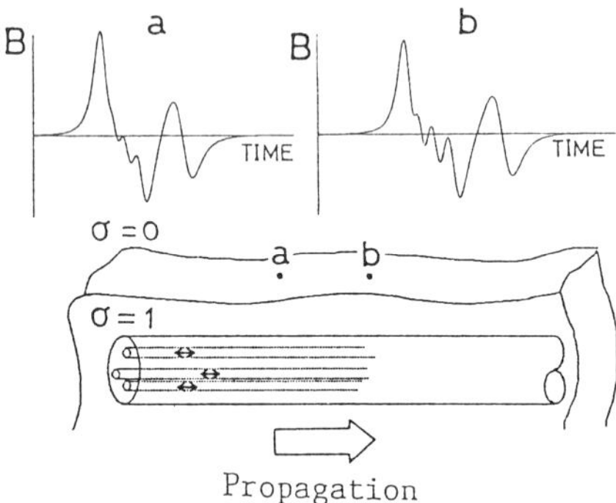

Fig. 1 Equivalent current dipole sources of compound action potentials of a nerve bundle and the produced magnetic field components normal to the surface of a semi-infinite volume conductor.

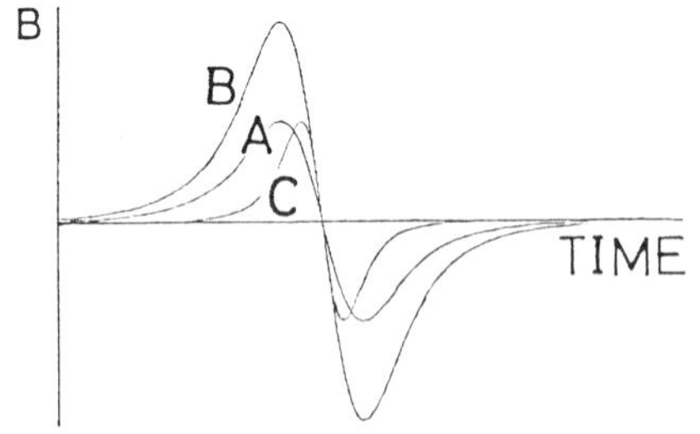

Fig. 2 Model waveforms. Velocities and the number of fibers are 20m/s, 10 for A, 20m/s, 20 for B, and 40m/s, 10 for C.

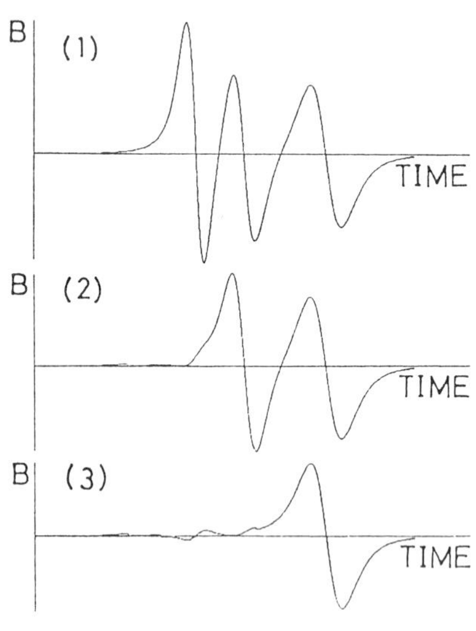

Fig. 3 Decomposition of waveforms for estimation of group velocities and the number of fibers. "Observed waveform" (1) consists of three wave components of which velocities are 50m/s 40m/s and 30m/s, and number of fibers 700, 500, 400, respectively. Subtracting the first wave component, the 2nd and 3rd wave components are obtained as show in (2). Finally, the 3rd wave component is obtained.

RESULTS AND DISCUSSION

The current sources are modeled by twin-dipoles. Each twin-dipole consists of two oppositely oriented dipoles which are located 0.01m apart from each other. The intensity of dipole moment is chosen 1.0×10^{-15} A·m. The nerve bundle is located 20mm under the surface. The measuring points a and b in Fig.1 are located 12mm anterior to the vertical plane which stands in the direction perpendicular to the boundary surface and passes the central axis of the nerve bundle. The distance between two observed points is 50mm. The model waveform is assumed to be generated by 10 sources which propagate at a constant velocity 20m/s. The sampling time is 1.0×10^{-5} sec.

Let us estimate both conduction velocities and the number of sources in the case shown in Fig. 3. "Observed waveform" (1) consists of three wave components of which velocities are 50m/s, 40m/s and 30m/s. The number of sources 700, 500 and 400, respectively.

The conduction velocities were correctly estimated, and the number of sources of each group was estimated 720, 510 and 390, respectively. The estimation error was around 3%, which was mainly due to the overlapping of waves.

The estimation error increases in increase of overlapping of wave components, and the preceding error affects on the estimation of the next wave. For assessment of the errors, we estimate conduction velocities and the number of sources from data simulated by a forward problem. For simplicity, we assume that a nerve bundle consists of three velocity groups, and each group contains 1000 nerve fibers.

The error in estimation of the number of sources was obtained for different combinations of group velocity, changing the distance between stimulus point and observing point.

The results are shown in Fig. 4, where estimation error for the first velocity group was plotted at each position. Conduction velocities of wave components are 70m/s, 50m/s and 30m/s for curve (I), 70m/s, 60m/s and 50m/s for curve (II), and 70m/s, 65m/s and 60m/s for curve (III).

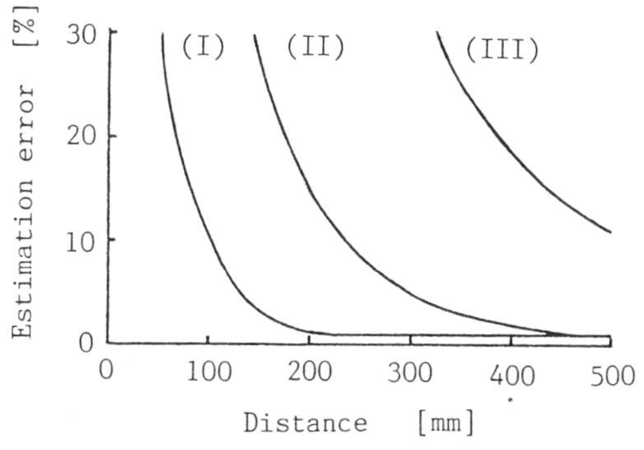

Fig. 4 Change of estimation error of the number of sources for the fast velocity group with the distance between stimulus point and observing point. Conduction velocites of wave components are 70m/s, 50m/s and 30m/s for curve (I), 70m/s, 60m/s and 50m/s for curve (II), and 70m/s, 65m/s and 60m/s for curve (III).

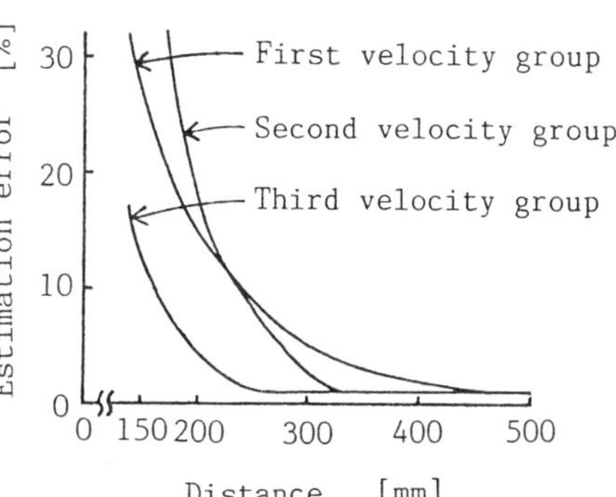

Fig. 5 Change of estimation error of the number of sources for curve (II) with the distance between stimulus point and observing point.

The estimation error of the first group is caused mainly by overlapping of the second and third wave groups. In accordance with decrease in distance, the estimation error increases. Whereas, the overlapping error can be ignored when the distance is large enough. The estimation error was around 1% at 500mm for curves (I) and (II).

In the case of curve (II), velocities of the first, second and third groups were obtained as shown in Fig. 5. The estimation error of the first velocity group affects on estimation of the second velocity group. The error becomes serious when the distance is shorter than 200mm. This is caused by overlapping of two group waves as shown in Fig. 6(a). The waveform which represents an approximately real wave pattern is shown in FIg. 6(b), where the overlapping error can be ignored since the distance is large enough.

The method proposed here is useful in estimating sources of the spinal cord and sources of short-latency evoked magnetic fields.

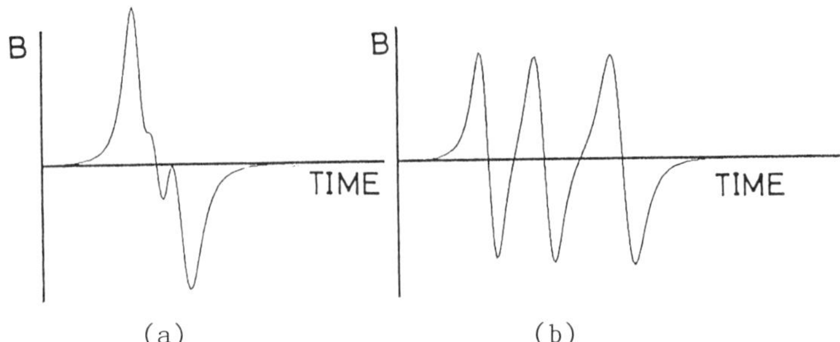

(a) (b)

Fig. 6 Overlapping of three group waves for curve (II). The distance is 150mm for (a) and 500mm for (b).

ACKNOWLEDGMENT

This work was supported in part by research grant from Ministry of Education, Science and Culture of Japan, 63850090.

REFERENCES

Barker, A. T., Brown, B. H. and Freeston, I. L., (1979), Modeling of an active nerve fiber in a finite volume conductor and its application to the calculation of surface action potentials. IEEE Trans. Biomed. Eng., vol. BME-26, pp.53-56.

Barker, A. T., Brown, B. H. and Freeston, I. L., (1979), Determination of of the distribution of conduction velocities in human nerve trunks. IEEE Trans. Biomed. Eng., vol.BME-26, pp.76-81.

Cohen, D., Hosaka, H., (1976), Magnetic field produced by a current dipole. J. Electrocardiology, 9(4) 409-417.

Wikswo, J. P., Jr., Barach, J. P., and Freeman, J. A., (1980), The magnetic field of a nerve impulse. First measurements. Science 208, 53-55.

Wikswo, J. P., Jr., (1985). Magnetic measurements on single nerve axons and nerve bundles. XIV ICMBE and VII ICMP, ESPOO, Finland.

SOURCE LOCALISATION FROM SOMATOSENSORY NEUROMAGNETIC DATA

R.J-M. Grognard and A.D. Seagar

CSIRO, Division of Radiophysics

P.O. Box 76, NSW 2121, Australia

INTRODUCTION

We are developing methods for determining the location of sources from their external neuromagnetic fields. The radial components of these fields are measured at an array of points over an arbitrarily shaped head. Some of these methods have been used to study the localisation information available in the measured somatosensory data of *Lim et al* (1989). We report here the main features of our method.

GEOMETRICAL MODEL OF THE HEAD

The shape of each head under study is measured directly from a plaster cast. We determine in a polar frame fixed to the head the distance from the origin $r(\theta, \varphi)$ of a point on the scalp at co-latitude θ and longitude φ (fig.1). The surface is sampled at a critical set of polar angles (θ_i, φ_j), which permits a truncated spherical harmonic series representing the surface to be obtained directly.

Our method rests on the following fundamental property of sets of functions which are approximations of the polar equation $r(\theta, \varphi)$ of an arbitrary head's surface.

Consider the set $\mathcal{S}_N$ of all functions $f(\theta, \varphi)$ which are linear combinations of spherical harmonics Y_n^m of order at most equal to N:

$$f(\theta, \varphi) = \sum_{n=0}^{n=N} \sum_{m=-n}^{m=+n} f_{nm} \, Y_n^m(\theta, \varphi). \tag{1}$$

If $f(\theta, \varphi) \in \mathcal{S}_N$, the (complex) coefficients f_{nm} are exactly given by the formula:

$$f_{nm} = \frac{2\pi}{2N+1} \sum_{i=1}^{N+1} A_i \sum_{j=0}^{2N} f(\theta_i, \varphi_j) \, [Y_n^m(\theta_i, \varphi_j)]^* \,, \tag{2}$$

where: $\varphi_j = 2\pi j/(2N+1)$, and the θ_i are such that the $\cos\theta_i$ are the roots of the Legendre polynomial of order $N+1$. The coefficients A_i are the corresponding Gaussian weights in the Gauss-Legendre quadrature formula of order $N+1$ (for an introduction to multi-dimensional quadratures consult *Stroud*, 1971). The asterisk denotes complex conjugation.

If we measure the finite set of radial distances $f(\theta_i, \varphi_j) = r(\theta_i, \varphi_j)$, on a given head,

Advances in Biomagnetism
Edited by S.J. Williamson *et al.*
Plenum Press, New York

equation 2 gives us the coefficients $r_{nm} = f_{nm}$. Equation 1 can then be used as a spherical harmonic approximation of order N to the polar equation of the head's surface.

Our method of finite spherical harmonic analysis differs from the current ones reviewed by *Brett* (1988) and the details will be published separately.

The base of the model is obtained by a smooth closure of the measured net which we determined from standard atlases of anatomy to coincide with the base of the brain. Obviously one would use more specific data if available, for instance from Magnetic Resonance Imaging.

The example of figure 1 is obtained from one of our plaster casts by using a truncated spherical harmonic expansion of order 16. Where this surface represents the accessible portion of the head, i.e. for $\theta \leq 90°$, it differs from it by less than 0.5 mm.

THE GRADIOMETER MEASUREMENTS

The model is used to determine the positions of the gradiometer adopted in the set of experiments reported in *Lim et al* (1989). They found that the set of points where the magnetic data were recorded differed from a spherical net by a typical standard error in position of the order of a millimetre.

Each gradiometer measurement B_{Grad} is accurately represented by a formula of the form:

$$B_{Grad}(\theta, \varphi) = \sum_{i=1}^{N} a_i B_r \left[r(\theta, \varphi) + h_i,\, \theta,\, \varphi \right], \qquad (3)$$

where there are $N = 8$ coils, the h_i are their respective distances from the point of contact of the gradiometer with the skull, and $B_r(r, \theta, \varphi)$ is the radial component of the magnetic flux density at the point (r, θ, φ). The a_i take values of plus or minus one, chosen so that the eight coils together approximate a third-order gradiometer. The axis of the gradiometer was taken to be normal to the head's surface.

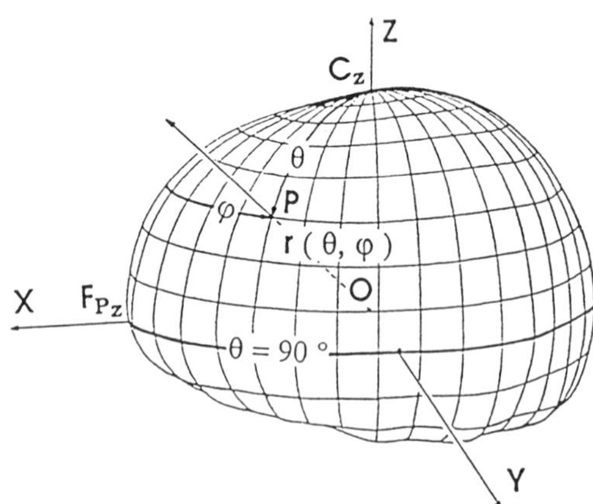

Figure 1. Polar coordinates for a skull: the plane OYZ is the plane of C_z, T_3 and T_4 (International 10-20 System); OX goes through F_{Pz}; the co-latitude θ of a point P is the angle (OZ, OP); its longitude φ is the dihedral angle between the plane OXZ and OZP. The grid of longitudes and co-latitudes represented on the figure has its nodes at the sampling points required for a finite spherical harmonic transform of order 16.

SOURCE LOCALISATION

Given that the set of points where our magnetic data are recorded differs little from a spherical net, our localisation algorithm uses the standard model of a radial magnetic field generated by a tangential element of current embedded in a uniformly conducting sphere.

Corrections due to the non-sphericity of the head have been estimated in a semi-analytic model based on truncated spherical harmonic expansions of head shape, sources and external magnetic fields. Provision is also made for inhomogeneities within the head in the form of domains with uniform conductivities and topologically equivalent to a sphere. This method is a generalisation of *Atkinson*'s method (1985) for solving Laplace's equation and will be published elsewhere.

The corrections to the position of the localised dipole for the cases reported in *Lim et al* (1989) are typically of the order of 1 mm. We base that conclusion mainly on three types of numerical experiments which will be presented in more detail in another publication. In order of complexity, these numerical experiments use: (i) a general analytic model of non-intersecting spherical interfaces between domains of uniform conductivities in arbitrary numbers and with an arbitrary topology; (ii) semi-numerical models based on ellipsoids; (iii) semi-numerical models based on finite spherical harmonic analysis. Whereas models of type (i) are suitable for computations on a personal computer the more realistic models of type (iii) require at least a 'mini-super-computer' such as our Convex 2.

The position and the tangential component of the element of current are obtained in relation to the spherical frame by an iterative algorithm based on the minimisation of the root mean square residual between the actual magnetic data and the predictions of the elementary spherical model. At the minimum the residual is about 20 fT and this is typically one order of magnitude below the maximum value recorded by the gradiometer. The noise performance of the SQUID system used by Lim was 23 fT, which was achieved using a 350 Hz bandwidth and averaging 1024 signals. The agreement between the minimum residual and the noise level suggests that there are no major systematic errors. It also confirms that the dominant noise source in the measurement is the intrinsic white noise of the SQUID.

For the component N19 from subject SC of *Lim et al* (1989), figure 2 displays the change in the residual when the assumed source is moved from its estimated position: (a) displays the variations under a radial motion; (b) and (c) display the variations under motion along a meridian and a parallel respectively.

Error estimates in the position of the source (see Table 1 in *Lim et al,* 1989) were calculated from the square root of the diagonals of the dispersion matrix (cf. *Kendall and Stuart,* 1977), which is in turn obtained from the second derivatives of the residual with respect to the free parameters. These estimates rely on a parabolic approximation to the curves in figure 2, which for curves (b) and (c) is clearly valid. However, curve (a) is hardly a parabola; the skewing observed is due to the rapid loss in sensitivity of a third-order gradiometer with its distance from the source.

The validity of the error estimates was investigated using a Monte-Carlo approach. Gaussian noise having a standard deviation of 20 fT was added to data simulated for a dipole at the minimum of the curves in figure 2. The resulting values were processed as before to yield an estimate of the dipole source. Elementary statistical methods applied to a set of 100 such experiments show a standard deviation of 2.0 mm in the radial direction and 1.5 mm in the two tangential directions. Although the radial distribution is skewed, the effect is too small at a 20 fT noise level to be significant. The tangential component of the dipole is attained with a standard deviation of 10% in its amplitude and of 5° in its orientation. The agreement between the error estimates yielded by the Monte-Carlo method and that based on second derivatives confirms that there is no bias in the measurements.

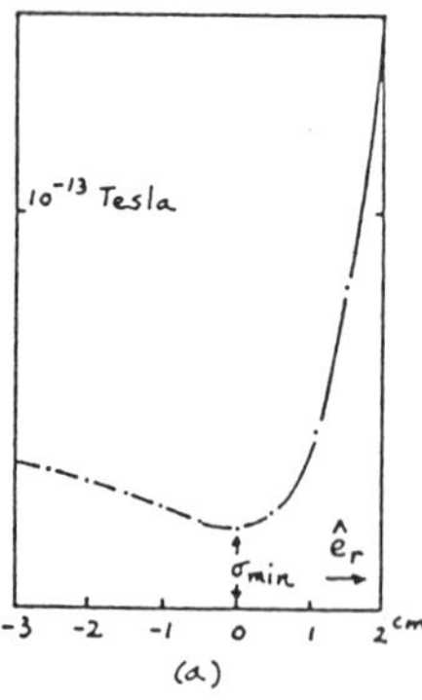

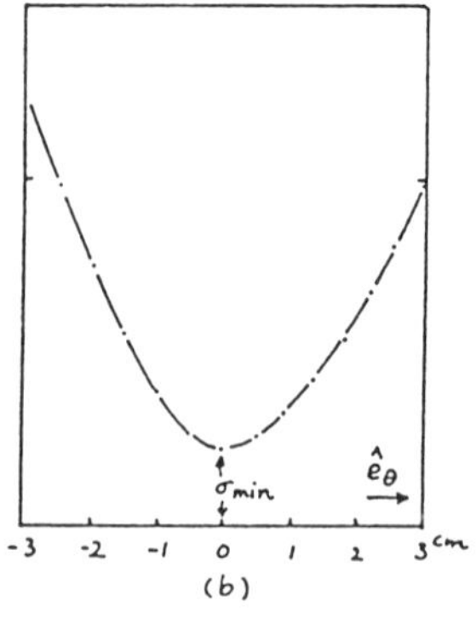

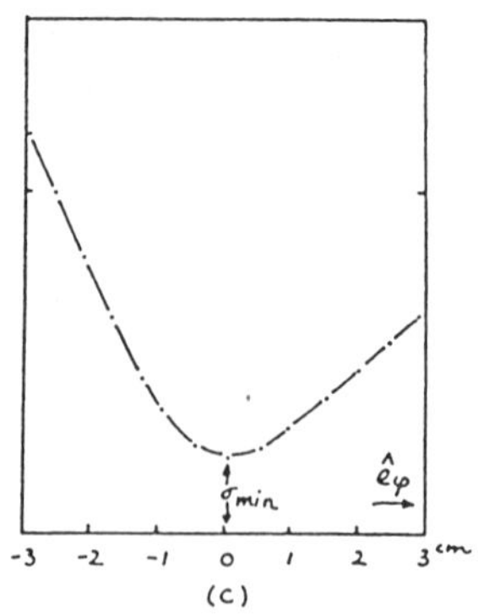

Figure 2. Variation of the residual:

$$\sqrt{\left(\sum_{i=1}^{81} |B_{Grad}^{measured}(P_i) - B_{Grad}^{model}(P_i)|^2\right) /81},$$

where the sum is extended over the set of 81 measured points. (a) the source is moved radially; (b) the source is moved along a meridian of constant longitude; (c) the source is moved along a parallel of constant co-latitude.

The results of our analysis on four subjects are presented in the table and figures of *Lim et al* (1989).

REFERENCES

Atkinson, K. E. 1985. *Algorithm 629: An integral equation program for Laplace's equation in three dimensions,* ACM Trans. Math. Soft. **11**, 85-96.

Brett, L. 1988. *Methods of spherical harmonic analysis,* Q.J.R.Astron.Soc. **29**, 129-155.

Lim, C. L., Rennie, C., Yiannikas, C., Gordon, E., Sloggett, G. J., Grognard, R. J.-M., and Seagar, A. D. 1989. *Short latency median nerve somatosensory evoked magnetic fields and electrical potentials,* Appearing elsewhere in these proceedings.

Kendall, M., & Stuart A. 1977. *The advanced theory of statistics, volume 1, distribution theory,* 4th ed., Charles Griffin, London, ch. 15.

Stroud, A. H. 1971. *Approximate calculation of multiple integrals,* Prentice-Hall, New Jersey.

SHORT LATENCY MEDIAN NERVE SOMATOSENSORY EVOKED MAGNETIC FIELDS AND ELECTRICAL POTENTIALS

C.L.Lim*, C.Rennie*, C.Yiannikas*, E.Gordon*,
G.J.Sloggett#, R.J-M.Grognard&, and A.D.Seagar&

*Neuroscience Unit, Westmead Hospital, Sydney, Australia
#CSIRO, Division of Applied Physics, Sydney, Australia
&CSIRO, Division of Radiophysics, Sydney, Australia

INTRODUCTION

Short latency somatosensory evoked potentials recorded with median nerve stimulation at the wrist have been widely used to assess pathology affecting the sensory pathways. The generator sites for some response components have been well established (P30) but there is still disagreement about others (N19, P22, N40). The corresponding somatosensory evoked magnetic fields are particularly suited to the study of cortical generator sites. Transient response studies to slow rates of median nerve stimulation have concentrated on peaks from 30 to 200 ms(1,2). Several wave components have been identified and attributed to sources in the primary and secondary sensory cortical areas SI and SII (3,4,5). Only a small number of studies have specifically examined short latency responses (6,7,8) and the results have been inconclusive. In this study we aimed to examine the early somatosensory magnetic equivalents to the electrical N19, P22, P30 and N40, assess the reproducibility of the findings and suggest potential sources for these signals.

METHODS

Somatosensory evoked responses were obtained from four normal volunteers by applying electrical stimuli at 2.3 Hz on the right median nerve at the wrist. The magnetic field was recorded in an unshieded hospital room by a 3rd order RF-SQUID gradiometer (CTF Systems Inc.). The recording was performed by placing the dewar nose normal to the scalp at each of the 81 points of a grid based on sub-division of an area bounded by Fz, Pz, F7 and T5 of the International 10-20 System (Fig.1). The responses passed through a 50 Hz filter and also a 50 to 400 Hz bandpass filter and were recorded up to 100 ms after stimulation. Two sets of 512 responses were recorded from each point. Measurements were made on the average of the two. Simultaneously, the scalp electrical potential was monitored from C3' in reference to shoulder. Two subjects were retested over a month later. In a separate session, SEPs were recorded with 40 electrodes placed at double the 10/20 System density mainly on the contralateral scalp.

The peak components were measured and isofield contour maps were obtained by interpolation. For source localisation head shape was measured and accurately characterised by a spherical harmonic expansion. It was found that for each case, the recording grid points differed from a best fitting spherical surface grid by a standard error of the order of a millimeter. The

Advances in Biomagnetism
Edited by S.J. Williamson *et al.*
Plenum Press, New York

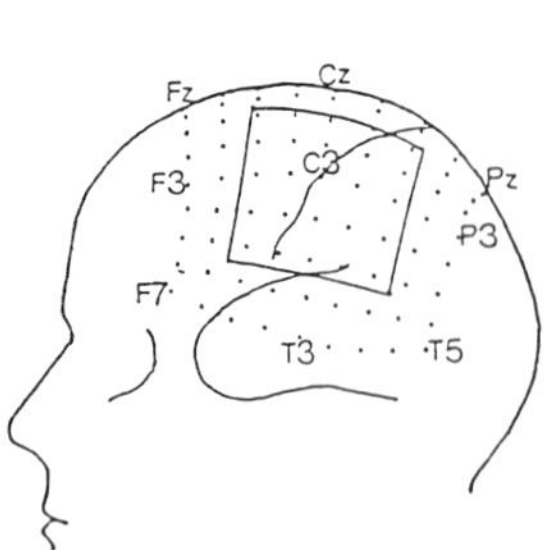

Fig.1 The locations of the 81 measurement points based on subdivision of the 10/20 System. Also shown is the 80 x 80 mm region centred at C3 that is depicted in fig.5.

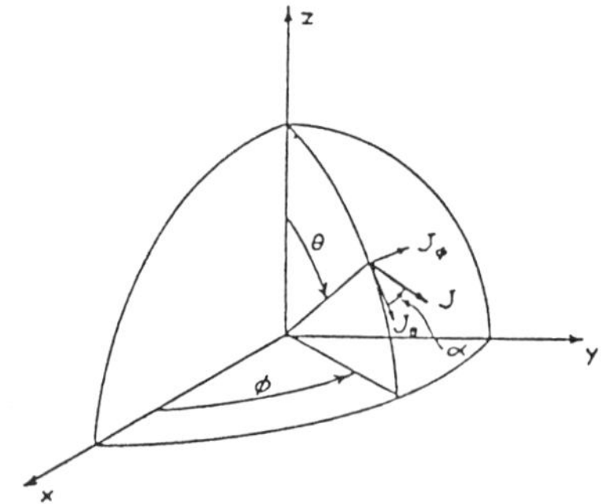

Fig.2 The coordinate system used in Table 1. The x axis passes through Fpz, the z axis through Cz, and T3 and T4 lie in the xy plane.

equivalent current dipole (ECD) localization was therefore performed by an iterative method with the conventional assumption of a dipole in a homogenous conducting sphere. Statistical estimates of location uncertainty were also determined (9).

RESULTS

An example of the recordings is shown in figure 3 where the components N19, P22, P30 and N40 are also illustrated. Across subjects the flux extrema ranged from 110 to 220 fT for N19, 110 to 180 fT for P22, 50 to 250 fT for P30 and 110 to 220 fT for N40. The isofield contour maps from another subject are shown in figure 4. The fields of N19 emerged from an area inferior and anterior to C3 and reentered superior and posterior to C3. The P22 field had reversed direction, and in all but one subject the patterns moved anterior to those of N19. The P30 and N40 distributions were similar to those of P22 and N19 respectively. The locations and their standard errors, depths, dipole

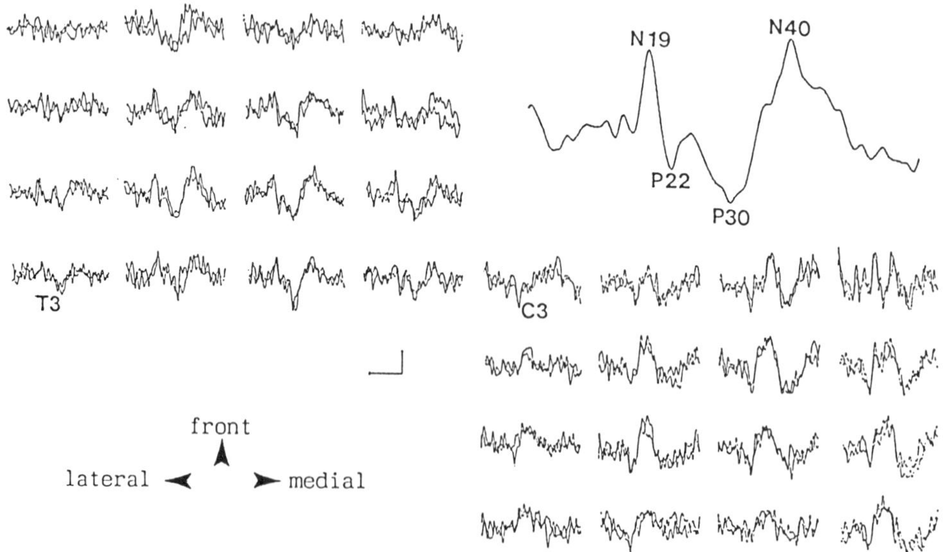

Fig.3 Superimposed magnetic responses taken from 32 grid points around the extrema in subject CK. An averaged trace is shown with the relevant peaks labelled. Upward deflection indicates emerging flux. The vertical calibration bar = 150 fT and horizontal bar = 20 ms.

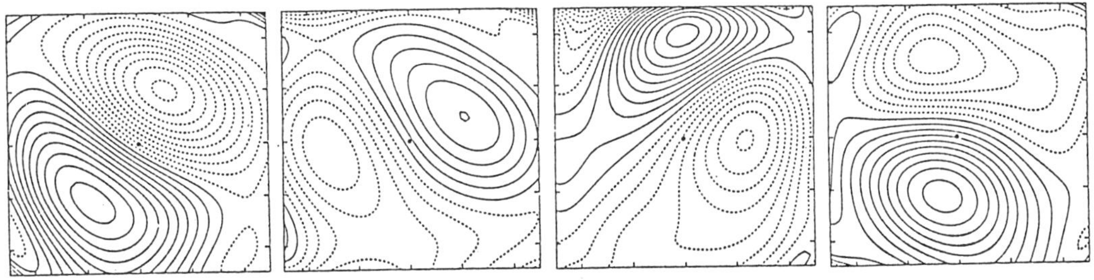

Fig.4 shows the isofield contour maps of N19, P22, P30 and N40 in subject SC. The maps are projected normally onto the plane tangential to the head surface at C3. Each of the 110 x 110 mm frames is centred at C3. Cz is in the upward direction and the front of the head is to the left. From left to right the contour steps are 11 fT, 31 fT, 5.7 fT and 11 fT. The solid contours indicate emerging flux.

moments and directions of the best fitting ECDs, according to the coordinate system shown in figure 2, are listed in table 1. The locations are also shown graphically in figure 5.

DISCUSSION

It is difficult to reach an optimal compromise between the number of sampling sites required for adequate spatial resolution and the number of trials needed to give a satisfactory signal to noise ratio. The grid spacing of about 18 mm used in this study is adequate for spatial resolution if we transpose the figure of 30 mm for median SEPs recommended recently by Spitzer et al (10) and take into account the SEF extremum separation generally being 60% of that of the SEP (6). As N19 and P22 have higher frequency content than later waves we used a higher upper cutoff frequency than most others. By averaging 1024 trials we obtained signal to noise ratios of up to 10. We found superimposed traces of separate trials useful in assessing signal reliability and helpful in detecting spurious errors. The retesting of two cases demonstrated response stability, giving us confidence that the error due to multi-sessional data collection in an unshielded hospital room was not excessive.

The depths of the four components in all subjects varied from 16 to 35 mm with a mean of 26 mm, not dissimilar to the range 25 to 30 mm estimated by Wood et al (6) in their two subjects and 12 to 30 mm by Huttunen et al (4) in a series of four. These depths are consistent with cortical sources.

As determined from table 1 the source locations of the four components in each subject were within 19 mm of each other and all lay in the vicinity of C3. This site has been shown by Sutherling et al (8) to be within 15 mm about the central sulcus.

In one of our cases (SC), the P30 dipole position was somewhat different from that found in the other subjects, perhaps reflecting an anatomical variation. However, the signal to noise ratio was small and so this finding should be treated as tentative. In the remaining three cases the ECDs of P30 were in close proximity to those of N19.

In three subjects, separations between N19 and P22 dipole locations were 9.5±1.8, 13.7±2.7 and 11.8±2.0 mm suggesting two distinct sources. Moreover, the equivalent current dipoles were directed towards each other and the field patterns place the P22 source anterior to that of N19 (Fig.5). These findings are consistent with the source of N19 being in the posterior bank of the central sulcus and the P22 arising pre-centrally in the motor strip. This supports the recent claim of Desmedt et al (11) based on their electrical potential distribution data.

Table 1. The equivalent current dipole localizations of four components in four subjects

	radius		x ±SE	y ±SE	z ±SE	depth	J	α
	(------		------	mm	------	------)	(nAm)	(°)
SC	90.9	N19	2.3 ±1.3	45.9 ±1.2	53.7 ±1.1	20.2	5.5	238
		P22	8.7 ±1.2	39.5 ±1.5	56.6 ±1.4	21.3	6.1	59
		P30	-8.4 ±1.9	34.6 ±1.7	62.5 ±2.1	19.0	2.4	106
		N40	2.6 ±2.2	42.2 ±1.7	52.2 ±2.2	23.7	6.0	265
EM	86.6	N19	-0.6 ±1.4	42.6 ±1.4	44.1 ±1.7	25.3	14.1	230
		P22	6.4 ±2.4	42.2 ±1.4	55.9 ±2.0	16.3	4.7	84
		P30	2.1 ±1.8	39.7 ±2.2	38.5 ±1.8	31.3	18.2	48
		N40	-5.9 ±1.8	44.3 ±1.6	43.1 ±1.8	24.6	10.1	226
JR	91.8	N19	-2.2 ±1.8	39.5 ±1.7	53.2 ±2.0	25.5	8.4	237
		P22	-5.3 ±1.8	36.8 ±2.2	55.2 ±2.1	25.2	7.1	45
		P30	-5.6 ±1.2	44.6 ±1.1	51.5 ±1.3	23.4	10.3	65
		N40	1.0 ±1.6	35.8 ±1.6	54.1 ±1.8	26.9	7.2	263
CK	90.7	N19	-6.6 ±1.0	36.0 ±1.2	42.0 ±1.3	35.0	22.7	217
		P22	-2.7 ±1.5	29.6 ±1.3	51.1 ±1.6	31.6	14.4	58
		P30	-3.5 ±1.0	39.6 ±1.4	41.0 ±1.3	33.6	25.9	53
		N40	-3.5 ±1.3	38.3 ±1.7	50.2 ±1.9	27.5	13.4	227

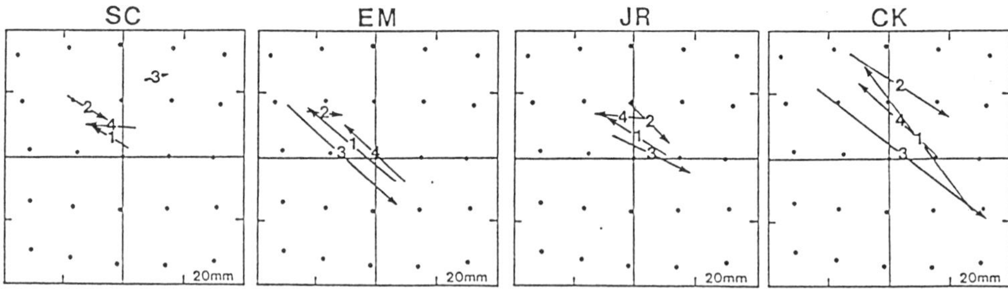

Fig.5 shows estimated positions of the equivalent current dipoles for all four subjects. The frames are centred at C3 and orientated as in fig.4. The locations of the best fit equivalent current dipoles associated with N19, P22, P30 and N40 are indicated by the numbers 1, 2, 3 and 4 respectively, and the magnitude and directions by arrows.

REFERENCES

1. L.Kaufman et al, Intern J Neuroscience, 1981;15:223-239.
2. D.Teszner et al, Il Nuovo Cimento, 1983;2D,2:429-437.
3. R.Hari et al, Electroenceph clin Neurophysiol, 1984;57:254-263.
4. J.Huttunen et al, Electroenceph clin Neurophysiol, 1987;66:391-400.
5. E.Kaukoranti et al, Exp Brain Res, 1986;63:60-66.
6. C.C.Wood et al, Science, 1985;227:1051-1053.
7. P.M.Rossini et al, Biomagnetism, 1987;178-181.
8. W.W.Sutherling et al, Neurology, 1988;38:1705-1714.
9. R.J-M.Grognard and A.D.Seagar. Source localisation from somatosensory neuromagnetic data. (submitted for publication in these procedings).
10. A.Spitzer et al, Electroenceph clin Neurophysiol, 1989;72:355-361.
11. J.E.Desmedt et al, Electroenceph clin Neurophysiol, 1987;68:1-19.

ON THE FRONTAL COMPONENTS OF SOMATOSENSORY SCALP RESPONSES TO MEDIAN NERVE STIMULATION: NEUROMAGNETIC DEMONSTRATION OF AN ANTERIOR, MIDLINE GENERATOR

Paolo M.Rossini*, Livio Narici**, Vittorio Pizzella#, Gian Luca Romani##, Raimondo Traversa*

* Dipartimento di Sanità Pubblica, II Università di Roma *"Tor Vergata"*, Roma, ITALY
** Dipartimento di Fisica, II Università di Roma *"Tor Vergata"*, Roma, ITALY
\# Istituto di Elettronica dello Stato Solido - CNR, Roma, ITALY
\#\# Istituto di Fisica Medica, Università *"G. D'Annunzio"*, Chieti, ITALY

INTRODUCTION

Studies on short-latency Somatosensory Evoked Potentials (SEPs) to median nerve stimulation, have focused mainly on parietal components peaking between 20 and 30 msec after stimulus delivery (waves N20 & P27; Desmedt & Cheron 1980). Some authors have suggested the existence of a single dipole located in the posterior bank of the central sulcus, being the unique generator source for pre- and postcentral SEP components (Broughton 1969). However, the advent of multichannel recording equipments and of brain mapping, have clearly shown that the central and frontal peaks of short-latency SEP have separate generators with respect to the parietal components (Giard et al 1986; Rossini et al 1987). This is particularly important for the frontal wave N30 which is supposed to reflect multiple sources embedded in pre-central and fronto-mesial non-primary motor areas (Rossini et al 1987,1989).

Neuromagnetic measurements of Somatosensory Evoked Fields (SEFs) to median nerve stimulation did invariably demonstrate a well organized dipolar structure, nicely interpretable on the basis of a unique post-central generator (Williamson & Kaufman 1982; Hari et al 1985; Narici et al 1987). In the present study, we demonstrate that a strictly frontal dipolar pattern is consistently present with two maxima on both the frontal lobes, during the build-up of the 'electric' N30 components. This pattern of field distribution is overlapping the "classical" one previously described on the parietal and temporal scalp regions. The dipole responsible for the frontal SEF is medially located, in a position compatible with the activation of the Supplementary Motor Area (SMA).

SUBJECTS AND METHODS

Three healthy volunteers were examined after having obtained their informed consent. SEPs have been recorded from 6 scalp electrodes glued with collodion on P4, C4, F4, P3, C3 & F3 positions of the 10-20 International System, with a common reference on the right earlobe. The four channel is fully described elsewhere (Romani & Narici, 1987) and is represented by four home-made Superconducting QUantum

Advances in Biomagnetism
Edited by S.J. Williamson *et al.*
Plenum Press, New York

Interference Devices (SQUIDs) with a noise level of about 45 fT $Hz^{-1/2}$. Each SQUID is coupled to a second derivative gradiometer with a baseline of 7 cm. Magnetic signals were acquired simultaneously to the electric ones. The tail of the dewar was placed perpendicularly to each scalp recording site, and up to 64 different scalp positions spanning from the vertex on both frontal districts were investigated. Post-stimulus analysis time was 90 ms. For each position 2000 artifact-free responses were averaged. In one subject data were replicated via a 9-channels system which became recently available.

When the isofield maps showed a clearcut dipolar pattern a least squares algorithm was utilized to calculate the best fitting equivalent dipolar source and to localize it tridimensionally (Romani & Narici, 1986).

Median nerve stimulation at wrist was settled with an intensity provoking a painless thumb opposition and with a repetition rate of 2.1 c/sec. This was a good compromise for eliciting an evident N30 wave on electric traces (this SEP component is known to easily fatigue with faster stimulus rates) in a relatively short time (Rossini et al 1987).

RESULTS

Fig. 1 represents the distribution of the scalp sites where SEFs were recorded; these covered the whole frontal districts with somewhat larger spread on the hemiscalp contralateral to the stimulated side.

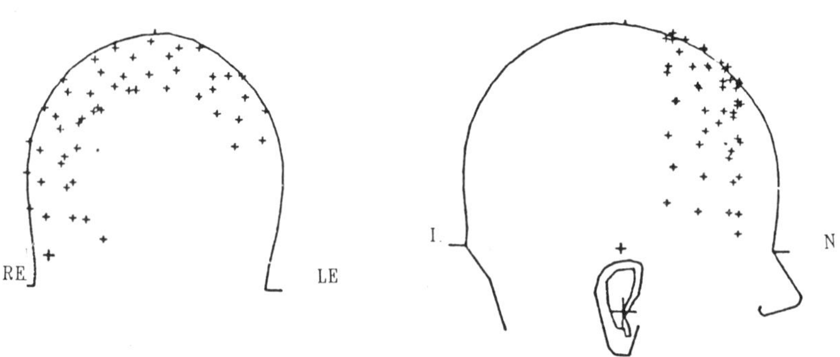

Figure 1 Position of the measured sites in the SEF records.

In all the examined subjects frontal SEPs were characterized by a widespread peak of negative polarity, which was bilobed in one case, whose major components was peaking around 30 ms. This wave, was on both the frontal districts, with an amplitude maximum on the parasagittal locations contralateral to the side of stimulation. The simultaneously acquired SEFs also showed clear components with latencies of about 30 ms (Fig. 2) and featuring two extrema on both sides of the frontal scalp (figs. 2 & 3).

When the least square algorythm for dipole localization was applied, an equivalent current dipole was found on the midline structures, at a depth of about 1.3 cm, with an antero-posterior or a postero-anterior direction (Fig. 3).

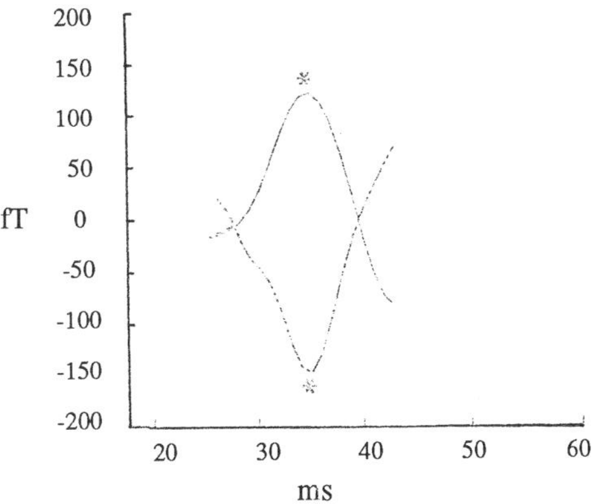

Figure 2 SEFs to left median nerve stimulation picked up at the two extrema on the left (dotted line) and on the right hemiscalp. Notice the phase reversal of the peak with a latency of about 32 ms (asterisks).

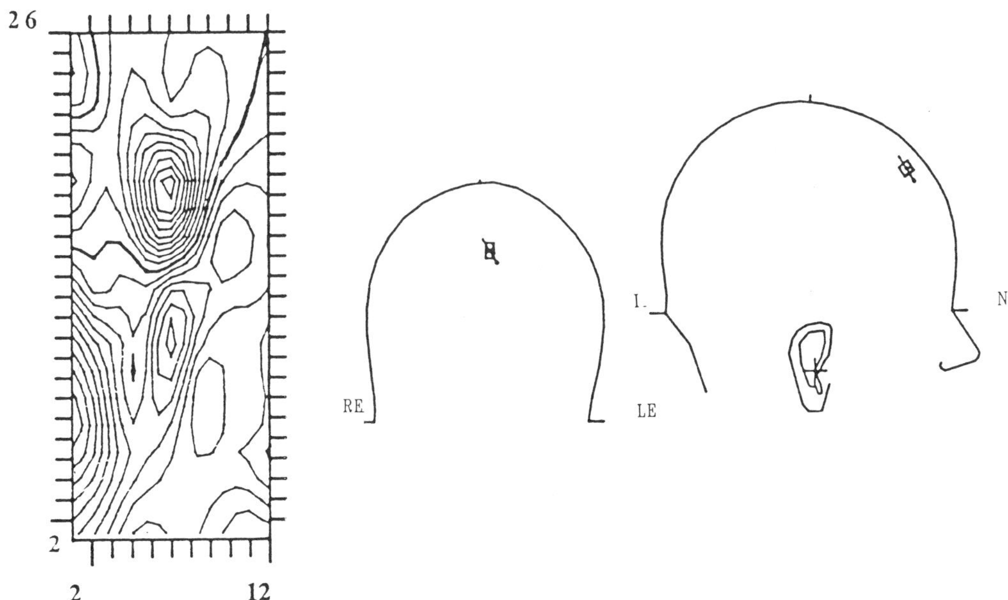

Figure 3 On the left: field distribution of SEFs. Coordinates are cartesian with the origin in the right ear canal, the X axis along the nasion (N)-inion (I) line and the Y axis along the vertex-ear line. On the right: Equivalent Current Dipole Location. The boxes represent the 95% confidence interval given by the fit.

It is noteworthy to consider that dense isofield lines were evident toward the rolandic and temporal boundaries of the examined head region, on the hemiscalp contralateral to the stimulated side (Fig. 3, left). This presumably reflects the anterior front of a strong dipole which is embedded in the sensorimotor cortices around the central sulcus. Therefore, the contribution of the frontal dipole, would have been entirely missed without a carefull search on both the frontal lobes, with an appropriate stimulus repetition rate.

DISCUSSION

Previous studies have repeatedly suggested that a wave at about 30 millisec latency -as recorded with SEPs- might be generated in frontal, parasagittal structures which include non-primary motor areas (Desmedt & Cheron 1980; Mauguiere et al 1983; Rossini et al 1987). However, a direct support to this hypotesis has never been provided, even if wave N30 was found to be altered in patients with an abnormal function of the Supplementary Motor Area (Rossini et al 1989). The present study prompts further support to the existence of a midline, frontal generator source responsible for SEPs and SEFs which are elicited after about 30 ms from median nerve stimulation at wrist. Non-primary motor areas in frontal lobes are the target for a cascade of sensory inputs in a "cortico-subcortico-cortical" reentry circuit which is relaying in the Basal Ganglia as well as in the Ventro-Lateral thalamic nuclei. Such a circuitry is possibly involved in sensorimotor integration for preparing the motor plans.

REFERENCES

Desmedt J.E., Cheron G. (1980): Central somatosensory conduction in man. Electroencephalogr. clin. Neurophysiol. 50: 382-403.

Broughton R.J. (1969): Average evoked potentials: method, results and evaluations, NSA SP-191, Gov.ment Print Off. 1, 79-84.

Deiber M.P., Giard M.H., Mauguiere F. (1986): Separate generators with distinct orientation for N20 and P22 somatosensory evoked potentials to finger stimulation. Electroencephalogr. clin. Neurophysiol. 65: 321-334.

Rossini P.M., Gigli G.L., Marciani M.G., Zarola F. and Caramia M. (1987): Non invasive evaluation of input output characteristic of sensorimotor cerebral areas in healthy humans. Electroencephalogr. clin. Neurophysiol. 68: 88-100.

Rossini P.M., Babiloni F., Bernardi G.,Stanzione P. and Urbano A. (1989): Abnormalities of short latency somatosensory evoked potentials in parkinsonian patients. Electroencephalogr. clin. Neurophysiol. 74.

Williamson S.J., Kaufman L. (1981) Evoked cortical magnetic fields. In: Erne' SN, Hahlbohm HD, Lübbig H (eds). Biomagnetism; Berlin, Walter de Gruiter.

Hari R. and Kaurokanta E. (1985): Neuromagnetic study of somatosensory system: principles and examples. Prog. Neurobiol. 24:233-256.

Narici L., Romani G.L., Salustri C., Pizzella V., Torrioli G. and Modena I. (1987): Neuromagnetic characterization of the cortical responce to median nerve stimulation in the steady state paradigm. Int. J. Neurosc. 32: 837-843.

Romani G.L. and Narici L. (1986): Principles and clinical utility of the biomagnetic method. Med. Prog. trough Technol. 11: 123-159.

Mauguiere F., Desmedt J.E., Courjon J. (1983): Astereognosis and dissociated loss of frontal or parietal components of somatosensory evoked potentials in hemispheric lesions: detailed correlations with clinical signs and computerized tomography scanning. Brain 106: 271-311.

SPATIOTEMPORAL MODELING OF SOMATOSENSORY EVOKED MAGNETIC FIELDS

Christoph Baumgartner (1,3), Daniel S. Barth (1,2), and William W. Sutherling (1)

Department of Neurology (1) and Psychology (2), University of California, Los Angeles, CA 90024, U.S.A.
Neurological University Clinic Vienna (3), Vienna, Austria

INTRODUCTION

Identification and localization of the neuronal sources generating somatosensory evoked responses is of both clinical and scientific interest. Localization of hand sensorimotor cortex is clinically important for patients undergoing surgical treatment of partial epilepsy, brain neoplasms and vascular malformations to avoid neurologic deficit. Electrophysiological techniques are required to localize sensorimotor cortex, as intraoperative visual inspection due to anatomical landmarks can be inaccurate in up to 50% of the cases (Wood et al., 1988). Usually, cortical stimulations or intraoperative evoked responses are used, but these techniques are time consuming and can increase operation time considerably. Thus, the improvement of non-invasive electrophysiological techniques for localization of sensorimotor cortex is warranted. Evoked responses are of scientific interest because exact location, time activity and interaction of its neuronal sources is still somewhat controversial (Allison et al., 1980).

Magnetoencephalography (MEG) helped to improve non-invasive localization of hand sensorimotor cortex and to resolve some ambiguities of evoked responses recorded in the scalp-EEG (Okada et al., 1984; Sutherling et al., 1988; Wood et al., 1985). Single equivalent dipole models were used as source localization procedures in these studies. There is, however, evidence that evoked responses are generated by at least two spatially separate generators (Allison et al., 1980). Thus, evoked neuromagnetic fields appear to be produced by multiple sources whose fields overlap both in space and time. We therefore applied new modeling techniques using a combined approach of multivariate statistical techniques and multiple dipole modeling, similar to methods previously proposed in a theoretical paper (Achim et al., 1988) and for analysis of visually evoked potentials (Maier et al., 1987), to study somatosensory evoked magnetic fields after median nerve stimulation.

METHODS

Evoked responses were recorded in the MEG after shock stimulation of the median nerve in 3 subjects. In two subjects suffering from partial complex seizures, evoked responses were also recorded from chronically

Advances in Biomagnetism
Edited by S.J. Williamson *et al.*
Plenum Press, New York

indwelling subdural grid electrodes. One subject was a healthy volunteer. Neuromagnetic recordings were performed with a seven channel magnetometer with dc-SQUIDs. The magnetometer was placed at 9 different overlapping positions to test reproducibility yielding 45 distinct measurement points. Two runs of at least 500 trials were performed to assess reproducibility.

Data analysis consisted of the following steps. We first applied principal component analysis (PCA) to identify the number of underlying neuronal sources. We then applied a physical model involving multiple dipoles fixed in space and varying in activity over time to estimate three-dimensional location, time activity and interaction of the neuronal sources producing the evoked responses. A more detailed description of the modeling procedures was presented elsewhere (Baumgartner et al., 1989). Finally, we compared the results obtained from MEG to those from ECoG.

RESULTS

In all 3 subjects the first two principal components explained over 90% of the system variance suggesting two neuronal sources underlying the evoked neuromagnetic fields. We therefore used two dipoles for the physical model. The results of PCA for Subject 1 are shown in Fig. 1B-E. The component loadings represent the spatial field pattern generated by the principal components and are shown in form of isofield maps (Fig. 1B). The component scores correspond to the time activities of the principal components (Fig. 1C). The contribution of a given principal component to the evoked neuromagnetic field can be calculated by multiplying the component loadings with the component scores (Fig. 1D). The first principal component explained 68% and the second 27% of the data variance. These field contributions sum up to the reconstructed data (Fig. 1E) which approximate the actual data very closely (Fig. 1A).

We then applied multiple source modeling using two dipoles. In all 3 subjects over 90% of the system variance could be explained by two dipoles fixed in space and varying in activity over time. The results of multiple source modeling for Subject 1 are shown in Fig. 1F-I. The spatial field patterns generated by the dipoles are shown in Fig. 1F. The time activities (Fig. 1G) show a positive and negative wave for each source with peaks corresponding to the N20-P30 component for the first dipole and to the P25-N35 component for the second dipole (Fig. 1H). The first dipole accounted for 60%, the second for 31% of the data variance. The field contributions of the individual dipoles can be calculated by multiplying the spatial field patterns with the time activities (Fig. 1H) and sum up to the reconstructed data due to the law of superposition (Fig. 1I). The reconstructed data are very similar to the actual data (Fig. 1A). The estimated source locations obtained agreed very well with the results obtained from ECoG. Although the results of PCA and multiple source modeling look similar there are some differences especially between component 2 and dipole 2 (Fig. 1B and F). This can be explained by the fact that PCA is a purely statistical technique bound only to mathematical constraints (e.g. orthogonality condition) without any physiological restrictions, whereas multiple source modeling is bound to a dipolar source configuration, but not to the orthogonality condition.

DISCUSSION

Our results indicate that multiple source modeling may be a useful tool for non-invasive localization of sensorimotor cortex in the MEG. However, the results should be viewed within the limitations of the procedure. PCA is a purely statistical technique without any physiological assumptions. The reconstructions obtained from PCA are not unique and any orthogonal rotation of the principal components yields an equivalent fit.

We applied several methods of rotation (varimax, oblimin, frequency domain rotation (Baumgartner et al., 1989)) which did not change the reconstructions significantly and thus enhanced the plausibility of our results. Nevertheless, PCA should be viewed more as a tool to determine the number of sources underlying the evoked response, rather than a method of making definitive inferences about source locations and field contributions. Multiple source modeling has the advantage that physiologically reasonable assumptions underlie this method. Our model permits investigation of the evoked response over its entire time domain and is not restricted to selected latencies given by peaks in amplitude as single dipole modeling (Okada et al., 1984; Sutherling et al., 1988; Wood et al., 1985). Thus, besides estimates of location also time course and interaction of the sources can be inferred. Two sources were sufficient to explain over 90% of the system variance in all subjects. One source

MEASUREMENT SITES AND DATA

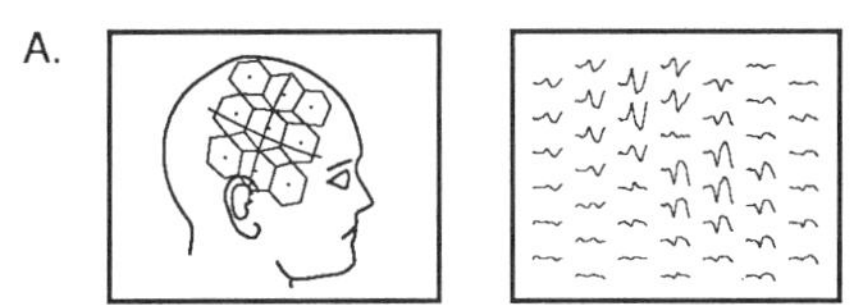

RESULTS OF PRINCIPAL COMPONENT ANALYSIS

B. C. D. E.

COMPONENT 1 X =

COMPONENT 2 X =

⊕ =

RECONSTRUCTED DATA

COMPONENT LOADINGS COMPONENT SCORES RECONSTRUCTION

RESULTS OF PHYSICAL MODEL WITH MULTIPLE DIPOLES

F. G. H. I.

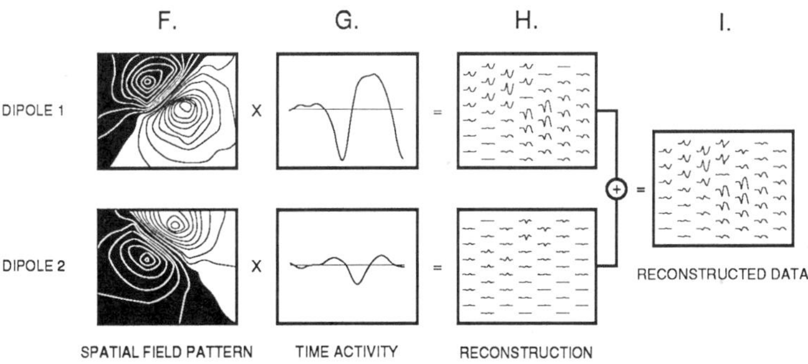

Fig. 1, Results for Subject 1. (A) Measurement sites and data. (B-E) Results of PCA, showing component loadings (B), component scores (C), field contributions of each principal component (D), and data reconstructed from first two principal components (E). (F-I) Results of multiple dipole model, showing spatial field patterns (F), time activities (G), field contributions (H), and data reconstructed from the two sources.

generated the N20-P30 component and the other the P25-N35 component (Fig. 1G). These results are in agreement with the literature suggesting at least two spatially separate generators, one located in the posterior bank of the central sulcus generating the the N20-P30 component and the other in the anterior portion of the crown of the postcentral gyrus near the central sulcus generating the P25-N35 component (Allison et al., 1980). The estimated locations agreed very well to the results obtained from ECoG. However, certain model assumptions of the multiple dipole model should be kept in mind when interpreting the results. First, the model is bound to dipolar source configuration. Dipole modeling is reasonable as the magnetic field generated by any source with equal number of positive and negative charges falls off like that generated by a dipole, at a distance which is large compared to the dimensions of the source. Second, the dipoles in our model were fixed at a given location, which imposes additional assumptions in modeling of propagation. However, as only highly synchronized activity in a large number of neurons is detected in MEG whereas localized activity tends to cancel out, this assumption seems to be justified to achieve a simple and yet reasonable model. Further studies in more subjects and further comparisons to the results of invasive recordings are needed to confirm our results.

ACKNOWLEDGMENTS

This research was supported by the Fonds zur Förderung der wissenschaftlichen Forschung Österreichs (Erwin Schrödinger Stipendium J246M and J334MED), by the Van-Swieten-Gesellschaft Österreichs (Hofrat Erwin Domanig Stipendium), by USPHS grants 1-R01-NS20806, 1-R01-NS00678 and 1-R01-NS22575 and by NSF grant BNS-86-57764, and the Whitaker Foundation.

REFERENCES

Achim, A., Richer, F., and Saint-Hilaire, J.M., 1988, Methods for separating temporally overlapping sources of neuroelectric data, Brain Topography, 1:22-28.

Allison, T., Goff, W.R., Williamson, P.H., and Van Gilder, J.C., 1980, On the neural origin of early components of the human somatosensory evoked potential, Prog. clin. Neurophysiol., 7:51-68.

Baumgartner, C., Sutherling, W.W., Di, S., and Barth D.S., 1989, Investigation of multiple simultaneously active brain sources in the EEG. J. Neurosci. Meth. (in press)

Maier, J., Dagnelie, G., Spekreijse, H., and Van Dijk, B.W., 1987, Principal component analysis for source localization of VEP's in man, Vision Res. 27:165-177.

Okada, Y.C., Tanenbaum, R., Williamson, S.J., and Kaufman, L., 1984, Somatotopic organization of the human somatosensory cortex revealed by neuromagnetic measurements, Exp. Brain Res., 56:197-205.

Sutherling, W.W., Crandall, P.H., Darcey, T.M., Becker, D.P., Levesque, M.F., and Barth, D.S., 1988, The magnetic and electic fields agree with intracranial localizations of somatosensory cortex, Neurology, 38:1705-1714.

Wood, C.C., Cohen, D., Cuffin, B.N., Yarita, M., and Allison, T., 1985, Electrical sources in the human somatosensory cortex: Identification by combined magnetic and electric potential recordings, Science, 227:1051-1053.

Wood, C.C., Spencer, D.D., Allison, T., McCarthy, G., Williamson, P.D., and Goff, W.R., 1988, Localization of human sensorimotor cortex during surgery by cortical surface recordings of somatosensory evoked potentials, J. Neurosurg., 68:99-111.

MAGNETIC LOCALIZATION OF SOMATICALLY EVOKED RESPONSES IN THE HUMAN BRAIN

J. Suk, J. Cappell, U.Ribary,T. Yamamoto*, & R. R. Llinás

Center for Neuromagnetism, Department of Physiology and Biophysics
New York University, New York, N. Y., 10016
*Dept. Otorhinolaryngology, Faculty of Medicine, Kyushu University
Maedashi, Fukuoka, 812, Japan

INTRODUCTION

In an earlier study (Penfield and Rassmussen,1950) the exposed human cortex was electrically stimulated and a map of associated anatomical regions was produced. Projections of contralateral anatomical regions were found in the primary somatosensory cortex (SI), with various body parts represented sequentially from the Sylvian fissure to the midline. More recently, magneto-encephalography (MEG) has been used to study somatosensory activity, initially by Brenner et. al. (1978). Since then, various aspects of somatosensory function have been studied using MEG techniques (see Hari and Kaukoranta, 1984; also Huttunen,1986 and Kaukoranta, 1986). Okada et. al. (1984) localized dipole sources of responses to thumb, index, little finger and ankle stimulation. Based upon the depth and position of the calculated sources, it was inferred that the sources lie on the posterior bank of the Rolandic fissure in SI. A fourteen channel cryogenic magnetometer system (BTi) was used in the present study to record the magnetic fields in order to locate the source of response to the tactile stimulation of the index, the thumb, and the little finger of the right hand in three subjects. The responses were measured from the contralateral side of the head. The location of the magnetic sources determined by the spherical model were then projected onto the Magnetic Resonance Image (MRI) of the individual subjects in order to determine the degree of correlation between the anatomy of each subject and the calculated source of the dipole (Yamamoto et. al, 1988).

METHODS

The recording system has previously been described (Yamamoto et al, 1988).The cryogenic magnetic recording system is located inside the magnetic shielded room (MSR) to reduce interference from external magnetic and rf noise. The system consists of two probes, each having seven recording channels. The location and orientation of the probes in relation to the head were recorded using a Probe Position Indicator (PPI), a system of two transmitters, one on each of the two probes and three receivers placed on each subject's head. PPI recorded probe positions using a head based coordinate system, defined by using three reference points; the nasion and the left and right periauricular points. PPI was also used to digitize a large surface of curvature of each subject's head, thereby determining the center and radius of the spherical model of the head to be used for dipole localization calculations.

Three normal male subjects were measured (age range 18-41). The stimulus, at a constant intensity and at a frequency of 250 Hz, was randomized among the three fingers to allow maximum consistency in experimental conditions. The interstimulus interval ranged from 400 to 600 msec. The stimulus was triggered at 100 msec, after the start of each recording window of 300 msec, for a duration of 100 msec. The stimulus was provided by vibrating Piezo electric buzzers. The data was later separated into three sets, one for each finger, to be averaged and analyzed for source location and response amplitudes. An analysis of variance (ANOVA) was used to evaluate statistically the significance of the differences found among the locations of the three sources in each subject.
MRI scans were then obtained for all of the subjects. The axis used for the dipole source location was specified on the MRI scans by landmarks at the periauricular points and the nasion point. This defined axis was then used as the plane for sectioning the MRI scans. We were then able to use the appropriate x, y, z data obtained from the MEG and directly superimpose it (after correcting the scale) onto the MRI scans.

RESULTS

Preliminary results from three subjects showed that the largest difference for source location occurred between the little finger and the thumb. In all cases, the source for the little finger was the highest in the vertical axis. Individual differences were most prominent in the location of the index finger. The ANOVA confirmed that the differences in source locations among the fingers were significant between 95% to 99%.

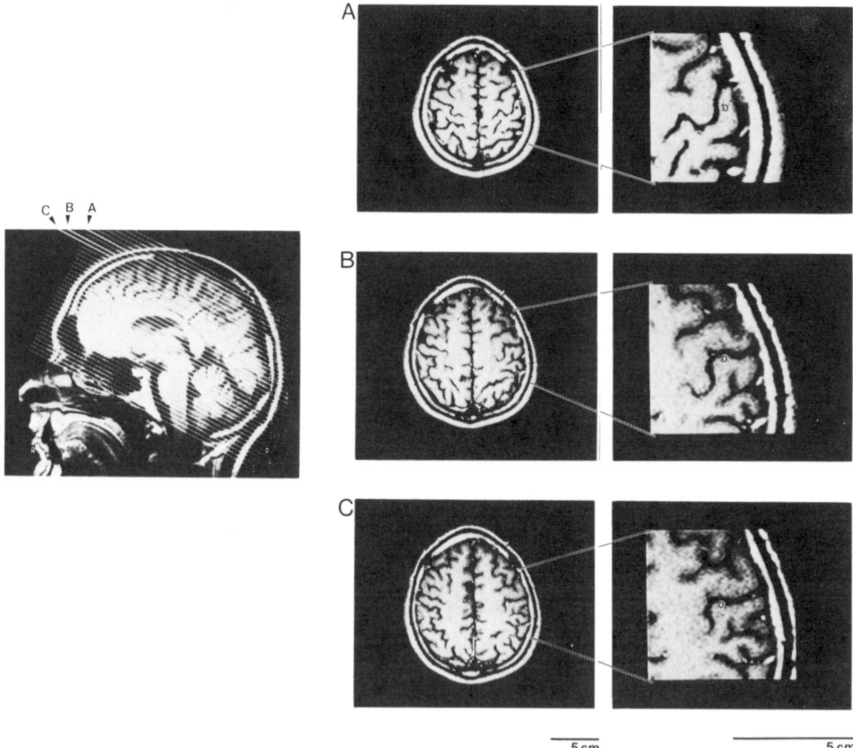

Fig. 1 *Subject UR*: The planscan of *axial* sections which correspond to A, B and C. (A) Section containing the source location of the little finger with corresponding area shown on a larger scale in the adjacent figure with location indicated by (O). (B) Section and large scale figure of area containing the source location of the thumb with location indicated by (O). (C) Section and large scale figure of area containing the source location of the index finger with location indicated by (O)

In figures 1 and 2, the plan of the MRI scan is first shown, with letters specifying the location of the slice which contains the dipole sources for the three fingers. The second figure A and B (C) of each set then shows that slice with the adjacent figure showing a magnification of the MRI with symbols depicting the deduced source locations. Each of the locations are depicted on axial and coronal slices which correspond to the x-y plane and the y-z plane, respectively. The locations of the sources all lie along the posterior bank of the Rolandic fissure on the post central gyrus with the little finger source location being the highest on the x-y plane and the most posterior in the y-z plane and the index and the thumb source locations being in close proximity of each other.

Comparing the amplitudes of the responses from the three fingers also showed significant and consistent differences. The thumb produced the largest response, the index being the second in amplitude, (in one of the subjects there was no significant difference between the index and the thumb) and the little finger being the smallest. This was true for all subjects although the degree to which the amplitudes differed varied among the subjects.

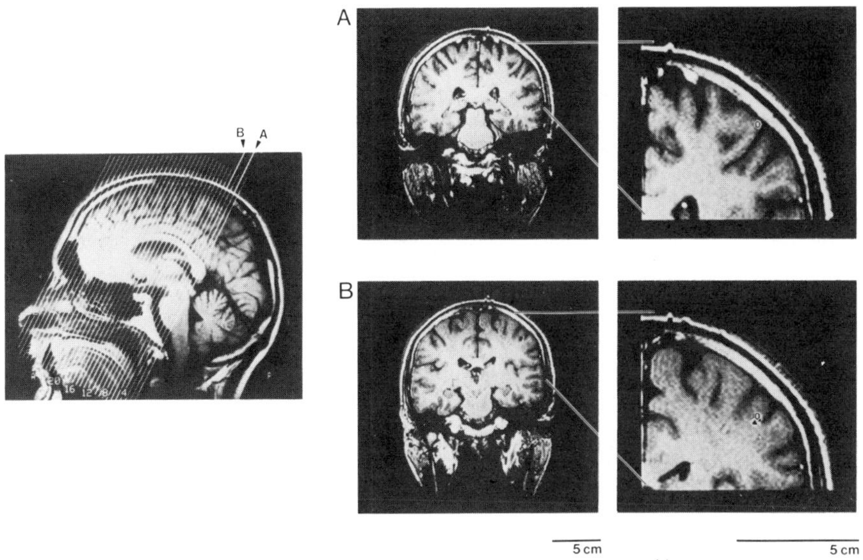

Fig. 2 *Subject UR:* The planscan of *coronal* sections which correspond to A and B. (A) Section containing the source location of the little finger with corresponding area shown on a larger scale in the adjacent figure. (B) Section and large scale figure of area containing the source locations of the thumb (O) and the index finger (▲).

DISCUSSION

These source location findings were found to be consistent with the organizational structure of the somatosensory cortex as described by Penfield and Rassmussen, (1950) as well as the dipole locations given by later magnetic field studies (Okada et. al., 1984). The correlation of dipole source location with the anatomical information of the MRI provided the first anatomical mapping of SI activity using noninvasive techniques. Furthermore, the use of a multichannel system allowed simultaneous recording from the minimum and maximum of the response field, providing sufficient data for source localization in a single trial. This made movement of channels within a session and the use of separate sessions for each finger unnecessary, eliminating those as sources of error as mentioned by Okada et. al. (1984).

The most parsimonious interpretation of the differences found in response amplitudes of the three fingers is that they have unequal projection areas in SI (Penfield and Rasmussen, 1950). However, a variation in areas stimulated due to different finger shapes, was not eliminated in these experiments. Another source of variation may be due to the possible rotation of the dipoles.

Ultimately, the high level of statistical significance (95 to 99%) of the data objectively demonstrates the degree of precision and reproducibility in these measurements and the correlations with the MRI scans further support the utility of combining MEG data with other imaging modalities.

REFERENCES

Brenner, D., Lipton, J., Kaufman, L., Williamson, S. J. (1978). Somatically evoked magnetic fields of the human brain. Science. 199, 81-83.

Hari, R. and Kaukoranta, E. (1985). Neuromagnetic studies of somatosensory system: Principles and examples. Progress in Neurobiology. 24, 223-256.

Huttunen, J. (1986). Magnetic cortical responses evoked by tactile stimulation of the middle finger in man. Pflügers Archiv. 407, 129-133.

Kaukoranta, E., Hämäläinen, M., Sarvas, J., and Hari, R. (1986). Mixed and sensory nerve stimulations activate different cytoarchitectonic areas in the human primary somatosensory cortex SI. Neuromagnetic recording and statistical consideration. Experimental Brain Research. 63, 60-66.

Kuriki, S., and Mizutani, Y. (1987). Magnetic responses evoked in cervical cord and brain by somatic stimulation. Biomagnetism '87 Tokyo Denki University Press, 50-57.

Okada, Y. C., R. Tanenbaum, S. J. Williamson, and L. Kaufman. (1984). Somatotopic organization of the human somatosensory cortex revealed by neuromagnetic measurements. Exp. Brain Res. 56, 197-205.

Penfield, W., Rasmussen, T. (1950). The Cerebral Cortex of Man. A Clinical Study of Localization of Function. Macmillan Company, New York.

Yamamoto, T., Williamson, S. J., Kaufman, L., Nicholson, C., Llinás, R. (1988). Magnetic localization of neuronal activity in the human brain. Proc. Natl. Acad. Sci. USA. 85, 8732-8736.

EVOKED AND SPONTANEOUS MAGNETIC ACTIVITY OF THE HUMAN SOMATOSENSORY CORTEX

J. Tiihonen, R. Hari, M. Kajola, and M. Hämäläinen

Low Temperature Laboratory, Helsinki University of Technology
02150, Espoo, Finland

INTRODUCTION

The generation sites of the somatosensory evoked responses, as well as those of the mu rhythm, have remained controversial. We have, therefore, recorded early somatosensory evoked magnetic fields (SEFs) with a good signal-to-noise ratio. We also measured spontaneous magnetic brain activity over the rolandic area, to find out whether it is possible to detect the magnetic counterpart of the electric mu rhythm and to locate its generators with respect to those of SEFs.

METHODS

SEFs were recorded over the right hemisphere on 7 subjects. The left median nerve was stimulated at the wrist with rectangular 0.3-ms constant current pulses, at interstimulus intervals (ISIs) of 200 - 220 ms and 500 - 520 ms. Spontaneous magnetic activity was recorded over the right rolandic area in 4 subjects.

We used a 7-channel first-order dc-SQUID gradiometer (diameter of measuring area 93 mm, field sensitivity 5 - 6 $fT/\sqrt{Hz}$; Knuutila et al. 1987). Signals were obtained from 21 - 49 locations, covering areas of about 10 cm x 20 cm. The recording passband was 0.05 - 2000 Hz for SEFs and 0.05 - 100 Hz for spontaneous activity; the signals were digitized at 8000 Hz and at 500 Hz, respectively. To analyze the topography of the spontaneous rhythm, four successive transients of a spindle were averaged. The averaged epochs were 200 ms in duration, including 100-ms periods before and after the transient. Averaging was started from such a recording location, where the polarity reversal could be seen between simultaneously measured signals. The zero level was determined as the mean value of the recording. The equivalent dipoles were found by a least-squares fit; a spherically symmetric volume conductor, fitting to the local radius of curvature of the head, was assumed.

RESULTS

SEFs typically consisted of a N20m peaking at 18 - 20 ms, a small P22m at 21 - 23 ms and a P27m at 29 - 31 ms (Fig. 1). The topography of N20m could be explained by a tangential current dipole in the central sulcus (probably in area 3b). On average, the equivalent dipoles of P27m were located 10 mm anteromedially to the sources of N20m. On the average, a decrease of ISI from 500 ms to 200 ms dampened the amplitude of P27m by 67%, and that of N20m by 24%, respectively.

Advances in Biomagnetism
Edited by S.J. Williamson *et al.*
Plenum Press, New York

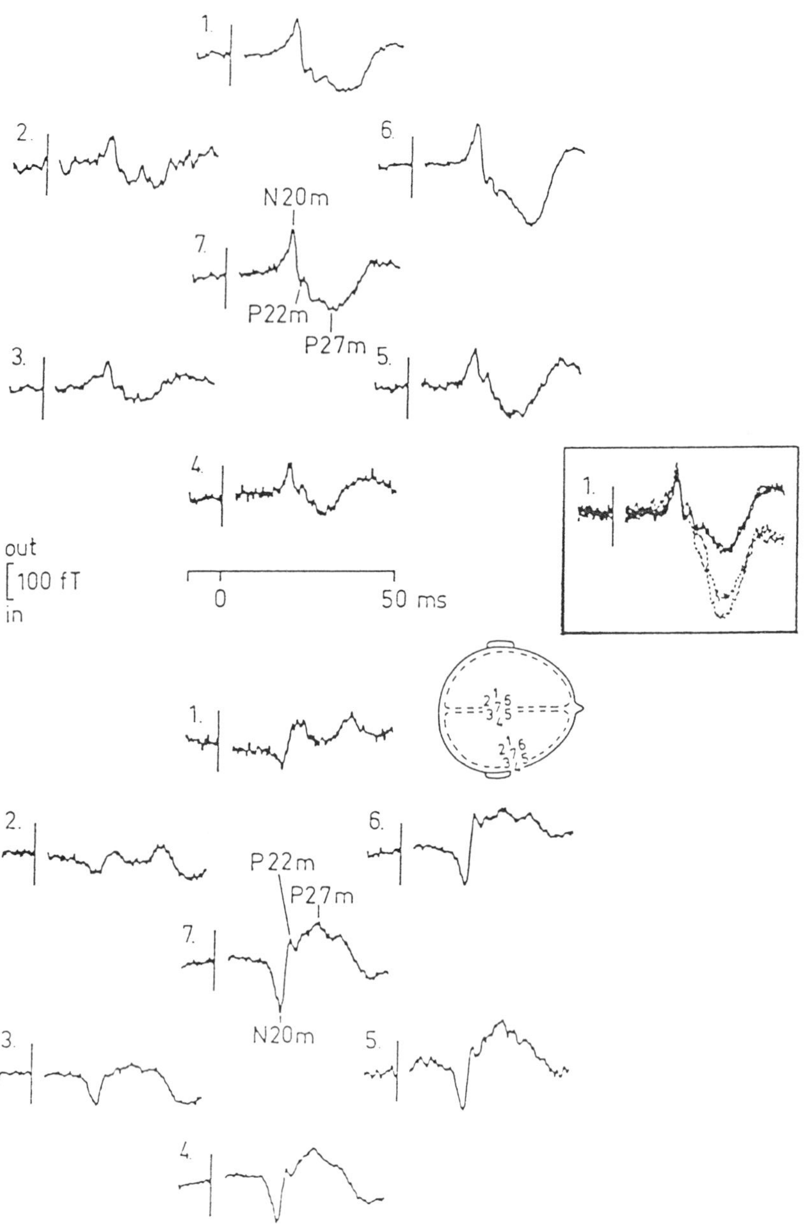

Fig. 1. Responses from the superior and inferior field extrema at the ISI of 200 - 220 ms in one subject. Polarity reversal is seen for all deflections (N20m, P22m, and P27m) between the upper and lower locations. In the insert, solid lines indicate two responses at the ISI of 200 - 220 ms and dashed lines at the ISI of 500 - 520 ms. Passband was 0.05 - 2000 Hz and about 1000 responses were averaged.

The frequency spectrum of the spontaneous rhythm contained peaks around 10 Hz and 21 Hz, and the activity had opposite polarity at the upper and lower ends of the central sulcus (Fig. 2). The measured field pattern could be satisfactorily explained by a current dipole located close to the source of N20m: in one subject the sites of the equivalent dipoles for mu and N20m did not differ at the 95% confidence level, and in the three others the source for mu was located 11 - 14 mm medial (along the central sulcus) to that of N20m (Fig. 3).

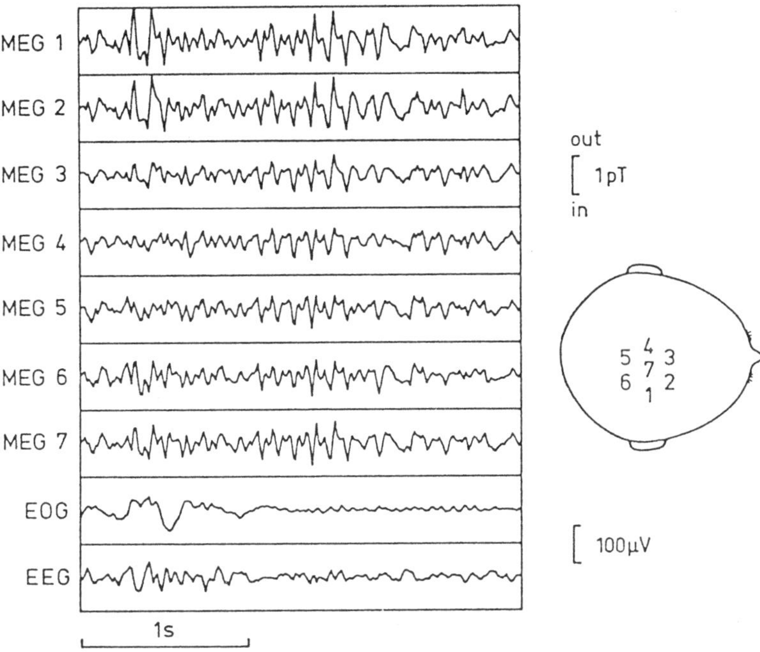

Fig. 2. Simultaneously recorded spontaneous brain activity of Subject 1: magnetic activity from 7 locations (MEG 1 - 7; see the insert), vertical electro-oculogram (EOG), and EEG from derivation C4 - P4 (10 - 20 system). The passband was 2 - 40 Hz.

DISCUSSION

Our low-noise instrument and wide recording passband allowed us to record early SEF components with a good signal-to-noise ratio. The N20m, P22m, and P27m deflections could be seen in all 7 subjects, but no earlier responses were observed. The electric P22 is generally believed to be generated by radial sources and, therefore, it was thought that its magnetic counterpart would be undetectable outside the skull. However, even a slight tangential component of source currents can generate a magnetic field, big enough to be measured with low-noise equipment and with adequate bandwidth. The location of its source suggests that P27m receives contributions from the anterior wall of the central sulcus. The different effect of ISI on N20m and P27m also implies that these responses are not generated by identical neural networks.

Mu activity had two different frequency components, and thus its characteristic comb shape may be composed of two superposed sinusoids (around 10 Hz and 21 Hz). Because magnetic mu was seen in all our four subjects, we consider mu rhythm a normal spontaneous brain rhythm, although infrequently seen in routine EEG. Kuhlman (1978) has suggested that mu rhythm is a consequence of the lack of somatosensory afferentation, as alpha rhythm is a sign of the absence of visual input, i.e., both rhythms would reflect 'idling' of the modality-specific sensory cortex, which obtains no input but is tuned ready for it. The location of the equivalent source of the magnetic mu close to the sources of N20m implies that the mu rhythm is generated mainly at the primary somatosensory hand projection area. In the somatosensory homunculus hand, and especially thumb, occupy a relatively large area, which may explain why somatosensory idling is seen mainly in the hand area.

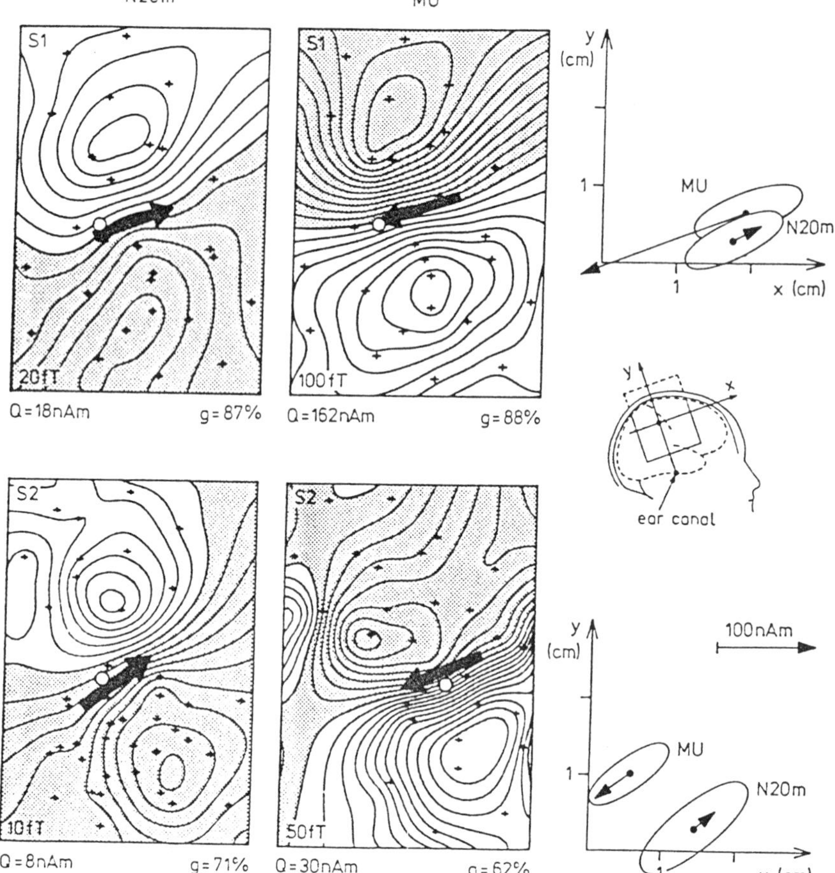

Fig. 3. Field maps for the N20m component of the SEF and for the largest transient of the averaged mu rhythm in two subjects (S1 and S2). The recording area and the coordinate system is shown in the insert. The y-axis connects the right ear canal to a midline point 30 mm posterior to vertex. The origin, indicated by the open circle in the maps, is located 40 mm lateral to the midline. The differences between the isocontour lines, the strengths of the dipoles (Q), and the goodness-of-fit values (g) are also indicated. On the right, the dots show the locations and the arrows the orientations of the equivalent dipoles. The 95%-confidence areas are indicated by the ellipsoids.

REFERENCES

Knuutila, J., Ahlfors, S., Ahonen, A., Hällström, J., Kajola, M., Lounasmaa, O.V., Vilkman, V., and Tesche, C., 1987, A large-area low-noise seven-channel dc SQUID magnetometer for brain research, Rev. Sci. Instrum., 58:2145.

Kuhlman, W. N., 1978, Functional topography of the human mu rhythm, Electroenceph. Clin. Neurophysiol., 44:83.

Tiihonen, J., Hari, R., and Hämäläinen, M., 1989, Early deflections of cerebral magnetic responses to median nerve stimulation, Electroenceph. Clin. Neurophysiol., 74: 290.

Tiihonen, J., Kajola, M., and Hari, R., 1989, Magnetic mu rhythm in man, Neuroscience, in press.

ECD TRACING FOR MIDDLE LATENCIES OF NEUROMAGNETIC RESPONSES TO RIGHT TIBIAL NERVE STIMULATION

Y. UCHIKAWA, T. HASEGAWA*, M. KOTANI*, K. KIDA**, H. YAMAMOTO**, and H. HOSAKA***
Department of Applied Electronic Engineering, Tokyo Denki University, Hatoyama, Saitama 350-03 Japan
* Department of Electronic Engineering, Tokyo Denki University Kandanishiki-cho, Chiyoda-ku, Tokyo 101 Japan
** Kochi Medical University, Nangoku-shi, Kochi 781-1 Japan
*** Nihon Koden Kogyo Company, Ltd., Ochiai, Shinjyuku-ku Tokyo 161 Japan

INTRODUCTION

Location and origin in the cortex for the electric sources of the eary components of somatosensory evoked potentials (SEPs) have been discussed[1,2]. Recently, the combined measurement of SEPs and somotosensory evoked magnetic fields (SEFs) elicited by median nerve stimulation were performed by Wood and coworkers[3] to test the previous discussions. In the middle and/or long latencies, however, it seems that there are also similar problems concerned with feature and localization of electric sources in the cortex. An aim of this paper is to show the new results of ECD tracing of the equivalent source localization in the cortex for the middle latencies of SEFs elicited by tibial nerve stimulation.

MEASUREMENT SYSTEM AND METHOD

SEFs have been measured in a nonmagnetically shielded room with a SQUID connected to a second order gradiometer with a base line of 3.2 cm and a coil of 2.48 cm diameter. In order to avoid and/or reduce the interference of magnetic noise coming from electronic devices, a wooden house to install subjects was set up in the distance of 20 m from data acquisition system.

Rectangular electric pulses of 0.2 ms duration were applied to tibial nerve of the right ankle through two electrodes of 5 mm diameter separated by 2 cm on the skin. A stimulation interval is 0.5 s. SEFs were recorded at 25 positions separated by 2 cm on the scalp as shown in the left panel of Fig.1. Magnetic field perpendicular to the scalp was measured over all positions. All magnetic data were digitized by 0.3 ms sampling interval and averaged by 500 measurements at one position. Band pass filter was used in the range of 1 to 30 Hz. The maximum rms amplitude of magnetic noise for a peak to a peak was 10 fT by 500 averages of signals in the range of 1 to 30 Hz.

RESULTS

1) Averaged magnetic time recordings

Fig.1 shows an example of the averaged magnetic time recordings of

Advances in Biomagnetism
Edited by S.J. Williamson *et al.*
Plenum Press, New York

SEFs on the mesial surface obtained by electric stimulation to tibial nerve of the right ankle. It can be seen that the upward (positive field) and the downward (negative field) deflections were elicited for latencies of 70 to 120 ms. The upward deflection indicates magnetic flux into the scalp. These deflections changed polarity between B3 and D3. Position of B3 is corresponded to Cz of international ten-twenty electrode system. For latencies of 80 to 100 ms, downward deflections were observed at A3 and B3. And D3 was the upward deflection. On the contrary, for long latencies of 100 to 120 ms, A3 and B3 were upward. D3 was downward.

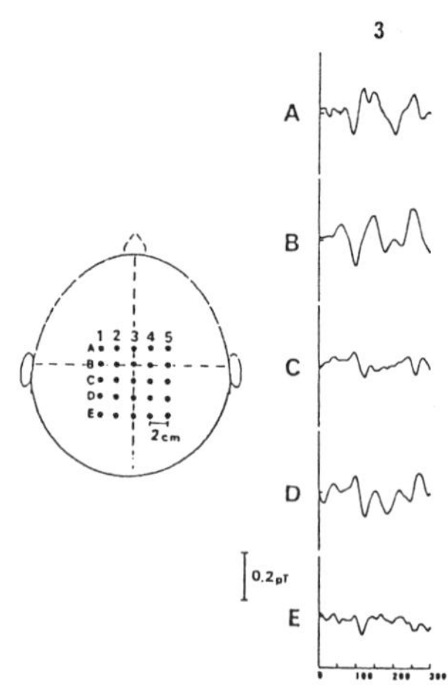

Fig.1 Averaged magnetic recordings of SEFs.

2) Isofield contour maps

Fig.2 shows the isofield contour maps for successive middle latencies obtained from the averaged magnetic recordings. Measurement positions are indicated by dots and letters in the leftside of Fig.1. Shades and broken lines indicate magnetic flux out of the scalp which is negative fields. The field distribution showed dipolar and/or dipolar-like feature with two extrema of opposite polarity for latencies of 75 to 115 ms between A3 and D3. Namely, polarity of magnetic field was negative on the precentral and was positive on the postcentral to a boundary of around Cz. At a latency of 80 ms, for instance, the extrema of magnetic field distribution showed that B3 is minimum of -121 fT and D3 is maximum of 80 fT, and it showed clockwise

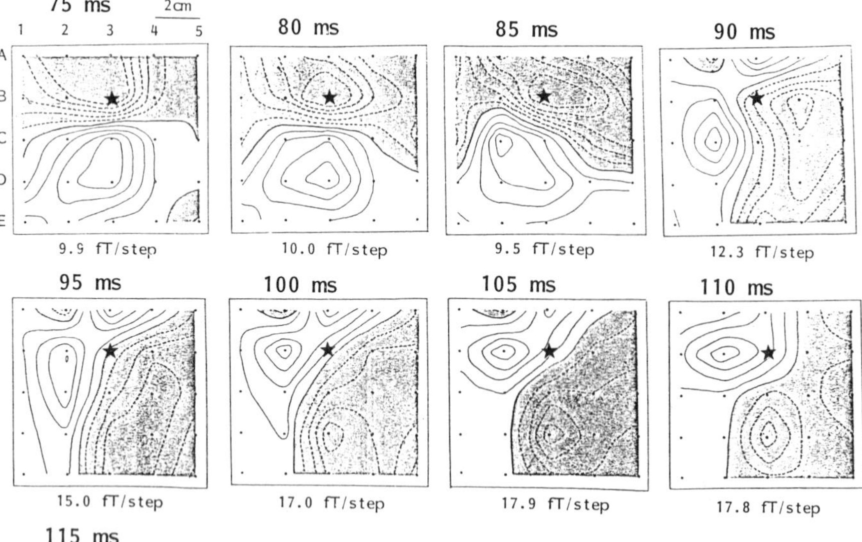

Fig.2 Isofield contour maps of SEFs on the scalp. Dots indicate the measurement positions and stars show the location of Cz.

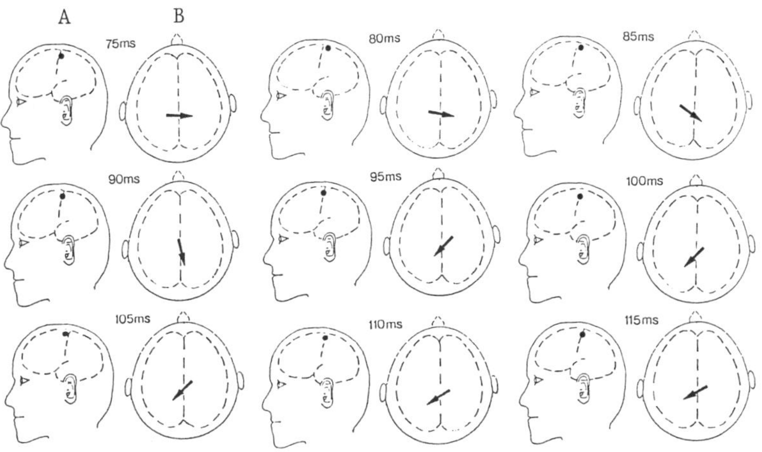

Fig.3 Location and direction of the calculated ECD in the cortex (panel A) and on the scalp (panel B).

rotation with lapse of latency in the neighborhood of postcentral gyrus of foot representing dipolar and/or dipolar-like feature. At a latency of 100 ms, extrema showed that B2 was maximum of 100 fT and D3 was minimum of about - 100 fT.

DISCUSSION

To trace the the equivalent source localization in the brain for the middle latencies of SEFs, we calculated ECD in a meaning of the best fit between experimental and theoretical distribution[4]. To compare the field distribution of model with the measured distribution, we used a criterion factor, $\sigma(t)$ minimizing by the best fit at each latency. $\sigma(t)$ is given by

$$\sigma(t) = \frac{\sqrt{N^{-1}\sum_j (B_{Ej}(t) - B_{Cj}(t))^2}}{B_{max}(t) - B_{min}(t)}$$

where N is a total number of measured position. $B_{Ej}(t)$ and $B_{Cj}(t)$ is a measured magnetic field and a calculated magnetic field at position j, respectively. $B_{max}(t)$ and $B_{min}(t)$ is a field extrema at a latency measured over all positions on the scalp.

When ECD was calculated, we set up a head model consisting of a homogeneous sphere of 10 cm radius by referring an image of X-ray computed tomography of a subject's head. Fig.3 shows the locations of ECDs in the cortex (panel A) and on the scalp (panel B) located in the center of arrows. Arrows represent the direction of ECD projected on to the measurement plane.

Results of ECD tracing were summarized as follows; ECDs localized at about 1 cm posterior from Cz and the contrary side of stimulation site on the mesial surface. Angle of clockwise rotation from latencies of

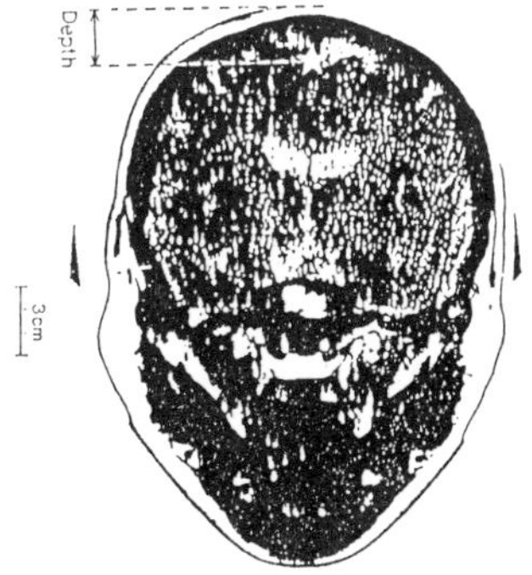

Fig.4 Location of ECD at 80 ms inserted into an image of X-ray computed tomography.

75 ms to 115 ms was 141 degree. The depth from the scalp was in the range of 19.7 to 24.1 mm and the strength of ECD was in the range of 3.79 to 4.52 nAm.

To test the validity of the location of the equivalent source in the cortex, an ECD at a latency of 80 ms representing the best dipolarity was selected. Fig.4 shows the location of ECD inserted to an image of X-ray computed tomography obtained from a subject's head (male, 22 years old). It can be seen that a calculated ECD is located at the depth of 19.7 mm from the scalp and is extended in the postcentral gyrus of the contrary side to the stimulation site correponding to foot representation. The direction of ECD is almost perpendicular to the surface of the cortex and it can be seen as a tangential source faced from the left to the right. This localization results is in a good agreement with a viewing point of foot representation of functional localization of the brain.

CONCLUSIONS

We have performed the measurement of somatosensory evoked magnetic field perpendicular to the scalp over 25 positions in a nonmagnetically shielded room with a SQUID connected to a second order gradiometer. The tibial nerve of the right ankle was stimulated electrically. Isofield contour maps for the middle latencies of 75 to 115 ms obtained from the averaged time recordings showed clear clockwise rotation on the mesial surface of the scalp representing dipolar and/or dipolar-like feature. A validity of the calculated equivalent source localization in the cortex by ECD tracing was confirmed by comparing the location of ECD with an image of X-ray computed tomography obtained from a subject's head.

ACKNOWLEDGEMENTS

We would like to thank Dr. Y.Ishiyama for making X-ray images at his hospital. This study has been supported by the grant of research from Center for Research, Tokyo Denki University.

REFERENCES

1. T.Allison, W.Goff, P.Williamson and J.Vangilder, On the neural origin of the human somatosensory evoked potential, Prog.clin.Neurophysiol., Vol.7, 51-68 (1980)
2. T.Allison, Scalp and cortical recordings of initial somatosensory cortex activity to median nerve stimulation in a man, Ann.N.Y.Acad. Sci., Vol.388, 671-678 (1982)
3 C.Wood, D.Cohen, M.Yarita, Electrical sources in human somatosensory cortex:Identification by combined magnetic and potential recordings, Science, Vol.227, 1051-1053 (1985)
4. S.N.Erne, H.P.Lehmann, M.Masselli and Y.Uchikawa, Biomagnetism: Application and theory, ed.by H.Weinberg, G.Stroink, T.Katilla, 126-131 (1985)

NEUROMAGNETIC LOCALISATION OF SENSORIMOTOR CORTEX SOURCES ASSOCIATED WITH VOLUNTARY MOVEMENTS IN HUMANS

D. Cheyne, R. Kristeva, W. Lang, G. Lindinger and L. Deecke

Neurological Clinic
University of Vienna
Lazarettgasse 14, 1090 Vienna, Austria

INTRODUCTION

Source localisation techniques based on neuromagnetic measurements and the concept of an equivalent current dipole source has proven to be a useful method for the study of discrete sources of electrical brain activity in humans. A great deal of success has been achieved in describing the functional organization of sensory input to the primary auditory, somatosensory and visual cortices using these methods (for a recent review see Romani and Rossini, 1988). Magnetic field changes have also been observed over the motor areas of the cerebral cortex prior to, and during self-initiated movements (Deecke et al., 1982; Hari et al., 1983; Cheyne and Weinberg, 1989) and the sources of these movement-related magnetic fields are presumed to arise, in part, from the primary motor cortex.

The representation of movement for different parts of the body has been shown to be organized in a somatotopic or "homuncular" fashion within the primary motor cortex in humans on the basis of electrical stimulation studies (Penfield and Rasmussen, 1968) and also on the basis of comparisons with somatotopic maps in the motor cortex of non-human primates (Lemon, 1988). In the present study, neuromagnetic fields accompanying voluntary movements of different body regions were measured over the contralateral motor areas in two subjects, with the hypothesis that sources localised for neuromagnetic fields associated with activity in the primary motor cortex should also reflect this functional organization.

METHODS

Magnetic fields accompanying self-paced movements of the right foot (dorsiflexion), right index finger (flexion), right hand (flexion about the wrist), and lower right face (unilateral contractions) were studied in two right-handed subjects. One subject also performed right thumb flexions. Magnetic recordings (bandpass 0.1-50 Hz) were taken from 30 to 90 positions over the left and central scalp using two 7-channel, 2nd-order gradiometer systems (BTi model 607) located in a magnetically shielded room (Vacuumschmelze, GmbH) with an overall noise level of about 15 $fT/Hz^{1/2}$ (above 1 Hz). Extensive care was taken to avoid head movement artifacts due to respiration by having subjects hold their breath 2-3 sec prior to, and during the movement. A 3-dimensional head coordinate system defined by the nasion and pre-auricular points, and the location of standard (International 10-20 system) electrode positions, were measured using a 3-D digitizing system. This system also recorded the position and orientation of the sensing coils during each measurement.

Epochs of 2 sec duration were triggered on the rectified surface EMG of the active muscles (1.5 sec pre-trigger) and averaged off-line after excluding artifact contaminated trials. Averages were filtered using a 10 Hz low-pass digital filter (-24 dB Butterworth). Isocontour mapping of selected time points (averaged over 40 msec intervals) was used to identify dipolar field patterns prior to, and during movement. Single current dipole sources were then fitted for chosen time periods using a least-squares fitting algorithm described by Harrop et al. (1987) taking into account both gradiometer geometry and orientation with respect to the head coordinate system.

Advances in Biomagnetism
Edited by S.J. Williamson *et al.*
Plenum Press, New York

RESULTS

In both subjects, slow magnetic fields were observed over the left and central scalp, beginning about 1 sec prior to movement, which became maximal in amplitude at EMG onset. These slow shifts reversed in direction over the region of the sensorimotor cortex with outgoing fields laterally and ingoing fields medially as shown in Fig. 1(a). A response is also seen during movement onset (80 to 130 ms following EMG onset) over the same region, larger in amplitude and of opposite direction. (A second, less consistent response was also observed at about 270 msec post EMG onset in some of the waveforms). Two time periods were chosen for further analysis: (1) the pre-movement period 70 to 30 ms prior to EMG onset, designated here as a "readiness field" (RF), and (2) the large movement-onset related response 90 to 130 ms after EMG onset, termed here a "movement-evoked field" (MEF).

Iso-contour mapping of both RF and MEF for all movements revealed dipolar field patterns reversing over the region of the central sulcus with the RF patterns being somewhat asymmetrical with larger amplitude outgoing maxima. These patterns are shown for index finger movements in Fig. 1(b). Comparisons of field topography for different movements indicated that these reversals shifted anteriorly and laterally for movements of the hand, thumb, finger and face, respectively, in accordance with the somatotopic representation of these body regions in the primary motor cortex. Fields recorded for foot movements, however, were generally smaller in amplitude and did not show a similar dipolar topography.

Least-squares fitting of single dipole sources for both RFs and MEFs resulted in source locations for hand, finger, thumb, and face movements as predicted from the field topography which accounted for 70 to 90 percent of the variance in the data (Table 1). Comparisons of fitted dipole locations for the RFs with the digitized 10-20 electrode positions suggest sources of superficial depths anteriorly directed and distributed over the lateral extent of the left hemisphere. Figure 2 illustrates the projected positions of RF and MEF source estimates together with digitized 10-20 system electrode placements in the head coordinate system. The RF source estimates can be seen to be distributed over the lateral extent of the left hemisphere in the vicinity of electrode position C3 which roughly overlies the precentral gyrus (Homan et al., 1987).

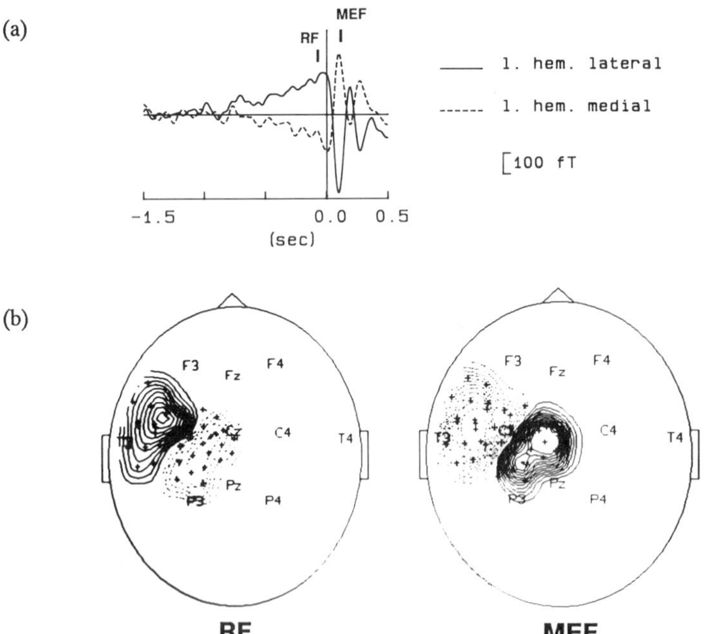

Fig. 1. (a) Neuromagnetic fields accompanying voluntary right index finger flexions measured over the lateral (solid trace) and medial (dashed trace) left hemisphere in subject 2. RF = readiness field; MEF = movement-evoked field. Upward deflection indicates flux out of the head. A vertical line at 0 sec indicates EMG onset. (b) Isocontour field maps for the RF and MEF intervals during index finger movements in the same subject . Contour steps are 26 fT. Dotted lines indicate flux into the head.

Table 1. Dipole Parameters for RF and MEF Source Estimates

	N	Q(nA-m)	X(cm)	Y(cm)	Z(cm)	R(cm)	% fit
Readiness field (RF)							
Subject 1							
hand	37	4.1	3.25	2.15	11.23	11.9	89%
index	27	4.3	2.87	3.03	10.12	10.9	80%
face	89	8.4	3.13	5.16	7.38	9.5	89%
Subject 2							
hand	39	12.2	3.08	2.03	10.59	11.2	80%
thumb	31	6.6	1.83	3.10	9.99	10.6	66%
index	41	7.8	1.90	4.43	9.16	10.4	88%
face	28	7.5	1.40	4.91	7.16	8.8	69%
Movement-evoked field (MEF)							
Subject 1							
hand	84	30.1	1.73	4.15	8.52	9.6	86%
index	77	32.5	1.65	3.56	7.67	8.6	72%
face	89	20.5	2.47	5.20	7.03	9.1	85%
Subject 2							
hand	35	36.1	1.72	2.91	9.15	9.8	72%
thumb	31	25.4	1.59	2.84	9.01	9.6	80%
index	41	31.6	0.98	3.41	9.11	9.8	87%
face	28	13.5	2.30	4.83	7.64	9.3	84%

N = number of recording positions; Q = dipole strength in current density; Positions are given in right-handed coordinate system with +x-axis through nasion and +y-axis through left pre-auricular point; R = radius; % fit = percent of observed variance accounted for by the theoretical field.

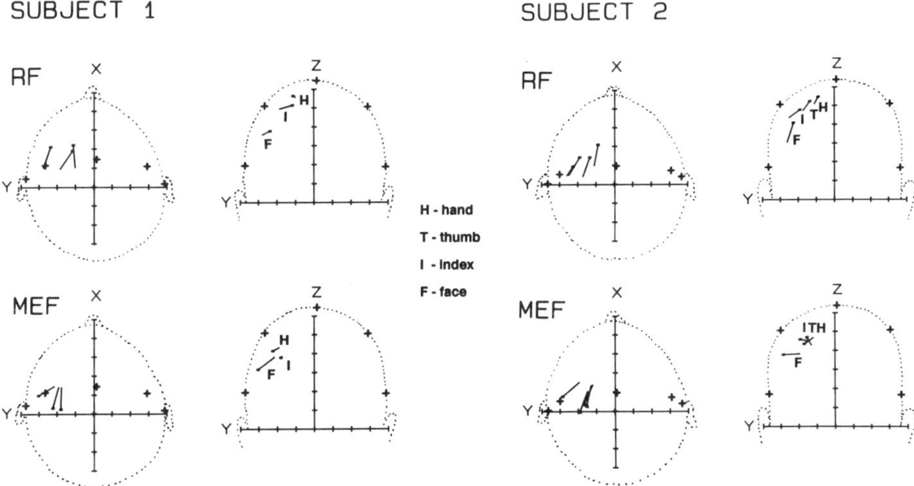

Fig. 2. Dipole locations for the readiness field (RF) and movement-evoked field (MEF) accompanying hand (H), index finger (I), face (F) and thumb (T) movements shown as projections in the head coordinate system as seen from above the head (x-y projection) and from the back of the head (z-y projection). Actual location is the midpoint of the dipole. Square heads indicate direction of negative pole. The 10-20 system electrode placements T3, C3, Cz, C4 and T4 (from left to right respectively) are indicated by crosses. Scale is 2 cm per division. Head outlines are drawn to provide perspective only.

Comparisons of the positions and radii for RF and MEF source estimates indicates that MEF sources were about 1 cm posterior and greater in depth than those for the RFs (with the exception of face movements in subject 2). MEF estimates for hand and thumb movements were in a similar location to that for finger movements. Similar fits could not be achieved for foot movements in either subject.

DISCUSSION

These results indicate that neuromagnetic recordings can be successfully used to identify current dipole sources associated with voluntary movement preparation within contralateral sensorimotor cortex. Least-squares estimated locations of equivalent dipole sources for the readiness field (RF) immediately preceding movement onset agree reasonably well with the known somatotopic representation of different body regions for movement, in accordance with the motor "homunculus" of Penfield (Penfield and Rasmussen, 1968), thus indicating that such sources may reflect localised activation of primary motor cortex related to movement execution. Equivalent sources can also be localised for a "movement-evoked" field (MEF) at about 110 msec after EMG onset within the same region. These MEF sources were greater in depth and slightly posterior to the pre-movement RF sources suggesting that the MEF may reflect activity in the posterior bank of the central sulcus related to early reafferent input resulting from the beginning of the movement. However, MEF sources for hand, finger and thumb movements were fitted to very similar positions, whereas the location for face movements corresponded to the pre-movement source location. Thus, MEF sources may also reflect to some degree the somatotopic organization of reafferent input to the cortex but were not somatotopically distributed in the same manner as the RF source estimates.

The inability to achieve clear results for foot movements may be explained by the representation of such movements at a greater depth along the mesial surface of the hemisphere. However, in the case of medially located sources, one should also consider the possibility of summation of additional field activity arising from the ipsilateral hemisphere which may also be present during unilateral movements (Cheyne and Weinberg, 1989). Additionally, fronto-medial motor structures which are also known to be active prior to movement (eg., supplementary motor area) may also contribute to field patterns near the vertex and may account for the observed asymmetry of the RF patterns. However, it is not known to what extent such asymmetry may be due to the orientation of sources in primary motor cortex which may be vertical or radial in orientation if they extend into the crown of the precentral gyrus itself.

Comparisons of equivalent dipole sources localised for movement-related fields with precise anatomical information is needed in order to clarify the exact nature of such sources. However, the present data indicate that one source of neuromagnetic fields preceding voluntary movements can be successfully localised within the region of the sensorimotor cortex and corresponds to the somatotopically organized output map of the primary motor cortex. Such measures may thus provide a useful, non-invasive, means of studying human sensorimotor function.

ACKNOWLEDGEMENTS

D. Cheyne was supported by an NSERC of Canada Postdoctoral Fellowship.

REFERENCES

Cheyne, D. and Weinberg, H., 1989, Neuromagnetic fields accompanying unilateral finger movements: readiness fields and movement-evoked fields, submitted for publication.

Deecke, L., Weinberg, H. and Brickett, P., 1982, Magnetic fields of the human brain accompanying voluntary movements: Bereitschaftsmagnetfeld, Exp. Brain Res., 48: 144-148.

Hari, R., Antervo, A., Katila, T., Poutanen, T., Seppaenen, M., Tuomista, T., Varpula, T., 1983, Cerebral magnetic fields associated with voluntary limb movements in man, Il Nuovo Cimento, 2(D): 484-494.

Harrop, R., Weinberg, H., Brickett, P., Dykstra, C., Robertson, A., Cheyne, D., Baff, M. and Crisp, D., 1987, The biomagnetic inverse problem: Some theoretical and practical considerations, Phys. Med. Biol., 32: 1545-1557.

Homan, R.W., Herman, J and Purdy, P., 1987, Cerebral location of International 10-20 system electrode placement, Electroenceph. clin. Neurophysiol., 66: 376-382.

Lemon, R., 1988, The output map of the primate motor cortex, Trends Neurosci., 11: 501-506.

Penfield, W. and Rasmussen, T., 1968, The cerebral cortex of man, Hafner, New York-London.

Romani, G.L. and Rossini, P., 1988, Neuromagnetic functional localisation: Principles, state of the art, and perspectives, Brain Topog., 1: 5-21.

MEASUREMENT OF NEUROMAGNETIC FIELDS

PRECEDING TRIGGERED AND SELF-PACED FINGER MOVEMENTS

Yoshinari Mizutani[*], Kazuhiko Okano[**], and Shinya Kuriki[***]

[*] Department of Information Engineering, Faculty of Engineering, Tohoku University, Sendai 980, JAPAN
[**] Department of Physiology, School of Medicine, Hokkaido University, Sapporo 060, JAPAN
[***] Research Institute of Applied Electricity, Hokkaido University, Sapporo 060, JAPAN

INTRODUCTION

In previous reports[1-5] slow magnetic field shifts preceding voluntary finger or foot movements were detected from the brain. It was considered that the magnetic fields were generated from the motor area, premotor area, or supplementary motor area of the cortex. The signal sources were estimated for the magnetic field accompanying different kinds of movements. Those magnetic fields were called movement-related magnetic fields that include readiness fields(bereitschafts magnetic fields) and motor fields. We have carried out measurements of neuromagnetic fields for the purposes of comparing the neuronal activity preceding triggered movement by a visual signal and nontriggered (self-paced) movement.[6]

METHODS

The subject was instructed to switch a key between an index finger and a thumb for two kinds of task. One task(50%) was a visual-triggered finger movement, which was a press of the key within 1 sec after the light of a red LED in front of the subject. Another 50% was a nontriggered (self-paced) movement, which was a press of the key after waiting for the nolight of LED more than 8 sec. The movement-task sequence was controlled by a microcomputer, and the two tasks were selected at random. The magnetic fields were measured in the environment without magnetic shielding using an rf-SQUID with a second-derivative gradiometer. The measurement frequency was limited from 0.1 to 20 Hz. To improve S/N ratio, averaging of more than 64 trials was carried out. The trigger of the averaging was the key-pressed time. Responses to the triggered movement later than 1 sec, and the self-paced movement less than 8 sec waiting, were rejected for averaging. The movement-related magnetic fields were recorded for two right-handed subjects and one left-handed subject.

Muscle activity was recorded from index dorsal interossei muscle with surface electrodes distanced 2 cm. The Electromyogram(EMG) was limited from 50 to 3k Hz, and full-wave rectified.

Advances in Biomagnetism
Edited by S.J. Williamson *et al.*
Plenum Press, New York

RESULTS AND DISCUSSION

Magnetic Fields

Figure 1 shows typical measured magnetic fields preceding and during key press movements for two subjects. Key-pressed time is indicated as 0 msec. The slow magnetic field shifts preceding the movements are observed at the contralateral hemisphere for the two kinds of key press. At the ipsilateral hemisphere distinct magnetic field shifts are not observed in the two subjects. The polarity of these slow magnetic shifts at the contralateral hemisphere is reversed between the upper and lower region of the head. In right-handed subject YM the magnetic field emerges from the lower region and re-enters into the upper region of the left hemisphere for both tasks. In left-handed subject KO the field emerges from the upper and re-enters into lower region of the right hemisphere. Thus the current-dipole sources oriented forward are estimated at around the motor area in both the subjects.

Figure 2 shows magnetic fields measured at various locations over contralateral hemisphere in subject KO. The slow shifts appear about 1 sec - 800 msec before the key-pressed time for the self-paced movement, whereas the slow shifts appear about 400 msec before the key-pressed time for the triggered movement. The triggered movement has about 500msec later onset of the magnetic shifts than the self-paced movement. Another subject YM also showed similar latency difference of the slow shift. However, the obserbed slow magnetic shifts were contaminated by background noise, i.e., other brain activities or movements of the head. Therefore, the distinct dipole estimation was difficult.

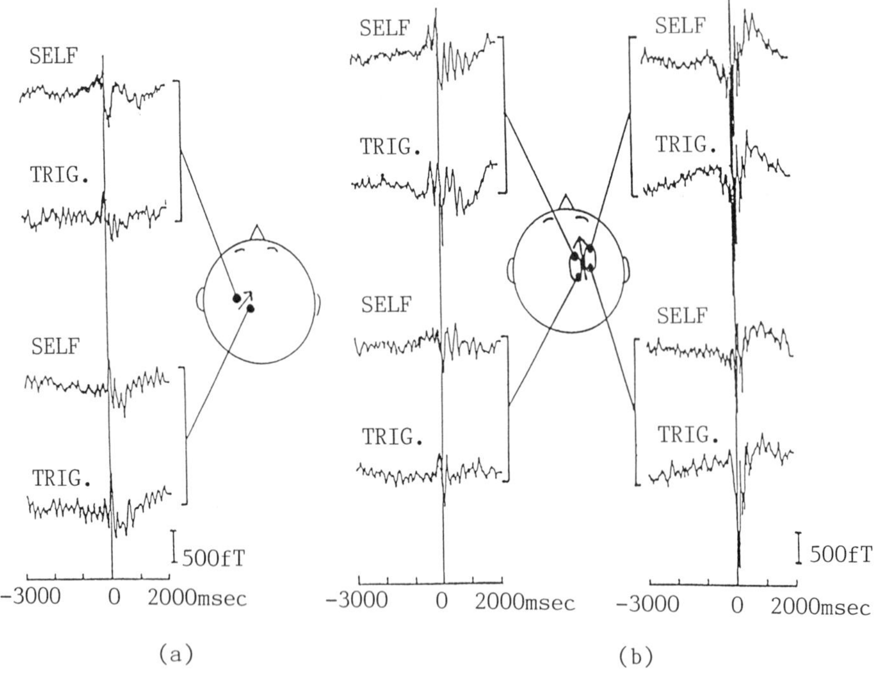

Fig. 1. Averaged magnetic fields measured at the contralateral hemisphere accompanying triggered and self-paced finger movements. (a)Responses in a right-handed subject YM, and (b)responses in a left-handed subject KO. Key-pressed time is at 0 msec. Upward deflection indicates the magnetic field out of the head. An arrow indicates the direction of a dipole source estimated from the slow magnetic shifts.

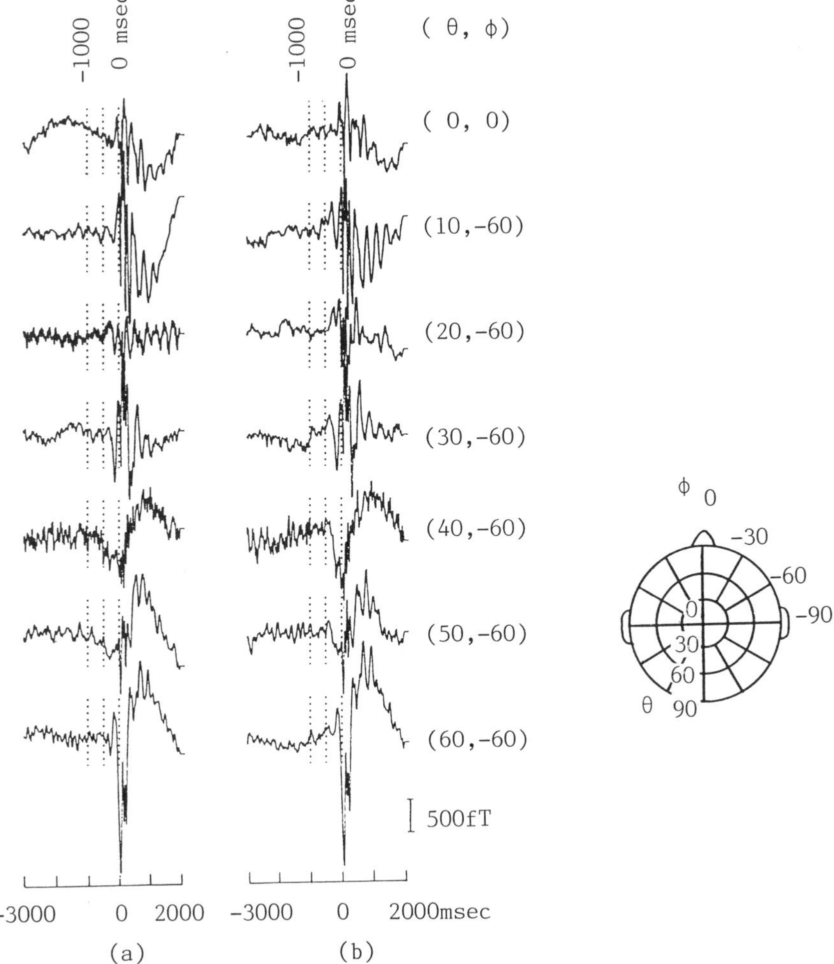

Fig. 2. Averaged magnetic fields measured at various locations over the contralateral hemisphere of subject KO accompanying (a)self-paced movement and (b) triggered movements. Key-pressed time is at 0 msec. Upward deflection indicates the magnetic field out of the head. Measuring portions are described by spherical coordinates. θ is the angle of declination from the z-axis, and ϕ is the angle of rotation from the mid sagittal plane.

EMG Potentials

Figure 3 shows typical EMG potentials measured at the hand preceding and during key press movements. Key-pressed time is indicated as 0 msec. It was observed that muscle activities began before the key-pressed time for both two kinds of task. In 20 trials of subject YM, the onset of muscle activities for the self-paced movement began 40-90 msec (average was 63 msec) before the key-pressed time(Fig.3(a)), and the onset for the triggered movement began 45-90 msec(average was 61 msec) before the key-pressed time (Fig.3(b)). There was no significant difference in the EMG onset between the triggered and self-paced movements. Therefore, about 500 msec difference in the onset of magnetic shifts is the difference in the onset of neural activities associated with two kinds of finger movements.

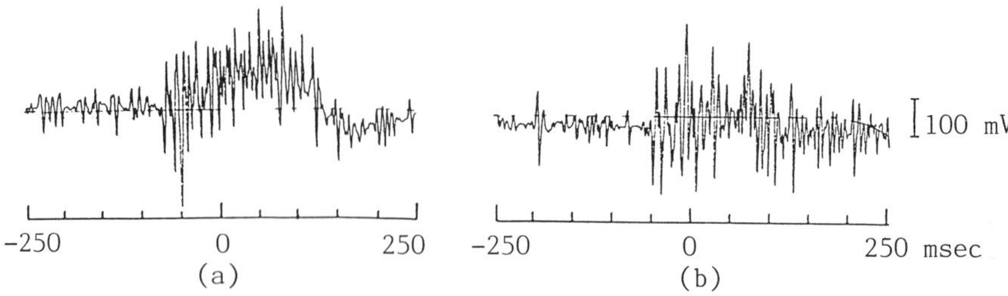

Fig. 3. EMG potentials measured at the hand accompanying the finger movement. (a)Response for self-paced movement, and (b) response for triggered movement. Key-pressed time is at 0 msec.

CONCLUSION

Different latencies of slow shifts preceding movements were observed in the magnetic fields associated with self-paced and triggered finger movements. The result suggests that the two movements have neural sources activated at around the motor area of the cortex at different times. Different states of readiness and pre-processings may be involved in the two kinds of finger movements.

ACKNOWLEDGMENTS

We are grateful to Prof.G.Matsumoto for helpful suggestions, and to Prof. M.Yamamoto and Dr.M.Nakao for helpful supports.

REFERENCES

1. L.Deecke, H.Weinberg, and P.Brickett, Magnetic fields of the human brain accompanying voluntary movement: bereitschaftsmagnetfield, Exp.Brain Res., 48:144 (1982).
2. L.Deecke, J.Boshert, H.Weinberg, and P.Brickett, Magnetic fields of the human brain(bereitschaftsmagnetfield) preceding voluntary foot and toe movements, Exp.Brain Res., 52:81 (1983).
3. R.Hari, A.Antervo, T.Katila, T.Poutanen, M.Seppänen, T.Tuomisto, and T.Varpula, Cerebral Magnetic fields associated with voluntary limb movements in man, IL Nuobo Cimento, 2D-2:484 (1983).
4. J.Boshert, R.F.Hink, and L.Deecke, Finger movement versus toe movement -related potentials: Further evidence for supplementary motor area(SMA) participation prior to voluntary action, Exp.Brain Res., 52:73 (1983).
5. L.Deecke,J.Boshert,P.Brickett, and H.Weinberg, Magnetoencephalographic evidence for possible supplementary motor area participation in human voluntary movement, in: "Biomagnetism: Application and theory," H.Weinberg, G.Stroink, and T.Katila eds., Pergamon Press, New York (1984).
6. K.Okano and J.Tanji, Neuronal activities in the primate motor fields of the agranular frontal cortex preceding visually triggered and self-paced movement, Exp.Brain Res., 66:155 (1987).

NEUROMAGNETIC LOCALIZATION OF LATE PAIN-RELATED FIELD SOURCES

R. Wakai[1,3], J. Joseph[1], E. Howland[2], M. Backonja[2,3], F. Potenti[2], O. Baffa[1], and C. Cleeland[2]

Biomagnetism Research Lab[1] and Pain Research Group[2]
Departments of Medical Physics[1] and Neurology[2]
University of Wisconsin, Madison, WI 53706
Middleton Veterans Hospital[3], Madison, WI 53705

INTRODUCTION

Since the early work of Chatrian et al. (1974), pain-related evoked potentials (PEPs) have been extensively investigated as possible physiological correlates of laboratory pain (see Chapman et al. 1979). The utility of PEPs is largely based upon studies which show that the amplitudes of the late potentials often correlate well with stimulus intensity and subjective report, and exhibit a consistent diminution when analgesic or behavioral pain control methods are introduced. It is also notable that for most types of stimulation, the dominant components of the evoked response occur at latencies near 150 and 250 ms (N150-P250), with largest amplitudes measured at the vertex. Hence, many studies have focussed specifically upon the N150-P250 as a likely correlate of laboratory pain.

A major obstacle to the use of PEPs is the problem of their interpretation. Some data suggest that the late PEPs correlate with pain perception; but it has never been established whether these potentials are pain specific or are due to the late processing of signals received via the fast conducting pathways, perhaps indicative of the attention or arousal level of the subject. Furthermore, the sources of many of these potentials are unknown. A knowledge of the pathways and substrates involved in the generation of late PEPs may be essential in resolving their true meaning. We report here the source localization of several pain-related magnetic field (PEF) components-- N90m, N150m, and P250m--using intracutaneous electrical stimulation of the finger.

METHODS

Three healthy male subjects participated in the study. Moderately painful intracutaneous electrical stimulation of the little finger of the nondominant hand was employed. The finger was prepared by removing the epidermis with a manually-rotated #2 dental drill, and attaching an electrode over the burr hole using EEG paste. This preparation was found to produce a

Advances in Biomagnetism
Edited by S.J. Williamson *et al.*
Plenum Press, New York

sensation of sharp, localized pain. The electric stimulator (Grass SD9) was set to output a 5 ms square pulse, and the voltage was adjusted until the subject reported a pain rating of four on a scale of zero to ten.

PEF measurements were made in a relatively quiet, unshielded environment, using a single-channel, asymmetric third-order SQUID gradiometer (CTF Systems, Inc.). The detection coil was 2.54 cm diameter, and the system noise was 35 $fT/(Hz)^{1/2}$, throughout the measurement bandwidth of 0.2- 40.0 Hz.

PEFs were recorded over the contralateral scalp at about 40 positions, arranged in a grid with 2.54 cm grid spacing. Two hundred trials were averaged at each position, using a random intertrial interval of 2.0 to 4.0 s. For each trial, a one-second time record was digitized, consisting of 250 ms prestimulus and 750 ms poststimulus data. PEPs at the vertex (referenced to the contralateral ear) were simultaneously recorded with the PEFs, in order to monitor the stability of the evoked response throughout the duration of the study. MRI scans were performed on two of the subjects. A tube of water, extending from the vertex to the preauricular point was placed on the subjects head during the scan in order to register the images to the PEF measurement grid.

RESULTS

Figure 1 shows the grid of averaged PEFs obtained from the right (contralateral) side of subject EH's head. The top row of the grid runs along the midline, and the midpoint of this row is at the vertex. The amplitudes of the N150m-P250m are very large--up to 700fT. The N150m-P250m reverses phase near the Sylvian fissure, and exhibits a marked asymmetry as is often observed for frontotemporal sources (Barth et al., 1986, Rose et al., 1987). PEP measurements revealed that the electric N150-P250 was largest at the vertex, as expected. In addition, we note that the top two rows of the grid show PEFs that appear morphologically similar to the N150m-P250m, but which have latencies that are significantly longer-- 190 and 330 ms. These components presumably arise from sources other than the N150m-P250m generators. In order to localize these components, a much larger region of the head would have to be measured. This was not attempted, in view of the time demands already placed upon the subjects.

Equivalent dipole fitting

Raw magnetic isofield contours at latencies of 90 and 150 ms are shown in Figure 2a-b. The contour for the 250 ms PEF was omitted because it is nearly identical, though opposite in phase, to the 150 ms contours. The fitting routine assumes a spherical local geometry for the head, with the radius estimated from MRI images of the subject. Corrections for the gradiometer baseline and the finite area of the gradiometer coils were taken into account.

Anatomical localization

The localizations obtained from the magnetic measurements were overlaid onto an MRI scan in order to anatomically localize

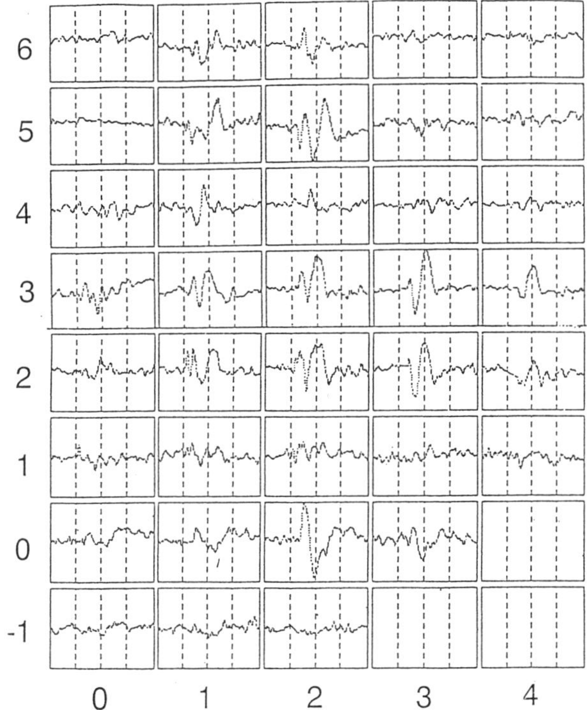

Figure 1. Grid of averaged PEFs from the right side of the head of subject EH. The top row runs along the midline, with the middle point of this row at the vertex. The left edge of the grid is towards to back of the head. The grid spacing is 2.54 cm. Each time record is 1 s, with 250 ms of prestimulus and 750 ms of poststimulus data.

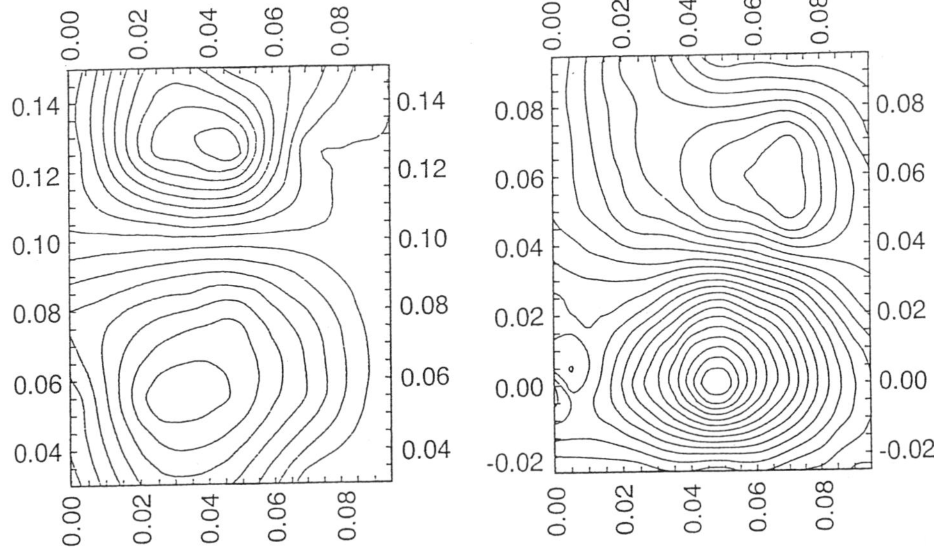

Figure 2. Magnetic isofield contours at latencies of a) 90 ms and (b) 150 ms. The origin is at the first column and the next to last row of the measurement grid of Fig. 1. Units are in meters.

the sources. The 90 ms component of the PEF is localized to the finger area of the primary somatosensory cortex at a depth of 2.3 mm below the scalp. The N150 and P250 are both localized to the frontal operculum at a depth 2.8 mm below the scalp. The locations of the N90 and N150-P250 obtained from all subjects are in good agreement, except for the depth of the P250 in subject FM, which was about 1 cm deeper.

DISCUSSION

The localization of the N150m-P250m to the frontal operculum is quite unexpected from electric measurements alone, which nearly always exhibit a maximum at the vertex. A likely explanation for this is that the N150-P250 arises from bilateral sources which summate to produce a maximum at the vertex.

Hari and co-workers have also localized PEFs to the frontal operculum using electrical stimulation of tooth pulp (Hari et al., 1983), but our results differ somewhat from theirs. In particular, both our electric and magnetic data exhibit strong deflections at 150 and 250 ms, while the magnetic data of Hari et al. do not. The largest component of their PEFs occurred at a latency of about 90-110 ms, and was localized to the frontal operculum. These differences may reflect the sensitivity of magnetic field recording to dipole orientation, which can be affected by details of the stimulus. In this regard, the late pain-related PEFs appear to contrast with the corresponding PEPs, which display a morphology that is relatively insensitive to the type of stimulation used.

In conclusion, we have localized late pain-related evoked fields corresponding to N90, N150, and P250. Our findings demonstrate that evoked field recording can be a valuable tool in the study of laboratory pain, and may lead to a better understanding of the late pain-related potentials and fields.

REFERENCES

Barth, D.S., Sutherling, W., Broffman, J., and Beatty, J. (1986), Magnetic localization of a dipolar current source implanted in a sphere and a human cranium, Electroenceph. and Clin. Neurophysiol., 63: 260-273.

Chatrian, G., Canfield, R.C., Lettich, E., and Black, R.G. (1974), Cerebral response to tooth stimulation in man, J. Dent. Res., 53: 1299.

Chapman, C.R., Chen, A.C.N., and Harking, S.W. (1979), Brain Evoked Potentials as Correlates of Laboratory Pain: A Review and Perspectives, in Advances in Pain Research and Therapy, vol. 3, ed. John J. Bonica et al., Raven Press, New York.

Hari, R., Kaukoranta, E., Reinikainen, K., Huopaniemi, T., and Mauno (1983), J., Neuromagnetic localization of cortical activity evoked by painful dental stimulation in man, Neurosci. Lett., 42: 77-82.

Rose, D.F., Sato, S., Smith, P.D., et al., Modeling the temporal region in patients with temporal lobe epilepsy (1987), Phys. Med. Biol., 32: 59-63.

MULTI-DIMENSIONAL VECTOR ANALYSIS OF EVOKED RESPONSES

J. Suk and D. Brenner

New York University, Center for Neuromagnetism
Department of Biophysics and Physiology
New York, N.Y., 10016

INTRODUCTION

We used model independent multi-dimensional vector analysis of evoked responses recorded with two seven channel magnetometers and multi-variate statistics to detect changes over time in the source distribution. Furthermore, we found visual inspection of the vectors' magnitude and direction a simple way to determine a responses' important features. Donchin (1966), working in time domain pioneered the application of multi-dimensional analysis to evoked potentials. Ilmoniemi et al., (1988) applied multi-dimensional analysis to magnetic recordings of spontanteous activity.

A vector can be constructed by using each magnetometer output as a component. The vector's magnitude squared is a measure of the total detected signal power. It depends on both the source strength and its distribution but it can be used for easily approximating the latencies and widths of a response's components. The vector's direction in fourteen dimensional space relates only to the distribution of neuronal activity and is independent of its total strength. By a cursory examination of its variation over time, one can tell whether the source distribution is relatively stable or changing rapidly. More sophisticated statistical analysis can be applied to test for small changes.

By remaining in the fourteen dimensional "signal" space as opposed to a smaller, "model" space, five dimensional in the case of the dipole model, one can make stronger inferences about source behavior as a functon of time or stimulus. After fitting data to a model, less information is available to test for differences between data sets. Furthermore, with model independent analysis, one need not be concerned over whether or not a particular model is appropriate or how it is put into practice, i.e. the computer algorithm. This is important in areas such as epilepsy where the question of an appropriate model is still being debated (Gloor, 1985). In evoked response experiments where the dipole model is, at least, partially appropriate (Gidok et al., 1988), both techniques can be used: modeling for determining the approximate source location and vector analysis for statistical testing for changes in the source distribution. We applied vector analysis to responses evoked by the stimulation of individual fingers. The results show that changes in the source distribution can be detected without using a model. Having used the dipole model to determine where the neural source is, we can now study the response's dynamics more closely.

METHODS

We analyzed somatically evoked responses taken with two seven channel probes (Biomagnetic Technologies Inc.). A 300 Hz vibratory stimulus of 100 msec duration was used. Piezo-electric stimulators were attached to the thumb, index and little fingers of a subject's right hand. For each subject, exploratory measurements were made to determine two probe locations from which good responses could be recorded by most channels for each finger stimulated. The probes were then centered over each maximum and checked for position prior to each recording session. Data were digitized at 350 Hz with a bandwidth of 1-50 Hz. Approximately 667 stimuli were applied in random order with random interstimulus intervals to each finger. After separating by finger, the signals were averaged for 100 msecs prior to and 200 msecs subsequent to stimulus onset. The vector powers and directions were calculated from the average response except for statistical analysis when the direction was calculated for each trial. Power is the sum of the squares of each component, i. e. channel output. Its direction can be thought of as similiar to direction in three dimensional space, as a set of ratios (cosines) between the vector length and its projection onto

Advances in Biomagnetism
Edited by S.J. Williamson *et al.*
Plenum Press, New York

each axis. Here, each channel is an "axis" and the projection of the vector onto each axis is simply the strength of that channel's response. Instead of trying to visually analyze all fourteen directional cosines, which defeats the whole purpose of the analysis, we looked at the vectors' direction relative to a reference direction arbitarily, choosen to be the direction of the responses' first maximum. The direction between the two vectors is calculated in the usual way:

$$\cos(\text{theta}) = \frac{\sum a_i b_i}{\sqrt{\sum a_i^2 \sum b_i^2}}$$

We then looked at the change in power and direction as a function of time.

Since our axes change if the probes are not returned to their exact locations for each recording session, care has to be taken in comparing the results across sessions. Therefore, we applied statistical analysis only to data taken during each run. Furthermore, since changes in amplitude do not necessarily relate to changes in source distribution, statistical analysis was performed only on the vector direction. We tested three cases for significance; The first was that the source distribution was different for each finger stimulated; Second, that the responses of two major responses, 100 msecs apart, are not mirror images of each other as suggested by the direction versus time plots; And third, that the distribution changes during the first major peak.

Multi-variate ANOVA was performed using SAS statisical software. We took a conservative approach by assuming that each single trial in each condition was statistically independent of every other trial rather than being correlated because they came from the same subject. This underestimated the significance of the results.

RESULTS

The vector power and direction relative to the direction at 163 msecs for thumb stimulation for one subject are shown in figures 1 a - b. The average response for each of the fourteen channels

Figure 1 a-b. Response power and phase for subject UR; thumb stimulation. The vector's direction is calculated relative to its direction at 163 msecs. The stimulus onset was at 100 msec.

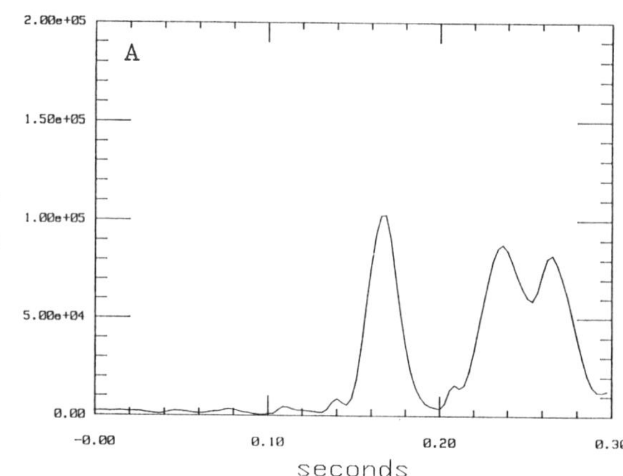

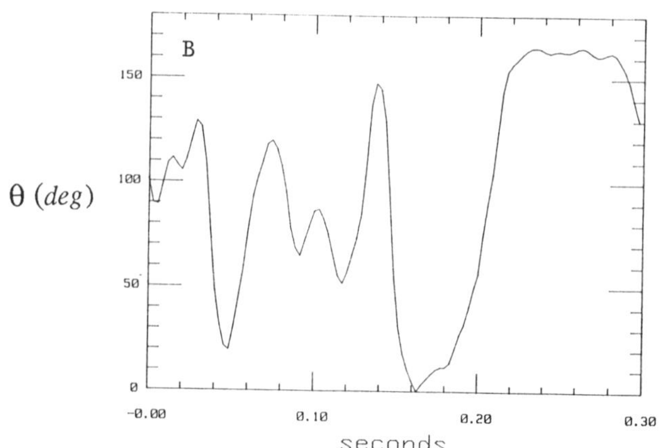

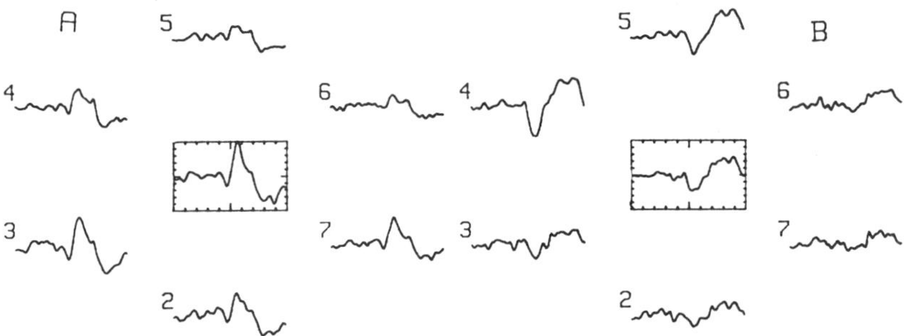

Figure 2. The responses of each of the fourteen channels, seven from each probe used to calculate the phase and power plots in figure 1. The x-axis is 300 msecs long. The y-axis goes from -150 fT to +150 fT.

used to calculate the phase and power in figure 1 is shown in figure 2. The power plot is typical of almost all the data analyzed, independent of subject, recording session or finger stimulated, a total of over 25 responses. However, there are significant changes in the absolute power of each peak and relative powers between peaks. Compare for example, figure 1a with figure 3a from the same subject, the same finger stimulated, but a different recording session. The peak at 163 msecs is 50% stronger, while the peaks at 237 and 266 msecs are 50% weaker. Occassionally we found responses with fewer or poorly defined peaks.

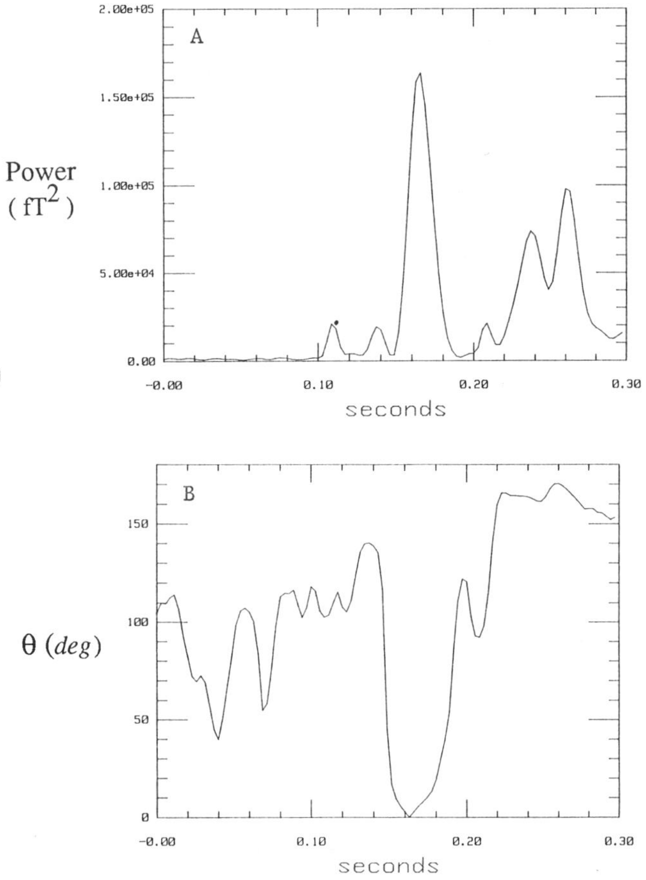

Figure 3 a-b. As in fig.1 except from a recording session one day later.

The phase plots show much less variabiltity, most of which can be related to low signal-to-noise ratios. The period between 150 and 180 msecs is always as seen in figure 1b. We detected no reliable responses prior to about 150 msec. The period between about 220 and 280 msecs shows more variability but is never exactly 180 degrees out of phase from the direction at 163 msecs. We investigated other reference directions The results suggest that at no time during the response are two vectors 180 degrees apart. Comparing figures 1 and 3 illustrates how little the phases relate to response power.

We tested for significance in the difference between response phases at 163 msecs for different fingers in three subjects. Surprisingly, only two subjects showed significance ($p < .0001$ and $p < .0002$) but this was consistent with the results of dipole localization in those subjects. In five cases, over three subjects and differing fingers, we found that the changes in phase between about 150 and 170 msecs, as seen in figure 1 and 3 b, are significant ($p < .025$ to $<.0001$). In comparing the distributions of two major peaks, at 163 and 263 msec, by reversing the direction of one of the vectors, we found significance differences at the .0005 level or lower in four cases . Two cases were not significance $p >.09$.

DISCUSSION

Viewing the power plots shows how easily they can be used to study the response morphology, peak amplitudes and peak latencies. For example, the peak at 260 msecs which shows up clearly in most of the power plots is barely visibile in much of the individual channel data and could be mistaken for noise. This is because summing the individual channels' response powers is a type of signal averaging improving the signal to noise ratio and the latency estimation.

The phase plots are strikingly similiar across subjects and trials. They show and statistical analysis confirms, that the source distribution is relatively constant during the first response peak. The distribution then changes rapidly over the next 25 or 30 msecs, again becoming relatively constant until the end of the response. To obtain the same results from the dipole model, it would have to be applied to each point in time. Then the time course of the dipole's position and orientation, four parameters, have to be studied, assuming that the information is available after the dipole model has been applied, not, for example, lost in a higher moment of the dipole expansion.

The statistical analysis confirmed that vector analysis can be used to study changes in source distributions during a response and across responses recorded with fixed probe positions. The ability to look at small changes in the source distribution independent of a model promises to be an important tool for research into physiological activity at the cortical level. The comparision of responses at 163 and 263 msecs is an example of what can be done. Although the approximately 180 degree shift in the vector direction suggests an off response occuring at the same location as the intial response, the statistics show that the sources of the two peaks are different, even though probably located in the same cortical region. Furthermore, the almost constant phase occuring after the on peak suggests that the cortex continues to note the existance of the stimulus and its termination using the same set of cells.

Finally, the finding of no significance for stimulating different fingers for one subject serves to remind us that large subject to subject variations do exist. This is easily seen on a gross anatomical scale by anyone who has looked at a few MRI images and is likely to be true on smaller scales as well.

ACKNOWLEDGEMENTS

We gratefully acknowledge the help and support of Bert Holland, Rodolfo Llinas, Yoshio Okada, and Steve Robinson.

REFERENCES

Godik, E.E., Gulyaev Yu. V., Matlashov A.N., Zhuravlev Yu. E., Lipovich A.Ya., and Tatatorin A. M., 1988, Dynamic maps of the neuromagnetic evoked fields. in: Biomagnetism '87 , K. Atsumi et al., ed., Toyko Denki University Press, Toyko.

Gloor, P., 1985, Neuronal generators and the problem of localization in electroencephalography: application of volume conductor to electroencephalography, J. Clin. Neurophys., 2:327.

Donchin, E., 1966, A multivariate approach to the analysis of average evoked potentials, IEEE Trans Bio-Med Eng., Vol. BME-13:131.

Ilmoniemi, R.J., Williamson, S.J., and Hostetler, W.E., New method for the study of spontaneous brain activity, in: Biomagnetism '87, K. Atsumi et al., ed., Denki University Press, Tokyo.

Suk, J ., Yamamoto, T., Ribary, U., and Llinas, R., 1989 , Magnetic localization of somatically evoked responses in the human brain, this conference.

Yamamoto, T., Williamson,.S.J., Kaufman, L. Nicholson, C., and Llinas, R., 1989, Magnetic localization of neuronal activity in the human brain, Proc. Natl. Acad. Sci., 85:8732.

IDENTIFICATION OF MULTIPLE SOURCES IN TRANSIENT VISUAL EVOKED NEUROMAGNETIC RESPONSES

C. Aine, J. George, P. Medvick, S. Supek, E. Flynn, and I. Bodis-Wollner[1]

Life Sciences and Physics Divisions, MS M882
Los Alamos National Laboratory, New Mexico 87545
[1]Mt. Sinai School of Medicine of the City University of New York, One Gustave Levy Place, New York, NY 10029

INTRODUCTION

Neuromagnetic measurements and associated modeling procedures must be capable of resolving multiple sources in order to localize and accurately characterize generators of visual evoked activity. Okada (1984) has estimated that a field pattern generated by two dipoles can be distinguished from that generated by a single dipole provided that the separation between the sources is greater than 1-2 cm, but there have been few attempts at modeling neurally generated field patterns with multiple, simultaneously active dipoles. The expanse of man's occipital cortex is estimated to be 150-250 cm^2 and invasive experiments with cats and monkeys suggest that this region most likely includes several discrete visual areas (e.g., Van Essen, 1985). It thus seems plausible that visual stimuli evoke activity from multiple discrete populations of neurons within visual cortical areas and that the application of appropriate modeling procedures to visually evoked neuromagnetic field data will resolve these populations.

We have examined several complex human neuromagnetic field distributions evoked by small area sinusoidal gratings presented to different locations in the visual field. Our results suggest the existence of multiple sources. The analyses we have utilized for resolving multiple sources in these studies differ depending on whether there was evidence of 1) two discrete asynchronous sources or 2) synchronous activation of two spatially discrete sources. In some cases we have observed field patterns which appear to be adequately modeled by a single source with its orientation and location evolving in time. This situation is examined in detail in a separate paper (George et al., this volume).

METHOD

Vertical sinusoidal gratings ($2^o \times 2^o$) of either 1 or 5 cycles per degree (cpd) were randomly presented to different spatial locations (e.g., central field, right field along the horizontal meridian, lower left and right quadrants) at a rate of approximately 1 per second while subjects maintained central fixation. Neuromagnetic responses from 6 right-handed subjects were monitored with a 7-channel SQUID-coupled gradiometer system in a magnetically shielded chamber. Neural responses were obtained from 42-112 sensor locations over occipital and parietal cortical areas while subjects lay prone on a table viewing a screen through a hole in the table. Left hemisphere recordings (frontal, temporal, parietal and occipital) were made while subjects lay on their right side; these data sets were kept separate from the posterior recordings to prevent potential confounds

Advances in Biomagnetism
Edited by S.J. Williamson *et al.*
Plenum Press, New York

due to small differences in the size of retinal image. Each condition was replicated at least three times resulting in averages containing at least 75 individual responses.

Field maps were constructed from amplitudes measured from the prestimulus baseline at 10 msec intervals. Least squares procedures were applied to fit a single dipole model to neuromagnetic distributions demonstrating two or more extrema of opposite polarity. Initial estimates of source locations were generated by bisecting the line segments connecting all possible pairs of positive and negative peaks apparent in contour maps of the data: peaks were defined as local extrema at least 40 fT (i.e. 2 x the noise level) greater or less than adjacent regions of the field map. A 2-dipole model was applied to the data if there was evidence of three or more peaks in the field distributions and/or the residual field maps obtained from single dipole fits (i.e., the difference between the empirical and theoretical field patterns) contained a dipolar field pattern. In some analyses, the percent of variance accounted for by the 2-dipole model was not significantly better than that achieved by a single dipole fit. The 2-dipole solution was considered reasonable if it accounted for at least 10% more of the variance than accounted for by the single dipole model.

RESULTS

Figure 1 illustrates that multiple sources can sometimes be resolved in MEG data by a careful examination of the temporal characteristics of neuromagnetic field patterns, without relying on modeling procedures. In the field maps for this subject (lower panels), the dominant feature from 120-170 msec was a high amplitude region of negative flux spanning left occipital and parietal regions. The top row of this figure compares waveforms

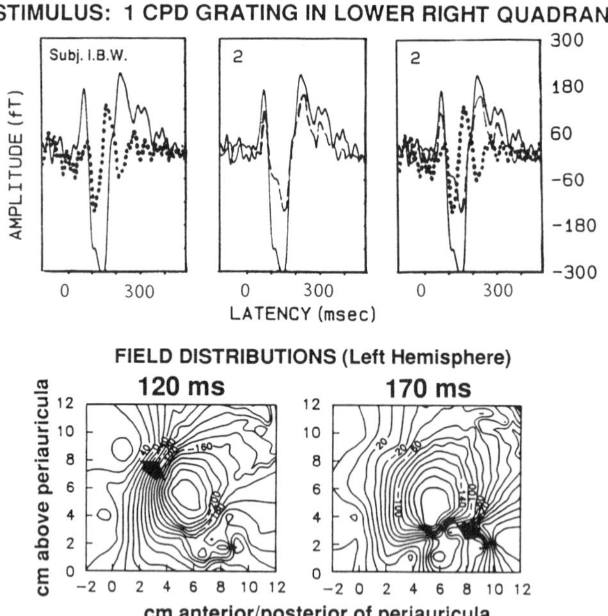

Figure 1. Sample neuromagnetic waveforms and field distributions recorded from the left hemisphere of one subject while gratings were presented in the lower right quadrant of the visual field. Stimulus duration was 400 msec. Each tracing represents an average of 100 individual evoked responses. The left periauricula is at x=0, y=-1 in the x-y surface plots.

from selected sensors to illustrate the temporal asynchrony of response components. The first two columns suggest that the broad negative peak seen in some waveforms from 120-170 msec is a composite of at least two different sources. The first column shows a weak negative peak which correlates with the first half of the broad negative wave. The second column reveals a second weak negative peak which correlates with the second half of the broad negative wave. The third column shows the two waveforms superimposed on the broad negative wave. At some locations, the 170 msec peak was positive while the first half of the negative wave (120 msec) remained negative. Such observations clearly suggest the existence of at least two discrete sources. The lower panels of the figure illustrate the field distributions at 120 and 170 msec. The 120 msec field map shows a small positive peak at x=1, y=9 and a much larger negative peak at x=6 and y=5; the arrow represents the approximate location of the equivalent current dipole. The field distribution at 170 msec reveals a different source location (arrow). Although cortical responses for stimuli near the midline could not be mapped while the subject was lying on his side, another data set collected from the posterior region of the head corroborated the existence of the 170 msec source.

Figure 2a displays neuromagnetic field distributions for another subject when the right visual field was stimulated along the horizontal meridian. These maps illustrate the resolution of two discrete synchronous sources using a modeling procedure based on Biot Savart Law, ignoring return currents. In the top row the measured (empirical) field distributions observed at 120 msec poststimulus are shown in the first column. Theoretical distributions calculated from a 2-dipole model are illustrated in the second column. Residual fields are illustrated in the third column. Component dipole fields of the 2-dipole model (Dipole 1 and Dipole 2) are shown in the bottom row. The best-fitting single dipole solution accounted for 48% of the variance. The residual field distribution, however, contained amplitudes at some sensor locations which were 3 times the noise level (standard deviation of prestimulus baseline = 23.6 fT across sensor locations) and a dipolar-like pattern still remained. A 2-dipole model was applied using several initial parameter estimates. The best-fitting solution accounted for 65% of the variance in the empirical field distribution (17% more than the single dipole solution) and the residual amplitudes were in the noise level (although note a remaining dipole-like distribution in the residual map). An examination of the component dipoles (Dipole 1 and 2) suggest some cancellation between the negative peak of Dipole 1 and the positive peak of Dipole 2 which resulted in an imbalance in the magnitude of the peaks in the empirical distribution.

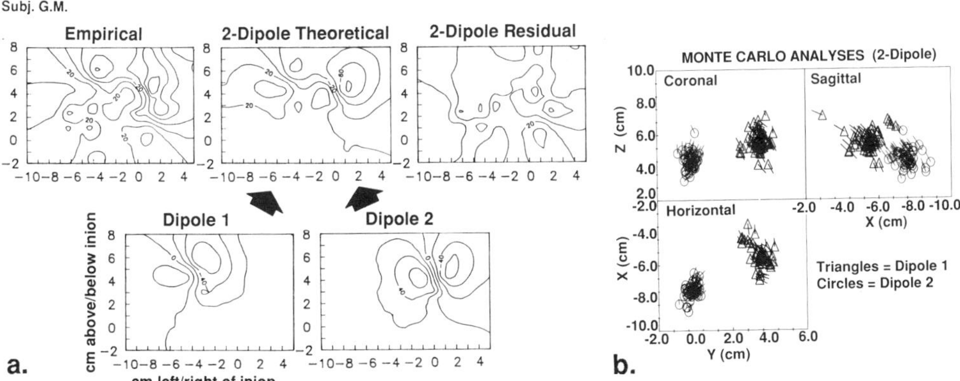

Figure 2a. Field distributions at 120 msec for one subject when a small sinusoidal grating was presented 7° along the horizontal meridian in the right visual field. A 2-dipole model was fit to the empirical field distributions. **b.** Monte Carlo simulations employing the 2-dipole model were performed on the field distributions above to assess the stability of the solutions.

Figure 2b illustrates the results of a Monte Carlo simulation based on 50 individual trials. This analysis is utilized to establish spatial confidence limits for the calculated source locations by randomly adding noise (SD=23.6 fT) to the calculated solutions (for details see Medvick et al., this volume). The results of the analysis are plotted in orthographic projections of the head volume using x-y-z head-centered coordinates consistent with those used in MRI scans. Note that these are not equivalent to the surface coordinates (Mercator projections) used in contour plots. In all views there is a clear separation between the calculated locations of dipole 1 and dipole 2 (triangles and circles, respectively). Note that the dipole solutions cluster, demonstrating the stability of the solutions. However, the extent of the clusters suggests a localization error of approximately +/- 1 cm, due to the low-amplitudes of features in the data.

The observation of multiple dipole sources is typical of field distributions evoked by stimuli along the horizontal meridian in the right visual field. Sources calculated for subject CA were strikingly similar to those presented above, with one source close to the midline and a second source ~5 cm lateral, although field maps were notably different. The field distributions reported above were also similar to data presented by Okada (1983; Fig. 12.9.4, pp. 447) when a 1 cpd grating was presented in a hemicircle of 5° radius in the right visual field. Okada's data suggest the existence of two sources in the left hemisphere: one source located close to midline and an additional source located more laterally .

DISCUSSION

In our visual studies, neuromagnetic field patterns measured from the head surface of occipital, parietal and temporal regions typically show evidence of multiple sources. We have found an examination of the temporal characteristics of field maps to be valuable in differentiating between multiple sources. When two sources are separated in time and space (e.g., Figure 1), tracking the rise and fall of peaks aids in determining which positive and negative peaks belong together. Multiple sources often have overlapping fields which result in complex field patterns. However, when complex field patterns are reduced to component sources, similarities across subjects may be more apparent than in the field distributions themselves. Finally, an analysis of the field distributions and of component sources can aid in locating sensors at which components may be temporally resolved in the waveform data.

ACKNOWLEDGEMENTS

This work was supported by the U.S. Army Research Institute, the Department of Energy contract W-7405-ENG-36 and the VA/LANL/UNM Magnetoencephalography Program.

REFERENCES

Okada, Y., 1983, Visual evoked field, in: "Biomagnetism: An Interdisciplinary Approach," S.J. Williamson, G.L. Romani, L. Kaufman, and I. Modena, eds., Plenum Press, New York.

Okada, Y., 1984, Discrimination of localized and distributed current dipole sources and localized single and multiple sources, in: "Biomagnetism: Applications and Theory," H. Weinberg, G. Stroink, and T. Katila, eds., Pergamon Press, New York.

Van Essen, D.C., 1985, Functional organization of primate visual cortex, in: "Cerebral Cortex, Vol. 3, A. Peters and E.G. Jones, Eds., Plenum Press, New York.

SPATIAL/TEMPORAL RESOLUTION OF MULTIPLE SOURCES:

PATHS OF ACTIVATION IN HUMAN VISUAL CORTEX

J. S. George, C. J. Aine, P. A. Medvick,and E.R. Flynn

Neuromagnetism Laboratory, MS-M882
Los Alamos National Laboratory, Los Alamos, NM 87545

INTRODUCTION

We have employed neuromagnetic mapping techniques to characterize neural responses evoked by sinusoidal gratings presented at various locations in the visual field. A primary goal of this work has been to localize the neurophysiological processes which underlie response components empirically defined in previous event-related potential (ERP) studies. Our analyses have focused on temporal as well as spatial tracking of sources because the combination permits more powerful inferences concerning the number and location of active neural sources (1-4).

This paper focuses on a sequence of evoked field maps obtained in one subject in response to a 1 cpd grating presented at 2° in the right visual field. Experimental procedures have been outlined in a previous paper (5). Field maps for each 10 msec interval were fit initially with a single dipole model. Because of difficulties in analytically tracking errors, Monte Carlo techniques were used to assess the uncertainty in source calculations due to measurement noise (6). Procedures utilized for data analysis in this paper do not account for errors in localization due to uncertainty of sensor position, however the experimental design insures that relative differences in source locations can be reliably determined.

RESULTS

Field maps obtained at representative time slices are illustrated in figure 1. These field maps are mercator (surface) projections with the inion located at the origin. From 90 - 140 msec the location and strength of field extrema appeared to systematically shift. A similar sequence was observed from 190-240 msec. At around 280 msec another discrete dipole-like source became apparent.

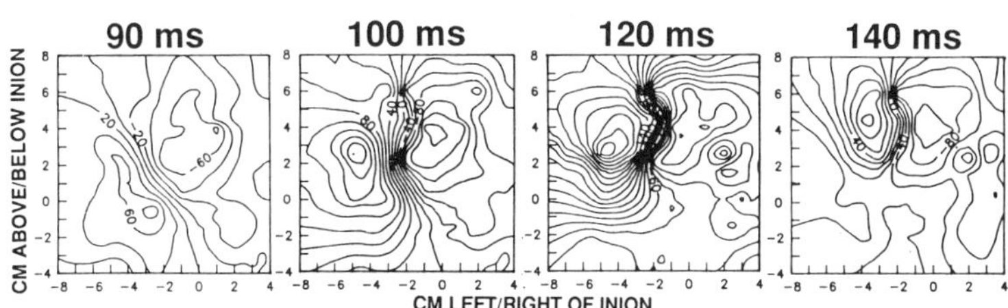

Figure 1. A series of evoked field maps from one subject in response to a 1 cpd sinusoidal grating presented at 2° in the right visual field. The inion is located at x=0, y=0.

Advances in Biomagnetism
Edited by S.J. Williamson *et al.*
Plenum Press, New York

Equivalent dipole source locations and scatter estimated from Monte Carlo analyses are illustrated in orthographic projections (figure 2). Noise estimated from the prestimulus baseline was added to amplitude measures for each sensor, and resulting distributions were fitted; recent studies by Kaufman indicate that brain noise is decreased during evoked activity, so our estimate is probably an upper limit. In this sequence, the application of 2-simultaneous dipole model fitting procedures (5) did not significantly improve the goodness of fit. Note the apparent path of activation suggested by successive apparent sources. In the head-centered coordinate system used for these studies, the -x axis is centered on the inion (a boney protrusion near the rear of the skull), the +y axis passes through a reference point on the left hemisphere ~2 cm above and in front of the ear canal, and the +z axis exits the top of the head. The scatterplot reliably illustrates the relative locations and confidence limits of calculated sources, however the error in absolute localization may be significantly larger.

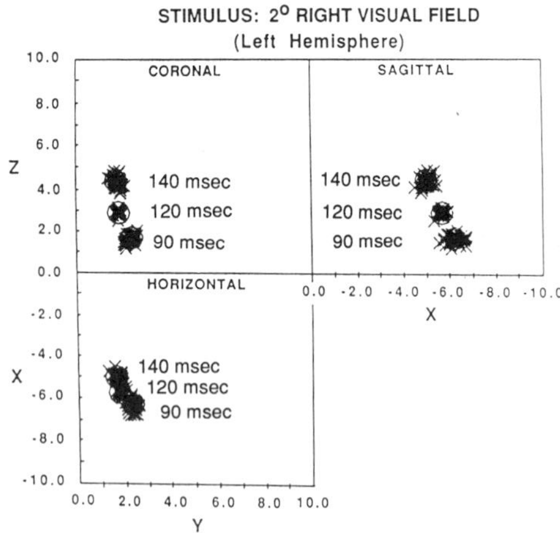

Figure 2. Monte Carlo error analyses for calculated sources at 90, 120 and 140 msec post-stimulus. An ensemble of 50 source calculations for each timepoint is illustrated.

Can field patterns observed from 90-140 msec be explained by the combination of two discrete, temporally overlapping sources? To address this question we compared three classes of source model. The first was the unconstrained single dipole model, fit to each individual map. The second was a single dipole model where dipole location and orientation was a weighted average of fitted parameters for 90 and 140 msec field distributions. This was a highly arbitrary analytical control and was not motivated by a physiological mechanistic hypothesis. The third was a double dipole model where the resulting distribution was a weighted linear combination of 90 and 140 msec theoretical distributions. This model assumed that the observed field distributions might reflect the asynchronous activation of two discrete, stationary neuromagnetic sources. The weighting ratio and field amplitude multiplier were adjusted to produce optimal fits in each case. Figure 3 compares goodness of fit measures between constrained single and double dipole sources over the range of times The single migrating (unconstrained) source model was the best explanation for observed intermediate field distributions. The linear constrained single source model performed better than the two source model, however this was probably fortuitous. Because the positive extrema did not overlap significantly in the 90 and 140 msec field distributions, the two source model did not reproduce the focal positive extremum experimentally observed at intermediate times.

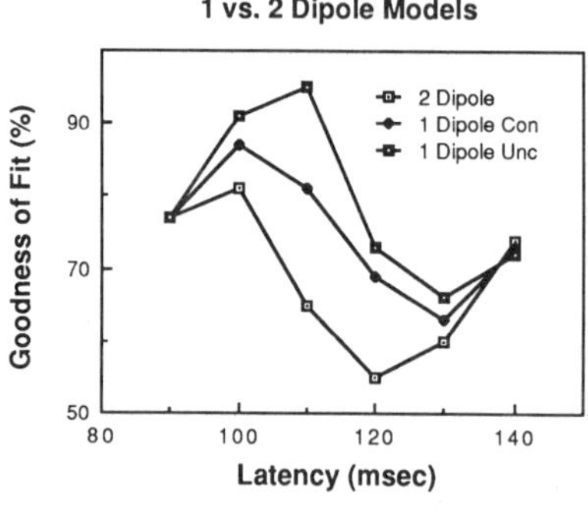

Figure 3. Computer modeling to account for the sequence of field maps observed from 90-140 msec. The graph compares an unconstrained single source model, a linearly constrained single source model, and a dual source model using 90 and 140 msec sources as linear basis sets.

Can three discrete, temporally overlapping sources explain the 90-140 msec evoked field distributions? Our modeling strategy was similar to that described above. 90 and 140 msec calculated sources were accepted as endpoints and the optimal single dipole fit for the 120 msec timepoint was accepted as the intermediate source. Table 1 compares the percent of variance accounted for by each of three models: the unconstrained single (migrating) source, and the linearly constrained single source and dual dipole models delimited by 90 to 120 and 120 to 140 msec equivalent sources. There was little

TABLE I. Three Source Constrained Fits
(percent of variance accounted for)

Latency	90	100	110	120	130	140 ms
original fit	_	92%	85%	_	66%	_
constrained 1 dipole	_	89%	85%	_	65%	_
constrained 2 dipole	_	89%	83%	_	65%	_

difference in goodness of fit between constrained single source and dual source models; the unconstrained single source model performed only slightly better, however this may reflect less than optimal selection of intermediate source parameters used in constrained fits. We obtained essentially the same results when the 110 msec single dipole fit was accepted as the intermediate source. From this analysis, we conclude that while the observed field distributions might reflect a continuously migrating focus of neural activation, the data are reasonably explained by three discrete, temporally overlapping sources.

Calculated neuromagnetic sources were located on magnetic resonance images (MRI). During imaging, oil-containing capsules were attached at reference locations to a bathing cap also worn during neuromagnetic data acquisition. By identifying the inion and left and right periauricular reference points in each slice series, it was possible to reconcile coordinate systems between volumetric series and with the neuromagnetic coordinate system. We estimate the accuracy of sensor location measurements used in this study to be +-.5 to 1.0 cm, better near the inion. Improved procedures will allow mm resolution. Even given this degree of uncertainty, suggested sources are anatomically reasonable. The 90 msec source appears to lie in or near the calcarine fissure (primary visual cortex). The 120 msec equivalent source is deeper, located near the anterior extent of striate cortex, possibly in area 18. The 140 msec source is more dorsal and may lie along the parietal occipital sulcus.

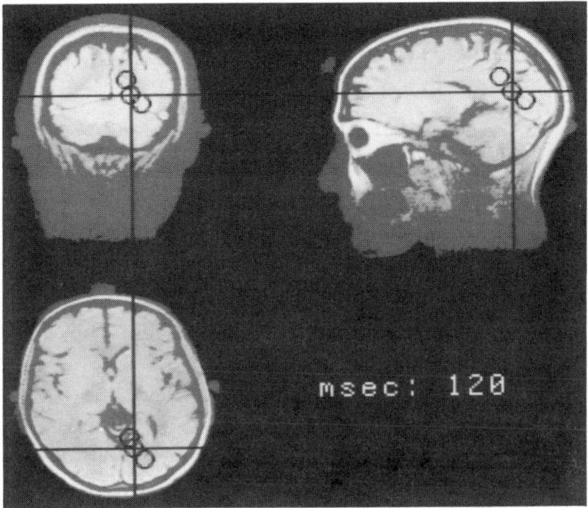

Figure 4. Neuromagnetic sources located on MRI. Calculated sources are indicated by circles; the 90 msec source is the lowest in all three views. Locations of selected slices are indicated by crosshairs. MRI data was acquired using volumetric acquisition techniques, producing a series of 32 contiguous slices at 4.5 mm thickness in each of three views. Slices were selected and pixel coordinates were calculated by software after reference points were identified. Silhouettes are provided as a visual coordinate reference.

DISCUSSION

We have begun to systematically apply these analyses to data from other subjects and for other stimulus conditions. The apparent migrating source associated with P1-N1 temporal components is observed across subjects. In some subjects, simultaneous source fitting procedures (5) were able to resolve multiple apparent sources at some time slices. In the example considered here, the apparent path of activation suggested by single source fits is slightly curved, and there are significant shifts in the orientation of the calculated source vector. In data from other subjects, paths are typically curved, suggesting that at least three discrete sources are required to account for observed evoked field distributions.

In our experience with the analysis of transient visual evoked response data it has proven necessary to develop procedures for the analysis of field distributions in which multiple sources are apparent. Multiple simultaneous source fitting strategies often produce a robust and surprisingly accurate model of observed field distributions when three or more peaks are apparent in an evoked response field map. However, within a single time slice the effective pairing of positive and negative peaks by the fitting algorithm may be arbitrary, a function of the starting estimates passed to the routine. While it is possible to generate a heuristic or combinatorial procedure to generate such starting estimates, there is no guarantee that goodness-of-fit measures will produce proper source assignments. In many cases it has proved possible to resolve such ambiguities by reference to field distributions at earlier or later times. If sources are asynchronous, it is often possible to assign pairings on the basis of temporal correlations between peaks of opposite polarity.

In the case considered here, there is no explicit evidence for multiple simultaneous sources. There are two dominant peaks in the evoked field maps, and the distribution at each time step is reasonably explained by a single dipole model. However, if the sequence of time slices is considered, the single (moving) dipole model suggests the existence of a focus of activation migrating across the cortical surface. This view is not supported by our knowledge of cortical anatomy and physiology derived from invasive studies of experimental animals. Instead, we would expect these experimental stimuli to activate a focal region of primary visual cortex, which might subsequently produce focal activation in secondary visual areas. Our analyses suggest that such a model can provide a reasonable explanation for the sequence of observed field distributions.

Our experimental observations clearly suggest the need for modeling strategies which account for a temporal sequence of spatial field maps by fitting a limited number of equivalent dipole sources. The locations of such sources, presumably determined by iterative nonlinear procedures, would remain fixed throughout the sequence. The strength (and possibly orientation) of each of the calculated sources would be allowed to vary as a function of time, and might be optimized using linear procedures. Algorithms incorporating these ideas are currently being developed in our laboratory.

ACKNOWLEDGEMENTS

This work was supported by the U.S. Army Research Institute, the Department of Energy contract W-7405-ENG-36 and the VA/LANL/UNM Magnetoencephalography Program.

REFERENCES

1. Scherg, M. , and Von Cramen, D. (1985) Two bilateral sources of the late VEP as identified by a spatio-temporal dipole model. Electroenceph. Clin. Neurophysiol. 62:32-44.

2. Scherg, M. , and Von Cramen, D. (1986) Evoked dipole source potentials of the human auditory cortex. Electroenceph. Clin. Neurophysiol. 65:344-360.

3. Maier, J., Dagnelie, G., Spekreijse, H., van Dijk, B.W. (1987) Principal components analysis for source localization of VEPs in man. Vision Res. 27:165-177.

4. Achim, A., Richer, F. and Saint-Hilaire, J. M. (1988). Methods for separating temporally overlapping sources of neuroelectric data. Brain Topography. 3:22-28.

5. Aine, C. J., George, J. S., Medvick, P. A. and Flynn, E. R. (This Volume) Resolution of multiple sources in the transient visual evoked neuromagnetic response.

6. Medvick, P. A., Lewis, P. S., Aine, C. J., and Flynn,E. R. (This Volume) Monte Carlo analysis of localization errors in magnetoencephalography.

A FREQUENCY DOMAIN TECHNIQUE FOR USING EVOKED MAGNETIC FIELDS TO TEST MULTI-STAGE MODELS OF SENSORY PROCESSING

M. P. Regan[1] and D. Regan[1,2]

1. Dept of Experimental Space Science, York University
2. Dept of Ophthalmology, University of Toronto. Dept of Psychology
BSB, York University, 4700 Keele St, Ontario, Canada, M3J 1P3

INTRODUCTION

One aim of neuromagnetic studies of human sensory pathways is to obtain data that can test quantitative models of these sensory pathways. The human auditory and visual pathways are composed of neurons, many of which can be modelled as a rectifier (Figure 1). Here we describe a method for characterizing one or more rectifiers arranged in a sequential or parallel/sequential order. The procedure is to calculate the response of such a neural model to an input that consists of the sum of two sinusoids. The calculation is repeated for each candidate model. Then the magnetic response of the brain to a sum of sinewaves input is measured, and the empirical result compared with the catalogue of theoretical predictions. We have published a preliminary catalogue (Regan & Regan, 1988) and are currently engaged in assembling a more extensive catalogue. The method allows a small population of specialized neurons to be isolated, and magnetic recording offers a precise localization of the selected neurons.

MATHEMATICAL BASIS OF THE TECHNIQUE

Note: P, Q are the amplitudes of the two input sinusoids and taken as positive. $k = Q/P$ $p = 2\pi *$frequency of the input of amplitude P, θ_p =phase, $q = 2\pi *$frequency of the input of amplitude Q, θ_q =phase, $x = (pt + \theta_p)$, $y = (qt + \theta_q)$ The constant of proportionality of the rectifier characteristic, $c = 1$.

Half-wave linear rectifier : response to one sinusoid

If the input voltage is given by $e(t) = Pcos(pt+\theta_p)$, then we can rewrite this as $F(x) = Pcos\, x$.
Then the output will be

$$f(x) = \begin{cases} Pcos\, x, & cos\, x \geq 0 \\ 0, & cos\, x < 0 \end{cases}$$

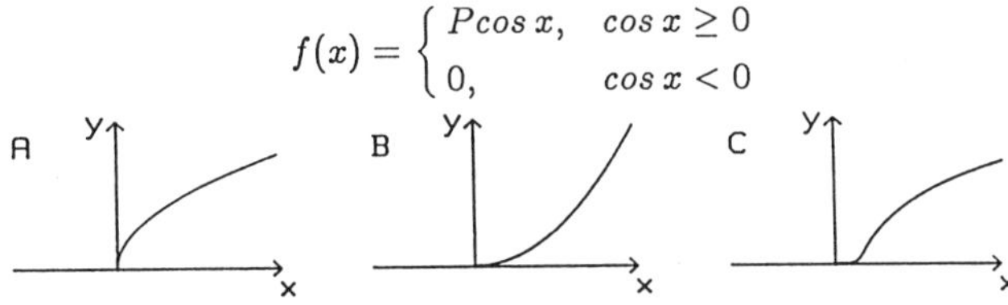

Figure 1 HALF-WAVE RECTIFIERS. Input is x, output is y. A, compressive. B, accelerating. C, initially accelerating then compressive as for the human visual contrast transducer function.

Advances in Biomagnetism
Edited by S.J. Williamson *et al.*
Plenum Press, New York

This can be expressed as the Fourier series,

$$f(x) = \frac{P}{\pi} + \frac{P}{2} cos\, x + \frac{2P}{3\pi} cos\, 2x - \frac{2P}{15\pi} cos\, 4x + \ldots$$

Half-wave Nth power rectifier : response to the sum of two sinusoids

If the rectifier is of the form $s = cr^N, r \geq 0$ and $s = 0, r < 0$ then the input to the rectifier is given by $e(t) = Pcos(pt + \theta_p) + Qcos(qt + \theta_q)$, or $F(x,y) = P(cos\, x + k\, cos\, y)$. Then we can consider the rectifier's output as the function $f(x,y)$ where

$$f(x,y) = \begin{cases} P^N(cos\, x + k\, cos\, y)^N, & cos\, x + k\, cos\, y \geq 0 \\ 0, & cos\, x + k\, cos\, y < 0 \end{cases}$$

$f(x,y)$ is bounded in the rectangle $(-\pi, \pi) * (-\pi, \pi)$ by $cos\, x + k\, cos\, y = 0$ and is an even function, so its Fourier expansion will be a cosine series given by

$$f(x,y) = \frac{1}{2} A_{00} + \sum_{m=1}^{\infty} \sum_{n=1}^{\infty} A_{\pm mn} cos(mx \pm ny) + A_{\pm 10} cos\, x + A_{\pm 01} cos\, y$$

where

$$A_{\pm mn} = \frac{2P^N}{\pi^N} \int_0^{\pi} cos\, ny \int_0^{arccos(-kcosy)} (cos\, x + k\, cos\, y)^N cos\, mx\, dx\, dy$$

since $f(x,y) = 0$ when $x > arccos(-k\, cos\, y)$.

An illustration of this is shown for N=1/2 in Figure 2.

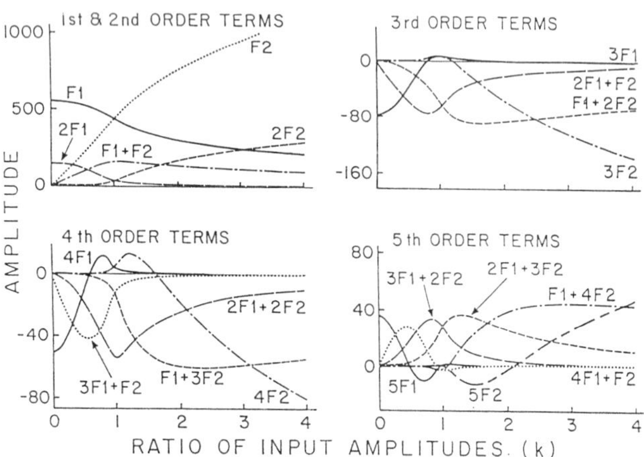

Figure 2 HALF-WAVE SQUARE ROOT RECTIFIER. Ordinates plot the amplitudes of frequency terms in the output of a half-wave square root rectifier whose input is the sum of two sinusoids, one of frequency F_1 and the other of frequency F_2. The amplitude (P) of the F_1 input is constant and the amplitude (Q) of the F_2 input is varied. Values of k are plotted along the abscissa, where $k = Q/P$.

Two or more rectifiers in series

These methods, first described by Bennett (1933), can be extended for a series of rectifiers, that may or may not have the same characteristic. If they are DC coupled, then the output of one rectifier is the input of the next, but AC coupling requires the deduction of the DC level which will vary with the value of k (Regan & Regan, 1988).

Two parallel rectifiers whose summed outputs pass through a third rectifier : the dichoptic or dichotic case

In this situation the input to one rectifier is a single sinewave of frequency $p/2\pi$, and the input to a second rectifier in parallel with the first rectifier is a single sinewave of frequency $q/2\pi$. Then the output from both rectifiers combine to form the input to the third rectifier.

The output of the first rectifier is $f(x)$ where

$$f(x) = \begin{cases} P\cos x, & \cos x \geq O \\ 0, & \cos x < 0 \end{cases}$$

with a D.C.-level of P/π. The output of the second rectifier is $g(y)$ where

$$g(y) = \begin{cases} Pk\cos y, & \cos y \geq O \\ 0, & \cos y < 0 \end{cases}$$

whose D.C.-level is Pk/π. To adjust for the D.C.-level, the input to the third rectifier will be the function

$$h(x,y) = f(x) - P/\pi + g(y) - Pk/\pi.$$

The output from the third rectifier is given by

$$H(x,y) = \begin{cases} h(x,y), & h(x,y) \geq 0 \\ 0, & h(x,y) < 0. \end{cases}$$

Hence the coefficients of the double Fourier series can be found, since

$$A_{\pm mn} = \frac{2P}{\pi^2}\int_0^{\pi} \cos ny \int_0^{\pi} H(x,y)\cos mx\,dx\,dy.$$

We have obtained plots of amplitude versus k for the cases of all three rectifiers being linear, or all three square root or all three thirdroot, the coupling being A.C. rather than D.C. Other cases such as mixed rectifiers (e.g. where nos.1 and 2 are thirdroot rectifiers and no.3 is a square law rectifier) are amenable to the same general mathematical treatment.

RESULTS

We have derived the family of curves that characterizes of single rectifiers of compressive, linear, accelerating and mixed nature. In particular, if the input is the sum of two sinusoids of frequencies F_1 and F_2 Hz, the output will consist of discrete terms of frequency $(nF_1 \pm mF_2)$, where n and m are zero or integral. If, now, the amplitude of one of the two inputs is held constant while the amplitude of the other input is progressively increased from zero, the several $(nF_1 \pm mF_2)$ terms can be described by a family of curves of response amplitude versus k, where k is the ratio of the two input amplitudes (Regan & Regan, 1988). Our approach can be applied to any rectifier whose characteristic function is continuous, has no hysteresis and is frequency-independent. We have also developed a method for obtaining the family of curves for sequences of similar or dissimilar rectifiers. Finally, we have derived the family of curves for the parallel/sequential case corresponding to dichoptic (visual) or diotic (auditory) stimulation.

Theoretical curves have shown that if only the first and second harmonic terms are taken into account the curves for quite different candidate nonlinearities may be rather similar. This is also the case even when low-order cross-modulation terms are additionally taken into account. But when consideration is extended to third and higher order terms, much sharper distinctions can be made between different candidate nonlinearities. As with a real fingerprint, the greater the possible number of points of similarity and points of disagreement, the greater the certainty with which different candidate owners of the finger can be confirmed or rejected. In our context, the shape of each $(nF_1 \pm mF_2)$ curve provides a point of similarity or point of disagreement.

DISCUSSION

Compared with the white noise (Wiener Kernel) time domain method for characterising nonlinear systems (Marmarelis & Marmarelis, 1978), the advantage of the technique described here is that at least some of the high order cross-modulation terms can readily be measured in practical physiological experiments, thus giving superior discrimination between candidate models in the catalogue. The reasons for this superior discrimination are as follows: [1] In some physiological cases the discrete components in the frequency-domain response have very narrow bandwidths. Therefore, because noise is distributed continuously along the frequency dimension, very little noise exists within the narrow bandwidth of any given response component, so that terms with small amplitudes may be recorded at excellent signal-to-noise ratios and many "points of similarity and difference" are available; [2] response components do not overlap along the frequency axis even when they are very closely spaced (though, of course, all components overlap in the time domain). Consequently, the major strength of this approach is its ability to reject physiologically-plausible models.

Results to date suggest that the family of, perhaps 20-30, $(nF_1 \pm mF_2)$ curves constitutes a sort of "fingerprint" of the responsible single or multi-rectifier nonlinearity. By using an ultra high resolution zoom-FFT technique (Regan, 1989) we have experimentally recorded up to twenty $(nF_1 \pm mF_2)$ terms in the brain response to sum-of-two-sinewave visual or auditory stimulus. By comparing the family of data curves with various families of curves calculated for competing neural models, it is possible to test models sharply against data. This approach is powerful in the sense that candidate models can be unequivocally rejected. This new approach offers a means of using neuromagnetic recording to test candidate neural models of sensory processing.

ACKNOWLEDGEMENTS

This work was sponsored by the U.S. Air Force of Scientific Research.

REFERENCES

Bennett, W. R. New results in the calculation of modulation products. Bell System Tech. J. 1933: 228-243 (1933).

Marmarelis, P. Z. and Marmarelis, V. Z. *Analysis of Physiological Systems. The White Noise Approach.* Plenum Press, New York (1978).

Regan, D. *Human Brain Electrophysiology: Evoked potentials and evoked magnetic fields in science and medicine.* New York: Elsevier (1989).

Regan, M. P. and Regan, D. A frequency domain technique for characterising nonlinearities in biological systems. J. Theoret. Biol., **133**, 293-317 (1988).

ULTRA-HIGH RESOLUTION ANALYSIS OF AUDITORY AND VISUAL BRAIN RESPONSES USING ZOOM-FFT

D. Regan [1,2] and M.P. Regan[1]

1 Dept of Experimental Space Science, York University
2 Dept of Ophthalmology, University of Toronto
Dept of Psychology BSB, York University, 4700 Keele St
Ontario, Canada, M3J 1P3

INTRODUCTION

According to the Gabor-Heisenberg uncertainty relation, the spectrum of a MEG recording can be obtained at a frequency resolution ΔF Hz of up to $\Delta F = (1/T)$, where T is the duration of the time series. In principle, therefore, a recording of duration 500 sec can be analyzed at a resolution of 0.002 Hz giving, for example, a plot of power versus frequency containing 100,000 lines for a recording of bandwidth DC-200Hz. In practice, however, commercial FFT analyzers give far poorer resolution typically 0.5 or 0.25 Hz for a DC-200Hz bandwidth. This limitation on frequency resolution has not previously been considered serious on the assumption that brain responses to repetitive sensory stimulation (e.g. flickering light or AM tones) consist of frequency components, each of which has a substantial bandwidth due to amplitude variability and latency jitter.

METHODS

We have implemented a nondestructive zoom-FFT technique over a wide bandwidth for obtaining the spectrum of a MEG recording with a frequency resolution up to the Heisenberg-Gabor limit (Regan, 1989).

RESULTS

Ultra-high resolution spectral analysis revealed ultra-fine detail in brain responses to repetitive stimulation. For example, the brain response to an auditory tone that was amplitude modulated at F Hz comprised discrete frequencies (harmonics of F). In Fig. 1A the bandwidth of the 2F Hz response was evidently no more than the 0.008 Hz resolution of the analyzer. When the recording duration was increased to 500 sec compared with the 160 sec of Fig.1 the analyzer's resolution increased to 0.002 Hz, but the 2F Hz response spike was still largely contained within one line, indicating that the bandwidth was no more than 0.002 Hz. Responses to visual stimulation were of similarly narrow bandwith.

The presence of F Hz harmonics in the response to an AM tone implies nonlinear processing because the auditory stimulus contained no power at F

Advances in Biomagnetism
Edited by S.J. Williamson *et al.*
Plenum Press, New York

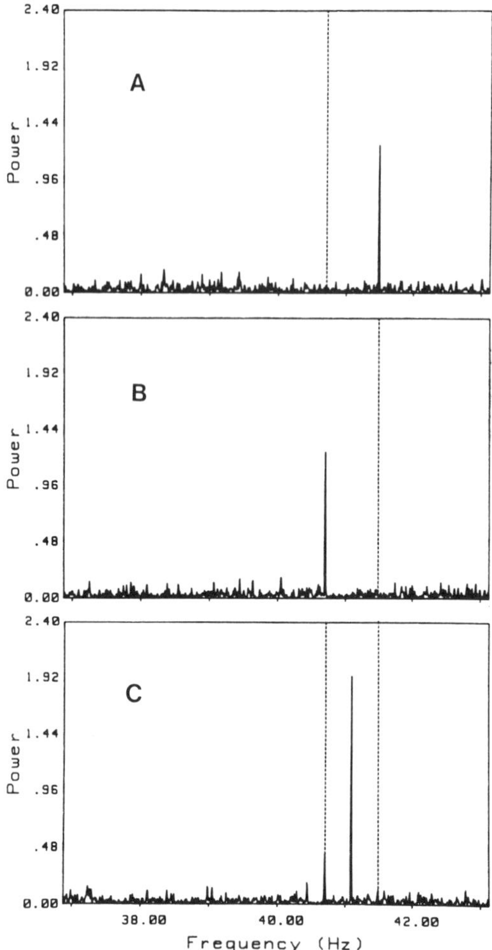

Figure 1 A small section of the MEG spectrum analyzed at a resolution of 0.008 Hz. A - 1000 Hz tone was modulated at F_1 = 20.742 Hz. The spike is at $2F_1$ = 41.484 Hz. B - subject's contralateral ear stimulated with a 1000 Hz tone amplitude-modulated at F_2 = 20.351 Hz. The spike is at $2F_2$ = 40.703 Hz. C - contralateral ear stimulated with the two tones simultaneously. The spike is at $(F_1 + F_2)$ = 41.093 Hz.

Hz or at its harmonics. We studied this nonlinearity by stimulating simultaneously with two tones that were amplitude-modulated at different rates F_1 Hz and F_2 Hz. Fig.1A shows the $2F_1$, response to F_1 Hz AM alone and Fig. 1B shows the $2F_2$ response to the F_2 Hz AM alone. When both tones were fed to the same ear the $2F_1$, and $2F_2$ Hz responses were suppressed and a nonlinear cross-modulation term of frequency $(F_1 + F_2)$ appeared (Fig. 1C). The behaviour of the $2F_1$, $2F_2$ and $(F_1 + F_2)$ terms was consistent with their generation by an the rectifier-like hair cell transducer function of the inner ear.

We have also used this two-sinewave approach in visual studies to isolate small subpopulations of cells (e.g. visual cortical cells tuned to a particular orientation). and are using MEG recording to localize these specialized neurons.

The rationale is as follows. A vertical grating counterphase-modulated at F_1 Hz (i.e. bright and dim bars exchange places $2F_1$ times per sec) preferentially stimulates cortical neurons that prefer vertically-oriented stimuli. A second superimposed F_2 Hz grating produces cross-modulation terms of frequency ($nF_1 \pm m F_2$) where n, m are zero or integral. But cross-modulation terms can only be produced by a neuron that "sees" both gratings. Therefore, the orientation bandwidths of neurons can be measured by altering the relative orientations of the gratings until cross-modulation terms attenuate by some criterion amount. A similar rationale can be used to measure spatial frequency tuning bandwidths, auditory tuning bandwidths and spatial discriminations (Regan, 1989).

DISCUSSION

The finding that brain responses evoked by repetitive sensory stimulation comprise discrete frequency terms (i.e. sinewave components) whose bandwidths are as narrow as 0.002 Hz implies that these brain signals are rather constant in amplitude and phase in the time domain, and that what seems to be response variability in low-resolution recordings is in reality mainly additive noise. Because brain noise is spread out through many (e.g. 100,000) lines while the signals are concentrated into single lines where the power per Hz is comparatively very high indeed, evoked responses can be recorded whose powers are many thousands of times less than the power of spontaneous brain activity. Signal-to-noise ratios (power) of evoked signals can reach several hundreds. The combination of ultra-high resolution spectral analysis with our recently-developed mathematical method for calculating the responses of multi-neuron models to sum-of-two-sinewave inputs (Regan and Regan, 1988, 1989a, b) offers a new means for quantitively investigating nonlinear processes in sensory pathways and for testing multi-neuron models of auditory and visual processing.

ACKNOWLEDGEMENTS

This work was sponsored by the U.S. Air Force of Scientific Research.

REFERENCES

Regan, D. (1989) *Human Brain Electrophysiology: Evoked potentials and evoked magnetic fields in science and medicine*, New York: Elsevier.

Regan, M.P. and Regan, D. (1988). A frequency domain technique for characterizing nonlinearities in biological systems. *J. Theoret. Biol..*, 133, 293-317.

Regan, M.P. and Regan, D. (1989a). Objective investigation of visual function using a nondestructive zoom-FFT technique for evoked potential analysis. *Can. J. Neurol Sci.*, 16, 168-179.

Regan, M.P. and Regan, D. (1989b). A frequency domain technique for using evoked magnetic fields to multi-stage models of sensory processing. Abstract, this meeting.

NEUROMAGNETIC MEASUREMENTS OF VISUAL RESPONSES TO CHROMATICITY AND LUMINANCE

J. Krauskopf,† G. Klemic, O.V. Lounasmaa,* D. Travis,† L. Kaufman, and S.J. Williamson

†Department of Psychology, New York University, New York, NY 10003, U.S.A.
Neuromagnetism Laboratory, Departments of Physics, Psychology, and
Center for Neural Science, New York University, New York, NY 10003, U.S.A.
*Low Temperature Laboratory,
Helsinki University of Technology, 02150 Espoo, Finland

INTRODUCTION

Psychophysical studies have demonstrated that there are three cardinal directions in color space which may be habituated independently (Krauskopf, J., Williams, D.R., and Heeley, D.W., 1982). Two are chrominance directions which we call "red-green" and "blue-yellow", and the third is the achromatic direction for luminance. After viewing modulations along one color axis, detection thresholds for that color direction increase, but thresholds for the other color or luminance are unaffected. Similarly, after exposure to luminance variations detection thresholds for luminance stimuli increase but those for either color direction do not. This implies that there are separate mechanisms in the brain for these specific colors and luminance. However electrophysiological experiments have not clearly identified these separate pathways. Cells in the lateral geniculate nucleus (LGN) signal for color and luminance simultaneously, though at different spatial frequencies (Derrington, A. M., Krauskopf, J., Lennie, P., 1984; see also DeValois, R. L., Devalois, K.K., 1975 for review of earlier results). Recent work on the striate cortex (Lennie, P., Krauskopf, J., Sclar, G., 1989) shows that there is no clear separation of color and luminance, even in the "blob" and "interblob" regions of layers II/III, although contrary conclusions were reached by Livingstone and Hubel (1984). Furthermore the habituation effects observed psychophysically have not been observed to occur at the LGN (Derrington et al., 1984) or the cortex (Lennie et al., 1989).

Recent antomical studies have revealed a multiplicity of retinotopic cortical areas (Van Essen, D.C., 1985) and it has been suggested that they serve some distinct purposes. Indeed, Zeki (1973) has proposed a special role for area V4 in the process of color. Magnetic methods are capable of locating regions of activity on the scale of cortical maps, therefore the present study was undertaken. We have used a 5-channel SQUID system with second order gradiometer detection coils, in a magnetically shielded room, to seek evidence of separate neuronal sources of response to color and luminance stimuli.

METHODS

Two classes of stimuli were generated by an AT type personal computer with a VGA board capable of displaying the stimuli by means of an Electrohome video projector which served to project the images onto a rear projection screen inside a magnetically sheilded room. One class of stimuli was maximally modulated along the red-green color axis, and the other was maximally

Advances in Biomagnetism
Edited by S.J. Williamson *et al.*
Plenum Press, New York

modulated along the luminance axis. In both cases the stimulus was a disc of 0.5 deg diameter presented in the lower-left visual field against a neutral surround. The red and green stimuli were made equiluminant with the neutral surround by means of flicker photometry for each subject. The luminance (black-white) stimuli were against the same neutral surround. Red, green, black, and white stimuli were presented in random order, each for a duration of 360 ms with an interstimulus interval of 600 ms. The magnetic field was measured at 60-65 positions over the occipital and parietal areas of the head.

RESULTS

Red and green responses were averaged together (*rg*) as were the black and white responses (*bw*). At least four temporal components of the neuronal response were detected for both classes of stimuli, with the fourth being an offset response occuring after the duration of the stimuli. This differs from EEG studies (Paulus et al. 1987) that reported an early negative component (87 ms) only for color stimuli and a later positive component (110 ms) for luminance stimuli. The latencies of *rg* responses in our study were consistently longer than *bw* response, typically by 10 - 20 ms, but this was found to be related to the amplitude of modulation along the *bw* axis, and the latencies became comparable when the luminance change in the *bw* condition was reduced to near threshold.

The results are shown in Figure 1. For the first subject, the peak *rg* responses occured at 88, 152, and 217 ms which we identify as P1, N1, and P2 respectively. Similarly the peak *bw* responses occured at 63, 142, and 205 ms. For the second subject the P1, N1, and P2 responses to *rg* were at 69, 127, and 182 ms and those to *bw* were at 50, 99, and 160 ms. A third subject showed similar though weaker responses. The field pattern at each of these latencies is shown in Figure 2. Most components show clear evidence for a dipolar pattern, with positive and negative extrema having comparable magnitudes. This suggests that the underlying neuronal activity may be well modelled by a single current dipole.

DISCUSSION

For subject A, the contour plots in Figure 2a show no apparent difference between chrominance and

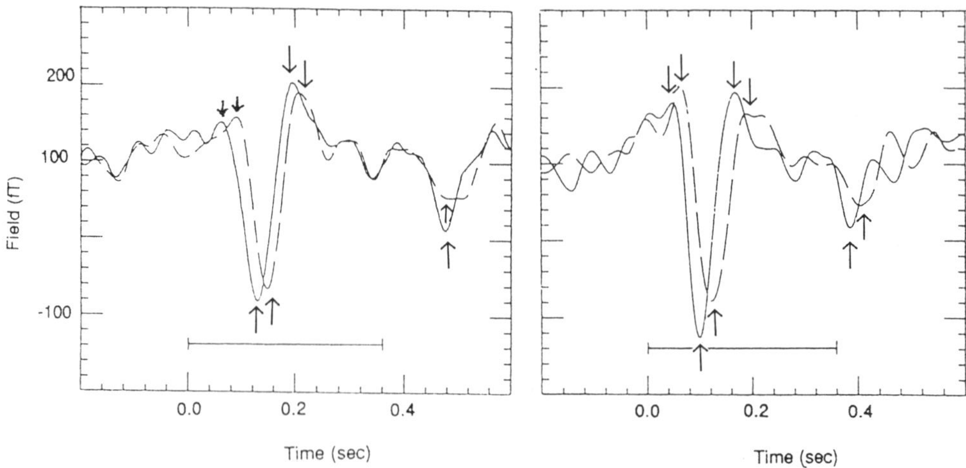

Fig.1. Average of 90 responses to *bw* (solid line) and to *rg* (dashed line) stimuli for two subjects. Stimulus duration is shown at the bottom, and components are marked with arrows. Bandwidth is 2-20 Hz.

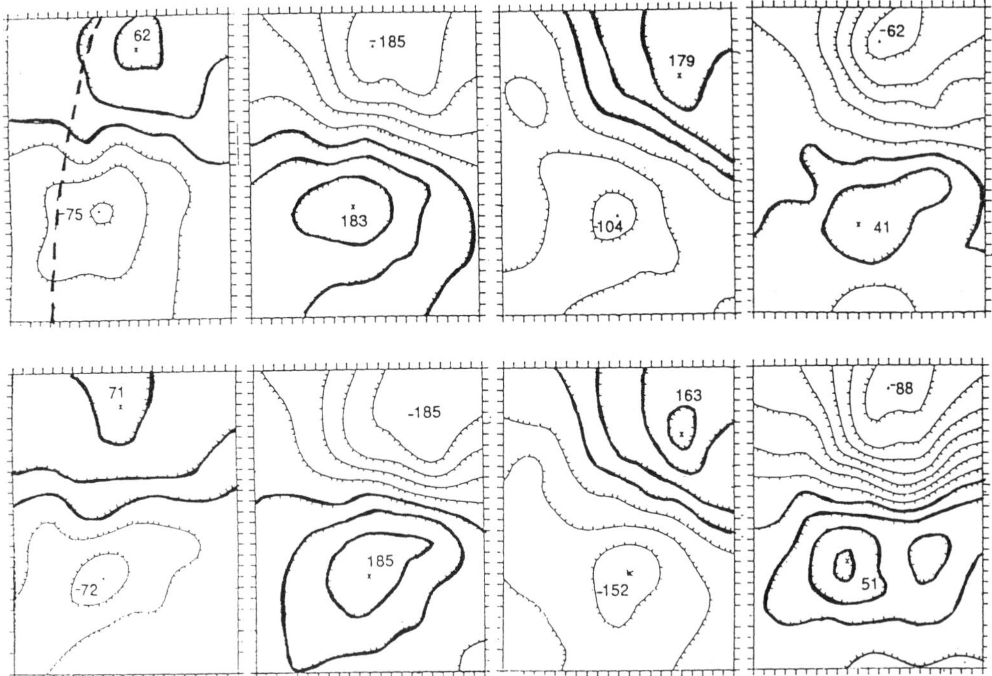

Fig. 2a. Isofield contour plot showing magnetic field pattern of cortical activity for P1, N1, P2, and offset responses to chrominance (top) and luminance (bottom) stimuli for subject A. Distance intervals between tics along the axes are 5 mm, amd the midline is indicated by the dashed line in the first plot. Field strengths at the extrema are given in femtotesla.

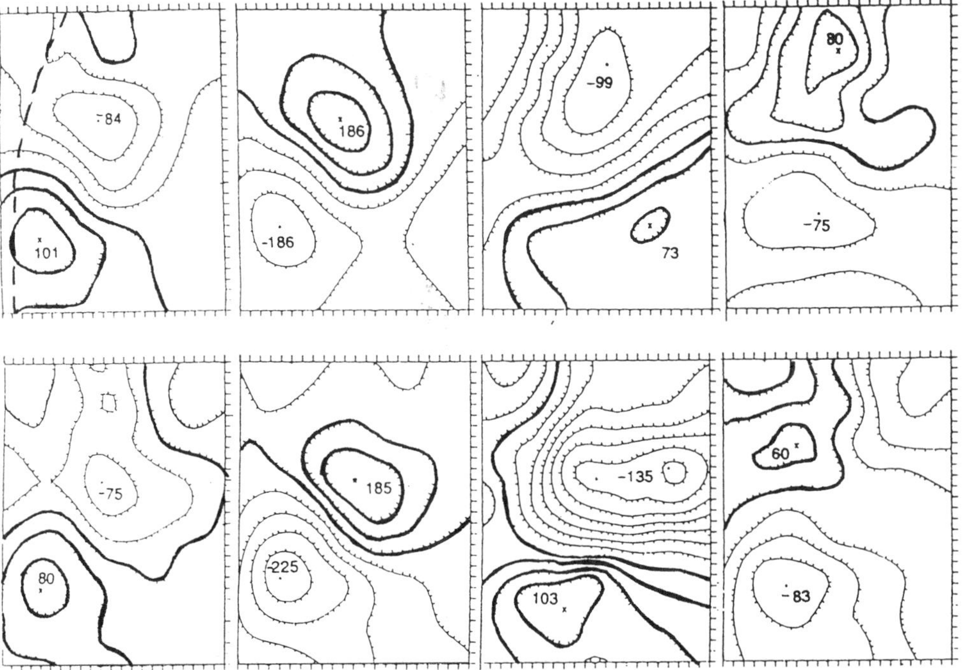

Fig. 2b. Same as Fig. 2a but for subject B.

luminance conditions. The same is true for the first two components of subject B, but the third component (P2) shows a clear difference in field patterns. The extrema for the luminance responses are laterally shifted from those for the chrominance response, but the midpoint between the extrema are only slightly displaced. Indeed the simplest way to describe the change in pattern is by a rotation of the source, as could occur in a subtle shift of neuronal activity across the curved cortical surface of a gyrus. The equivalent current dipole source rotates clockwise by about 50 degrees. This difference in neuronal population provides evidence for separate spatial processing of chrominance and luminance information. The fact that no such separation is seen for subject A could be due to a difference in cortical topology and is not necessarily a contradiction. More studies are called for to support this conclusion.

ACKNOWLEDGEMENTS

We thank Bruce Luber, Irene Martin, Robert Picardi and Jia Zhu Wang for their assistance. Research was supported in part by Air Force Office of Scientific Research Grants F49620-88-K-0004 and F49620-86-C-0131 and 86-0334, and NIH grant EY06638.

REFERENCES

Derrington, A.M., Krauskopf, J., Lennie, P. (1984). Chromatic Mechanisms in Lateral Geniculate Nucleus of Macaque. *J. Physiol.* 357: 241-265.

DeValois,R.L., DeValois,K.K. (1975). Neural Coding of Color. In: *Handbook of Percecption Vol. 5.* Carterette E.C., Friedman, M.P., Eds., Academic Press New York, pp.117-166.

Hari, R., Joutsiniemi, S.-L., Sarvas, J. (1988) Spatial resolution of neuromagnetic records: Theoretical calculations in a spherical model. *Electroencephalography and clinical Neurophysiology* 71: 64-72.

Krauskopf,J., Williams,D.R., Heeley,D.W. (1982). Cardinal Directions of Color Space. *Vison Res.* 22: 1123-1131.

Lennie, P., Krauskopf, J., Sclar, G. (1988). Chromatic Mechanisms in Striate Cortex of Macque., *in preparation.*

Livingstone, M.S. and Hubel, D.H. (1984). Anatomy and physiology of a color system in primate visual cortex, *J. Neurosci.* 4: 309-356.

Paulus, W.M., Plendl, H., Krafczyk, S., (1988). Spatial dissociation of early and late colour evoked components. *Electroenceph. clin. Neurophysiol.* 71: 81-88.

Van Essen, D.C. Functional Organization of Primate Visual Cortex. In: *Cerebral Cortex, Vol.3, Visual Cortex.* Peters,A. and Jones, E. eds. Plenum Press. New York, pp. 259-329. 1985

Zeki, S.M. (1973). Color coding in rhesus monkey prestriate cortex. *Brain Research, 53: 422-427.*

BRAIN ACTIVITY RELATED TO SPATIAL VISUAL ATTENTION

B. Luber, L. Kaufman, and S.J. Williamson

Neuromagnetism Laboratory
Departments of Psychology and Physics and Center for Neural Science
New York University, New York, NY 10003, U.S.A.

INTRODUCTION

When attention is directed toward one location in the visual field, electrical potentials evoked by stimuli at that location are enhanced relative to when attention is directed elsewhere (Eason et al., 1969, VanVoorhis and Hillyard, 1977). This enhancement begins about 100 msec after stimulus onset, and components both positive and negative over the next 200 msec are affected. These results led Hillyard and Mangun (1986) to propose that attention modulates a mechanism at the thalamic level which gates neural activity along the pathway which includes the lateral geniculate nucleus in the thalamus and the striate cortex. However, Harter and Aine (1984) suggested that the modulation of ERP components by spatial attention is due to activity in a second visual pathway, following a route which passes through the superior colliculus in the midbrain, the pulvinar nucleus of the thalamus, and the parietal cortex. This proposal was based on anatomical and physiological research on cats and macaque monkeys. Conclusions drawn from ERP research about these theories can only be tentative, given that the poor spatial resolution of scalp electrode measurements often makes it difficult to determine the neural origins of effects of spatial attention on the activity of the brain. In this study, we made use of the high spatial and temporal resolution afforded by measuring the brain's magnetic field in locating the places where focused spatial attention modulates activity in the cerebral cortex.

METHODS

Three paid right-handed subjects with normal vision, two female and one male, were employed in this experiment. A visual stimulus containing either 2 or 4 parallel vertical bars within a square field 1 deg on a side was presented in random sequence above the horizontal meridian, either 5 deg to the left or to the right of a central fixation point. The bars were alternating black and white, each slightly less than one order of magnitude below and above a background gray luminance of 0.68 cd/m^2. The 4-bar pattern had a 20% probability of occurrence. All bar patterns were presented for 34 msec with a random ISI of 1100 msec mean and 250 msec SD. Stimuli were generated using a Commodore Amiga computer, and projected into a magnetically-shielded room with an Electrohome color projection system. The subject was seated facing the projection screen and was instructed to maintain fixation on a small cross while attending to either the right or left field. Subjects depressed a button whenever the 4-bar pattern appeared in the field to which attention was being paid. Presentations continued until at least 100 stimuli had occured on each side. This procedure was then repeated, with the subject instructed to attend to the stimuli in the other field.

Magnetic field measurements were made using a multisensor probe incorporating 5 SQUID-based second-order gradiometers, each having a 1.5 cm coil diameter and a 3.4 cm baseline between adjacent coils. The outputs of the SQUID electronics were bandpassed between 0.1-50 Hz and then sampled by an HP9000 Model 350 computer at a rate of 128/sec. Sampling began 100 msec before stimulus onset and continued over a 700 msec recording epoch. Recorded data were digitally filtered from 2-30 Hz, and recorded epochs were averaged selectively by stimulus location across

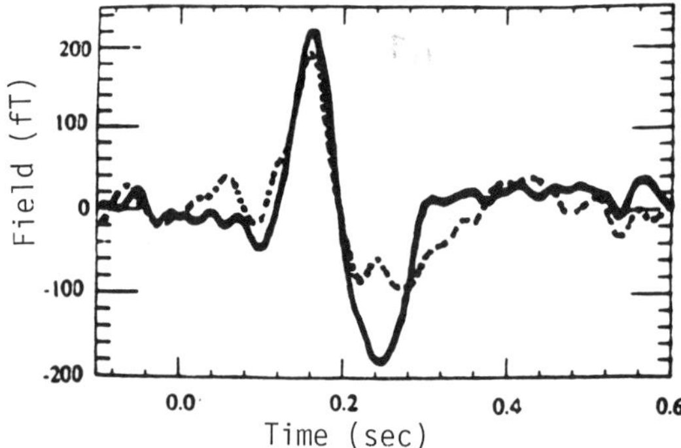

Fig. 1. Time courses of averaged responses to stimuli in the right visual field in attended (solid line) and unattended (dashed line) conditions, obtained over the occipital area of the scalp. Stimulus onset is at 0 seconds.

both 2 and 4 bar patterns. Reaction time and accuracy data were also recorded and analyzed.

Measurements were made over the entire posterior region of each subject's head. In the case of subject SS, recordings were made from 34 probe positions, resulting in 170 spatially separate measurements. For subjects BR and JV, 48 and 19 probe positions were used, providing measurements from 240 and 95 locations, respectively. Sensor positions and orientations relative to a head-based coordinate system were determined by the PPI system (Biomagnetic Technologies, Inc.).

Isofield contour maps were constucted in the following way. Magnetic field amplitudes at a selected instant in time were retrieved from the averaged data along with their associated sensor positions. Data from across the occipital and parietal regions of the scalp were transferred onto a two-dimensional surface using an azimuthal equal distance projection. According to this scheme, the midpoint between periauricular positions of the head was taken as the center of a sphere; and distances from this origin along any great circle were indicated by the same distances from the origin across the flat graph. These data were used by a program which performs Laplacian and spline interpolations and generated isofield contour maps.

RESULTS

Typical time series of responses to the attended and unattended stimuli presented in the right visual field are shown in Figure 1 for subject SS. There is a strong resemblance between the field patterns and response strengths for both the attended and unattended stimuli until about 200 msec after the onset of the stimulus. Between 200 and 360 msec, the strength of response to the attended stimulus is strongly enhanced relative to the response to the unattended stimulus. This is a common feature of the difference in waveforms between attention conditions in all three subjects: early similarity in amplitude up to about 150 to 210 msec after stimulus onset, followed by increasingly marked differences in amplitude and, in some cases, component structure, over the next 150-200 msec.

Examples of contour maps are given in Figures 2 and 3. Figures 2a and 2b represent the field patterns 150 msec after stimulus onset for the attended-right and unattended-right location, respectively for subject SS. There is no significant difference between main features of the patterns. Overall pattern and field amplitudes reflect similar underlying neural activity at this latency. This is to be contrasted with Figures 2c and 2d, which represent the field for the same situation at a latency of 252 msec. At this time, field amplitudes in the attend case are much larger and contribute to a more well-defined structure than in the unattended condition.

Figure 3 presents data analogous to Figure 2, this time for subject BR's responses to stimuli in the left visual field. Field patterns at 173 msec latency are quite similar over attended and unattended conditions. At 228 msec, this situation changes, once again with field amplitudes in the attended case (3c) much larger than in the unattended (3d).

In Figures 2c-d and 3c-d it can be seen that the fields, while remaining strong, have become difficult to interpret in terms of a simple dipolar pattern. This is true of the field maps for all three subjects over the 200-350 msec range. Strong peaks often emerge over parietal and temporal regions many centimeters from occipital locations where earlier peaks occurred. While it is difficult to interpret these field patterns in terms of dipolar sources, their widespread nature does suggest extrastriate neural activity. It is interesting to note that the time at which the field patterns begin to become increasingly complex appears to be quite similar to the onset latency of attention effects.

Further analyses revealed other properties of the spatial attention effect on neural activity. The data can be averaged not only by spatial position, but also by the identity of the stimulus as a target or a non-target. The resulting waveforms show no differences in responses until about 275 msec after stimulus onset. Neural activity modulated by spatial attention prior to this latency does not discriminate between target and non-target stimuli, implying that the effect is solely due to spatial location.

CONCLUSIONS

Using a similar paradigm in the auditory domain (Curtis, Kaufman and Williamson, 1988), components with sources in the primary auditory cortex as early as 100 msec reveal strong effects of attention. Unlike that study, here attention did not strongly affect the neuromagnetic response to visual stimuli until about 150-210 msec after stimulus onset. This is well after at least the first component of cortical response has occured. Furthermore, analyses of target/non-target stimuli imply that the manipulation of spatial location alone modulates responses at least until 275 msec. These results suggest that in this study mechanisms of spatial attention have their effect on cortical processing over a period of 100 msec or more, beginning only after that processing has been underway for as long as 100 msec. This result was not found by VanVoorhis and Hillyard (1977). In grand average waveforms over twelve subjects, they found that a similar manipulation of spatial attention resulted in the enhancement of ERP components as early as 100 msec after stimulus onset. One

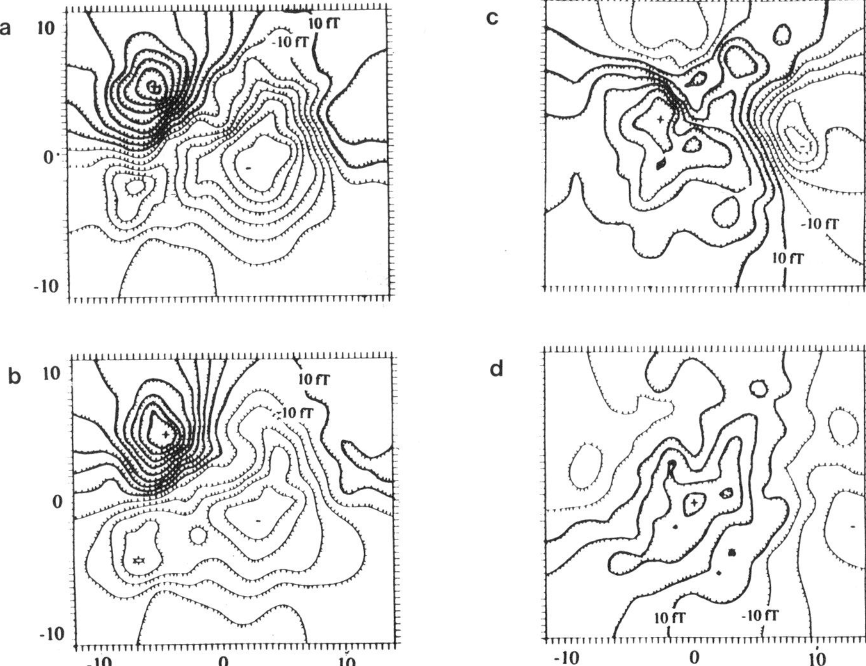

Fig. 2. Isofield contour maps over occipital area of subject SS for: 150 ms field pattern when (a) attended and (b) unattended; 252 ms field pattern when (c) attended and (d) unattended. The origin of each projection is approximately on the midline (which extends vertically along x=0) of the scalp about 3 cm above the inion. Isofield contours are drawn in 20 fT increments and distances are in cm. An extremum of the emerging field is indicated by +.

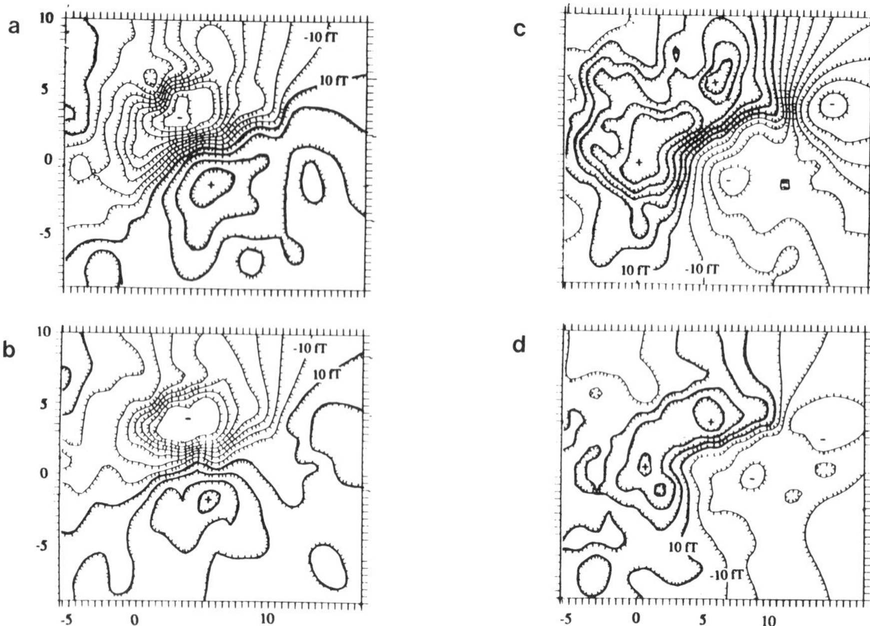

Fig. 3. Same as in Figure 2, for subject BR. Field patterns at 173 ms when (a) attended and (b) unattended; and at 228 ms when (c) attended and (d) unattended.

major difference in the two studies is that luminance increments were used in stimuli in the Van-Voorhis et al. research, while stimuli of approximately constant luminance were used in this study. Entoptic stray light from these increments could contaminate ERP data with unintended responses from other regions of the retina, including the fovea. We suggest the effect of this parameter requires further investigation. Of course, since scalp electrodes may be more sensitive to relatively distant sources than is the magnetic field measuring instrument, the early effects of attention may well be due to activity of sources far from the visual areas. Both alternatives need further study.

ACKNOWLEDGEMENTS

We thank G. Sperling and B.J. Schwartz for helpful discussions. This research was supported in part by Air Force Office of Scientific Research Grants F49620-88-K-0004 and F49620-88-C-0131.

REFERENCES

Curtis, S., Kaufman, L., and Williamson, S.J. (1988). Divided attention revisited: selection based on location or pitch. In: Atsumi, K., Kotani, M., Ueno, S., Katila, T., and Williamson, S.J., Eds., *Biomagnetism '87.* Tokyo Denki University Press, Tokyo, pp. 138-141.

Eason, R., Harter, M., and White, C. (1969). Effects of attention and arousal on visually evoked cortical potentials and reaction time in man. *Physiology and Behavior* 4, 283-289

Harter, R.H., and Aine, C.J. (1984). Brain mechanisms of visual selective attention. In: Parasuraman, R., and Davies, R., Eds., *Varieties of Attention.* Academic Press, New York, pp. 293-321.

Hillyard, S.A., and Mangun, G.R. (1986). The neural basis of visual selective attention: A commentary on Harter and Aine. *Biological Psychology* 23, 265-279

Van Voorhis, S., and Hillyard, S.A. (1977). Visual evoked potentials and selective attention to points in space. *Perception and Psychophysics* 22, 54-62.

TEMPORAL VARIABILITY OF THE NEUROMAGNETIC EVOKED FIELD: IMPLICATIONS FOR HUMAN PERFORMANCE ASSESSMENT[1]

G.W. Lewis, L.J. Trejo, P. Naitoh*, M.H. Blankenship, and M. Inlow

Navy Personnel Research and Development Center
San Diego, CA 92152-6800, USA
*Naval Health Research Center, P.O. Box 85122
San Diego, CA 92138-9174, USA

INTRODUCTION

One major asset of magnetoencephalography (MEG) and resulting signal averaged neuromagnetic evoked fields (EF) is that of determining field maps and localizing neural source generators. Averaging of many single epochs, most often required for such localization, maximizes signal strength, but minimizes signal changes or variability. An area of research of considerable interest to us is that of assessing short term temporal changes in brain processing and their possible relationships to individual differences and job performance. There appears to be a direct relationship between neuroelectric evoked potential (EP) variability and on-job performance. Low performers show greater intra- and inter-subject EP variability than do high performers (Lewis, 1983). Previously, we have found relationships between EF variability, as measured by the group coefficient or variation (CV=SD/MN) for average EF amplitudes, and on-job performance in military personnel (Lewis, Trejo, Nunez, Weinberg, & Naitoh, 1988). The present research reexamines a portion of, and augments, the EF data presented in our earlier paper (Lewis, et. al., 1988). Here we examine EF trial-to-trial variability (TTV), not the CV based on group averages. This paper will report that substantial decreases in the TTV and the EF occurred relatively early during a 10-minute recording period, and that groups of high- and low-performing individuals differed in the size and time course of these changes.

METHOD

Recording of evoked fields and the measurement of job performance were the same as those reported earlier (Lewis, et. al., 1988). Briefly, the performance measures were obtained by a supervisor rating questionnaire one month after the recording of the EFs. Job performance criteria included job knowledge and performance, military knowledge and performance, reliability, and motivation level. Each subject (15 male military personnel mean age: 21 +/- 1.93 years) was rated as "high", "satisfactory", or "low" on each criterion and was later placed into one of two groups (HIGH or LOW). Assignment to the HIGH group (N = 10) was made if the subject received a "high" mark on all four criteria and to the LOW group (N = 5) if he received less than a "high" mark on any criterion. In our earlier paper (Lewis,

[1]The opinions expressed in this paper are those of the authors, are not official, and do not necessarily reflect the views of the Navy Department.

Advances in Biomagnetism
Edited by S.J. Williamson *et al.*
Plenum Press, New York

et. al., 1988), we discussed the homogeneity of the subject sample, of which the current subjects were part. The subjects were male, similar in age, had been in the military for four years, and were selected for security positions. We also discussed the validity of using supervisor ratings as criteria. The correlation between the ratings and military rank two years later was 0.79 ($p < .0002$).

Each subject viewed an appearing-disappearing black-and-white checkerboard stimulus (binocular, central fixation) which subtended 5° visual angle. Checks subtended 23 minutes each (1.3 cycles/degree). The stimuli were presented for 10 msec with a variable inter-stimulus interval of 500 to 1500 msec. Three intensities (34, 6, 64 cd/m^2) were presented in the same sequence for each subject. Background luminance was 3 cd/m^2.

The EF data were obtained with a single-channel DC biomagnetic system (Biomagnetic Technologies, Inc. (BTi), model 600B), line filtered (Quantum Design, Synchronous Capacitor Filter, model 640S), bandpassed (0.1-40Hz), and digitized at 256 Hz. The data reported in this paper were a subset of EF data acquired serially from twelve sites located in four columns at 2 and 4 cm lateral to the midline on each hemisphere and at 3, 5, and 7 cm anterior to the inion. The two sites which were analyzed were located at 4 cm lateral to the midline and 3 cm anterior to the inion, approximating the location of 01 and 02 in the 10/20 system (Jasper, 1958). These sites were selected because of earlier analyses showing correlation between EF amplitude and job performance, and that sensory EPs and EFs correlate with higher-order cognitive processing which is required for complex behavior and performance. The EFs were recorded with 256 msec of pre-stimulus and 512 msec post-stimulus activity and stored as single spochs on a computer system (Masscomp 5500). All EF data were viewed as single epochs prior to storage and rejected on line, if artifacts were present.

The single epochs were averaged in 3 blocks of 6 epochs each for a total of 18. Block 1 corresponded to epochs 1-6, block 2 to epochs 7-12, and block 3 to epochs 13-18. For each block, EFs were ensemble averaged and the TTV was computed. Resulting average EF and TTV waves were segmented into five contiguous pre-stimulus and ten contiguous post-stimulus windows of about 50 msec width. The TTV was computed as the variance over trials in the block for each point along the waveform. The resulting metric was left as variance through all windowing and subsequent statistical analyses. Mean values where discussed or plotted, were the square root (standard deviation), expressed in femtotesla (fT) units. Sample amplitude and TTV data from one subject appear in Figures 1A and 1B.

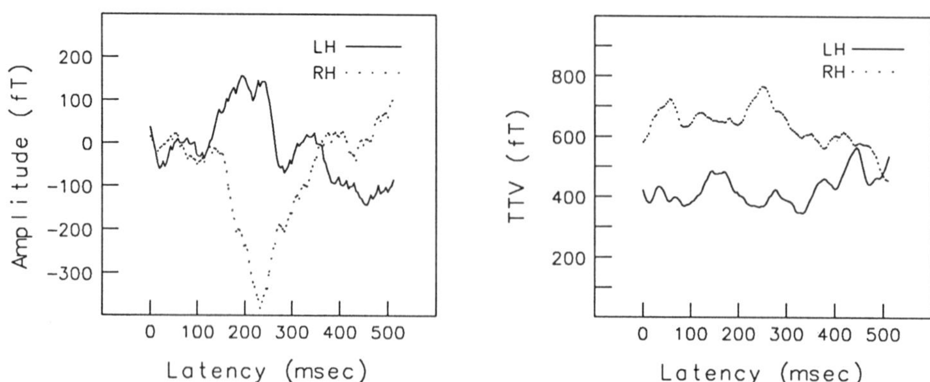

Figure 1. A. Average EF and B. TTV for one subject. LH: left hemisphere, RH: right hemisphere.

RESULTS

The TTV values of five pre-stimulus windows and ten post-stimulus windows were input to separate repeated measures analyses of variance. Reported probabilities have been corrected for possible violations of compound symmetry (Geisser & Greenhouse, 1958). Factors were blocks (3), groups (2), intensity (3), recording site (2), and window (10). Of particular interest was the interaction between blocks of epochs and the two performance groups. In order to test for group differences, due to spontaneous MEG activity, we analyzed the five pre-stimulus windows by analysis of variance. No statistically significant group or group interactions were found for the EF pre-stimulus data [block-by-group ($F(2,26) = 0.323$, $p < .727$]. The main effect for site was statistically significant [$F(1,13) = 16.58$, $p < .001$] as well as block [$F(2,26 = 4.54$, $p < .040$].

Analyses of variance for the post-stimulus conditions showed that the intensity factor was not statistically significant. Mean TTV values for the 34, 6, and 64 cd/m^2 stimuli were 661, 599, 574 fT respectively (corresponding amplitudes were 173, 155, and 160 fTrms). Therefore the intensity factor was treated as a stimulus sequence (time-on-task) factor. Significant main effects were found for blocks [$F(2,26) = 10.68$, $p < .002$] and recording site [$F(1,13 = 17.63$, $p < .001$]. Mean TTV values for the sites were 480 and 722 fT for the left and right hemisphere sites, respectively. A two-way interaction was found for block-by-group [$F(2,26) = 4.44$, $p < .036$].

Figure 2 shows the mean TTV values of the block main effect and the block-by-group interaction. The LOW group shows greater TTV than does the HIGH group over the three blocks, the group differences being 31%, 25%, and 22% for blocks 1, 2, 3, respectively. Between blocks 1 and 2, TTV in the LOW group decreased about 3 times more than in the HIGH group (105 vs. 34 fT). Block-by-stimulus sequence interaction were 778, 591, 598, 614, 614, 560, 574, 592, and 564 fT which corresponded to blocks 1, 2, 3 for sequences 1, 2, 3, respectively. Greatest TTV change occurred between the first and second block, first sequence, and remained somewhat constant for the remainder of the testing session (about 10 minutes).

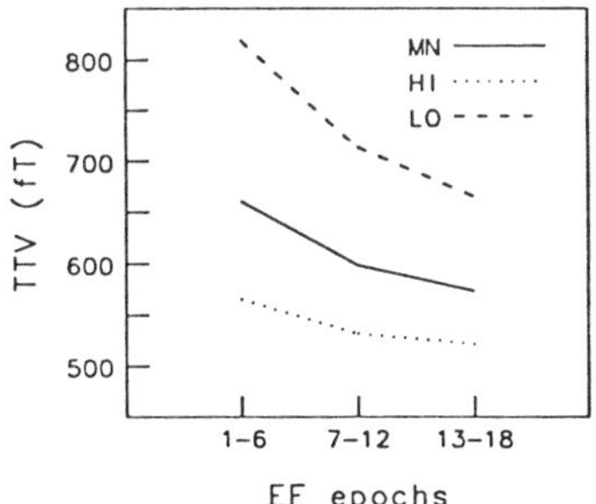

Figure 2. Mean TTV values collapsed over windows, sites, and sequence (intensity) of the main effect for blocks and the block-by-group interaction.

DISCUSSION

Individuality and the constancy and variability in brain activity have been noted for more than 50 years (Travis & Gottlober, 1936; Rubin, 1938). Callaway (1975) has discussed evoked potential variability, cognitive variability and individual differences at length. He refers to a comment by Dodge (1924) which may be appropriate to the current research, "variations are not artifacts to be statistically lumped and treated as though they were errors of measurement, but they represent realities which might well be quite as significant as the conscious aims of measurement in which they occurred." Evoked field TTV measures may make as large a contribution to describing individual differences in brain processing as that of traditional signal averaged EF amplitude measures. The results of this study support the notion that TTV is inversely related to on-job performance and suggest that TTV may change as a function of individual differences and time-on-task. Even though the TTV of the LOW performers decreased more than that of the HIGH performers from block 1 to 2, their overall TTV remained higher over the entire testing situation. We have no reason to believe that if more EFs were obtained from the LOW performers over a longer period of time, that their TTV would decrease to that of the HIGH performer group. Variability of EF activity may represent individual differences in adaptation to the testing situation, differential attention being paid to the stimulus over time, or differential decay of an orienting response. Such factors may reflect more general behavior and job performance.

The EF data being reported here were among the first to be recorded from an operational military environment, and with a single channel SQUID system. Recording limitations, due in part to the requirement of not interferring with training or operations did restrict the precision of data recording, however did provide a unique opportunity to address relationships between EF data and job performance.

Our earlier paper (Lewis, et. al., 1988) described relationships between EF amplitude and performance, and suggested that variability at the group level (coefficient of variation) may contribute to the between-group performance differences which we found. In the current paper, we explored in more detail, the variability associated with single epoch EF recordings from two sites. We acknowledge that two sites represent limited assessment of brain variability and performance relationships, and that our results may be specific to the particular sites which we analyzed. Further research will explore both EF amplitude and TTV measures with wider spatial distribution. We have recently integrated a five channel MEG system (BTi, model 605) into our laboratory. This system may improve the assessment of temporal aspects of EF components which may be spatially distributed. In a recent review paper, Hari & Lounasmaa (1989) suggested that investigating spatiotemporal relationships in brain processing may be among the most important contributions which could be made by the MEG.

REFERENCES

Callaway, E. (1975). Brain electrical potentials and individual psychological differences. Grune & Stratton, New York.

Dodge, R. (1924). Problems of human variability. Science 59, 263.

Geisser, S., & Greenhouse, S.W. (1958). An extension of Box's results on the use of the F distribution in multivariate analysis. Annals of Mathematical Statistics 29, 885-891.

Hari, R., & Lounasmaa, O.V. (1989) Recording and interpretation of cerebral magnetic fields. Science 244, 432-436.

Jasper, H. (1958). The ten-twenty electrode system of the International Federation. Electroencephalography and Clinical Neurophysiology 10, 371-375.

Lewis, G.W. (1983). Event related brain electrical and magnetic activity: Toward predicting on-job performance. International Journal of Neuroscience 18, 159-182.

Lewis, G.W., Trejo, L.J., Nunez, P., Weinberg, H., & Naitoh, P. (1988). Evoked neuromagnetic fields: Implications for indexing performance. In: Atsumi, K., Kotani, M., Ueno, S., Katila, T., & Williamson, S. (Eds.) Biomagnetism '87, 6th International Conference on Biomagnetism. Tokyo Denki University Press, Tokyo, pp. 266-269.

Rubin, MA (1938). A variability study of the normal and schizophrenic occipital alpha rhythm, Journal of Psychology 6, 325-334.

Travis, L.E., & Gottlober, A. (1936). Do brain waves have individuality? Science 84, 532-533.

CROSSMODAL INTERACTIONS OF AUDITORY STIMULUS PRESENTATION ON THE VISUAL EVOKED MAGNETIC RESPONSE

C. Busch[1], G. Wilson[2], C. Orr[1], and A. Papanicolaou[3]

1) Systems Research Laboratories, Inc., Dayton, OH
2) Armstrong Aerospace Medical Research Lab, WPAFB, OH
3) Division of Neurosurgery, Univ. of Texas, Galveston, TX

INTRODUCTION

Alterations in electrical potentials have previously been used to demonstrate crossmodal interactions in cortical functioning among several sensory modalities. Measuring electrical potentials recorded at the vertex in response to auditory, tactile, electric and visual stimuli, Davis et al. (1972) reported significant reductions in the peak-to-peak amplitude measures of the N1-P2 evoked potentials (EPs) when either an intramodal or crossmodal stimulus was presented 500 ms prior to the test stimuli. However, these results are of limited interpretive utility due to the susceptibility of EPs to the effects of non-zero reference values and volume conduction of activity (Nunez, 1981). Thus, it was not possible to separate the relative contributions of multiple, simultaneously activated, cortical regions to the recorded response using electroencephalography (EEG).

Magnetoencephalography (MEG), however, due to its more discrete spatial resolution and its specificity to source, provides a unique opportunity for examining crossmodal interactions at the primary sensory cortices. Recently, Huttunen et al. (1987) combined both electrical and magnetic recording techniques to further assess sensory convergence and reported that the more spatially select magnetic measures failed to substantiate interactions of the auditory and somatosensory systems at the level of the primary projection areas. The purpose of this study was to evaluate visual and auditory modality interactions at the visual cortex by capitalizing on the relative advantages of MEG.

METHODS

Visual evoked magnetic field (EF) maxima in response to a flashed checkerboard pattern (duration, 20 ms; rate, 1/s) were identified for nine male subjects (one ambidextrous, eight dextrous; ages 22 to 30) using a single channel DC SQUID (BTI Model 601). Projected to the subject via mirrors, the pattern subtended a visual angle of 3.65 degrees horizontal and 3.95 degrees vertical (check size .3 degrees) and a small diode at the center provided a point for visual fixation. During EF mapping, no generalized pattern of hemispheric laterality for visual processing was noted; although, individual subjects frequently evidenced higher amplitude responses in one hemisphere relative to the other. Therefore, all subsequent recordings were obtained from over the dominant N1m maximum in either the left (5 subjects) or right (4 subjects) occipital regions as determined by that individual's response strength. MEG measures were obtained from within a double-walled magnetically shielded chamber with a shielding factor of 250 at 1.9 Hz. EF responses were notch-filtered at 60 Hz and bandpass filtered at 1 to 30 Hz using a Grass amplifier (Model P511). Data were digitized at a 1000 Hz rate for 100 ms pre-stimulus, 400 ms post-stimulus and stored for off-line analyses using a Masscomp 5400 Laboratory Computer.

Averages of 50 responses time-locked to the presentation of the visual stimulus were recorded during six different experimental conditions, each repeated 2-3 times, in a different random order for each subject. They were: (1) the Flash condition involving a 1/s presentation of the checker-board pattern, (2) the Audio condition during which a brief audio stimulus (10 ms rise, 3 ms fall, 65 dB SPL) was presented to the subject binaurally at a 1/s rate, (3) the Alternate condition consisting of the visual and audio stimuli presented alternately at 0.5 s intervals, (4) the Simultaneous condition with coincident onset of both visual and audio stimuli presented at 1/s, (5) the Flash-Audio condition wherein the onset of the visual stimulus preceded the onset of the audio stimulus by 50 ms, and (6) the Audio-Flash condition during which the audio stimulus preceded the visual by 50 ms.

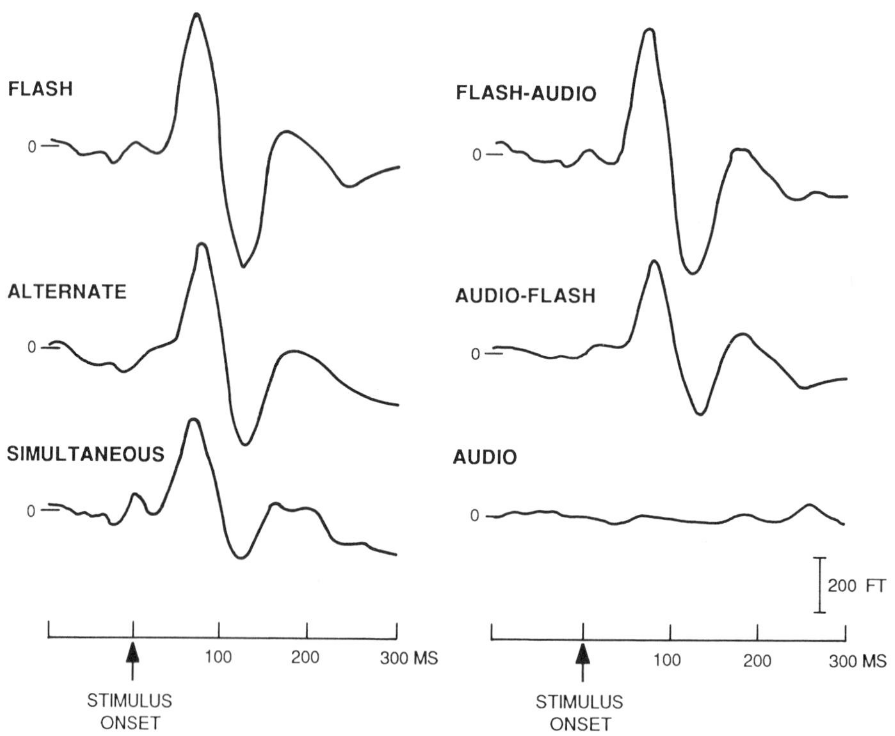

Figure 1. Averaged waveforms of one subject's responses during each experimental condition.

RESULTS

The occipitally recorded EF waveforms produced by the visual stimulus were characterized by two prominent peaks corresponding to the N1m and P2m components. In all cases, these components were clearly identifiable and their peak amplitudes, adjusted to base-line by subtracting the mean value of the 100 ms pre-stimulus period from each post-stimulus data point, constituted the dependent measure in the analyses. There were, however, no measurable peaks evident in signals obtained in response to the audio stimulus per se; therefore the Audio condition measures were not included.

Figure 1 illustrates the averaged EF responses of one subject. To assess the reliability of the measures across conditions, the average peak values obtained for four subjects during repeated recordings were compared using a Pearson product moment correlation. Results yielded a coefficient of .94, thus indicating that, for individual subjects, the relative mean values obtained during the different experimental conditions were highly consistent.

Analyses of the EF results were performed using two separate repeated measures ANOVAs for the N1m and P2m components, respectively. Results of the N1m evaluation indicated a significant main effect for condition ($F = 2.96$, $p < .03$) and effects tests showed that the amplitude obtained during the Simultaneous and the Audio-Flash conditions were significantly reduced compared with Flash or Flash-Audio responses. Analysis of the P2m component amplitudes also indicated a significant main effect for condition ($F = 2.74$, $p < .045$). Post hoc examination revealed that both the Alternate and Simultaneous conditions yielded lower amplitude responses than did the Flash condition. To normalize for intersubject variability in absolute peak values, the percentage change in each condition relative to the Flash condition was also calculated. The average percent reductions during each condition are shown in Figure 2.

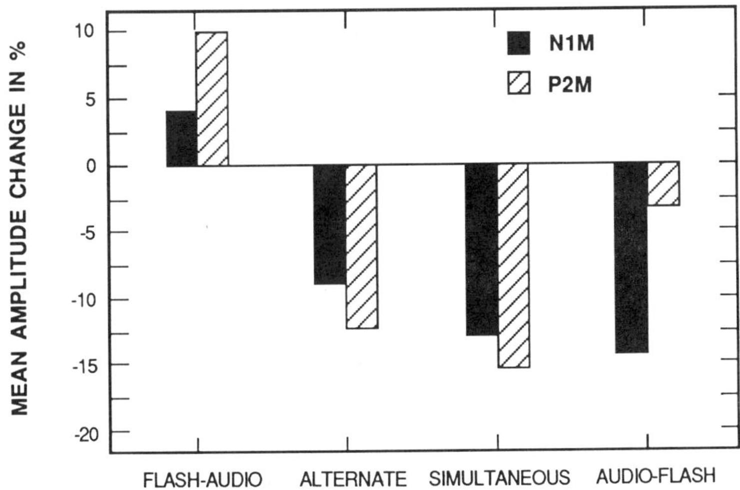

Figure 2. Crossmodal interactions; mean amplitude changes in the N1m and P2m components. Bars indicate percent amplitude differences of the responses from the Flash condition.

DISCUSSION

Reductions in the amplitude of the vertex-recorded visual evoked response after auditory stimulation have been interpreted as demonstrating convergence of sensory information (Davis et al., 1972). However, in the case of electrical potentials, it is not possible to separate cortical activity generated in the primary sensory areas from that activity simultaneously generated at more distant locations, thus the relative contributions cannot be assessed. By utilizing MEG technology for this study, it was possible to evaluate the interactions of auditory and visual stimulation at the visual projection area.

The implications of the amplitude decrease observed in the N1m and P2m components of the visual EF during the Simultaneous, Alternate and Audio-Flash conditions are two-fold. First, they suggest that audio-visual crossmodal interactions may be observed at the visual projection areas. Since there were no auditory EFs observed for any subjects during the Audio-alone condition, the reductions in the visual response appear to indicate a convergence of the sensory information rather than simply a summation response. Second, the relative timing of auditory and visual presentations appears to be critical in determining effects. Davis et al. (1972) reported a degradation in the second visual EP when an auditory or a visual stimulus was presented 500 ms prior. In the realm of crossmodal pairing, this corresponds to the Alternate condition in this study which also resulted in comparable reductions. Similar reductions were also observed during simultaneous crossmodal stimulus presentations and when auditory stimulation occurred just prior to the visual stimulation. However, no changes were noted when auditory stimulation followed 50 ms after visual. Although no intramodal stimulus pairs were included in this design, previous investigations conducted in this laboratory have shown no differences in the amplitudes of the visual EF components when stimuli were presented at either a 1/s or a 2/s rate. Thus, no reductions would be predicted, at least during the Alternate condition.

The degradation of responses due to attentional shifts or non-specific changes in arousal cannot be ruled out as a contributing factor in the present study; however, the implementation of behavioral controls during future experiments should help resolve this issue. Additional research will also be necessary to better delineate the exact neuronal processes underlying these results. For instance, it remains to be determined if the observed response attenuation reflects a true reduction in response strength or results instead from the rotation of the source vector thus giving the appearance of strength reductions. Such investigations are currently in progress in this laboratory. One conclusion, however, is clear. MEG represents a uniquely advantageous technique for evaluating crossmodality response interactions while circumventing some of the problems inherent in EEG.

REFERENCES

Davis, H., Osterhammel, P., Weir, C. & Gjerdingen, D., 1972, Slow vertex potentials: Interactions among auditory, tactile, electric and visual stimuli. EEG, 33: 537-545.

Huttunen, J., Hari, R. & Vanni, S., 1987, Crossmodal interaction is reflected in vertex potentials but not in evoked magnetic fields. Acta Neurol. Scand., 75: 410-416.

Nunez, P., 1981, "Electrical Fields of the Brain", Oxford Press, New York.

SCALP DISTRIBUTION OF MAGNETIC FIELDS GENERATED BY HORIZONTAL EYE MOVEMENTS AND EYE BLINKS

M.T. Oakley, G. Sullivan, S.B.W. Roeder*, E.R.Flynn

Biomagnetism Group Los Alamos National Laboratory, Los Alamos, NM 87545

*San Diego State University, San Diego, CA 92182

INTRODUCTION

Eye movements are known to produce artifacts in the electroencephalogram (EEG) and in the magnetoencephalogram (MEG) which can result in substantial distortions of the morphology of sensory-evoked waveforms (Antervo et al., 1985; Katila et al., 1981; Vaughan, 1969). Some studies are more susceptible to these artifacts. For example, certain studies require peripheral presentations of visual stimuli which tend to evoke unwanted, foveating eye movements, from untrained subjects. The application of MEG to neurological diagnosis and basic neuroscience research requires the assessment of possible contamination of surface-recorded electromagnetic fields (ERFs) by time-locked ocular and myogenic activity such as eye movements and eye blinks. Three types of electrical potentials associated with eye movements have been identified; the antecedent slow activity (Kurtzberg and Vaughan 1977), the spike potential (Riemslag et al., 1988) and the lambda wave (Gaarder et al.,1964). The spike potential (SP) has maximal amplitude near the orbital regions and seems to originate in the oculomotor neurons innervating the ocular muscle units (Riemslag et al., 1988). However, the retino-corneal potential which has been the primary concern of eye movement artifacts in evoked potential studies (Vaughan Jr., 1969) also contributes to the spike potential. Lambda waves have been recorded in the occipito-parietal scalp locations of humans (Barlow and Ciganek,1969) both following eye movements made over an illuminated structured field and by a pattern displacement across a stationary retina (Remond and Lesevre, 1971) suggesting that the potential is a response to visual image movement. Some types of activity associated with eye movements can be separated out. Muscle activity (Riemslag et al., 1988) and potentials associated with displacement of the retina (Eason et al., 1983) increase as the deflection angle increases; thus magnetic response associated with these two types of activities should also increase with increasing eye deflection. Lambda waves can be dissociated from muscle and corneo-retinal activity by comparing equivalent eye movements in light and dark.

METHODS

Subjects made horizontal eye movements (left and right) and eye blinks under light and dark conditions. The degree of eye displacement from a center fixation point was 6 and 14 degrees along a horizontal meridian (8 degrees for one subject) in the light condition and approximately 14 degrees in the dark condition. The dark condition served as a control to help delineate ocular and lambda activities. In the light condition, the eye

Advances in Biomagnetism
Edited by S.J. Williamson *et al.*
Plenum Press, New York

movements were prompted by a small beam of light emitted by a fiberoptic cable; in the dark condition the prompting stimulus was a faint tone beep. The duration of both stimuli was 800 msec. Prestimulus interval which served as a baseline was 100 msec. Twenty passes for each type of eye movement were averaged on-line. Two replications were obtained for a total of 40 passes. Neuromagnetic activity was recorded over both hemispheres. A 7-channel, SQUID-coupled, 2nd order gradiometer located in an aluminum and mumetal magnetically shielded room was used.

RESULTS

The peak latency of deflections associated with horizontal eye movements was approximately 400 msec after the onset of the prompting stimulus; the amplitude ranged from 300 fT near the orbits to 180 fT at posterior locations (Fig.1). Several polarity inversions are apparent in this figure (a negative magnetic field is directed inwards). (1) Near the orbital regions rightward and leftward movements produced deflections of opposite polarity. However, over the temporal, parietal and occipital areas the polarity of deflection was independent of the direction of movement. (2) Horizontal eye movements produce an inversion above and below the eye; however, the extrema for left eye movement are closer together than extrema for the right eye movement. (3) Another inversion is evident over the temporal region.

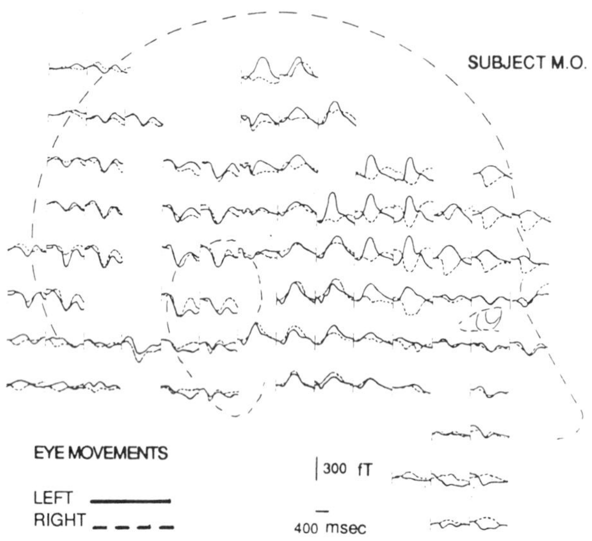

Figure 1. Magnetic fields associated with horizontal eye movements over the right hemisphere. Eye deflection was 8 degrees.

Larger eye deflections produced deflections of larger amplitude. However, over posterior areas the magnetic fields generated by the different degree of eye deflection were either the same or even larger for the smaller eye deflection. The direction of eye movement did not affect the polarity of magnetic fields obtained from the parietal and occipital areas. Responses associated with horizontal eye movements made in the light and dark conditions shown in Fig. 2 indicate the absence of later (400 msec) activity over the posterior region when eyes move in the dark. This figure also shows primary sensory responses evoked by the timing stimuli which peak out at about 150 msec. Eye blinks (Fig.3) generated magnetic fields over the entire scalp. Near the orbits of the eyes the magnitude of the signal was about 1200 fT and declined with distance. At posterior regions the magnitude of response was about 60 fT. The magnetic fields reversed polarity along the midline above the nasion.

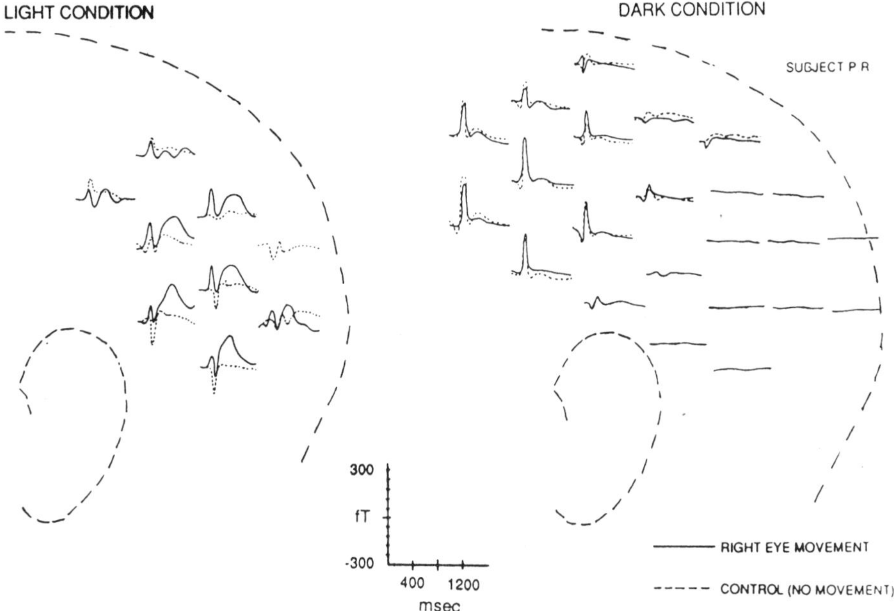

Fig. 2. Comparison of magnetic fields associated with horizontal eye movements made in the light and dark. Light flash elicited a sensory response at 150 msec and a lambda wave at 400 msec over the occipito-parietal cortex (left panel); auditory prompting stimulus elicited sensory response over the temporal region at 150 msec (right panel). Notice the absence of activity over the posterior region in the dark condition. Eye deflection was 14 degrees.

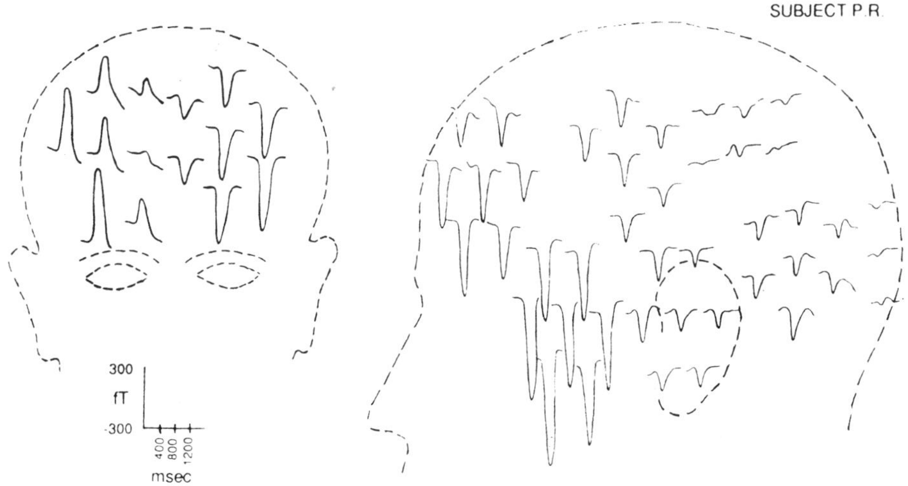

Fig. 3. Magnetic fields associated with eye blinks made in the light condition.

DISCUSSION

Magnetic fields associated with horizontal eye movements and eye blinks can be detected over the entire scalp and thus can significantly contaminate activity evoked by sensory stimuli. The sources responsible for this activity differ across the scalp. The difference in magnitude of the response as a function of degree of eye movement displacement suggests that near the orbits of the eyes and over temporal areas the activity is generated either by ocular muscles (Riemslag, 1988), by the displacement of the eye (Katila et al., 1981), or a combination of both mechanisms. Katila et al. calculated the magnetic field distribution of horizontal eye movements based on the assumption that the magnetic field is due to two current dipoles one in each eye in equivalent locations. Their calculations, compared with empirical data in which subjects performed horizontal eye movements of 55-60 degrees, suggest that the magnetic field is due to two horizontal current dipoles. Our data are consistent with Katila's interpretation. In addition, our data show that horizontal eye movements of much smaller lateral deviation produce detectable magnetic fields over scalp areas far removed from the orbital regions. However, there seems to be considerable variability across subjects. Comparing magnetic responses generated by eye movements made in darkness vs movements made over a lighted source suggests that magnetic fields obtained at posterior scalp regions reflect neural responses generated by the pattern displacement across the retina (lambda wave). Magnetic fields generated by eye blinks have been recorded by Antervo et al (1985). Our data show similar field distributions near the orbits of the eyes which, in accordance with Antervo et al., suggests that the primary current source of the blink potential is the corneo-retinal potential. The pattern of eye blink activity was not consistent across subjects. In one instance, eye blinks produced larger magnetic fields over the forehead and zero at locations posterior to the external canthi of the eyes.

In conclusion, the magnetic fields generated by eye movements obtained in this study and by others (Antervo et al., 1985; Katila et al., 1981) shows that MEG records are succeptible to eye movement contamination at virtually any scalp area. Although the magnitude of the response at areas far removed from the orbital regions is relatively weak, the artifact caused by eye movements can contaminate later components assumed to be associated with higher cognitive function. Due to individual differences it is very difficult to predict the field distribution of the eye movement artifact.

This work was supported by the U.S Army Reasearch Institute, the Department of Energy contract W-7405-ENG-36 and the Veterans Administration. The authors wish to thank D. Valdez and W. Madland for technical assistance.

REFERENCES

Antervo A., Hari R., Katila T., Ryhanen T., Seppanen M. (1985). EEG, 61:247-253.

Barlow JS., Ciganek L. (1969) EEG, 26:183-192.

Eason R.G., Flowers L., Oakley M. (1983) Beh. Res. Meth. and Instr., 15:13-21.

Gaarder K., Krauskopf J., Graf V., Kropfl W., Armington JC. (1964). Science, 146:1481-83.

Katila T., Maniewski R., Poutanen T., Varpula T. (1981) J. Appl. Phys., 52:2565-71.

Kurtzberg D., Vaughan HG Jr., (1977). In JE Desmedt (Ed), Visual evoked potentials in man: new developments, pp.314-31, Clarendon Press, Oxford.

Remond A., Lesevre N. (1971). EEG, 30:250.

Riemslag FCC., Van der Heijde GL., Van Dongen MMMM., Ottenhoff F. (1988). EEG, 70:281-287.

Vaughan HG Jr. (1969). NASA, Washington, DC.

A MODALITY-SPECIFIC NEUROMAGNETIC P3

J.D. Lewine, S.B.W. Roeder, M.T. Oakley, D.L. Arthur, C.J. Aine, J.S. George and E.R. Flynn

Neuromagnetism Laboratory, Mail Stop M715, Los Alamos National Laboratory Los Alamos, New Mexico, 87545

INTRODUCTION

Several studies indicate that in cases of psychopathology and alcoholism the amplitude and/or latency of endogenous, scalp-recorded P3 potentials elicited by rare events are abnormal (e.g., Roth et al., 1980; Polich, 1984). The P3 complex may normally be a valuable index of cognitive processing (see Donchin and Coles, 1988) and identification of the neural generator(s) of this response would thus provide valuable insight into both normal and abnormal information processes.

Several laboratories have recorded magnetic field correlates of P3 potentials evoked by visual and auditory stimuli. Data of Okada et al., (1983) from a mapping study of a visually evoked magnetic P3 are consistent with a hippocampal source, but attempts to localize the generator(s) of the auditory magnetic P3 have been unsuccessful. In an effort to independently confirm, extend, and clarify previous results, the surface topographies of magnetic P3-like complexes evoked during the performance of auditory and visual detection tasks were examined.

METHODS

Magnetic fields evoked during performance of auditory and visual detection tasks were recorded in the Los Alamos shielded room via a seven sensor, second-order gradiometer system (BTi). Data were collected at a digitization rate of 1KHz and filtered on-line with a bandpass of 0.1 - 50 Hz. The data were subsequently subjected to low pass (40Hz) digital filtering. In nine cases recordings were made at a minimum of eight dewar placements per hemisphere. Scalp potentials were often simultaneously recorded from Pz, Cz, and Fz locations. Electro-ocular artifacts were monitored and data from trials contaminated by eye-blinks or movements were rejected from further analyses.

Four auditory and four visual test blocks were administered at each dewar location. For the auditory test blocks, individual stimuli were 100 msec tone pips with a frequency of 1000 or 3000 Hz. The subject's task was always to count the number of target, 3000 Hz stimuli that occurred during a 2-3 minute interval during which a sequence of 125 stimuli was presented. Stimuli were presented with a random inter-stimulus-interval of 750-1250 msec. For half of the auditory test blocks given at each dewar placement, the 3000 Hz tone occurred with a probability of .20, whereas for the remaining auditory test blocks it occurred with a probability of .80. The procedures for visual testing were identical to the above except the target was a centrally-fixated 4 cycle/degree horizontal grating whereas the non-target stimulus

Advances in Biomagnetism
Edited by S.J. Williamson *et al.*
Plenum Press, New York

was a 4 cycle/degree vertical grating. Each subject participated in 1-2 dewar placements per 1-2 hr test session.

RESULTS

By comparing physiological activity evoked by presentation of counted, target stimuli in the two probability conditions within each modality, it was possible to identify those components of the P3 complex specifically associated with the probability manipulation, uncomplicated by a comparison across physically different stimuli (e.g., 1000 versus 3000 Hz tones) or task conditions (counted versus not counted).

Each of nine subjects demonstrated a clear probability dependent modulation of the amplitude of the evoked electrical and magnetic P3 components. However, for four additional subjects for which only left hemisphere data were obtained, a neuromagnetic P3 could not be identified. On the one hand, in three of these instances the electrical P3 complex was absent, of low amplitude, or of unstable amplitude across test sessions, but for the forth subject, a magnetic P3 was absent despite the existence of a robust and stable electrical P3.

When present, the auditory magnetic and electrical P3 components had peak latencies between 280-330 msec. In the visual modality the P3 complexes had peak latencies between 380-450 msec. Figure 1 provides examples of averaged auditory and visual magnetic field and electrical potential waveforms for target stimuli. Figure 2 provides example, iso-field contour maps based upon difference-waves (20% probability - 80% probability). The presented maps are for the "time slices" corresponding to the peak of that subject's electrical P3 as identified in the electrical difference-wave. Although iso-field patterns were highly individualistic, field extrema were invariably separated by 10-24 cm (arc length). Also, auditory and visual patterns for the same subject were always disparate.

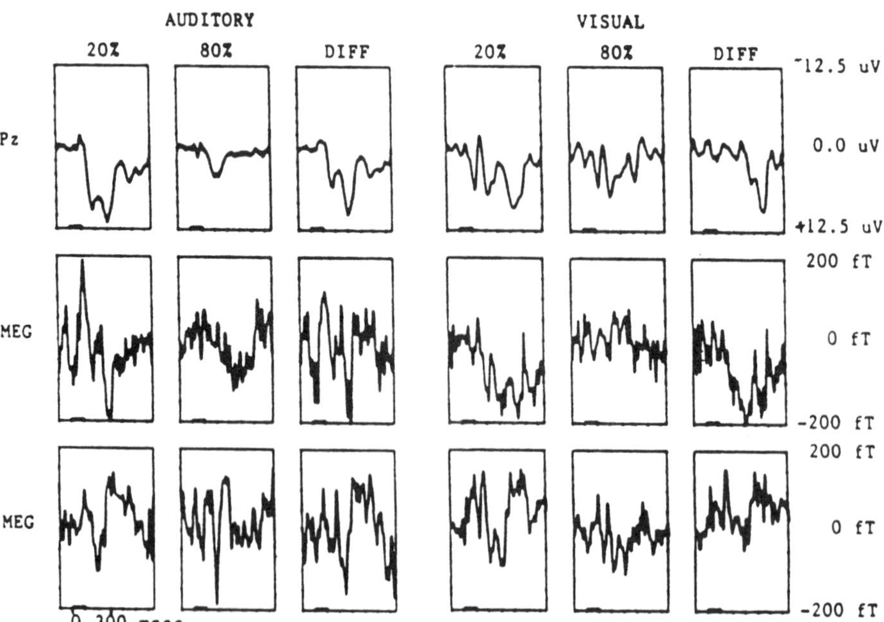

FIGURE 1: One subject's Pz electrical and example MEG waveforms derived from target trials where the target probability was 20% or 80%. Difference waves are also shown.

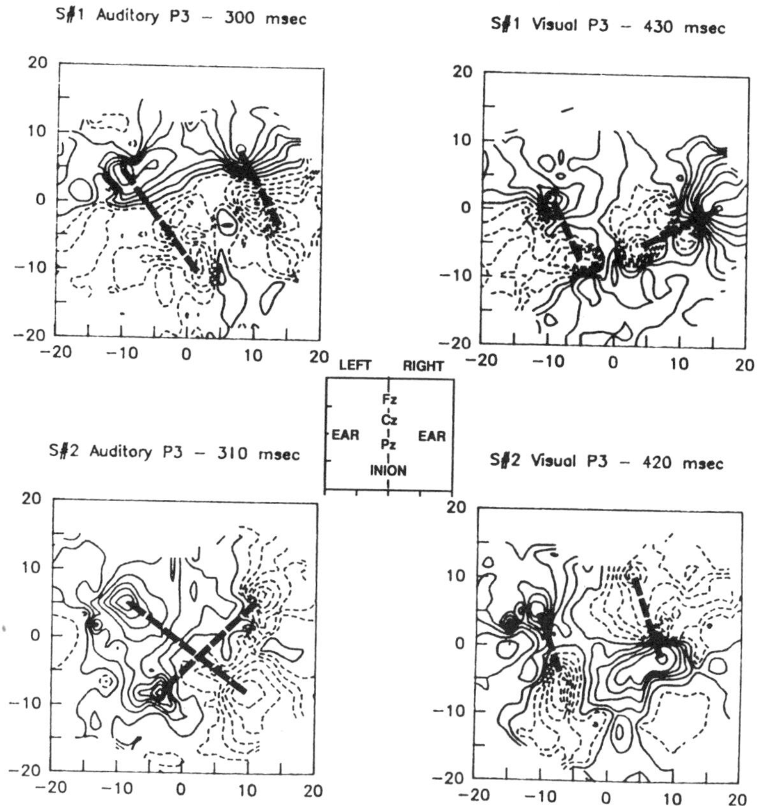

FIGURE 2: Iso-field contour maps for two subjects. Maps are top-down surface projections. Thin dashed lines are for entering flux, the solid lines are for exiting flux. Lines are separated by 25fT. The thick dashed lines link extrema believed to reflect the same generator.

DISCUSSION

A key observation in this study was the high degree of variability in evoked magnetic responses. Not all subjects displayed a neuromagnetic P3 and when neuromagnetic P3 responses were identifiable, iso-field maps revealed marked hemispheric asymmetries and inter-individual differences. For example, the polarities of seemingly corresponding extrema were opposite in some subjects (e.g., right anterior visual extremums for subjects #1 and #2) This indicates that the orientation of the magnetic P3 generators are variable from subject-to-subject. If the same basic region is responsible for P3 generation across subjects, it is likely that spatially displaced pyramidal cells within the region display widely disparate orientations.

Given the observation that field extrema were always separated by a minimum of 10 cm, coupled with the fact that auditory and visual iso-field patterns were different for the same subject, the most parsimonious explanation of the data is that the auditory and visual magnetic P3 are generated at distinct, but nearby, deep temporal lobe sites. One possibility is that slightly different cell clusters within the hippocampus are responsible for generation of the P3 complex identified here. For the one available case where magnetic resonance images of the subject's brain were available **and** the evoked field patterns were exceptionally simple, a dual-source, "least-squares" field-pattern fitting algorithm, modeled that subject's P3 data (>75% of the variance accounted for) with a point-source current dipole in each hippocampus. This result is consistent with previous neuromagnetic data of Okada and colleagues and also consistent with invasive intracranial data, obtained by both UCLA and Yale research groups (Halgren et al., 1986; McCarthy et al., 1989), which indicate limbic generation of large amplitude (100-200 uV) P3-like potentials.

On the other hand, a straightforward hippocampal interpretation of the current data must be viewed with caution. First, magnetic resonance imaging data are currently lacking on several subjects and in many cases dual source models positing one equivalent current dipole in the hippocampus of each hemisphere are insufficient to fully account for observed field patterns. That is, field patterns were often complex and possibly indicative of the activity of multiple generators within each hemisphere. Secondly, while the magnetic data indicate modality specificity for the magnetic P3 field patterns, the Yale group (McCarthy et al., 1989) failed to find any modality specificity in the spatial gradient of P3-like, intracranially recorded limbic field potentials. This descrepancy may reflect limited spatial sampling in the intracranial experiments, or alternatively, it may indicate that the observed modality specificity in the field patterns is a consequence of non-limbic generators. Thirdly, and of equal import, the large separation of field extrema could reflect extended and/or multiple shallow sources rather than deep sources. It is clear that final clarrification of these issues must await the development of sophisticated multiple-source, temporal-spatial modeling procedures and additional invasive and non-invasive data.

Some final notes of caution concern the generalizability of these results. The magnetic P3 component described here has been characterized on the basis of a very limited functional manipulation (stimulus probability) and the results may not be indicative of P3 complexes elicited in other situations. Furthermore, and perhaps more importantly, a description of the generators of the observed magnetic P3 is likely to provide only limited insight into the nature of the generators of the electrical P3. Neuromagnetic P3 iso-field patterns were rarely consistent with generation by elements appropriately oriented for the production of a maximal electrical response at Pz. This, coupled with the inability to find any neuromagnetic correlates of a robust P3 electrical response in one subject, suggests that the vertex electrical response reflects generators beyond those contributing to the magnetic response and that some of the generators of the electrical response are unfavorably oriented for identification via the employed magnetoencephalographic techniques. Nevertheless, the data suggest that magnetoencephalography can serve as a non-invasive tool for the analysis of the functional organization of the temporal lobe.

ACKNOWLEDGEMENTS

The authors wish to thank D. Valdez for technical assistance. This work was supported by the United States Army Research Institute and United States Department of Energy contract W-7405-ENG-36.

REFERENCES

Donchin, E. and Coles, M.G.H., 1988, Is the P300 component a manifestation of context updating? Behav. Brain Sci., 11:357.

Halgren, E., Stapleton, J.M., Smith, M., and Altafullah, I., 1986, Generators of the human scalp P3(s). In: "Evoked Potentials", R.Q. Cracco and I. Bodis-Wollner, eds., Alan R. Liss, New York.

McCarthy, G., Wood, C.C., Williamson, P.D., and Spencer, D.D., 1989, Task-dependent field potential in human hippocampal formation. Journal of Neuroscience, in press.

Okada, Y.C., Kaufman, L., and Williamson, S.J., 1983, Hippocampal formation as a source of endogenous slow potentials. Electroencephalogr. Clin. Neurophysiol. 55:417.

Polich, J., 1984, P300 latency reflects the cognitive effects of personal drinking history in normals and individuals at risk for alcoholism. Psychophys., 21:521

Roth, W.T., Horvath, T.B., Pfefferbaum, A., and Kopell, B.S., 1980, Event-related potentials in schizophrenia. Electroencephalogr. Clin. Neurophysiol., 48:127

CORTICAL RESOURCE ALLOCATION DURING MENTAL ROTATION DETERMINED BY MAGNETO- AND ELECTRO- ENCEPHALOGRAPHY

G. Wilson[1], C. Busch[2], A. Papanicolaou[3],
C. Oliver[2], and C. Orr[2]

1) Armstrong Aerospace Medical Research Lab, WPAFB, OH
2) Systems Research Labs, Dayton, OH
3) Div. of Neurosurgery, U. of Texas, Galveston, TX

INTRODUCTION

Of the many electrophysiological techniques employed for the assessment of cortical resource allocation, the probe paradigm has been especially useful. This technique involves the ensemble averaging of evoked responses to task-irrelevant probe stimuli presented to subjects actively performing a cognitive task. Based on the limited resources hypothesis of neuronal functioning, this methodology assumes that: (a) as task demands increase, the proportion of available cortical resources allocated to that task also increases, resulting in a concomitant decrease in the system's capacity to respond to a simultaneously presented probe stimulus, and (b) reductions in the amplitude of the probe evoked response index the reallocation of resources for performance of the primary task. The utility of this method for evaluating hemispheric lateralization of functions in a variety of cognitive tasks has been previously demonstrated (for review see Papanicolaou and Johnstone, 1984). However, conclusions concerning relative hemispheric dominance that are based solely on the results of evoked potentials (EPs) have the added assumption that the measured electrical activity was indeed generated within the hemisphere over which it was recorded, an interpretation which can be problematic due to the conductive properties of the electrical potentials (Nunez, 1981).

Employing the probe paradigm, and using simultaneously obtained EPs and regional cerebral blood flow (rCBF) measures, Papanicolaou et al. (1987) reported a right hemisphere superiority for processing visuo-spatial information. During performance of a mental rotation task, greater rCBF increases and a greater degree of reduction of the P2 peak in the probe EP to a light flash were observed in the right parietal areas compared to the left. The primary purpose of the present study was to replicate and extend those findings using simultaneously recorded EPs and magnetic evoked fields (EFs) obtained from the occipital regions using the same task stimuli and the same basic experimental design. Additionally, a second experiment was conducted to evaluate changes in electrical EPs and magnetic EFs to an auditory probe during the spatial rotation task. By exploiting the relative advantages of magnetoencephalography (MEG), including its greater spatial resolution of components and its resistance to distortions from volume conduction of the signal or non-zero reference values (Williamson & Kaufman, 1981, 1987), the location of a component source within a specific hemisphere can be verified.

Advances in Biomagnetism
Edited by S.J. Williamson *et al.*
Plenum Press, New York

METHODS

Experiment 1

Six right-handed male volunteers, 21 to 40 years of age, participated in the study. EPs were recorded from the O1 and O2 electrode sites and EFs were recorded from previously determined N1m and P2m maxima at homotopic regions over the left and right occipital regions in response to a flashed checkerboard probe stimulus. Linked ears served as the reference for the EP electrodes, and an additional electrode on the subject's mandible served as ground. Electrode impedances were maintained below 5 kohms throughout the experiment. EF measurements were made using a single-channel DC SQUID (BTI) coupled to a second-order gradiometer with a 5 cm baseline and a 2 cm coil diameter. Both MEG and EEG data were notch-filtered at 60 Hz and bandpass filtered from 1.0 to 30 Hz using Grass amplifiers. The data were digitized at a 200 Hz sampling rate for 0.5 s (100 ms pre-stimulus and 400 ms post-stimulus intervals).

The probe stimulus was a full-field checkerboard pattern flashed for 20 ms at a rate of 1.2/s. The checkerboard subtended a visual angle of 3.65 degrees horizontally and 3.95 degrees vertically with each check subtending an angle of 0.30 degrees. A small diode at the center of the pattern provided a point for visual fixation. The task stimuli were geometric figures patterned after those of Shepard and Metzler (1971). Two averages, each comprised of 100 responses, were randomly obtained during each of three different conditions, at each maxima. The probe condition involved presentations of the checkerboard pattern alone. The control condition involved presentations of 40 randomly chosen pairs of the task stimuli, with instructions to the subject to attend to and count the superimposed probe stimuli and press a button on every fifth probe. The task condition involved 80 stimulus pairs and subjects were instructed to mentally rotate one of the figures in each pair, determine if the figures were the same or different, and press the appropriate button. Therefore, the control and task conditions were closely matched in terms of stimuli and response requirements, but differed in the cognitive processing demands.

Experiment 2

Four right-handed male subjects (ages 24 to 30) participated in the second experiment in which an auditory probe (600 Hz, 65 dB tone), instead of the visual probe, was presented during the same three conditions of the spatial rotation task. MEG signals were recorded from the previously mapped N1m and P2m auditory maxima, while concurrent EEG signals were recorded from electrode sites C3 and C4. All other experimental parameters were identical to those used in the first experiment.

RESULTS AND DISCUSSION

Experiment 1

The EF and EP waveforms to the visual probe were similar and were characterized by prominent N1 and P2 components with average latencies of approximately 140 ms and 200 ms, respectively. Baseline-to-peak amplitude measurements were made for each peak and constituted the primary dependent measure in subsequent statistical analyses. Four separate 2 (hemispheres) by 3 (conditions) repeated measures analysis of variance (ANOVA) tests were performed for each peak in each signal type.

Electrically, the results obtained from the occipital areas mirrored those previously reported concerning parietally recorded EPs. There was a bilateral reduction of the probe N1 amplitudes (Figure 1A) during the task

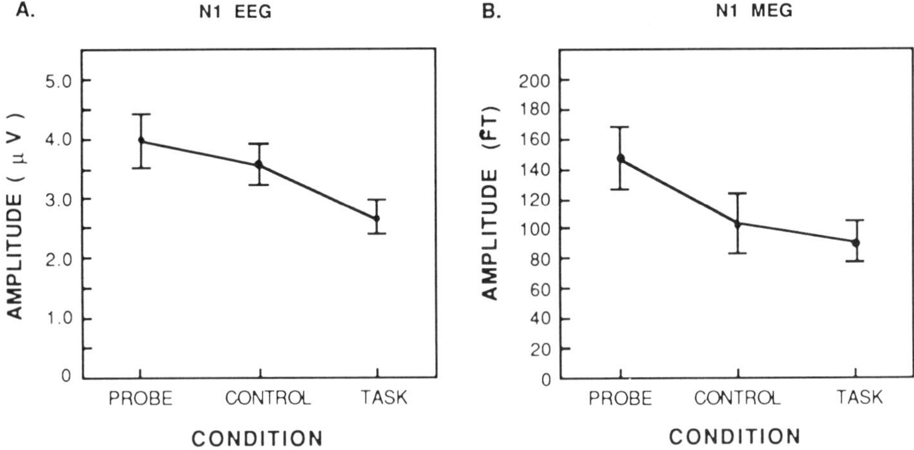

Figure 1. Mean amplitudes (± standard error) for the N1 peak in (a) the electrical EPs and (b) the magnetic EFs.

condition ($F = 6.37$, $p < 0.01$), most likely due to attentional shifts, as has been reported under similar conditions (Hillyard, Munte & Neville, 1985). In contrast, electrical P2 amplitudes (Figure 2A) displayed a greater decrease in the right hemisphere than in the left during the mental rotation task ($F = 4.35$, $p < 0.04$), suggesting right hemisphere dominance for task performance.

Magnetically, the probe N1m amplitudes (Figure 1B) also reduced bilaterally during the task ($F = 9.7$, $p < 0.004$) in a proportion nearly equal to that exhibited in the EP data (N1 = 33%, N1m = 37% amplitude reductions from probe to task conditions). This suggests that both the magnetic and the electrical measures were indexing the same underlying neural functions. Task-related attenuations were also observed in the P2m

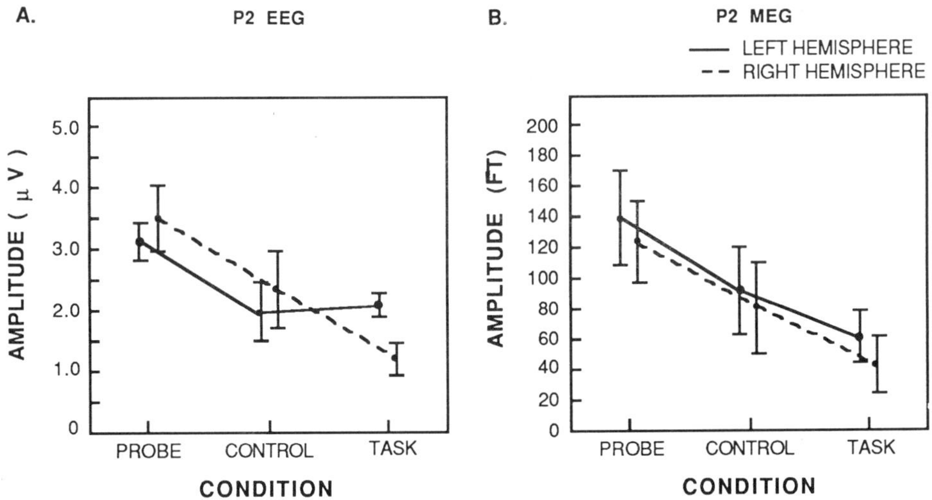

Figure 2. Mean amplitudes (± standard error) in the P2 peak in the left (solid line) and right (dashed line) hemispheres in (a) the electrical EPs and (b) the magnetic EFs.

component (Figure 2B), irrespective of the hemisphere from which it was recorded ($F = 4.86$, $p < 0.03$), suggesting that the allocation of resources was equivalent across hemispheres. Proportionally, the decreases during the task (compared to the probe condition) in the left and right hemisphere EF responses and the right hemisphere electrical P2 response were comparable (P2m left = 56%, P2m right = 64%, P2 right = 67%). Thus, the divergence between the electrical and magnetic measures occurred only with respect to the smaller amplitude attenuation in the left hemisphere electrical P2 compared to the probe condition (P2 left = 33%). Since the more spatially sensitive MEG measures evidenced a bilateral reduction in the P2m during the task condition, the implications are that: (a) in the occipital area resource allocation is bilaterally symmetric and, (b) the lateralization of function reflected in the EEG measures may result from asymmetric right hemisphere resource allocation occurring at more anterior locations.

Experiment 2

There were no significant differences in either the electrical EPs or the magnetic EFs to the auditory probe during the three task conditions. There was, however, a significant performance difference between the two experiments. The subjects in the visual probe experiment were able to complete significantly more comparisons ($M = 144.17$) than the subjects in the auditory probe experiment were able to complete ($M = 64.25$) ($t = -6.313$, $p < 0.001$). There were no differences, though, in the number of errors.

SUMMARY

There are two general results from the visual probe phase of this study. First, the observed reductions in amplitude in both the magnetic N1m and the P2m components were dependent on the complexity of the information processing, indicating that MEG is a viable method for evaluating complex cognitive processing. Second, the observed differences in the MEG and EEG measures suggest that the electrical P2 component reflects neural activity from multiple sources and, further, that the asymmetric cortical resource allocation associated with visuo-spatial processing does not occur in the occipital regions. Research aimed at clarifying this issue is currently in progress in our laboratory.

REFERENCES

Hillyard, S.A., Munte, T.F., & Neville, H.J., 1985, Visual-spatial attention, orienting and brain physiology, in: "Attention and Performance XI," M.I. Posner & O.S. Marin, eds., Erlbaum, Hillsdale, NJ.

Nunez, P., 1981, "Electrical Fields of the Brain," Oxford University Press, New York.

Papanicolaou, A. & Johnstone, J., 1984, Probe evoked potentials: Theory, method and application. Intern. J. Neuroscience, 24: 107-131.

Papanicolaou, A., Deutsch, T., Bourbon, G., Will, K., Loring, D., & Eisenberg, H., 1987, Convergent evoked potential and cerebral blood flow evidence of task-specific hemispheric differences. Electroenceph. Clin. Neurophysiol., 66: 515-520.

Shepard, R. & Metzler, J., 1971, Mental rotation of three-dimensional objects. Science, 171: 701-703.

Williamson, S. & Kaufman, L., 1981, Magnetic fields of the cerebral cortex, in: "Biomagnetism," S. Erne, H. Hahlbohm, & Lubbig, H., Eds., Walter de Gruyter, Berlin.

Williamson, S. & Kaufman, L., 1987, Analysis of neuromagnetic signals, in: "Methods of Analysis of Brain Electrical and Magnetic Signals", A. Gevins & A. Remond, Eds., Elsevier, Amsterdam.

ALPHA SUPPRESSION RELATED TO A COGNITIVE TASK

Barry J. Schwartz, Carlo Salustri*, Lloyd Kaufman, S. J. Williamson

Neuromagnetism Laboratory
Departments of Psychology and Physics and Center for Neural Science
4 Washington Place, New York University, New York, NY 10003

INTRODUCTION

Is the visual cortex involved in manipulating mental images as well as visual stimuli? This question may now be amenable to a direct test.

When subjects are in a resting but alert state, alpha activity (8-12 Hz) predominates in the spontaneous EEG. It has been reported (Kaufman and Locker, 1970; Pfurtscheller, et al., 1977, 1987) that alpha activity diminishes coinciding with presentation of visual stimuli and that the duration of this alpha supression is much longer than that of the classic evoked response. In this paper we report that MEG activity during a visual memory task shows a dramatic amplitude reduction in the alpha range lasting 500 to 2000 msec, following which the amplitude recovers despite continuous visual fixation on the display.

Recent evidence argues against the general idea that alpha arises from simultaneously active "generators" that become desynchronized during arousal, causing partial self-cancelation of their fields. Microelectrode studies using dogs (Lopes Da Silva and van Leeuwen, 1978) suggest that alpha originates in small areas of visual cortex and spreads over relatively short distances. Recent magnetoencephalography (MEG) studies (Chapman, et al., 1984; Ilmoniemi, et al., 1988) showed that alpha spindles have multiple sources in occipital and perhaps in parietal areas.

The accuracy provided by MEG for localizing neuronal activity in sensory cortex (Yammamoto, et al, 1988) suggests that alpha suppression can be localized specifically to visual cortex. To test this hypothesis we used a combination of two classic paradigms: Sternberg's memory matching task (Sternberg, 1969) and Shepard's mental rotation task (Shepard and Metzler, 1971). Both tasks require a search of memory for representations of visual images, and performance in each case is indexed by systematic differences in choice reaction time (RT). We observed alpha suppression and averaged responses. In this paper we present data from one 41 year old male subject. These results are similar to those obtained with 6 other subjects. Data analysis from other subjects will be described in detail in subsequent publications.

METHODS

The subject, seated on a chair in a magnetically shielded room, maintained fixation on a small cross and viewed a sequence of three irregular polygon shapes on a dark background in the lower right quadrant of his visual field. Each shape was seen outlined in white for 1 sec followed by a 0.3 sec dark interval; 3.0 sec after the disappearance of the last image a fourth "probe" shape was presented for only 0.1 sec. In one block of trials ("choice reaction time", CRT) the subject pressed one of two buttons after seeing the probe, indicating whether it belonged in the memory set or was new. In a second block of trials ("simple reaction time", SRT) the subject simply had to press one button as soon as he saw the probe shape. In this task, the subject still had to attend to the whole sequence of visual shapes in order to know which one required a response. Each block consisted of a sequence of 30 trials.

The component of the magnetic field normal to the subject's head was recorded over posterior and parietal areas at 65 different locations by means of a 5-channel SQUID-based Neuromagnetometer (Williamson, et al., 1983; Buchanan, et al., 1988) The outputs of the SQUIDs were bandpassed between 0.1 - 50 Hz. Each recording epoch lasted 7 sec, 3 sec prior to and 4 sec following the onset of the (100 msec) visual probe.

Visual evoked potentials were extracted after digitally filtering the MEG between 1 and 20 Hz and then averaging over the 30 recording epochs. Alpha activity was isolated by filtering each epoch of data between 8 and 12 Hz, and computing the variance across the 30 trials in each block as a function of time for each SQUID channel. This variance is the mean square field (power), which excludes the average evoked response. Temporal changes in this variance are due to changes in amplitude, not to coherence across the epochs. An examination of single trial data shows that alpha activity (filtered from 8 to 12 Hz) is not time-locked stimulus onset.

RESULTS

Our results show that MEG power in the alpha band undergoes a systematic reduction during the performance of visual memory-search tasks. Alpha power for CRT trials is sharply suppressed for about 1500 msec. For SRT trials, suppression lasts for about 500 msec, beginning at the time of probe stimulus onset. Both tasks require subjects to attend to all visual stimuli. The duration of evoked responses for both tasks are typical of sensory evoked responses, on the order of 100 msec. Alpha suppression and RT's, on the other hand, are on the order of 500 msec to 1500 msec.

The RT for the SRT task coincides with the minimum of its alpha power curve, about 500 msec after the onset of the probe. Suppression of alpha power for CRT trials is significantly longer in duration. At 1200 msec after stimulus onset, the alpha power is half way through its recovery back to its *baseline* level. RT for the CRT task occurs during its recovery phase (Figure 1). The longer duration of the suppression in the CRT task is consistent with the interpretation that the visual cortex is engaged during a search of memory.

The distribution of alpha power over the scalp prior to and following the suppression is quite

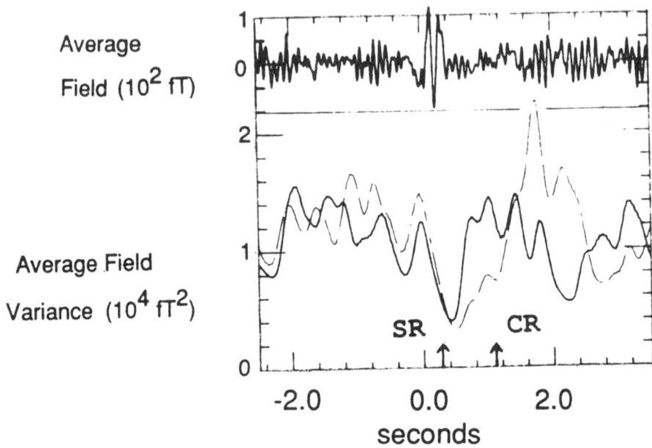

Fig. 1. A representative plot of variance across epochs. The darker trace is the SR condition, the lighter trace is the CR condition. Reaction times are indicated by arrows. An averaged evoked response is shown for comparison of its time span.This evoked field is a grand average of 10 groups of 30 trials for all 5 sensors, as it was impossible to obtain a sharply defined evoked field averaging only 30 trials.

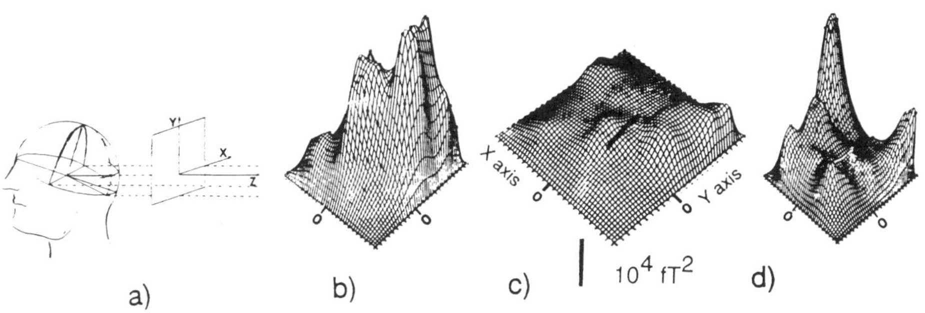

Fig. 2. (a) Distribution of average alpha power across the posterior scalp portrayed by an azimuthal equal distance projection. Equal distances across the surface of a spherical representation of the head from the center of projection map onto equal distances across a flat plane. The x-axis corresponds to a horizontal line normal to the midline, the y- axis to a vertical parallel to the midline. (b) Distribution of average *baseline alpha*, defined as the average alpha power observed within a 200 msec interval 100 msec prior to presentation of the visual probe in the CRT condition. (c) Distribution of alpha power averaged over a 100 msec interval centered on the moment of maximum suppression. The locations of the midlines are indicated by the short lines in these graphs. (d) Distribution of the ratio of residual to baseline alpha, which defines the *relative alpha suppression.*

similar, showing a correlation of 0.81 over 65 measured positions ($p < 0.001$). There is less of a similarity in distribution over the scalp during the time maximum suppression.

To characterize the suppression of alpha activity during mental *imagery*, the magnitude of average alpha power was plotted as a function of position over the posterior scalp (Fig. 2 a-d). The average power within a 2 sec interval 200 msec prior to presentation of the probe stimulus represents the *baseline*, which has a peak in the right hemisphere about 5 cm above the inion and 5 cm to the right of the midline. It is important to note that the distribution changes during maximum suppression, with overall reduction in activity most pronounced in the vicinity of the midline. Figure 2d represents the proportional change in alpha power, or the ratio of b) to c) at each location over the scalp. If the suppression of alpha were global and uniform, this surface would be flat. Instead, the relative suppression is greatest in a band about the midline above the inion and below the vertex. The pattern of relative suppression is consistent with changes of limited extent and near the surface of visual cortex.

The temporal pattern of alpha suppression for SRT and CRT tasks is very similar for seven subjects, with individual differences in reaction time and mean duration of suppression. Interestingly, there are large and stable individual differences in the magnitude of power in alpha among subjects, differences which remain constant over the months involved in our observations. There are also individual differences in local patterns of alpha distribution for the three subjects whose fields have been extensively mapped. Individual differences in the strength and distribution of alpha cannot be attributed to differences in skull thickness (Leissner, Lindholm, and Petersen, 1970), since thickness of the skull has a negligible effect on magnetic fields. Instead, they must be attributed to underlying brain anatomy and neural function.

When alpha is suppressed, beta activity (16-24 Hz) does not show an increase, contrary to some predictions. In fact, there is a correlated *decrease* in beta power during alpha suppression. The distribution of beta power across the scalp is not the same as that of the alpha band. For this subject, BS, one percent of the of variance in the beta distributions could be accounted for by the alpha distributions. Partly independent neuronal populations must be responsible for spontaneous activity in these two bandwidths, although both populations exhibit suppression when subjects search visual memory.

CONCLUSIONS

These data support the hypothesis that power within the alpha and beta bands is systematically reduced during the performance of a mental task involving the matching of memories of visual images. The source of this reduction appears to be in the visual cortex, a finding that is consistent with local cerebral blood flow studies (Roland and Frieberg, 1985).

Although the field pattern of alpha appears to be suppressed over a widespread area on the occipital scalp, a more local pattern of suppression is clearly superimposed on it. Functionally, this suppression is correlated not merely with visual attention, but more specifically with the task of visual memory search, since its duration varies with task and also correlates with RT. We believe the above procedure will prove useful for direct tests of hypotheses about the roles of various areas of the brain during different types of mental acts.

ACKNOWLEDGEMENTS

Supported in part by Air Force Office of Scientific Research Grants F49620-88-K-0004 and F49620-86-C-0131. C. Salustri is partially supported by Associazione Italiana Ricerche Neurologiche (ARIN).
* Permanent address: Istituto di Elettronica dello Stato Solido (CNR), via Cineto Romano 42, I-00156 Rome, Italy.
We thank Arthur Robinson and John P. Snyder for advice about azimuthal equal distance projections, and Jia Zhu Wang and Irene Martin for assistance with software development.

REFERENCES

Buchanan, D.S., Paulson, D., and Williamson, S.J. (1987). Instrumentation for clinical applications of neuromagnetism. In: Fast, R.W., Ed., *Advances in Cryogenic Engineering* Vol. 33, Plenum Press, New York, pp. 97 - 106.

Chapman, R.M., Ilmoniemi, R.J., Barbanera, S., and Romani, G.L. (1984). Selective localization of alpha brain activity with neuromagnetic measurements. *Electroenceph. clin. Neurophysiol.* 58, 569-572.

Costa Ribeiro, P., Williamson, S.J., and Kaufman, L. (1988). SQUID arrays for simultaneous magnetic measurements: calibration and source localization performance. *IEEE Trans. Biomed. Engr.* BME-35, 551 - 560.

Kaufman, L. and Locker, Y. (1970). Sensory modulation of the EEG. *Proc. 78th Annual Conv. Amer. Psychol. Assoc.*, 179-180.

Leissner P., Lindholm, L.-E. and Petersen, I. (1970). Alpha amplitude dependence on skull thickness as measured by ultrasound technique. *Electroenceph. and clin. Neurophysiol., 29*, 392-399

Lopes Da Silva, F.H. and van Leeuwen, S. (1978). The cortical alpha rhythm in dog: The depth and surface profile of phase. in *Architectonics of the Cerebral Cortex*, M.A.B. Brazier and H. Petsche, Eds. (Raven Press, New York, 1978), pp. 319-333.

Pfurtscheller,G. (1988). Mapping of event-related desynchronization and type of derivation *Electroenceph. clin. Neruophysiol 70*, 190-193.

Pfurtscheller,G. and Aranibar,A. (1977). Event-related desynchronization detected by power measurements of scalp EEG. *Electroenceph. clin. Neruophysiol 42*, 138-146.

Roland, P.E. and Frieberg, L. (1985). Localization of cortical areas activated by thinking. *J. Neurophysiol. 53*, 1219-1243.

Shepard, R.N. and Metzler, J. (1971). Mental rotation of three dimensional objects. *Science, 220*, 632-634.

Sternberg, S. (1969). Memory scanning: mental processes revealed by reaction time experiments. *Amer. Scientist, 57*, 421-457.

VISUALIZING AND RHYMING CAUSE DIFFERENCES IN ALPHA SUPPRESSION

L. Kaufman, M. Glanzer,* Y.M. Cycowicz, and S.J. Williamson

Neuromagnetism Laboratory,
Departments of Psychology and Physics and Center for Neural Science
*Department of Psychology
4 Washington Place, New York University, New York, NY 10003, U.S.A.

INTRODUCTION

The alpha rhythm of the EEG is strongest over the occipital region, and the visual cortex is apparently a major contributor (Chapman et al., 1984; Vvdensky et al., 1987; Williamson, et al., 1989). Since behavioral evidence suggests that the visual cortex may also be involved in mental imagery (cf. Shepard and Metzler, 1971), we set out to determine if forming mental images produces changes in the occipital alpha rhythms of the MEG. It has been demonstrated that scanning memory for visual forms causes changes in alpha activity originating in visual cortex (Kaufman, Schwartz, Salustri, and Williamson, 1989). However, this study did not control for a possible effect of mental effort *per se*, since scanning visual memory was compared only with a condition in which subjects merely responded as soon as they saw a visual form. To prove that changes in alpha accompanying the processing of visual images is due to such processing and not to mental effort, it is necessary also to provide a non-visual cognitive task that is approximately as difficult as that of forming mental images.

There are precedents for this type of experiment. For example, visual imagery is accompanieds by changes in occipital alpha activity of the EEG (Golla, et al., 1943), but performance of a language-related task does not have so apparent an effect (Slater, 1960). However, the use of non-visual tasks, e.g., memorization and classifying words, may affect the alpha activity (Pfurtschuller, 1988), so it is unclear that changes in alpha activity provides an unambigous indication of processes entailing mental imagery.

Farah (1988) presented words to subjects who responded either by forming mental images of objects represented by the words, or by simply reading them. This did result in a difference in amplitudes of the occipital event related potentials elicited by the words, but the number of electrodes used in this study was not sufficient to permit identification of the location of the sources of the potential changes.

Using cerebral blood flow (CBF) techniques, Roland and Friberg (1985) found extensive activation of posterior regions of the brain during mental imagery, but no increase in CBF when subjects did mental arithmetic or engaged in a cognitive task entailing the scanning of memory to determine if tones had been previously heard. Since suppression of alpha originating in the occipital cortex accompanies the search of visual memory (Kaufman, et al. 1989), we sought in this experiment directly to compare the effects of forming mental images of objects represented by words with those of finding words in memory that rhyme the same visual presented words. The hypothesis tested is that forming rhymes of visually presented words will affect alpha suppression differently than does forming a mental image.

Advances in Biomagnetism
Edited by S.J. Williamson *et al.*
Plenum Press, New York

METHODS

Our word stimuli were drawn from a large population of words composed of words that represent easily imaged objects and also abstract words which subjects find difficult to respond to by forming images. On each trial subjects saw 24 sequentially presented words. These were constructed from the master list and were composed either of all imageable words or half imageable words and half abstract words. The latter were used in trials where subjects had to search their memories and find words that rhymed with the presented words. Alternatively, when viewing all imageable words subjects were instructed to form mental images of the objects represented by the words. Since only 12 of the 24 words used in the rhyming task were imageable, subjects were exposed to twice as many rhyming trials as imaging trials. By combining 12 responses (corresponding to 12 imageable words) from each of two rhyming trials, we were able to determine if imageable words produce different responses under the two different conditions. Subjects pressed a button to indicate when they had either formed and image or found a ryhme. Finally, subjects were also shown lists of 24 nonsense words to which they responded by pressing a button as soon as they were seen. Comparing the reaction times (RTs) in the imaging and rhyming task permits assessment of the relative difficulties of the two tasks as compared to the simpler control task of merely observing the appearance of a nonsense word.

The word stimuli were generated by an Amiga 100 computer and projected by an Electrohome video projector onto a screen in a magnetically shielded room. Subjects inside the room maintained fixation on a point on the screen which was reflected by mirrors to the subject. The words were presented 7 sec apart for 200 msec each.

Subjects were seated on a kneeling stool and leaned forward with their heads on a vacuum cast while they looked downward into a mirror to see the screen. A probe containing a 5-sensor SQUID-based Neuromagnetometer® (Biomagnetic Technologies, inc.) was placed at the occipital area of the scalp over the right or left hemisphere near the region where alpha rhythm is strongest. The five detection coils detected the field at five different places normal to the posterior portion of the head.

With the coils placed near the scalp the subject performed the rhyming task for two blocks of stimuli, then they performed the imaging task, and finally, the control task both for only one block of stimuli. Measurements of the MEG were recorded for 6 seconds for each word stimulus, beginning 2 second before the stimulus appeared and extending 4 seconds afterwards. This was follow by one more second with no recording to provide a total interstimulus interval of 7 seconds. The outputs of all five channels of the SQUID electronics were bandpass filtered from 0.1-50 Hz and then applied to an HP 9000 model 350 computer for analysis. Also, RTs corresponding to the time of button press were stored for each trial, and then averaged later within each experimental condition.

All epochs were digitally bandpassed from 8 to 12 Hz before computing the average response and the variances about the averages. The variance represents brain activity that is not coherently related to the presentation of the visual stimulus. The variance is actually the power (mean square field) of the spontaneous activity in the alpha band. Thus we will use the term 'alpha power' to describe the results.

Four young adult subjects, two female and two male, served in this experiment.

RESULTS

Figure 1 shows alpha power as a function of time for the three conditions: imaging task with imageable words, rhyming task with imageable and non-imageable words, and control task with the nonsense words. The suppression of alpha in all cases started at the time of word presentation. In general, there is a short-lived (about 0.5 sec) suppression of alpha under all conditions. However, this initial suppression effect is supplemented, in the imaging condition only, by an additional period (about 1 sec) of suppression. The initial effect may be related to a shift in generalized arousal level, while the supplementary suppression probably reflects the role of visual cortex in forming images. Although rhyming is also a cognitive act, there is no suppression of occipital alpha other than described here as the initial suppression effect. This same effect is present in the control condition.

The foregoing results are generally true for all four subjects. However, there were strong individual differences in the average magnitude of alpha activity accross subjects as well as positions at which the field was measured. The latter differences among probe recording positions over the occipital scalp reflected both differences in alpha power as a function of probe position, and also differences in the magnitude of suppression, which was strongest in the vicinity of the midlines of all subjects. The difference in the magnitude of the suppression between positions is related to the distance between the detection coil and the "source" whose activity is suppressed when subjects form images. It is evident that RTs for the imaging and rhyming tasks are essentially the same for all subjects, while the RT for the control task is about one half of the for the other two tasks. This is offered as evidence for the approximately equal difficulty of the rhyming and imaging tasks.

Mean Reaction Time (sec)

Subject	Imaging	Rhyming	Control
STF	0.958	1.740	0.686
LS	1.490	0.876	0.575
JB	1.176	1.177	0.582
BOR	1.085	1.139	0.663

Since the duration of suppression in the rhyming task is short as compared with that for the imaging task, and that the RT is comparable to that of the imaging task, it is clear that changes in occipital alpha reflect only the effects of imaging, and do not reflect the language-related rhyming task. Assuming that both rhyming and imaging require about the same amount of attentional effort, we also conclude that the prolonged suppression of alpha during imaging is not due to changing levels of attention.

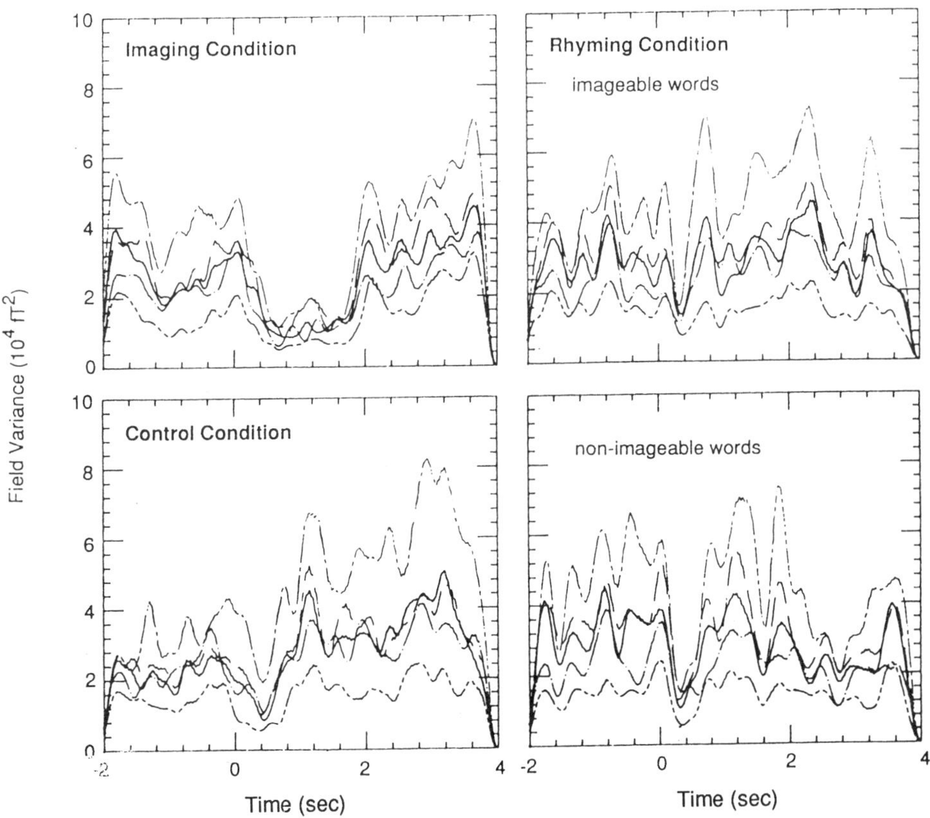

Fig. 1. Alpha power of subject LS for the three conditions. The five curves in each condition represent the five sensors. At time zero the word stimuli appears on the screen.

CONCLUSIONS

We have found that power within the alpha band is reduced when subjects form mental images. Since Kaufman et al. (1989) showed that activity of sources in visual cortex is suppressed when visual memory is scanned, it is posible that visual cortex is also affected during the imagery task of the present study. Two different processes are apparently involved. These are the so-called *initial effect*, and the subsequent prolonged suppression associated with imagery. The initial effect appears to be ca general process, since it acompanies all tasks, but the second order prolonged effect may be modality specific.

We also conclude that alpha suppression is not due to attentional differences since we assume that in both cases, imaging and rhyming, the subject has to attend in order to perform the tasks. The fact that prolonged suppression occurs only for imaging tasks is consistent with the conjecture, which we are now testing, that language related tasks have effects similar to that describe for imagery here, but occurring elsewhare in the brain.

ACKNOWLEDGEMENTS

We thank B. Schwartz for his assistance with this project. This research is supported in part by Air Force Office of Scientific Research Grants F49620-88-K-004 and F49620-86-C-0131.

REFERENCES

Chapman, R.M., Ilmoniemi, R., Barbanera, S., and Romani, G.L. (1984). Selective localization of alpha from brain activity with neuromagnetic measurements. *Electroenceph. clin. Neurophysiol.* 58, 569 - 572.

Fara, M.J. (1988). Is visual imagery really visual? Overlooked evidence from neuropsychology. *Psychological Review vol 95: 307-317*

Golla, F., Hutton, E.L., and Gray Walter, W.G. (1943). The objective study of mental imagery. I. Physiological concomitants. *J. Mental Sci.* 75, 216-223.

Kaufman L., Schwartz B., Salustri C., Williamson S.J. (1989). Modulation of spontaneous brain activity during mental imagery. *submitted for publication.*

Pfurtcheller, G. Steffean, J. Naresch, H. (1988). ERD mapping and functional topography: Temporal and spatial aspects. In: Pfurtscheller, G. and Lopes da Silva, F.H., Ed., *Functional Brain Imaging,* Hans Huber Publishers, pp. 117-130.

Roland, P.E. and Frieberg, L. (1985). Localization of cortical areas activated by thinking. *J. of Neurophysiology, 53, 1219-1243.*

Shepard, R.N., and Meltzer, J. (1971). Mental rotation of three-dimensional objects. *Science,* 171, 701-703

Slatter, K.H. (1960). Alpha rhythem and mental imagery. *Electroenceph. clin. Neurophysiol.* 12, 851-859.

Vvedensky V.L., Guntovoy, K.G., Ilmoniemi R.J., and Kajola M. (1987). Determination of the sources of the magnetic alpha thythm of man. *Human physiology* 13, 934-939 [in Russian].

Williamson, S.J., Wang, J-Z., and Ilmoniemi, R.J. (1989). Method for Locating Sources of Human Alpha Activity. This conference.

PHASE RELATIONSHIPS IN SYNCHRONOUS MAGNETIC AND ELECTRIC ALPHA ACTIVITY IN THE PARIETO-OCCIPITAL AREA OF THE HUMAN BRAIN

V.L.Vvedensky, K.G.Gurtovoy, A.P.Grebenkin,
S.P. Naurzakov, V.I.Ozhogin, S.Yu.Shabanov

Kurchatov Institute of Atomic Energy, 123182, Moscow
USSR

INTRODUCTION

Previous combined EEG-MEG measurements of the human alpha-rhythm showed clear difference between magnetic and electric signals, so large, that their Fourier-spectra were different (Hughes, 1976, Carelli, 1983). This can be due in part to positioning of electrodes and coil, so that MEG and EEG were sensitive to different sources. In order to establish relationships between magnetic and electric fields generated by presumably the same process we tried to find signals least different in EEG and MEG. We chose experimental setup which was expected to suit best our aim.

METHODS

Experiments were performed in the center for neuromagnetic studies of the Kurchatov Institute. This includes wooden house with aluminium shielded room, resting on separate basement, inside. Data acquisition system consists of personal computers. Tangential magnetometer (Vvedensky et al., 1985) is used for magnetic measurements and standard EEG equipment for electric recordings. The experiments were performed under standard conditions - subject sitting with closed eyes. The magnetometer measured field directed across midline and was positioned just above the bipolar pair of electrodes oriented along midline. The pair separated by 4 cm was fixed 2 cm to the right from midline where the strongest magnetic signal is observed for our subjects. The arrangment is shown in Fig.1. This setup was considered to be appropriate for the proposed study of a source of alpha-rhythm generating both high amplitude electric and magnetic signals. For subject whose data are presented in this paper the location of electrodes shown in Fig.1 is the place of steep longitudinal gradient of phase for electric alpha-rhythm. This was established in a separate experiment with three electrodes for EEG fixed at 3 cm from each other along midline. Phase shift of about 30° is observed between oscillations in frontal and rear pairs of this triple electrode arrangement. This probably means that we observed on EEG the same processes as discussed by Walter et al. (1966) for P4-O2 lead. Another experiment when magnetometer was rotated above

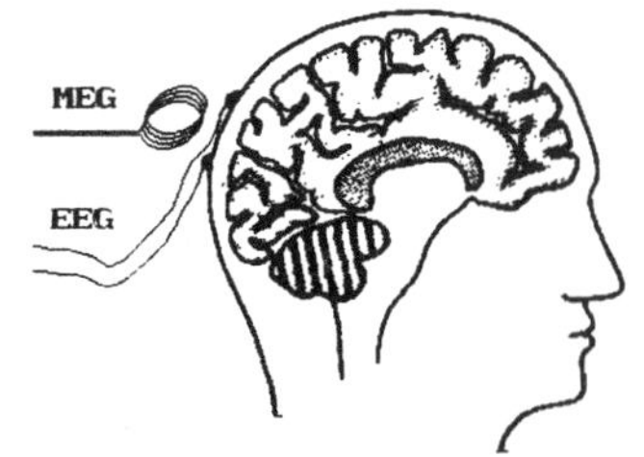

Fig.1. Schematic presentation of the pickup coil and electrodes arrangement

the electrodes did show that magnetic field there is directed across midline. Usually we made simultaneous EEG and MEG records 8 sec long with sampling time 4 ms. The signals were analog filtered in 1 - 100 Hz band and for MEG in 1 - 30 Hz for EEG. Complex coherence between MEG and EEG was computed in 8 to 13 Hz frequency band fór 256 samples. The window of analysis was sliding in 100 ms steps through the whole record. The phase angle of the coherence which represents phase difference between EEG and MEG oscillations reflecting physical time delays for the processes in the cortex.

RESULTS

Contrary to our expectations, signals measured in our setup on three subjects were quite different in EEG and MEG although generally of the same frequency around 10 Hz. The time course of EEG and MEG amplitudes was usually different. The peaks of electric and magnetic oscillations were often shifted in time for tens of milliseconds. It was difficult to extract any clear correlation in the case of unstable rhythm. When alpha-rhythm was stable for several seconds one can see different types of EEG - MEG relationships. The general observation is that behavior of the rhythm tend to be stable for a second or several seconds and then switches quickly to a new regime. This evolution in behavior is best displayed in the record presented in Fig.2. Switches from in-phase to 180° out-of-phase regimes and back coincide here with appearence of EEG spindles. Gradual change of phase lag in the end of the record means different frequencies of EEG and MEG. Similar difference is seen on the record presented in Fig.3. In the first half of the record EEG and MEG are of the same frequency although slightly shifted in phase. Later EEG only switches to a lower frequency (10.2 Hz

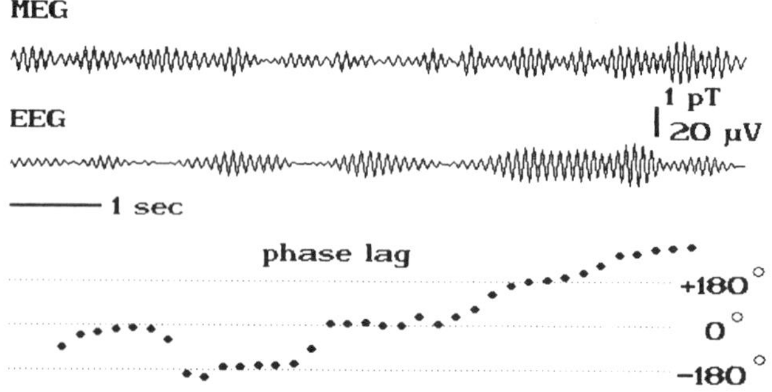

Fig.2. Simultaneous MEG and EEG (8-13 Hz) and phase shift of MEG in respect to EEG. Frequency of magnetic rhythm is 10.7 Hz.

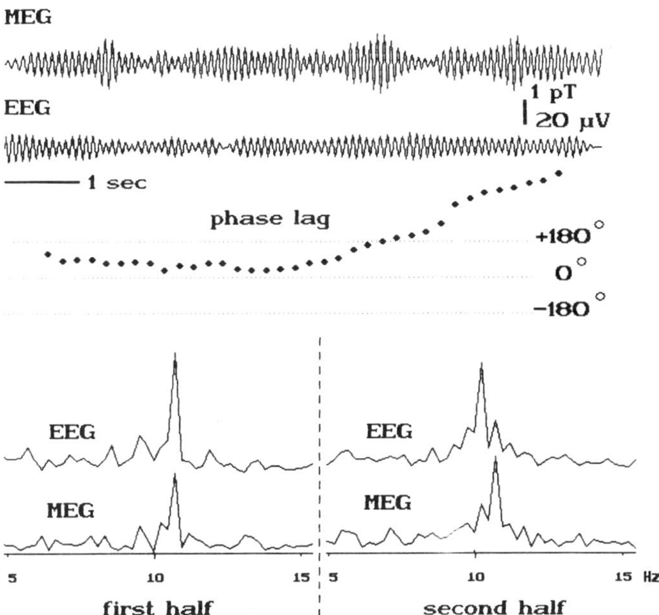

Fig.3. Simultaneous MEG and EEG records Fourier-spectra for the beginning and the end of the records. The decrease in the EEG frequency in the second half is evident.

instead of 10.7 Hz) as seen from the Fourier-spectrum and keeps it for at least 4 seconds. Nevertheless most of the time (about 95% of the total) EEG and MEG frequencies are the same. Strong signals (2 pT, 20 µV) often happen to be in phase, although with gradual variations for +/-10 ms. For several seconds EEG or MEG may have stable lag and then return to in-phase regime as is shown in Fig.4. An interesting observation was made in an experiment when triple electrode arrangement was used together with magnetometer positioned above the middle electrode. When stable 30° phase shift was present between EEG signals from frontal and rear pairs of electrodes the MEG signal first happened to be in phase with one EEG lead and later switched to be in phase with another EEG lead. The period of phase stability was about 2 seconds.

DISCUSSION

Our results show that we can observe fine structure of alpha-rhythm in restricted area of the head. The sources of considerable strength are distinguishable by the phase or even frequency of oscillations. One can investigate separately their behavior under different conditions. The area under study is clearly distinct as a source of alpha-rhythm with well defined properties. The accumulated evidence from many subjects shows that magnetic field of the alpha-rhythm is strongest in the parieto-occipital part of the head and is directed across midline, while gradient of electric potential is directed along midline and is largest just in this place. This probably

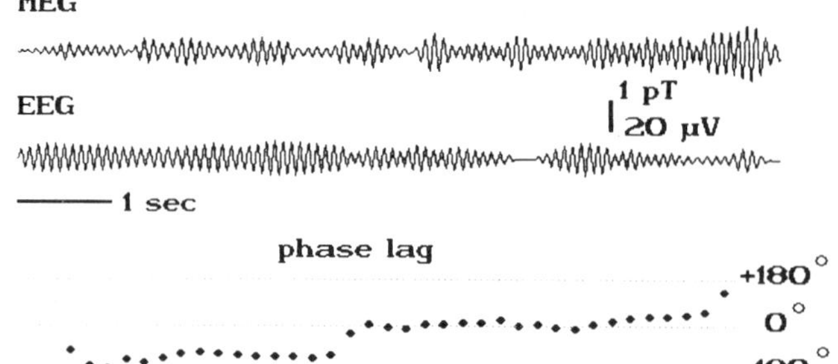

Fig.4. Records displaying two different epochs of alpha-rhythm. EEG and MEG are phase-shifted in the beginning and later switch to the in-phase regime.

implies the common process generating alpha-rhythm in this area on both EEG and MEG. On the other hand we see that even strong "electric" and "magnetic" generators can behave quite different in the same area. This poses definite limitations on the geometric structure of these sources in the cortex because they have to keep certain orientation and occupy extended portions of cortical surface to generate strong and stable signals. We expect that real layout of the sources in this area can be established provided multichannel recording of both EEG and MEG as well as map of fissures from MRI scan were available. If some averaging procedures were to be used in such a study one should keep in mind the observed changes in the regime of the rhythm. Selective averaging over time periods of constant phase shift is to be used.

ACKNOWLEDGEMENTS

We thank D.M.Marcishevsky for assistance in experiments and R.P.Marqui and J.C.J.Sobrino for help in calculations.

REFERENCES

Carelli, P., Modena, I., Ricci, G.B., Romani, G.L. (1983). Magnetoencephalography. In: Biomagnetism: An Interdisciplinary Approach. Plenum Press, New York, London, pp. 469-482.

Hughes, J.R., Hendrix, D.E., Cohen, J., Duffy, F.H., Mayman, C.I., Scholl, M.L., Cuffin B.N. (1976). Relationship of the magnetoencephalogram to the electroencephalogram. Normal wake and sleep activity. Electroenc. clin. Neurophysiol. 140, p.261

Vvedensky, V.L., Naurzakov, S.P., Ozhogin, V.I., Shabanov, S.Yu.(1985). Measurement of the tangential component of the magnetic field associated with rhythmic activity in the human brain. In Biomagnetism: Application and theory. Pergamon Press, New York. pp.57-60.

Walter, D.O., Rhodes, J.M., Brown, D., Adey, W.R. (1966). Comprehensive spectral analysis of human EEG generators in posterior cerebral regions. Electroencephal. clin. Neurophysiol. 120, pp.224-237.

DISTRIBUTION OF PHASE FOR ALPHA-RHYTHM MEASURED BY MULTICHANNEL MAGNETOMETER OVER OCCIPITAL HEAD

K.G.Gurtovoy, M.J.Kajola , V.L.Vvedensky

Kurchatov Institute of Atomic Energy, Moscow, USSR

Low Temperature Laboratory, Helsinki University of Technology, 02150, Espoo, Finland

INTRODUCTION

Electric alpha-rhythm of a human being displays definite phase relationships between different areas of the head, most often opposite phases in the occipital and frontal lobes (Nunez, 1981). Similar relationships for magnetic rhythm are not established yet. It is known that magnetic oscillations over occipital head are in phase provided magnetometer coils are no more then 3 cm apart (Vvedensky et al., 1988). Opposite-phase signals can be observed in magnetometers positioned 12 cm apart (Ilmoniemi et al., 1987). We tried to get a more detailed picture on the distribution of phase for magnetic alpha-rhythm.

METHODS

Alpha-rhythm was measured with the 7-channel SQUID-magnetometer in Otaniemi shielded room (Knuutila et al.,1987). The data recorded from three magnetometer positions for one subject are reported here. Positions of pickup coils, measuring radial field component, are shown in Figs. 1, 2 and 3. We computed phase differences for oscillations in every channel in respect to channel of highest amplitude in a manner similar to (Gurtovoy et al. this volume). Field maps in hexagonal area under magnetometer were computed through interpolation in 12 ms steps.

RESULTS

In general the field is similar to what is usually observed for alpha-rhythm: it is strongest in the parieto-occipital part of the head and directed across midline. For radial component this means that right and left regions are observed where the signals are in opposite phases. For our subject such simultaneous signals (channels 2 and 3 versus 5 and 6 in Fig.1.) are seen at the left magnetometer position only. The amplitudes of the field are usually highest in channels 2 and 3 or channels 5 and 6. The signals are smaller in channels 1 and 4. This distribution of amplitude is well in accord with data obtained in two other measurements on another subjects

Advances in Biomagnetism
Edited by S.J. Williamson *et al.*
Plenum Press, New York

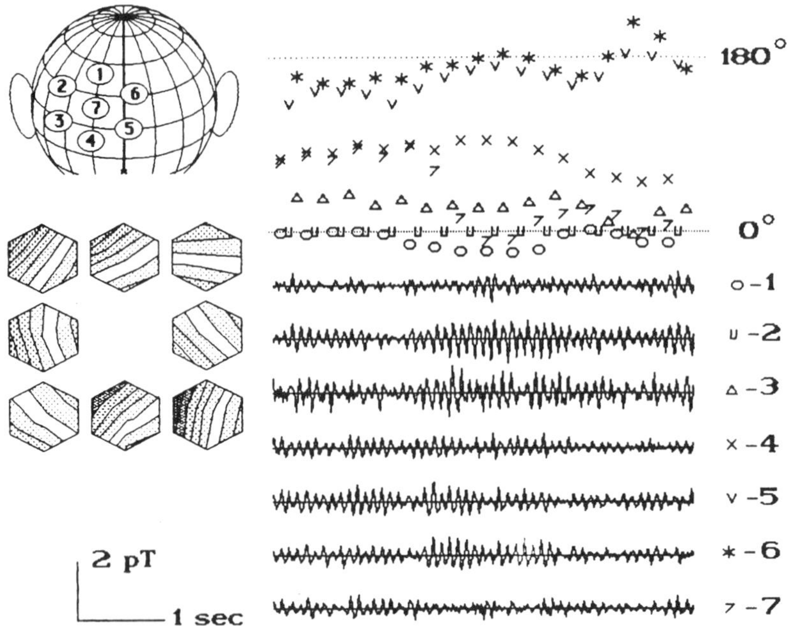

Fig.1. Simultaneous records of alpha-rhythm (5-25 Hz) in 7 channels and the calculated phase differences for each channel in respect to the channel number 2. The phase lags for different channels are indicated by different symbols on the upper plot. The position of the magnetometer over the head is presented on the left (inion is shown as cross, vertex as pole, coordinates drawn with 20° step). Evolution of the field distribution in the hexagonal area under magnetometer is shown in 12 ms steps for one period. Time runs clockwise. Field difference between two adjacent hatched areas is 0.15 pT.

(Vvedensky et al 1987, 1988). Phase relations between the signals in different channels reflect evolution with time of the spatial distribution of harmonic signal. When these relations are stable the evolution is repetitive. Characteristic sequences of the field maps during one period of the rhythm are shown in Figs.1, 2 and 3. The scenario is specific for every position of the magnetometer. At the right position the phases are close which means that field distribution is stable. This is shown in Fig.3, where sudden change in the phase distribution is also present. In the beginning of the record field behavior is similar to what is observed at the central position. The signals at the central position display gradual shift in phase from channels 5 and 6 through channels 1, 4, 7 to channels 2 and 3, see Fig.2. At the maps this looks like extrema of the field are permanently running from the right to the left under magnetometer. The 180° phase reversal implies equivalent source underneath channel 7 at the left magnetometer position. The field map seems to rotate in this area which implies 90° "phase- shifted" source in close proximity. We analyzed records several minutes long at the every position of the magnetometer. The described features of magnetic alpha-rhythm for this subject are stable over extended

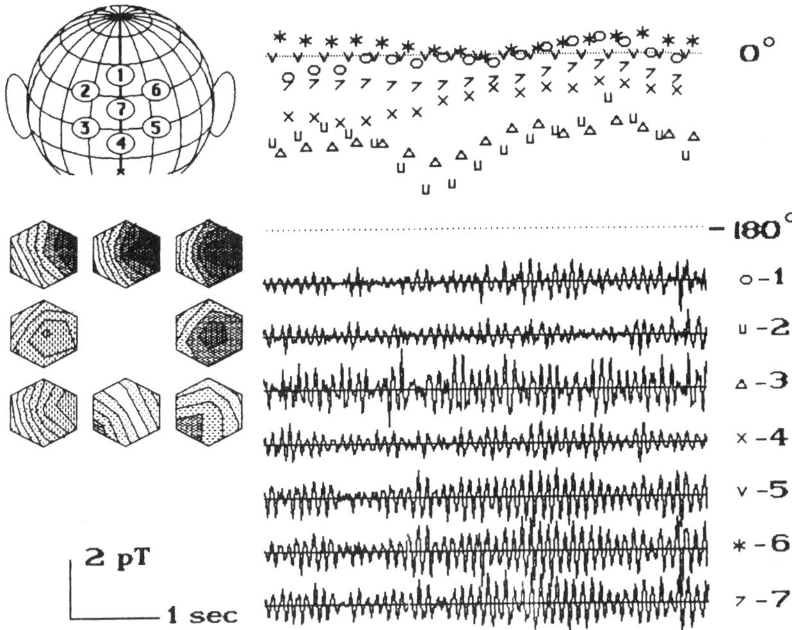

Fig.2. Same as in Fig.1 at the central position of the magnetometer. Reference channel 5.

periods of time. This implies stability of internal state of the subject, although at times we observed different behavior of the rhythm. We recorded 10 Hz alpha-rhythm with the second harmonics comparable in strength with the first. We could also observe "disintegration" of the alpha-rhythm probably due to the drowsiness of the subject. This manifested itself as appearence of supplementary peaks in the Fourier-spectrum. These peaks at roughly 9, 6 or 4 Hz remain after disappearence of 10 Hz component.

CONCLUSION

We consider as important that we can see two correlated and distinguishable sources of high amplitude alpha-rhythm in the occipital head and can start research on their relationship under different conditions. In spite of difference in behavior these sources are located close by, so they are a good object for study of their mutual interaction under different conditions. The interesting observation is obvious left-right asymmetry in the location of these sources inside the head. This can be important prompt in search for appropriate stimuli affecting those sources.

ACKNOWLEDGEMENTS

The authors are greatly indebted to prof. O.V.Lounasmaa and prof. V.I.Ozhogin for reviewing the manuscript and to N.E.Chumakov and S.Yu.Shabanov for help in calculations.

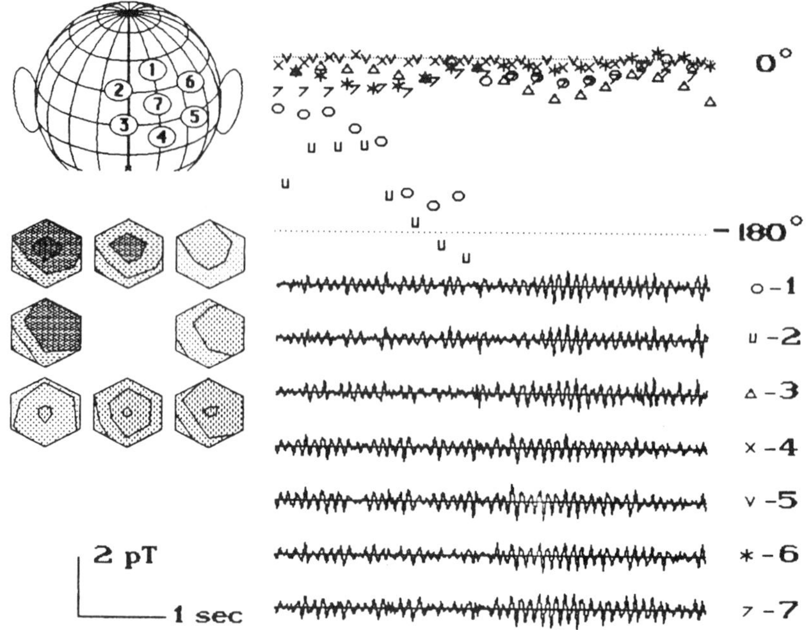

Fig.3. Same as in Fig.1 for the right position of the magnetometer. Reference channel 5.

REFERENCES

Ilmoniemi, R.J., Williamson, S.J., Hostetler, W.E. (1987). New method for the study of spontaneous brain activity. In Biomagnetism'87, Tokyo Denki University Press, Tokyo, pp.182-185.

Knuutila, J., Ahlfors, S., Ahonen, A., Hallstrom, J., Kajola, M.J., Lounasmaa, O.V., Vilkman, V., Tesche, K., (1987). Large-area low-noise seven-channel DC SQUID magnetometer for brain research. Rev. Sci. Instr., 58(11), pp.2145 -2156.,

Nunez, P.L. (1981). Electric fields of the brain. Oxford University Press, New-York, Oxford. Chapter 7.

Vvedensky, V.L., Gurtovoy, K.G., Ilmoniemi, R.J., Kajola, M.J. (1988). Determination of sources of the human magnetic alpha-rhythm. Human Physiology (USSR) 13, pp.400-404.

Vvedensky, V.L., Gelman, E.B., Gurtovoy, K.G., Naurzakov, S.P., Ozhogin, V.I., Shabanov, S.Yu., (1987). Study of spontaneous activity of the human brain with a tangential neuromagnetometer: 1. Occipital alpha-rhythm. In Biomagnetism'87, Tokyo Denki University Press, Tokyo, pp.190.

COHERENCE ANALYSIS OF ALPHA RHYTHM MEG MEASURED SIMULTANEOUSLY AT TWO POSITIONS

N. Kasai, H. Kado, M. Higuchi*, M. Nakanishi, K.Chinone**, M. Koyanagi

Electrotechnical Laboratory, 1-1-4 Umezono, Tsukuba 305 Japan
*Tsukuba University, 1 Ten-nohdai, Tsukuba 305 Japan
**Seiko Instruments Inc.

INTRODUCTION

The alpha rhythm of brain activity is a simple and outstanding rhythm which is observed within the frequency band between 8 and 13 Hz and is dominant in the occipital area[1]. From EEG studies, it has been revealed that the rhythm is widely distributed over the scalp between frontal and occipital regions. Ozaki et al. analyzed the alpha rhythm using power- and cross-spectrum [2]. They found that there were two components of alpha activity; one component has maximum power in the bilateral occipital areas and has rather high frequency. The other component appeared dominantly in the central area and has lower frequency.

MEG is expected to be superior to EEG in spatial resolution and phase delay. However it is difficult to study a spontaneous activity using a single channel SQUID. We have developed two channel DC-SQUID magnetometer system to study spontaneous activity. Vvedensky et al [3] showed that detection of the tangential component of the magnetic field due to brain activity was useful in the study of alpha rhythm. We have measured simultaneously tangential components of alpha rhythmic field at two positions over a head and analyzed them by power- and cross-spectrum.

MEASUREMENT

The 2 channel DC-SQUID magnetometer system has two parallel and 10 cm apart stages for two integrated DC-SQUID magnetometers (ch1 and ch2). The pick-up coil of the DC-SQUID magnetometer is 8x8 mm^2 rectangular coil. The noise level was about $30fT/\sqrt{Hz}$ above 10 Hz. The SQUID magnetometers were located tangentially to scalp. The measuring points were shown in Fig. 1. The lines in the figure show the pairs of simultaneous measuring positions.

We examined 4 male subjects (aged 26-44). MEGs at each SQUID pick-up coil were simultaneously aquisited during 100 sec. The analog band pass filter (6.7-15Hz) was used. EEG was simultaneously measured at two positions (near C3 and C4) in all sessions. Each reference electrode was at ear lobes. We divided one session into 40 epochs of 5sec duration by overlapping 2.5 sec with the following epoch. Off-line power and cross-spectral analyses were performed on every epoch of these MEG and EEG in each session.

RESULT

The power spectra of MEG in the frequency range from 7 to 14 Hz at 16 positions around the head were obtained by averaging the power spectra over about 40 epochs. The frequency and amplitude of alpha rhythmic field varied in time. Our system has only two

Advances in Biomagnetism
Edited by S.J. Williamson *et al.*
Plenum Press, New York

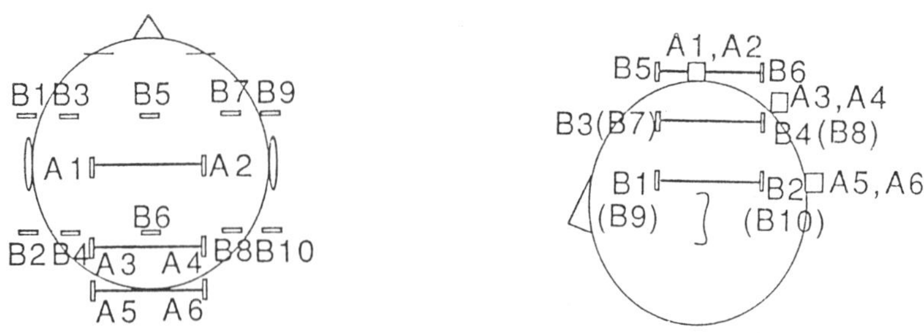

Fig.1 measured points.
The pair positions where MEGs are detected simultaneously by the two channel DC-SQUID system are connected by the bar.

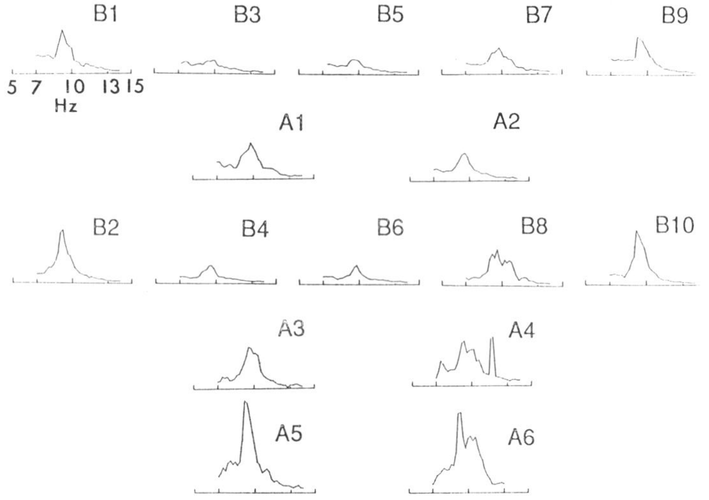

Fig.2 Power spectrum of MEG in the frequency range 7-14 Hz. The power spectrum was normalized by the total power of EEG measured simultaneously at near C3 and C4, in order to compare the spectra measured at different time each other

SQUIDs. We could not directly compare alpha rhythmic fields at different positions except pair positions. Measured MEGs had some correlations with measured EEG in corresponding session. The power spectrum of MEG was normalized by total power of corresponding EEG to obtain the spatial distribution of alpha rhythmic field. The power of alpha rhythmic field was strong at bilateral occipital area. It was weak at central and parietal areas. The peak frequency in the alpha rhythmic frequency range fluctuated about 1Hz in time and the peak of the power spectrum has about 1Hz width. One of subjects has the power spectrum in which has multiple peaks at several positions. The normalized power spectrum of one of subjects are shown at 16 positions in Fig.2 .

There was a tendency that the power spectrum of simultaneously measured MEGs at a pair of positions had the same peak frequency independently of the position. We can suppose that the alpha rhythmic sources at different position act with same frequency. In order to investigate the sources in more detail, the phase difference between alpha rhythmic fields at ch1 and ch2 was estimated using cross-spectrum between them. We assumed that the frequency of alpha rhythmic field was the peak frequency in the cross-spectrum in the range 8-13Hz. If it had more than single peaks , the frequency of the peak with highest amplitude was assumed as alpha rhythmic field frequency. The frequency differed in each epoch. The phase differences at the alpha rhythmic frequency in each epoch are obtained as histograms. The examples of the histograms and corresponding configurations of pick-up coils are shown in Fig.3. The phase differences appeared randomly from $+\pi$ to $-\pi$ when ch1 and ch2 were located at bilateral hemispheres (A-type). The phase difference concentrated at zero or π when ch1 and ch2 were located at front and rear position of head (B-type).

DISCUSSION

We could not observe the clear spatial distribution of high frequency and low frequency components of alpha rhythmic field, though subjects displayed high frequency and low frequency alpha rhythmic field depending on the time.

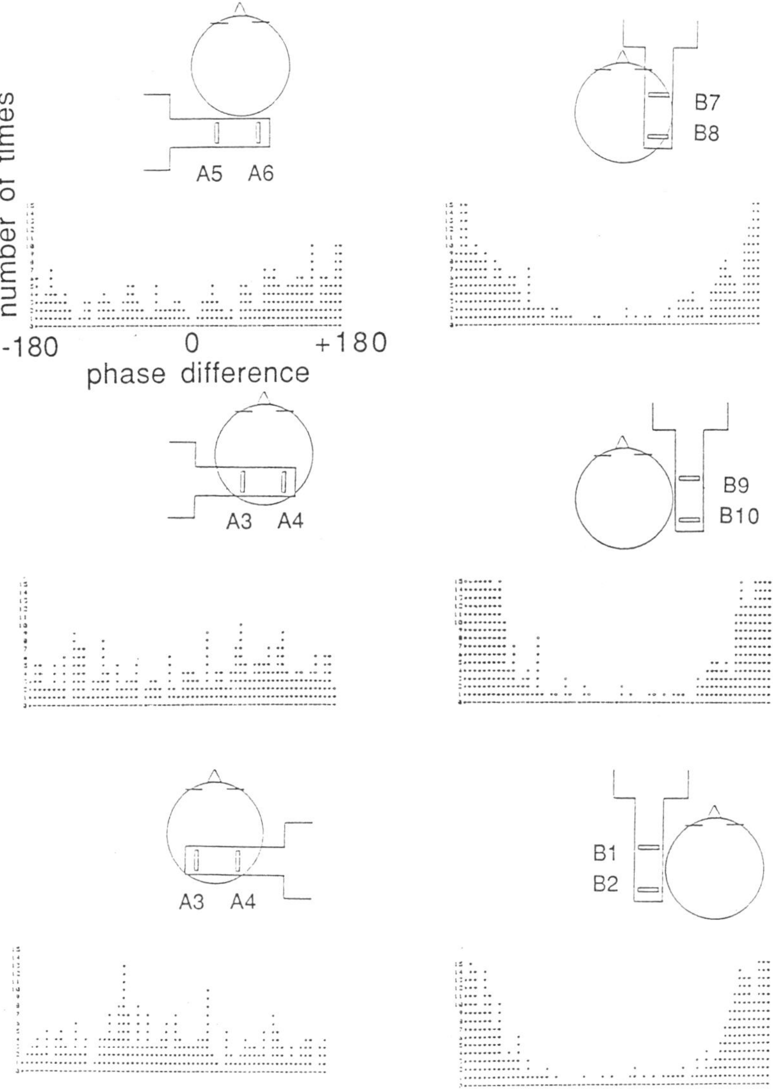

Fig.3 Phase difference between alpha rhythmic fields detected simultaneously at pair positions.
The phase differences appeared randomly from $+\pi$ to $-\pi$ when ch1 and ch2 DC-SQUID magnetometers were located at bilateral hemispheres (A-type). The phase difference concentrated at zero or π when ch1 and ch2 were located at front and rear position of head (B-type). This suggests that the sources of alpha rhythmic field are not synchronized over bilateral hemisphere and that the sources which are distributed over frontal and occipital areas in a hemisphere are synchronized .

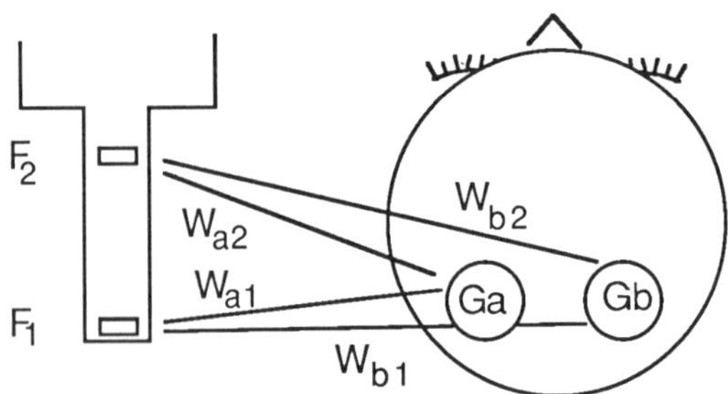

Fig.4 A model of the spatial relationship between signal sources and sensors.

The phase differences between alpha rhythmic fields detected at different positions show the correlation. If the phase difference is always constant, all sources are synchronized. The results of A-type suggest that the sources of alpha rhythmic field are not synchronized over bilateral hemisphere.The results of B-type suggest that the sources which are distributed over frontal and occipital areas in a hemisphere are synchronized .

It is noticed that SQUID detects not only the signal from the sources just under the SQUID pick-up coil but also the signal from the sources apart from the coil. When we assume, for example, two generators of the alpha rhythm as shown in Fig. 4, the phase differences between MEGs detected by two SQUIDs are considered as follows. The spatial relationship between sources and sensors is shown in Fig.4 and the Fourier transform of signals detected by sensors F1 and F2 are expressed as follows:

$$F1=Wa1Ga+Wb1Gb \quad F2=Wa2Ga+Wb2Gb$$

where Ga and Gb are the Fourier transform of source signals, and W.. are weights function of distance from generator to sensor.The cross spectrum of F1 and F2 is;

$$\begin{aligned} S12 &= F1^*F2 \\ &= Wa1Wa2|Ga|^2+Wb1Wb2|Gb|^2+Wa2Wb1GaGb+Wa1Wb2GaGb \\ &= A0+(A1+A2)\cos P_{ab} + j(A1-A2)\sin P_{ab} \end{aligned}$$

where $A0=Wa1Wa2|Ga|^2+Wb1Wb2|Gb|^2$, $A1=Wa2Wb1|G_{ab}|$ and $A2=Wa1Wb2|G_{ab}|$. P_{ab} is the phase difference between source signals and G_{ab} is cross spectrum of Ga and Gb. The phase difference between signals detected by two sensors is expressed as ;

$$P_{12}=\tan^{-1}\{(A1-A2)\sin P_{ab}/[A0+(A1+A2)\cos P_{ab}]\}$$

When A1 is equal to A2, the phase differences between signals detected by two sensors is equal to zero or π. The phase difference between source signals is always not equal to zero independently of the source configuration, when the phase difference between detected signals with sensors is not equal to zero.

The speculation that the sources act independently to each others does not change by this consideration of source configuration from the result of A-type. Even if the sources act independently each others, we could get the results like that of B-type if the SQUID coils configuration against sources satisfied the condition A1=A2 .

By our measuring system, only MEGs at two different positions were simultaneously detected. In order to decrease the uncertainty of normalized power spectrum due to the fluctuation of the frequency and amplitude of the spontaneous activity in time, it is necessary to use a multi-channel SQUID magnetometer system covering whole head.

REFERENCE

1) D.Lehmann, H.Ozaki and I.Pal,"EEG alpha map series; brain micro-states by space-oriented adaptive segmentation",Electroenceph. Clin. Neurophysiol.,67:271(1987)

2) H.Ozaki and H.Suzuki, "Transverse relationships of alpha rhythm on the scalp", Electroenceph. Clin. Neurophysiol., 66: 191(1987)

3) V.L.Vvedensky, E.B.Gelman, K.G.Gurtovoy, S.P.Naurzakov, V.I.Ozhogin and S.Yu.Shabanov, "STUDY OF SPONTANEOUS ACTIVITY OF THE HUMAN BRAIN WITH A TANGENTIAL NEUROMAGNETOMETER: 1. OCCIPITAL ALPHA-RHYTHM", Proc. Biomag. '87: 190(1988)

METHOD FOR LOCATING SOURCES OF HUMAN ALPHA ACTIVITY

S.J. Williamson, J.-Z. Wang, and R.J. Ilmoniemi*

Neuromagnetism Laboratory, Departments of Physics and Psychology and Center for Neural Science, New York University, New York, NY 10003, U.S.A.
*Low Temperature Laboratory, Helsinki University of Technology
02150 Espoo, Finland

INTRODUCTION

Alpha activity is commonly defined as electrical fluctuations between 8 and 13 Hz that can be detected on the occipital scalp and are attenuated by visual stimuli. While projections from brain stem play a role in its generation (c.f. Steriade and Llinás, 1988), evidence for the cortical origin of these electrical signals has been obtained from studies of potentials at various depths within the cortex of animals. Lopes da Silva and van Leeuwen (1978) suggest that alpha sources originate in different epicenters from which activity spreads across cortex in several directions. Previous magnetic studies on humans of the covariance between the EEG and magnetic recordings with a single sensor indicate sources deep within the occipital lobe (Carelli et al., 1983). Studies with a four-sensor system (Vvedensky, Ilmoniemi, and Kajola, 1986) indicate that there are time series of the rhythm lasting for typically 1 sec during which the oscillation period is constant. We call these time series *spindles*, whether or not occurring in the sleeping state. Ilmoniemi, Williamson, and Hostetler (1988) using a 14-sensor system found that the magnetic field pattern during a spindle appears relatively stable, indicating that its source is a specific configuration of neurons. Moreover, an analysis of the time-invariant spatial pattern based on a 14-dimensional signal space indicates it is possible to distinguish between most of the sources of the observed spindles. In other words, the human alpha rhythm represented by the spindles is generated by a large number, or possibly a continuum, of different source configurations. We introduce the term *alphon* for the neuronal excitation producing a spindle. The purpose of the present study is to develop a technique to determine the locations in the human brain of alphons and to characterize the orientation and strength of their equivalent current dipole moments.

METHODS

Two dewars, each containing seven dc-SQUID sensors (Biomagnetic Technologies, inc.) were positioned over the left and right occipital areas to record magnetic activity. The detection coils were second-order gradiometers with 1.5-cm diameter and 4-cm baseline, and the sensor noise level was about 20 fT/√Hz for most channels, while one or two exhibited noise as high as 50 fT/√Hz. Individual sensors were calibrated with a relative accuracy of better than 1%. With the subject prone and alert, recordings within the bandwidth 0.5-50 Hz were made for 16-sec epochs of spontaneous activity with eyes closed. The total level of instrument and subject noise was determined with eyes open. Data were digitally filtered in the bandwidth 8-13 Hz, and a computer routine was used to spot those segments of the time-series where the rms amplitude within the middle 12 seconds of the epoch significantly exceeds the noise level.

Advances in Biomagnetism
Edited by S.J. Williamson *et al.*
Plenum Press, New York

A spindle was defined by a time-series where signals in all the sensors are coherent and can be attributed to a single source. The criteria were: (1) the peak rms amplitude averaged across 14 sensors exceeds 500 fT; (2) this mean amplitude across sensors exceeds 200 fT for at least 3 oscillations before and after the peak; (3) the period between zero crossings is stable to within 5% throughout the duration; and (4) field polarity reverses between the two probes, to ensure that the source lies somewhere between them. To ensure accuracy in locating each alphon, it was important to achieve a high signal-to-noise ratio, because only a small area of the field pattern is measured. By positioning the probes so that field extrema of the individual spindles are close by, the source positions in three dimensions can be determined without need to move the dewars. The accuracy of this "fixed position" technique when probes are placed directly over the extrema has been analyzed by Costa Ribeiro et al. (1988) who considered the cases of a single probe with 5 or 7 sensors and two probes with 7 sensors each. However, this is the ideal situation, since determining the positions and fields of the two extrema is sufficient to determine all 5 dipole parameters (Williamson and Kaufman 1981). If both extrema are not within the areas of the probes, accuracy in location greatly diminishes. Therefore it was essential to maximize the signal-to-noise ratio, and so the best estimate for the mean amplitudes of each spindle was obtained from elements of the covariance matrix computed across the time-series of the spindle.

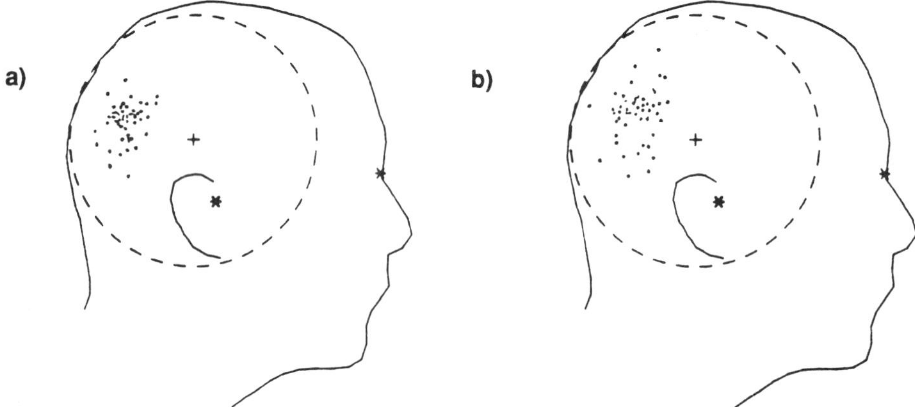

Fig. 1. Sagittal view of deduced alphon positions for those producing spindles with (a) one field extremum lying within the area of a probe and (b) neither extremum lying within the area of a probe. Nasion and periauricular points: $*$; center of sphere model for posterior head: +; subject: S.

Positions and orientations of individual sensors relative to a head-based cartesian coordinate system was determined by the Probe Position Indicator (PPI) method (Buchanan et al. 1987). This system is indexed to the periauricular points and nasion, with the origin placed midway between the former. This method, together with data from the 14-sensor system, has been shown to provide 3-mm accuracy in determining the location of a current dipole at a depth of about 4 cm in a conducting sphere, model head, and human auditory cortex (Yamamoto et al., 1988). The set of 14 mean values for each spindle was used to determine the location of the current dipole best representing its source, using a minimum chi-square criterion. The subject's head was modeled as a sphere, whose center of curvature was determined by digitizing the shape of the occipital and parietal areas of the scalp using PPI and determining the least-squares fit with a sphere. Preliminary studies indicated that strongest spindle amplitudes were detected with the probes placed over right and left occipital scalp, about 4-8 cm above the inion and displaced symmetrically by about 6-8 cm to left and right of the midline. Signals were generally very weak directly over the midline or farther than 9 cm to either side of the midline, in agreement with measures of relative covariance (Carelli et al., 1983; Chapman et al., 1984). Strong alpha rhythm generally exhibited field extrema of opposite polarity over left and right hemisphere, indicating that the corresponding alphons lie near the midline. Each alphon was modeled by a current dipole, so its center of activity could be characterized by 5 parameters specifying location, orientation in the plane tangent to the sphere, and strength.

We found that the variety of alphons for a given subject was so diverse that very few of the spindles provided extrema that simultaneously appeared within the areas of the two probes. This remained true when the probes were placed at various asymmetrical positions over left and right hemispheres with one further from the inion or midline than the other. The deduced positions for a set of about 100 alphons of a subject are shown in Fig. 1, where those providing an extremum within the area of one probe (a) are compared with a nearly equal number whose extrema lie outside (b). The greater scatter in the latter case is due in part by less accuracy in localization. The uncertainty in position (95% confidence) for the former case is typically about 0.8 cm in radial position and 1.3 cm in distance above the midline. Most alphons lie within 2 cm of the midline. Similar results were obtained for a second subject. Measurements over many days produced on the average 1-2 spindles meeting the criteria during each 12-second analysis period. These source positions are in a tighter cluster and lie much shallower than the average positions estimated on the basis of relative covariance measurements (Carelli et al., 1983; Chapman et al., 1984). Visual inspection of our time-series showed on the order of 5 times more spindle features that did not meet our present criteria for defining a spindle.

The deduced dipole orientations were generally within 30 deg of the longitudinal fissure (Fig. 2a). When probes were placed on either side of the midline so the line joining them makes an angle of 45 deg with the midline, spindles could not be detected. This justifies our primary reliance on data obtained with the probes placed above the inion at the same distances, or at distances differing by no more than 5 cm. Since extracranial magnetic fields arise from intracellular currents, the source of the field most likely is an aligned population of cortical neurons. The most conspicuous preferentially aligned population is that of the pyramidal cells. In this case the orientation of the current dipoles indicates that alphons are largely confined to the floor and/or ceiling of the calcarine fissure, which is aligned approximately perpendicular to the longitudinal fissure. The few dipoles tipped as much as 20 deg may well have contributions from neurons in the longitudinal fissure as well. We cannot rule out the possibility that alphons also occur within the parietal-occipital fissure. Indeed, the fact that many are located rather high above the inion suggests this to be the case.

The remaining parameter of interest is alphon strength. Fig. 2b illustrates the distribution of current dipole moment for about 100 alphons. A remarkable feature is that all of the alphons have similar strengths, with a typical rms moment of about 40 nA·m. The cutoff of the distribution at low strengths may be influenced in part by our minimum-field criterion for identifying a spindle. This effect merits additional study, but in any event the narrowness of the distribution argues that the alphon is a characteristic excitation, involving about the same number of neurons no matter where it occurs. The deduced alphon strength is sensitive to the choice for the center of curvature of the sphere modeling the posterior head. If the midpoint between the periauricular points is used instead, the amplitude decreases to about 20 nA·m.

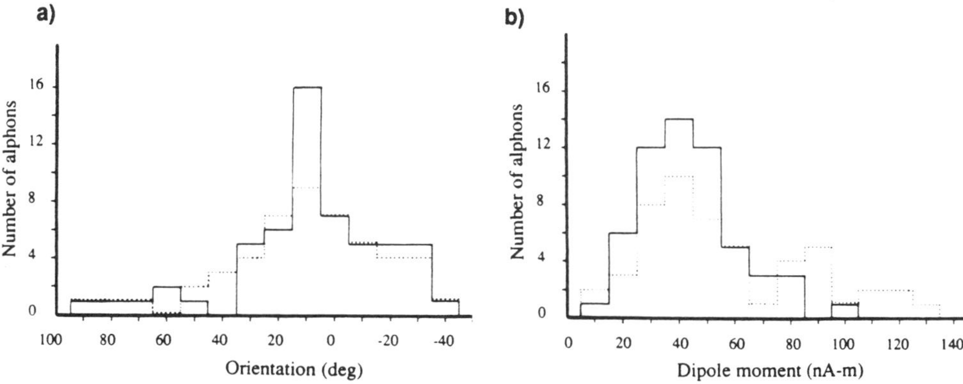

Fig. 2. a) Distribution of alphon orientation in the tangent plane, with positive angles measured clockwise from the inion-vertex line. b) Distribution of alphon strength. Solid curves describe about 50 alphons where an extremum lies within the area of a probe, dashed curve about 50 where an extremum does not. Subject: S.

An alphon strength of 40 nA·m is only an order of magnitude stronger than a typical sensory evoked response. Considering estimates for postsynaptic currents in pyramidal cells, an area of cortex of only a few square millimeters, corresponding to 10^5 coherently active pyramidal cells, is required to account for an alphon. This area is considerably smaller than deduced on the basis of the cited relative covariance measurements, but is consistent with electrophysiological studies (Lopes da Silva and van Leeuwen, 1978).

CONCLUSION

The picture that emerges from this work is that magnetic alpha rhythm arises from many discrete sources oscillating one after another, and occasionally overlapping temporally. Alphons giving rise to the observed activity are clustered near the midline, extending to a depth of several centimeters. Dipole orientations are nearly parallel to the longitudinal fissure indicating that the underlying neuronal activity is largely confined to cortical areas within calcarine fissure or perhaps parietal-occipital fissure. Deduced source strengths are consistent with each alphon extending across only a few square millimeters of cortical area.

ACKNOWLEDGEMENTS

We thank Dr. D.S. Buchanan for calibrating the sensors, P. Fusco for technical help, and L. Kaufman and D. Brenner for helpful discussions. The work was supported in part by Air Force Office of Scientific Research Grants F49620-86-C-0131 and F49620-88-K-00004.

REFERENCES

Buchanan, D.S., Paulson, D., and Williamson, S.J., 1987, Instrumentation for clinical applications of neuromagnetism, in: *Advances in Cryogenic Engineering, Vol. 33*, Fast, R.W., Ed., Plenum Press, New York, pp. 97-106.

Carelli, P., Foglietti, V., Modena, I., and Romani, G.L., 1983, Magnetic study of the spontaneous brain activity of normal subjects, *Il Nuovo Cimento* 2D, 538-546.

Chapman, R.M., Ilmoniemi, R.J., Barbanera, S., and Romani, G.L., 1984, *Electroenceph. clin. Neurophysiol.* 58, 569-572.

Costa Ribeiro, P., Williamson, S.J., and Kaufman, L., 1988, SQUID arrays for simultaneous magnetic measurements: calibration and source localization performance. *IEEE Trans. Biomed. Engr.* BME-35, 551-560.

Ilmoniemi, R.J., Williamson, S.J., and Hostetler, W.E., 1988, New Method for the study of spontaneous brain activity, in: *Biomagnetism '87*, Atsumi, K., Kotani, M., Ueno, S., Katila, T., and Williamson, S.J., Eds., Tokyo Denki University Press, pp. 182-185.

Lopes da Silva, F.H., and Storm van Leeuwen, W., 1978, The cortical alpha rhythm in dog: the depth and surface profile of phase, in: *Architectonics of the Cerebral Cortex*, Brazier, M.A.B., and Petsche, H., Eds., Raven Press, New York, pp. 319-333.

Steriade, M., and Llinás, R.R., 1988, The functional states of the thalamus and the associated neuronal interplay, *Physiol. Revs.* 68, 649-742.

van Rotterdam, A., Lopes da Silva, F.H., van den Ende, J. Viergever, M.A., and Hermans, A.J., 1982, A model fo the spatial-temporal characteristics of the alpha rhythm, *Bull. Math. Biol.* 44, 283-305.

Vvedensky, V.L., Ilmoniemi, R.J., and Kajola, M.L., 1986, Study of the alpha rhythm with a 4-channel SQUID magnetometer, *Med. & Biol. Eng. & Computing* 23, Suppl. Part 1, 11-12.

Williamson, S.J., and Kaufman, L., 1981, Evoked cortical magnetic fields, in: *Biomagnetism*, Erné, S.N., Hahlbohm, H.-D., and Lübbig, H., Eds. de Gruyter, Berlin, pp. 353-402.

Yamamoto, T., Williamson, S.J., Kaufman, L., Nicholson, C., and Llinás, R., 1988, Magnetic localization of neuronal activity in the human brain, *Proc. Natl. Acad. Sci. USA* 85, 8732 - 8736.

NEUROMAGNETIC IMAGING OF SYNCHRONIZED MU ACTIVITY

L. Narici[1], G. Iori[1], I. Modena[1], G.L. Romani[2], G. Torrioli[3], R. Traversa[4], and P.M. Rossini[4]

[1] Dipartimento di Fisica & [4]Dipartimento di Sanità Pubblica - Università di Roma "Tor Vergata"; [2] Istituto di Fisica Medica - Università di Chieti [3]Istituto di Elettronica dello Stato Solido - CNR - Roma

INTRODUCTION

Sensory stimulation at certain frequencies was shown to elicit EEG and MEG (MagnetoEncephaloGraphic) responses persisting longer than one second after the stimulation. Such responses have been described as a consequence of a process of synchronization of bioelectrical spontaneous activities in the brain with a specific frequency content, but otherwise uncorrelated (*Narici et al 1987a*).

In this paper we present new results achieved with this technique. We performed a neuromagnetic study on healthy subjects under somatosensory stimulation of the median nerve at wrist, recording magnetic fields over the parietal and parieto-frontal regions of the side contralateral to the stimulated wrist. Aim of the work was to identify the source(s) of the synchronized activity in this sensory modality, possibly following their time evolution, and to obtain evidences for the underlying spontaneous activity responsible for the synchronized responses.

METHODS

We studied four male subjects, 25 to 30 years old, right handed. The magnetic measurements have been performed with the four channel neuromagnetic detector in use at the Istituto di Elettronica dello Stato Solido in Roma. This device, fully described elsewhere (*Romani et al. 1985*), features four home made rfSQUIDs, with 7 cm baseline second order gradiometers, and a noise of about 45 fT $Hz^{-1/2}$, operating in an unshielded enviroment.

The median nerve was stimulated following the 'train' paradigm (*Narici et al 1987a, Narici 1988*) consisting in delivering bursts of stimuli (about 800 ms duration) at a specific rate, separated by non-stimulated periods (about 1200 ms duration). Preliminary measurements were carried out to find the 'resonant' rate (the burst rate at which the following responses were consistently stronger than at any other rate of stimulation). The experiment was then carried out at such a rate. The subjects were asked to keep their eyes closed during the measurements, however test were carried out and showed no differences between the responses in the open/closed-eye conditions

In order to allow for a good resolution in reconstructing the field spatial distribution over the parietal and parieto-frontal regions, scanning the sensor over about 15 position was required, measuring the field in about 60 scalp sites. The scanning procedure, described in detail elsewhere (*Romani and Narici 1986*), followed a pre-determined grid printed on a plastic cup weared by the subjects. To monitor the stationarity of the response two electric leads (from pre- and post-rolandic positions) have been monitored and acquired during all the measurement sessions.

Advances in Biomagnetism
Edited by S.J. Williamson *et al.*
Plenum Press, New York

The magnetic measurements were analogically filtered with a flat-delay filter of the Bessel type (48 dB/octave) in a 1-100 Hz bandwidth and then stored on a computer (HP1000) at a rate of 256 Hz for successive off-line analysis

RESULTS

We have been able to identify in each subject a stable 'resonant' rate. Across all the examined subjects such frequency was found to range between 5.5 Hz and 8 Hz. The maps constructed from time traces digitally filtered between 1 Hz and 40 Hz did not show easibly recognizable and cyclic structures (an example of these maps is shown in Fig. 1a). Fourier analysis showed that the frequency content at the 'resonant' rate was clearly dominant, and that another activity at about twice this rate was clearly measurable on most of the parietal region (see Fig. 1b). Once these two activities were recognized, filtering the traces in a 1 Hz band with a zero-phase shift digital filter (centered on the activity's rate) allowed to discriminate and study their distribution. The former response, at the 'resonant' rate,

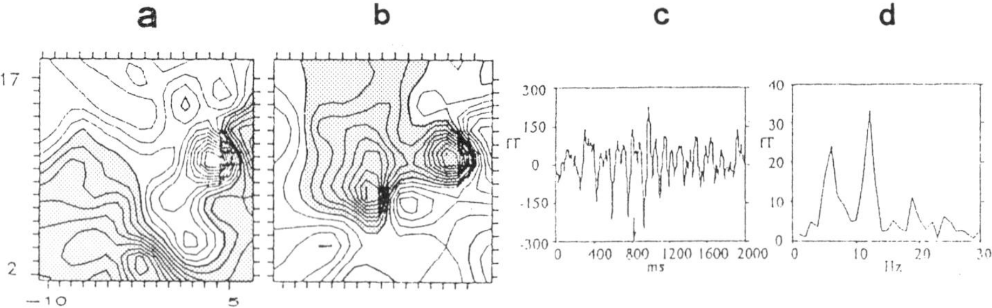

Figure 1 (a,b) Scalp field distributions of a subject under somatosensory 'resonant' stimulation. The maps have been constructed from responses filtered in a 1-40 Hz bandwidth at latencies corresponding to 140 ms (a) and 220 ms (b) after the delivery of the last stimulus. Coordinates are cartesian with the origin on the right ear canal, the x axis along the nasion -inion line and the y axis along the ear canal-vertex line. Units are cm. Interval between isofield lines is 15 fT (c,d) Response (c) and frequency spectrum (d), in the non stimulated period, as measured at position X = 2.7 cm, Y = 4.8 cm [250 averages].

featured a complex repetitive spatial structure, with a four-pole (negative-positive-positive-negative) distribution across the rolandic fissure, up to the frontal region (Fig. 2a). This whole distribution reversed synchronously every ≈ 80 ms (≈ 6 Hz) and still appeared more then one second after the end of stimulation. The latter response, on the other hand, featured a weaker distribution but strongly dipolar, similar to the N20 distribution (Fig. 2b), reversing every ≈ 40 ms (≈ 12 Hz), and appearing until well after the end of the stimulation. We interpreted this distribution as generated by a single Equivalent Current Dipole (ECD), and carried out the localization routine, based on a least squares algorhythm, at those latencies showing field maxima after each inversion of polarity. The routine provides the coordinates and strength of the ECD together with the 95% confidence interval (*Romani and Narici 1986*). In Fig. 3 we show six positions of the ECD during the stimulation and four in the non-stimulated period, together with the strength at the same latencies. The stationarity of the source is striking. The four pole distribution, showing a very high time and phase coherence, has been interpreted as generated by an extended source with two well separated foci of activity. Accordingly, we tried a 'double-ECD' localization for each latency showing a maximum of the field and found consistently one parietal ECD and a frontal one, both stationary for almost 1 s after the end of the stimulation (Fig. 4).

DISCUSSION

The results of the localization for the 12 Hz activity (Fig. 3), but also simple visual inspection of the distribution of the 12 Hz activity (Fig 2b) clearly suggest to position its

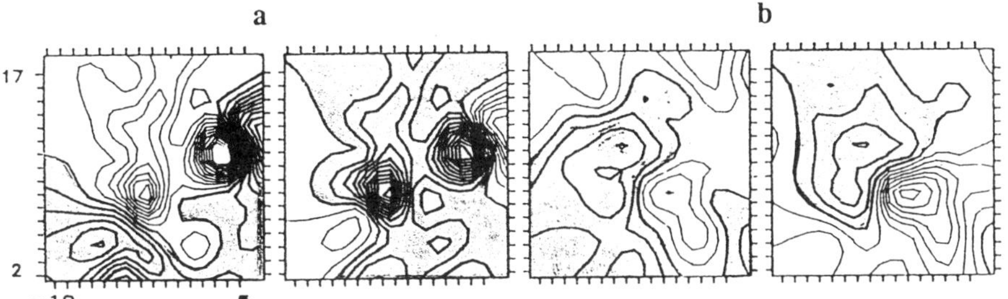

Figure 2 Scalp field distributions (same latencies as in Fig. 1) of a subject under somatosensory 'resonant' stimulation. The map has been constructed from responses filtered in 1 Hz bandwidth centered at 6 Hz (a) and 12 Hz (b). Coordinates are as in Fig. 1. Interval between isofield lines is 5 fT

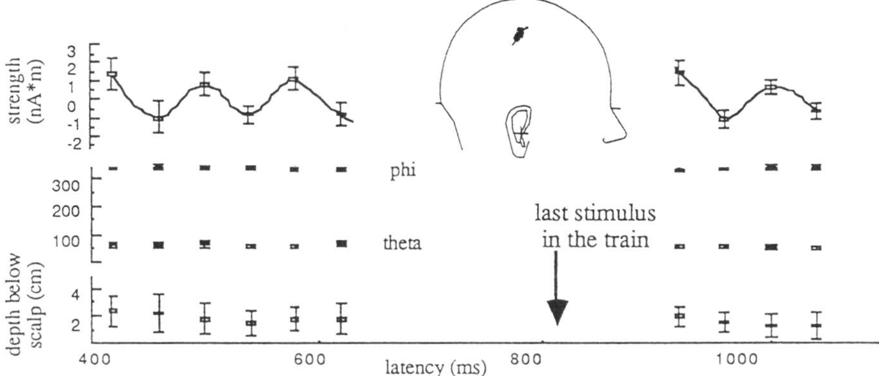

Figure 3 Strength (top) and angular coordinates (center) and depth below the scalp (bottom) of the location of the ECD of the 12 Hz activity (Fig. 2b) at ten different latencies, 6 during the stimulated period, four after the end of the stimulation. The latencies are measured from the beginning of the stimulation. The errors represent the 95 % confidence interval given by the fit. The angular coordinates are theta (latitude, zero at the vertex) and phi (longitude, zero at the right ear canal). Note the stationarity of both position and strength, over the whole period and during all the phase inversions. In the insert is shown the lateral view of three localizations of the ECD (at 480ms, 960 ms, 1040 ms after the beginning of the stimulation), with the 95% confidence interval.

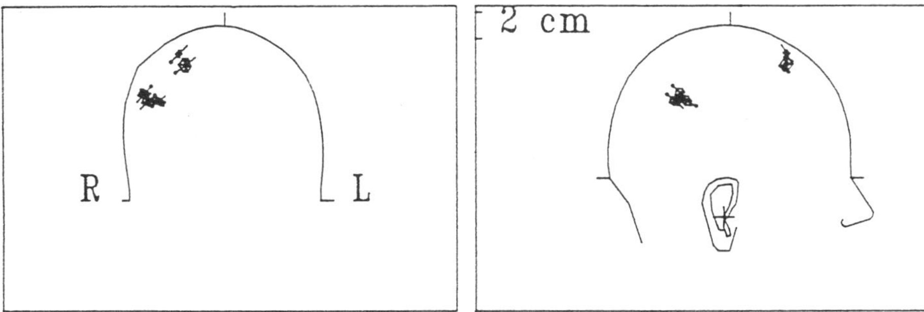

Figure 4 Localizations of the two concurrent ECDs of the 6 Hz activity (Fig. 2a) at three different latencies, from about 400 ms after the beginning of the stimulation, to 1030 ms (corresponding to 220 ms after the end of the stimulation). The boxes represent the 95 % confidence interval given by the fit.

generator in the sensorimotor brain areas circumscribing the central sulcus contralateral to the stimulation side. A probable candidate for this activity is the mu (or rolandic alpha) rhythm. This rhythm has been described since the early fifties (*Gastaut et al 1952, Chatrian et al. 1959*) with a small intrinsic amplitude, in a position slightly shallower than the one of the early somatosensory evoked responses, unaffected by opening or closing the eyes, and with a restricted localization. More recently Kuhlman (1978) localized with depth electrodes techniques the generator of the rhythm in the sensorymotor areas. Our results are in agreement with an ECD in this location, which is also similar to the one of the N20 peak of the somatosensory evoked fields (*Hari and Kaukoranta 1985, Narici et al. 1987b, Rossini et al. 1988*). We can therefore suggest that the 12 Hz activity is the mu-rhythm synchronized by the stimulation and therefore brought in evidence even if, as in the presented case, the rhythm was not measurable in the on line EEG or MEG. Furthermore we can suggest that the rhythm share at least partially the same generators than the short latency somatosensory evoked activities. The cyclic appearance of the rhythm spatial structure for more then one second, up to 600 ms in the non-stimulated period is very impressive. The stationarity of the source appreciated in Fig. 3 seems to indicate that the synchronized rhythm is generated in the same small region for a long interval of time, so that either all the 'mu-generators' are circumscribed in a very small region of the cortex, or the synchronization mechanism does not diffuse in the studied time window.

The four-pole distribution (Fig 2a) appears cyclically with a ≈ 160 ms period and it is detectable for longer than the 12 Hz activity, most probably due to its larger amplitude. The spatially stationary parietal and frontal generators (Fig.4) with a very good time locking would therefore suggest the presence of a single clock, possibly thalamic. It should be stressed that the double dipole hypotesis has to be considered with extreme caution, due to the non uniqueness of the inverse problem solution. Nevertheless it remains that the actvity *is* time locked, extends from parietal to frontal regions and seems to be much stronger (and therefore 'focused') around two separate positions.

The presented work underlines the usefulness of this method, and prompts for new measurements to verify the genesis of the two, sinchronous, ECDs, possibly two end-stations of cortical relays, driven by the same deep clock. Furthermore measurements of the sychronizability of the cortex of patients with synchronization problems (i.e. epilepsy, multiple sclerosis) might provide clinically relevant information.

REFERENCES

Chatrian G.E., Petersen M.C. and Lazarte J.A., 1959, The blocking of the rolandic wicket rhythm and some central changes related to movement. Electroenceph. clin. Neurophysiol. 11: 447-510.

Gastaut H., 1952, Etude èlectrocorticographique del la rèactivitè des rhythmes rolandiques. Rev. Neurol. 87: 176-182.

Hari R. and Kaukoranta E., 1985, Neuromagnetic studies of somatosensory system: principles and examples. Progress in Neurobiol. 24: 233-256.

Kuhlman W.N. (1978) Functional topography of the human μ-rhythm. Electroenceph. clin. Neurophysiol 44: 83-93.

Narici L., Romani G.L., Salustri C., Pizzella V., Modena I. and Papanicolau A.C., 1987a, Neuromagnetic evidence of Synchronized Spontaneous Activity in the brain following repetitive sensory stimulation. Inter. J. Neuroscience 32: 831-836.

Narici L., Romani G.L., Salustri C., Pizzella V., Torrioli G. and Modena I., 1987b, Neuromagnetic characterization of the cortical response to median nerve stimulation in the steady state paradigm. Inter. J. Neuroscience 32: 837-843.

Narici L., 1988, Synchronization of brain activity revealed by neuromagnetic measurements. In K. Atsumi, M. Kotani, S. Ueno, T. Katila and S.J. Williamson (Eds.) *Biomagnetism '87* , Tokyo Denky University Press - Tokyo - pp. 42-49.

Romani G.L., Leoni R., Salustri C. "Multichannel instrumentation for biomagnetism." In H.D. Hahlbohm, Lübbig H (Eds.) SQUID85: Superconducting Quantum Interference Devices and their Application, Walter De Gruyter, Berlin-New York, pp. 918-932, 1985.

Romani G.L. and Narici L., 1986, Principles and clinical validity of the biomagnetic method. Medical Progress through Technology 11: 123-159.

Rossini P.M., Narici L., Romani G.L., Traversa R., Cecchi L., Cilli M., Urbano A., 1989, Short latency somatosensory evoked responses to median nerve stimulation in healthy humans: electric and magnetic recordings. Int. J. Neurosci. 46: 67-76.

SLEEP SPINDLES IN MAGNETOENCEPHALOGRAPHY AND ELECTROENCEPHALOGRAPHY

Nobukazu Nakasato, Keisaku Hatanaka*, Kaoru Seki, Takashi Yoshimoto and Hisashi Kado**

Division of Neurosurgery, Institute of Brain Diseases, Tohoku University School of Medicine, Sendai 980, JAPAN
*ULVAC JAPAN, Ltd., Hagisono, Chigasaki 253, JAPAN
**Electrotechnical Laboratory, Tsukuba 305, JAPAN

INTRODUCTION

Sleep spindles are one of the characteristic EEG transients of sleep. They are found at a frequency range of 12.5-16.0 Hz and primarily at the vertex. This important pattern, however, is poorly understood neurophysiologically and its origin remains controversial. A previous neuromagnetic study (Hughes et al., 1976) indicated there are few sleep spindles in MEG recordings, however, we observed many MEG spindles above the central vertex (Nakasato et al., 1988). We also indicated that sleep spindles were under three distinct conditions:(i) when they were detected simultaneously in MEG and EEG, (ii) when they were detected alone in MEG without comparable EEG activity, (iii) when they were detected alone in EEG without comparable MEG activity. In this study, we measured the MEG at larger number of point over the scalp to show the spatial distribution of sleep spindles in MEG.

METHODS

In three normal health males, MEG and EEG recordings were obtained simultaneously without the aid of magnetic shielding. For MEG measurements, we used a single channel dc-SQUID with a second order gradiometer (BTi, 601 Biomagnetometer). The ambient noise level under control conditions was below 25 $fT/\sqrt{Hz}$ above 6 Hz. Subjects lay on a non-magnetic table with their eyes closed and were instructed to try not to move. The pickup coil was positioned over the wide area of the scalp around Cz. MEG was measured at one site in one session. After completion of the session, the MEG and EEG were drawn on chart paper. Then we counted the number of spindle bursts in the MEG and EEG recordings by visual observation.

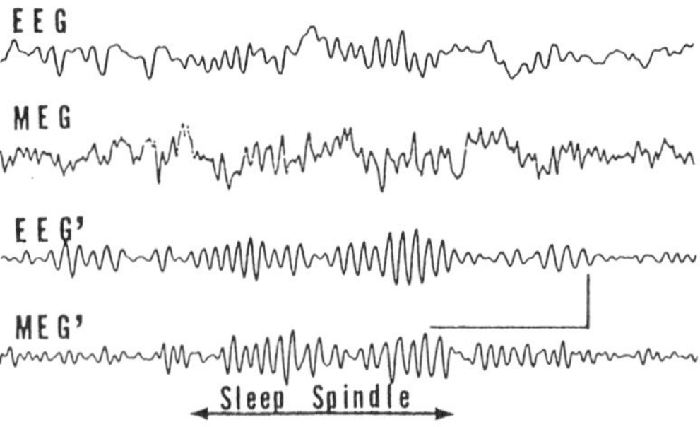

Fig. 1. An example of a spindle burst detected simultaneously in MEG(Cz) and EEG(Cz-A2). Recording bandwidth of EEG and MEG were 0.5-30Hz and 1-30Hz respectively. For analysis, bandwidth of EEG' and MEG' were 10-16Hz. Calibration: 1s, 100μV(EEG), 1.2pT(MEG), 50μV(EEG'), 600fT(MEG').

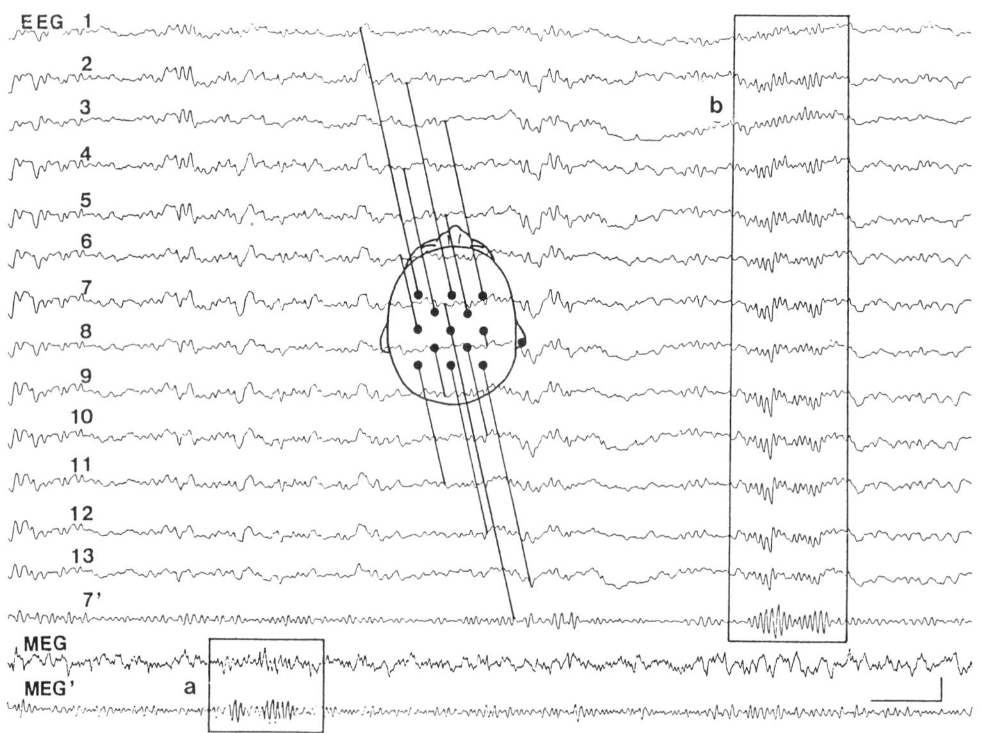

Fig.2. Difference in the time of appearance of spindle bursts in EEG and MEG. (a) an example of a sleep spindle burst detected alone in MEG without comparable EEG activity. (b) an example of a sleep spindle burst detected alone in EEG without comparable MEG activity. EEG 7 & 7': Cz-A2.
EEG 1-13: bandwidth 0.5-30Hz; Cal. 100μV, 1s.
EEG 7' : bandwidth 10-16Hz; Cal. 50μV, 1s.
MEG (Cz): bandwidth 1-30Hz; Cal. 1.2pT, 1s.
MEG'(Cz): bandwidth 10-16Hz; Cal. 600fT, 1s.

RESULTS

Data were recorded for 46±14 minutes including the time of awakeness and sleep in each session. Sleep spindles were under three distinct conditions stated in INTRODUCTION(Fig. 1, 2). MEG spindles were detected over wide area of scalp. They were most frequent near the central vertex (Fig. 3).

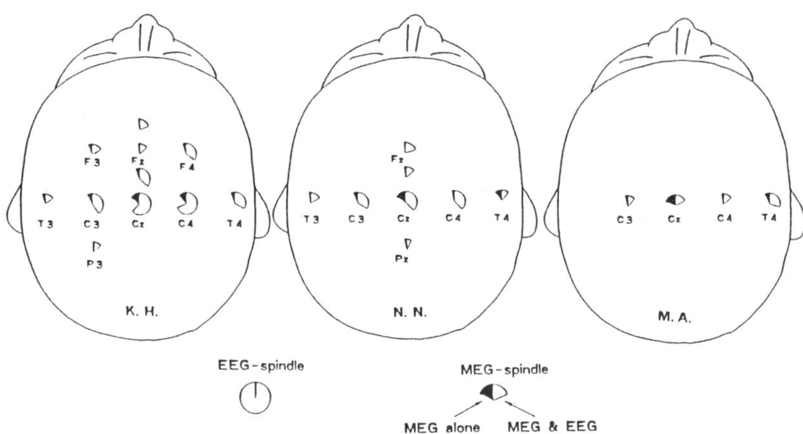

Fig.3. Spatial distribution of spindle bursts in MEG. Whole circle (100%) indicates the number of total EEG spindles in each session (n=247±61 in subject K.H., n=205±45 in subject N.N., and n=91±15 in subject M.A.). White sector indicates the number of sleep spindles recorded simultaneously in both MEG and EEG. Black sector indicates sleep spindles detected alone in MEG without comparable EEG activity.

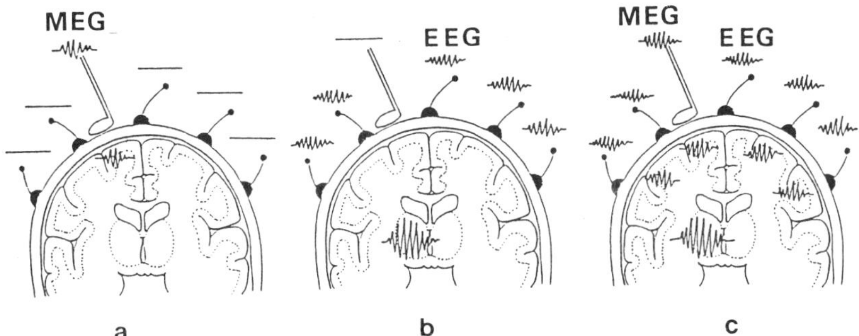

Fig.4. A hypothesis to explain difference in the time appearance of spindle bursts in EEG and MEG. a) If sleep spindle activity is confined to a small portion of cortex, it may be detectable by the MEG but undetectable by scalp EEG. b) If sleep spindle is active in deeper structure such as thalamus, it may be detectable by EEG over wide area of scalp owing to volume conduction but undetectable by MEG. c) If the wide area of cortex is activated by spindle in the deeper structure, spindle bursts are detectable by both MEG and scalp EEG.

DISCUSSION

We measured MEG and EEG simultaneously and observed MEG sleep spindles over wide area around the vertex. It has long been known that sleep spindles in the EEG are concentrated around the vertex and our result is consistent with this finding. However, in order to explain difference in the time appearance of spindle bursts in EEG and MEG, a new hypothesis is necessary (Fig. 4.). In this hypothesis, following two problems are to be considered: (i) The field spread of extracellular current (volume current) inside the head is significant as a source of EEG, but the contribution of volume current to the MEG is probably small(Okada, 1983). (ii) In EEG, the influence of the electrical conductivity of the skull and scalp is significant(Cooper et al., 1965). On the contrary, MEG is not influenced by conductivity of those tissues, and may provide more spatial information than EEG. If electrical activity is involved to only small volume of cortex, it may be detectable by MEG but undetectable by EEG. In fact, previous reports (Caderas et al., 1982) have shown that sleep spindles appear earlier from intracerebral recordings at superior frontal cortex than from scalp electrodes. Such findings are rich in implications for the interpretation of our own data.

In conclusion, the difference of time appearance of sleep spindle in EEG and MEG may contribute to explanation the difference between sources of EEG and MEG.

ACKNOWLEDGEMENTS

This work was supported in part by Grant-in-Aid for Scientific Research #63440053 from the Ministry of Education, Science and Culture of Japan, and the Nakatani Electronic Measuring Technology Association of Japan. We thank T.Otsuka, M.Koyanagi, N.Kasai and M.Nakanishi for their encouragement throughout this work.

REFERENCES

Caderas, M., Niedermeyer, E., Uematsu, S., Long, D.M., and Nastalski, J., 1982, Sleep spindles recorded from deep cerebral structures in man. Clin. Electroenceph., 13:216.

Cooper, R., Winter, A.L., Crow, H.J. and Walter, W.G., 1965, Comparison of subcortical, cortical and scalp activity using chronically indwelling electrodes in man. Electroenceph. Clin. Neurophysiol., 18:217.

Hughes, J.R., Hendrix, D.E., Cohen, J., Duffy, F.H., Mayman, C.I., Scholl, M.L., and Cuffin, B.N., 1976, Relationship of the magnetoencephalogram to the electroencephalogram. Normal wake and sleep activity. Electroenceph. Clin. Neurophysiol., 40:261.

Nakasato, N., Kado, H., Nakanishi, M., Koyanagi, M., Kasai,N., Niizuma, H., Yoshimoto, T., and Suzuki, J., 1988, Magnetic detection of sleep spindles in normal subjects. The 3rd Congress of Japan Biomagnetism and Bioelectromagnetics Society, June 3-4, Tokyo.

Okada, Y.,1983, Neurogenesis of evoked magnetic field, in: "Proc. NATO advanced study institute on biomagnetism," Plenum, New York, pp399-408.

MAGNETOENCEPHALOGRAPHY IN EPILEPSY RESEARCH AND ITS PERSPECTIVES

Marshall Balish and Susumo Sato

Neurophysiology Unit, Clinical Epilepsy Section, Medical Neurology Branch
National Institute of Neurological Disorders and Stroke, National Institutes
of Health, Bethesda, Md.

INTRODUCTION

Magnetoencephalographic studies of patients with epilepsy are still in their infancy, and the clinical value of magnetoencephalography (MEG) is uncertain [see Sato and Smith (1985) and Sato et al. (1987) for overviews]. The possible importance of such studies derives from an understanding of some simple clinical and epidemiologic data on epilepsy. Epilepsy occurs in about 0.5% of the population of the United States, and 10% to 20% of the patients do not respond to medical therapy. Many of the more than 300,000 patients with intractable epilepsy may be helped by surgical therapy. Currently, however, no more than several thousand patients per year are considered for epilepsy surgery, and fewer are operated on. Patients are generally considered good candidates for epilepsy surgery if they are refractory to medical therapy and if a concurrence of information from several sources points to a safely resectable (usually single) epileptogenic zone (Porter, 1984). Information from computed tomography (CT) or magnetic resonance imaging (MRI) is typically combined with information from functional testing, including neuropsychological testing, and, perhaps most importantly, electroencephalographic (EEG) examinations in an attempt to localize the epileptogenic focus. In many patients, this information is inconclusive, and invasive testing must be performed, including prolonged monitoring with implanted depth or subdural electrodes or intraoperative recording from the cortical surface, called electrocorticography (ECoG). For certainty of localization, depth (or subdural) recordings of seizures are considered by many the gold standard. These procedures are not without risk, and are technically difficult, time consuming, and costly.

The disadvantages of these procedures highlight the need for improved, noninvasive techniques to localize the epileptogenic focus. MEG is a noninvasive procedure, but it remains to be seen if it will provide sufficiently certain localizing information to supplant the invasive methods. This is the crux of the clinical question. Several groups have been exploring this question, each using somewhat different techniques. We will give an overview of the approach that we use and describe some of our results. In addition, we will relate our results to the work of others in the field. Finally, we will outline the limitations of present techniques and directions for further work

PATIENTS AND METHODS

We studied patients with focal epilepsy, most of whom were being evaluated for surgical treatment of their epilepsy. A seven-channel magnetometer manufactured by Biomagnetic Technologies Inc (BTI) with a second order gradiometer linked to DC-coupled SQUIDs is presently used, although a single-channel magnetometer was used in earlier studies (Rose et al.,1987a). Data acquisition hardware is linked to a Hewlett-Packard HP300 computer, and we currently employ data acquisition software supplied by BTI. A Mcdonnell Douglas "3Space" head digitizer was used in our earlier studies to obtain the head shape; currently, we use the probe position indicator (PPI) of the BTI system. The EEG is simultaneously monitored typically using both bipolar and referential leads covering the area of interest. One or two 21-channel EEG machines (Nihon-Kohden model 4321B) are used with typical filter settings of 1 to 70 Hz for EEG channels. MEG channels are also filtered at 1 to 100 Hz. The MEG and EEG channels are digitized (256 Hz,12 bits for spontaneous activity) and then stored on the HP300 computer. The digitized signals are also stored on video tape, using a Biomedical Monitoring Systems, Inc. (BMSI) Tape-32 unit, for future review. Measurements are performed in a magnetically shielded room. In some patients, EEG recording of epileptiform transients is also performed with closely spaced electrodes for EEG comparison. For these measurements, we also use data acquisition software provided by BTI.

The EEG and MEG are always measured simultaneously. For spontaneous activity (i.e., spikes), a manual triggering mode allows the physician to collect epochs (3-sec window) of data surrounding epileptiform discharges. During a typical session, multiple events are recorded at each magnetometer position and multiple magnetometer positions are recorded. We typically record from at least 5 magnetometer positions, yielding at least 35 measuring points. Events are evaluated visually and those with identical EEG appearance at different magnetometer locations are subjected to further analysis, including contour mapping and dipole fitting.

Visual analysis is used to group spike types for "single spike mapping" (Sato et al., 1985). Recently, software, including BTi's data editor, has been used to supplement the visual analysis, allowing classification of signals for further analysis. For localization, we generally assume a spherical model with volume currents, although in regions expected to show gross departure from sphericity, we have used more exact models (based on boundary-element analysis). Software for analysis was developed at NIH and subsequently compared to BTI's more computationally efficient software for contouring and dipole fitting (which uses a least squares fit to a homogeneous spherical model).

Many patients in whom we have performed MEG spike localization have had subsequent ECoG or prolonged monitoring with subdural electrodes. Information from these studies has been used to validate MEG localization.

RESULTS

An important observation is that spike discharges vary in configuration, with some disparity between EEG and MEG. Thus, we have recorded very similar EEG spikes with dissimilar MEG spikes, similar MEG spikes with dissimilar EEG spikes, and similar EEG spikes with and without MEG spikes. Rather than simply averaging spikes, which would potentially result in loss of information, we have selected comparable individual events (based on visual analysis of EEG signals) at each MEG recording position. We have reported the findings of several patients recorded and analyzed in this fashion (Rose et al., 1987b). In one of the patients reported, for example, interictal discharges were evident in right temporal regions on the EEG; these were of varying shapes and distribution and accompanied by MEG. At least six EEG spike types were distinguished and magnetic signals sampled at several magnetometer positions. The magnetic signals for each spike type were mapped and showed a dipolar pattern. Two spikes were localized in the frontal lobe and four spikes in the temporal lobe. EEG spike maps based on 73 closely spaced electrodes showed a single peak of negativity for the temporal spikes and a dipolar pattern for the frontal spikes. ECoG showed active frontal and temporal discharges, confirming the MEG data, as well as the EEG data.

We have now examined 28 epileptic patients since installation of the shielded room, and preliminary analysis on 12 of these patients who have had surgery confirms a good match between MEG predictions and the results of ECoG.

DISCUSSION

We have observed, especially in patients with discharges from the temporal lobe, that the dipolar pattern of the MEG signal is frequently asymmetric. We have shown that this results in part from departure of the local geometry from sphericity (Rose et al., 1987a). Another important factor arises from volume currents, which play a significant role in regions where there is departure from sphericity (Rose et al., 1989b). When recording from these regions, the magnetometer may not be truly tangential to the surface of the brain and thus may record radial as well as tangential components of a current dipole.

We have shown good agreement between MEG localization of epileptiform discharges and intraoperative ECoG. Similarly, locations of implanted dipoles appear to be well localized by MEG. For analysis of interictal discharges, we have taken the path of "single spike localization" in hopes that spatiotemporal patterns might be better explored than in techniques employing spike averaging. An obvious limitation of our method is that we have only a seven-channel magnetometer so that in general we must choose comparable spikes at each magnetometer location and combine this information for subsequent localization. An important point relates to the fact that we are assuming a single dipole source for each event. In general, the epileptogenic area, and certainly the discharging area as measured by ECoG, are not as restricted as this, and there is probably a zone of abnormal discharging tissue. It would be helpful if the extent and location of this zone were delineated by MEG measurements. It is certainly possible that if enough events are mapped with our "single spike technique" this epileptogenic zone will be delineated. We hope to test this hypothesis.

OTHER STUDIES

Other groups studying epilepsy with MEG have employed somewhat different analysis techniques. Sutherling et al. (1988) have typically averaged interictal discharges at each magnetometer location and estimated dipole locations (using either least-squares routines or routines dependent on interpeak distance in field maps). They have noted good agreement between MEG dipole localization of averaged spikes in nine patients with partial seizures and localization based on invasive EEG recording. They also have mapped the MEG fields of partial seizures in four patients (Sutherling et al., 1987) and have found good agreement between MEG-estimated source localization and, in two patients, findings from depth electrode recordings.

Ricci et al. (1987) have used a technique based on the relative covariance of MEG and EEG signals. They examined the frequency components of each signal, identified "abnormal components" in each, and then filtered the original signals with a narrow filter centered on this abnormal frequency. They then mapped the relative covariance of the filtered MEG and EEG signals, looking for dipolar maps. They employed least-squares fit routines to a spherical head model to localize those sources with dipolar maps. They reported their findings in 13 patients in whom MEG localization agreed with other localizing information, although few patients had undergone invasive studies for confirmation of localization.

LIMITATIONS AND FUTURE DIRECTIONS

Most studies, regardless of analysis techniques, have shown at least promising agreement between MEG localization and localization based on other supporting information. In spite of this, we are still far from answering the question of its clinical value. There are still several limitations of MEG that must be overcome:

1. Technical limitations include the limited number of channels presently available in commercial magnetometers. This precludes measuring large regions simultaneously and limits the spatiotemporal resolution of present studies. Magnetometers with 20 or more channels are just now becoming available and will hopefully improve localization; multichannel instruments will also reduce the time required for studies.

2. Conceptual problems include the simplistic modeling assumptions typically used in analyzing clinical data. In most work we have discussed, the generator of interictal discharges is modeled as a current dipole. It is clear from surface EEG recordings that the epileptogenic zone is not in general a small region; hence, models employing distributed source currents may be more realistic, although they may require more powerful analysis

hardware. It must also be determined when simple head models (i.e., homogeneous spherical models) are adequate for localization and when more sophisticated models will provide adequate localizing information. This is already being actively pursued. Techniques to combine information from EEG and MEG studies are presently being explored and may be very important to clinical studies. These techniques may need to be perfected in order for MEG to play a role in localization in epileptic patients with rare interictal events, for example.

Overall, MEG studies of epileptic patients are promising. They suggest that MEG can provide accurate three-dimensional localizing information in selected patients. However, there are limitations that must be overcome before MEG can be expected to be fairly evaluated and used on a routine clinical basis.

REFERENCES

Porter, R.J., 1984, Epilepsy: 100 Elementary Principles. WB Saunders, London.

Ricci, G.B., Romani, G.L., Salustri, C., et al., 1987, Study of focal epilepsy by multichannel neuromagnetic measurements. Electroencephalogr. Clin. Neurophysiol., 66:358-368.

Rose, D.F., Sato, S., Smith, P.D., and White, J., 1987a, Modelling the temporal region in patients with temporal lobe epilepsy. Phys. Med. Biol., 32:69-63.

Rose, D.F., Sato, S., Smith, P.D., et al., 1987b, Localization of magnetic interictal discharges in temporal lobe epilepsy. Ann. Neurol., 22:348-354.

Sato, S., Rose, D., and Porter, R., 1985, Single spike mapping. In :Weinberg, H., Stroink, G., and Katila. T., eds., Biomagnetism : Application and Theory. Pergamon Press, New York, pp. 261-263.

Sato, S., Rose, D., Smith, P., et al., 1987, Magnetoencephalography: Contribution to presurgical evaluation for temporal lobectomy. In: Wolf, P., Dam, M., Janz, D., and Dreifuss, F.E., eds., Advances in Epileptology, Vol. 16. Raven Press, New York, pp. 295-299.

Sato, S., and Smith, P.D., 1985, Magnetoencephalography. J. Clin. Neurophysiol., 2:173-192.

Sutherling, W.W., Crandall, P.H., Engel, J., et al., 1987, The magnetic field of complex partial seizures agrees with intracranial localizations. Ann. Neurol., 21:548-558.

Sutherling, W.W., Crandall, P.H., Cahan, L.D., and Barth, D.S., 1988, The magnetic field of epileptic spikes agrees with intracranial localizations in complex partial epilepsy. Neurology, 38:778-786.

RECENT DEVELOPMENTS

ON THE PHYSIOLOGICAL BASIS OF MAGNETOENCEPHALOGRAPHY (MEG)

Yoshio C. Okada

Magnetophysiology Laboratory, Department of Physiology and Biophysics, New York University Medical Center, New York, NY 10016

INTRODUCTION

This review discusses some of the progress made in recent years toward understanding the nature of generators of MEG signals. Attempts to rigorously relate cellular currents to an MEG signal have forced us to examine in detail the ways by which various currents in the volume conductor can give rise to such a signal. We will first consider this issue theoretically to elucidate how various currents may contribute to the MEG signal, then consider the magnitudes of their contributions determined in a particular experimental paradigm, namely in the in vitro preparation of turtle cerebellum, in order to make some general inferences about the nature of generators of MEG signals.

NATURE OF GENERATORS OF MEG SIGNAL: THEORETICAL CONSIDERATIONS

In evoked response paradigms one may assume that MEG signals arise from a non-ohmic transmembrane current (impressed current J^i) produced by conductance changes in the neuronal membrane. It produces an ohmic current J_i in the active cells (intracellular current), an ohmic current J_e in the interstitial space adjacent to the walls of active cells (extracellular current), an ohmic current in the non-active passive cells in the region surrounding the active tissue and an ohmic current farther out in the volume conductor. These ohmic currents are collectively called the volume current J^v. The current in the volume conductor everywhere can be expressed as $J = J^i + J^v = J^i - \sigma \nabla \Phi$, where σ is the conductivity of the intra- or extracellular space and Φ is the electrical potential in the volume conductor. The J^i itself does not produce an MEG signal at distances greater than the dimension of neurons, because the equivalent dipole moment of each impressed current element is small due to thinness of the membrane and because an ensemble of radially symmetric J^i's tend to mutually cancel their magnetic fields (Swinney and Wikswo, 1980; Plonsey, 1981). That is, the generators of MEG signals are all volume currents perturbed by conductivity boundaries in the head.

Advances in Biomagnetism
Edited by S.J. Williamson *et al.*
Plenum Press, New York

It has been shown that the magnetic field **B** due to the volume current $\mathbf{J}^v$ in an isotropic, piecewise homogeneous volume conductor is given by:

$$\mathbf{B} = \frac{\mu_o}{4\pi}\int_V \frac{\nabla'\times\mathbf{J}^v}{R}dV' - \frac{\mu_o}{4\pi}\int_S \frac{\mathbf{n}\times\mathbf{J}^v}{R}dS$$

where μ_o is the permeability of free space, R is the magnitude of the position vector between the field point and each source point, **n** is the normal unit vector at each point on the surfaces separating regions of differing electrical conductivities, dS is the surface element and the prime operation refers to the source coordinates (Plonsey, 1981, eq. 17; Wikswo, 1979). This equation separates the sources of the **B** field into the $\mathbf{J}^v$ within the open volume of each homogeneous region and the transverse to each boundary surface separating regions of differing conductivities. This separation of sources clearly brings out one important property of MEG signal; i.e. the volume current $\mathbf{J}^v$ away from conductivity boundaries does not produce any magnetic field, contrary to one's intuition, because $\nabla'\times\mathbf{J}^v = \nabla'\sigma\times\nabla'\Phi = 0$ everywhere locally in any isotropic homogeneous volume. The $\mathbf{J}^v$ in such a medium produces a **B** field only when the $\mathbf{J}^v$ transverse to the boundary surface is non-zero. Boundaries are thus crucial in the generation of MEG signals.

The surface currents can be classified into three categories. The first consists of the intra- and extracellular currents, $\mathbf{J}_i$ and $\mathbf{J}_e$, that are transverse to the inner and outer walls, respectively, of active cells, i.e. of those cells whose membranes contain generators of $\mathbf{J}^i$. These currents are collectively called the primary current $\mathbf{J}^p$ (Tripp, 1983) and they are the primary source of MEG signal. Often, it is believed that the $\mathbf{J}_i$ and $\mathbf{J}_e$ as defined above produce **B** fields of opposing polarity. One comes to this erroneous conclusion by noting the opposing directions of the $\mathbf{J}_i$ and $\mathbf{J}_e$ and by assigning the opposite polarities to their **B** fields. One should recall, however, that the $\mathbf{J}^v$ away from a membrane does not produce any magnetic field. The **B** fields are produced by the discontinuity of these currents along active membranes. Contrary to one's intuition, the fields from these surface currents in fact <u>add</u>, because the cross product term between the normal vector directed outward from an active membrane and $\mathbf{J}^v$ has the same direction for both $\mathbf{J}_i$ and $\mathbf{J}_e$.

The picture of the primary generators can be further simplified. As discussed in Okada (1983), the MEG signals are expected to be predominantly due to cells which have so-called "open field" morphologies (Lorente de No, 1947). These cells can be modeled as cylindrical core conductors (Llinas and Nicholson, 1974). For cylindrically symmetrical core conductors, the primary current generator of the MEG signal can be equivalently represented as a sum of current dipoles chained along the length of the core conductors (Plonsey, 1981; Tripp, 1983). We believe that this representation of the primary generators is sufficiently general in interpreting the MEG signals and thus used this model in analyzing our data. At large measuring distances, the equivalent primary generator may be simply represented as an opposing pair of current dipoles when the pattern of current sink and source is symmetrical as in the case of an action current in an axon and as a single current dipole when the pattern is asymmetrical as in case of a synaptic input at one end of a dendrite (Okada, 1983). It is important to note that these equivalent representations include the boundary effect. For example, a current dipole **Q**, which is defined as $\mathbf{Q} = \mathbf{J}dv$, takes into account the presence of an active membrane. Thus, its magnetic field is non-zero, even though **J** is a volume current. An apparent paradox arises if one forgets the implicit role of the boundary (cf. Tripp, 1983).

The second category is the volume current along outer and inner walls of non-active membranes, i.e. those membranes in which $\mathbf{J}^i = 0$. The contribution of these currents should be negligible, since the currents on the opposite sides of a passive membrane should have the same direction and, therefore, should produce

B fields of opposite polarity. Note that the field is determined by the cross product of **n** and $\mathbf{J}^v$ with **n** directed outward from the membrane. Consequently, the membrane boundaries in the tissue outside of an active region can be ignored and this region can be treated as a homogeneous medium for our purposes.

The third category is the surface current along the boundaries separating large or thick regions of differing conductivities, e.g. along the skull-cerebrospinal fluid boundary or the interface between an anoxic and a normoxic region. The potential across this boundary is continuous as in the second category. This type of surface current may contribute significantly to the MEG signal outside the head, the amount of contribution depending on the geometry of particular boundaries (cf. Huang et al., this volume). They give rise to the so-called secondary sources at such an interface that is defined as $D\sigma\mathbf{n}\Phi$, where $D\sigma$ is the difference in conductivity across the boundary, the unit vector **n** is normal to the boundary and Φ the electrical potential at the interface (Geselowitz, 1967).

NATURE OF CURRENT GENERATORS: EXPERIMENTAL EVALUATION

In the past two years we have succeeded in experimentally evaluating the relative contributions of the intra- and extracellular currents along active membranes and the secondary current generators at interfaces separating large regions of different conductivities. Here we summarize our principal results. See Okada et al. (1988) for the experimental detail.

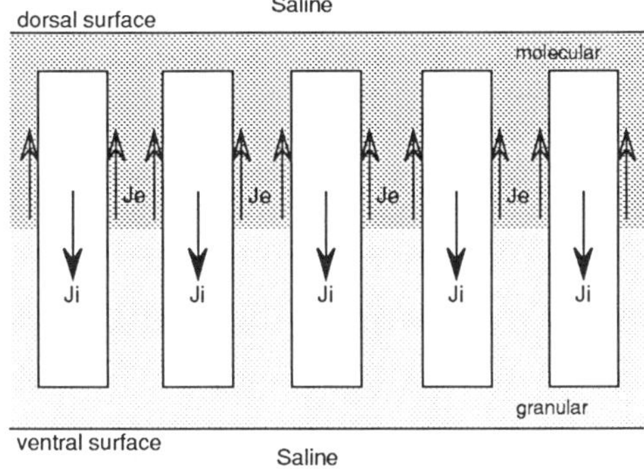

Fig. 1.

Figure 1 schematically shows the cross-sectional picture of the turtle cerebellum immersed in a large bath of physiological saline. This cerebellum, viewed from the top of the bath, has a set of cells perpendicular to cerebellar surface. They are here all represented by core conductors which extend over the depth of the cerebellum.

Consider that the climbing fibers are stimulated. Their axons synaptically terminate on the lower third of the Purkinje cell dendrites near the soma, producing an impressed current $\mathbf{J}^i$ in this dendritic zone. The $\mathbf{J}^i$ produces an intracellular current $\mathbf{J}_i$ in these active neurons and an extracellular current $\mathbf{J}_e$ in the surrounding region. In this case, we need to determine the MEG signals that can be produced by $\mathbf{J}_i$ summed over all the active neurons, by $\mathbf{J}_e$ along the outer walls of these active neurons, by the $\mathbf{J}_e$ at the boundary between the cerebellum and saline and by the $\mathbf{J}_e$ at the conductivity boundary between the molecular and granular layers.

We used the following formulations to estimate the contributions of these generators of the MEG signal. First, a coarse-grain approximation was made for the intra- and extracellular spaces (Nicholson, 1973). That is, the discontinuity across these two domains were smoothed out and they were considered to coexist in the same space - they were considered to form a bi-domain (Roth et al., 1988). $\nabla\cdot(\mathbf{J}_e + \mathbf{J}_i) = 0$ by the conservation of charge. Thus, $\nabla\cdot\sigma_e\nabla\Phi_e = \nabla\cdot\mathbf{J}_i = -I_m$ where I_m is the current source-density (Nicholson, 1973). According to this formulation, we could experimentally estimate J_i and J_e from the measured values of σ_e and Φ_e. To simplify the experimental analysis, a large volume of tissue (2 x 3 mm^2 x 1 mm thickness) was nearly uniformly activated, so that we could consider the one-dimensional version of this equation, parallel to these principal core conductors.

The stimulation of one peduncle with a brief electrical stimulus (50 μs) was found to produce activity mostly in the ipsilateral side of the cerebellum. The mapping of the evoked extracellular response (Okada and Nicholson, 1987) showed that the activity was nearly uniform over a surface area of 5-6 mm^2. Thus, the laminar potential measurements were carried out at the potential extremum within this active tissue to determine $\Phi_e(z)$ as a function of depth z. In our most recent study, we have measured σ_e as well as Φ_e for the same cerebellum, and estimated J_i from the one dimensional equation: $J_i(z) = -J_e(z) + J_e(0)$, where $J_e(0)$ is the current at the boundary between the cerebellum and saline on the ventral side. Now, the **B** field can be produced by both $J_i(z)$ and $J_e(z)$, since they are the surface currents along the inner and outer walls of the active neurons. Furthermore, the **B** fields due to $J_i(z)$ and $J_e(z)$ add, even though these currents are directed oppositely, as mentioned earlier.

Their **B** fields were calculated by applying the Biot-Savart law to the net dipole moments Q_i and Q_e associated with $J_i(z)$ and $J_e(z)$, respectively, summed over the entire active tissue and to the total net dipole moment $Q_{total} = Q_i + Q_e$ where, for j = i or e,

$$Q_j = \int_A dA \int_0^L J_j dz$$

This formulation ignored the differences in depth of the dipoles chained along the longitudinal axis of the core conductors, since the measuring distance (17 mm) was very large compared to the thickness (1 mm) of the cerebellum. The area A and thickness L of the active tissue were determined experimentally as in our earlier study (Okada and Nicholson, 1987).

In addition to the currents along active membranes, the **B** field can be thought of as produced by the boundaries between the molecular and granular layers and at the cerebellar surface. To estimate their contributions, we modeled the turtle cerebellum by a rectangular box whose dimensions were 5 x 5 x 1.08 mm with a boundary separating the molecular and granular layers at a depth of 630 μm from the dorsal surface. The conductivities of the molecular layer, granular layer and the saline were experimentally determined (Okada et al., unpublished) and found to be 0.30, 0.19 and 1.27 Siemens/m, respectively. We then applied the boundary element method to solve for **B** for this geometry (cf. Huang et al. this volume).

These analyses have enabled us to explicitly calculate the component of the **B** field normal to bath surface (Bz) that should be due to each of the dominant contributors. Figure 2a shows the predicted field due to the J_i alone and that due to the combined contributions of J_i and J_e. Fig. 2b indicates the fields associated with the secondary sources produced by the primary current generators, separately for J_i and J_e. The sum of the Bz fields due to the primary and secondary sources is compared with the measured Bz field in Fig. 2c. These calculations are parameter-free predictions. That is, all the parameters (e.g. σ_e, Φ_e and size of active tissue A) needed for the calculations were obtained experimentally within each cerebellum.

Several results are noteworthy. First, the measured Bz field is closely related to the J_i in temporal waveform. Second, the J_i contributes to the Bz field much more than the J_e. This result may depend on the geometry of regions of differing conductivities adjoining the active tissue and, thus, some care should be taken in generalizing this result. Third, the boundary effect can produce a magnetic field that is even larger than that due to the primary sources.

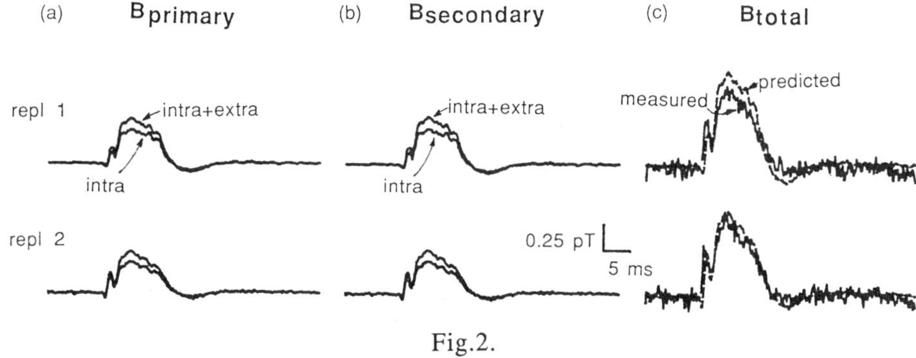

Fig.2.

The contribution of secondary sources is especially strong in our preparation, since the thinness of the cerebellum makes the secondary sources very proximal to the primary source and the conductivity ratio across the cerebellar surface is large. However, secondary sources may play a significant role even for the MEG signal from the human head when similar conditions prevail as in the case of cortical sources, for example, where the primary sources are close to the pial surface and the ratio of conductivity may be comparable to the turtle cerebellum at the boundary between the cerebral cortex and the cerebrospinal fluid. The effect of secondary source is to simply (in this case) increase the amplitude of the field due to the primary sources, without distorting the waveform. Lastly, the predicted MEG signal agrees surprisingly well with the magnitude of the measured field, considering that there was no free-parameter in these predictions. This last result suggests that all the dominant generators of the MEG signal were taken into account in our analysis.

CONCLUSION

In one case study we have demonstrated that the MEG signal is directly related to the intracellular current, with the signal predominantly coming from intra- rather than extracellular current generators. The secondary sources at conductivity boundaries may play significant roles when the boundary is close to the primary generator and the conductivity ratio across the boundary is large. The results for the turtle cerebellum suggests that the MEG signal measured non-invasively from the humans may also be directly related to the intra-neuronal currents.

ACKNOWLEDGEMENT

I wish to thank my colleagues (Drs. Nicholson, Chan, Tranchina, Huang and Lopez) for making this research possible and also wish to acknowledge the generous support from National Institute of Neurological Disorders and Stroke (R01-NS21149).

REFERENCES

Geselowitz, D.B. 1967. On bioelectric potentials in an inhomogeneous volume conductor. Biophys. J., 7:1-11.

Geselowitz, D. B. 1970. On the magnetic field generated outside an inhomogeneous volume conductor by internal current sources. IEEE Trans. Mag., MAG-6:346-347.

Huang, J. C., Okada, Y. C. and Nicholson, C. 1989. Conductivity boundaries may produce stronger magnetic fields than the primary current source: Comparison of three analytical methods. This Conference.

Llinas, R. R. and Nicholson, C. 1974. Analysis of field potentials in the central nervous system. In: A. Remond, (ed.), Handbook of Electroencephalography and Clinical Neurophysiology. Elsevier, Amsterdam, 61-85.

Lorente de No, R. 1947. Action potential of the motoneurons of the hypoglossus nucleus. J. Cell. Comp. Physiol., 29:207-287.

Nicholson, C. 1973. Theoretical analysis of field potentials in anisotropic ensembles of neuronal elements. IEEE Trans. BME-20:278-288.

Okada, Y. C. 1983. Neurogenesis of evoked magnetic fields. In: S. J. Williamson, G.-L. Romani, L. Kaufman and I. Modena, (eds.), Biomagnetism: An Interdisciplinary Approach, Plenum, New York

Okada, Y.C. and Nicholson, C. 1987. Currents underlying the magnetic evoked field in the cerebellum. In: K. Atsumi, M. Kotani, S. Ueno, T. Katila, and S. J. Williamson, (eds.), Biomagnetism '87. Tokyo Denki Univ. Press, Tokyo, 198-201.

Okada, Y. C. and C. Nicholson. 1988. Magnetic evoked field associated with transcortical currents in turtle cerebellum. Biophys. J. 53:723-731.

Plonsey, R. W. 1981. Generation of magnetic fields by the human body (theory). In: S. N. Erne, H.-D. Hahlbohm, and H. Lubbig, (eds.), Biomagnetism, Walter de Gruyter, Berlin, 177-205.

Roth, B. J. and Wikswo,. J. P. Jr 1985. The magnetic field of a single axon: a comparison of theory and experiment. Biophys. J., 48:93-109.

Swinney, K. R. and Wikswo, J. P. Jr. 1980. A calculation of the magnetic field of a nerve action potential. Biophys. J. , 32:719-732.

Tripp, J. 1983. Physical concepts and mathematical models. In: S. J. Williamson, G.-L. Romani, L. Kaufman and I. Modena, (eds.), Biomagnetism: An Interdisciplinary Approach, Plenum, New York, 101-139.

Wikswo, J. P. Jr. 1978. The calculation of the magnetic field from a current distribution: Application to finite element techniques. IEEE Trans. MAG-14:1076-1077.

Woosley, J. K., Roth, B. J. and Wikswo, J. P. Jr. 1985. The magnetic field of a single axon: a volume conductor model. Math. Biosci. 76:1-36.

APPLICATION OF A MULTICHANNEL MEG-SYSTEM IN TEMPORAL LOBE EPILEPSY

H. Stefan[1], S. Schneider[2], K. Abraham-Fuchs[2], J. Bauer[1], H. Feistel[3], U. Neubauer[4], W. J. Huk[4]

1 Department of Neurology, University Erlangen-Nürnberg
2 Medical Engineering Group, Siemens AG
3 Department of Nuclear Medicine, University Erlangen-Nürnberg
4 Department of Neurosurgery, University Erlangen-Nürnberg

INTRODUCTION

Magnetic field measurements in partial epilepsy may improve the localization of epileptic activity. Measurements in patients with epilepsy have already been demonstrated in various studies using single or few channel biomagnetic systems (Barth et al. 1984, Ricci et al. 1985, Rose et al. 1987, Sutherling et al. 1987, Sato et al. 1987, Vieth et al. 1988). Our study was performed to evaluate measurements with a multichannel biomagnetic system (KRENIKON / Gudden et al. 1989, Hoenig et al. 1989) on the basis of standard presurgical procedures in patients with pharmacoresistant epilepsies.

METHOD

Multichannel recordings with up to 31 magnetic channels were performed in 10 patients with pharmacoresistant temporal lobe epilepsies. Simultaneously to MEG, EEG (scalp-,sphenoidal- and foramen ovale electrodes) was recorded during withdrawal of antiepileptic drugs. An MEG recording lasted five to ten minutes. From the MEG locations of epileptic sources were reconstructed by the moving dipole algorithm. Biomagnetic source localization was carried through with an iterative nonlinear optimization algorithm. The model of a current dipole immersed in a homogeneous sphere was used. The sphere was fitted to the patients brain with aid of an MR-image. Source locations were correlated with anatomic brain structures from 3D MR-images. Further to presurgical evaluation intensive video-EEG-monitoring including sphenoidal-, foramen ovale electrodes and interictal and ictal 99m TC-HMPAO SPECT measurements were performed. Intraoperative ECoG was recorded. In one case electric activity subsequent to the epileptic focus could be localized from the MEG after noise reduction by means of a spatio temporal correlation technique (Abraham et al. 1989).

Advances in Biomagnetism
Edited by S.J. Williamson *et al.*
Plenum Press, New York

RESULTS

From 10 recorded patients analysis of 8 patients showed that at least in 7 patients a lobar congruence or even an intra lobar congruence was found. The comparison of the findings concerning EEG, MRI, SPECT and ECoG (in case of operated patients) is shown in the table.

<u>Table1</u> Comparison of the results of different investigation techniques; r = right, l = left, + = ECoG performed, SI = increased signal intensity in MRI, inf. mes. = inferior mesial temporal.

Case-no.	EEG Sp,FO	ECoG Op	MRI	SPECT	MEG
1	inf.mes.l.	+	astrocytoma	inf.mes.l.	inf.mes. (hippoc.)
2	temp. r.	+	angioma	temp. r.	surrounding tissue angioma
3	temp. r.	+	cyst	temp. r.	surrounding tissue cyst + inf.mes.post. + lat. temp.
4	inf.mes.l.	+	normal	temp. l.	temp.
5	inf.mes.l.	+	hippocam-pus l.(SI)	temp. l.	mid-line region
6	temp. r.		normal	temp. r.	temp.
7	temp. r.	+	sylvian fissure r. (SI)	temp. r.	temp.
8	temp. r.	+	angioma	temp. r.	surrounding tissue angioma temp.

Intraoperative ECoG was performed in 5 cases which was in agreement with the preoperative localization results. In one case the focal epileptic activity was localized inferior mesial temporal at the hippocampus; in 3 cases at the surrounding tissue of an angioma (2, 8) or cyst (3). In 3 patients the magnetic source localization showed focal activity in the area of sylvian fissure (4, 6, 7). During the presurgical evaluation positive findings were seen 60 % to 100 % for the different investigation techniques.

In case 8 the interictal EEG showed focal epileptic activity temporal posterior right and inferior mesial right. At seizure onset rhythmic polyspike activity was recognized temporal right inferior mesial. MRI disclosed an angioma temporal right. The primary activity within the interval of a spike complex was localized from the MEG near the edge of the angioma. Subsequent to the focal epileptic activity two further centres of electric activity could be localized with the method of spike averaging by spatio-temporal correlation, which are interpreted as propagation of the epileptic activity (Fig.1 and 2).

In animal experiments cortical travelling waves have been observed (Petsche and Sterc 1967) indicating that potential fields of epileptic activities are not stationary. Interictal epileptic activity in the EEG often is widely dispersed and it is not definitely known if such abnormalities originated at the recording side or had been propagated there (Rossi 1973, Lieb et al. 1978). Therefore more information than obtained by means of EEG recordings regarding movement of epileptic foci would be

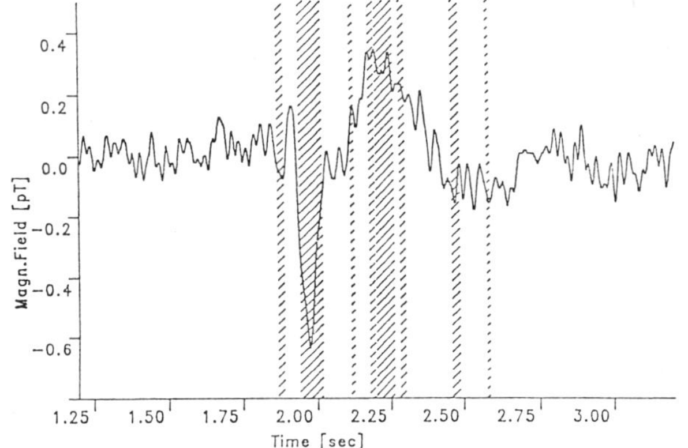

Fig.1.
Averaged spike-wave event (magnetic channel); time intervals in which dipoles were localized are shaded.

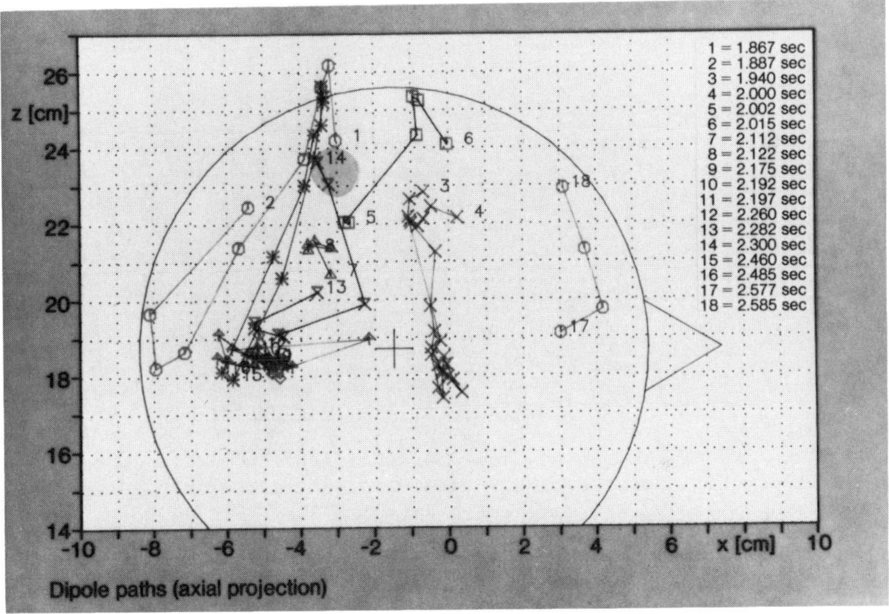

Fig.2. Dipole propagation, begin and end of each localized interval is given by the points 1 to 18, with the corresponding times during the spike-wave event shown above.

desirable for presurgical evaluation. Barth et al. (1984) observed changes in the magnetic field patterns within averaged spike wave events which indicate the possibility of propagation of epileptic activity and which could be interpreted as sequential sources due to deep-superficial propagation (Sutherling and Barth 1989). Our results obtained by means of high resolution Multichannel MEG and intracranial foramen ovale EEG recordings reveal the total activation process during the whole spike wave complex.

CONCLUSION

Comparison with standard presurgical investigation procedures and intraoperative ECoG shows that MRI correlated current source localization by means of multichannel recordings offer important clinical advantages e.g.:

1. Non- or only minor invasive focus localization even of deeper sources in the temporal lobe using combined MEG/scalp-EEG or invasive EEG recordings. The error derived from system analysis is below 1 cm for superficial sources and about 2 cm for deep sources.

2. Considerable shortening of the time of investigation (data acquisition time mean 10 minutes per hemisphere; total investigation 1 - 2 hours including EEG recording).

3. Localization of a single event is possible.

Recognition of repeated movement of deep sources of epileptic activity in the human brain by means of combined MEG/EEG recordings was performed for the first time.

REFERENCES

Abraham et al., 1989, to be published.

Barth D.S., Sutherling W., Engel J.R., Beatty J.: Neuromagnetic evidence of spatially distributed sources underlying epileptiform spikes in the human brain, Science 223, 293 - 296, 1984.

Gudden F., Hoenig H.E., Reichenberger H., Schittenhelm R., Schneider S.: A multi-channel system for use in biomagnetic diagnosis in neurology and cardiology: principle, method and initial results, Electromedica 57, 1989.

Hoenig H.E., Daalmanns G., Folbert W., Reichenberger H., Schneider S., Seifert H.: Biomagnetic multi-channel system with integrated SQUIDs and first order gradiometers operating in a shielded room, Cryogenics, 1989.

Lieb J.P., Woods S.C., Siccardi A., Crandall P.H., Walter D.O., Leake B.: Quantitative analysis of depth spiking in relation to seizure foci in patients with temporal lobe epilepsy, Electroencephalography & Clin. Neurophysiol. 44, 1978, 641 - 663.

Petsche H., Sterc J.: The significance of the cortex for the travelling phenomenon of brain waves. Electroen. & Clin. Neurophys. pp: 11 - 22, 1968.

Ricci G.B., Leone R., Romani G.L., Campitelli F., Buonomo S., Modena I.:3-D neuromagnetic localization of sources of interictal activity in cases of focal epilepsy. In: Weinberg H., Stroink G., Katila T. (eds) Biomagnetism: Application and Theory. Pergamon, New York pp: 304 - 310, 1985.

Rose D.F., Sato S., Smith P.D. et al.: Localization of magnetic interictal discharges in temporal lobe epilepsy, Ann. Neurol. 22, 1987, 354.

Rossi G.F.: Problems of analysis and interpretation of electrocerebral signals in human epilepsy. A neurosurgeon's view. In MAB Brazier (ed) Epilepsy: Its phenomena in Man Acad Press, New York, pp: 259 - 285 (1973).

Sato S., Rose D.F., Kufta C.V.: Localization of interictal spikes using a seven-channel magnetometer, Biomagnetism, Proc. 6, Int. Conf. on Biomagn., Tokyo Univ. Press: pp 206, 1987.

Schneider S., Abraham-Fuchs K., Daalmaans G., Folbert W., Hoenig H.E., Reichenberger H., Röhrlein G., Seifert H., Wirth A.: Development and performance of a multichannel system for studies of biomagnetic signals of brain and heart, this conference.

Sutherling W.W., Crandall P.H., Engel J.R., Darcey T.M., Cahan L.D., Barth D.S.: The magnetic field of complex partial seizures agrees with intracranial localizations. Ann. of Neurol. Vol. 21, No. 6: 548 - 558, 1987.

Sutherling, W.W. and Barth D.S.: Neocortical propagation in temporal lobe spike foci on magnetoencephalography and electroencephalography. Ann. Neurol. 25: 373 - 381, 1989.

Vieth J., Stefan H., Meyer C., Grummich P., Hauk D., Üllein T., Schüler P.: Herdbefunde im MEG und EEG in: Epilepsie 87 Hrgb. E.G. Speckmann u. D.G.Palm 394 - 398, Einhorn Presse Verlag 1988.

MAPPING OF MEG AND EEG IN NORMALS AND EPILEPTIC PATIENTS

Kholodov Yu.A., Gorbach A.M., Verkhlutov V.M.,
Maragey R.A., Konyshev V.A.

Laboratory of Electromagnetic Neurophysiology
Institute of Higher Nervous Activity & Neurophysiology
Academy of Sciences, Moscow, USSR

INTRODUCTION

Using the EEG-mapping a frontal and occipital extrema of alpha-rhythm in the human were found, their location being constant in different subjects (Lehmann, 1971, 1987). In order to study the individual variability of EEG and MEG and to localize a sources of the brain rhythms we have mapped the electric and magnetic fields of the human brain in alpha-frequencies for healthy adults and in theta- and delta-frequencies for patients suffering from epileptic seizures.

METHOD

We used the technique of magnetic field measurements by second-order SQUID-magnetometer with noise level equal to 40 fT/Hz reported preliminary (Gorbach, 1987) for both 16 healthy volunteers and 13 patients. In each case we obtained the interpolated maps of the distribution of MEG-amplitude spectrum in corresponding frequencies. During MEG measurements the subjects were lying on the bed in the dim room in the resting state with closed eyes. The MEG measurements took about 3 hours per day for 3 days. A distribution of both the EEG-amplitude spectrum and the instant amplitudes of normal EEG digitally filtered in alpha-range were interpolated over 16 points. A special algorithm for dynamic review of the latter was used. Using the image processing and analysis system (Pericolor 2001, Numelec, France) the 16 chanels of filtered EEG and film consisted of 512 isopotential maps were simultaneously displayed. To contrasting the low-amplitude areas of the maps we used the non-linear colour scale.

In the study of alpha-activity the subjects were right-handed normals (10 men and 6 women) between 20 and 30 years of age. They were divided into 2 groups. In first group the MEG measurements were carried out over 40 points (3 subjects, preliminary mapping), in second that it was done over 60-150 points (13 subjects, detail mapping). In the case of patients the MEG study was carried out in 2 groups. The first group consisted of patients of both sexes between 16 and 29 years of age with preliminary diagnoses "petit mal" (2 patients) and "focal epilepsy" (3 patients). The second group consisted of 7 children, being 10-15 years old, suffering from epileptic seizures of perinatal origin. For 2 patients we have repeated the map

Advances in Biomagnetism
Edited by S.J. Williamson *et al.*
Plenum Press, New York

ping of the MEG and EEG amplitude spectrum a year after the first one. The patients were also tested by the Luria's neuropsychological test of personality (Luria,1973) for analysis of topology of the intrahemispherical disfunction and the deficiency of the interhemispherical interaction. This part of the research was done at the Institute of Pediatry and Surgery of Ministry of Health of the USSR. Thus a double blind control was held in our study. Using the correspondance of MEG points on the helmet and its edges with nasion, inion, meatus and canthus we carefully estimated the probable localization of sources in the certain structures of the brain.

RESULTS

The magnetic field maps in alpha-range in normal subjects showed a few powerful extrema of different intensity in the temporo-parieto-occipital areas (see Fig. 1, left) and was stable for 3 days till month. In 2 patients the maps in theta-range have not changed after a year.

A multiple of magnetic field extrema of alpha-activity confirmed the existence of multiple sources in this frequence range. The spatial distribution of these extrema was found to be symmetrical in relation to the midline of the head, and charachterized by significant amplitude gradients. By using the dipole-like distributions of the magnetic field the sources of alpha-rhythm have been localized within s. calcarina and s. parieto-occipitalis of the cortex. We did not find the magnetic field extrema in the precentral or the frontal areas where EEG-extremum have been observed in some subjects. The position of the EEG-extrema at the amplitude spectrum distribution coincided with the MEG-extrema in the occipital areas.

In most cases the dynamic review of the isopotential maps of the instant EEG-amplitudes revealed radial or spiral waves. Each spiral wave had center which was formed by rotation of the null isopotential line around its intrinsic point and migrated from one area to another. We have found no more than one center per each hemisphere in both the central and the occipital areas. The appearence of spiral waves coincided with begin of the spindle in most leads. Their rotation directions variated from one spindle to another, from one subject to other. But in the case of one center per each hemisphere the directions were opposite every time in different hemisphere. Then we observed the confluence of the isopotential lines of both centers along the midline of the head in frontal and precentral areas with their subsequent distortion and annihilation. These features are charachteristic of the autowaves in the active media concluding a heart tissue (Allesie et al., 1973).

Whereas the routine EEG in 7 ill children revealed widespread theta-activity (diffusing type) the localization of the epileptic sources as a result of the MEG-mapping in delta- and theta-ranges (see fig. 1, right) was found to coincide with the lesion foci revealed by the neuropsychological tests which accuracy for some cortex areas is about 2 cm.

DISCUSSION

The analysis of the revealed individual differences of the spatial distribution of the magnetic field extrema allowed us to divide the subjects into three groups and to propose the hypothesis concerning correspondance of these groups to known variants of the position of the s. calcarina and the s. parieto-occipitalis in the human brain (Blinkov, 1955).

The absence of the extrema of the magnetic field in the precentral and the frontal areas may be explained either by the low spatial sensitivity of the method or the absence of the powerful sources in these areas. The des-

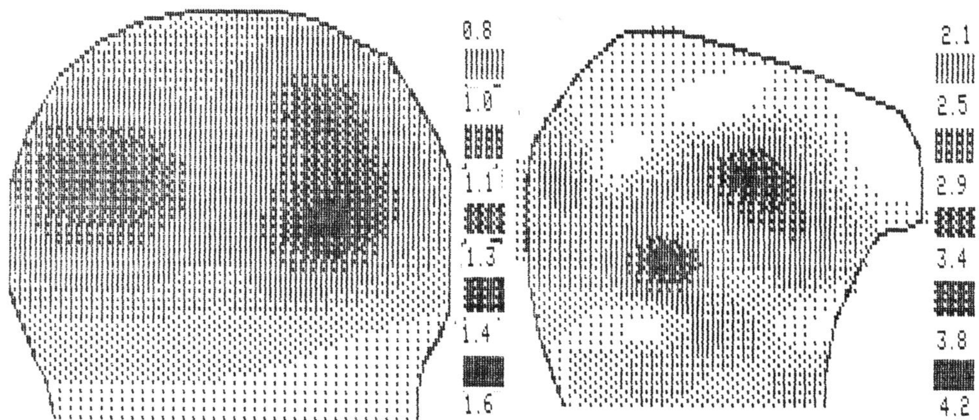

Fig.1 Left: Amplitude-spectrum distribution of MEG in alpha-range(9.0-11.0 Hz) at occiput in normal subject.
Right: Amplitude-spectrum distribution of MEG in delta-range (3.4-4.6 Hz) at right hemisphere in ill. Field in pT.

cribed spiral waves of the potential relief is assumed to be due to the morphofunctional organization of the given EEG. Such organization is characterized by sequential activation of the pools of cortex columns (f. e. within the walls of the s. parieto-occipitalis) in certain spatial order through the thalamo-cortex and cortex-cortex projections that results in the rotation and center migration. As null isopotential line devides the negative sites from positive ones its rotation could be modeled by switching of the groups of tangential equivalent dipoles located in TPO areas. This explains the existance of magnetic field extrema in alpha-range in the vicinity of these areas. Confluence of isopotential lines in frontal areas may explain the appearence of frontal electric extrema as conducted from parietal and occipital sources.

The radial and spiral scanning described have a pivot and consequently may indicate the actual source of generation of alpha-rhythm as compared to an idea of united circuit of the EEG waveforms where it is not possible to distinguish its origin (Dubikajtis, 1982). The finding of the centers of radial scanning in TPO areas may argue in favour of hypothesis concerning the involving of the certain scanning mechanisms to consequent cyclic excitation of spatially separated sensor areas of the cortex, the afferent flow being quantized with rate of alpha-rhythm. Thus the magnetic and electric fields distributions obtained could be generated by tangentially or radially oriented sources lying within the s. calcarina and by tangentially oriented sources lying within the s. parieto-occipitalis, their orientation being opposite in both hemispheres.

In the coming the comparison of the experimental and model maps of the EEG and MEG will allow to say about electromagnetic tomography method as a new that of function studies.

REFERENCES

Allessie, M., Bonke, F., Schopman, F., 1973, Circus movement in rabbit muscle as a mechanism of tachycardia, Circul. Res., 33:54-57.

Blinkov, S. M., 1955, The features of an architechture of human brain, Moscow, p. 155.

Gorbach, A. M., 1987, Method of recording of human brain magnetic field, J. Higher nervous activity, 37:587-590.

Dubikajtis W. W., 1982, The probable significance of short-term processes of spatio-temporal organization of EEG in relation to psychic activity formation, J. Human physiology., 5:757-764.

Lehmann, D., 1971, Multichanel topography of human alpha EEG fields, EEG & Clin. Neurophysiol., 31:439-449.

Lehmann, D., Ozaki,H., Pal,I., 1987, EEG alpha map series: brain microstates by space-oriented adaptive segmentation, EEG & Clin. Neurophysiol., 67:271-288.

Luria, A. R., 1973, The principles of the neuropsychology, Moscow Univ., M., p. 374.

Williamson, S. J., Kaufman, L., 1981, Magnetic fields of cerebral cortex, in: W. de Gruyter, Biomagnetism.,B.-N.Y., pp. 353-402.

TEMPLATE ANALYSIS ON INTERICTAL NEUROMAGNETIC DATA FROM CASES OF FOCAL AND GENERALIZED EPILEPSY

G.B. Ricci*, S.N. Erne'**, C. Del Gratta#, M. Peresson*, V. Pizzella, G.L. Romani##, G. Torrioli

Istituto di Elettronica dello Stato Solido - CNR. Via Cineto Romano 42, 00156 Roma, ITALY
*Dipartimento di Scienze Neurologiche, Universita' di Roma *"La Sapienza"*, Roma, ITALY
**Physicalisch-Technische Bundesanstalt Institut Berlin, FRG
#Supported by grant by CITEC S.p.A., Roma, ITALY
##Istituto di Fisica Medica, Universita' *"G. D'Annunzio"*, Chieti, ITALY

INTRODUCTION

The investigation of partial (focal) epilepsy by neuromagnetic measurements has provided significant results on the localization of epileptogenic foci related to intercritical activity (Barth et al., 1982; Chapman et al., 1983; Barth et al., 1984; Ricci et al., 1985). It has been demonstrated, however, that quite often the morphology of epileptic signals is not unique (Rose et al., 1987). This may be interpreted in terms of various neural groups simultaneously active but underlying different *firing* process. If we do not consider quasi-rhythmic activity, for which the best analytical approach remains the Relative Covariance Method (RCM) (Chapman et al., 1983), it would be particularly useful to identify a procedure that permits to reliably select epileptic signals (spikes, sharp waves, spike-and-wave complexes), and to eventually carry out a source localization procedure from the magnetic field distribution over the scalp relative to each of the selected epileptiform signals, henceforth referred to as epileptic complexes. An automatic selection procedure would be of great help also in the investigation of more complex diseases like, for instance, generalized epilepsy. In these pathologies the lack of simultaneity, which so far characterizes all neuromagnetic measurements, even those carried out with the largest systems today available, is one crucial drawback, the other being the variety of different signals that are usually recorded also during intercritical periods. For these reasons, the neuromagnetic study of cases of generalized epilepsy has been so far limited to simple morphological approaches, with no attempt to carry out source localization. with the unique exception of a recently reported study (Ricci et al., 1988) of photoconvulsive response, which may be referred to as one possible manifestation of generalized epilepsy (Jeavons and Harding, 1975).

In the present paper we describe the use of a newly developed template analysis for an automatic selection of epileptic complexes. The analysis has been carried out on electroencephalographic (EEG) recordings during interictal periods, and has permitted to obtain isofield maps illustrating the distribution of the magnetic field over the scalp in correspondence of the selected complex. From these maps a source

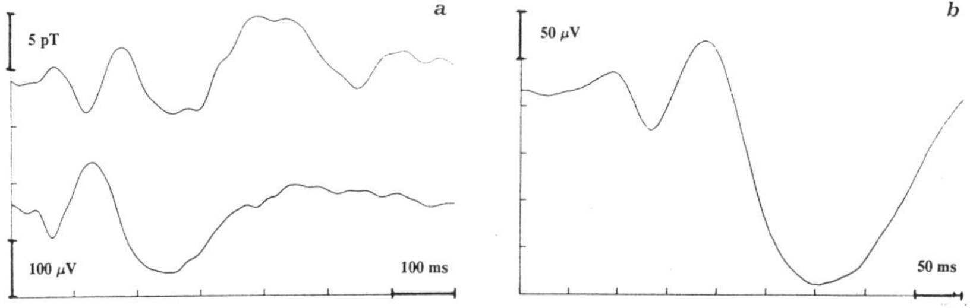

Fig. 1. a) EEG signal (up) recorded from F_3-A_1 and simultaneous MEG signal recorded over the temporal area (subject EG). b) Template selected from the specified derivation.

Advances in Biomagnetism
Edited by S.J. Williamson *et al.*
Plenum Press, New York

localization procedure has been carried out both in one case of focal epilepsy and in two cases of generalized epilepsy.

MATERIALS AND METHODS

In order to facilitate the template investigation, the selected patients were all presenting spikes, sharp waves, and/or spike-and-wave interictal activity. All patients were studied using the 4-channel neuromagnetometer in use at the Istituto di Elettronica dello Stato Solido - CNR in Roma (Romani et al., 1985), and a 16-channel GRASS EEG amplifier (Ag-AgCl electrodes, positioned according to the 10-20 system). Detailed magnetic mapping was carried out for each patient according to the individual pathology: approximately 40 to 50 measuring sites in localized activity (one patient, EG), whereas about 120 sites were explored in generalized epilepsy (two patients, LC and GS). This site distribution typically covered the whole scalp, with the exception of very frontal positions where large artifacts from eye movements might occur. All EEG and MEG signals were acquired in a recording bandwidth from 0.5 to 40 Hz, successively A/D converted at a rate of 256 Hz, and finally stored onto a disc for off-line processing.

The procedure followed for the template analysis was executed in two steps: i) a search for a pathological complex was performed by the operator on the raw EEG signals from a specific derivation. A sequence of "similar" complexes was selected by eye and then averaged to get the template waveform. Evidently this step - which uniquely depends on the operator's skillness - is crucial in that the whole subsequent procedure relies on this choice. ii) the correlation between the template and all the EEG recordings (from the same derivation) is evaluated and, if its value is larger than a preset threshold (typically 0.85-0.9), the corresponding MEG epoch is averaged. In this way a set of averaged MEG signals is obtained in correspondence of all, or part of, the measuring sites, to be used for investigating the field distribution over the scalp relatively to the selected pathological complex. The same procedure may be repeated for other significant pathological events.

RESULTS

Results of a template study carried out on a case of focal epilepsy are shown in Fig.1. The upper part of the figure (a) shows original EEG and simultaneous MEG traces containing an epileptic complex, particularly evident in the raw EEG. The template analysis performed on the EEG signals obtained from derivation F_3-A_1, provided the template reported in (b). After selection of EEG complexes having a correlation with the template larger than 0.85, the corresponding magnetic complexes were averaged for all measuring sites. Typically, about 20 to 30 MEG complexes were averaged at each position, and from these data a sequence of isofield maps was obtained. Fig.2 shows eight maps from this sequence at time instants corresponding to the most significant events, among which we point out the *spike*, and the two maxima of the slow deflection (*wave*), at a latency of about 130 ms, 200 ms, and 300 ms from the beginning of the template, respectively. It is worth remarking that two dipolar-like field distributions characterize the initial and final part of the sequence, and that these two patterns are relatively stable for few tens of milliseconds. In the "central" part of the sequence, however, a more complex field distribution is observed which cannot be simply interpreted in terms of an Equivalent Current Dipole (ECD). In order to understand whether or not another source was active during the specified part of the sequence, a least squares fit with an ECD

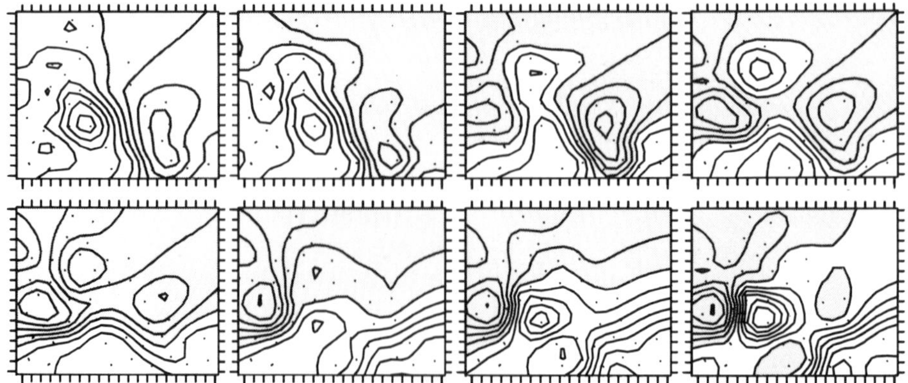

Fig. 2. Isofield contour maps obtained at latencies from 130 to 300 ms from the beginning of the template, every 25 ms. Isofield step is 220 fT. Units are in centimeters. The origin of the coordinate system is 2 cm above the left ear canal whereas the negative abscissae point toward the left eye corner.

was carried out both for the first and for the last maps. The three-dimensional localizations of the ECDs accounting for the two field distributions at 130 (α) and 300 ms (β) are reported in Fig.3a,b,c) and clearly show two different sources responsible for the two selected events in the pathological complex. In particular, a deeper and more posterior source is identified for the first component (α), whereas a shallower and more frontal source might be responsible for the second one (β).

In consideration of the relative "stability" in time of the two fitted distributions, a similar analysis was carried out also for the maps immediately following the first and preceding the second: in this way it was possible to extrapolate a theoretical map accounting for the residual distribution of the two ECDs in correspondence of the "central" map at about 200 ms, and to subtract the extrapolated distribution from it. The result is shown in Fig.3d, where again the residual distribution has a nice dipolar character. By fitting this last pattern a third ECD is identified, at a location also shown if Fig. 3a,b,c) (γ). This source is relatively shallow (depth 1.2 cm) and is located in between the other two, but closer to source (β). We stress, however, that this source is clearly distinct from source (β) as the contribution of this last source has already been subtracted from the map.

A template analysis was also carried out for two cases of generalized epilepsy, and a complete description of this study will be reported in a longer paper (Ricci et al., in preparation). We briefly resume here the main results obtained for one of the subjects (GS). Fig. 4 shows in (a) an example of simultaneously recorded EEG (F_4-C_4) and MEG signals from subject GS, and in (b) the selected template. The scalp distribution of the measuring sites is shown in (c). Four isofield maps ($\alpha,\beta,\gamma,\delta$) obtained averaging the magnetic samples corresponding to this template are reported in Fig. 4d, at latencies (390,510,660,780 ms) which identify some of the positive and negative peaks in (b). The maps clearly show reproducible dipolar patterns. The ECD localization carried out for each map provided four equivalent generators located only in two different positions, as illustrated in Fig.4e. We want to stress that the ECDs corresponding to the positive peaks of the template (α,γ) have almost coinciding positions, and the same occurs for the other two sources (β,δ).

DISCUSSION

The use of an automatic selection of pathological signals offers the advantage of an objective criterion, substantially independent of the human factor, the choice based on it being limited to the very first selection of the complex to be used as a template. Furthermore, by adequately increasing the threshold of correlation during the automatic selection process, it is possible to rigorously identify "very" similar complexes and, consequently, obtain reliable field distributions.

The results obtained in the case of focal epilepsy clearly show that sequential events, i.e. a *spike* followed by a slow *wave*, are most likely originating from two distinct cortical areas, far apart one from the

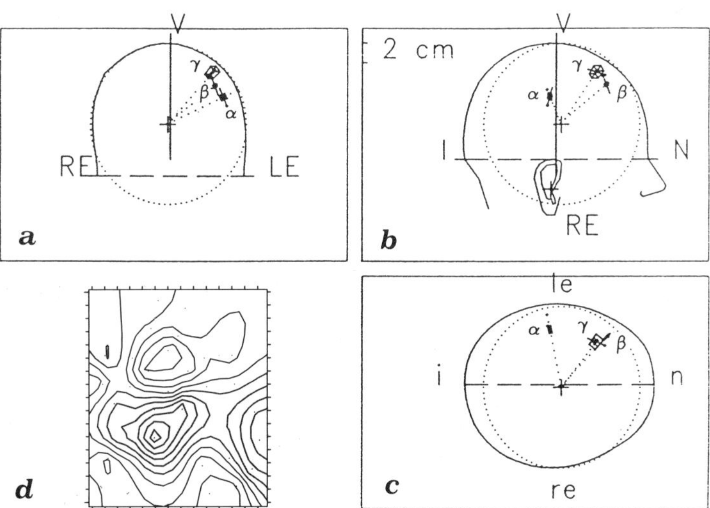

Fig. 3. a,b,c) 3D localization of the ECDs accounting for the measured field distributions at 130 ms (α), 305 ms (β), and for the "residual" distribution at 205 ms (γ) shown in d).

other. Moreover, a third generator might be operative when the first source is not completely over and the second one is not yet fully active. For what concerns the reported results on one of two studied subject suffering by generalized epilepsy, it has been possible to identify two reproducible clearcut dipolar distributions, and to obtain experimental evidence for periodic activation of two sources, at different depths, the first being most likely subcortical, whereas the second one at a cortical level. Preliminary results (not reported here) obtained in the second case (LC) again provided evidence for identification of focal activity in a frame typical of generalized EEG epilepsy. The preliminary results so far achieved show promise of interesting application of the procedure to complex pathologies, and, in perspective, to the study of critical events.

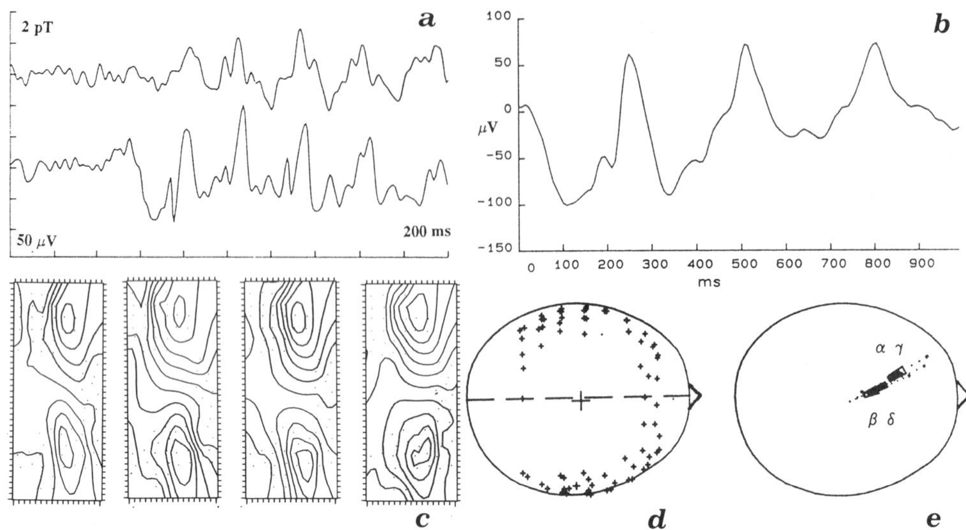

Fig. 4. a) EEG signal (up) recorded from F_4-C_4 and simultaneous recorded MEG signal (subject GS). b) Template selected from the specified derivation. c) Four isofield maps at latencies 390,510,660,780 ms, respectively. Units are in centimeters and the origin of the coordinate system is at 2 cm above the right ear canal. The isofield step is 260 fT. d) Scalp distribution of the measuring sites. e) Three-dimensional localization of the ECDs accounting for the four isofield maps. Note that the sources at 390 ms (α) and 660 ms (γ) are almost coinciding, and the same occurs for the other two at 550 ms (β) and 780 ms (δ).

REFERENCES

Barth, D.S., Sutherling, W., Engel Jr. J and Beatty, J. (1982). Neuromagnetic localization of epileptiform spike activity in the human brain. Science, 218, 891-894.

Chapman, R.M., Romani, G.L., Barbanera, S., Leoni, R., Modena, I., Ricci, G.B. and Campitelli, F. (1983). SQUID instrumentation and the relative covariance method for magnetic 3-D localization of pathological cerebral sources. Nuovo Cimento, 38, 549-554.

Jeavons, P.M., and Harding, G.F.A., 1975, "Photosensitive Epilepsy. A review of the literature and a study of 460 patients", William Heinemann Books, London.

Ricci, G.B., Leoni, R., Romani, G.L., Campitelli, F., Buonomo, S. and Modena, I. (1985). 3-D neuromagnetic localization of interictal activity in cases of focal epilepsy. In: Weinberg, H., Stroink, G. and Katila, T., Biomagnetism: Applications and Theory, Pergamon Press, New York-Toronto, 304-310.

Ricci, G.B., Chapman, R.M., Erne', S.N., Modena, I., Narici, L., Pizzella, V., Romani, G.L., Salustri, C., Torrioli, G., Buonomo, S., Cilli, M., Peresson, M., 1988, Topographic study of stimulated fields and potentials in photosensitive epileptic patients, in: "Biomagnetism87", K. Atsumi, M. Kotani, S. Ueno, T. Katila, S.J. Williamson, eds., Tokyo Denki University Press, Tokyo.

Romani, G.L., Leoni, R. and Salustri, C. (1985). Multichannel instrumentation for biomagnetism. In:Hahlbohm, H.D. and Lubbig, H., SQUID85: Superconducting Quantum Interference Devices and their Applications. Walter de Gruyter, Berlin-New York, pp. 918-932.

Rose, D.F., Smith, P.D. and Sato, S. (1987). Magnetoencephalography and epilepsy research. Science, 238, 329-335.

COMPARISON OF DYNAMIC SPATIOTEMPORAL FIELD STRUCTURES OF DORSOLATERAL FRONTO-CENTRAL SEIZURES AND HAND SENSORIMOTOR CORTEX

William Sutherling (1), Christoph Baumgartner (1,3),
Terrance M. Darcey (4), and Daniel S. Barth (1,2)
Department of Neurology (1) and Psychology (2),
University of California, Los Angeles, CA 900224, U.S.A
Neurological University Clinic Vienna (3), Vienna Austria
Neurology Service, VA Hospital, West Haven, CT (4)

INTRODUCTION

Among the most difficult diseases to diagnose accurately and treat effectively are diseases of brain function. A prototype brain disease which manifests symptoms of many diseases of brain function is frontal lobe epilepsy. Frontal lobe epilepsy usually is considered a focal disease; however, in patients uncontrolled by anticonvulsant medication, frontal lobe seizures often are difficult to localize for surgical excision. This could be due to large areas of seizure cortex which overlap non-resectable areas of normal function or to inaccurate localization because of rapid propagation or complex electric fields.

Dipole methods applied to MEG and EEG have successfully localized dynamic brain function in validation studies. MEG and EEG mapping with high time resolution could reduce the problem of propagation. Mapping with MEG and EEG with high spatial resolution could reduce the problem of interpretation of complex electric fields by reducing ambiguity. Due to the success of dipole methods in localizing epileptic spikes, we applied dipole methods to the frontal lobe seizure and compared it with a controlled focal biological source, the somatosensory evoked response (SER), to determine if the frontal seizure was a focal disease.

METHODS

We mapped MEG, EEG, electrocorticograph (ECoG), and depth electrodes (SEEG) for frontal seizures in 3 patients and SERs to shock stimulation of the contralateral median nerve at the wrist in 3 patients (Sutherling et al. 1987, 1988). We localized the centroids of seizures and SERs using single equivalent dipole modeling both by the peak separation method (Williamson and Kaufman 1981) and by least squares modeling (Barth et al., 1986, Darcey et al., 1980).

RESULTS

Figure 1 shows the SER maps in MEG, EEG, and ECoG in one patient with frontal seizures using coordinates centered on the C3 scalp electrode position which lies within about 1.5 cm from central fissure (Jasper 1958). At 22 milliseconds post-stimulus, MEG shows amplitude peaks which are perpendicular to and about 1/3 closer together than the peaks in EEG, with appropriate polarities. The underlying source current strength from single equivalent dipole modeling using least-squares procedure was similar for MEG and the tangential component of EEG. The spatial pattern of the MEG and EEG

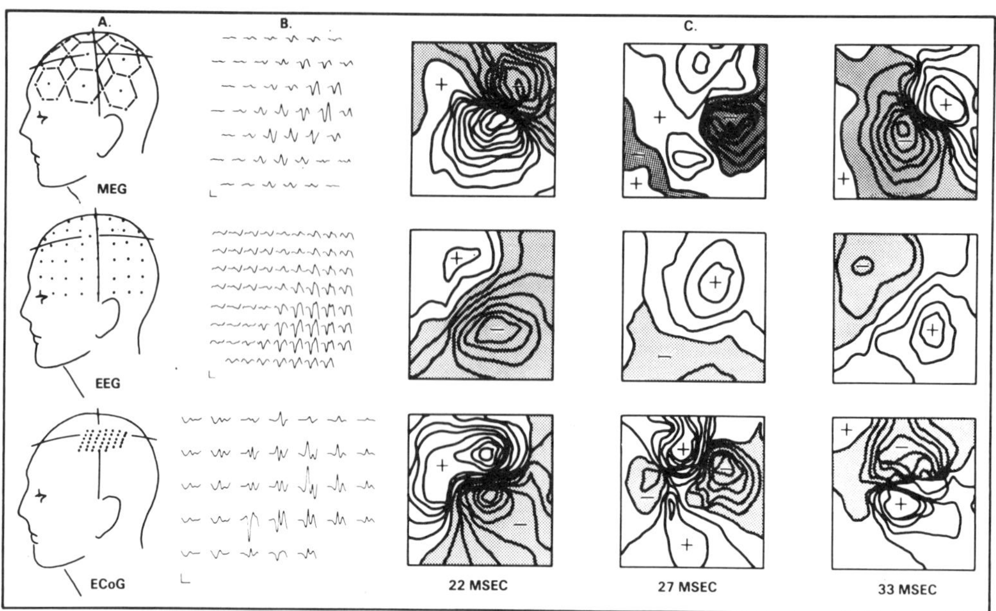

Figure 1. SER maps (Patient #1). Mean dipole localization for MEG-EEG combination was about 3 millimeters from central fissure, similar to ECoG localization, confirmed by cortical stimulations.

map set is repeated at 33 msec. More than 90% of the variance of these map sets is explained by the fields of a single current dipole. These findings make it likely that the source of underlying current measured by both these procedures is a single focal electrically active cortical region, likely in the posterior bank of the central fissure, slightly behind the scalp landmark of C3, (Wood et al., 1985). The ECoG map has polarities and orientation like the EEG map. Similar maps patterns and locations in relation to the C3 or C4 were shown in the other 2 patients. The mean localization of MEG and EEG together was about 3 millimeters from central fissure, similar to ECoG accuracy and confirmed by cortical stimulations.

Figure 2 shows maps sets of a frontal lobe seizure at the peak and trough of a 40 millisecond sinusoidal seizure cycls in MEG and EEG. Only two out of ten maps over this cycle showed an orderly tangential dipolar pattern in both MEG and EEG. The frontal seizure shows appropriate relations between the MEG and EEG and repetition of the pattern similar to the SER in Figure 1. This makes it likely that the maps sets of the frontal seizure are produced by an electrically active focal cortical region which is small compared with the distance from the MEG coil or EEG electrode to the brain, analogous to the SER. The location of the electric current source of the maps sets of the frontal seizure is anterior to the vertical line through T3 (and C3 which lies on the same vertical column of electrode positions), indicating that the location of the center of seizure cortex is likely anterior to sensorimotor cortex.

This patient previously had SEEG which indicated left lateral frontal seizure onset but did not prove focality. Based on the implied focality of the frontal seizure from MEG and EEG mapping, this patient had chronic ECoG seizure mapping which revealed a focal zone of seizure origin near Broca's area which was determined by speech arrest without comprehension deficit using cortical stimulations (Sutherling et al. 1989). Patient had two-thirds reduction of seizure frequency after focal excision of most of seizure focus immediately adjacent to Broca's area.

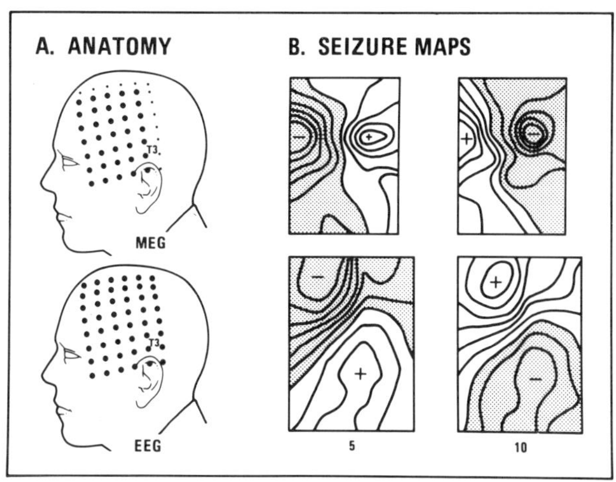

Figure 2. Frontal seizure maps (Patient #2). Localization estimate from dipole methods indicates focal area in inferior-posterior frontal cortex, adjacent to Broca's area, confirmed by ECoG and cortical stimulations.

DISCUSSION

The similarity of the frontal seizure maps to the SER maps and the relative location between their deduced current sources are important converging lines of evidence that this frontal lobe seizure arose from a focal cortical region which warranted further invasive presurgical evaluation. This conclusion has clinical and scientific implications.

First, visual analysis of the routine scalp EEG voltage versus time tracing showed largest signals in the superior frontal region above the current source deduced from both the MEG and EEG and above the ECoG focal zone of seizure origin directly in front of Broca's area. Non-invasive mapping of MEG and EEG implied a different location of the seizure zone than classic visual analysis. High spatiotemporal resolution was essential to identify the orderly field patterns of the map set. The temporal resolution of mapping at millisecond intervals helped eliminate the ambiguity of propagation and complex electric fields which are serious problems in localization of frontal lobe seizure disorders. Without high temporal resolution, the complementary dipolar patterns in MEG and EEG might not have been detected, since they occurred for only about 20% of the time during the seizure. The widespread, global sampling using high spatial resolution of the MEG and EEG combination and dipole methods helped reveal the simplicity at one time of a complex electric tracing, also reducing a problem in accurate localization.

Second, the combination of MEG and EEG in a "map set" had a similar utility in the unknown frontal seizure as in the known SER in determining focality. Since the MEG measures primarily currents tangential to the skull, in this region of the head, MEG indicated that there was probably one focal electric current source that had a large tangential component rather than two widely separated radial current sources, or large region.

Third, the visual comparison between a known, controlled focal biological source, the SER, and an unknown, uncontrolled pathological cortical activity, the seizure, further supported focal functional anatomy of the frontal lobe seizure and indicated the relative location of a reliable landmark, the central fissure. This knowledge is essential for planning of surgical excision.

The deductions from the MEG and EEG map sets, in context of the clinical hypothesis, focused a subdural electrode chronic ECoG grid evaluation to successfully localize a complicated, dynamic seizure disorder for successful focal excisional surgery. This patient likely would not have had further intracranial evaluation if there had not been converging evidence to support focality.

The human frontal lobe seizure is a serious medial problem. Frontal lobe seizures are frequently difficult to control by anticonvulsant medication but also difficult to localize for surgical excision of the seizure focus. Frontal lobe epilepsy is likely to affect a larger clinical population in the future due to head injury in trauma from motor vehicle accidents (Rasmussen 1963). Non-invasive localization using MEG and EEG to focus intracranial mapping could improve localization of a complicated disease of dynamic brain function.

The human frontal lobe seizure also is interesting scientifically. Frontal lobe seizures manifest some of the most complex stereotyped behaviors known, documented by patient reports of "forced thought" without specific content (Sutherling et al., 1987; Penfield and Kristiansen 1951), laughter without subjective humor (Sutherling et al., 1987), and sexual automatisms (Spencer et al., 1983). Further studies of frontal lobe seizures could suggest strategies to map the functional anatomy of some automatic component parts of complicated behaviors.

ACKNOWLEDGEMENTS

Supported by NINCDS grants NS20806, NS22575, BNS8657764, Epilepsy Foundation of America, Forschungsförderungsfon Österreichs (J246M,J334MED)

REFERENCES

Barth D.S., Sutherling W., Broffman J., Beatty J., 1986, Magnetic localization of a dipolar current source implanted in a sphere and a human cranium, Electroenceph clin Neurophysiol, 63:260.

Darcey T.M., Ary J.P., Fender D.H., 1980, Methods for location of electrical sources in the human brain, Prog Brain Res, 54:128.

Jasper H.H., 1958, The ten-twenty electrode system of the International Federation, Electroenceph clin Neurophysiol, 10:367.

Penfield W.G., Kristiansen K., 1951, Epileptic Seizure Patterns, Charles C. Thomas, Springfield, Illinois, 104.

Rasmussen T., 1963, Surgical therapy of frontal lobe epilepsy, Epilepsia, 4:181.

Spencer S.S., Spencer D.D., Williamson P.D., Mattson R.H., 1983, Sexual automatisms in complex partial seizures, Neurology, 33:527.

Sutherling W.W., Crandall P.H., Engel J., Darcey T.M., Cahan L.D., Barth D.S., 1987, The magnetic field of complex partial seizures agrees with intracranial localizations, Ann. Neurol., 21:548.

Sutherling W.W., Crandall P.H., Darcey T.M., Becker D.P., Levesque M.F., Barth D.S., 1988, The magnetic and electric fields agree with intracranial localizations of somatosensory cortex, Neurology, 38:1705.

Sutherling W.W., Risinger M.W., Crandall P.H., Becker D.P., Baumgartner C., Cahan L.D., Wilson C., Barth D.S., Levesque M.F., 1989, Focal functional anatomy of dorsolateral fronto-central seizures, Neurology, in press.

Williamson S.J., Kaufman L., Magnetic fields of the cerebral cortex, 1981, In: Erne S.N., Hahlbohm H.D., Lubbig H., eds, Biomagnetism, Berlin: Walter de Gruyter, 353.

Wood C.C., Cohen D., Cuffin B.N., Yarita M., Allison T., 1985, Electrical sources in the human somatosensory cortex: Identification by combined magnetic and electric potential recordings, Science, 227:1051.

PRE- AND POSTOPERATIVE MAGNETOENCEPHALOGRAPHY IN PARTIAL EPILEPSY.

A CASE STORY

A.Sabers, J.Roenager and The Hvidovre Epilepsy Surgery Group, K.Saermark*, C.K.Bak*, J.Lebech* and K.B.Mikkelsen*

Hvidovre Hospital, Copenhagen, 2650 Hvidovre
*Technical University of Denmark,Lyngby, DK-2800 Lyngby, Denmark

INTRODUCTION

Magnetoencephalographic (MEG) recordings of spontaneous brain waves have in recent years been repeatedly applied in examinations of pathological activity in epileptic patients with the aim of a (3-D) localization of epileptic foci.In particular, Ricci et al. (see, e.g. Ricci et al. 1981,1985a,1985b) have used MEG-recordings in the examination of numerous epileptic patients. In their analysis of the experimental data they use the relative covariance method (see, e.g. Chapman 1989) for the detection of epileptic foci. In a number of cases they also determine a focus on the basis of an observed spatial distribution of spikes. The latter method was first used by Barth et al. (1982,1984) and was also used in Sutherling et al. (1985). In the present paper we present some results of an MEG examination of an epileptic patient for whom a conventional preoperative test battery had already documented a left hemisphere frontotemporal epileptogenic focus. The MEG data were recorded before operation as well as after operation. The results of an analysis based on a relative covariance method are in agreement with the already documented focus.

THE CASE

A 32 years old male with medically intractable partial epilepsy, with complex partial seizures,underwent surgery (left side uncohippocampectomy), in February 1988. The preoperative test battery included extracranial EEG recordings with standard provocations, supplemented with zygomaticus and sphenoidal recordings, CT and NMR scans of the brain, ictal and interictal SPECT scans and neuropsychological and psychiatric examinations. A Wada test was performed to locate the dominant hemisphere. Most of these conventional preoperative tests showed focal abnormalities in the left frontotemporal region. Additionally, MEG examinations were performed 3 months before and 10 months after the operation. Postoperative the patient was seizure free. The medical treatment was unchanged during the observation period.

Advances in Biomagnetism
Edited by S.J. Williamson *et al.*
Plenum Press, New York

METHODS

The magnetoencephalographic recordings were taken by means of a BTI 7 channel second order gradiometer SQUID-system located at a magnetic quiet location. At the time of the postoperative examination the system had been equipped with a Probe-Position-Indicator system (PPI) which allows for a digitization of the head shape as well as for an automatic recording of the actual measuring position relative to a coordinate system fixed relative to the head of the subject. This facility was not present at the preoperative examination. Simultaneously with the MEG conventional EEG recordings from surface electrodes were taken (preoperative 7, postoperative 10 electrodes). The time epoch for the recordings was in all cases 120 s. Preoperative a sampling frequency of 100 Hz was used and a total of 13 measuring positions (91 MEG recordings) was used. Postoperative the sampling frequency was raised to 200 Hz and a total of 16 measuring positions (112 MEG recordings) was used. The combined MEG/EEG data were analyzed in several ways. First of all, a spectral density analysis was performed using a maximum entropy method. This analysis was, for each recording, performed on 40 subsections of 3 s duration and was, further, combined with axonometric plots to study the time dependence of the observed frequencies and with contour plots in order to look for indications of source location(s). Secondly we applied a relative covariance analysis using (most of) the EEG channels as reference channels. Again this was done in the hope of obtaining evidence for source localization. Thirdly, a trained neurophysiologist inspected the recordings for epileptogenic signals.

RESULTS

In Fig. 1a,b we show compressed spectral arrays for MEG-data. For the preoperative MEG data,Fig.1a,the spectral density analysis shows several frequencies in the 2-9 Hz band, the presence of a 14 Hz signal and a weak 17 Hz signal. The signals in the 2-9 Hz band are consistent with the simultaneously recorded EEG signals; the 14 and 17 Hz signals are also present in the EEG recordings, however, only as very low amplitude signals.Applied to the postoperative data, Fig.1b, the spectral analysis shows that the 14 Hz signal has disappeared nearly completely, whereas the signals in the band 2-7 Hz are considerably reduced in strength, but to some extent still visible. The 17 Hz signal is still present in the postoperative data.

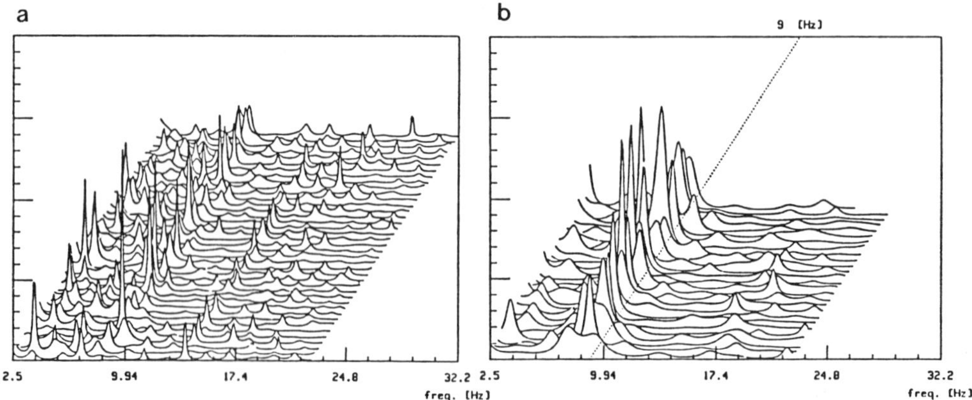

Fig. 1a,b. Compressed spectral array. a:pre-operative, b:post-operative.

The relative covariance was calculated for each of the 7 MEG channels referenced to a simultaneously measured EEG channel. In turn 5 EEG channels were used for the preoperative data and 8 for the postoperative data. The data were first filtered in the frequency bands: 1-30 Hz, 2-8 Hz and 12-16 Hz. Contour plots for the relative covariance consistently, i.e. across the EEG channels used as reference channels, show a dipole-like structure in a left hemisphere, frontotemporal region when the preoperative data are used, but not when the postoperative data are used. This is also true for the contour plot based on the data filtered in the band 12-16 Hz. In Fig.2 we show a contour plot for the relative covariance with the EEG electrode T3 as reference channel and for 2-8 Hz bandpass filtered preoperative data.

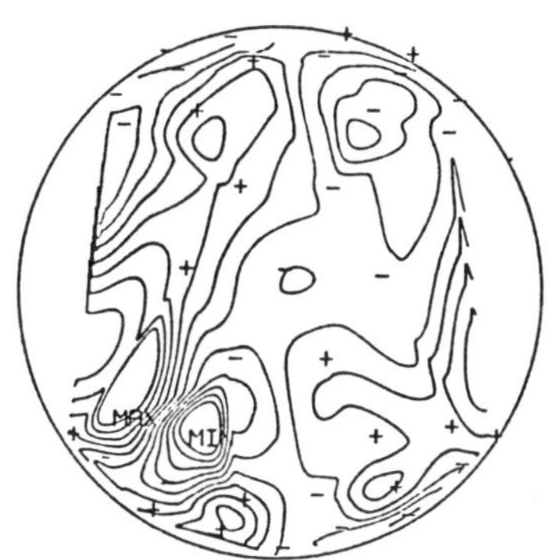

Fig. 2. Contour plot of the relative covariance viewed from the top of the scalp with nasion to the left and inion to the right. 2-8 Hz filtered data.(BTI contour program).

Finally, a contour plot based on the value of the spectral density at the fixed frequency 14 Hz again shows the dipole-like structure in the same left hemisphere, frontotemporal region. It should be noted that in this case no EEG reference channel enters in the calculations.

CONCLUSION

The analysis of the MEG data indicate a left hemisphere frontotemporal focus in agreement with results obtained by means of the conventional methods for locating epileptic foci. The relative covariance method thus seems to be a useful tool in clinical diagnostic work.

REFERENCES

Barth, D. S., Sutherling, W., Engel, J. and Beatty, J., 1982, Neuromagnetic Localization of Epileptiform Spike Activity in the Human Brain. Science, 218: 891-894.

Barth, D. S., Sutherling, W., Engel, J. and Beatty, J., 1984, Neuromagnetic Evidence of spatially distributed Sources underlying Epileptiform Spikes in the Human Brain. Science, 223: 293-296.

Chapman, R. M., 1989, The Relative Covariance Method, in: Advances in

Biomagnetism. Functional Localization: A Challenge for Biomagnetism. S. N. Erne and G. L. Romani, World Scientific, Singapore.

Ricci, G. B., Romani, G. L., Modena, I., Barbanera, S., Leoni, R. and Carelli, P., 1981, Magnetic Recording (MEG) in Epilepsy. Electroenceph. clin. Neurophysiol., 52: S95.

Ricci, G. B., Leoni, R., Romani, G. L., Campitelli, F., Buonomo, S. and Modena, I., 1985a, 3-D Neuromagnetic Localization of Sources of Interictal Activity in Cases of Focal Epilepsy, in: Biomagnetism: Applications and Theory, H. Weinberg, G. Stroink and T. Katila eds., Pergamon Press, New York.

Ricci, G. B., Romani. G. L., Modena, I., Buonomo, S., Leoni, R. and Persson, M., 1985b, Multichannel Neuromagnetic Measurements in Focal Epilepsy, Electroenceph. clin. Neurophysiol., 61: S34.

Sato, S., Rose, D. F. and Kufta, C. V., 1988, Localization of Interictal Spikes Using a Seven-Channel Magnetometer, in: Biomagnetism '87. 206-209. K. Atsumo, M. Kotani, S. Ueno, T. Katila, S. J. Williamson, eds., Tokyo Denki University Press, Tokyo.

Sutherling, W., Barth, D. S. and Beatty, J., 1985, Magnetic Fields of Epileptic Spike Foci:Equivalent Localization and Propagation, in: Biomagnetism: Applications and Theory, H. Weinberg, G. Stroink and T. Katila, eds., Pergamon Press, New York.

MULTIPLE SOURCE MODELING OF THE HUMAN EPILEPTIC SPIKE COMPLEX IN THE MAGNETOENCEPHALOGRAM

Christoph Baumgartner (1,3), William W. Sutherling (1), Shi Di (1,2), and D.S. Barth (1,2)

Department of Neurology (1) and Psychology (2),
University of California, Los Angeles, CA 90024, U.S.A
Neurological University Clinic Vienna (3), Vienna, Austria

INTRODUCTION

Interictal spikes are a common characteristic of human focal epilepsy. These spikes are of both clinical interest as they can help to localize the epileptic focus as well as scientific interest as they provide evidence of altered cortical excitability. As localization by the scalp-EEG is not always conclusive and invasive techniques like stereotaxically placed electrodes or subdurally implanted grid or strip electrodes bear medical risks (e.g. infection, subdural hematoma or intracranial bleeding), new non-invasive techniques are required for the study of the epileptic spike complex. Investigation of the epileptic spike complex with the magnetoencephalogram (MEG) has shown initial promising results and good agreement with localizations obtained from invasive recordings (Barth et al., 1984; Ricci et al., 1987; Rose et al., 1987; Sutherling et al., 1988). Single dipole modeling was applied in these studies as source localization method. However, as evidenced from recordings of the surface of the brain, epileptiform discharges vary both in space in time within an extended epileptogenic zone (Graf et al., 1984) and the interictal spike complex is thus clearly not generated by a single equivalent dipole. In fact, the magnetic field recorded in the MEG often appears to be produced by multiple sources whose fields overlap substantially both in space and time. We therefore applied new modeling techniques using a combined approach of multivariate statistical techniques and multiple dipole modeling, similar to methods previously proposed in a theoretical paper (Achim et al., 1988) and for analysis of visually evoked potentials (Maier et al., 1987), to study the human epileptic spike complex in patients with focal epilepsy.

METHODS

Data were selected from 7 patients with focal epilepsy in which interictal spikes had been recorded in the MEG. A single channel neuromagnetometer (second-derivative gradiometer, coil diameter 24 mm, coil baseline 32mm; Biomagnetic Technologies Inc., San Diego, California) in an unshielded environment was positioned normal to the head in a matrix spaced 2cm centered on the location of the interictal spike as determined by the scalp-EEG. The data were filtered with a bandpass of 1 to 35 Hz and digitized (256 Hz, 12 bits). At least 15-20 MEG spikes were averaged for each measurement location using the EEG spikes as trigger (Barth et al., 1984).

Data analysis consisted of the following steps. First, we applied principal component analysis (PCA) in order to identify the number of brain sources producing the epileptic spike complex and to get a rough estimate of their contributions to the measured magnetic fields. We then applied a physical model involving multiple dipoles fixed in space and varying in activity over time and thus estimated three-dimensional location, time course and interaction of the brain sources generating the epileptic spike complex. A more detailed description of this method has been presented elsewhere (Baumgartner et al., 1989).

RESULTS

PCA indicated that in 3 patients, two sources produced the epileptic spike complex, whereas in the other 4 patients, a single source appeared to generate the spike complex. The results of PCA for Patient 1 are shown in Fig. 1B-E. Each principal component is uniquely represented by component loadings, representing its spatial field pattern (Fig. 1B) and by component scores, representing its time activity (Fig. 1C). The field contributions of each principal component (Fig. 1D) can be calculated by multiplying the component loadings with the component scores and add up to the reconstructed data (Fig. 1E).

We then applied physical modeling to the data using two dipoles in the first 3 patients, and one dipole in the other 4 patients. In all patients at least 75% of the data variance could be explained by one or two dipoles. The results for Patient 1 are shown in Fig. 1F-I. As the dipoles were fixed in space and varied in activity over time, the magnetic field pattern generated by each individual dipole remains constant over time (Fig. 1F) and is multiplied by its time activity (Fig. 1G) to calculate the field contributions of this dipole (Fig. 1H). These field contributions sum up to the reconstructed data (Fig. 1I) due to the law of superposition. The estimated locations of the sources were 26mm and 38mm beneath the scalp in the anterior and midtemporal region. The time activities of the dipoles in this particular patient indicated that two components of the spike complex are generated by two spatially distinct neuronal populations. Both PCA (Fig. 1E) and multiple source modeling (Fig. 1I) could reproduce the actual data set (Fig. 1A) very closely and explained over 85% of the data variance. Although the results of PCA and multiple source modeling look similar, there are some differences which are reflected especially in the spatial field patterns (Fig. 1B and F). This can be explained by the fact that PCA is bound to purely mathematical restrictions (component extraction, orthogonality condition), but not to any physiological assumptions, whereas the multiple source model is not bound to orthogonality, but to a dipolar source configuration.

DISCUSSION

Our results indicate that multiple source modeling may be useful to study the complex interactions of multiple simultaneously active neuronal sources within the epileptogenic zone in the MEG. However, our results should be interpreted within the limitations of the procedure. PCA is a purely statistical technique and the underlying assumptions (component extraction, orthogonality condition, no unique solution) are bare of physiological reality. We also applied different methods of rotations of the principal components (Baumgartner et al., 1989), which did not change the results significantly and thus enhanced plausibility of our results. Nevertheless, PCA should mainly be regarded as a tool to estimate the number of brain sources underlying the epileptic spike complex, rather than making definitive inferences about the sources. In our patients one or two principal components were sufficient to explain a significant amount of the system variance and could reproduce the data closely (Fig. 1A and 1E). Physical modeling has the advantage that neurophysiological rather than statistical assumptions (as in PCA) underlie the model and that location and time course of the brain sources can be estimated. Usually, one or two dipoles were sufficient to explain a significant amount of the system variance. In contrast to single dipole modeling, which is restricted to selected time slices, given for instance by amplitude peaks (Barth et al., 1984; Ricci et al., 1987; Rose et al., 1987; Sutherling et al., 1988), our multiple source model allows

MEASUREMENT SITES AND DATA

A

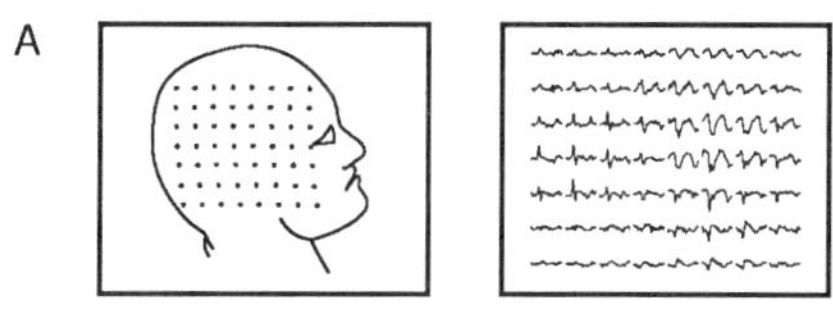

RESULTS OF PRINCIPAL COMPONENT ANALYSIS

B C D E

COMPONENT 1 X =

COMPONENT 2 X =

RECONSTRUCTED DATA

COMPONENT LOADINGS COMPONENT SCORES RECONSTRUCTION

RESULTS OF PHYSICAL MODEL WITH MULTIPLE DIPOLES

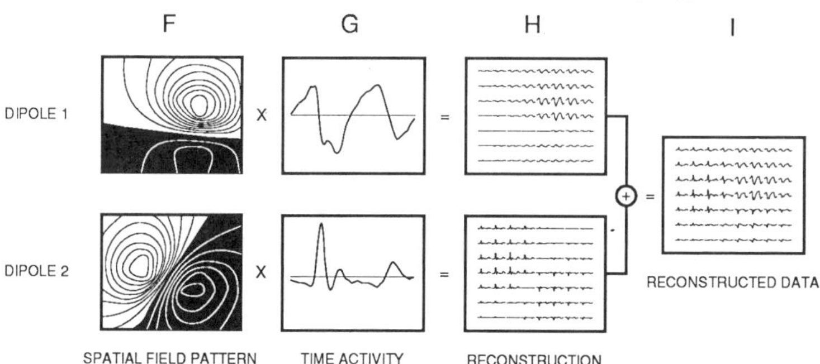

Fig. 1, Results for Patient 1. (A) Measurement sites and data. (B-E) Results of PCA, showing component loadings (B), component scores (C), field contributions of each principal component (D), and data reconstructed from the first two principal components (E). (F-I) Results of the multiple dipole model, showing spatial field patterns (F), time activities (G), field contributions (H), and data reconstructed from the two sources.

investigation of time activity and interactions of the neuronal sources producing the epileptic spike complex over the entire time domain. In some patients, our results indicated that two components of the spike complex seem to be generated by spatially distinct neuronal sources (Fig. 1F-H). Recordings from the surface of the brain show that interictal epileptic discharges usually arise from an extended epileptogenic zone and vary both in space and time (Graf et al., 1984). Modeling of such complex activity with a few dipoles may seem an oversimplification. However, the dipole concept is justified by the fact that the magnetic field generated by any source with an equal number of positive and negative charges falls off like that generated by a dipole, at a distance which is large compared to the dimensions of the source. Thus, dipoles should be regarded as convenient mathematical abstractions rather than as real neuronal elements. The concept of fixing the dipoles in space does not allow modeling of rapid spread of epileptic activity. However, MEG is sensitive primarily to highly synchronized activity of a large number of neurons, whereas localized activity tends to cancel out. Thus, our model may give a good and yet sufficiently simple approximation of the synchronized events within the epileptogenic zone. Further confirmation of our procedure is needed by direct comparison to the results obtained from ECoG and depth electrode recordings.

ACKNOWLEDGMENTS

This research was supported by the Fonds zur Förderung der wissenschaftlichen Forschung Österreichs (Erwin Schrödinger Stipendium J246M and J334MED), by the Van-Swieten-Gesellschaft Österreichs (Hofrat Erwin Domanig Stipendium), by USPHS grants 1-R01-NS20806, 1-R01-NS00678 and 1-R01-NS22575 and by NSF grant BNS-86-57764, and the Whitaker Foundation.

REFERENCES

Achim, A., Richer, F., and Saint-Hilaire, J.M., 1988, Methods for separating temporally overlapping sources of neuroelectric data, Brain Topography, 1:22-28.

Barth, D.S., Sutherling, W.W., Engel, J., and Beatty, J., 1984, Neuromagnetic evidence of spatially distributed sources underlying epileptiform spikes in the human brain, Science, 223:293-296.

Baumgartner, C., Sutherling, W.W., Di, S., and Barth D.S., 1989, Investigation of multiple simultaneously active brain sources in the EEG. J. Neurosci. Meth. (in press)

Graf, M., Niedermeyer E., Schiemann, J., Uematsu, S. and Long, D.M., 1984, Electrocorticography: Information derived from intraoperative recordings during seizure surgery. Clin. Electroenceph., 15:83-91.

Maier, J., Dagnelie, G., Spekreijse, H., and Van Dijk, B.W., 1987, Principal component analysis for source localization of VEP's in man, Vision Res. 27:165-177.

Ricci, G.B., Romani, G.L., Salustri, C., Pizella, V., Torrioli, G., Buonomo, S., Peresson, M. and Modena, I, Study of focal epilepsy by multichannel neuromagnetic measurements, 1987, Electroenceph. clin. Neurophysiol., 66:358-368.

Rose, D.F., Sato, S., Smith, P.D., Porter, R.J., Theodore, W.H., Friauf, W., Bonner, R., and Jabbari, B., 1987, Localization of magnetic interictal discharges in temporal lobe epilepsy, Ann. Neurol., 22:348-354.

Sutherling, W.W., Crandall, P., Cahan, L.D., and Barth, D.S., 1988, The magnetic field of epileptic spikes agrees with intracranial localizations in complex partial epilepsy, Neurology, 38:778-786.

A METHOD TO SEPARATE CONTRIBUTIONS OF DIFFERENT FOCI IN INTERICTAL EPILEPTIC ACTIVITY

R. Stehr, Ch. Lefèbre, D. Janz, W. Scheuler, S. N. Erné*, L. Trahms*, and J. Wedemeyer*

Universitätsklinikum Rudolf Virchow, D-1000, Berlin, W.-Germany
*Physikalisch- Technische Bundesanstalt, Institut Berlin, D-1000 Berlin, W.-Germany

INTRODUCTION

So far in MEG studies of epilepsy the main attention has been devoted to patients, showing only a single focus. However, in many patients with pharmacoresistent epilepsy, who are candidates for neurosurgical therapy, a clear unifocal picture of the interictal activity is not found. More probably, the interictal electric and magnetic activity can be referred to a number of separated generators. In order to localize these foci by MEG, it is necessary to extract their contribution out of the measured magnetic activity.

Here a method is presented to reach this goal, which is based on an analysis of EEG-traces, recorded in parallel with the MEG. It applies to evaluations of sharp potentials as well as to rhythmic epileptic activity. The total number of foci, which can be separated by this technique, mainly depends on the number of EEG channels used. To illustrate this procedure, we present the extraction of a dipolar pattern out of a more complicated field distribution.

As a side aspect of possible practical relevance this procedure might provide some information about causal interdependence between foci.

PROCEDURE

As a prerequisite it is necessary that in parallel to the MEG measurements two or more EEG channels are recorded. On the basis of previously performed standard EEG analysis the positions of the electrodes of the auxiliary EEG channels have to be carefully selected to get a maximum differentiation of the activity due to different sources.

As the first step in this procedure the pathological intervals of one of the electric derivations are identified: (a) In the case of sharp potentials this is usually done by comparing the recordings with a selected template known to be pathological (1). (b) Rhythmic activity is identified by an analysis of the power spectrum. After bandpass-filtering, for each interval of 0.125 s weak and noisy parts are suppressed by discriminating signal intervals with an rms-value S below a certain threshold.

Advances in Biomagnetism
Edited by S.J. Williamson *et al.*
Plenum Press, New York

Then the correlated parts of the signal of a second EEG derivation are calculated for every time interval selected. The ratio of this rms-value S_2 and S_1 will be computed for each selected event. (The index refers to the EEG channel number.)

The result of this procedure is equivalent to the relative covariance(2):

$$R = S_1/(S_2{*}a_{1,2}),$$

where $a_{1,2}$ is the Correlation Coefficient

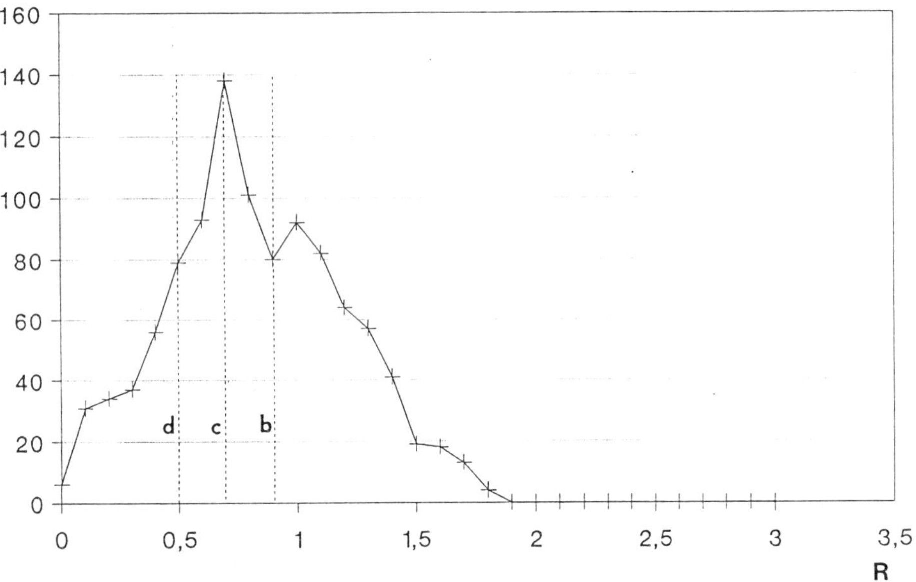

Fig.1 Number of events depending on the ratio R as described in the text. R is calculated from the deviations FP2-PZ and T4-PZ, recorded from an epileptic patient in the BMSR. The dashed lines mark the right border of the range of R used to construct fig.2b-d.

The statistical distribution of R for all of the selected time intervals gives some insight into the nature of the underlying process. Fig.1 shows such a distribution based on rhythmic activity, filtered between 3 and 4 Hz.

The width of the distribution indicates, that several generators with varying amplitudes are active. One single generator would lead to a very narrow peak, broadened by noise only and positioned around one value of R, which depends on the chosen EEG-derivations. Several generators with constant amplitudes would yield a number of distinct narrow peaks. Every interval of R values in the wide distribution reflects a different state of the generator ensemble.

The wings refer to events where the activity is dominated by a part of the generators. Thus, from magnetic recordings, belonging to these events, a field distribution can be constructed, that shows the field of these sources. Provided, that a sufficient large number of pathological events has been recorded to ensure statistical validity, the field of a single source can be isolated in this way.

EXPERIMENTAL APPLICATION

The procedure is illustrated in the following example. It refers to recordings of epileptic interictal activity, recorded in the Berlin Magnetically Shielded Room with a commercial 7-channel first-order-gradiometer. From Fourier-analysis pathological activity had been identified as rhythmic activity between 3 and 4 Hz.

The magnetic field distribution of this activity over the right hemisphere as obtained by the relative covariance method is shown in fig.2a. Evidently, the pattern does not reflect the magnetic field of a simple dipolar source. In terms of the diagram of fig.1, this field pattern represents the activity of the entire distribution of intensity ratios R.

In the following figure, the magnetic field due to a fraction of the whole set of events is displayed: Fig.2b-d reflect the magnetic field corresponding to the events left of the dashed lines in fig.1. The decrease of the threshold of the ratio leads to a structural change of the field pattern. This becomes evident by the gradually vanishing of the field in one region, denoted by A in fig.2a, upon decreasing of the threshold for R. In fig.2d, a clearly bipolar pattern has emerged, that reflects the field of a simply structured source. Here, a localisation under the assumption of a dipolar source becomes admissible. It leads to a location as indicated in fig.2d at a depth of 3.8 cm, which is in a good agreement with the CT-localisation of a hamartom.

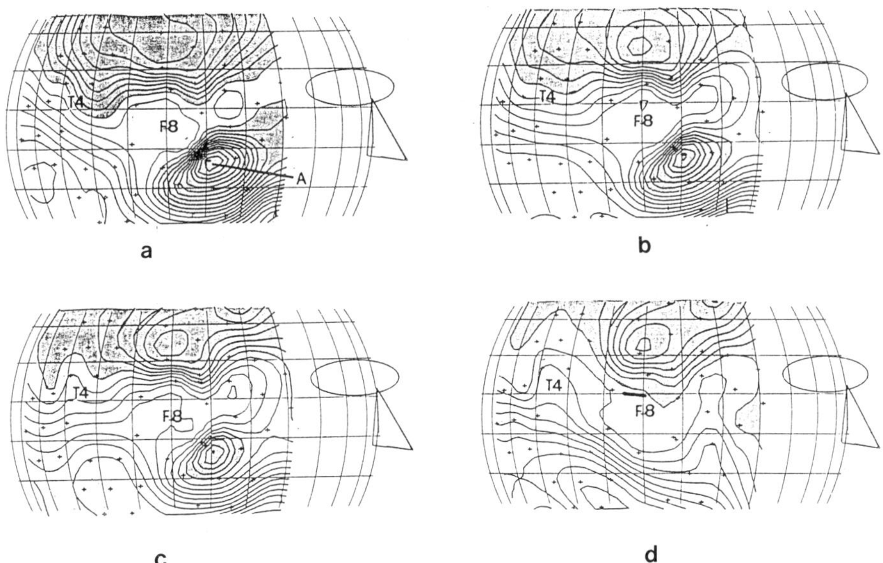

Fig.2a-d Isofield contours over the right hemisphere of an epileptic patient. For fig.2a the whole pathological part of the recordings has been used. Fig.2b-d were constructed with an decreasing number of selected events as indicated by the dashed lines in fig.1. Contour lines 1.5 pT/mV steps (unit due to normalisation on EEG activity).

Applying the same procedure to the right wing of the distribution in fig.1, we did not obtain a comparing simple structure, but a pattern similar to that of fig.2a. This indicates that the total sources ensemble remains active.

DISCUSSION AND CONCLUSION

In the shown example two activation states could be selected by this method: The activity of one isolated generator and the activity of a compound generator including the isolated one. The calculated distribution of selective EEG intensities together with the obtained magnetic maps suggest some more speculative aspects of the relationship between the two activation states:

a) The isolated generator acts as a leading focus, but other activity is not always triggered by this focus. In this case, the other foci need the activity of the leading focus only as a necessary condition for their own activity.

b) Other activity, which contains the leading focus always triggers the isolated generator. This generator is able to fire independently but it never triggers other activity. In this case, the activity of the leading focus is not a necessary but a sufficient condition for activity of the isolated focus.

To keep the example simple, we used only two electric derivations. In principle, the amount of information obtained by this method depends on the number of electric derivations. One may expect that a more extended application of this method will allow a separation of complex activity in MEG analysis.

REFERENCES

(1) Sato, S., Douglas, R., Roger, P.: In: Weinberg, H., Stroink, G., Katila, T. (eds.): Biomagnetism: Applications and Theory. London: Pergamon Press, 261-263, 1982

(2) Chapman, R.M., Romani, G.L., Barbarena, S., Leoni, R., Modena, I., Kaufman, L. and Campitelli, F.: Lett. Nuovo Cimento, 38, 549-554, 1983

ISCHEMIC AND EPILEPTIC LESIONS MEASURED BY AC- AND DC-MEG

J. Vieth, G. Sack, P. Schueler, P. Grummich and S. Schneider +)

Dept. exp. Neuropsychiatry, University of Erlangen,
+) SIEMENS AG Medical Engineering Group, Erlangen
Erlangen, Federal Republic of Germany

INTRODUCTION

The MEG (7 channel system) only was used to show alterations or missing of auditory evoked magnetic field responses caused by brain infarction in the auditory cortex (Leinonen and Joutsiniemi, 1989). And TIAs up to now only could be localized by the PET scan in a reliable way (Vyska et al. 1983). We wanted to find, if the AC-MEG is able to locate spontaneous pathological activity produced by ischemic lesions and especially by TIAs.

In addition: Shortly before and during epileptic seizures DC-potential shifts could be found (Stodiek and Wieser, 1987). So we asked, if direct coupled (DC) MEG shifts also can be found during ictal or interictal epileptic activity.

METHODS

Single channel MEG was recorded on the skull at 30 to 40 points with a BTi DC-SQUID (2nd order gradiometer, unshielded room, measuring point distance 2-3 cm) and a recording time of 2-3 minutes of artifact free data for each point coming successively to a total positioning and recording time of 4 to 5 hours. The EEG was recorded using a point distance of 3-6 cm. Ten patients were investigated (2 infarctions, 6 TIAs, 2 hemorrhages). The filtered pathological slow wave activity was analyzed using the relative covariance method (Chapman et al., 1987). The source model was the single current dipole, the volume conductor model an appropriate sphere. The dipole was located using the angle between the extrema in the map (Williamson and Kaufman, 1981).

Multichannel MEG was recorded in two patients (infarction and TIA) with a SIEMENS 31 channel DC-SQUID system (1st order axial gradiometer, sensor coil diameter and measure point distance 3 cm on a flat plane, outer diameter of sensor array 20 cm, 26 channels selected, shielded room; Gudden et al. 1989). The recording time was 5 minutes. A multichannel system not only reduces the recording time substantially but provides coherent data. Thus, the single current dipole in an appropriate sphere was directly estimated from the simultaneously obtained data using a least mean square fit of the measured field maps. The filtered data were analyzed by selecting typical slow activity sections. Also an automatic selection was used (Abraham-Fuchs et al. unpublished).

The direct coupled (DC) MEG was recorded with the single channel system in

Advances in Biomagnetism
Edited by S.J. Williamson *et al.*
Plenum Press, New York

a few positions in 2 patients with continuous epileptic seizures, in 1 patient with interictal epileptic activity, and in 2 patients using hyperventilation as a provocative method. Possible magnetic artifacts as movements of the head, eye bulbs and lids, the jaw and the hairs (Cohen et al. 1980) were studied in two subjects. In all other measurements mechanisms were avoided to produce artifacts or they were evoked for comparison.

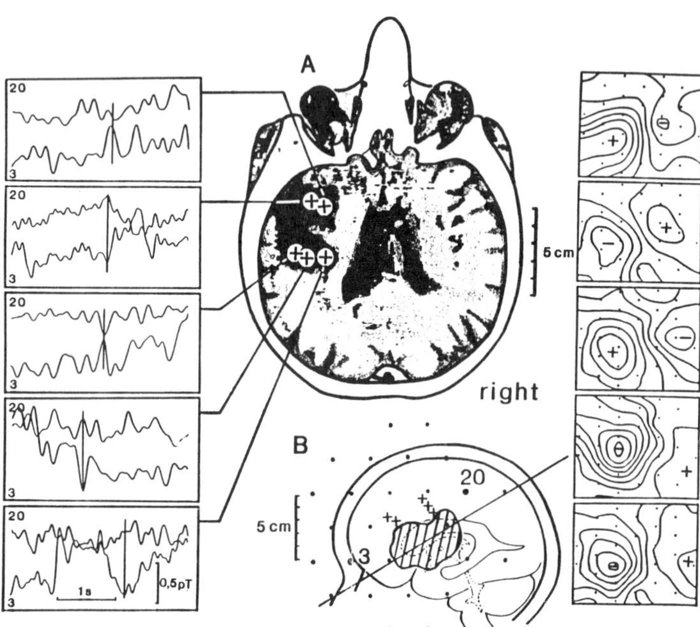

Fig. 1. Examples of locations of estimated current dipoles from simultaneously obtained MEG data of 26 channels of pathological activity around a brain infarction. Distinct data points and maps with two extrema are shown. Left column: Raw MEG data of two channels (20 and 3, with high pathological amplitude near the extrema of the maps). The time is marked (vertical line) at which the isocontour maps (right column) were calculated and from which the dipoles were estimated by dipole fit. Right column: Isocontour maps at the marked time in the corresponding row of the left column. The extrema are indicated by plus (field out of the head) and by minus, steps between isocontour lines are 50 fTesla. A: MRI slice (partly redrawn) containing the infarction on the left hand side. Crosses indicate the projections of the centers of the estimated current dipoles connected to the related data in the left column by lines. B: Drawing of the midline MRI section with projections of ventricles and the infarction. The slice of A is marked by a line, the points of the measuring matrix by dots (channel 3 and 20 are indicated), the infarction is marked by a hatched area and the projections of the centers of the estimated dipoles by crosses.

RESULTS

In the patients with brain infarctions - verified by CCT - the MEG dipole obtained by the relative covariance method could be located in the area near to the lesion. In the patients with hemorrhages the maps show a distorted dipole pattern, which might be an indication for more than one dipole. In the patients with TIAs - even several days after the TIA symptoms - a MEG dipole could be located in a brain region corresponding to the former clinical symptoms, whereas standard EEG, CCT and MRI did not show a lesion.
In multichannel recordings the isocontour maps were much smoother than those obtained by successive recording with a 1 channel system. Timely successive data points revealed spatially successive dipoles in the vicinity of the lesion (distinct examples: Fig. 1) but also in some distance, clustering together in sections.

Observing carefully precautions to avoid or detect DC-MEG artifacts we found interictal epileptic activity accompanied by DC-MEG shifts. In addition ictal behavioral, EEG-, and AC-MEG activity was preceded 10-20 sec by a DC-MEG shift similar to the DC potential shifts found by Stodiek and Wieser (1987). All possible artifacts mainly were much smaller than the ictal DC shifts or could be distinguished very well from the DC shifts. In one subject during strong hyperventilation (17 mm Hg endtidal CO_2 level) for some days very large DC-MEG shifts were found in a small area with a reversal of the DC- polarity. In this area in addition in the standard EEG during hyperventilation also small epileptic spikes and an accentuated delta wave activity occorred. The MRI did not show any lesion. In one patient seizures provoked by strong hyperventilation were accompanied by large DC-MEG shifts.

DISCUSSION

This study shows that focal slow wave pathological activity produced by ischemic lesions - including TIAs - can be located by the AC-MEG. Recently available multichannel MEGs allow the investigation of the spatial distribution of the dipoles in time. This distribution might indicate the region involved. But since activity not only was found near the lesion the area involved might be larger - depending on the case - or the separation of the pathological activity from the non pathological activity must be improved.
This study also shows that ictal and interictal epileptic activity can be accompanied by pronounced MEG-DC shifts, which can be distinguished very well from existing and possible artifacts. During hyperventilation the DC-MEG also could serve to detect locally increased excitability. The DC-MEG thus provides new information related to epileptic activity that compliments the AC-MEG and EEG records.

ACKNOWLEDGEMENTS

We are grateful for collaboration to the pediatricians U. Brandl and D. Wenzel, to the neurologist B. Neundoerfer and to the epileptologist H. Stefan, all Erlangen, and to the neuromagnetism group of NYU, New York for providing us (Dept.exp.Neuropsychiatry) with the basic dipole fit software.

REFERENCES

Chapman, R. M., Romani, G. L., Barbanera, S., Leoni, R., Modena, I., Ricci, G. B., and Campitelli, F., 1983, SQUID Instrumentation and the relative covariance method for magnetic 3D localization of pathological cerebral sources. Lettere al Nuovo Cimento, Ser.2, 38: 549-554.

Cohen, D., Palti, Y., Cuffin, B.N., Schmid, S.J., 1980, Magnetic fields produced by steady currents in the body. Proc. National Acad. Sci. 77: 1447-1451.

Gudden, F., Hoenig, H. E., Reichenberger, H., Schittenhelm, R., Schneider, S., 1989, Ein Vielkanalsystem zur biomagnetischen Diagnostik in Neurologie und Kardiologie: Prinzip, Methode und erste Ergebnisse. Electromedica 57: 2-7.

Leinonen, L., Joutsiniemi, S. L., 1989, Auditory evoked potentials and magnetic fields in patients with lesions of the auditory cortex. Acta Neurol. Scand. 79: 316-325.

Stodiek, S. R. G., Wieser, H. G., 1987, Epicortical DC changes in epileptic patients. In: "Advances in Epileptology Vol.16," P. Wolf, M. Dam, D. Janz, and F. E. Dreifuss, eds., Raven Press, New York.

Vyska K., Kloster, G., Feinendegen, L. E., Heiss W. D., 1983, Regional perfusion and glucose uptake determination with 11C-methyl-glucose and dynamic positron emission tomography. In: "Positron Emission Tomography of the Brain," W.-D. Heiss and M.E. Phelps, eds., Springer-Verlag Berlin Heidelberg New York pp. 169-180.

Williamson S.J., Kaufman, L., 1981, Magnetic fields of the cerebral cortex. In: "Biomagnetism," S. N. Erne, H. D. Hahlbohm, and H. Luebbig, eds., Walter de Gruyter, Berlin, New York, pp 353-402.

NEUROPATHOLOGICAL DYNAMICS OF MAGNETIC, AUDITORY STEADY-STATE RESPONSES IN ALZHEIMER'S DISEASE

U. Ribary, R. Llinas, A. Kluger*, J. Suk and S. H. Ferris*

Department of Physiology & Biophysics and Department of Psychiatry*
New York University Medical Center, New York, N.Y 10016 USA

INTRODUCTION

The steady-state auditory mid-latency response in humans is maximal in amplitude and sinusoidal in form in response to repetitive auditory stimulation between 35 and 45 Hz (Galambos et al., 1981). This has been reported in both, EEG and MEG studies. MEG data reported single dipoles in the temporal lobe of cortex in humans after an auditory 40Hz stimulation (Maekelae and Hari, 1987), which were believed to be a part of a thalamo-cortical loop becoming resonant at 40 Hz (Weinberg et al., 1988). Recently, our EEG/MEG studies suggested two dipoles in thalamo-cortical areas, indicating that more than one generator must be involved in the 40Hz response (Ribary et al., 1989a and 1989b). Moreover, these dipoles seemed to be more rigerously in phase in controls than those observed in psychiatric patients.

A number of various neurotransmitter systems (e.g. monoamine and ACh systems), whose activities are altered in psychiatric patients, seem to influence thalamo-cortical systems and are expected to change the pattern of the 40 Hz response. In our earlier studies with depressed patients, the first MEG study on psychiatric patients (Ribary et al., 1987), we reported various changes in the dynamics of the EEG and MEG 40 Hz response over time (Ribary et al., 1989a and 1989b). In the case of Alzheimer's disease (AD), degeneration of cholinergic neurons, leading to deficits in central cholinergic functions in various brain areas, play a major role in the cognitive loss in AD (Scheibel et al., 1986), and suggests that an altered 40 Hz response observed in these patients may relate to such synaptic abnormalities.

METHODS

The 14-multichannel neuromagnetic measuring system (BTi) consists of a magnetically shielded room, two cryogenic dewars with 7 magnetic sensors each and a probe position indicator (PPI) to determine the position and orientation of the sensors with respect to the head (Yamamoto et al., 1988).

MEG data of the 40 Hz auditory evoked response were analysed in a pilot study, consisting of 4 male patients (65-80 years old), with severe dementia, and were compared with 4 older control subjects matched for age and sex. Both groups were diagnosed after various clinical and cognitive tests, including MRI and PET. The experiment was set between 10am and 2pm. Subjects were asked to lie on a bed with their eyes closed and listen to the tone presented. MEG recordings were done from 30-35 positions over the right hemisphere during 3 sessions of 50 sec each with a bandpass filter of 1-100 Hz. The stimuli consisted of a 12 msec duration 250 Hz tone with a rise and fall time of 0 msec, presented binaurally at repetition rates of 40 Hz. In order to avoid magnetic artifacts, the sound was conducted to the subject through plastic tubing and earpiece with an output of approximately 60 dB from a transducer placed outside of the shielded room. MEG data were filtered offline between 25-55 Hz and with a notch-filter at 60 Hz. 500 epochs of 100 msec intervals and 4 cycles were averaged. The steady-state response was mapped over all positions and analyzed at 1 msec steps, such that the dynamic component of the response may be determined, depending on the distribution of amplitudes and phase shifts over the head over time, as well as the source localization at various time points. For source localization analysis a single dipole model was used (Yamamoto et al., 1988), indicating an estimation of a vectorproduct of complex, multidipolar sources responsible for a changing phase reversal over time.

Advances in Biomagnetism
Edited by S.J. Williamson *et al.*
Plenum Press, New York

RESULTS

Preliminary results from earlier EEG 40 Hz studies with Alzheimer patients (Ribary and Weinberg, unpublished) showed amplitude values that were approximately 3 times smaller than those from control subjects. There was also less activity in the right frontal and temporal lobe and enlarged phase shifts in right frontal/frontal temporal areas.

The sinusoidal auditory evoked MEG data in control subjects indicated a stereotyped temporal pattern of magnetic activity over the hemisphere as seen in subject oc001 (Fig.1). It consisted of a positive-negative field sequence which rotated from dorso-posterior to ventro-anterior cortical areas in a continous phase shift manner over parietal, temporal and frontal areas during half a cycle (12.5 msec).

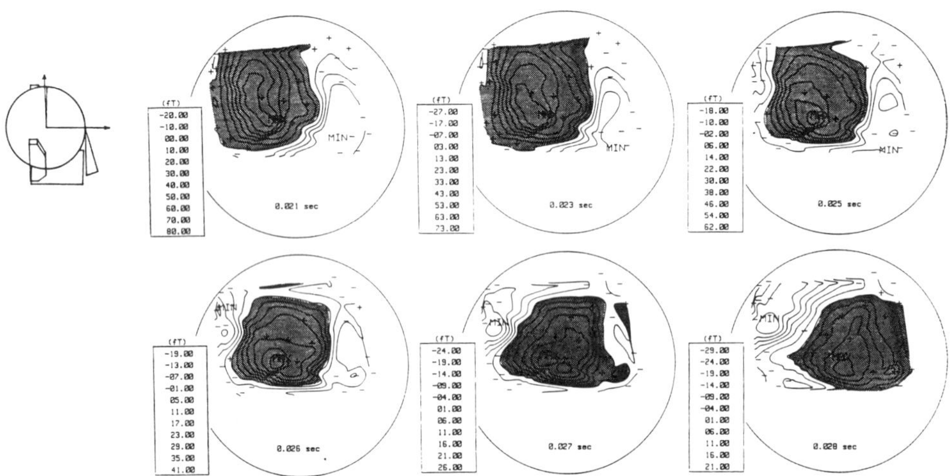

Fig.1. Isofield maps of magnetic 40Hz activity in an older control subject oc001. Top farleft: orientation of the head, top from left to right and bottom from left to right: magnetic Isofield maps between 21 and 28 msec. The contour lines correspond to the levels (fT) as indicated in the box beside the map.

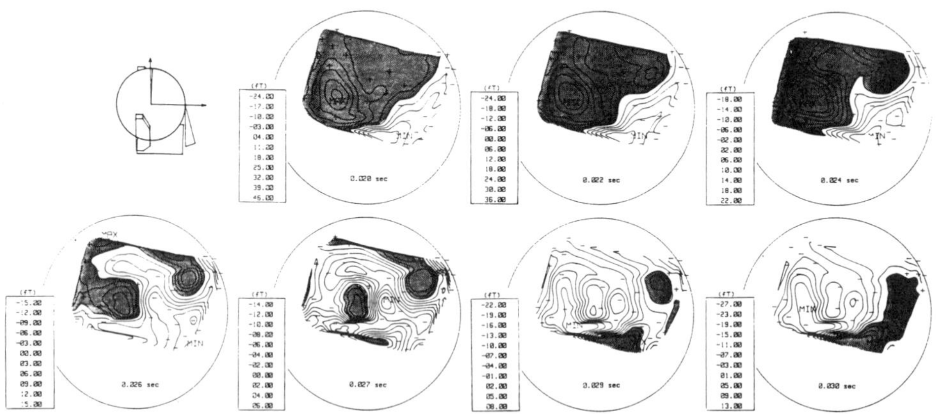

Fig.2. Isofield maps of magnetic 40Hz activity in an older Alzheimer patient op002. Top farleft: orientation of the head, top from left to right and bottom from left to right: magnetic Isofield maps between 20 and 30 msec. The contour lines correspond to the levels (fT) as indicated in the box beside the map.

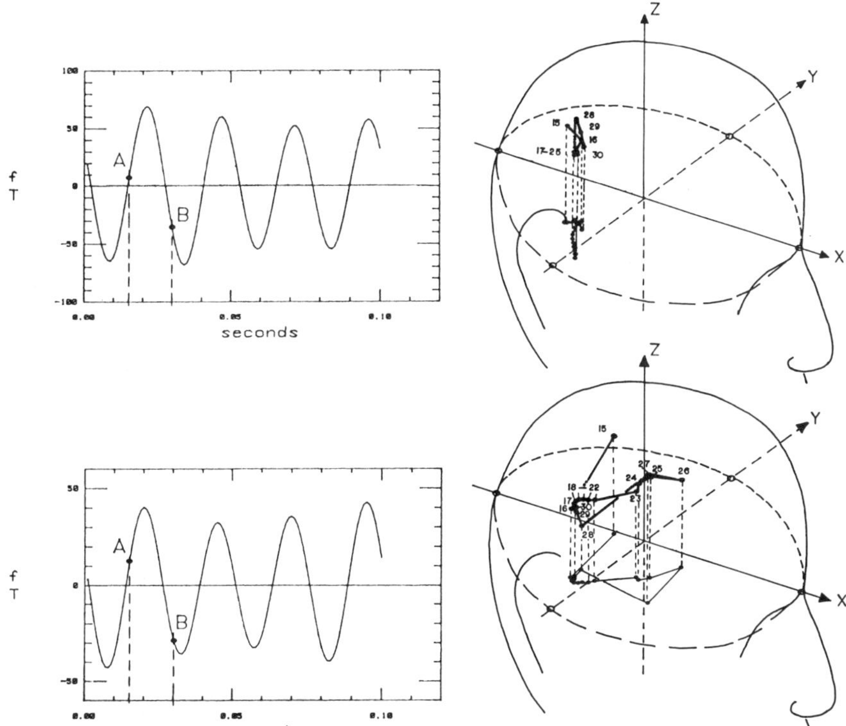

Fig.3. Source localization of magnetic 40Hz activity in an older control subject oc001 (top row) and in an older Alzheimer patient op002 (lower row). Left: 40Hz response; points A and B indicate time interval where dipole localization was done. Right: 3-dimensional localization of complex sources between 15 and 30 msec (thick line) and projection to xy-plane.

This was consistent in all control subjects. The largest amplitudes for this activity was found over temporal cortex, varying between 40 and 80 fT among all subjects. Source localization was done over the time interval from A to B, between 15 and 30 msec (Fig.3), over the maximum positive peak found in temporal areas, when the rotation over the hemisphere was observed. Source analysis indicated a summation of sources within cortical and subcortical areas, focused in temporal regions (Fig.3). The highest correlation coefficient for these dipole fits were found for subject oc001 between 0.87 and 0.95, but source estimates remained the same in other subjects. In Alzheimer patients, decreased magnetic fields over time, a reduction of the rotational speed of their response and a distortion of the dynamics over frontal areas was observed, as seen in subject op002 (Fig.2). This was largely due to increased phase shifts over the hemisphere and to a lower activity in fronto-pariotemporal areas. These observations remained the same among all patients, even though these areas may vary slightly in size across individuals. The maximum response was located more posterior to temporal areas (Fig.2) as compared with control subjects and reached levels between 30 and 50 fT among all patients. Source localization was done over this maximum positive peak between time points A and B (Fig.3), again during the time when the rotational response was observed. Estimated sources (correlation: 0.87-0.94) were more distributed over a larger area within thalamo-cortical systems. The correlation for the source estimates was lower in the other patients, but the tendencies of the results remained the same.

DISCUSSION

Our MEG data indicate that the dynamics of the auditory evoked 40 Hz response over the head and over time is altered in Alzheimer's disease. The data further support our previous findings with depressed patients, that more than one generator must be involved in the 40 Hz response and that these generators are more in phase in controls than in psychiatric patients (Ribary et al., 1989a).

The stereotyped dynamic pattern of magnetic activity over the right hemisphere in control subjects, consisting of a rotation of a positive-negative field sequence was due to a continuous phase shift over these areas. These findings were consistent in all control subjects and correlated with our earlier EEG and MEG data, obtained from younger and older control subjects (Ribary et al., 1989a and 1989b). The distribution of phases and amplitudes over the hemisphere and over time determined the speed and the pattern of the rotational response. The largest response was found over temporal cortex. In addition, source localization, using a single-dipole model, indicates that this magnetic wave reflects a complex, time locked sequence of network activations involving most probably thalamo-cortico-thalamic pathways, with a focus on temporal areas. The estimate of each single dipole correlates to a vectorproduct of various active sources and indicates a complex interaction over time within those areas. In Alzheimer patients, a general decrease in magnetic fields over time was observed. In fronto-pariotemporal brain regions, certain areas showed an increased phase shift and a lower magnetic activity, which were resposible for the pathological dynamic pattern over the hemisphere. The size of these areas seems to vary among patients, indicating that the size of these "abnormal" areas might be correlated to the severity of Alzheimer's disease. In addition, source localization indicated a disturbance of interactions within thalamo-cortical areas and an activation over larger brain regions. These findings correlate to other studies with respect to changes in thalamo-cortical systems in AD. One of the most pathological indicators of AD is neuronal degeneration, especially of dendrites, with a decrease in cortical volume and increase in ventricular space. In later stages, these findings can be widespread throughout the brain, but more focal involvement of subcortical structures is characteristic of earlier stages of the disease (Marco and Randels, 1984). Limbic structures in the medial temporal region are among the first to be affected, including entorhinal cortex, hippocampus and amygdala (Damasio and Hoesen, 1986; Scheibel et al., 1986). In addition, electrical components of the auditory evoked P-300 response were altered in AD showing decreased amplitudes in pariotemporal areas (Maurer et al., 1988).

We hypothesize, that in control subjects, there is an increased synchronization of cortical 40Hz activity, driven by subcortical areas, with a focus on the activated sensory area during an auditory 40 Hz stimulation. In Alzheimer patients, the cortical 40Hz activity is more desynchronized and is spread over a wider sensory area, due to the neuropathophysiological parameters as described above.

Our preliminary results show that the MEG-technology can be usefully applied in psychiatric patients. In connection with the 40Hz response, the MEG technique could be a powerful tool to study the dynamics of pathological brain function in mental illnesses. However, more studies, more subjects and more sophisticated analysis procedures are necessary, in order to analyse the various parameters of the neuropathological response in more detail, including a statistically significant set of patients to generate a comprehensive clinical study.

REFERENCES

Damasio, A.R. and Hoesen, G.W. (1986) Neuroanatomical correlates of amnesia in Alzheimers's disease. In Biological Substrates of Alzheimer's disease, A.B.Scheibel, A.F.Wechsler and M.A.B.Brazier, eds., NY.Academic Press, pp. 65-71.

Galambos, R., Makeig, S. and Talmachoff, P.J. (1981) A 40 Hz auditory potential recorded from the human scalp. Natl. Acad. Sci., USA, 78: 2643-2647.

Maekelae, J.P. and Hari, R. (1987) Evidence for cortical origin of the 40 Hz auditory evoked response in man. Electroencephalogr. Clin. Neurophysiol., 66: 539-546.

Marco, L.A. and Randels, P.M. (1984) Neurobiology of cognitive deterioration. In Alzheimer's disease and related disorders, W.E.Kelly, ed., Springfield: C.C.Thomas, pp. 26-80.

Maurer,K., Dierks, T. and Ihl, R. (1988) Topographic mapping of auditory evoked P300 in psychiatric disorders. In Functional Brain Imaging, G.Pfurtscheller and F.H. Lopes da Silva, eds., Hans Huber Publisher, Toronto, Canada, pp. 187-192.

Ribary, U., Weinberg, H., Brickett, P., Ancill, R.J., Holliday, S. and Johnson, B. (1987) Imaging of EEG and MEG for the estimate of sources in the human brain responsive to antidepressant drugs. Soc. Neurosci. Abstr. 13,1268.

Ribary, U., Weinberg, H., Cheyne, D., Johnson, B., Holliday, S. and Ancill, R. (1989a) EEG and MEG (magnetoencephalography) mapping for indexing pathological changes in human brain. European J. Neurosci. Suppl., in press.

Ribary, U., Weinberg, H., Johnson, B., Ancill, R. and Holliday, S. (1989b) EEG and MEG mapping of the 40Hz auditory evoked response in depressed patients. Submitted.

Scheibel, A.B., Wechsler, A.F. and Brazier, M.A.B. (1986) Biological Substrates of Alzheimer's disease, NY.Academic Press, 1986.

Weinberg, H., Cheyne, D., Brickett, P., Gordon, R. and Harrop, R. (1988) An interaction of cortical sources associated with simultaneous auditory and somesthetic stimulation. In Functional Brain Imaging, G.Pfurtscheller and F.H. Lopes da Silva, eds., Hans Huber Publisher, Toronto, Canada, pp. 83-88.

Yamamoto, T., Williamson, S., Kaufman, L., Nicholson, C. and Llinas, R. (1988) Magnetic localization of neuronal activity in the human brain. Proc. Natl. Acad. Sci., 85, 8732-8736.

THE USE OF FLASH AND PATTERN EVOKED FIELDS IN THE DIAGNOSIS OF ALZHEIMER'S DISEASE

R A Armstrong, B Janday, A Slaven, G F A Harding

Clinical Neurophysiology Unit
Department of Vision Sciences
Aston University
Aston Triangle, Birmingham B4 7ET

INTRODUCTION

Alzheimer's Disease (AD) is the commonest form of presenile and senile dementia and currently affects about 1.3 to 6.2% of the population over 65 (Mortimer, 1983). The dementia is of insidious onset and takes a gradually progressive course involving short term memory impairments, cognitive disturbance and ultimately results in a mute inattentive patient incapable of caring for him or herself (DSM-III-R, 1980). The average duration of the disease from onset to death is 5 years but much longer durations are possible e.g. up to 30 years.

AD is notoriously difficult to diagnose clinically. Neither CT, PET nor EEG can diagnose AD definitely. However, in a recently published protocol using visual evoked potentials (VEP), (Wright et. al. 1986) subjects with AD exhibited a normal P100 component of the evoked response to a pattern reversal stimulus and increased latency of the P2 component to diffuse light flashes. The P100 may originate in the primary visual cortex area B17 via the geniculo-calcarine pathway while the flash P2 may originate in association areas via a cholinergic tectal pathway (Wright et. al. 1987). It may be advantageous to record neuromagnetic evoked fields to the same stimuli because of the possibility that the signals originate deeper in the calcarine fissure where the pathological changes characteristic of AD may be more pronounced (Mann, 1985). The purpose of this study is to use the neuropathological data as a foundation for the evoked magnetic field studies. We now a) show that the pathology of AD is more pronounced in the visual association areas B18/19 than in B17 b) present evidence that the magnetic signals to flash and pattern may originate in B18/19 and B17 respectively and 3) present normative magnetic data to flash and pattern stimuli from 50-90 years of age that could be used in a diagnostic test for AD.

METHODS

Neuropathological Techniques

The hallmark lesions of AD are senile plaques (SP) and neurofibrillary tangles (NFT) (Brun, 1983). SP are 5-200μm lesions comprising a central core surround by dystrophic neurites while NFT are silver positive, hairlike hooks or loops in the cytoplasm of the pyramidal cells.

The density of SP and NFT was measured in B17 and B18/19 of silver stained coronal sections of calcarine cortex in 18 clinically diagnosed and neuropathologically verified cases of different disease onset and duration. SP and NFT were counted in vertical transects of 250 x 125μm contiguous samples, the long diameter being parallel to the pia, and extending from pia to white matter. The density of SP and NFT were compared between brain regions and between cases of presenile (< 65) and senile (> 65) onset.

Table 1. The density of SP and NFT in B17 and B18 in 18 cases of AD with correlations with age at death and disease onset (* $P < 0.05$, ** $P < 0.01$)

		Mean density (per mm^2)		Correlation Coefficients		
		Presenile	Senile	Age at death	Onset	Duration
	B17	13	6*	-0.61**	-0.70**	0.13
SP	B18	18	9*	-0.35	-0.46	0.11
	B17	12	3*	-0.52 *	-0.26	-0.31
NFT	B18	35	11*	-0.55 *	-0.34	-0.15

Magnetic data (Mapping)

Mapping of flash and pattern evoked fields was made on 3 normal subjects with a single channel dc SQUID (BTI) second order gradiometer. 20-35 points were mapped on a grid with a separation of 2cm and using the inion as a reference point. The magnetic signal was band passed (1-30Hz and power line notch) before digital conversion. Light flashes of intensity 68 cd/m^2 were produced by a Grass PS22 stroboscope while pattern stimuli (field size 15°, subtense 1.5°) and reversing at 2Hz were produced by an optical projection system (Drasdo, 1976). Full field binocular stimulation was used for flash and pattern while right half and quarter fields were also used for pattern. 64-128 responses were recorded from each point on the scalp with a 500 ms baseline. Source localisation for pattern data was made as described previously (Janday and Swithenby, 1988).

Magnetic data (normative study)

Full field, binocular magnetic fields were recorded from 45 seated subjects at a point 6-9 cm above the inion. Subjects were between 50 and 90 years of age without apparent neurological or ophthalmological disease. Recording and stimulus conditions were as described above.

RESULTS

The neuropathological study (Table 1) indicated 1) that SP and NFT density in B17 and B18 was negatively correlated with age at death of the patient and 2) the density of SP + NFT was greater in B18 than B17 particularly in younger cases with more extensive pathology.

The neuromagnetic data (Fig 1) gave quarter field pattern reversal localisation above and below the calcarine fissure consistent with a source in B17 (error parameter 0.26-0.34). The flash P2 responses were more complex and did not indicate a single localised source but the field contours were consistent with sources outside B17 in the visual association areas.

Normative values for the P100m pattern reversal component and the flash P2m component are shown in Table 2. Standard deviations are in general larger for the magnetic components compared with corresponding VEPs. In addition, both the pattern reversal and flash components show a pronounced trend of increasing latency with age.

DISCUSSION

The neuropathological data indicate that the different visual areas vary in the extent of the pathological changes characteristic of AD with B18/19 being more severely affected than B17. VEP studies on presenile AD patients show a normal pattern response but a delayed flash response (Harding et. al. 1985) which may be attributable to variation in pathological development in the occipital cortex. In addition, animal lesion experiments and the study of human subjects with local brain lesions suggest that different aspects of visual information are transmitted by separate channels as early as the optic nerve. Evoked potential and psychophysical studies suggest that high temporal frequencies and patterned stimuli are processed by the normal geniculocalcarine pathway while low temporal frequencies and luminance discrimination are processed by a tectal pathway from the superior colliculus and pulvinar to the visual association areas B18/19 (Wright, et.al.1987).

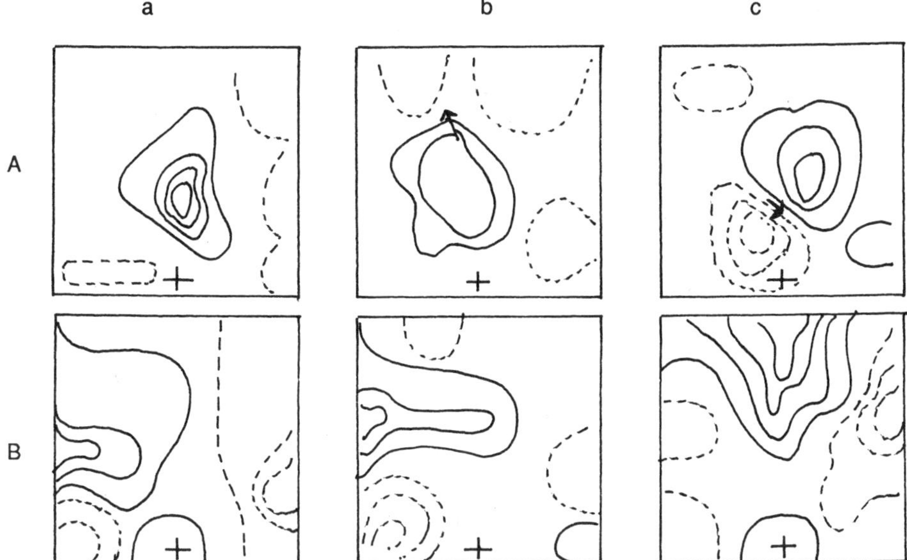

Fig 1 The measured magnetic fields for A. Pattern reversal P100m for one subject a) right hemifield b) upper right quarter field c) lower right quarter field and B. Flash P2m (100 ms) for three subjects. Lines are plotted a 100fT intervals with the zero contours omitted. Solid lines indicate positive Bz, crosses mark the inion and arrows the position of fitted dipoles.

Although the data from the magnetic mapping are not extensive enough for conclusive localisation they are consistent with localisations of sources to flash and pattern stimuli in B18/19 and B17 respectively, areas differentially affected by AD pathology. These localisations may be reflected in the differential responses of the VEP to flash and pattern stimuli shown in AD subjects (Harding et. al.1985; Wright, et. al. 1987).

There may be advantages to recording neuromagnetic fields in addition to the VEP in AD subjects since the signals may reflect, to a greater extent, activity of tangential sources in brain fissures where

Table 2. Normal values for the latency of the magnetic visual evoked field to flash and pattern stimuli.

Age group (years)	Pattern reversal P100 (ms)	Flash P2 (ms)
50-9	108 ± 7.9	106 ± 9.7
60-9	114 ± 15.1	115 ± 15.5
70-9	119 ± 16.6	119 ± 9.1
80-9	153.5 ± 5	125 ± 19.7

the development of SP and NFT is more pronounced (Armstrong et. al. 1989). To establish a diagnostic protocol using neuromagnetic recording requires normative data of suitable quality to be established for flash and pattern . Although our present data are limited in that they are recorded from a single position on the skull and vary more between subjects in different decades than the corrresponding VEP (Harding and Wright, 1986) it is likely that normative magnetic data of sufficient quality can be recorded for use in a diagnostic protocol for AD.

REFERENCES

American Psychiatric Association, 1987, Diagnostic criteria from DSM-II.

Armstrong R.A., Myers, D. and Smith, C.U.M. 1989, Further studies on the pattern of senile plaques in Alzheimer's Disease with a hypothesis on the colonization of the cortex. NeuroSci. Res. Comm. 4: 17.

Brun, A. 1983, An overview of light and election microscope changes. In: "Alzheimer's Disease. The Standard Reference" (Ed by B. Reisberg) pp 37-45, MacMillan, London and New York.

Drasdo, N.,1976, A method of eliciting pattern specific responses and other electrophysiological signals in human subjects. B.J. of Physiol. Optics, 31:14.

Harding, G.F.A., Wright, C.E. and Orwin, A. 1985, Primary presenile dementia. The use of the visual evoked potential as a diagnostic indicator. B.J. of Psych. 147: 533.

Harding, G.F.A. and Wright, C.E. 1986, Visual evoked potentials in acute optic neuritis. In: Optic Neuritis. (Ed. by R.F. Hess and G.T. Plant) pp 230-254 Cambridge University Press.

Janday, B.S. and Swithenby, S.J. 1988, Investigation of the pattern reversal response by combined MEG and EEG measurement. Electro and Clin. Neurophysiol. 70: 132P.

Mann, D.M.A. 1985, The neuropathology of Alzheimer's Disease: a review with pathogenetic aetiological and therapeutic considerations. Mechanisms of Aging and Development. 31: 213.

Mortimer, J.A. 1983, Alzheimer's disease and senile dementia: Prevalence and Incidence. In: "Alzheimer's disease. The Standard Reference" (Ed. by B. Reisberg) pp 141-148, MacMillan, London and New York.

Wright, C.E., Harding, G.F.A. and Orwin, A. 1986, The flash and pattern VEP as a diagnostic indicator of dementia. Doc. Ophthalmol. 62: 89.

Wright, C.E., Drasdo, N. and Harding, G.F.A. 1987, Pathology of the optic nerve and visual association areas: information given by the flash and pattern visual evoked potential and the temporal and spatial contrast sensitivity function. Brain, 110: 107.

OBJECTIVE EVIDENCE OF TINNITUS IN AUDITORY EVOKED MAGNETIC FIELDS

M. Hoke, H. Feldmann*, C. Pantev, B. Lütkenhöner,K. Lehnertz, W. Kumpf*

Institute of Experimental Audiology, and *ENT Clinic
University of Münster, Münster
Federal Republic of Germany

INTRODUCTION

Tinnitus, or ringing in the ear, often is a very distressing symptom which can be associated with various diseases of the middle and inner ear (e.g. M. Menière, acoustic trauma, sudden hearing loss) or general diseases (e.g. arteriosclerosis). Its incidence is very high (~15%), and in 0.5-1%, tinnitus has a severe effect on the ability to lead a normal life. Apart from a minority of cases in which a real (internal) sound source exists ("objective tinnitus"), "subjective" tinnitus consists in purely subjective auditory sensations which could be evaluated so far only by psychoacoustic methods. All attempts to detect the pathophysiological processes underlying tinnitus in auditory evoked potentials (AEP) or in the electroencephalogram (EEG) have failed so far, which does, however, not rule out that certain components contributing to the AEP or EEG are affected by tinnitus. In view of the great number of individuals who are unable to lead a normal life and the ineffectiveness of current tinnitus therapy it is highly desirable that some method be devised to objectively assess the existence of tinnitus and to determine its representation in the central nervous system. Hence it was natural to study whether the magnetic signals of the brain reveal an interference with tinnitus, owing to the high spatial resolution offered by neuromagnetic measurements.

MATERIAL AND METHODS

The auditory evoked magnetic field (AEF) in response to tone-bursts (carrier frequency 1000 Hz, duration 500 ms, rise /decay time 15 ms, interstimulus interval 4 s, intensity 60 dB HL) was measured in 25 patients suffering from unilateral tinnitus, and in 40 normal-hearing individuals without tinnitus. Both groups matched largely in age (tinnitus group: median 39 y, quartiles 33 and 56 y; non-tinnitus group: median 36 y, quartiles 26 and 46 y) and hearing loss at the test frequency (tinnitus group: 5 dB (0 dB, 10 dB); non-tinnitus group: 0 dB (0 dB, 5 dB)). AEF were measured over the hemisphere contralateral to the side of stimulation at the anterior field maximum in an electrically and acoustically, but not magnetically shielded room (overall noise level 30-50 fT/!Hz) with a single-channel DC SQUID (BTi) equipped with a second-order gradiometer. Average waveforms were computed from 96 stimulus-related magnetoencephalogram (MEG) epochs (sampling frequency 250 Hz, bandwidth 0.1-40 Hz), and, in some individuals, from 96 EEG epochs, simultaneously recorded between vertex and contralateral earlobe. Amplitudes and latencies of waves M100 and M200 (AEF) and their electric counterparts N100 and P200 were off-line evaluated (for more details, see Hoke et al., 1989).

RESULTS

While the mean amplitudes of waves M100 and M200 do not differ significantly in the non-tinnitus group, wave M200 is missing or only very poorly developed in the tinnitus group, and the amplitude of wave M100 is distinctly augmented as compared to the normal group. Student's t-test for paired data revealed a high level

Advances in Biomagnetism
Edited by S.J. Williamson *et al.*
Plenum Press, New York

of significance ($p < 0.001$) for the differences of the mean amplitudes of corresponding waves of both groups as well as for the differences of the mean amplitudes of waves M100 and M200 in the tinnitus group. The mean latencies of wave M100 are not significantly different in the two groups, but the mean latency of wave M200, when developed, is significantly prolonged in the tinnitus group ($p < 0.002$). Plotting the individual values of the amplitude ratio M200/M100 versus age (Fig. 1) shows that the amplitude ratio decreases with increasing age in the normal group, while no dependence on age of the amplitude ratio is evident in the tinnitus group. Linear regression analysis revealed that the regression coefficient of the tinnitus data is not significantly different from 0, whereas that of the normal data differs significantly ($p < 0.05$). Simultaneously recorded AEP showed only an uncharacteristicallly prolonged mean latency of wave P200 with unchanged mean amplitudes of N100 and P200.

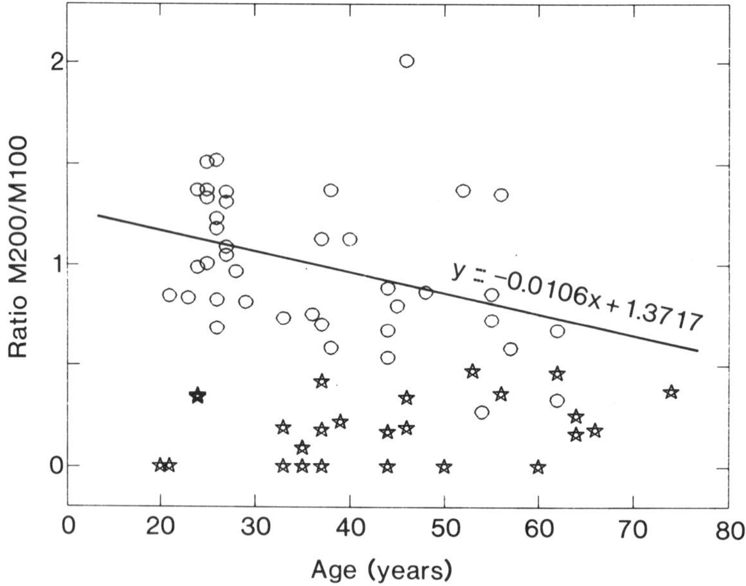

Fig. 1. Individual amplitude ratios M200/M100 of the normal group ( ) and the tinnitus group (*) plotted as a function of age (From Hoke et al., 1989)

We have also been able to trace the process of tinnitus remission in one exemplary case of acute tinnitus (noise trauma) (Pantev et al., 1989). During the period of recovery from tinnitus, the waveforms underwent a remarkable reorganization. Initially wave M100 was considerably augmented and wave M200 was totally missing, whereas at the end of the study both waves had quite regular shapes and amplitudes (Fig. 2). As evident from the upper panel of Fig. 3, the amplitude of wave M100 decreased continuously with time elapsed since the noise trauma from its initial value of 570 fT, asymptotically approaching a value of 180 fT (mean and standard deviation for tinnitus patients are according to Hoke et al. (1989) 436 ± 105 fT, for non-tinnitus individuals 275 ± 137 fT). The decrease of the amplitude of wave M100 was accompanied by a recovery of wave M200 from an initial value of 0 (the amplitude of M200 is assumed to be zero if this wave is not detectable) to a final value of 190 fT (mean and standard deviation for the tinnitus group according to Hoke et al. (1989) 77 ± 69 fT, for the non-tinnitus group 252 ± 100 fT). The temporal development of the amplitude ratio M200/M100 is shown in the middle panel of Fig. 2. The amplitude ratio recovered from 0 to a normal value of 1.1 (1.17 according to Hoke et al., 1989).

DISCUSSION

The results reported here suggest that at least one component of the cortical auditory evoked response with a latency of approximately 200 ms interacts with tinnitus. We explain the diminution or disappearance of wave M200 by a pathologically enhanced spontaneous activity in the generator population of that particular component, causing the generator population to be less or not at all responsive to external stimuli. Waves M100 and M200, which are probably generated by different processes, are assumed to have basically monophasic waveforms of opposite polarity. Wave M200 is supposed to be broader than wave M100, and its deflection is supposed to begin before wave M100 assumes its maximum, so that both waves partially overlap in non-tinnitus individuals. Only if wave M200 is significantly diminished or if it has totally diasappeared then wave M100 will be seen in its full shape. The enhanced spontaneous activity is supposed to be initiated by (probably multiple) exogenous or endogenous noxes or noxious events. If such an event occurs only once or extremely rarely (e.g., acute noise trauma), then the spontaneous activity may recede, allowing a normal generation of wave M200 as seen in Fig. 2. If, however, noxious events happen very frequently or even permanently, then the pathological neural activity cannot recede and eventually becomes manifest. That circumscribed enhanced spontaneous activity in the auditory cortex indeed exists in tinnitus patients has already been described before (Hoke, 1988).

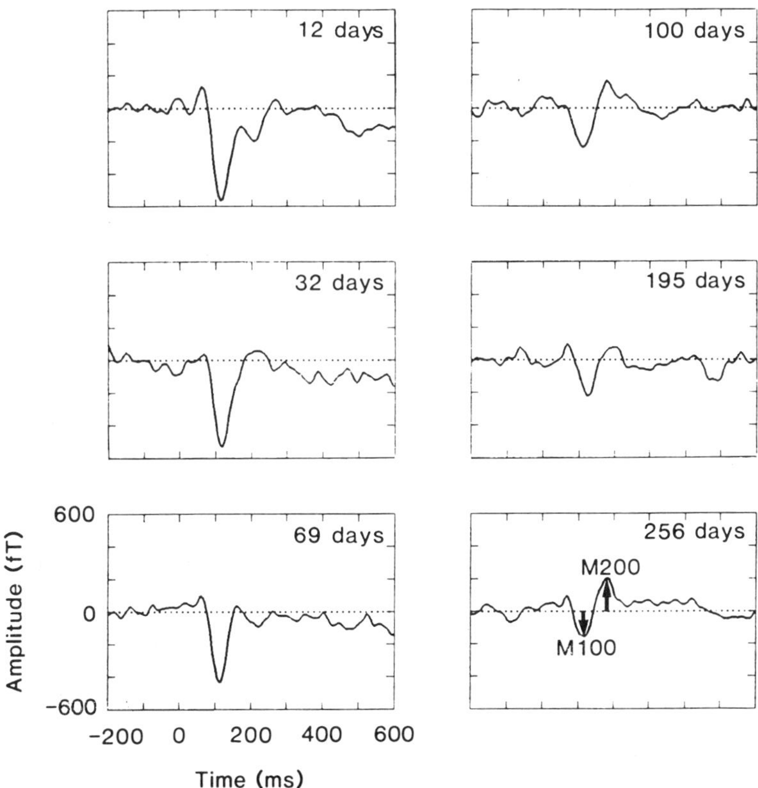

Fig. 2. Averaged waveforms of the auditory evoked magnetic field recorded over the supralateral surface of the right cerebral hemisphere at the anterior field maximum. The waves M 100 and M200 are indicated by arrows in the lower right panel of the figure (From Pantev et al., 1989).

The strong correlation between the amplitude ratio M200/M100 and the clinical manifestation of tinnitus points to two important applications: Besides its usefulness for studying mechanisms of tinnitus pathophysiology, AEF measurements might become an invaluable clinical tool for the objective assessment of tinnitus and an objective control of tinnitus therapy.

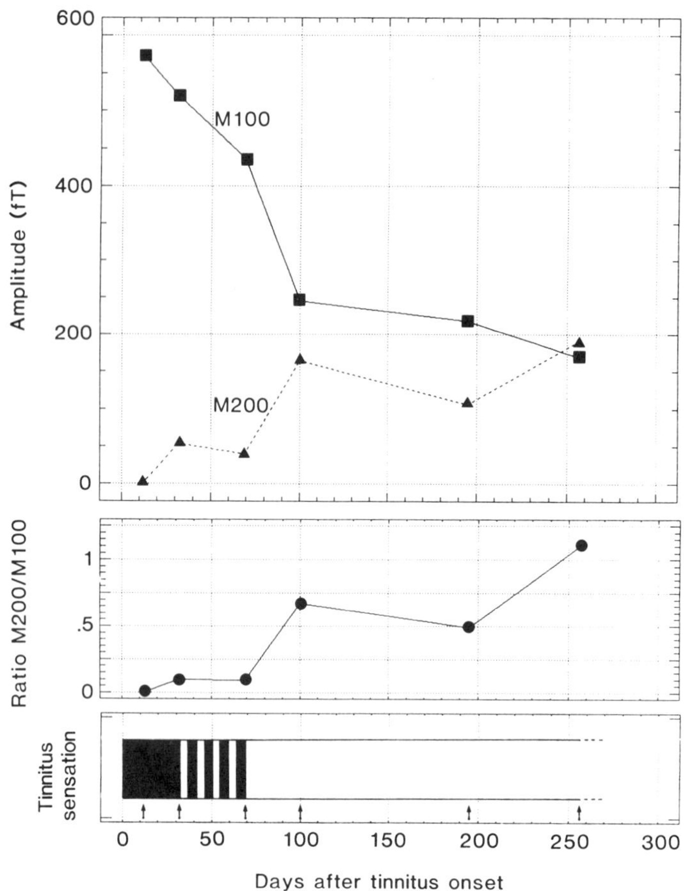

Fig. 3. Amplitudes of waves M100 and M200 (top) and amplitude ratio M200/M100 (middle) as a function of time since tinnitus onset. The subjective sensation of tinnitus is indicated at the bottom (black field: permanent tinnitus; vertical bars: intermittend tinnitus; blank field: no tinnitus) (from Pantev et al., 1989)

REFERENCES

Hoke, M. (1988) SQUID-based measuring techniques - A challenge for the functional diagnostics in medicine. in: "The Art of Precise Measurement in Physics and Medicine", B. Kramer, ed., Verlag Chemie, Weinheim: 287.

Hoke, M., Feldmann, H., Pantev, C., Lütkenhöner, B., Lehnertz, K., 1989, Objective evidence of tinnitus in auditory evoked magnetic fields, Hearing Res. 37, 281.

Pantev, C., Hoke, M., Lütkenhöner, B., Lehnertz, K., Kumpf, W., 1989, Tinnitus remission objectified by neuromagnetic measurements. Hearing Res., 40: 261.

MAGNETIC OBSERVATION OF SPREADING CORTICAL DEPRESSION IN ANAESTHETIZED RABBITS

A.R. Gardner-Medwin[*], N. Tepley[+o], G.L. Barkley[+], J. Moran[+o], S. Nagel-Leiby[+], R.T. Simkins[+] and K.M.A. Welch[+]

[*]Physiology Dept., University College, London WC1E 6BT, UK
[+]Neurology Dept., Henry Ford Hosp., Detroit, MI 48202, USA
[o]Physics Dept., Oakland University, Rochester, MI 48309, USA

INTRODUCTION

Spreading depression (SD) is a profound disturbance of the environment of brain cells that occurs as a stereotyped response to several types of strong stimulation or trauma (for reviews see e.g. Bures et al., 1974; Nicholson & Kraig, 1981). It can propagate in some circumstances in a non-decrementing, regenerative, wave through susceptible tissue at speeds of 2-5mm/min, causing transient disturbances of function at each site for a minute or more. There are many points of similarity between the characteristics of SD in animals and the disturbances associated with classical migraine in man (Leao & Morrison, 1945; Milner, 1958; Gardner-Medwin, 1981; Lauritzen & Olesen, 1984). Magnetic fields associated with SD were first demonstrated using isolated tissue from the turtle cerebellum (Okada et al. 1988). We have studied fields during propagation of SD through the cerebral cortex of the anaesthetised rabbit. Such studies are of interest primarily because they may offer points of comparison with magnetic events studied during migraine in man (Tepley et al., 1989).

METHODS

Rabbits (1.5-2kg) were anaesthetized with urethane (750 mg/kg) and chloralose (40 mg/kg) through an ear vein. After induction, a non-magnetic plastic cannula was inserted into the vein for maintenance of anaesthesia, using 10%-20% of the initial dose every 1-2hrs to maintain surgical anaesthesia. The trachea was cannulated to facilitate normal breathing and a circular opening (5.5mm dia.) was made in the skull and dura, centred approximately 5mm left of the midline and 5mm behind the coronal suture. A perspex cylinder (3mm height, 8mm outside dia.) was glued to the skull over the opening, with cyanoacrylate gel. A silicone rubber cap, moulded with silicone inflow and outflow tubes, fitted tightly over the cylinder to form a chamber. This was flushed with saline (147 mM NaCl + 3mM KCl). Single propagating waves of SD were initiated by replacing the fluid in the chamber with 150mM KCl, usually for 2min, followed by washout. SD was verified by voltage recording at a subdural electrode (0.5mm dia. Ag/AgCl, approximately 6mm in front of the chamber), held with bone wax in a second (2mm) burr hole in the skull. The animal was grounded through an Ag/AgCl electrode in neck muscle. Cable ran to a battery operated pre-amplifier at 1m distance.

Measurements (DC-50Hz) were made with a 7 channel, DC-coupled SQUID magnetometer (BTI Model 607) in a magnetically shielded room. The head was positioned on paper cushions with the chamber uppermost. The hexagonal array of

Advances in Biomagnetism
Edited by S.J. Williamson *et al.*
Plenum Press, New York

18mm diameter magnetometer coils was positioned with the central coil measuring the axial (vertical) field over the chamber, 20-25mm from the brain. Peripheral coils were centred at 21.5mm radius around this point, measuring fields 7° inclined to the vertical, at about the same height. Peripheral coils are identified by orientation from the cup: 0° = anterior, 90° = right, etc. Fluctuation analysis was carried out by calculating the standard deviation of the signal within 0.5s segments.

The fluid inflow was led to the chamber through a 3m length of fine Tygon tube, from a tap controlled manually inside or outside the shielded room. Outflow was collected (without dripping) in a beaker close to the animal's head. Non-magnetic materials and cables were selected and/or degaussed to minimise artefacts from respiratory or other movements. In one experiment, field changes were measured with deliberate horizontal movements of the animal on a sliding table. At the different coils, the changes varied from 0-2pT per cm of movement, reflecting the pattern of steady fields around the head and equipment. An experimenter sat in the room during most recording sessions to monitor and record, with an event marker, any animal movements. Undetected movements could not have exceeded about 1mm. Magnetic signals with cardiac or respiratory frequency were not visible under normal conditions.

RESULTS

Satisfactory magnetic recordings were made with 10 episodes of SD in 5 animals. A typical set of magnetic and voltage recordings is shown in Fig.1A. The changes of magnetic field were slower to develop and lasted longer than the local voltage shifts. The most consistent component developed gradually from 150-250s after KCl application (350s from the start of Fig. 1A), reaching a maximum 200-300s later. Orientation was positive (out of the head) in the right posterior quadrant (90-180°) and negative in the left anterior (270-360°). Measurements 400s after KCl application, pooled for all data in these quadrants, gave mean shifts of 1.32 pT ($\pm$ 0.82 s.d., n=20, P<.001: 2-tailed t test) and -0.82 pT ($\pm$ 0.80 s.d., n=20, P<.001). Shifts in the other two quadrants and at the centre were inconsistent in sign and not statistically significant overall.

These magnetic shifts were in a very low frequency domain, at which the shielded room is less efficient at screening out interference than at higher frequencies. The bottom traces in Fig. 1A (X,Y,Z,G) show signals from the artefact rejection channels on the magnetometer, recorded far from the brain. Magnetic events in the principal traces could sometimes be identified as due to external artefacts (e.g. around t=650s in this record). The main shift associated with the SD did not have correlates in these control traces. Transient artefacts were also seen occasionally at times of injection of fluid into the chamber, and with movements (e.g. of the jaws or ears) that occurred sometimes with light anaesthesia. These artefacts were generally readily identifiable.

In addition to the slow magnetic field shifts associated with SD, we found variations during the experiments of the level of fluctuations of magnetic field around its mean value. These are illustrated in Fig. 1B, for the same magnetic data shown in Fig. 1A. There was a drop in the standard deviation of the field measurements on most channels around 350-700s in the record (230-580s after KCl application). This was about the same time as the slow magnetic shifts. The pattern of changes of fluctuation level was less consistent in relation to SD, and may in at least some cases have been due to changes in brain arousal mechanisms. For example, sudden drops in fluctuation level occurred sometimes at the time of KCl application and sometimes at other times without any evident precipitating stimulus.

DISCUSSION

The magnetic fields from the rabbit cortex (1-2pT) were smaller and slower in time course (ca. 200-300s) than those described by Okada et al. (1988), which were up to 8pT with components lasting as little as 5s. Several factors are relevant to the comparison.

The rabbit hemisphere extends from the cup for 10-25mm in different directions. This means that new tissue continues to be invaded by a single wave of SD for 500s or more, eventually affecting tissue within the sagittal (midline) sulcus and down the lateral aspect of the brain. SD does not cross from one hemisphere to the other (Bures et al., 1974). The rabbit has a smooth cortex, unlike man, but in geometry it resembles a single human gyrus.

During SD, the same sequence of brief local events affects different pieces of tissue in turn. The magnetic measurements sum almost uniformly from this tissue, and therefore change only slowly as the amount and orientation of affected tissue alters. A situation in which the amount of affected tissue would change rapidly is where SD is

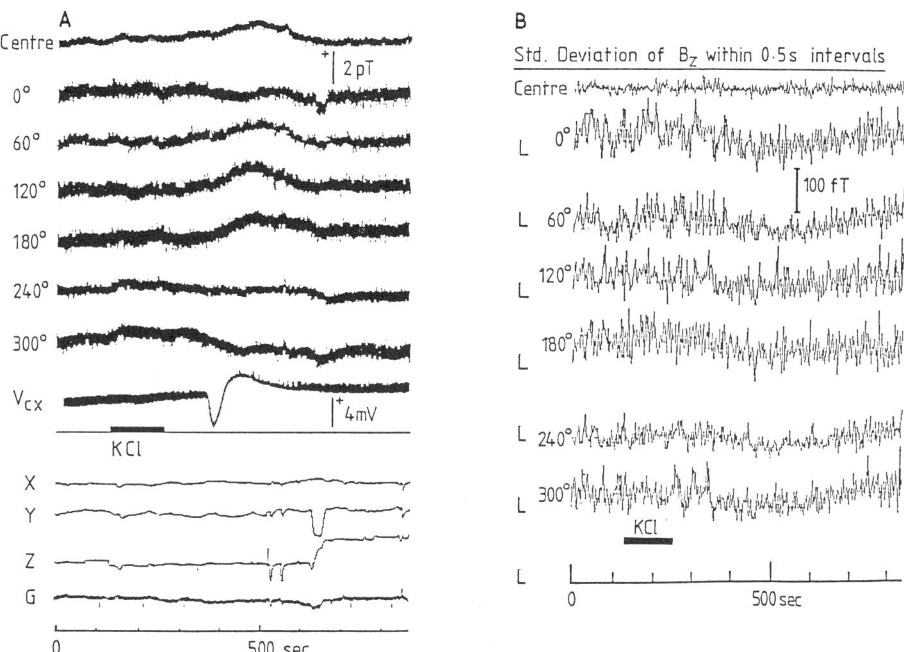

Fig. 1. (A) Magnetic and electric signals during SD elicited with a solution of KCl (bar) applied to the left hemisphere of the cerebral cortex of an anaesthetised rabbit. Top 7 traces are magnetic fields perpendicular to the skull, from above the initiation site and from 21.5mm distant, anterior (0°) and at specified angles. Vcx: voltage at an electrode on the cortical surface. X,Y,Z,G: magnetic signals from distant coils, for monitoring magnetic disturbances of external origin. Calibration: 2pT (+ = outward) for top 7 traces. (B) Measurements of the standard deviation of the top 7 records in A, calculated for 0.5sec intervals. Calibration: 100fT from origins shown at left. The normal characteristics of SD can be seen from the voltage recording (Vcx), 6mm anterior from the chamber. A biphasic (negative - positive) voltage shift occurred with sudden onset 240s after KCl application. The latency reflects the time for initiation of SD in the cup, plus propagation from cup to recording site. The same pattern occurs at different times at different distances from the cup. A drop in amplitude of the normal voltage fluctuations is visible in the record at the time of SD, due to a depression of the local brain activity for 200-300s.

initiated synchronously in a sufficient bulk of tissue. This may have been the case in the experiments of Okada et al. (1988), where electrical stimulation was used. It is not certain that SD, if it occurs in man during migraine, would be synchronously initiated over such an area, several mm across. This would probably be necessary (within a sulcus to obtain optimal orientation) before SD would give rise to rapidly changing magnetic signals comparable to those of Okada et al. (1988). SD was initiated in our experiments at a region of cortex parallel to the skull. Symmetry dictates therefore that we do not see any field during the initiation of SD, only once the SD reaches regions of different orientation or fails to spread symmetrically.

The intracellular current flow during the acute phase of SD is away from the zone affected, probably principally in glial cells (Gardner-Medwin, 1981). The component that may be capable of producing the greatest magnetic fields is that flowing perpendicular to the cortical surface towards deeper tissue, which for symmetry reasons only produces magnetic fields for cortex within a sulcus (Okada et al., 1988). The changes observed in this study may be at least partly due to the spread of SD into the sagittal sulcus, producing a leftward current dipole and field components that are positive (outwards) towards the back of the head (180° in Fig.1A) and negative at the front (0°). The fields also contain a positive component on the right of the head (90°), which may arise from propagation in other regions.

The small amplitude of our signals compared with those of Okada et al. (1988) may be due partly to the less favourable electrical conditions in intact tissue, compared to a tissue bath. Intracellular current flow can, in a tisue bath, return by relatively low resistance and long current loops through the surrounding saline, producing conditions for substantial magnetic fields. In intact tissue, a larger fraction of the current will return through the local extracellular space, running parallel to the intracellular current and cancelling out the magnetic fields.

The reduced level of higher frequency magnetic fluctuations (1-50Hz) that we observed in some experiments may have been partly caused by SD, since local reductions in neural activity and voltage fluctuations occur in the tissue. The variable time relation between the changes and the induction of SD suggests, however, that the decreases of the level of fluctuations could have been be due to arousal, not to SD itself. This possibility requires further investigation.

REFERENCES

Bures J., Buresova O. & Krivanek J., 1974, Mechanisms and applications of Leao's spreading depression of electrical activity, Academia, Prague.

Gardner-Medwin A.R., 1981, Possible roles of vertebrate neuroglia in potassium dynamics, spreading depression and migraine, J. exp. Biol., 95:111-127

Lauritzen M. & Olesen J., 1984, Regional blood flow during migraine attacks by Xe-133 inhalation and emission tomography, Brain, 107:447-461

Leao A.A.P. and Morrison R.S., 1945, Propagation of spreading cortical depression, J. Neurophysiol., 8:33-45

Milner P.M., 1958, Note on a possible correspondence between scotomas of migraine and spreading depression of Leao, EEG clin. Neurophys., 10:705

Nicholson C. and Kraig R.P., 1981, The behaviour of extracellular ions during spreading depression. In: The application of ion-selective electrodes, T. Zeuthen, ed., Elsevier, Amsterdam

Okada Y.C., Lauritzen M. and Nicholson C., 1988, Magnetic field associated with spreading depression: a model for the detection of migraine, Brain Res., 442:185-190

Tepley N., Barkley G.L., Moran J., Simkins R.T. and Welch K.M.A. Observation of spreading cortical depression in migraine patients. This volume.

OBSERVATION OF SPREADING CORTICAL DEPRESSION IN MIGRAINE PATIENTS

N. Tepley[*+], G.L. Barkley[*], J.E. Moran[+], R.T. Simkins[*], K.M.A. Welch[*]

Neuromagnetism Laboratory, Department of Neurology
Henry Ford Hospital, Detroit, MI 48202 USA

[+]Department of Physics, Oakland University, Rochester, MI 48309, USA

Introduction

Spreading cortical depression (SCD) in animal models was first described by Leao [1] in 1944. SCD, although never observed spontaneously in humans, has been implicated in migraine for a variety of reasons: 1) the marked dilation of pial blood vessels accompanying SCD [2], 2) the slow propagation speed of 3 mm/min which is comparable to the motion of migraine scotomata [3] and 3) the cerebral blood flow anomolies observed in migraine with aura which are also similar to those seen during SCD [4]. SCD is not observable by surface EEG, but Okada et al [5, 6] produced SCD in isolated turtle cerebellum by electrical stimulation and recorded biphasic slow magnetic waves. They suggested SCD should be observable by MEG in humans. We report here the results of studies on migraine patients, normal subjects and patients suffering non-migraine headaches.

Methods

Twelve migraine patients were studied using a BTI model 607 seven channel Neuromagnetometer® in a magnetically shielded room. The sensor in all cases was placed at the temporal-parietal-occipital junction on the side for which the patient reported more frequent headaches or the headache in progress. Each patient was monitored continuously for 20-60 minutes. Filter settings were either 0 to 50 Hz or 0.1 to 50 Hz. Patients included nine having migraine with aura and three having migraine without aura. Two of each type were studied during spontaneous attacks. Three patients were studied after exposure to known triggering agents (perfume, cheese, caffeine) or activity (exercise). Eight controls and three patients with tension headaches and one with headache due to an Arnold-Chiari malformation were also studied.

During prolonged neuromagnetic monitoring, even in a shielded room, a variety of artifacts usually occur. As sources of artifact were identified a number of precautions were taken: 1) The ambient magnetic field was

Advances in Biomagnetism
Edited by S.J. Williamson *et al.*
Plenum Press, New York

recorded continuously from the reference gradiometer and three reference magnetometers and data contaminated by excessive magnetic noise were excluded from analysis. 2) At the beginning of each study, the subject performed movements including eye opening and closing, various head and eye movements and swallowing, and the resulting artifactual signals were stored for later comparison to the data. The subject was observed throughout the study and similar movements were noted with an event-marker so that movement artifact could be excluded. In addition, Data Period Analysis (DPA), [7] a modification of known EEG analysis techniques described by Hjorth [8] was used to identify various changes in arousal state and to distinguish them from the suppression of neuronal activity associated with SCD. DPA determines the fraction of the magnetic energy occurring in waveforms of various periods. It is quicker to use and with careful interpretation is more useful than the power spectrum. DPA samples selected "windows" of arbitrary duration and identifies, at each instant of time, the dominant frequency component present. This produces a spectrum of these components, in contrast to Fourier transform which produces a time averaged spectrum.

Results

In patients with migraine with aura, signals believed to be associated with SCD were observed in both cases monitored during attack and in four of seven studied interictally. In two patients with migraine without aura, such signals were found in both studied during attacks and in one studied after a failed attempt to trigger an attack. Comparable signals were not found in eight control subjects or in four patients with non-migrainous headache. These signals have two features: 1) Usually biphasic waves less than ten seconds long with amplitudes ranging from 800 fT to 13 pT. Successive waves had different morphology with respect to the seven detectors suggesting that they arose from different cortical locations. A pair of these waves (band width 0.1 to 50 Hz) detected during migraine with aura is shown in Fig. 1. These waveforms may represent the onset or offset of depolarization in a sulcus where neurons are nearly tangential to the scalp, optimum for giving rise to measurable fields. 2) A ten minute or longer drop in signal amplitude as shown in the top trace of Fig. 2. Also shown

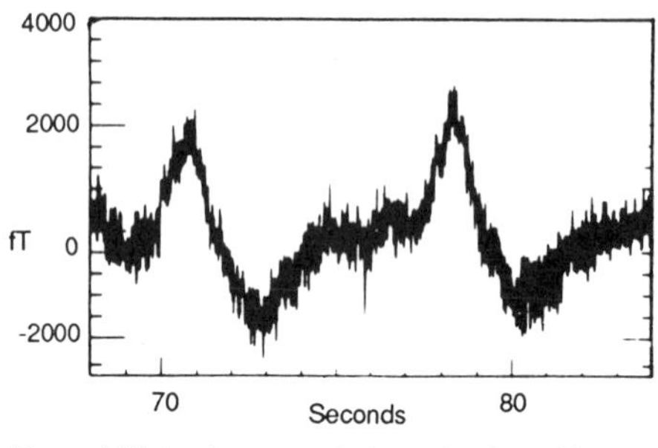

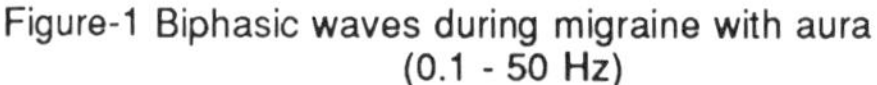

Figure-1 Biphasic waves during migraine with aura (0.1 - 50 Hz)

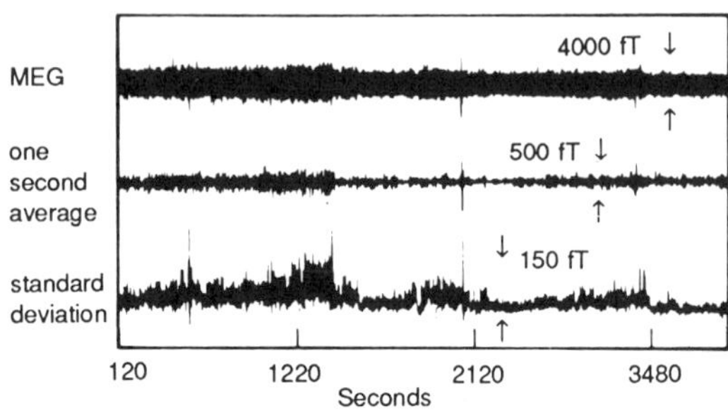

Figure-2 Fifty-six minute migraine study (0.1 - 50 Hz).

are one second averages of this data and standard deviations of these averages. Larger standard deviation is indicative of larger amplitude spontaneous activity. To identify the various changes in activity as being either changes in alertness or SCD we performed DPA as shown in Fig. 3. This DPA shows that in the interval from 2250 to 2410 seconds there is a generalized suppression of activity at all periods (hence frequencies) compared to the baseline interval from 120 to 240 seconds during which the patient was

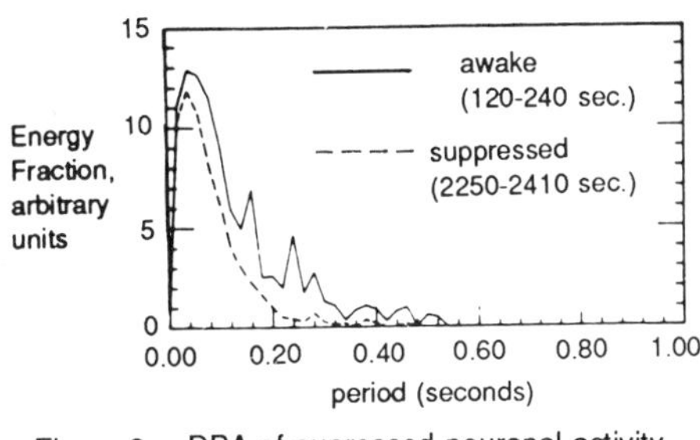

Figure-3 DPA of supressed neuronal activity.

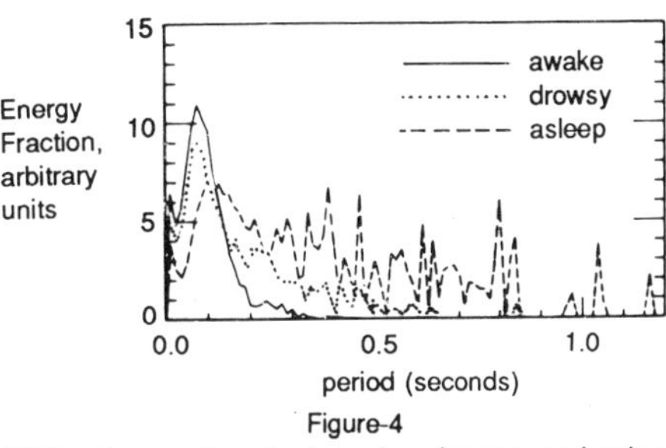

Figure-4 DPA's of normal patient awake, drowsy, and asleep.

known to be awake. This DPA should be compared to that for a normal subject as she becomes drowsy and finally falls asleep (Fig. 4). There is a progressive increase in long period activity and loss of short period (alpha rhythm) activity with drowsiness and sleep. (Note: DPA plots indicate waveform periods, twice the interval between zero crossings).

Comparison with rabbit model

We also applied DPA analysis to MEG data from a rabbit model where SCD can be reliably produced by infusing KC1 onto the cortex (see accompanying paper [9]). Figure 5 shows MEG data from one rabbit run (band width 0.1 - 5.0 Hz). As can be seen, neuronal suppression starts almost immediately after KC1 infusion, but the depolarization wave, as detected by ECoG, arrives at the electrode placed some distance from the infusion site at a later time. Average and standard deviation plots are qualitatively similar to those shown in Fig. 2. DPA, shown in Fig. 6, used a time window selected to emphasize frequencies faster than one Hz. As one would expect in SCD, DPA shows a suppression at all frequencies, and is qualitatively similar to the DPA shown in Fig. 3 which we believe represents spontaneous SCD in a migraine patient. Similar DPA patterns of suppression at all frequencies were obtained 13 runs (both AC and DC coupled) on five rabbits.

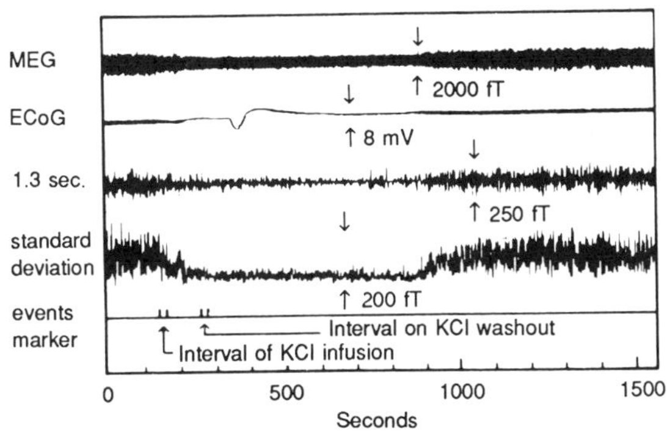

Figure-5 Study of induced SCD in a rabbit (0.1-50 Hz).

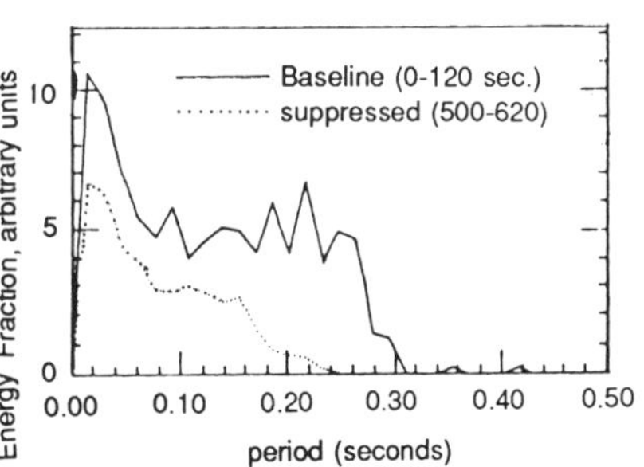

Figure-6 DPA of SCD in a rabbit.

Conclusions

Reproducible neuromagnetic signals consisting of long duration biphasic field shifts and suppression of ongoing background activity has been observed in migraine patients but not in patients suffering other forms of headache or normal controls. Similar suppression of activity has been observed in rabbits in which SCD was induced and confirmed by ECoG. The large biphasic waves in humans which we interpret as arising from a sulcus do not occur in the rabbit where the cortex is lissencephalic. While we are encouraged that this data may represent the first observation of spontaneous SCD in migraine, we caution that these findings come from a relatively small number of patients and controls.

We find it of interest that SCD seems to occur between attacks in some migraine patients. This may suggest a fundamental physiologic difference between migrainous and non-migrainous individuals. We are continuing to investigate this finding.

Further confirmation of this work would suggest that MEG may play an important role in the diagnosis of migraine and in the evaluation of various treatments. We propose to extend these studies to other maladies for which there is some evidence that SCD may occur such as head trauma and stroke.

Acknowledgement

The authors wish to acknowledge the contribution of Dr. A.R. Gardner-Medwin in carrying out the rabbit model studies refered to in the paper.

References

1. Leao, A.A.P., 1944, Spreading cortical depression of activity in the cerebral cortex, J Neurophysiol, 7:379-390.

2. Leao, A.A.P., Morrison, R.S, 1945, Propagation of spreading cortical depression, J Neurophysiol, 8:33-45.

3. Milner, P.M., 1958, Note on a possible correspondence between scotomas of migraine and spreading depression of Leao. EEG Clin Neurophysiol, 10:705.

4. Lauritzen, M., 1987, Cortical spreading depression as a putative migraine mechanism, Trends Neurosci, 10:8-13.

5. Okada, Y.C., Nicholson, C., 1988, DC-coupled single trial measurements of the magnetic field during spreading depression in the cerebellum. In: Biomagnetism '87, Atsumi K, Kotani M, Ueno S, Katila T, Williamson SJ (eds.), Denki University Press, London, 1988, pp. 202-205.

6. Okada, Y., Lauritzen, M., Nicholson, C., 1988, Magnetic field associated with spreading cortical depression: a model for the detection of migraine, Brain Research, 442:185-190.

7. Moran, J.E., Tepley, N., (submitted for publication) Data Period Analysis - a rapid method for recognizing changes of alertness in MEG and EEG data.

8. Hjorth, B., 1970, EEG analysis based on time domain properties. EEG Clin Neurophysiol 29:306-310.

9. Gardner-Medwin, A.R., Tepley, T., Barkley, G.L., Moran, J., Nagel-Leiby, S., Simkins, R.T., Welch, K.M.A., Magnetic observation of spreading cortical depression in anesthetized rabbits. This volume.

COMPARATIVE STUDY OF TRANSMEMBRANE POTENTIAL AND MAGNETIC EVOKED FIELD DUE TO APPLIED ELECTRIC FIELD IN THE TURTLE CEREBELLUM

L. Lopez, Y.C. Okada, C.Y. Chan*, C. Nicholson

Department of Physiology and Biophysics, New York University Medical Center, New York, NY 10016
*Department of Physiology, CUNY Medical School, New York, NY 10031

INTRODUCTION

The application of a uniform electric field to an in vitro preparation allows the selective polarization of definite regions of the neurons oriented parallel to the axis of the field (Chan & Nicholson, 1986). Thus, in the isolated turtle cerebellum, it is possible to depolarize the somatic region of the Purkinje cells (Pc) , while hyperpolarizing the superficial side of their dendrites, by means of an electric field directed from dorsal to ventral surface (d-v), and vice versa. We have used this method in order to measure the contribution of sodium (Na) and calcium (Ca) conductances to the magnetic evoked field (MEF). In a previous paper (Okada et al., 1988c) we have shown that it is possible to record both MEF and extracellular potential (EP) in response to pulsed applied electric field. In the present study, a comparison with the intracellular recording was carried out to ascertain the ionic basis of the MEF and EP. Sinusoidal electric fields were also used in order to apply the field along known directions, by avoiding capacitative properties of the membranes, and to provide a sufficient amount of depolarization to directly activate Na and Ca conductances. We made bath applications of specific drugs to block these conductances as well as synaptic transmissions.

METHODS

The turtle cerebellum was isolated and placed in Ringer solution (in mM: NaCl 100, KCl 5, $NaHCO_3$ 40, $CaCl_2$ 3.5, $MgCl_2$ 3.5, Glucose 20, bubbled with 95% O_2 and 5% CO_2). The orientation of the tissue was vertical so that the Pc axes were oriented parallel to the electric field, which was applied by means of two Ag/AgCl plate electrodes (4 x 1 cm.). We used both square wave (300-1000 μsec) and sinusoidal wave (4-10 Hz). The magnetic field produced by the neural elements oriented along the dorso-ventral (d-v) axis was recorded at the field extrema, with an asymmetric second order gradiometer coupled to a DC-SQUID (Okada et al., 1988b). The EP was measured by means of conventional glass micropipettes referred to Ag/AgCl ground electrode. The response to sinusoidal field was recorded with two electrodes, the stimulus artefact in the recording electrode was removed by subtracting the output of the second electrode that recorded only stimulus artefact. The intracellular recordings were performed together with the EP recording, the latter being the common element in the two sets of experiments. The transmembrane potential (TMP) was recorded with conventional glass micropipette, connected to an active bridge amplifier provided with current injection circuit (Chan et al, 1988). The sinusoidal artefact cancellation was achieved with subtraction of the stimulus artefact sensed by the extracellular electrode from the output of the intracellular electrode positioned at the same depth about 100 μm apart.

Advances in Biomagnetism
Edited by S.J. Williamson *et al.*
Plenum Press, New York

RESULTS

Pulsed field. The first component of the EP (1.4 ms) was negative in the granular layer and positive in the molecular layer. The second component (3.4 ms), which had much longer duration, was also negative in the granular layer and reversed its polarity at a location more dorsal (by about 100 μm) than the first component. We compared the laminar potential

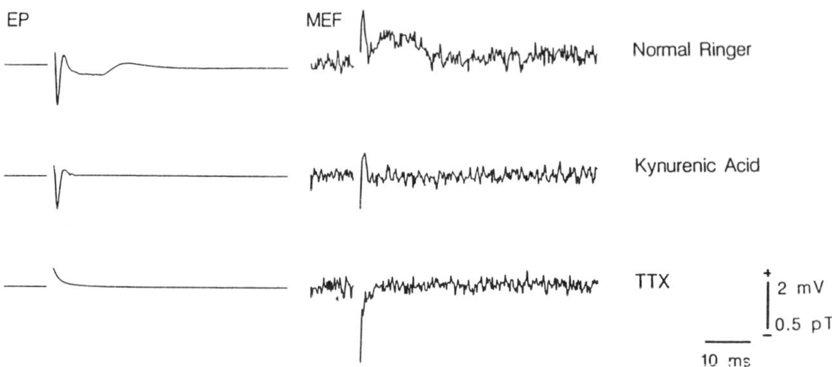

Fig. 1 . Responses to the square applied electric field. The field was applied from ventral to dorsal surface, at twice the threshold for the 1.4 ms component. EP: the recording electrode was placed in the Pc layer, (500 μm from ventral surface). MEF: probe position at field extremum 20 mm above the center of the cerebellum. (Kyn.A 7 mM, TTX 1μM). Outward MEF is positive.

profiles produced by the electric field and by a local peduncle stimulus. The second component in both cases reversed at the same depth and its waveform was very similar for both stimulations. The intracellular recording from a Pc dendrite showed a climbing fiber (cf) response at 3.4 ms; at the soma the direct activation of the Pc was seen at 1.4 ms. These latencies are consistent with direct activation and monosynaptic transmission in turtle. The corresponding MEF for both components was consistent with currents flowing from the soma to the dendrites of Pc (Fig. 1). Interestingly, these responses showed much lower threshold and higher amplitude if a d-v field was applied, that is if the ventral sides of the core conductors were depolarized. By administration of Kynurenic Acid (Kyn.A), which is known to specifically block the synaptic transmission mediated by excitatory amino-acids (Cochran, 1983) the second component was abolished, while the first component remained unchanged. This component could be blocked only by addition of tetrodotoxin (TTX).

Sinusoidal field. The asymmetry of activation for the two directions of the field could be clearly demonstrated with this stimulus pattern. In response to d-v stimulation two components were seen that resembled the responses to the pulsed field as far as polarities, latencies and amplitudes were concerned. The TMP showed Na spikes time-locked to the first component of the EP, followed by a post-synaptic complex spike, comparable to the intracellular response to the pulse., After administration of 8 mM Kyn.A, this second component was completely abolished (Fig. 2). In response to the v-d field (Fig. 3), the TMP recordings showed high threshold calcium spikes at the distal dendrite (cell A) that cannot be well recorded at the somatic level (cell B). The extracellular recording showed a high threshold biphasic response that changed after Kyn.A administration, the negativity being abolished and substituted by a positivity that was both TTX and Mn^{++} sensitive. This component has not been clearly recorded magnetically, possibly due to the fact that the Ca spikes, in phase with v-d field, do not have a good synchronization, at least at 2-5 Hz, stimulation.

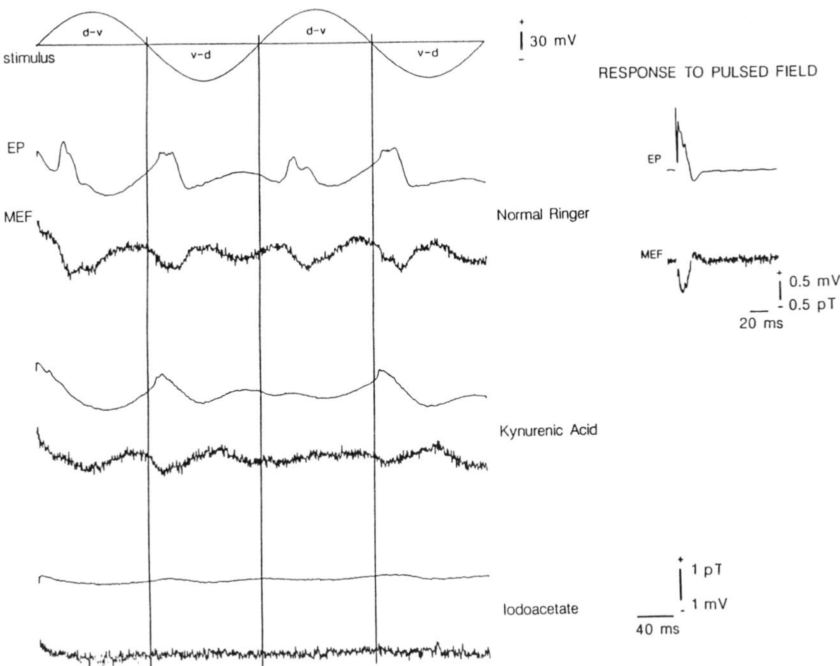

Fig. 2. Response to sinusoidal field (4 Hz). EP: recording electrode was placed at ~700 μm from ventral surface, note the polarity reversal of the post-synaptic component. MEF: probe 20 mm above the cerebellum at the rostral field extremum. Kyn.A (7 mM) abolished the response to d-v field, Iodoacetate (20 mM) abolishes all responses.

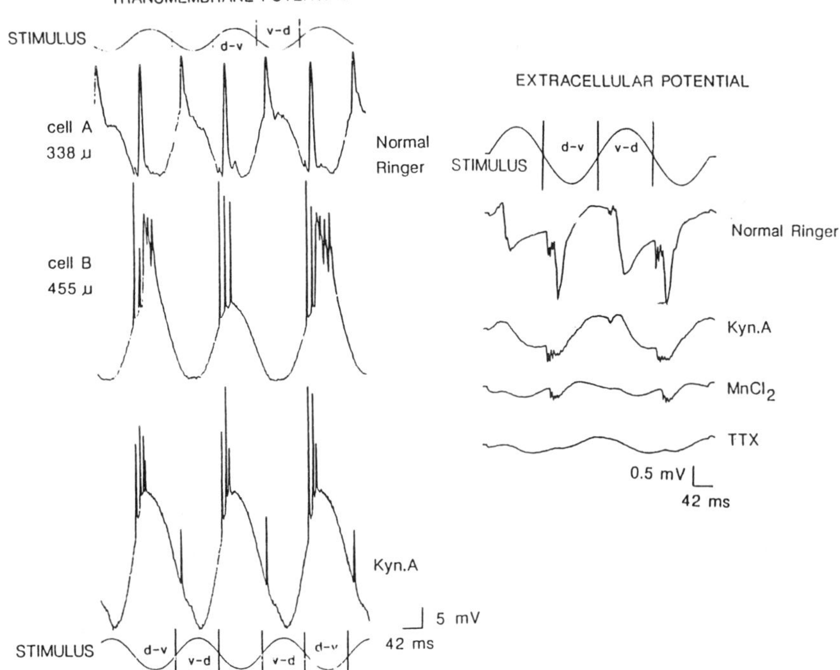

Fig. 3. TMP: The two recordings at distal Pc dendrite (cell A) and soma (cell B) both show a climbing fiber response to d-v field, which is abolished after bath application of Kyn.A (8 mM). cell A shows a better response to v-d field. EP: electrode position Pc layer. Kyn.A 7 mM, $MnCl_2$ 10 mM, TTX 1 μM

DISCUSSION

In this study we have correlated the MEF to the ionic currents directly activated by the applied electric field. In this preparation, all the neuronal circuits maintain their integrity. Five populations of cells can be considered as cable elements oriented parallel to the field: Pc, stellate cells, Golgi cells, the ascending portion of the granular cells and climbing fibers. For this reason, a correlation between MEF, EP and the intracellular Pc recording is needed to better understand what currents contribute to the waveforms described above. Our results show that d-v pulsed and sinusoidal fields elicit not only directly activated TTX-sensitive but also Kyn.A-sensitive post-synaptic responses in the EP and MEF recordings. The laminar potential profile confirms that the extracellular current sinks for both these responses lie close to the somatic region. The TMP recordings clearly show that the TTX-sensitive component is due to Na-spikes generated in the somatic region of the Pc. The Kyn.A-sensitive component is due to post-synaptic activation of the Pc through direct activation of the climbing fibers. In response to v-d sinusoidal fields we saw a Kyn.A-sensitive component in the EP plus a Kyn.A-insensitive component that can be due either to directly activated Ca currents or to inhibitory post-synaptic potentials. Failure to respond to picrotoxin administration indicates that this component is not inhibitory. The responses of the dendritic portion of the Pc can be obtained only with v-d sinusoidal field and, based on their morphology, they are mediated by Ca conductances.

The comparison of the three types of responses clearly showed that Na and Ca conductance changes which generate intracellular currents can give rise not only to the extracellular potential, but also to the magnetic evoked field. This correlation is important in understanding the ionic origin of the magnetic fields recorded from human brain.

ACKNOWLEDGEMENTS

Supported by NINDS grant NS21149

REFERENCES

Chan C.Y, and Nicholson C., 1986, Modulation by applied electric field of Purkinje and stellate cell activity in the isolated cerebellum. J. Physiol. (London), 371, 89-114.

Chan C.Y., Hounsgaard J., and Nicholson C., 1988, Effects of electric fields on transmembrane potential and excitability of turtle cerebellar Purkinje cells in vitro, J. Physiol. (London), 402, 751-771.

Cochran S.L., 1983, Kynurenic acid: competitive agonist of excitatory synaptic transmission? Neurosci. Lett. Suppl. 40, S68.

Okada Y.C., and Nicholson C., 1988a, Magnetic field associated with transcortical currents in turtle cerebellum, Biophys. J., 53, 723-731.

Okada Y.C., Lopez L., and Nicholson C,1988b, Origin of the magnetic evoked field produced by applied electric field in the isolated turtle cerebellum. Soc. Neurosci. Abs., 14 .

Okada Y.C., Lauritzen M., Nicholson C., 1988c, Magnetic field associated with spreading depression: a model for the detection of migraine. Brain Res. 442, 185-190, .

CONDUCTIVITY BOUNDARIES MAY PRODUCE STRONGER MAGNETIC FIELDS THAN THE PRIMARY SOURCE: COMPARISON OF THREE ANALYTICAL METHODS

J.-C. Huang, Y. C. Okada and C. Nicholson

Department of Physiology and Biophysics
New York University Medical Center, New York, NY 10016

INTRODUCTION

Conductivity boundaries distort the current in a volume conductor such as the human head. This distortion may significantly alter the electric potential and magnetic field on the surface of a volume conductor (e.g.scalp)(Ueno, 1983; Hämäläinen and Sarvas, 1989; Cuffin, 1982; Meijs et al., 1989). The magnetic field **B** and electrical potential on any given surface of a volume conductor is given by the following formulas (Geselowitz, 1970; Barnard et al., 1967a, b):

$$\mathbf{B} = \frac{\mu_0}{4\pi}\int_V \mathbf{J} \times \nabla\left(\frac{1}{R}\right) dv + \frac{\mu_0}{4\pi}\Delta\sigma \int_S \Phi \nabla\left(\frac{1}{R}\right) \times d\mathbf{S} ,$$

$$\Phi = \frac{1}{4\pi\bar{\sigma}}\int_V \mathbf{J} \cdot \nabla\left(\frac{1}{R}\right) dv + \frac{1}{4\pi\bar{\sigma}}\Delta\sigma \int_S \Phi \nabla\left(\frac{1}{R}\right) \cdot d\mathbf{S} ,$$

where μ_0 is the permeability of free space, **J** represents an equivalent impressed current density due to current generators such as neurons in the brain, R is the distance from each volume element dv (or surface element dS) to the observation point, $\Delta\sigma$ is the difference in electrical conductivity across boundary s, $\bar{\sigma}$ is the average conductivity at the boundary. In these equations, the first term represents the primary source contribution and the second term the boundary effects where the integral is over the surface of each boundary.

We evaluated the possible contribution of conductivity boundaries to the Φ and **B** for an isolated turtle cerebellum immersed in saline. The cerebellum is a lissencephalic oblate spheroid. This simple geometry enabled us to apply three analytical methods to evaluate the relative contribution of the boundary between the cerebellum and the saline to the surface potential and magnetic field outside the bath. We found that secondary sources at the boundary may produce a magnetic field and electrical potential that are identical in temporal waveform but as much as 2-3 times in magnitude as those that may be produced by the primary neuronal current source. (See Huang et al., 1989, for detail.)

METHODS

We considered the cerebellum (5 mm diameter and 1 mm thick) to be vertically immersed in a large bath of physiological saline at a depth of 10 mm (referred to the center of the cerebellum). The neuronal current source evoked by an

Advances in Biomagnetism
Edited by S.J. Williamson *et al.*
Plenum Press, New York

external stimulation was modeled by a single 10 nA·m current dipole (Q) placed along the center axis of the cerebellum, perpendicular to the cerebellar surface. We calculated the electrical potential at the potential extremum on the bath surface (V) and the component of the **B** normal to bath surface at its field extremum (Bz) due to Q and those that are due to the distributed set of secondary sources at the boundary between the cerebellum and saline. To calculate V and Bz, we first determined the potential Φ on the surface of the cerebellum embedded in an infinite ohmic medium, ignoring the bath surface, since it was relatively far away compared to the cerebellar thickness. The three methods were used to calculate Φ: (1) method of images, (2) method of integral equation (boundary element method) and (3) method of the Poisson equation. The comparison of results from these three methods enabled us to validate our analytical and numerical solutions for Φ. Then, we used the boundary element method to determine V and Bz due to Q and secondary current dipoles $(\sigma_{out}-\sigma_{in})\phi\mathbf{n}$ on the cerebellar surface, where $\mathbf{n}$ is a unit vector normal to the cerebellar surface, directed from the cerebellum (σ_{in}) to the outer conducting medium (σ_{out}) of saline (Geselowitz, 1970).

RESULTS

For the method of images the cerebellum was represented as an infinite slab of conductivity σ_{in} and thickness of d=a+b embedded in an infinite volume conductor of conductivity σ_{out} (Fig. 1A). The potential on the two surfaces were calculated from the following equation deduced for this geometry:

$$\Phi = \frac{Q}{4\pi\sigma}\sum_{n=0}\left(\frac{\Delta\sigma}{2\sigma}\right)^{2n}\frac{1}{[2nb+(2n+1)a]^2} + \frac{Q}{4\pi\sigma}\sum_{n=1}\left(\frac{\Delta\sigma}{2\sigma}\right)^{2n-1}\frac{1}{[2nb+(2n-1)a]^2},$$

where the primary source Q was oriented toward the positive x-direction and the was located at a distance a from surface S1 and b from surface S2 . When $\sigma_{in} < \sigma_{out}$, the image dipoles have the same orientation as the primary source. But, when $\sigma_{in} > \sigma_{out}$, their directions alternate. Note that $\Phi = \Phi_{primary}$ when $\sigma_{in} = \sigma_{out}$ as it should be when there is no conductivity boundary and $\Phi = 2\Phi_{primary}$ as it should be when the slab approximates a semi-infinite volume conductor (i.e., $\sigma_{out}= 0$, a is small and b is large).

For the boundary element method, we represented the cerebellum by a rectangular box (5 x 5 x 1 mm) of a conductivity σ_{in} with the primary source Q in its center (Fig. 1B). The surrounding saline had a conductivity σ_{out}. The Φ on the boundary was obtained by solving the Fredholm's equation numerically (Barnard et al., 1967a, b), by representing it in a matrix form and by utilizing the Jacobi's iterative algorithm. The solution for our problem was stable, since the matrix of the linear system of equations was non-singular with its eigenvalues less than unity. Each surface was divided into 20 x 20 boundary surface elements (each element being 0.25 mm x 0.25 mm) in order to minimize calculation errors. We varied the boundary element size to ascertain the accuracy of our solution.

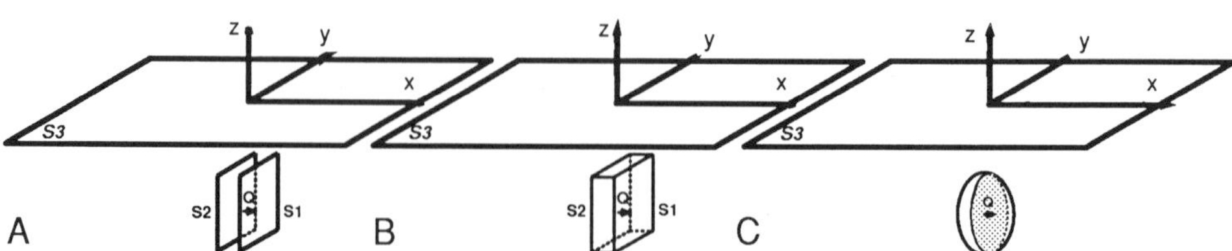

Fig. 1. Diagram of the three models used to represent the turtle cerebellum.

For the third method, we obtained a closed-form analytical solution to the Poisson equation for an oblate spheroid of a conductivity σ_{in} embedded in an infinite conducting medium of a conductivity σ_{out} with the primary source represented by a current dipole Q (Fig. 1C):

$$\Phi_{\zeta_a} = -\frac{1}{4\pi\sigma_{in}}\frac{1}{c^2}\sum_{n=0}^{\infty} j(-1)^n(2n+1)\left[Q_n(j\zeta_a) + \frac{(\sigma_{in}-\sigma_{out})Q_n(j\zeta_a)P_n(j\zeta_a)}{\sigma_{out}P_n(j\zeta_a) - \sigma_{in}\frac{P_n'(j\zeta_a)}{Q_n'(j\zeta_a)}Q_n(j\zeta_a)}\right]\cdot P_n(j\xi)P_n'(j\zeta_0)$$

where P_n and Q_n are associated Legendre functions, P' and Q' are their derivatives, $c^2 = a^2 - b^2$ (a=2.5 mm and b=0.5 mm are the major and minor axes of the spheroid) and ζ and ξ are coordinates of the oblate spheroid. This solution specializes to the equation given by Berry (1956) for the case $\sigma_{out} = 0$ and $\sigma_{in} = 1$.

$$\Phi_{\zeta_a} = -\frac{1}{4\pi}\frac{1}{c^2}\sum_{n=0}^{\infty} j(-1)^n(2n+1)\left[Q_n(j\zeta_a) - \frac{Q_n'(j\zeta_a)}{P_n'(j\zeta_a)}P_n(j\zeta_a)\right].P_n(\xi)P_n'(j\zeta_0)$$

Cuffin and Cohen (1977) obtained expressions for the **B** field for an oblate spheroid for the case $\sigma_{out} = 0$. The Φ calculated at the potential extremum P of each model cerebellum was 16.2, 16.2 and 16.2 mv for the methods of image, integral equation and Poisson equation, respectively, for the case where Q(10 nA-m) was 0.2 mm from the center of the cerebellum toward P and $\sigma_{in} = 0.1$ Siemens/m and $\sigma_{out} = 0.1$ S/m. The Φ at P was 3.9, 3.9 and 3.7 mV when $\sigma_{in} = 0.1$ S/m and $\sigma_{out} = 1.0$ S/m and 23.2, 23.3 and 23.7 mV when $\sigma_{in} = 0.1$ S/m and $\sigma_{out} = 0.01$ S/m for these three methods, respectively. The profile of the potential away from the extremum also showed a comparable degree of similarities. The good agreement among the three methods shows that the cerebellum was sufficiently thin to be accurately modeled by either an infinite slab or a rectangular box as well as by an oblate spheroid. Moreover, this result demonstrates that the numerical methods as well as the analytical formulas we derived were correct.

The V and Bz calculated for the rectangular model of the cerebellum were 4.6 mv and 3.85 pT, respectively, for the contribution due to the primary source located in the center of the box and 10.4 mv and 8.71 pT for the contribution due to the boundary, for experimentally determined values of $\sigma_{in} = 0.20$ S/m (extracellular conductivity) and $\sigma_{out} = 1.33$ S/m (conductivity of physiological saline at 21°C)

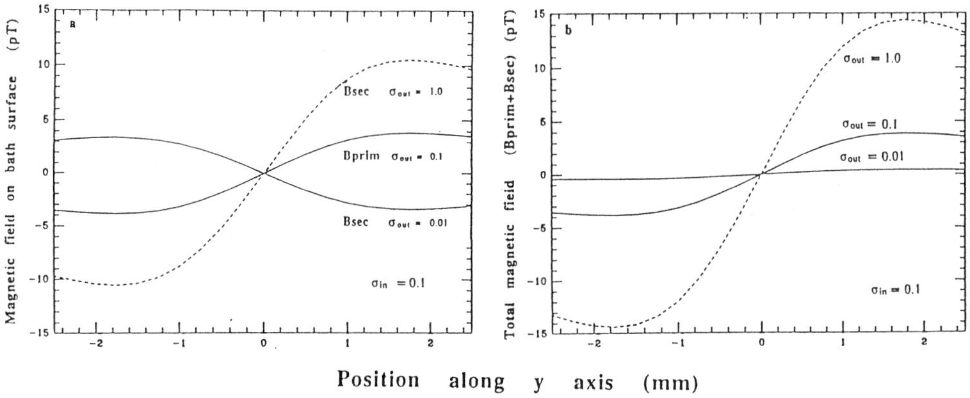

Fig. 2. Relative contributions of primary and secondary sources to the magnetic field on the bath surface.

(Okada et al., 1989). The results clearly show that the secondary sources may produce V and Bz that are larger than those due to the primary source for the values of conductivities and dimensions of the model cerebellum that are in accord with our experimental preparation.

Figure 2 shows the **B** field produced by the secondary sources (B_{sec}) on the large surfaces (S1 and S2) of the rectangular box, in comparison with the magnetic field (B_{prim}) produced by the primary source (a current dipole of 10 nA-m) in a model cerebellum of $\sigma_{in} = 0.1$ S/m. It demonstrates that the B_{sec} is as much as 2-3 times the B_{prim} when $\sigma_{out} = 10\sigma_{in}$ and almost the same but of the opposite polarity when $\sigma_{out} = \sigma_{in}/10$. The total combined field is significantly enhanced when the outer conductivity is higher and almost null when it is lower, by a factor of ten. The result is identical for the electrical surface potential. This example illustrates possible profound effects on the magnitude of the magnetic field one measures in various preparations when a primary source is close to a boundary.

DISCUSSION

Our result raises the possibility that secondary sources may significantly enhance or diminish the magnetic field and electrical potential due to primary neuronal currents. A detailed analysis of this implication (Huang et al., 1989) shows that indeed the secondary sources may produce a significant amount of field at boundaries of, for example, ischemia or edema. However, the cortical sulci can be ignored because they are less than 5 mm in normal human brains.

ACKNOWLEDGEMENT

This research was supported by NINDS grant NS21149.

REFERENCES

Barnard, A. C. L., Duck, I. M., and Lynn, M. S., 1967a, The application of electromagnetic theory to electrocardiology. I. Derivation of the integral equations. Biophys. J., 7:443-462.

Barnard, A. C. L., Duck, I. M., Lynn, M. S., and Timlake, W. P., 1967b, The application of electromagnetic theory to electrocardiology. II. Numerical solution of the integral equations. Biophys. J., 7:463-491.

Berry, P.M., 1956, N,M space harmonics of the oblate spheroid. Ann. N.Y. Acad. Sci., 65:1126-34

Cuffin, B.N., and Cohen, 1977, Magnetic fields of a dipole in special volume conductor shapes. IEEE Trans. Biomed. Eng., BME 24:372-381.

Cuffin, B.N., 1982, Effects of inhomogeneous regions on electric potentials and magnetic fields. J. Appl. Physics, 53:9192-9197.

Geselowitz, D. B., 1970, On the magnetic field generated outside an inhomogeneous volume conductor by internal current sources. IEEE Trans. Mag., MAG6:346-347.

Hämäläinen, M. S., and Sarvas J., 1989, Realistic conductivity geometry model of the human head for interpretation of neuromagnetic data. IEEE Trans. Biomed . Eng. . BME-36:165-171.

Huang, J.C., Nicholson, C. and Okada, Y.C., 1989, Distortion of magnetic evoked fields and surface potentials by conductivity differences at boundaries in brain tissue. submitted for publication.

Meijs, J. W. H., ten Voorde, B. J., Peters, M. J., Stok, C. S. and Lopes da Silva, F. H., 1988, The influence of various head models on EEGs and MEGs, in: "Functional Brain Imaging", G. Pfurtscheller and F. H. Lopes da Silva, eds., Springer-Verlag, Berlin, in press.

Okada, Y. C., Rice, M. E., Tranchina, D. and Nicholson, C., 1989, Inhomogeneity in electrical conductivity. in prep.

Ueno, S., Wakisako, H., and Matsuoka., S., 1983, Determination of the spatial distribution of abnormal EEG and MEG from current dipole in inhomogeneous volume conductor. Il Nuovo Cimento, 2D:558-566.

IN VIVO NEUROMAGNETIC STUDY OF NORMAL AND PATHOLOGICAL INTRACELLULAR CURRENT IN RAT CORTEX

Shi Di (1,2,3), Christoph Baumgartner (1,4), William W. Sutherling (1), and Daniel S. Barth (1,2)

Department of Neurology (1) and Psychology (2), University of California, Los Angeles, CA 90024, U.S.A.
Mental Health Institute (3), Beijinq Medical Univ., China.
Neurological University Clinic Vienna (4), Vienna, Austria

INTRODUCTION

The magnetoencephalogram (MEG) may be used to localize and study synchronized cellular currents during physiological and pathological cortical activities in animal and man. However, a detailed interpretation of the magnetic responses requires an understanding of the relationship between the cellular currents and the resultant electric and magnetic fields. Based on the theoretical prediction that MEG fields are induced predominantly by intracellular currents (Cohen and Hosaka, 1976; Barth et al., 1986; Okada,Y.C., 1987), MEG animal studies, combined with electrical measurement, may provide valuable information for understanding the neurogenesis of cortical responses.

In the present rat *in vivo* study, we attempt to combine current source-density (CSD) of laminar electrical recording with neuromagnetic measurement to obtain complementary information about the spatially and temporally organized cellular currents within local neural networks in the normal direct cortical response (DCR), and to extend this knowledge to the summed intracellular currents associated with electrically evoked interictal penicillin spikes (EIIS).

METHODS

The normal DCR and the penicillin interictal studies were carried in two separate animal groups. Both the DCR and EIIS were produced by biphasic pulses (0.5 ms per phase; 1 mA; Grass Model S8 Stimulator with Grass Model SIU7 Constant Current Stimulus Isolation Unit) applied to the surface of the temporal cortex using a gold coaxial rod under computer control at a rate of approximately one per second. The penicillin focus was produced by microinjection of penicillin G potassium (100 I.U.; 1000 I.U./μl) at approximately 0.5 mm below the cortical surface at a site 1 mm dorsal to the stimulating electrode. Recording of the EIIS was commenced after 15-20 min, when regular spontaneous penicillin spikes were established. Laminar recording of field potentials of DCR or EIIS was performed simultaneously at successive depths from a 4 electrode array. The electrode array was positioned immediately dorsal to the stimulation site and the interval between depth recordings was 100 um.

Advances in Biomagnetism
Edited by S.J. Williamson *et al.*
Plenum Press, New York

Figure 1 shows the experiment setting. All data were subjected to current source-density (CSD) analysis. The extracranial neuromagnetic field was measured with a 7 channel second derivative superconducting gradiometer (Model 607, Biomagnetic Technologies Inc., San Diego). Both the field potential and the magnetic response were amplified (0.1-100 Hz bandpass), digitally sampled (1024 Hz, 250 ms, 12 bits) and averaged over 100 stimulations. (for detail, please refer to Barth and Sutherling, 1988; Barth et al., 1989).

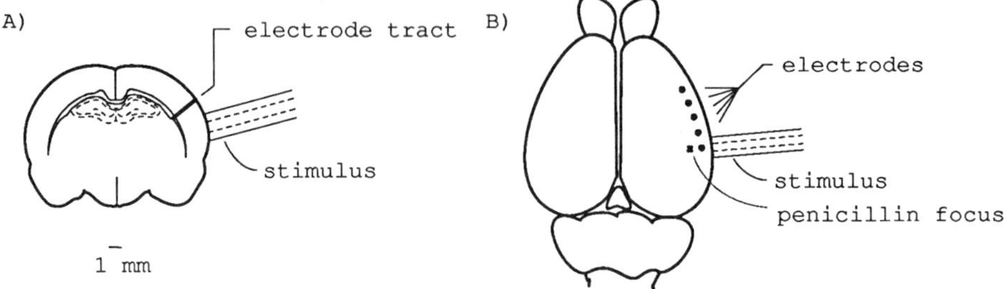

Fig. 1. Coronal (A) and dorsal (B) view of rat cortex showing locations of the stimulating and recording electrodes. An array of 5 parrallel electrodes (1 mm spacing) was inserted perpendicular to the cortical surface to 26 depths (100 µm increments) for field potential mapping. A gold coaxial stimulating electrode (2 mm O.D.) was pressed lightly against the temporal cortical surface to deliver current pulses eliciting the DCR and EIIS. Penicillin was injected right above the center of stimulating probe.

RESULTS

The cortical stimulation elicited a highly stereotyped laminar DCR complex with 4 major temporal components (DCR-P1,N1,P2,N2; Fig.2A). Although field potentials generally reversed polarity between the surface and depth of the cortex, the changing of the waveform throughout the depth suggested that there were differently timed neural elements at different layers active during DCR. CSD analysis of the field potential further indicated the locations of extracellular sinks and sources of each component(Fig. 2B). DCR-P1 was produced by a source at the surface with a complementary sink at a depth of approximately .75mm ; DCR-N1 was produced by a paired sink and source in layers I-IV and V-VI respectively; DCR-P2 had sources both in the surface and depth, while DCR-N2 was mainly generated by the deep source. All four temporal components of electrical DCR complex produced measurable magnetic fields (Fig. 2C). The magnetic DCR profile suggested that the intracellular currents directed toward the cortical surface during positive waves (DCR-P1,P2) and away from the surface during negative components (DCR-N1,N2). In order to evaluate assumptions relating the electrical field potential to extracranial magnetic fields, a computer simulation was created. The simulation model was composed of 7 parallel (1 mm spacing) current dipoles perpendicular to the lateral surface of the temporal cortex. Dipoles were calculated based on the information obtained from the field potential recodings (for detail, please refer to Barth and Sutherling, 1988). The center dipole corresponded to the laminar electrode nearest to the stimulation site. The three dipoles rostal to this location corresponded to the remaining laminar electrode sites in the recoding array. The same three dipoles were repeated caudally, based on the assumption that the cortex was activated symmetrically about the stimulation site. Though with minor differences, the simulation was very close to recorded neuromagnetic fields (Fig. 3).

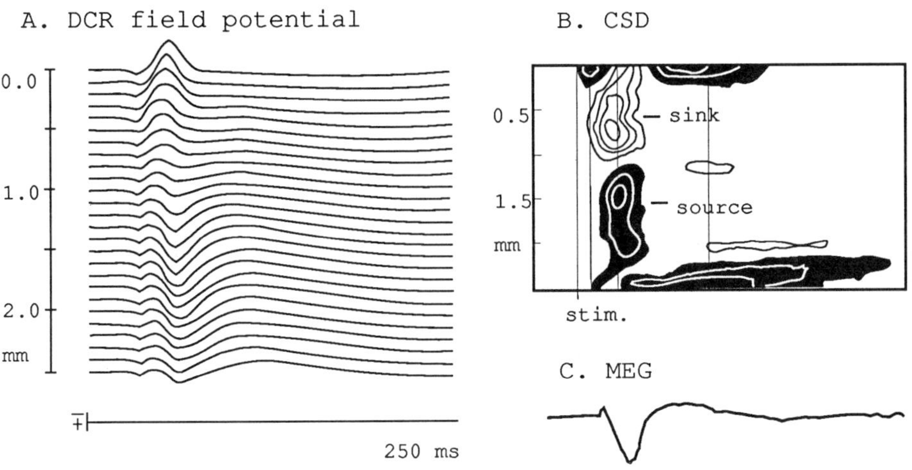

Fig. 2. DCR study. A: Laminar distribution of field potential. B: CSD profile indicates the locations of extracellular current sources (dark background) and sinks (light background). The approximate peak latencies of the DCR-P1, DCR-N1 and DCR-P2 are marked in the maps with thin vertical lines. DCR-N2 was too weak to appear in the isocontour map. C: MEG complex.

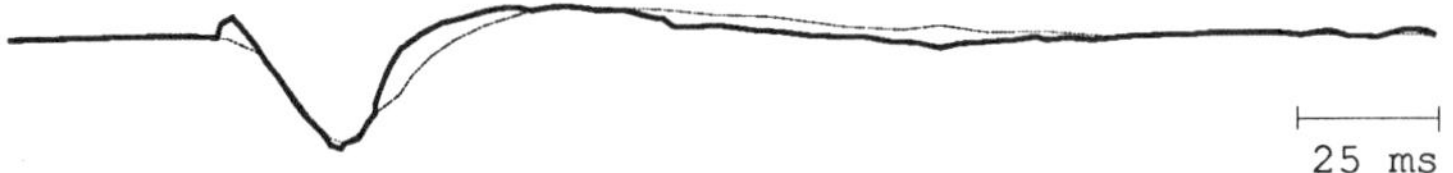

Fig. 3. The estimated intracellular current (light trace) and measured MEG pattern (dark trace) of DCR complex were very similar.

A similar CSD pattern was seen in the sinks and sources of the electrically evoked interictal penicillin spikes. However, based on our present data, the intracellular currents estimated from CSD do not match those actually measured by magnetic field recording for the penicillin interictal spikes (Fig.4).

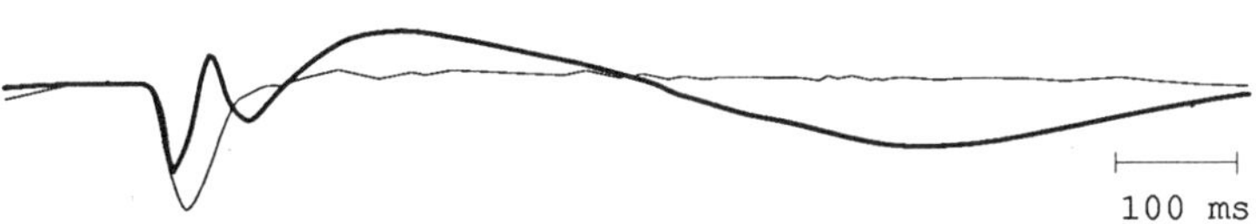

Fig. 4. MEG complex of penicillin interictal spikes (dark trace) revealed multiphasic components. The estimated intracellular current (light trace) is superimposed.

DISCUSSION

In the study of normal DCR, current source-density and neuromagnetic analysis consistently reflect laminar interactions among different neuronal populations which are activated by cortical stimulation. These data suggest that two major neuronal generators located in the different cortical depths, the supragranular pyramidal neurons and the infragranular pyramidal neurons, form a excitatory intracortical circuit. The recorded electric and magnetic waveforms can be explained by their spatial and temporal pattern of transmembrane currents.

Electrical measures of interictal penicillin spikes suggest that the same neural circuits are responsible for pathological discharge. However, the magnetic fields predicted from the model differed from measured fields. The reasons for these differences are unclear and may be a combination of several factors. In the study of magnetic and electric responses in vitro hippocampal slices (Tesche et al, 1988), discrepancies between these two measurements were also reported, suggesting that accurate interpretation of the magnetic measurement requires a more realistic numerical model. In the present study, the apparent discrepancy of electrical and magnetic measurement in the penicillin model of epilepsy is particularly interesting, since the studies of normal DCR have demonstrated their complementary characteristics in the similar experiment setting. It should be noted that the application of one dimensional CSD analysis is based on the assumption that the population of cells participating in the responses are synchronously and uniformly activated. This situation is only approximately true for the DCR, and especially EIIS, measured here, where potential changes are confined primarily along an axis perpendicular to the cortical surface but where there is also a measurable decrease in potential with recording tracks progressively further from the stimulation site. Furthermore the differences may reflect a greater complexity of neural involvement in and around the penicillin focus, requiring a more comprehensive physiological model to predict interictal neuromagnetic fields.

Further studies are in progress in our laboratory to improve our understanding and analysis of spatial and temporal interactions in neocortex both in normal and pathological situation, which will provide more detailed information about the underlying mechanisms of neuromagnetic fields.

ACKNOWLEDGMENTS

This research was supported by USPHS grants 1-R01-NS22575 and 1-R01-NS20806, NSF grant BNS-86-57764.

REFERENCES

Barth, D. S., Sutherling, W. W. and Beatty, J., 1986, Intracellular currents of interictal penicillin spikes: Evidence from neuromagnetic mapping, Brain Res., 368:36-48.

Barth, D. S., Sutherling, W. W., 1988, Current source-density and neuromagnetic analysis of the direct cortical response in rat cortex, Brain Res., 450:280-294.

Barth, D. S., Di, S. and Baumgartner, C., 1989, Laminar cortical interaction during epileptic spikes studied with principal component analysis and physiological modeling, Brain Res., 13-35.

Cohen, D. and Hosaka, J., 1976, Magnetic field produced by a current dipole, J. Electrocardiol., 9:409-417.

Okada, Y. C., Lauritzen, M. and Nicholson, C., 1987, Magnetic field associated with neural activities in an isolated cerebellum, Brain Res., 412:151-155.

Tesche, C. D., Krusin-Elbaum, L. and Knowles, W. D., 1988, Simultaneous measurement of magnetic and electric responses of in vitro hippocampal slices, Brain Res., 462:190-193.

CONTRIBUTION MAPS IN MAGNETOCARDIOGRAPHY

Adriaan van Oosterom, Thom F. Oostendorp, Geertjan Huiskamp

Laboratory of Medical Physics and Biophysics
University of Nijmegen
Nijmegen, The Netherlands

INTRODUCTION

The study reported on in this paper is an example of the so-called 'forward', or 'simulation' studies. Similar such studies were reported on within a decade of the appearance of the first report on the measured cardiac magnetic signals[1]. One of these early studies[2] included an extensive characterization of the heart's electrical activity as represented by numerous electrical dipole sources and an inhomogeneous torso model comprising several compartments of differing, homogeneous conductivity, having a realistic shape as deduced from standard anatomy textbooks.

Our study follows essentially the same approach, the textbook geometry having been replaced by actual, measured geometry of an individual subject, ensuring an accurate relationship between source and field points. The source model used is the classical uniform current dipole layer description of the sources associated with ventricular depolarization. Consequently the simulated wave forms are restricted to the QRS interval. A similar study based on standard, realistic rather than actual, measured geometry was previously reported on by Peters et al[3].

The new model has been recently shown to be capable of accurately simulating observed ECG data[4]. Here it will be demonstrated that the formalism used for describing the genesis of the ECG may be easily extended to the genesis of the MCG. In the analysis of the formalism related to the ECG a new concept was introduced: that of the contribution map[4,5]. In this paper this concept will be extended to magnetic data. It will be demonstrated that magnetic contribution maps are complementary to the corresponding electrical contribution maps.

THEORY

The Source Model

The source model used in our studies is the classical model associated with ventricular depolarization: the uniform double layer[6]. Whereas the 'actual' double layer coincides with the depolarization wave front spreading through the ventricular wall, a completely equivalent double layer is used which coincides with the part of the ventricular surface S_h at which the cells below have been depolarized at each time instant

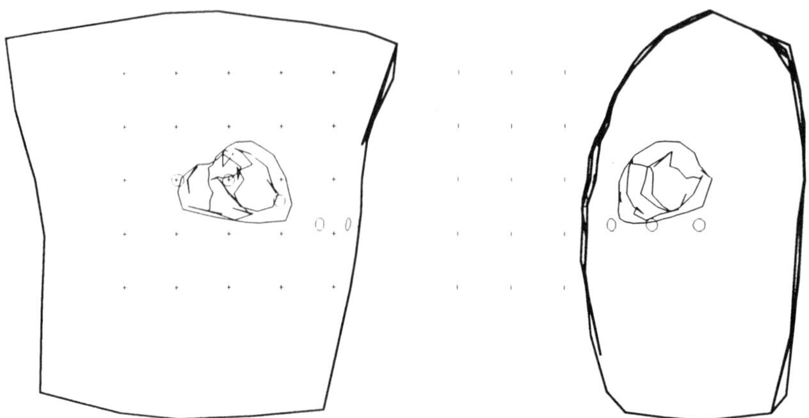

Fig. 1 Left: frontal and right: tranverse view of the torso contour, the heart position, the positions of the standard leads V_1 to V_6 and the gradiometer.

considered. S_h represents the closed surface bounding the ventricles. For the potentials this equivalence follows from standard solid angle theory[7]. For the magnetic field the equivalence was first formulated by Rush[8].

The Volume Conductor

The secondary sources which arise from the passive currents within the volume conductor may be computed from equivalent double layer sources situated at the interfaces between regions of differing conductivity. These secondary sources affect both the electrical potentials and the magnetic field. Their strengths may be derived from the solution of the associated forward problem for the electrical potentials[2,3].

In our ECG study the geometry of torso surface, ventricular surface, ventricular cavities and lung surfaces have been derived from NMR measurements, taken on a healthy subject on which the electrode positions have been accurately documented[4]. In the present MCG study the field points are on a plane parallel to the anterior thorax at a regular grid (6×6 cm^2), the centre of which coincides with the position of lead V_2. A frontal and a tranverse view of the torso contour, the heart position and the positions of the standard leads V_1 to V_6 are shown in Fig. 1.

The Genesis of the ECG

The genesis of the ECG based on our model can be expressed as

$$V(y,t) = \int_{S_h} A(y,x)H(t-\tau(x))dS(x) \tag{1}$$

in which $V(y,t)$ is the potential at time t within the QRS interval at torso point y,
$A(y,x)$ represents the transfer from elementary double layer sources $dS(x)$ at the heart surface S_h to torso points y,
$\tau(x)$ is the local depolarization time at x,
H is the Heaviside step function which switches on the elementary sources at $dS(x)$ from $\tau(x)$ onward.

The quality of the simulation based on a specific choice of the activation function $\tau(x)$ and a transfer function $A(y,x)$ computed from the measured geometry has been dis-

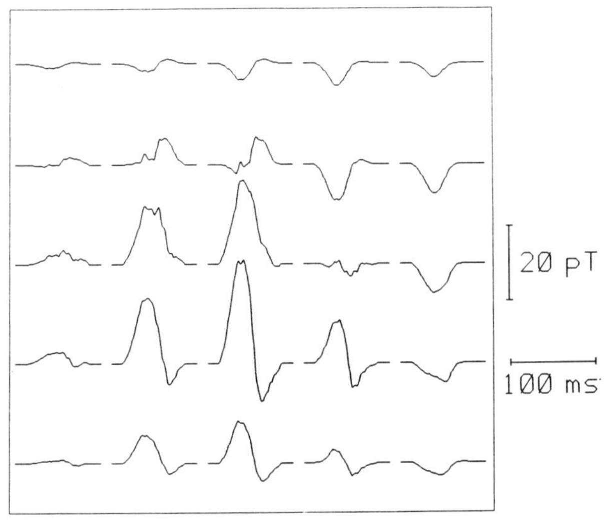

Fig. 2 Simulated MCG QRS wave forms at the grid points.

cussed elsewhere[4]. The activation function $\tau(x)$ used is documented in [9].

The Genesis of Magnetic Data

In this study one and the same model is postulated for the electrical and the magnetic signals. Accordingly, the MCG may be computed from

$$M(y,t) = \int_{S_h} B(y,x)H(t-\tau(x))dS(x)\,, \tag{2}$$

which follows from the fact that any component M of the magnetic field resulting from an elementary source at $dS(x)$ is a linear combination of its primary field and that of the secundary sources, which in turn depend linearly on the primary source strength. Hence the function $B(y,x)$ represents the total effect of the elementary source $dS(x)$. The computation of the function $B(y,x)$ has been carried out using the described geometry and conductivity values of 0.6, 0.04 and 0.2 ℧.m^{-1} for, respectively, the ventricular cavities, the lungs and the remaining torso (including the ventricular walls). The double layer strength was put at 40 mV.

An obvious complication in the application of (2) stems from the fact that observed basic magnetic data are components of a vector field. Hence the particular component considered has to be specified. In the results presented the data $M(y,t)$ represent simulations of the output of a second order gradiometer positioned at the grid points orthogonal to the plain mentioned. The diameter of the pick-up coils is 2.9 cm, the distance between succesive coils of the gradiometer used is 6 cm (see Fig. 1). For each of the loops at each of the field points a mean value $\tilde{B}$ of the magnetic inductance B over the loop considered has been computed using numerical integration. The corresponding gradiometer output can be expressed as

$$G(y,x) = \tilde{B}(y_1,x) - 2\tilde{B}(y_2,x) + \tilde{B}(y_3,x)\,,$$

the subindex denoting each of the three loops of the gradiometer. The observed (simu-

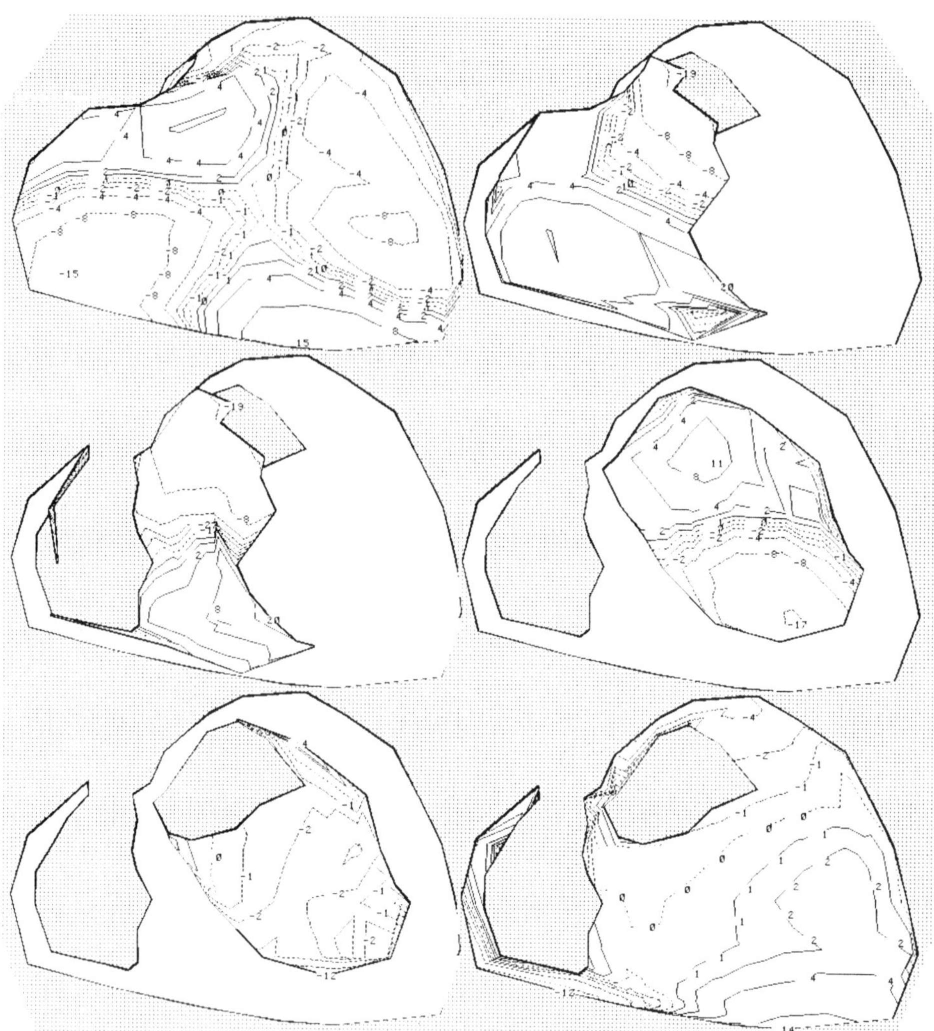

Fig. 3 Magnetic contribution map related to a field point lying directly over standard lead V_2. Ventricular aspects are shown from one and the same anterior view. These are (from left to right, from top to bottom) : anterior epicardium, endocardium right ventricle, septum right ventricular cavitiy, septum left ventricular cavity, endocardium left ventricle, posterior endocardium. Contributions are in units 0.1 pT.cm^{-2}. Drawn lines indicate positive values, dashed lines negative ones. Successive isofunction lines differ by a *factor* of two. Integers shown should facilitate the identification of individual isofunction lines.

lated) gradiometer output M(y,t) can be expressed as

$$M(y,t) = \int_{S_h} G(y,x)H(t-\tau(x))dS(x)\,. \tag{3}$$

Contribution Maps

The function $A(y,x)$ in (1) for fixed observation points y represents the contributions to the potential of elementary sources $dS(x)$ once activated. For any fixed y_0 $A(y_0,x)$ may be plotted on S_h, e.g. by using isofunction lines. Such maps have been

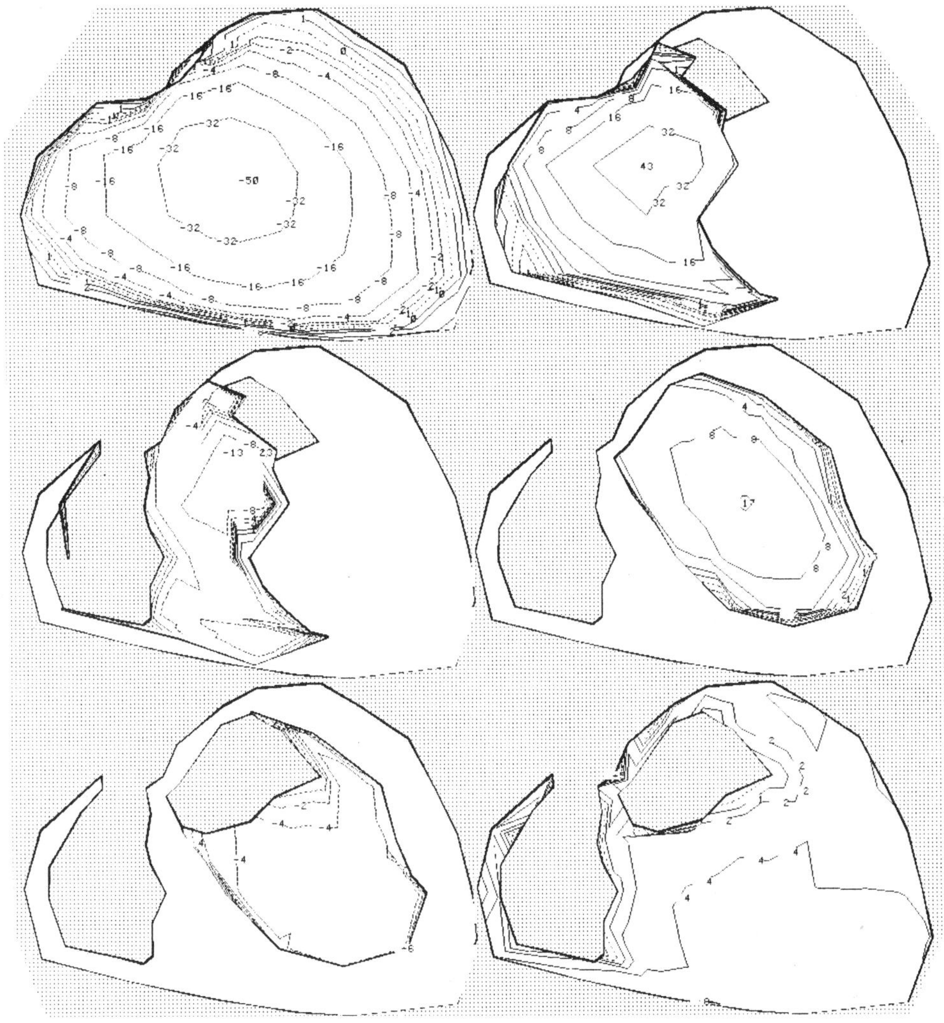

Fig. 4 Electrical contribution map related to lead V_2. Contributions are in units 10 $\mu V.cm^{-2}$. Remaining legend as in Fig. 3.

named 'contribution maps' [4,5]. Similarly, the function $G(y_0, x)$ represents the contribution to the magnetic measurement M of all elementary sources $dS(x)$ and may be plotted on (the same) heart surface.

RESULTS

The QRS waveforms of the MCG simulated at the grid from the assumed function $\tau(x)$ and the computed $G(y, x)$ are shown in Fig. 2. The magnetic contribution map of a field point lying directly over standard lead V_2 is shown in Fig. 3. The corresponding (electrical) contribution map of lead V_2 is shown in Fig. 4. Similar such electrical contribution maps, related to leads V_1, V_3, V_6, V_l, V_f and to a back electrode, are included in the paper introducing the contribution maps[4].

DISCUSSION

The results shown in Fig. 2 clearly demonstrate that the model used is capable of generating 'realistic' MCG wave forms. The model has been previously shown to be capable of very accurately simulating the ECG data[4].

The magnetic contribution map shown in Fig. 3 may be compared to the corresponding electrical contribution map shown in Fig. 4. This comparison reveals the fact that the magnetic and the electrical contributions are complementary in the following sense: areas where the electrical contribution map shows high magnitudes are accompanied by near zero magnetic contributions and vise versa. This effect is of course, in a qualitative manner, demanded by the orthogonality of the electrical and the magnetic fields generated by an elementary current dipole.

Whereas the electrical contributions tend to fall off rapidly for the deeper lying surfaces (e.g. the septum), the corresponding magnetic contributions seem to be relatively large. For a full comparison of the 'potentials' of magnetic and electrical methods the entire functions $G(y, x)$ and $A(y, x)$ should be analyzed. Matrices containing the discretized versions of G and A are available on request.

REFERENCES

1. G. R. Baule and R. McFee, Detection of the Magnetic Field of the Heart, *Am. Heart. J.*, 55: 95-96 (1963)
2. B. M. Horacek, Digital model Studies in Magnetocardiography, *IEEE Trans. Magn.*, MAG-9: 440-444 (1973)
3. M. J. Peters, M. J. M. Swennenhuis, A. van Oosterom and J. J. Wevers-Henke, The Influence of Inhomogeneities on the Cardiac-Magnetic-Field-Distribution, *Il Nuovo Cimento*, 2: 324-339 (1983)
4. A. van Oosterom and G. J. Huiskamp, The Effect of Torso Inhomogeneities on Body Surface Potentials Quantified Using 'Tailored' Geometry, *J. Electrocardiol.*, 22: 53-72 (1988)
5. A. van Oosterom an G. J. Huiskamp, The Silent Zones of the ECG Quantified, in: Electrocardiology 88, H. Abel (edt), Elsevier Science Publ.: 251-255 (1989)
6. A. van Oosterom, Cell models-Macroscopic Source descriptions, in: Comprehensive Electrocardiology, P. W. Macfarlane and T. D. Veitch Lawrie (edts):155-179 (1988)
7. A. van Oosterom, Computing the Depolarization Sequence at the Ventricular Surface from Body Surface Potentials, in: Pediatric and Fundamental Electrocardiography, J. Liebman, R. Plonsey and Y. Rudy (edts), Martinus Nijhoff, Boston:75-89 (1987)
8. S. Rush, On the Independence of Magnetic and Electric Body Surface Recordings, *IEEE Trans. Biomed. Eng.*, BME-22: 157-167 (1975)
9. G. J. Huiskamp, A. van Oosterom, The Depolarization Sequence of the Human Heart Surface Computed from Measured Body Surface Potentials, *IEEE Trans. Biomed. Eng.*, BME-35: 1047-1058 (1988)

HIGH RESOLUTION MAGNETOCARDIOGRAPHY, SOURCE LOCALIZATION AND MULTICHANNEL MAGNETOMETRY

Günter Albrecht, Martin Burghoff, Frank Gießler, Wolfgang Haberkorn*, and Hannes Nowak

PTI Jena, Academy of Sciences of the GDR, Helmholtzweg 4, Jena, 6900, GDR;
*ZWG Berlin, Academy of Sciences of the GDR, Rudower Chaussee 6, Berlin, 1199, GDR

INTRODUCTION

High resolution magnetocardiography (HR MCG) is a new and promising method of studying heart activity. One of the most interesting clinical applications of HR MCG is the localization of pathological cardiac sources which has often been demonstrated (Erné, 1985, Fenici et al., 1985, Katila et al., 1987). For the localization appropriate source and thorax models are needed.

The diagnostic power in spatial source localization is promising for the promotion of MCG into clinical application as Schmitz reported in 1987. Such investigations are very time-consuming when using one channel devices. Therefore, in our unshielded laboratory a sensitive multichannel dc SQUID magnetometer has been put to use.

METHOD

The source model used by us is based on the multipole theory. For the magnetic induction generated by the primary current density $\vec{j}_p$ we obtained the representation

$$\vec{B}(\vec{r}) = \text{rot}\ \vec{A}(\vec{r}),$$

$$\vec{A}(\vec{r}) = \frac{\mu_o}{4\pi}\,\text{Re}\sum_{n=0}^{\infty}\sum_{m=0}^{n}(\vec{\alpha}_{nm} + i\vec{\beta}_{nm})\,X_n^m,$$

$$\vec{\alpha}_{nm} + i\vec{\beta}_{nm} = \gamma_{nm}\int dv'\ \vec{j}_p(\vec{r}')\ r'^{\,n}\ P_n^m(\cos\vartheta')\ e^{im\varphi'},$$

$$\gamma_{nm} = (2 - \delta_{m,0})\ \frac{(n-m)!}{(n+m)!},\quad X_n^m = P_n^m(\cos\vartheta)\ e^{-im\varphi}\ /\ r^{n+1}$$

where r, ϑ, φ are spherical coordinates, P_n^m is the associated

Advances in Biomagnetism
Edited by S.J. Williamson *et al.*
Plenum Press, New York

LEGENDRE function of the first kind and $\vec{\alpha}_{nm}$, $\vec{\beta}_{nm}$ are the multipole coefficients. The first two terms are the contributions of the current dipole and the current quadrupole (Katila, 1983). For the localization of the pathological cardiac sources we applied the expansion up to the current octupole. The thorax was approximated by the conducting half-space model. For the localization, the component of the magnetic field normal to the surface of the half space was used. We used the model described above for the localization of the atrioventricular accessory conducting pathway in patients with ventricular preexcitation (Wolff-Parkinson-White syndrome) as reported by Burghoff et al.(1988). By taking into account the octupole terms, the accuracy of the localization could be improved, whereas the computing time was doubled.

The HR MCG recordings were made with a dc thin-film SQUID from the University of Jena in connection with a well-balanced second order gradiometer. The measurement conditions, an unshielded room of the biomagnetic laboratory in Jena, were similar to the ones reported by Fenici et al. (1985). Fenici was able to report sufficient measurements within the PR-interval in an unshielded hospital laboratory. Our single channel device is described in more detail by Nowak et al.(1988). The input sensitivity of the system is about 20 fT $Hz^{-1/2}$ for white noise. The measurements were based on the extended Saarinen grid (49 measurement points). A special software procedure with artefact rejection and averaging technique was developed. The results are given in the next paragraph.

Measurements with a single channel device have several disadvantages. Therefore, to overcome such problems we designed a 5-channel device using dc thin film SQUIDs. The antenna system is shown in Fig. 1. The diameter of every gradiometer is 20 mm, the baselength 55 mm. With a special construction it is possible to balance the gradiometers without removing the system from liquid helium. We achieved balances better than 10^{-4} and sensitivities of about 20 fT $Hz^{-1/2}$ for each gradiometer. MCGs measured with this device are demonstrated in Fig. 2. This 5 channel device enables us to reduce the recording time substantially and to

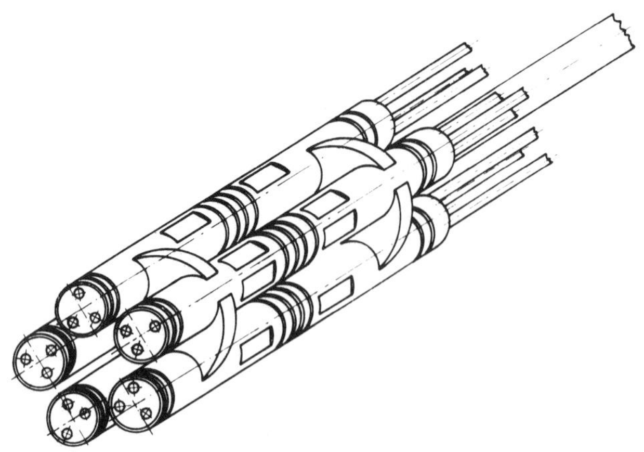

Fig. 1. The Jena 5-channel device

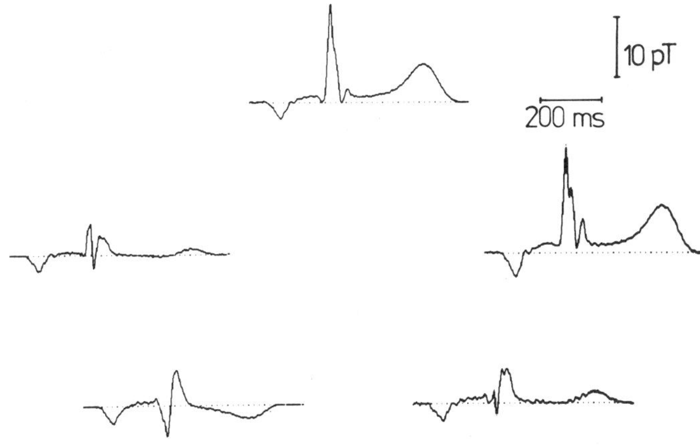

Fig. 2. Simultaneous 5 MCGs of a normal subject

look at simultaneous events from different points. This device will be used for source localization.

RESULTS

Using the single channel device described above measurements were taken in 23 patients with WPW syndrome. The localization procedure was carried out over a time interval from beginning of the preexcitation to the end of the ventricle excitation. For every time point the position of the source and the multipole components were obtained. In Fig. 3 the dipole strength is shown for one of the patients. The maximal dipole strength is designated as 100 %. The two peaks (arrows) which occur before the main heart activity are caused by the preexcitation. For the examined time interval (466 ms to 486 ms) the calculated multipole positions up to the octupole are shown in Fig. 4. The left part is with the plane of the measurement grid and the right one with the depth. The additional activities are within the time of 466 ms to 486 ms. The preexcitations occur in the area of B5-B6-C5-C6. The

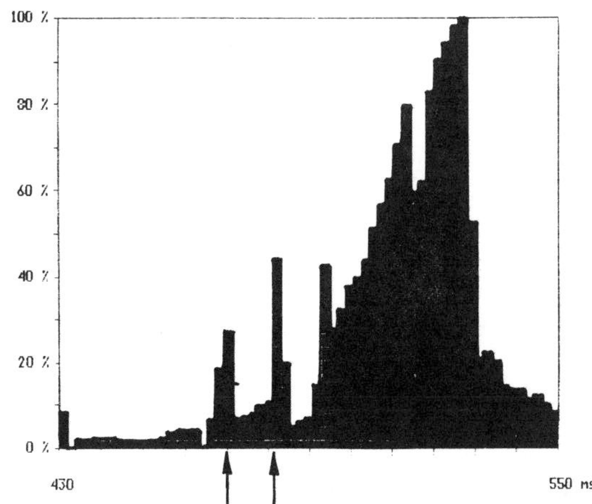

Fig. 3. Relative dipole strength of a patient with WPW syndrome

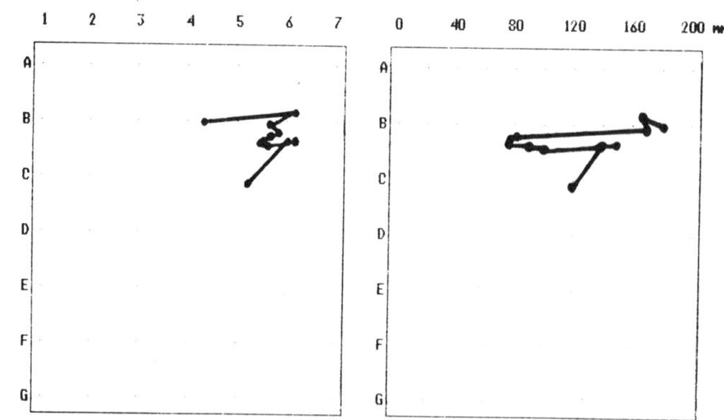

Fig. 4. Position of the sources of the preexcitation, the same patient as in Fig. 3

earliest excitation belongs to 468 ms in the vicinity of B6. To evaluate the localization procedure the comparison of the results with those of other methods is necessary. For our WPW patients such investigations are under way.

ACKNOWLEDGEMENTS

We thank Prof. K.-H. Berthel, Dr. G. Kirsch and their colleagues from the University of Jena for their advice. We are also grateful to H. Garlipp and U. Mänz.

REFERENCES

Burghoff, M., Haberkorn, W., and Albrecht, G.,1988, Localization of cardiomagnetic field sources based on the multipole expansion, in: Proc. 20th Int. Symp. L.T.P., in press.

Erné, S.N., 1985, High resolution magnetocardiography: modeling and source localization, in: Proc. XIV ICMBE, 1447.

Fenici, R.R., Masselli, M., Erné, S.N., and Hahlbohm, H.-D., 1985, Magnetocardiographic mapping of the P-R interval phenomena in an unshielded hospital laboratory, in: Biomagnetism: Applications & Theory, Edited by H. Weinberg et al., Pergamon Press, New York, 137.

Katila, T.E., 1983, On the current multipole presentation of the primary current distributions, Il Nuovo Cimento 2D., 660.

Katila, T., Montonen, J., Mäkijärvi, M., Nenonen, J., Raivio, M., and Siltanen, P., Localization of the accessory cardiac conduction pathway, in: Biomagnetism'87, Edited by K. Atsumi et al. Tokyo Denki University Press, 274.

Nowak, H., Albrecht, G., Berthel, K.-H., Burghoff, M., Haberkorn, W., Zach, H.-G., 1988, Biomagnetic measurements in unshielded environment, in: Advances in Biomedical Measurement, Edited by E. R. Carson et al., Plenum Press, New York and London, 161.

Schmitz, L., 1987, Magnetocardiography: the clinician's point of view, in: Biomagnetism'87, Edited by K. Atsumi et al., Tokyo Denki University Press, 66.

DYNAMIC MAGNETIC STUDY OF THE HEART CONDUCTION SYSTEM

Yu. Zhuravlev, A. Lipovich, A. Matlashov, E. Godik, Yu. Gulyaev

Institute of Radioengineering and Electronics
USSR Academy of Sciences
Moscow, USSR

INTRODUCTION

Since the first PR-segment high resolution MCG recordings attempts have been made to extract the His-Purkinje system (HPS) activity [1]. The main problem is that the HPS signal superimposes with the atrial repolarization activity. In some works the characteristic ramp pattern in PR-segment has been explained mainly by the atrial repolarization [2].

New features have been demonstrated by analysing instantaneous isofield maps [3]. The dynamic changes of the observed field patterns unlikely could be explained by only the atrial repolarization activity. To extract the HPS-produced pattern from the measured magnetic maps several different subtraction techniques have been applied [3,4].

Our current object is to investigate the problem how to separate the HPS and the atrial repolarization field patterns during PR-segment on the base of anatomical and physiological knowledge. At the same time spatial and temporal behavior of the magnetic field is analysed which can reduce the ambiguity when separating several electrical sources [5]. First, modelling assumptions are presented then some results are discussed.

SOURCE MODELLING

The detailed three-dimensional HPS model has been proposed in [6]. One of the basic assumptions was that the left bundle branch (LBB) contribution is significantly more than that of the right one (RBB) and increases as the LBB depolarization front moves away from the AV-node.

The anatomical data concerning the heart conduction system [7] enable us to propose an alternative electric model. The LBB thickness in its wide part (width approx. 1 cm) is only 0.1-0.2 mm. The RBB has an oval cross-section with the average diameter of 1-1.5 mm. Thus the cross-section areas of the LBB and RBB are comparable. There are reasons to believe the total cross-section area of the LBB to be approximately the same in all its parts. This in turn means that: 1) the LBB and RBB contributions to the generated magnetic field are probably comparable, especially when taking into account that the RBB may be closer to the chest surface; 2) there are no significant changes of the total ECD amplitude when moving away from the AV-node. To estimate

Advances in Biomagnetism
Edited by S.J. Williamson *et al.*
Plenum Press, New York

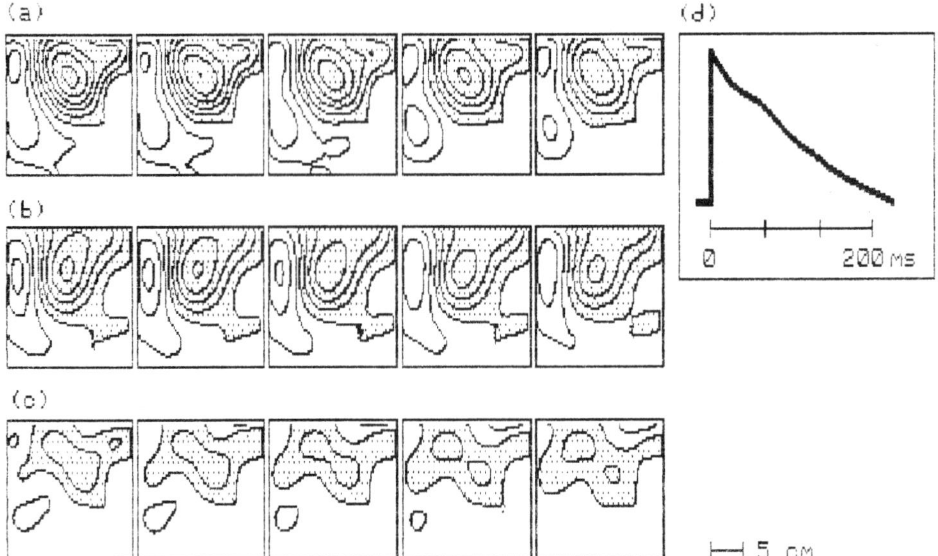

Fig. 1. Isofield contour maps illustrating the atrial repolarization simulation based on the optimized transmembrane action potential waveform. (a) The original map sequence. (b) The simulated sequence. (c) The difference between (a) and (b). Time interval between maps is 10 ms. The first map in each group corresponds to the time instant 50 ms before the QRS onset. Step on isocontour plot is 400 fT. (d) The optimized TAP waveform used to simulate the atrial repolarization (in arbitrary units).

the source amplitude we used linear current density value of 35 mA/m for myocardium fibers in longitudinal direction [8] and fiber cross-section areas discussed above. Calculation yields 50-70 nA·m for the LBB and 90-100 nA·m for the His bundle. If we assume source depth to be 9 cm the recorded component of the magnetic field should not exceed 0.2 pT.

METHOD

The PR-segment magnetic field analysis requires also the description of the atrial repolarization contribution. For this purpose one can use the known transmembrane action potential (TAP) waveforms of the isolated atrial tissue [9]. We assume the whole atrial myocardium to be homogeneous and consisting of the same contractible tissue. The source current density at each point is proportional to the local TAP gradient. Since the source region is thought to be homogeneous the instantaneous repolarization signal amplitude at each measurement point is the weighted sum of all the previous depolarization signal values, the weights being proportional to the TAP time derivatives for the appropriate time instants. Starting with these assumptions one can try to separate de- and repolarization signals in measured data.

INSTRUMENTATION

Magnetic measurements have been carried out by dc-SQUID second-order gradiometer (5 cm baseline, 2.8 cm coil diameter) in unshielded environment. The normal component of the heart magnetic field has been recorded. The measurement band was 0.01-130 Hz, the total system noise level was 15 fT/$\sqrt{\text{Hz}}$.

For anatomical referencing of the measuring grid (36 points, 20x20 cm) we used the frontal X-ray picture. About 100 cycles have been averaged at each point. Magnetic maps were then constructed with 2.5 ms intervals. Signal averaging and digital data processing were performed by personal computer.

RESULTS AND DISCUSSION

We examined high resolution MCG's of seven normal subjects. The observed isofield map sequences demonstrated spatial and temporal dynamics of the magnetic field during PR-segment similar to those obtained by Erne et al.[3].

To describe quantitatively the atrial repolarization signal during the last 50 ms before the QRS onset we applied a simple procedure based on the previously discussed considerations. The TAP waveform was simulated as realisticaly shaped curve dependent on six variable parameters. They were fitted to approximate the final part of the measured PQ-segment curve using its previous part. The best parameter set is the one which permits to fit the curves at all locations. The time instant separating these two parts corresponds to the end of atrial depolarization and was also determined by our procedure.

Then we attemted to restore further temporal dynamics of the repolarization process at each measurement point and constructed corresponding magnetic field maps to subtract them from the measured distributions. Unfortunately the simulated patterns differed from the measured maps more than could be explained by only the HPS activity. This is illustrated in Fig. 1. It should be noted however that the corresponding simulated TAP waveform (Fig. 1 (d)) may contain useful information concerning electrophysiological properties of the atrial tissue.

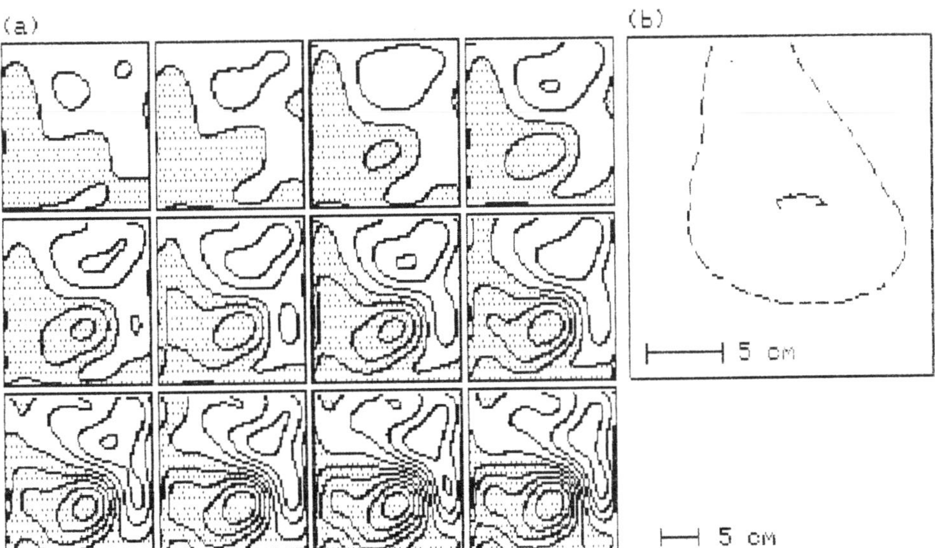

Fig. 2. Subtraction of the atrial repolarization assumed to be a spatially stable pattern changing in time as a whole. (a) Isofield contour maps after subtraction. Time interval between maps is 5 ms. The first map corresponds to the time instant 50 ms before the QRS onset. Step on isocontour plot is 50 fT. (b) Bidimesional ECD pathway on the real size heart siluette.

Probably the failure to obtain "good" patterns by this algorithm is explained by its sensitivity to the presense of additional (non-atrial) signals during PQ-segment, in particular, magnetic susceptibility contribution produced by blood flow in the earth magnetic field. We found the corresponding field maximum to be about 0.2 pT. Any kind of filtering also may influence the results of this algorithm due to signal shape changes. May be further improvement of the instrumentation and software methods will make this algorithm acceptable.

Another procedure was used to subtract the atrial repolarization patterns. The basic assumption was that this pattern changes in time but its spatial distribution is the same for all time instants. We chose a measurement point at the upper left part of the map (subject's right) far from the possible location of the HPS magnetic field pattern and ascribed its temporal behaviour to all the points of the grid starting from the time instant 50 ms prior to the QRS onset. Each calculated curve was then subtracted from the corresponding original one and a new map sequence was constructed for this time interval (Fig. 2 (a)). The resultant patterns have dipolar structure. The ECD pathway shown in Fig. 2 (b) suggests that the electrical source may be connected with the HPS activity.

REFERENCES

1. D. E. Farrell, J. H. Tripp and R. Norgren, Magnetic study of the His-Purkinje conduction system in man, IEEE Trans. Biomed. Eng., BME-27: 345-350 (1980).
2. M. Leifer, N. Capos, J. Griffin and J. Wikswo, Atrial activity during the PR-segment of the MCG, Il Nuovo Cimento, 2D:266-279 (1983).
3. S. N. Erne, R. R. Fenici, H.-D. Hahlbom, J. Korsukewitz, H. P. Lehman and Y. Uchikawa, Magnetocardiographic study of the PR segment of normals, in: "Biomagnetism: Applications and theory", H. Weinberg, G. Stroink and T. Katila, eds., Pergamon Press, New-York (1985).
4. G. Stroink, C. Purcell, R. Lamothe, R. Merritt, B. M. Horacek and B. J. ten Voorde, Body surface potential and magnetic mapping, in: "Biomagnetism'87", K. Atsumi, M. Kotani, S. Ueno, T. Katila and S. J. Williamson, eds., Tokyo Denki University Press (1988).
5. E. Godik, Yu. Gulyaev, A. Matlashov, Yu. Zhuravlev, A. Ya. Lipovich and A. Taratorin, Dynamic maps of the neuromagnetic evoked fields, in: "Biomagnetism'87", K. Atsumi, M. Kotani, S. Ueno, T. Katila and S. J. Williamson, eds., Tokyo Denki University Press (1988).
6. S. N. Erne, H. P. Lehmann, M. Masselli and Y. Uchikawa, Modelling of the His-Purkinje heart conduction system, in: "Biomagnetism: Applications and theory", H. Weinberg, G. Stroink and T. Katila, eds., Pergamon Press, New-York (1985).
7. A. F. Sinjov and L. D. Krymsky, "Surgical Anatomy of the Conduction System of the Heart", Meditsina, Moscow (1985).
8. D. E. Roberts and A. M. Scher, Effect of tissue anisotropy on extracellular potential fields in canine myocardium in situ, Circ. Res., 50:342-351 (1982)
9. H. Gelband and H. Bush, Electrophysiological properties of the isolated atrial tissue, Circ. Res., 30:293-300 (1972).

EVALUATION OF TECHNIQUES USED TO EXTRACT

HIS-PURKINJE SYSTEM SPATIAL DISTRIBUTIONS

R. Lamothe[†], G. Stroink[†‡] and C.J. Kafer[‡]

Depts. of Physics[†], and Physiology and Biophysics[‡]
Dalhousie University
Halifax, N.S., Canada, B3H 3J5

INTRODUCTION

The development of a numerical model of the human His-Purkinje system (HPS) and the availability of an atrial model has allowed us to calculate magnetic field maps (MFM) and body surface potential maps (BPSM) as a function of time during the PR-segment. With these maps we have investigated techniques used to extract the HPS signal from the atrial component in the PR-segment. The two methods studied are a time average representation of atrial repolarization (AR) and a Karhunen-Loève (K-L) expansion of the repolarization maps. The use of these two analysis techniques have relied, in whole or in part, on two assumptions which relate to the behavior of the AR source throughout the PR-segment. First, the AR source amplitude must be constant and secondly the source distributions must not move in time (fixed spatially). In particular the first assumption is addressed in this paper. Work to date using the time average representation technique has relied on this assumption. Originally it was believed that this assumption could be relaxed for the K-L expansion technique. However studies on simulated evoked potentials (Wood et.al., 1984) suggest that using this technique can result in over- or under-subtraction of primary components when a second source is also present.

METHODS

Isomagnetic and isopotential spatial distributions of PR-segment events were generated using a heart model with atrial and ventricular chambers, and newly developed conduction system (Kafer, 1988). Maps representing PR-segment activity in an interval of 44 ms before R-on were obtained by adding late AR and conduction system maps generated with the model.

From a set of early AR maps, a characteristic repolarization pattern was generated by computing the mean of this set of repolarization maps (Erné et.al., 1983, ten Voorde et. al., 1988). This average of early AR events was subtracted from the combination maps of late AR plus HPS activities to extract the HPS spatial distributions. The early AR maps were also used to generate an orthogonal set of eigenmaps (by K-L expansion techniques) to represent AR (MacAulay et.al., 1985, Lamothe et.al., 1987a&b). Using these eigenmaps,

Advances in Biomagnetism
Edited by S.J. Williamson *et al.*
Plenum Press, New York

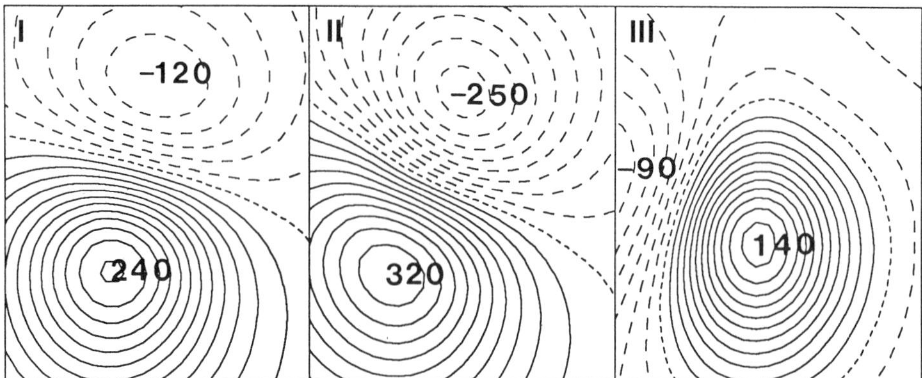

Figure 1. Isomagnetic field maps of the original HPS model data (panel I) during early bundle branch activity (t=–24 ms), the residual map after subtraction of the average map from the combination of AR plus HPS (panel II) and the residual map resulting from a fit of the first MCG eigenmap to the combination map (panel III). A 7×8 grid of 4 cm spacing was used for the model calculations. Units are in fT.

the component of AR present in the combination maps can be extracted.

Each technique used is expected to extract the AR component from the combination maps and reveal, as a residual map, the HPS component. These residual maps were compared to the original HPS model maps to determine if the HPS source was successfully separated from the AR signal in the combination maps.

RESULTS AND DISCUSSION

Presented in figure 1 are isomagnetic field simulation results. In panel I the original HPS pattern obtained from the model is shown. Corresponding to t=–24 ms before onset of ventricular activation, this particular map represents conduction through the early bundle branches. In panels II and III are the results of the attempt to extract this same HPS pattern from the combination map using the time average representation of AR (panel II) and applying the first K-L expansion eigenmap (panel III). Similar results are obtained in both the MFM and BSPM simulations. Subtraction of the average map gives a pattern which seems similar to the original HPS pattern, however its magnitude is substantially larger. The K-L technique yields a map not at all similar to the original HPS pattern at this time instant.

In Table 1 we present computations of the square root of the mean signal power (RMSP) present in the original and extracted maps for three representative time instances: His bundle (t=–44 ms), early bundle branch (t=–24 ms) and late bundle branch activities (t=0 ms). We were able to discern from this data that both techniques failed to extract the appropriate AR component present in the combination maps. We noted that the RMSP in the average AR map is larger than in the original late AR maps used to form the combination maps. The RMSP of the component of AR extracted from the combination maps using the first K-L eigenmap is, in this case, smaller than in the original AR maps. These incorrect subtractions of the AR components gave RMSP in the difference maps which were

Table 1. Root mean signal power (RMSP) of the original late AR maps and HPS maps at three different times in the HPS activation sequence : His bundle (t=–44 ms), early (t=–24 ms) and late (t=0 ms) bundle branch activities. Times are given relative to a theoretical Q-wave onset. These are to be compared to the AR representations and the results of extracting these from the combination maps according to the time average and K-L expansion techniques. Units are in fT/μV for the MFM and BSPM respectively.

Time	Original data		Time average method		K-L expansion method	
(ms)	Model AR maps	Model HPS maps	Average AR	Combination less average AR	First AR eigenmap fit to combination	Combination less fit
–44	331/14.9	4/.3	349/15.6	17/.6	330/14.7	3/0.3
–24	281/12.8	96/3.3	349/15.6	151/5.7	204/10.3	49/2.4
0	216/10.0	165/4.8	349/15.6	266/9.6	102/6.5	101/3.2

either larger (time average method) or smaller (K-L expansion method) than in the original HPS component present in the combinations. The analysis above demonstrates that either method, generally used to analyse maps with more than two sources present, can lead to erroneous results.

In search of a methodology which can be applied successfully to extract the HPS signals from the PR-segment the model predictions were studied more closely and compared with the available BSPM and MFM subject data. Although the atrial model (Macchi, 1973) predicts correctly the atrial field distributions, the calculated AR extrema of 3.5 pT and 0.1 μV in isomagnetic and isopotential maps respectively are too large and consequently were multiplied by a factor of 0.19. The simulation results presented in figure 1 and table 1 used these scaled AR patterns. The rate of change of extrema in this scaled sequence of AR maps was 5.0 fT/ms (isomagnetic) and 0.15 μV/ms (isopotential) and represented AR amplitudes which decreased throughout the PR-segment by an amount greater than in actual data.

Further simulations were completed using AR maps which were nearly constant in amplitude. With the time average method it was now possible to recover the HPS component in the combination maps. However, the K-L expansion results did not change. We have found that this technique does not work because of mathematical artifacts resulting from the non-orthogonality between the AR eigenmaps and the HPS source. This result was independent of the amplitude and rate of change of amplitude of the AR source.

One common feature of all simulations (whether amplitude of AR is constant or not) was that the time average representation of AR and the K-L expansion technique did not give the same residual patterns. This observation does not agree with real subject data results. When using either technique to extract the HPS spatial distribution from subject data, we have found that both techniques gave consistently similar distributions (Lamothe et. al., 1987a&b). For this reason some subtle changes in the AR pattern with time were explored further.

Both techniques also rely on the assumption that the AR source does not move during the PR-segment. This assumption was not absolutely satisfied in model data and certainly not in real data. For several subjects, the isomagnetic field maps of AR show a gradual motion of the zero contour lines through the PR-segment. A simulation of such a motion in the patterns using the original model data shows that under such circumstances both analysis techniques result indeed in similar residual patterns, as observed with real data. We therefore conclude, that to complete this work, further model simulation should include an AR source which is not fixed spatially.

ACKNOWLEDGEMENTS

This work has been funded by grants from the Natural Science and Engineering Research Council of Canada, the Medical Research Council of Canada and the Nova Scotia Heart Foundation.

REFERENCES

S.N. Erné, R.R. Fenici, H.-D. Hahlbohm, W. Jaszczuk, H.P. Lehmann, and M. Masselli, 1983, High-resolution isofield mapping in magnetocardiography, *Il Nuovo Cimento*, 2D(2):291–300.

C.J. Kafer, 1988, *Characteristics of Electrocardiographic and Magnetocardiographic Recordings of Human His-Purkinje Activity Investigated by Means of a Computer Model*, PhD thesis, Dalhousie University.

R. Lamothe, G. Stroink, and M.J. Gardner 1987a, High-resolution magnetocardiographic studies of the PR-interval, in: *13th Canadian Medical and Biological Engineering Conference*, 177–178, CMBES, Halifax, Nova Scotia.

R. Lamothe, C. Purcell, and G. Stroink 1987b, Magnetocardiographic and body surface potential detection of spatial features of the human His-Purkinje system, in: *Proceedings of the 9th Annual Conference of the IEEE Engineering in Medicine and Biology Society*, 172–173, IEEE, Boston, USA.

C. MacAulay, G. Stroink, and B.M. Horacek, 1985, Analysis of MCG spatial maps during the PR-interval, *Med. & Biol. Eng. & Comp.*, 23(SUPPL.2):1479–1480.

E. Macchi, 1973, *Digital-computer Simulation of the Atrial Electrical Excitation Cycle in Man*, PhD thesis, Dalhousie University.

B.J. ten Voorde, M.J. Peters, G. Stroink, and R.L. van der Wieken, 1988, High resolution magnetic mapping of PR-interval phenomena of normal subjects, *Med. & Biol. Eng. & Comput*, 26:130–135.

C.C. Wood and G. MacCarthy, 1984, Principal component analysis of event-related potentials: Simulation studies demonstrate misallocation of variance across components, *Electroenceph. Clin. Neurophysiol.*, (59):249–260.

MAGNETOCARDIOGRAPHIC LOCALIZATION OF A PACING CATHETER

R.R. Fenici, G. Melillo, A. Cappelli, C. De Luca, M. Masselli
Clinical Physiology - Cardiovascular Biomagnetism Unit, Catholic University, Rome, Italy

INTRODUCTION

Magnetocardiographic mapping during cardiac endocardial pacing was initially attempted by us, in patients undergoing invasive electrophysiological study for clinical reasons, in order to ascertain the reliability of the biomagnetic method in localizing a dipolar source placed in the human heart (Fenici et al 1985,1986a,b,c). Subsequently similar results have been reported, with measurements carried out in two patients with permanently implanted pacemakers (Schmitz 1988) and in animals (Costa Monteiro et al 1987). Here we report present results of an ongoing systematic research, carried out in our catheterization laboratory to quantify the accuracy of MCG localization of a catheter pacing different sites of the heart.

METHODS

10 patients were magnetically studied so far (table 1), all of them undergoing invasive EPS for diagnostic purposes. In all subjects significant conduction abnormalities were ruled out by ECG, Holter monitoring and EPS. All subjects had given informed consent and were already acquainted with magnetic mapping procedures. Cardiac pacing was carried out with impulse intensity of twice the diastolic threshold and duration of 1 or 2 milliseconds. In order to reduce the mapping time during EPS, only 16 to 25 grid points were mapped for 20 to 30 seconds each. In order to minimise localization errors linked to respiration, MCG recordings were carried out during held expiration.

MCG mapping was performed with a RF-SQUID based single channel instrumentation and protocols previously described in detail (Fenici et al 1985-87). The measurements reproducibility was tested by repeating MCG mapping of the field generated by the same catheter placed in a tank (55x40x15 cm.) filled with saline solution. For each tank experiment, grid sizes as well as amplitudes and duration of the

Advances in Biomagnetism
Edited by S.J. Williamson *et al.*
Plenum Press, New York

pacing impulses were identical to those used in individual patients during the invasive EPS. The latter procedure was carried out to compare the clinical MCG findings with the field pattern generated by the same artificial source placed in a semi-infinite space with homogeneous conductivity. For MCG source localization an Equivalent Current Dipole (ECD) inverse solution was used (Fenici et al 85-87). Fluoroscopic imaging of the pacing catheter in the patient heart was independently obtained with digital processing of orthogonal X-ray projections. Radiopaque references were placed on the chest surface and in the oesophagous to define the position and size of the heart with respect to the MCG recording grid.

Table 1. Localization accuracy of a pacing catheter in 10 pts.

PATIENT	**PACING SITE**	**LOCALIZATION ERROR (mm.)**			
		X	**Y**	**Z**	**3D**
BRRI62	RV Apex	7	19	0	20
COGI70	RA Lat Med	0	0	9	9
FELA33	RV Sept	2	5	5	7
FRFA25	RA Ant	3	7	2	8
TEMO66	Cor. Sinus	13	13	9	20
ERPO63	RV Apex	0	5	4	6
MABA62	RV Apex	1	19	3	19
FIEG59	RV Apex	6	1	0	6
FAPE61	RV Apex	2	9	0	9
ANNA32	RV Apex	2	0	18	18

RESULTS

When attempting MCG mapping under cardiac pacing, commercial intracardiac electrocatheters induced rhythmic, rate-dependent artefacts, due to the presence of ferromagnetic materials. This drawback, which obviously impeded the recording of good quality MCGs, was overcome by manufacturing custom non ferromagnetic electrocatheters specially designed for different electrophysiological purposes (patented). Thereafter MCG localization of the pacing catheter was successful in 10/10 investigated cases, being the average localization error 12.2 +/- 5.8 (SD) mm, in the three dimensions (table 1). Best accuracy was found on the frontal plane (X and Y) being the average bidimensional error 8.8 +/- 7 (SD) mm. A slightly larger error was found on the sagittal plane (Y and Z), mean 11 +/- 6 (SD) mm. The magnetic field distribution generated in the tank was typically dipolar. Its polarity was reversed by changing the polarity of the pacing dipole. The localization error on the frontal plane was 2.6 +/- 2.4 mm (on the x axis) and 2.3 +/- 2.6 (on the y axis), apparently increasing with the size of the pacing dipole.

DISCUSSION

The accuracy of MCG 3D localization of cardiac sources can be affected by several methodological factors, such as movements of the source itself in respect of the recording grid due to physiological activities, sequential mapping procedure, inadequate model for inverse solution. Nevertheless we have found that the MCG is effective in localizing preexcitation pathways with an uncertainty range of less than 15 mm in the three dimensions. In this study we have tried to independently calibrate the localization power of the MCG by decreasing the number of uncontrolled variables. However the average 3D localization error observed in patients, with this magnetic pacemapping technique, was still within the range of about 15 mm, even with atrial pacing (Fig.1). In contrast the localization accuracy in the tank was much higher. This demonstrates that, due to biological variables, best 3D localization accuracy obtainable in humans with sequential MCG mapping is in the order of 10 to 15 mm, whereas the biomagnetic localization power by itself is surely higher. Simultaneous mapping with multichannel systems will surely improve the accuracy of the method, which could be helpful to drive an ablation catheter as closer as possible to an arrhythmogenic target (Fenici and Melillo, this Conference). However, looking forward to such future clinical application, the major drawback to overcome for a routine use of MCG as a catheter driving method, will be the fast presentation of the biomagnetic "functional" images on realistic 3D images of the patient's heart.

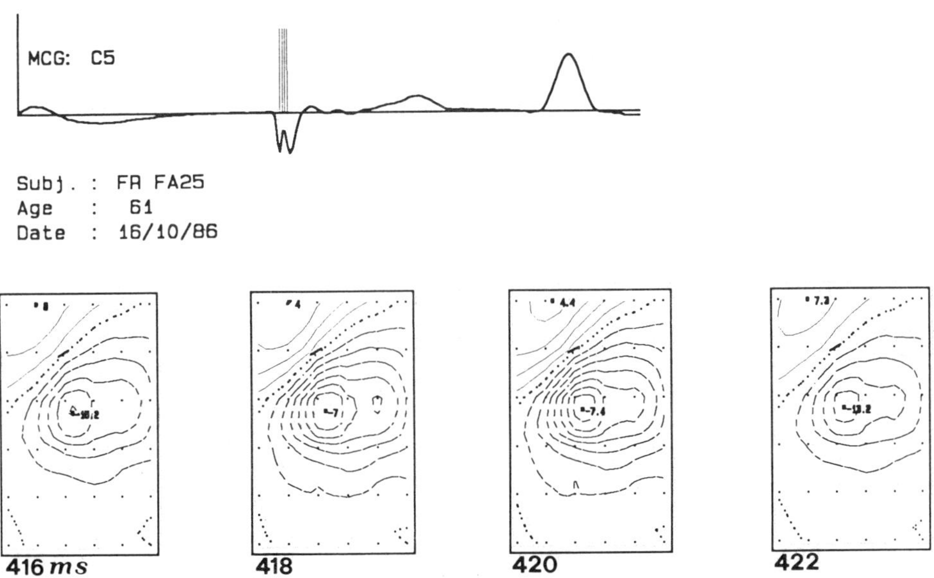

Fig. 1. Patient FRFA25: localization of a catheter pacing the anterior wall of the right atrium (3D error: 8 mm.).

ACKNOWLEDGEMENTS

Partially supported by grants: CNR n. 85.01473.57, CNR n. 86.00062.04, CNR n. 88.00503.04 and Italian Ministery of Education (60%), 1986-88.

REFERENCES

Costa Monteiro E., Bruno A.C., Louro S.R.W., Costa Ribeiro P., Fonseca Costa A., 1987, On the accuracy of source localisation in cardiac measurements. Phys. Med. Biol. Vol 32, N. 1: 65.

Fenici R.R., Masselli M., Lopez L., Sabetta F.,1985, First simultaneous magnetocardiographic and invasive Kent bundle localization in Man. New Trends in Arrhyt. Vol I, N.3: 455.

Fenici R., Masselli M., 1986a, Magnetocardiography: Perspectives in clinical application. In Proc of the IEEE Engineering in Medicine and Biology Society 8th Annual Conf., Vol 1: 439.

Fenici R., Masselli M., 1986b, Magnetocardiography: Localization of accessory pathways. In Proc of the IEEE Engineering in Medicine and Biology Society 8th Annual Conf., Vol 1: 437.

Fenici RR, Masselli M, Lopez L., Sabetta F., 1986c, Simultaneous MCG mapping and invasive electrophysiology to evluate the accuracy of the Equivalent Current Dipole inverse solution for the localization of human cardiac sources. New Trends in Arrhythmias, Vol. II, N.2: 357.

Fenici R.R., Masselli M., Lopez L., Melillo G., 1987, Catheter ablation of cardiac arrhythmias: MCG localization of electrocatheters and arrhythmogenic foci, New Trends in Arrhyt. Vol III, N.4: 723.

Fenici R.R., Masselli M., Lopez L., Melillo G., 1989c, Clinical Magnetocardiography. Localization of arrhythmogenic structures. In Advances in Biomagnetism Functional Localization: A challenge for Biomagnetism. I.S.I, Erne' S.N., Romani G.L. (eds.), World Scientific:102.

Fenici R.R., Masselli M., Lopez L., Melillo G., 1989b, Clinical Value of Magnetocardiography. In Electrocardiography and cardiac drug therapy. Hombach V., Hilger H.H. (eds.), Kluver Academic Publishers, Dordrecht/Boston/London:239.

Fenici R.R., Melillo G., Biomagnetic imaging in the cardiac catheterization laboratory. (this Conference).

Schmitz L., Oeff M., Erne' S.N.,1987. Magnetocardiography: Localization of arrhythmogenic areas in the human heart. In Biomagnetism 1987. Atsumi K, Katila T, Kotani M, Williamson SJ, Ueno S (eds). Tokyo Denki University Press:66.

MAGNETOCARDIOGRAPHIC LOCALIZATION OF KENT BUNDLES

Riccardo Fenici, Guido Melillo, Alessandra Cappelli, Claudio De Luca, Mariella Masselli.
Clinical Physiology - Cardiovascular Biomagnetism Unit - Catholic University - Rome, Italy

INTRODUCTION

First MCG recording in one patient with WPW was reported by Erne' and Fenici (1984). Since then several preliminary measurements have been published (Fenici et al 1985-88; Katila et al 1988; Novak el al 1988; Oeff et al 1989), demonstrating the accuracy of MCG to localize Kent type accessory pathways. Here we report present results of our ongoing perspective study carried out to interprete the MCG patterns and to compare the respective localization power of electrocardiographic and magnetocardiographic criteria.

MATERIALS AND METHODS

32 patients, all affected by Wolff-Parkinson-White (WPW) syndrome have been studied so far. MCG mapping was performed with a RF-SQUID based single channel instrumentation and protocols previously described in detail (Fenici et al 1985-89). The measurements reproducibility was tested by repeating MCG mapping in different recording sessions, with the same and/or different gradiometers and with different extension of the recording grid. In all subjects an electrocardiographic classification was independently attempted with the criteria proposed by Gallagher et al (1978) and with the algorithm of Milstein et al (1987). In 13/32 subjects, in whom invasive electrophysiology was clinically required, conventional catheter mapping (Gallagher, 1987) was used to localize the accessory pathway. In 1/32 patient cryosurgical ablation of a left sided Kent bundle was necessary. A detailed description of magnetic and intraoperative mapping in this case has been reported in a previous paper (Fenici et al 1988).

RESULTS

Typical dipolar magnetic field patterns of cardiac preex-

Advances in Biomagnetism
Edited by S.J. Williamson *et al.*
Plenum Press, New York

citation (Fenici et al 1986) were reproducibly found in 29/32 subjects and reproducible MCG localization of Kent bundles with equivalent current dipole (ECD) inverse solution was successful in 29/32 investigated cases (3D average uncertainty: 14 mm.). Septal/paraseptal accessory pathways were found in 17/29 patients (fig.1 B, C). Free wall (lateral or posterolateral) pathways were found in 13/29 patients (7/13 left, fig. 1D; 6/13 right, fig. 1A). In one case the localization was unsatisfactory because the degree of preexcitation was insufficient and the field during the delta wave was partially covered by the environmental noise. In two cases the preexcitation field pattern was reproducibly quadrupolar, thus proper source localization, impossible with the ECD model, was achieved only with current multipole inverse solution (Fenici and Melillo, this Conference). Significant interindividual reproducibility of the MCG pattern was found in patients with similar Kent bundle's localizations. Ajmaline and/or Flecainide induced normalisation of atrioventricular conduction provided additional information about the respective three- dimensional localization of normal and abnormal conduction pathways. This is helpful to infer the site of insertion of the accessory pathway with respect to the interventricular septum (Fenici et al 1987-88).

In 12/29 cases a discrepancy was found between MCG and both ECG criteria. In 8/29 cases a discrepancy was found between the two ECG classification criteria, being MCG in agreement with Gallagher in 2/8 cases, with Milstein in 3/8, and discordant with both in the remaining 3/8 cases. In all cases in whom the discrepancy was found, catheter endocardial localization was always in agreement with the magnetic imaging of the preexcitation pathways.

DISCUSSION

Although it is difficult to define what the "gold standard" is to test the accuracy of any closed chest technique used for non invasive localization of accessory pathways (Gallagher 1987), preliminary comparative investigations with invasive methods and surgical experience have demonstrated that the localization uncertainty of the biomagnetic method is well within the accuracy required for successful surgery of cardiac preexcitation (Fenici et al 1985-1989, Guiraudon et al 1986, Katila et al 1988, Oeff et al 1989).

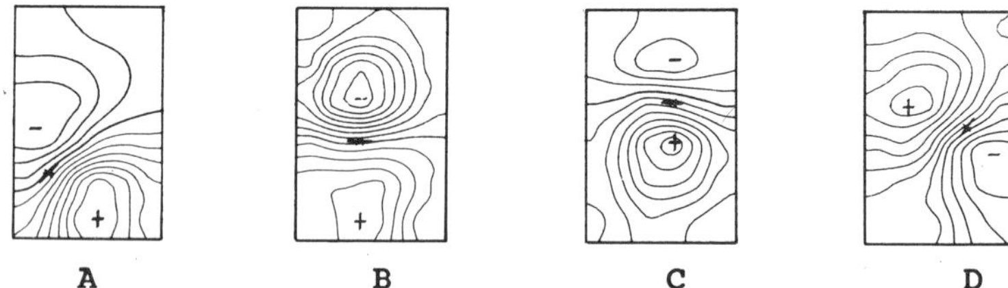

Fig. 1. Four different types of magnetic field distribution during delta wave: **A**) Right free wall, **B-C**) Septal/Paraseptal, **D**) Left free wall.

The results of the present study indicate that MCG can properly classify preexcitation patterns which are indefinable or wrongly localized with the ECG. On this basis at present in our laboratory the first approach to the study of WPW patients is non invasive. Trans-oesophageal atrial pacing is used for risk assessment and magnetocardiography for the localization of the preexcitation site. Invasive electrophysiology is indicated only when a more detailed analysis of arrhythmogenic mechanisms are required in risk patients, refractory to medical treatment and candidates for surgical ablation. As catheter mapping, although accurate, remains a qualitative localization method, it cannot be assumed as a goldstandard for MCG validation in WPW patients. However further experience in combining MCG mapping with catheterization procedures should confirm our opinion that the MCG localization capability could be used in combination with ablation procedures (Fenici et al 1986-89). Notwithstanding the MCG localization power will be clinically proficient only when a "quasi real time" presentation of the localization images will be available interactively, in the operation and catheterization rooms, to dynamically guide antiarrhythmic interventions.

ACKNOWLEDGEMENTS

Partially supported by grants: CNR N. 88.00503.04, contract Elettronica S.p.A./IMI (law n. 46, 17/02/82) and Italian Ministery of Education (60%) 1986-88.

REFERENCES

Erne' S.N., Fenici R.R.,1984, The present state of Magnetocardiography . In Collan H., Berglund P., Krusius M., (eds), Proc. of the Tenth International Cryogenic Engineering Conference, Helsinki, Butterworth, Westbury House: 329.

Fenici R.R., Masselli M., Lopez L., Sabetta F., 1985a, High resolution magnetocardiography: electrophysiological and clinical findings. In Proc. of the XIV ICMBE and VII ICMP, Espoo, Finland: 1475.

Fenici R.R., Masselli M., Lopez L., Sabetta F., 1985b, First simultaneous MCG and invasive Kent bundle localization in man. New Trends in Arrhythmias, 1: 455.

Fenici R.R., Masselli M., 1986, Magnetocardiography: localization of accessory pathways (WPW). In Proc of the IEEE Engineeering in Medicine and Biology Society 8th Annual Conference, Dallas, Nov. 7-10: 433.

Fenici R.R., Masselli M., Lopez L., 1987, Magnetocardiographic localization of arrhythmogenic sources. PACE, Vol.10, PartI: 600.

Fenici R.R., Masselli M., Lopez L., Melillo G., 1988, Magnetocardiographic localization of arrhythmogenic tissue. In Biomagnetism '87, Proceedings of the 6th International Conference on Biomagnetism. Atsumi K., Katila T., Kotani M., Williamson SJ., Ueno S. (eds). Tokyo Denki University Press: 282.

Fenici R.R., Masselli M., Lopez L., Melillo G., 1989a, Clinical value of Magnetocardiography. In Electrocardiography and cardiac drug therapy. Hombach V., Hilger H.H. (eds). Kluwer Academic Publishers, Dordrecht/Boston/London: 239.

Fenici R.R., Masselli M., Lopez L.,, Melillo G., 1989b, Clinical Magnetocardiography: Localization of arrhythmogenic structures. In Advances in Cardiomagnetism Functional localization: A challenge for Biomagnetism. World Scientific: 102.

Fenici R.R., Melillo G.,1989c, Biomagnetic Imaging in the Cardiac Catheterization Laboratory. (This Conference).

Gallagher J.J., Pritchet E.L.C., Sealy W.C., Kasell J., Wallace A.G. 1978, The preexcitation syndromes. Prog. Cardiovasc. Dis. 29:285.

Gallagher J.J., 1987, Localization of Accessory Atrioventricular Pathways: What's the Gold Standard", PACE, Vol.10, Part I,: 583.

Guiraudon G.M., Klein G.J., Sharma A., Jones D., McLellan D., 1986, Surgery for Wolff-Parkinson-White syndrome: further experience with an epicardial approach. Circulation, 74: 525.

Katila T., Montonen J., Marijarvi M., Nenonen J,. Raivio M., Siltanen P., 1988, Localisation of the accessory cardiac conduction pathway. In Biomagnetism '87, Proceedings of the 6th International Conference on Biomagnetism. Atsumi K., Katila T., Kotani M., Williamson S.J., Ueno S. (eds). Tokyo Denki University Press: 274.

Oeff M., Erne' S.n., 1989, Invasive measurements to validate magnetic localization of ventricular preexcitation in Wolff-Parkinson-White Syndrome. In Advances in Cardiomagnetism Functional localization: A challenge for Biomagnetism. World Scientific: 62.

Milstein S., Sharma A.D., Guiraudon G.M., Klein G.J., 1987, An algorithm for the electrocardiographic localization of accessory pathway in the Wolff-Parkinson-White Syndrome, PACE, Vol.10, Part I: 555.

Novak H., Albrecht G., Burghoff M., Kirsch G., 1988; MCG measurements in WPW patients. (personal communication).

APPLICATION OF A BIOMAGNETIC MULTICHANNEL SYSTEM TO THE COMPARATIVE LOCALIZATION OF ACCESSORY CONDUCTION PATHWAYS IN PATIENTS WITH WPW SYNDROME

K.Abraham-Fuchs,A.Weikl*,S.Schneider,W.Moshage*,
G.Röhrlein,A.Wirth,K.Bachmann*,R.Schittenhelm

Siemens Medical Engineering Group, Erlangen, Germany
*Med.Clinic II with Polyclinic, University of Erlangen

INTRODUCTION

The accessory pathway of patients suffering from a WPW syndrome can be localized from the MCG as an electric dipolar activity just before the onset of the R-wave (Fenici 1987, Katila 1987, 1987a). The multichannel biomagnetic system (KRENIKON) for the first time offers the possibility to obtain and evaluate sets of coherent data with sufficient channels and covering a sufficiently large area to allow for the localization from one single transient biomagnetic event. The number of SQUID channels is 31, the axial 1.order gradiometers cover a circular area of 20cm diameter. In this paper we will make use of this advantage and compare the localization of accessory pathways as well as normal AV-His excitation from the unaveraged signal of one heart cycle with the results obtained from averages over many heart cycles. Furtheron we will study the influence of respiration gating on the localization from averaged data. We propose some criteria derived from physiological knowledge for the automated rating of equivalent current dipole(ECD) results.These criteria are applied to the automated localization of heart excitation pathways. In patients with different excitation pathways, the relative location of the pathways is compared.

METHOD

In order to study the accessory pathway, ten patients with WPW syndrome were examined with the multichannel biomagnetic system. The data were bandpass-filtered from 0.016Hz to 250Hz with an analogue filter,data acquisition rate was 1000hz. The zero-signal assumption within the T-P interval provides for an automated bias correction.To allow for averaging of several heart cycles,data were acquired typically for 2 to 5 minutes. Biomagnetic source localization was carried through with an iterative nonlinear optimization algorithm (Williamson 1982). The model of an equivalent current dipole (ECD) immersed in the homogeneous halfspace was used. The ECD is not in all cases an optimal source model for accessory pathway activity (Katila 1987, Gonelli 1987), but it was supposed to be adequate for the comparative studies under consideration. The patient is lying supine, the angle between measured field component and halfspace surface (parallel to the torax surface)is taken into account for the inverse solution.The iterative localization procedure is run automatically over the time interval of interest.At every sampled data point an ECD is localized. The validity of the resulting equivalent sources is

Advances in Biomagnetism
Edited by S.J. Williamson *et al.*
Plenum Press, New York

automatically checked by several criteria:

1) The deviation of the measured field map and the map produced by the equivalent current dipole must not exceed a predefined threshold.
2) The location of the dipole must be within anatomically defined limits, e.g. within the heart volume with MCG evaluations.
3) The distance of successive dipole locations must not exceed a value which is defined by the sampling interval and the maximum possible conductance velocity of the activated tissue, plus the maximum systematic error.
4) The location of the electrical activity should be stable within the conductance velocity limit mentioned above and within a time interval defined by the typical duration of action potentials of the type of tissue under consideration.
5) Where possible, upper and lower limits can be defined from electrophysiology for the strength of the equivalent dipole result.

RESULTS

By this automated scheme, dipoles were localized every 1msec, starting from the end of the P-wave until the R maximum. ECDs which are valid according to the above criteria were found within the total duration of the delta wave in most WPW patients, only in two out of the ten cases valid dipoles could only be found at the end of the delta wave interval. The delta wave activity is analysed by assuming that the first deviation of the electric or magnetic signal from the zero line after the P-wave corresponds to the beginning of ventricular excitation at the end of the accessory pathway. The later phase of the delta wave reflects the spreading excitation of the ventricular myocardium near the accessory bundle. Since the current within the accessory bundle might be too weak to be localized from the MCG, and the myocardial excitation in the late delta wave can not necessarily be described by a simple ECD model, there is still an ongoing discussion about which time instant in the delta wave allows the best localization of the accessory bundle. But this discussion is not the object of this paper, we only state that we have found an ECD pathway within the delta wave interval which could

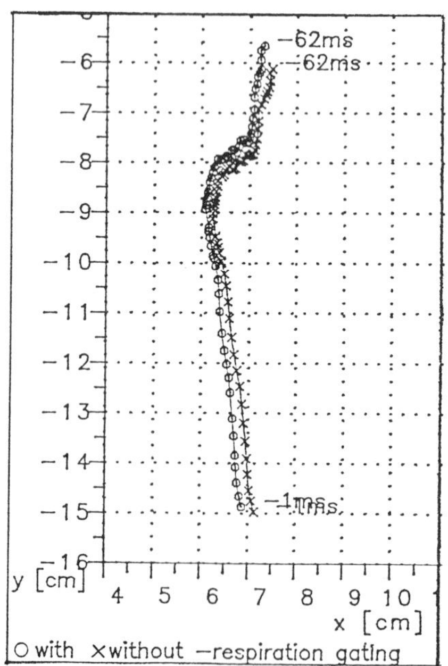

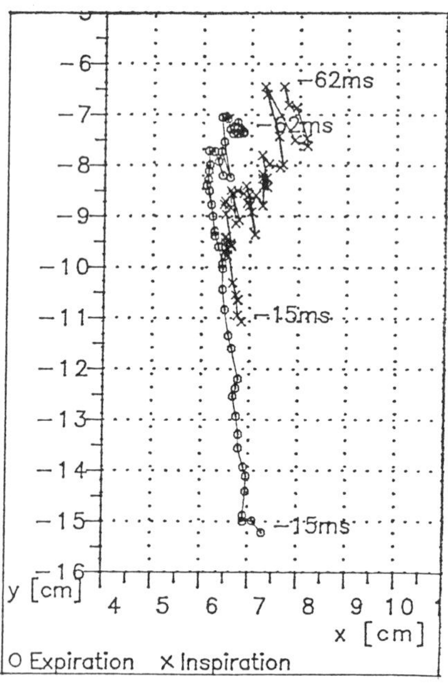

ECD pathways during delta wave, frontal projection:

Fig.1 Comparison of averaging with and without respiration gating

Fig.2 Comparison of expiration and inspiration phase

be related to an area between atria and ventricles and the upper ventricular myocardium in all patients, within the expected localization error of 0.5 to 2cm (Fenici 1987, Katila 1987).

Figures 1,2 and 3 present the ECD results in time and space as follows: The path of the ECD in time is marked by successive crosses or circles on a continuous curve, in this case the time interval between each marker is 1msec. The path of the dipole in space is shown in a frontal projection, where the y-axis points in direction of the body axis, from feet to head, the x-axis points from the right to the left shoulder, (x=0,y=0) is at the jugulum,and the z-axis points from the patient's back to the front. To the upper right of the starting and end point of each dipole path the time (in msec) relative to the R -maximum is printed. Only frontal projections of the ECD paths are shown here, the conclusions drawn therefrom are in accordance with the 3D paths of the ECD. In fig.1, the localization results from data of the same patient are compared without and with respiration gated averaging: first all 247 delta-wave -cycles out of the 5 minute recording were averaged (dipole locations marked with crosses), second only the delta-wave cycles falling in the expiration phase were averaged (a total of 89 averages, circle-marked curve). We can see from fig.1 that the influence of the respiration gating is small, there is a systematic shift of the whole ECD path of about 2 to 4mm. This is in accordance with the predominance of the expiration phase, and is reflected in the fact that MR images of the heart acquired without respiration gating are usually of sufficient quality.

The "worst case" -influence of the respiration movement can be estimated from the comparison of a heart cycle falling in the expiration phase and another one falling in the inspiration phase. This is shown in fig.2, where the dipole paths of one unaveraged delta-wave cycle for the two respiration phases are compared, from the same data set as the results in fig.1. The locations differ typically 2cm, in the late delta wave (15 msec before R-maximum) the difference is even more than 4cm.

The influence of averaging on the accuracy of the ECD localization can be

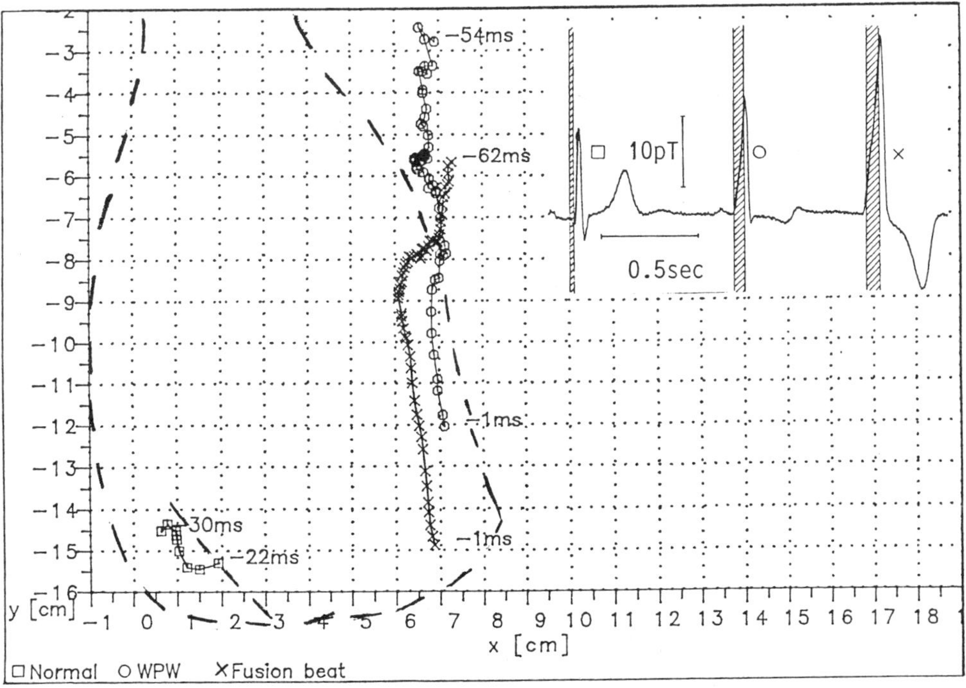

Fig.3 Comparison of ECD pathways in 3 different heart excitation cycles: MCG time signal and ECD pathways (frontal projection) during the shaded time intervals. (Heart contour determined from MR image)

estimated from the comparison of the circle-marked curves in fig.1 and 2. Both curves are localized from the same type of delta-wave heart excitation, in fig.1 from 89 averages, in fig.2 unaveraged. The curves follow essentially the same pathway, yet with the averaged data, the ECD path is much smoother. The higher topological variance of the ECD path from the unaveraged data corresponds well with the localization error estimated from the influence of noise (Abraham-Fuchs 1988).

In fig.3, we present the results from one patient who had randomly alternating excitation of three types: normal, WPW cycle (delta wave preceeded by a P-Wave), and a fusion beat (delta wave without P-Wave). The different types of heart cycles were automatically recognized and averaged by means of a spatio-temporal correlation algorithm.Fig.3 shows the ECD results and the magnetic signal of the three corresponding heart cycle types.The time intervals corresponding to the ECD paths are marked with a shaded area. The ECD path of the fusion beat is located nearer to the septal region than the ECD path during the maximum preexcited beat. This corresponds to the mixture of conduction via accessory pathway and the AV node in the fusion beat. Normal excitation was localized after separation from the atrial activity by means of a Karhunen-Loeve expansion (Stroink 1986, Erne1983, 1985). The resulting ECD pathway is interpreted,from it's time relative to the R maximum and it's location, rather as the beginning of septal excitation than His-Purkinje activity.The contour of the heart and the end of the septum have been determined from a frontal MR image and are indicated in fig.3 by the broken line.

CONCLUSION

The localization accuracy, as assessed by the coherence of successive dipole locations,improved with the number of averaged heart cycles according to the known dependence of the inverse solution on the signal-to-noise ratio (Abraham-Fuchs 1988).Yet with delta wave activity,the localization accuracy is sufficient with unaveraged data, at least in the middle and late delta wave. This is important, since the accessory pathway is not always stable over many heart cycles, and localization from averages of different heart cycles may be erroneous. In the contrary, averaging of at least 20 heart cycles, better 100 cycles, is recommended for the localization of AV-His -activity, according to the very low signal level of this activity.

REFERENCES

Abraham-Fuchs;Schneider;Reichenberger;(1988) "MCG inverse solution: influence of coil size, grid size,number of coils,and SNR" IEEE Tr.Biomed.Eng.35/8,573

Erne,S.N.;Fenici,R.R.;Hahlbohm,H.D.;Masselli,M.;Lehmann,H.P.;Trontelj,Z.; (1983) "High-Resolution Recordings of the PR-Segment in Magnetocardiography" Il Nuovo Cimento; 2D,N.2; 248-254

Erne,S.N. (1985) "High resolution MCG: modeling and sources localization Med. and Biol. Engeneering and Computing 8/85, 23/1,1447-1450

Fenici,R.R.;Maselli,M.;Lopez,L.;Melillo,G.; (1987) "Magnetocardiographic localization of arrythmogenic tissue" 6th Int.Conf.Biomag.,Tokyo, p.140

Gonelli,R.S.;Sicuro,M.;Agnello,M.; (1987) "Use of the current multipole model for the cardiac source localization in normal subjects" 6.Int.Conf.Biomagnetism, Tokiyo 8/1987; 162-163

Katila,T.;Maniewski,R.;Maekijaervi,M.;Nenonen,J;Siltanen,P.;(1987) "On the accuracy of source localization in cardiac measurements" Phys.Med.Biol.32/1,125

Katila,T.;Montonen,J.;Maekijaervi,M.;Nenonen,J.;Raivio,M.;Siltanen,P.(1987a) "Localization of the extra cardiac conduction pathway" 6.Int.Conf.Biomagnetism, Tokiyo 8/1987; 136-137

Stroink;MacAulay;tenVoorde;Montague;Horacek;(1986)"High-resolution magnetocardiographic field mapping and analysis" 8.Conf.Eng.Med.Biol.Soc.,445

Williamson,S.J.,Romani,G.L.,Kaufman,L.,Modena,I. (1982) "Biomagnetism:An interdisciplinary approach"New York,Plenum Press

DETECTION OF ACCESSORY PATHWAY IN PATIENTS WITH WPW SYNDROME BY MEANS OF THE ISOMAGNETIC MAP AND MRI

Masahiro Nomura, Yutaka Nakaya,
Katsusuke Watanebe, Mariko Katayama,
Akemi Takeuchi, Kazuya Fujino,
and Hiroyoshi Mori

The Second Department of Internal Medicine, School of Medicine, The University of Tokushima, Tokushima, Japan 770

INTRODUCTION

The current source is expected to be localized more exactly with a magnetocardiogram (MCG) than with an electrocardiogram (ECG). In the present study, the isomagnetic map at the time of the delta wave and a gated magnetic resonance imaging (MRI) were compared to assess the usefulness of the magnetocardiogram (MCG) in localizing a position of the accessory pathway (Kent bundle). Spach and Benson reported that the analysis of the T wave was as useful as that of the QRS wave in predicton of the pre-excited sites of the ventricle.[1,2] Therefore, we examined the repolarization wave in order to localize the site of an accessory pathway in WPW syndrome, because the repolarization abnormality might be detected more precisely by the MCG.[3] Our results showed that the analysis of the repolarization waves of the MCG was as useful as the delta wave to detect the site of an accessory pathway.

SUBJECTS AND METHODS

MCG were recorded at 36 points on the anterior chest wall in 8 cases with Wolff-Parkinson-White (WPW) syndrome using SQUID system with the second derivative gradiometer. The location of the accessory pathway determined by these methods was compared with the findings obtained by the body surface map and electrophysiological studies. Three patients had accessory pathway in the left ventricular free wall (left free wall type), 4 in the right ventricular free wall (right free wall type) and 1 in the intraventricular septum (septal type). Fig. 1 shows the recording sites of the MCG. A 2.5 x 2.5 cm rectangular grid system consisting of six horizontal (A-F) and six vertical (1-6) lines were used with xyphoid process serving as a reference point (E-2) for the grid. As a time reference, lead II ECG was recorded at a paper speed of 200 mm/sec simultaneously with the MCG. These patterns were inputted by an image scanner (NEC PC-IN 502) and transferred to the video RAM of a computer (NEC PC-9801). Amplitudes of these waves were measured from the beginning of the QRS waves of lead II ECG at an interval of 2 msec, and the data were converted to real values of density of the magnetic flux and the electrical potential. The isomagnetic maps during QRS and T

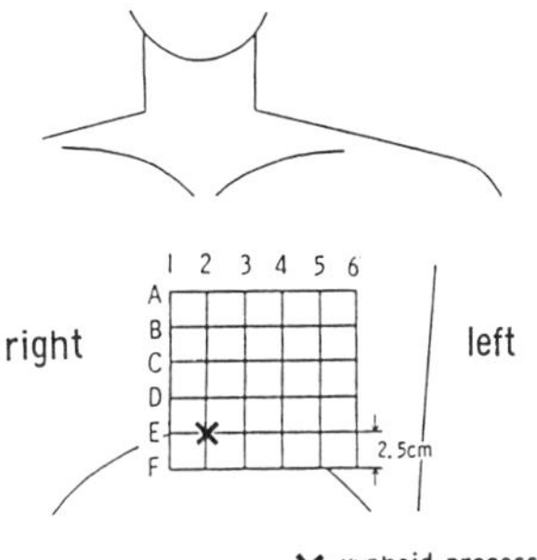

Fig. 1 Recording sites for MCG

waves were constructed based on these records every 2 msec from the biginning of the QRS waves of lead II. The isomagnetic and isopotential lines were drawn at the intervals of 1×10^4 pTesla and 0.1 mV, respectively. The distance between the current source supposed to originate from the accessory pathway and the detector coil was calculated mathematically. Location of an accessory pathway was estimated based on these calculated data and was compared with that estimated by the MRI findings. Body surface isopotential maps were constructed based on the simultaneously recorded unipolar chest lead ECG at 87 sites around the thorax with multiplexed data recording system (Fukuda Densi, VCM-3000).

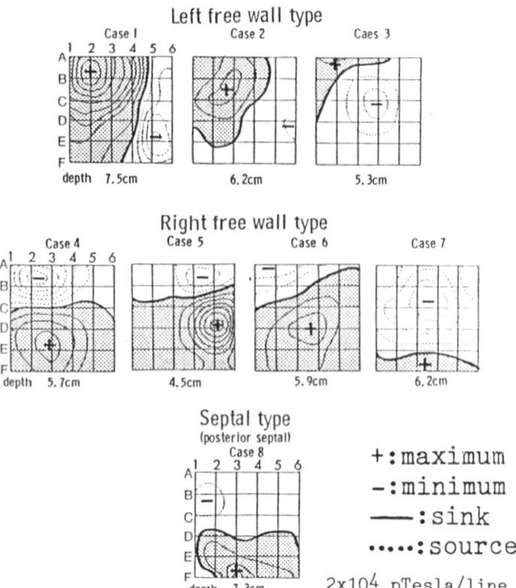

Fig. 2 Isomagnetic maps at 40 msec after the onset of the delta wave

RESULTS

1) Isomagnetic maps of WPW syndrome

Fig. 2 shows the isomagnetic maps at 40 msec after the onset of the delta wave in 8 patients. In left free wall type, the isomagnetic map showed that a maximum was located more superiorly than a minimum, and a dipole directed rightwards was deduced according to "the Biot-Savart Law". In right free wall type, a minimum was located more superiorly than a maximum, and a dipole directed leftwards was deduced. In septal type, a minimum was located more superiorly than a maximum.

2) Location of the accessory pathway and gated MRI

Supposing that the electric current source is a single dipole, location of the current dipole might be estimated by the positions of the maximum and minimum in the isomagnetic map.[4] Fig. 3 shows the isomagnetic (panel a) and the body surface isopotential maps (panel b) at 40 msec after the onset of the delta wave. From Fig. 3 a, the location of the accessory pathway was calculated at 3.8 cm leftward from the median line and 4.2 cm upward from the xyphoid process. The depth of the accessory pathway was calculated at 7.5 cm below the detector coil. Fig. 4 shows the gated MRI in the same patient as in Fig. 3. These findings agreed well with those of the isopotential map (Fig. 3 b), in which the accessory pathway was also predicted to be at the anterior free wall of the left ventricle.[5]

Fig. 5 shows the isomagnetic (panel a) and the body surface isopotential maps (panel b) at 40 msec after the onset of the delta wave. The location of the accessory pathway was calculated at 1.1 cm leftward from the median line and 4.3 cm upward from the xyphoid process. The depth of the accessory pathway was calculated at 5.7 cm below the detector coil. Fig. 6 shows the gated MRI in the same patient as in Fig. 5. From the isopotential map (Fig. 5 b), the accessory pathway was also predicted to

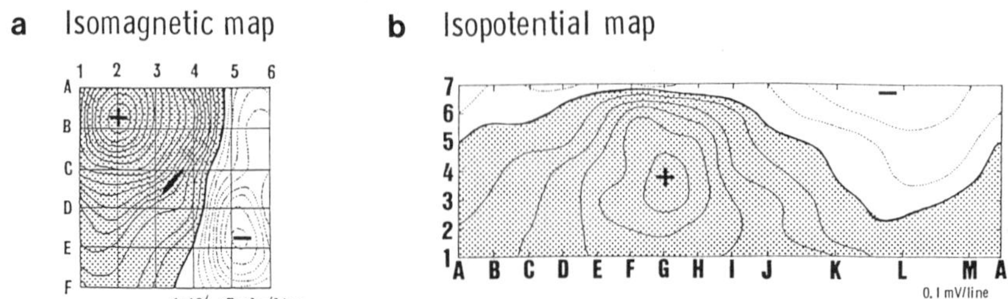

Fig. 3 Isomagnetic and isopotential maps (left free wall type)

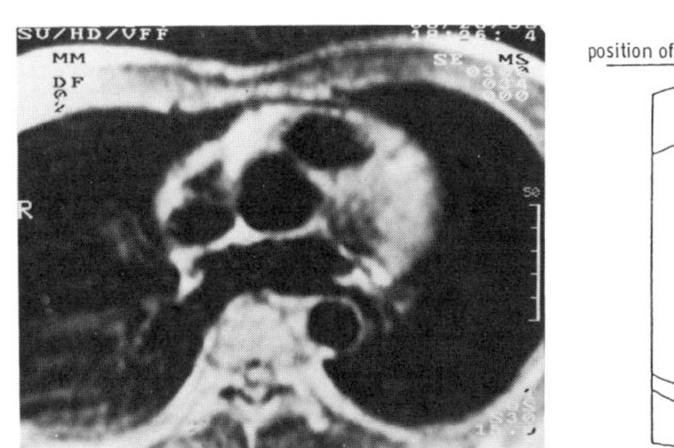

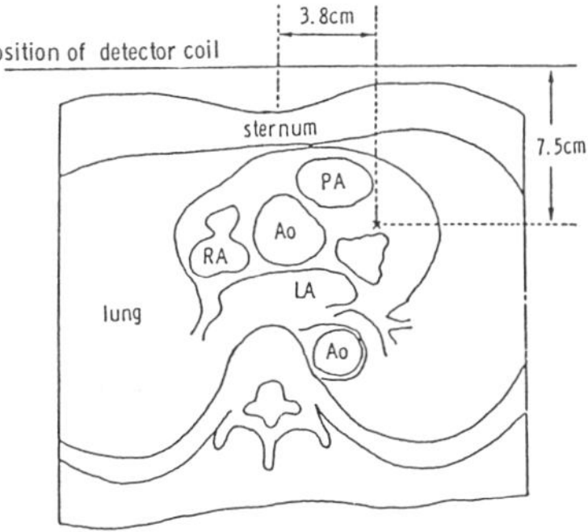

Fig. 4 Gated MRI of a same patient as in Fig. 3

be located at the anterior free wall of the right ventricle.

In the present study, locations estimated by the analysis of the isomagnetic map at 40 msec after the onset of the delta wave agreed well with the findings obtained by the body surface isopotential map.[5]

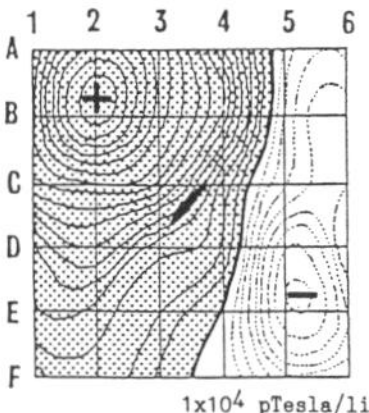

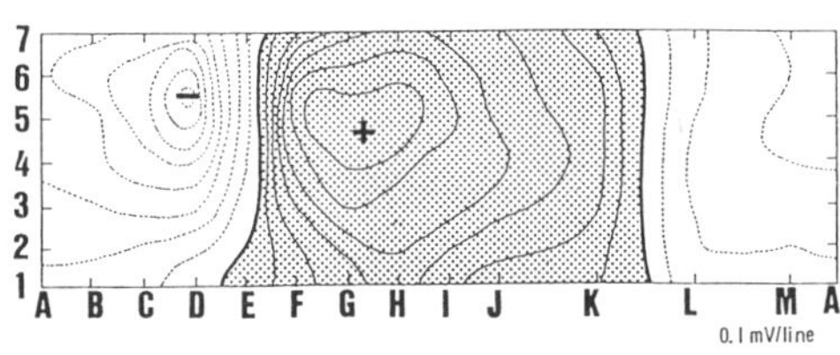

Fig. 5 Isomagnetic and isopotential maps (right free wall type)

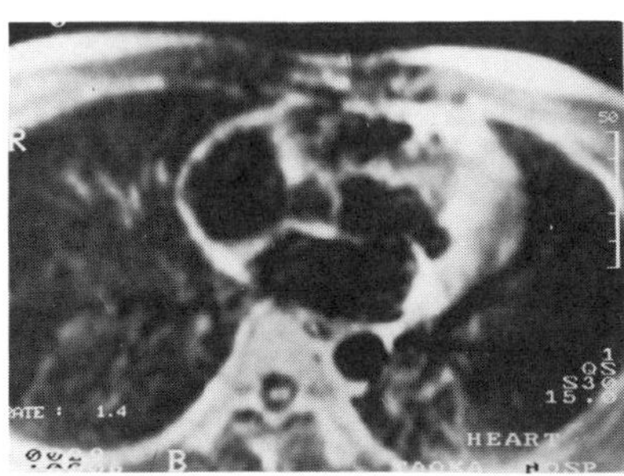

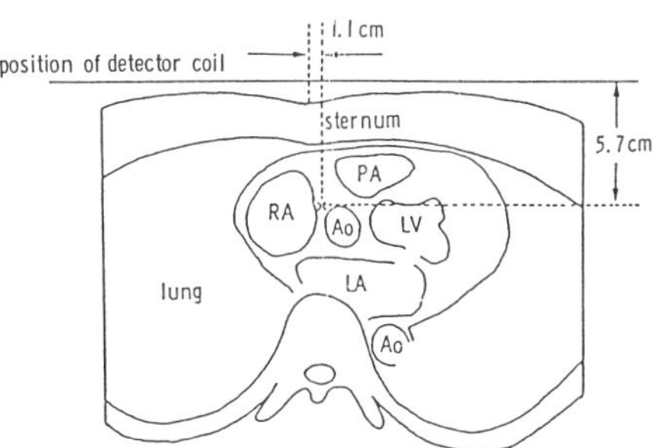

Fig. 6 Gated MRI of a same patient as in Fig. 5

3) Repolarization phase of WPW syndrome

Fig. 7 shows the isomagnetic (panel a) and isopotential maps (panel b) at the peak of the T wave of the lead II of the standard ECG of the same patient as in Fig. 3. From the isomagnetic map, a single current dipole directed leftward is deduced similarly to the isopotential map. From Fig. 7 a, the position of the repolarization vector is located at 3.0 cm leftward from the median line and 5.0 cm upward from the xyphoid process. The depth of this current dipole was calculated at 5.8 cm below the detector coil, which agreed well with the site deduced by the delta wave.

Fig. 8 shows the isomagnetic (panel a) and isopotential maps (panel b) at the peak of the T wave of the lead II of the standard ECG of the same patient as in Fig. 5. The isomagnetic map shows two minimum at the left upper and lower portions, indicating two current dipoles, one of which directed rightwards. But, from the isopotential map, only the single

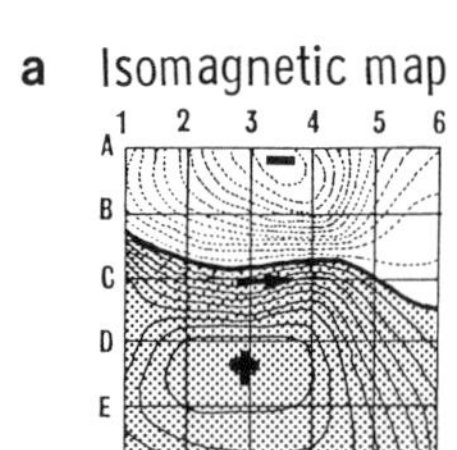

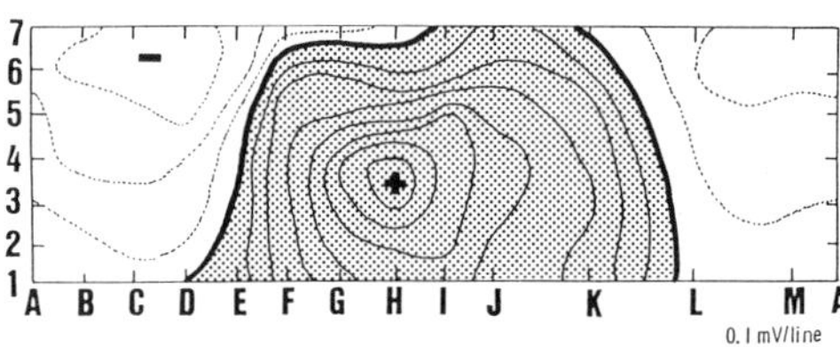

Fig. 7 Isomagnetic and isopotential maps at the repolarization phase

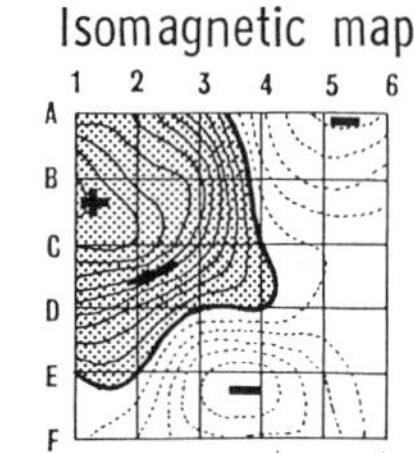

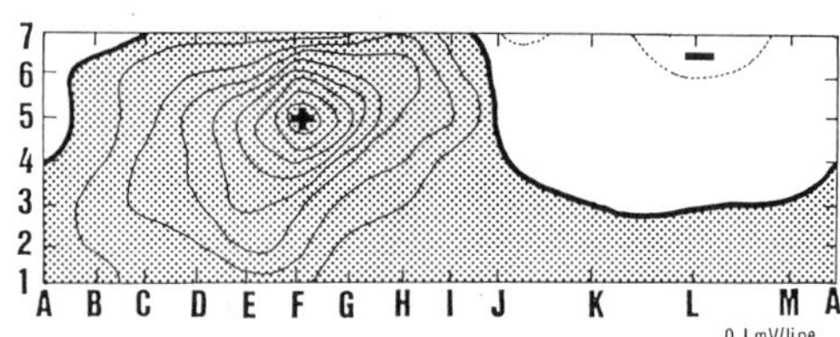

Fig. 8 Isomagnetic and isopotential maps at the repolarization phase

current dipole can be deduced. From Fig. 8 a, the repolarization vector directing rightwards is located at 0.8 cm leftward from the median line and 3.8 cm upward from the xyphoid process. The depth of this current dipole was calculated at 6.7 cm below the detector coil.

DISCUSSION

The present study shows that we can predict the three-dimensional location of the current dipole by the combined use of the isomagnetic map and gated MRI. We also examined whether we could predicte the location of the pre-excited site of the ventricle from the analysis of the isomagnetic map at the repolarization phase. Local inhomogeneity of the electromotive force is difficult to detect from the isopotential map.[3] Usually single dipole is deduced from the isopotential map as a summation of these localized current sources.[3] However, multiple dipoles are easily estimated by the analysis of the repolarization wave of the isomagnetic map as shown in Fig. 7 a. In the present study, some cases showed opposing pairs of dipole in the isomagnetic map at the peak of the T wave; one directed leftwards expressing a normal repolarization, and the other directed rightwards expressing presumably a repolarization of the myocardium excited by an impulse coming through an accessory pathway. Location of the current dipole determined by the analysis of the isomagnetic map at the peak of the T wave was quite similar as those determined by the isomagnetic map at 40 msec after the onset of the delta wave. These results suggest that the location of the accessory pathway could be predicted also by the analysis of the isomagnetic map at the ventricular repolarization phase.

CONCLUSION

MCG was useful to determine the location of the accessory pathway complementally with body surface mapping and other methods. In addition, the isomagnetic maps at the repolarization phase was as useful as those at the delta wave in detecting the site of the accessory pathway in patients with WPW syndrome.

REFERENCE

1.MS.Spach et al: Circ Res 15:103-118, 1978
2.DW.Benson et al: Circulation 65:1259-1268, 1982
3.H.Mori and Y.Nakaya: CV World Report 1:78-86, 1988
4.SJ.Williamson and L.Kaufman: Biomagnetism '81:353-402, 1981
5.T.Iwa and T.Magara: Jpn Circ J 45:1192-1198, 1981

ECG AND MCG STUDIES ON THE HIS-PURKINJE ACTIVITY IN A CASE OF CONGENITAL HEART BLOCK

M. Leiniö, J. Montonen, M. Mäkijärvi*, K. Mäkiniemi, J. Nenonen, T. Katila and P. Siltanen*

Laboratory of Biomedical Engineering, Department of Technical Physics, Helsinki University of Technology, SF-02150 Espoo, Finland, *Cardiovascular Laboratory, First Department of Medicine, Helsinki University Central Hospital, SF-00290 Helsinki, Finland

INTRODUCTION

Non-invasive detection of the His-Purkinje (HP) activity could be useful in clinical practice, e.g. in determining the actual site of atrio-ventricular (A-V) block or in evaluating the effect of anti-arrhythmic drug therapy on heart conduction system. The HP activity from body surface was first measured electrically by Berbari et al. (1978). First magnetic study of the HP conduction system was reported by Farrell et al. (1980). The HP activity was described as a ramp like structure in the P-Q interval. Fenici et al. (1985) reported magnetic His-Purkinje studies with invasive ECG reference. In normal subjects the overlapping atrial activity causes serious interference with the HP-signal. To avoid this overlapping, Mäkijärvi et al. (1985) investigated patients with total A-V block. However, in these studies the accurate timing was difficult because intracardial reference ECG was not available.

We report here a study of a patient with congenital total A-V block at the level of the A-V node. In this ideal case the HP signal can be recorded practically without disturbance of the atrial activity and the true waveform of the HP signal is revealed. Results of the invasive ECG, the standard 12-lead ECG, the high-resolution (HR) ECG, the HR MCG and the HR ECG mapping studies are given.

METHODS

The patient was a 21 yr. old male with a congenital total A-V block. He was examined because of symptomatic bradycardia and tachycardia attacks and syncope. He underwent the routine clinical evaluation, the standard 12-lead ECG and the biplane chest X-ray. In the electrophysiological (EP) study, the site of the total block was found at the level of A-V node. The HP signal was recorded invasively.

The HR ECG was recorded using 8 bipolar leads. The recording time was 10 minutes. The HR ECG mapping was performed at 36 locations according to the standard MCG grid, a row of 6 locations was measured at a time. The HR ECG measurements were made in an electrically shielded room. The sensitivity in the HR ECG measurements was $\leq 1\mu V_{p-p}$, the sampling frequency 2000 Hz and the frequency band 0.05 – 300 Hz.

The HR MCG recordings were made using the standard MCG grid with one extra column at the left. One channel DC-SQUID instrumentation with a first order gradiometer was utilized. The MCG measurements were performed in the Otaniemi magnetically shielded room. The sensitivity of the MCG measurements was $4.5\,\mathrm{fT}/\sqrt{\mathrm{Hz}}$. The sampling frequency and the bandwidth were similar to the HR ECG recordings. The recording time was two minutes. The signals were averaged both manually and automatically using cross correlation and noise checking. Only QRS complexes without overlapping atrial activity on the HP signal were selected for analysis.

RESULTS

The invasive EP study revealed a clear biphasic His spike 50 ms before the QRS onset (Fig. 1). The standard 12-lead ECG showed total dissociation of atrial and ventricular activations. In the HR ECG recordings the HP activity was best visible in the orthogonal z-lead (precordial-subscapular) (Fig. 2).

The HP activity was detectable both in the HR ECG and MCG maps. The activity started 35 – 45 ms before the QRS onset and showed curvy, ramp like patterns. The maximum amplitude of the field in the HR MCG measurements was about 0.2 pT. The field pattern was approximately dipolar (Fig. 4). The amplitude of the electric HP signal was 5 μV at maximum. In the ECG contour maps, the field pattern during the HP activity was also dipolar.

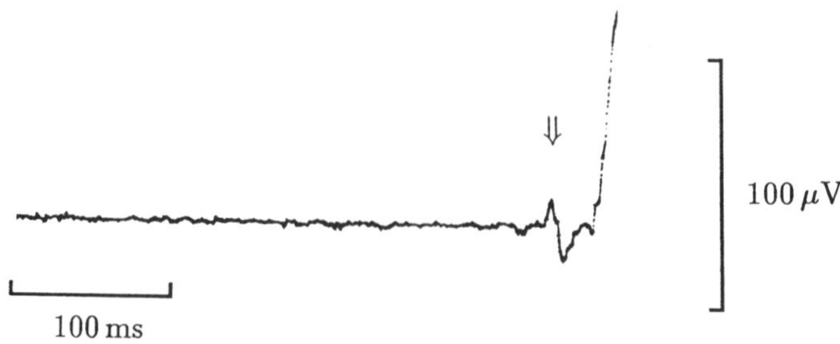

Fig. 1. His spike (arrow) recorded during invasive electrophysiological study.

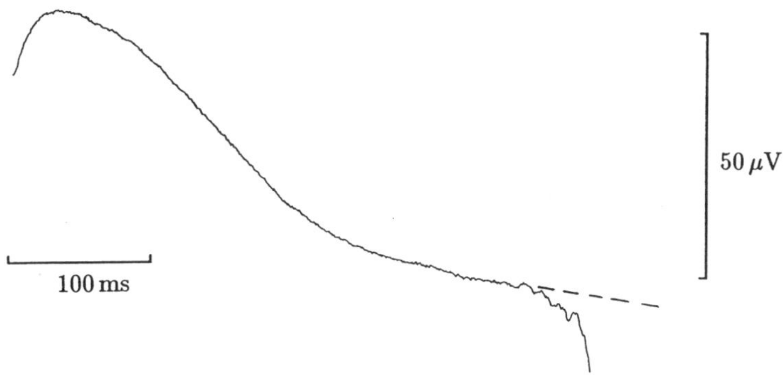

Fig. 2. Averaged high-resolution ECG z-lead recording before the QRS complex. (The dashed line shows the supposed continuation of the pre His signal)

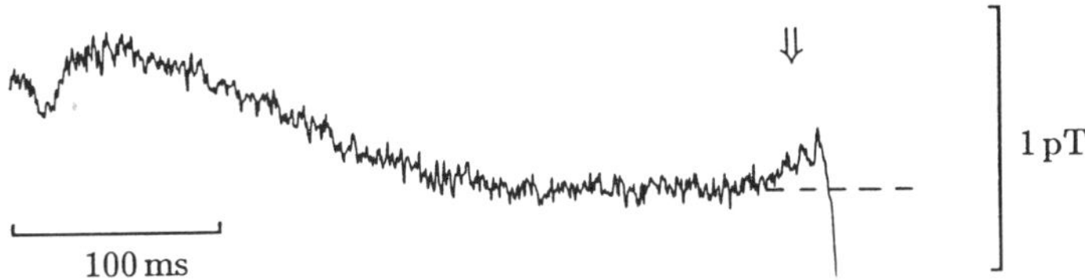

Fig. 3. Averaged high-resolution MCG recording before the QRS complex from the location C 3. Arrow shows the time instant of the field pattern in Fig. 4. (The dashed line shows the supposed continuation of the pre His signal)

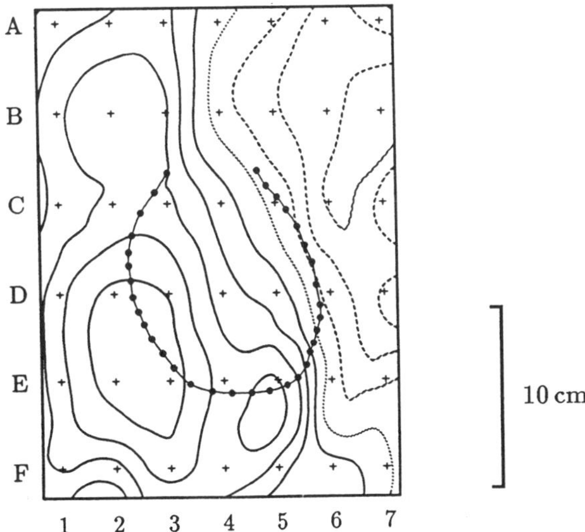

Fig. 4. MCG map showing dipolar field during His-Purkinje activity. The time instant of the field pattern has been marked by arrow in Fig. 3. The difference between isocontour lines is 0.03 pT.

DISCUSSION

In the present case of congenital heart block, we were able to study the HP activity with minimum interference by adjacent signals. Our study confirms the ramp like morphology of the magnetic HP signal. The heart of the patient was enlarged and the conduction system located exceptionally deep. The His Bundle (HB) was situated 8 cm below the anterior chest wall according to the EP study. Correspondingly, the signals measured were slightly smaller than in normal subjects.

The asymmetry of the magnetic field pattern during the HB activity influenced the results of source localization. Calculated localization was compared with invasive EP localization. Using a current dipole source model in a half infinite conducting space the error of the calculated depth was small (< 1 cm), but the deviation on the frontal projection was much bigger (≈ 3 cm). The localization calculated from the ECG map did not give good results.

The HP activity was detectable by all the non-invasive methods mentioned above. However, the signal is weak and its detection requires very sensitive instrumentation. Only in a few locations it was possible to detect the magnetic HP activity in real time and averaging had to be used to improve the signal to noise ratio. In the clinical use the high sensitivity and low noise needed is not easy to obtain.

REFERENCES

D. E. Farrell, J. H. Tripp and R. Nordgren, 1980, *Magnetic study of the His-Purkinje conduction system in man*, IEEE Trans. Biom. Eng., **BME-27**, pp. 345-350.

R. R. Fenici, M. Masselli, L. Lopez and F. Sabetta, 1985, *First Simultaneous Magnetocardiographic and Invasive Recordings of the P-R Interval Electrophysiological Phenomena in Man* Med. & Biolog. Eng. & Comp., **23** (S2), pp. 1483-1484.

M. Mäkijärvi, R. Maniewski, I. Derka, J. Puurtinen, T. Katila and P. Siltanen, 1985, *High-Resolution MCG Study on Heart Conduction System*, Med. & Biolog. Eng. & Comp., **23** (S2), pp. 1485-1486.

HIGH-RESOLUTION MAGNETOCARDIOGRAPHIC MAPPING OF PRE-EXCITATION IN WOLFF-PARKINSON-WHITE SYNDROME

M. Mäkijärvi*, J. Nenonen, M. Leiniö, J. Montonen, K. Mäkiniemi, T. Schulman, T. Katila and P. Siltanen*

Laboratory of Biomedical Engineering, Department of Technical Physics, Helsinki University of Technology, SF-02150 Espoo, *Cardiovascular Laboratory, First Department of Medicine, Helsinki University Central Hospital, SF-00290 Helsinki, Finland

INTRODUCTION

We have studied 10 Wolff-Parkinson-White (WPW) syndrome patients using high-resolution magnetocardiographic (HR-MCG) mapping, standard 12-lead ECG and invasive electrophysiologic study (EPS). The ventricular pre-excitation caused by abnormal conduction via an accessory pathway (AP), seen as a so-called delta-wave prior to the QRS complex, was characterized by studying the morphology of the QRS and the delta-wave in the measured ECG and MCG signals. For all patients, EPS was performed to determine the conduction properties and the location of the AP. The site of the pre-excitation was also localized using the HR-MCG mapping and the results were compared to the invasive results. For a surgical operation or catheter ablation therapy, the site of the AP should be determined with a reasonable accuracy. Non-invasive methods, such as the HR-MCG, would be helpful in minimizing the duration and discomfort of invasive catheter mapping and in some cases could even replace it. Studies of WPW patients have been previously reported by Erné et al. (1985) and first simultaneous catheter and MCG mapping was done by Fenici et al. (1985).

METHODS

The HR MCGs were measured in the Otaniemi magnetically shielded room using a one channel DC-SQUID gradiometer system. The recordings were performed at 42 locations according to the standard MCG grid, with an extra row on the left. The magnetic field component perpendicular to the anterior plane was measured, and the average sensitivity of the system was about 5 $fT/\sqrt{Hz}$. The frequency band was limited to 0.03–300 Hz, the sampling frequency was 2000 Hz and a 12-bit A/D conversion was used. The recorded data was processed off-line in an HP1000 minicomputer

Advances in Biomagnetism
Edited by S.J. Williamson *et al.*
Plenum Press, New York

using a semi-automatic averaging program based on the cross-correlation algorithm for correct time alignment.

The 12-lead ECG measurements and the invasive EPS were carried out at the hospital. A surgical operation to cut the AP was performed for two patients. The morphological studies were done for the ECG and HR-MCG delta-wave and QRS deflections.

The computer localizations were performed using three different source models, based on the current multipole expansion: the current dipole (CD), the current multipole (CM) and the magnetic dipole (MD) model (Katila et al. 1987). The volume conductor model used in these computations was a homogeneous conducting halfspace with a plane boundary.

The computed results were compared to the EPS results in 8 cases and intra-operative mapping studies in 2 cases. MCG measurement locations were marked with lead balls and biplane chest X-ray pictures were taken. Calculated localization results were positioned into these X-ray pictures. The results were compared to biplane drawings made from catheter and electrode positions on the fluoroscopy screen during EPS.

RESULTS

Morphology. The signals generated by the pre-excitation were always clearly detectable in HR-MCG. The morphology of the delta-wave and the QRS was depending on the site of the AP. This also reflected as different field patterns within the measurement area. In general, posterior and left sided APs generated monopolar patterns while the fields caused by septal and right sided APs were more dipolar. A typical monopolar field pattern in the case of a posterolateral AP is shown in Fig. 1.

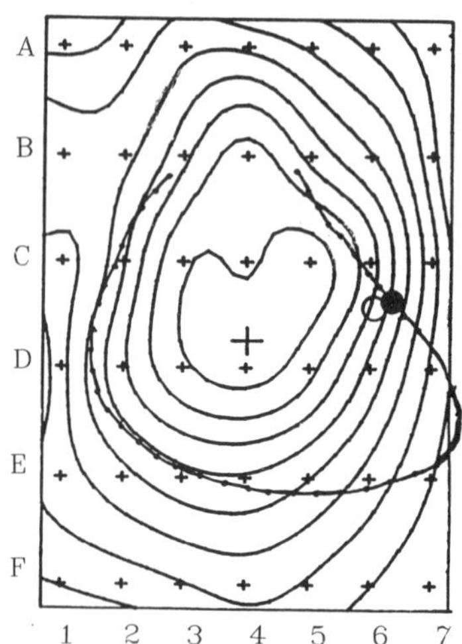

Fig. 1. The MCG field pattern during the delta-wave and the localization results in the case of a left posterolateral AP. Continuous lines indicate positive field values, and the difference between the isocontour curves is 1.0 pT. This patient was surgically operated and the result is marked by an open circle. The calculated result of the HR-MCG (the MD model) is shown with a filled circle. The three-dimensional difference between the calculated result and the result of intra-operative mapping was 1 cm.

Localization. According to the results of EPS, one patient had multiple right sided APs, three had posteroseptal APs and six had left lateral or left posterior APs. The obtained depths of the APs varied between 90–125 mm from the skin. In these ten cases the average three-dimensional distances between the invasive catheter localization of the atrial end of the AP and the computed estimation of the ventricular pre-excitation site were 3.1 cm for the MD, 3.8 cm for the CM and 7.7 cm for the CD model. The corresponding average distances of the source depth were 1.1 cm (MD), 2.1 cm (CM) and 5.1 cm (CD). An example of the computed localization compared to the result of the intra-operative study in the case of a left posterolateral AP is shown in Fig. 1.

DISCUSSION

The present most reliable pre-operative localization of the site of the AP is obtained by invasive catheter mapping. The best accuracy of this method is about 1 cm. In this study, we have tried to localize the ventricular pre-excitation site which usually differs 1–2 cm from the atrial end of the AP. According to the overall accuracy, the results of the HR-MCG mapping technique were comparable to the corresponding EPS results, in the two operated cases even slightly better. Although the location of the AP turned out to be very deep in all cases studied, the MD and CM models were able to estimate the depth well. On the other hand, the CD localizations were always too anterior. This happened even in cases of dipolar field patterns and is presumably due to the deep location of the AP.

The failure of the CD model was most notable in cases of left lateral or left posterior APs (6/10) with strongly nondipolar field patterns. On the frontal projection, the HR-MCG localizations results were usually too cranial and too much to the left. This is partly due to the downward shift in the heart position caused by deep inspiration during the X-ray study, compared to the HR-MCG mapping situation when patient breaths normally. This effect was verified with cineangiogram, too. In addition, the source models should be further developed and all available non-invasive data (the 12-lead ECG, the HR-MCG and ECG mapping) should be combined to obtain a more reliable non-invasive localization.

REFERENCES

Erné, S. N., 1985, *High Resolution Magnetocardiography: Modeling and Sources Localization*, Med. & Biolog. Eng. & Comp., **23** (S2), pp. 1447-1450.

Fenici, R. R., Masselli, M., Lopez, L. and Sabetta, F., 1985, *High Resolution Magnetocardiography: Electrophysiological and Clinical Findings*, Med. & Biolog. Eng. & Comp., **23** (S2), pp. 1475-1478.

Katila, T., Maniewski, R., Mäkijärvi, M., Nenonen, J., and Siltanen, P., 1987, *The accuracy of source localisation in cardiac measurements*, Phys. Med. Biol. 32(1), 125-131.

ANALYSIS OF HIGH RESOLUTION MCG RECORDINGS OF PATIENTS WITH VENTRICULAR TACHYCARDIA

J. Montonen, M. Leiniö, K. Mäkiniemi, M. Mäkijärvi*, J. Nenonen, T. Katila, and P. Siltanen*

Laboratory of Biomedical Engineering, Department of Technical Physics
Helsinki University of Technology, SF-02150 Espoo, Finland
* Cardiovascular Laboratory, First Department of Medicine
Helsinki University Central Hospital, SF-00290 Helsinki, Finland

INTRODUCTION

Selection of patients prone to sustained ventricular tachycardia (VT), by detecting abnormal cardiac electric micropotentials called late potentials (LP), from high resolution (HR) ECG recordings has recently become to clinical practice. Observation of magnetic late field (LF) signals, corresponding to electric LP:s, was first reported by Ernè et al. in 1983.[1] Since then only few studies have been published on late fields.

In this study, using methods based on high pass filtering, the applicability of HR MCG recordings for the detection of LF:s is for the first time compared with HR ECG recordings. The HR MCG measurements (noise level $<10\ \mathrm{fT}/\sqrt{\mathrm{Hz}}$) were performed over the whole standard MCG-grid[2]. In the analysis, however, the emphasis is laid on a 3×3 minigrid whose upper right corner is situated at the location C3. Such a grid area, with an outer diameter of less than 13 cm, can easily be covered with a multichannel instrumentation, nowadays commercially available.

The results suggest that the identification of the VT patients can be made at least as efficiently on the base of HR MCG data as on the base of HR ECG data. This supports the possibility to use the new magnetic multichannel systems, when available for clinical studies, also for VT measurements. Because no electrodes are needed, a quick and fluent screening of the VT patients would be possible.

METHODS

The HR MCG recordings of seven (7) patients with clinically documented VT and seven (7) normal controls (N) were analysed and the results were compared with corresponding data from HR ECG measurements.

Advances in Biomagnetism
Edited by S.J. Williamson *et al.*
Plenum Press, New York

The component of the magnetic field perpendicular to the frontal plane was measured in the Otaniemi magnetically shielded room utilizing a first order gradiometer and a dc-SQUID with a sensitivity about 4 $fT/\sqrt{Hz}$. The HR MCG data from a square 3×3 minigrid lying just above the heart with edge locations C3, C5, E3 and E5 was used in the analysis. Comparative surface potential HR ECG measurements, including orthogonal x-, y-, and z-leads were done in an electrically shielded room at HUCH with an instrumental noise level below 1 μV_{p-p}. Both electric and magnetic recordings were made in a frequency band from 0.03 to 300 Hz and the data were transferred via an 2 kHz A/D converter to an HP1000 minicomputer for signal processing. The QRS complexes from each measurement location were automatically but selectively averaged.

To enhance the possible LF signals and to automatically determine the duration of the QRS complex the following procedures were applied both to averaged and non-averaged HR MCG complexes: First, 25 Hz, 40 Hz, 60 Hz, and 80 Hz Chebyshev infinite impulse response high pass filters with about 80 dB attenuation were separately applied to time inverted and non-inverted QRS complexes. From each filtered signal an envelope (ENV) curve was calculated using a Hilbert transform.[3] Next, the beginning, the end, and the duration of the QRS complex were determined from the ENV curves by a computer algorithm. Finally, the average amplitude of the ENV curves during the last 40 ms, 50 ms and 60 ms intervals of the QRS complex and during the whole QRS complex were calculated. These values are called ENV40, ENV50, ENV60 and ENVQRS, respectively. A corresponding procedure was performed on the HR ECG recordings with the exception that the envelope curve was replaced by a root mean square (RMS) curve obtained from filtered x-, y-, and z-leads using a method proposed by Simson.[4] To compare results obtained with different high pass filter cut-off frequencies and with different ENV values, the ratio of the average value in N and VT groups (N/VT or VT/N) of the quantity under consideration was calculated.

RESULTS

The durations of the QRS complexes calculated from the averaged MCG recordings were found longer in the VT group than among the normal controls. Almost the same VT/N ratio was obtained with all cut-off frequencies, the 25 Hz giving the largest one (see Fig. 3). The QRS durations calculated from the non-averaged MCG recordings were only slightly longer in the VT group than in the N group. Calculated from the HR ECG recordings, the results were similar to those in the magnetic case, but the corresponding VT/N ratios of the QRS durations were even larger. The largest VT/N ratio from the averaged electric recordings was also reached with a 25 Hz high pass filtering (see Fig. 3).

A low amplitude signal after the fundamental QRS complex was detected by visual inspection both from the averaged and the non-averaged MCG complexes of three VT patients (see Fig. 1). When a 25 Hz high pass filtering was applied the largest N/VT ratios of the ENV values were obtained both for the averaged and the non-averaged data. The use of ENV60 values after 25 Hz high pass filtering gave the largest of all N/VT ratios: 3.9 for the averaged and 2.7 for the non-averaged data (see Fig. 4). The corresponding results obtained from the HR ECG recordings were again

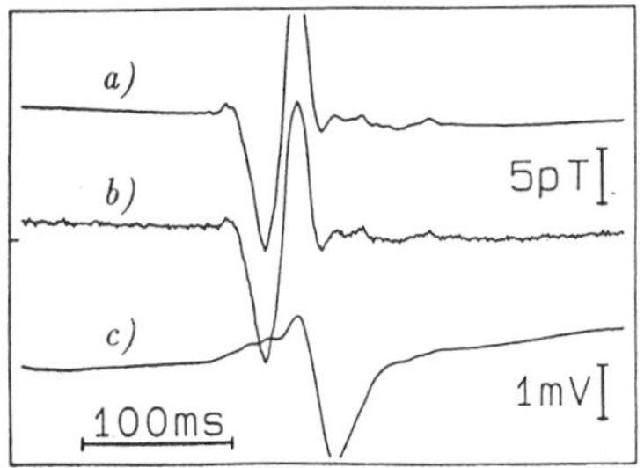

Fig 1. *a) An averaged MCG complex of a VT patient from the grid location D5 and b) a corresponding non-averaged MCG complex. c) An ECG II lead measured simultaneously for timing.*

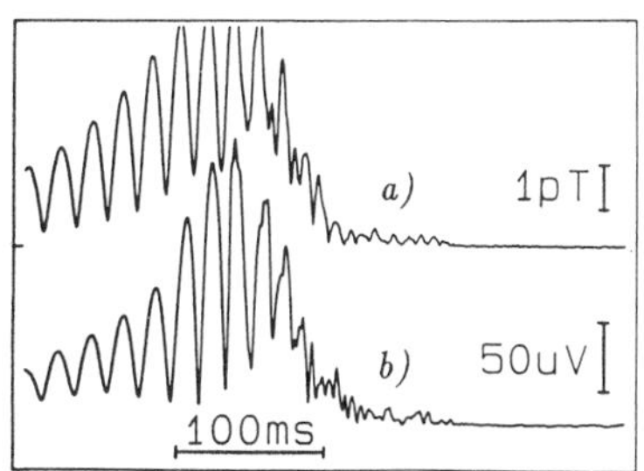

Fig 2. *a) The envelope complex of the averaged MCG curve (a) in Fig. 1, calculated after 25 Hz high pass filtering. b) The corresponding electric RMS complex of the same VT patient.*

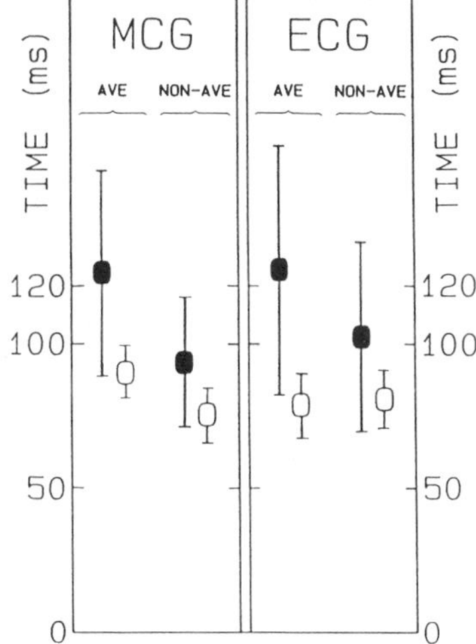

Fig 3. *Durations of the QRS complexes calculated from the power spectra of the 25 Hz high pass filtered complexes. Results from averaged and non-averaged MCG and ECG data are shown. One standard deviation has been marked.*

• = *VT patient;*

○ = *normal control.*

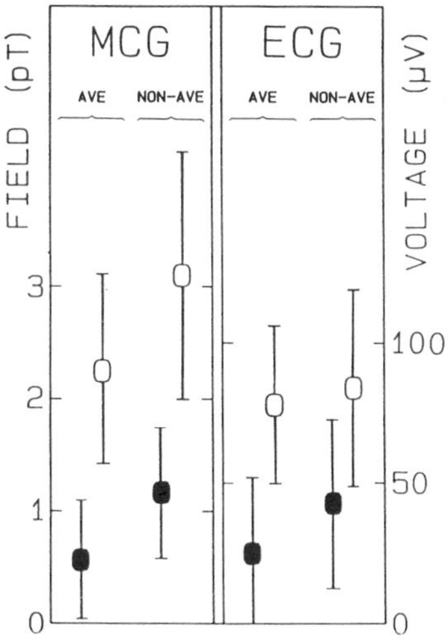

Fig 4. *The average values of the power spectra from the last 60 ms of the QRS complexes when 25 Hz high pass filtering was used. Results from averaged and non-averaged MCG and ECG data are shown. One standard deviation has been marked.*

• = *VT patient;*

○ = *normal control.*

similar to the results from the magnetic data: RMS60 values calculated from 25 Hz high pass filtered data and RMS60 values calculated from 40 Hz high pass filtered data gave the largest N/VT ratios for averaged and non-averaged data, respectively. However, the N/VT ratios reached both from averaged and non-averaged electric data were usually smaller than the corresponding ratios calculated from the magnetic data. For example, the averaged RMS60 values calculated after the 25 Hz filtering led to the best ratio of only 3.1 in the electric case. (See Fig. 4).

DISCUSSION AND CONCLUSION

In this study, the duration of the QRS complexes of the VT patients, calculated from the envelopes of the 25 Hz high pass filtered HR MCG recordings, was found in the average to be longer than 120 ms, which is considered pathological in the clinical intepretation of standard ECG recordings. A close morphological resemblance of the envelopes calculated from the filtered HR MCG recordigs and the RMS curves obtained from the HR ECG recordings was observed (see Fig. 2). The average ENV60 value calculated after the 25 Hz high pass filtering was essentially lower in the VT group than in the case of the normal controls. For the patient data analysed, this difference in the magnetic ENV values was even more distinquished than in the corresponding electric RMS values. Further, it was observed that within one standard deviation, the ENV60 values of the N and VT groups did not overlap even in the case of non-averaged data. It was, however, also observed that the duration of the fundamental QRS complex in the HR MCG recordings of three out of the seven VT patients was shorter in duration than the main QRS complex in the ECG II lead measured simultaneously (see Fig. 1). This unexpected feature, which was not observed in the case of of the normal controls, can to some extent be explained by the use of the minigrid covering only a limited area and it may also be due to the fact that only one component of the magnetic field was measured.

This study supports the possibility to identify VT patients on the basis of a quick and completely non-invasive magnetic mapping made above the heart.

REFERENCES

1. S.N. Erne, R.R. Fenici, H.-D. Hahlbohm, W. Jaszczuk, H.P. Lehman, and M. Masselli, High-Resolution Magnetocardiographic Recordings of the ST Segment in Patients with Electrical Late Potentials, Il Nuovo Cimento 2D, 340-345 (1983)
2. M. Saarinen, P. Siltanen, P.J. Karp, and T.E. Katila, The Normal Magnetocardiogram: I Morphology, Ann. Clin. Res. 10(S21), 1-43 (1978).
3. J. Montonen, T. Katila, M. Leiniö, S. Madekivi, M. Mäkijärvi, J. Nenonen, and P. Siltanen, Time and Frequency Domain Analyses of Cardiac Micropotentials, in: "Proc. of the 6th Internat. Conf. on Biomagn.", K. Atsumi, M. Kotani, S. Ueno, T. Katila, and S.J. Williamson, Eds. Tokyo Denki Univ. Press, Tokyo, (1988).
4. M.B. Simson, Use of Signals in the Terminal QRS Complex to Identify Patients with Ventricular Tachycardia After Myocardial Infarction. Circulation 64, 235-242, (1981).

DETECTION OF MAGNETIC ATRIAL FLUTTER WAVES

IN ISOLATED RABBITS HEARTS

P. Costa Ribeiro, A.C. Bruno, E. Parente Ribeiro, J.S. do Carmo

Departamento de Fisica, Pontificia Universidade Catolica
Caixa Postal 38071, Rio de Janeiro, RJ, 22453, Brasil

E. Costa Monteiro and A. Fonseca Costa

Instituto de Biofisica da UFRJ, Ilha do Fundão, Rio de Janeiro, RJ, Brasil

INTRODUCTION

The non-invasive character of Magnetocardiography and it's ability to monitor electrical phenomena place the MCG technique in a very good position for studying arrhythmias like flutter and fibrillation. Although these arrhythmias have long been studied, there are still questions about depolarization current patterns (Boineau et al., 1984). The periodicity of flutter, contrasting with the more chaotic behavior of fibrillation, places the former as more suitable for analysis using a one channel system. Models of reentry currents models are more commonly used to explain flutter, but the existence of ectopic foci is not completely ruled-out in some forms of such arrhythmia.

METHODS

Atrial flutter was induced in isolated rabbit hearts. After decerebration and thoracothomy the hearts were extracted and maintained in perfusion (Langendorf system) with a Tyrode solution ($NaCl$, glucose, $NaHCO_3$, KCL, NaH_2PO_4, $MgCl_2$ and $CaCl_2$), bubbled with a 95% O_2 - 5% CO_2 gas mixture.

Flutter was induced by adding acetylcholine (22×10^{-7} molar) to the Tyrode solution and submitting the heart to a rapid pacing (Alessie et al, 1984). For this purpose an electric stimulator delivering pulses of 20 Hz, 3 ms of duration and 20 Volts amplitude was used. It was easier to induce flutter in the atrial region under the right atrial appendage. The rapid rhythm could be easily interrupted by stopping the supply of acetylcholine to the nutrient solution of cardiac tissue. This procedure leads to the return of normal electric activity of the heart, and the tachyarrhythmia can be again produced.

The isolated heart (2x3cm) was immersed in a 4 cm depth cylindrical container with a volume conductor consisting of 2 liters of a conducting nutrient solution in

Advances in Biomagnetism
Edited by S.J. Williamson *et al.*
Plenum Press, New York

order to attenuate the influence of volume limits (Eghrari et al, 1983). The heart was positioned in the center of the solution container near the upper surface.

Magnetic signals were measured using a second order symmetric flux transformer (base line = $4\,cm$ and diameter = $1.6\,cm$) coupled to a commercial RF SQUID.

Electrical measurements were performed using glass extracelular electrodes immersed in the solution. This was used as a time reference for averaging the magnetic signal.

The signals were filtered with a bandwidth from 0.5 to 100 Hz by a Wavetek filter, model 852. In the computer, the signals were submitted to a signal average procedure in order to obtain isofield contour maps using bi-cubic spline functions. The proximity of the rabbit's heart to the pick-up coil produced a strong magnetic signal and therefore no magnetic shield was used. The magnetic signal was recorded as a function of time over 25 points of a $1\,cm$ spacing square grid, on a parallel plane distant 1.5 cm from the volume conductor surface.

RESULTS AND DISCUSSION

Fig.1 shows a typical tracing (F waves) of the magnetic field and the electric potential detected simultaneously during a flutter episode induced in an isolated rabbit heart. A strong atrioventricular block was obtained with our experimental protocol, leading to a large number of F waves compared to QRS complexes (8:1). A rapid flutter rhythm was obtained with this method (between 8 - 12 Hz, around 600 beats per minute).

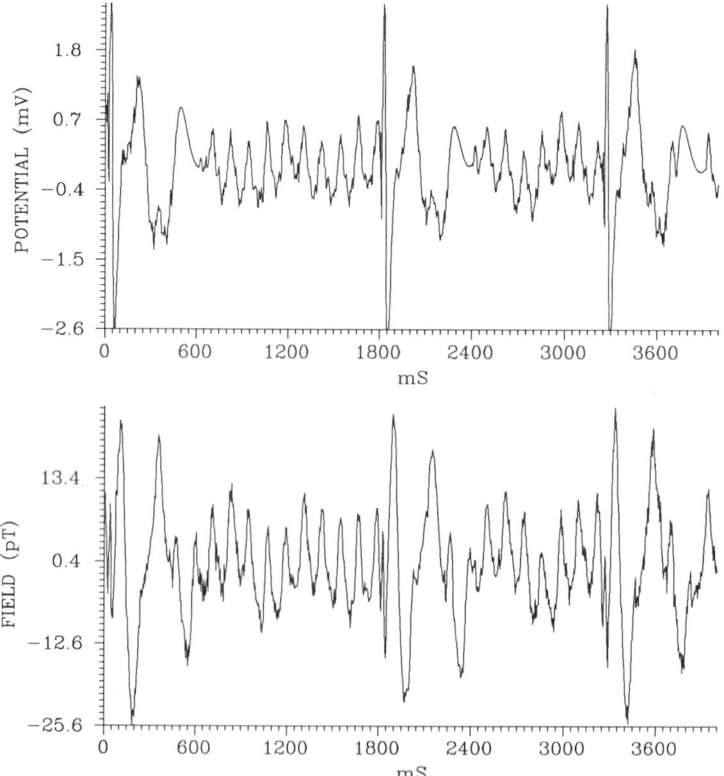

Fig.1 Electrical (ECG) and magnetical (MCG) recordings during an episode of flutter.

Ten isolated rabbit hearts were used for atrial flutter experiments. One of the sustained flutter episodes persisted for a sufficient time to enable mapping the magnetic F waves using a 5x5 grid. The isofield maps obtained after data processing were not always bipolar, preventing the identification of an equivalent dipole whose motion could be associated with the reentry current. A possible explanation for this difficulty is a gradual change of the depolarization path between the beginning and the end of measurements made over the grid.

An alternative approach is to look for the properties of the magnetic signal produced by a circular motion. A simple model for this motion will represent it as a constant intensity electric dipole (constant amount of excited atrial tissue) moving around a circle with constant speed (uniform conduction velocity).

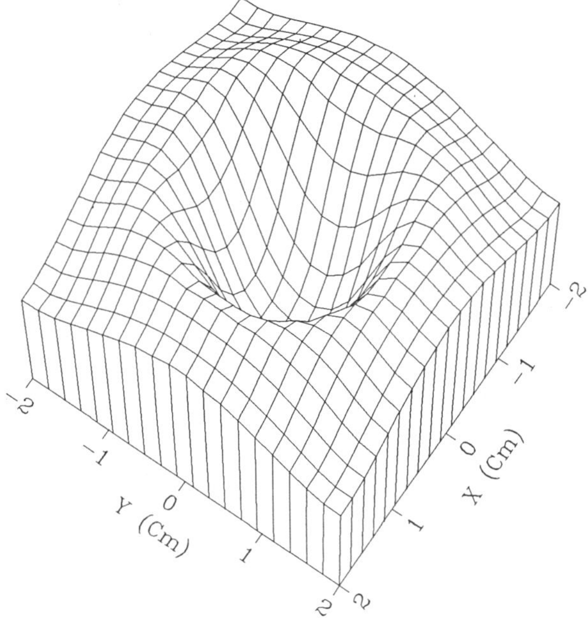

Fig.2 Simulation graph of the amplitude of oscilating z component of the magnetic field as a function of the magnetic sensor position measured over a current dipole moving around a circle of 0.8 cm radius, 1 *cm* sensor-source distance and 0.8 *cm* radius of detecting coil.

The main property of this motion is the existence of a zero AC field point over the circle's center. When moving away in any direction from the circle's center the amplitude of the oscilating z component of the magnetic field goes through a maximum then decreases again. Fig. 2 shows the amplitude of this oscilating z component of the magnetic field as a function of the measurement point in a 3D graph generated by a current dipole moving around a circle. The parameters used for simulation approximate the experimental results obtained. A maximum appears with a circle of 1.5 *cm* radius centered at the zero amplitude point.

The amplitude of a magnetic 10 Hz experimental F wave (digitally filtered with a bandwith of 8 to 12 Hz) is plotted in a similar graph in Fig.3. A minimum with a near zero value is observed over the atrium's position ($x = 0.2$; $y = 0.8$). The intensity of the signal goes through a maximum and then decreases when moving the detector in any direction away from the minimum.

The lack of cylindrical symmetry observed in the experimental results (Fig.3) is possibly explained by a non-uniform amount of excited tissue around the reentry

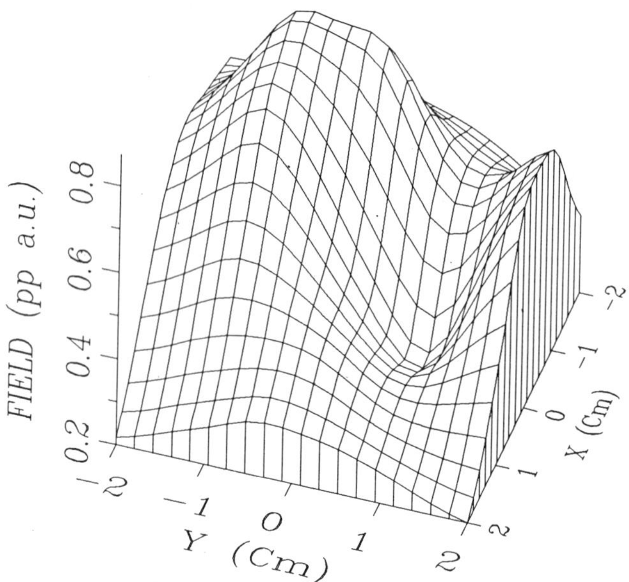

Fig.3 X and Y give the detector position coordinates in cm; Z gives the amplitude of the magnetic F waves.

path, as normally found by invasive electrodes measurements (Alessie et al,1984). The existence of maxima of different intensities, depending on the direction of measurement, was already present at the beginning of the experiment when looking for the minimum point as a preliminary measurement to test the validity of the model.

These preliminary results show the possibility for magnetocardiography to recognise the mechanism of flutter by a noninvasive method. More experiments are being made to confirm this finding.

AKNOWLEDGEMENTS

The autors would like to thank I.R.Eghrari for first discussions on flutter detection, J.Zimmerman for helpful comments, A. Scalabrini and Serviço de Informática do Instituto do Coração for useful discussions and providing literature. This work has been partialy supported by FINEP, IBM of Brazil and CAPES.

REFERENCES

Allessie, M.A., Lammers, W.J.E.P., Bonke, I.M, and Hollen, J., 1984, Intraatrial reentry as a mechanism for atrial flutter induced by acetylcholine and rapid pacing in the dog, Circulation 70 : 123.

Boineau, J.P., Wylds, A.C., Autry, L.J., Schuessler, R.B., Miller, C.B., 1984, Mechanisms of Atrial Flutter as Determined From Spontaneous and Experimental Models, in : "Tachycardias: Mechanisms, Diagnosis and Treatment," M.E. Josephson and H.J.J. Wellens, eds., Lea & Febiger, Philadelphia.

Eghrari, I.R., Costa Monteiro, E., Costa Ribeiro, P., von der Weid, J.P., Oliveira, P.M., Paes de Carvalho, A., 1983, On the influence of the volume conductor in Magnetocardiography : an experimental approach, Il Nuovo Cimento, 2D : 346.

THE MAGNETIC FIELD OF ISOLATED RABBIT HEART

R.S. Gonnelli*, G.F. Durin*, A. Sanmartino° and E. Rosettani°

* Dipartimento di Fisica, Politecnico di Torino, Torino, Italy
° Istituto di Medicina e Chirurgia Cardiovascolare, Universita' di Torino, Torino, Italy

INTRODUCTION

Direct measurement of the magnetic field and the electric potentials produced by an isolated mammalian heart in ideal conditions (absence of volume currents) is a unique tool for the assessment of the presence of electrically silent magnetic sources postulated by Wikswo et al (1982) and recently supported by some theoretical models in bidimensional (Roth et al.,1988) and in three-dimensional geometry (Gonnelli and Agnello, 1988). On the other hand, this experiment leads to special technical problems which can be partially overcome by the use of small mammalian hearts.
In this paper we present the first measurements of the magnetic field of isolated rabbit hearts.

MATERIALS AND METHODS

Electric and magnetic data were collected from 5 "in vivo" and then isolated and perfused rabbit hearts. In most of the experiments isolated hearts were completely immersed in horizontal position into a conductive solution in order to simulate, in the same thoracic anatomic position, the ideal condition of homogeneous conducting slab medium. Electric signals were detected at the 6 standard bipolar leads for "in vivo" hearts and by electrodes completely immersed at appropriate positions inside the conductive solution for isolated hearts.
For all measurements a single channel second-order symmetric gradiometer with a pick-up coil diameter of 1.6 cm, a baseline of 5 cm and a sensitivity of about 50 fT/√Hz was used for magnetic signal detection. Analog magnetic and electric signals were filtered between 0.3 and 100 Hz and data acquisition was performed at a frequency of 1 KHz by a 12 bit A/D converter. Magnetic maps were detected at 25, 30 or 36 positions.
After the measurement of "in vivo" electric and magnetic signals, rabbits were killed by a blow on the head and the isolated hearts were rapidly cannulated and perfused through the aorta with an oxygenated modified Tyrode solution using an adapted Langendorff perfusion equipment. The composition of the solution was: NaCl 137 mm., KCl 2.7 mm., $CaCl_2$ 2.7 mm., $NaHCO_3$ 12 mm., NaH_2PO_4 1.8 mm., $MgCl_2$ 0.5 mm., glucose 5.5 mm. (Brusca and Rosettani, 1973) and it was oxygenated with pure oxygen in a closed circuit. The pH was frequently checked and maintained at 7.33 ± 0.07. In order to reduce the magnetic noise, the perfusion set was placed at more than 3 meters from the cryogenic dewar and the solution was maintained at

Advances in Biomagnetism
Edited by S.J. Williamson *et al.*
Plenum Press, New York

(38 ± 1)°C using a jacketed warming coil for a re-heating of the solution just before the connection of the perfusion line to the aorta. In Fig.1 a schematic drawing of the perfusion experimental setup is shown. A special plexiglass support designed to perform movements in two perpendicular directions for a very precise positioning of the heart under the gradiometer was used. Its initial positioning was realized using a laser beam collimator. In experiments with isolated hearts immersed in the conductive solution a large tank was firmly fixed to the x-y moving support and the electric signals were detected by copper electrodes completely immersed inside the solution at appropriate positions in order to realize an orthogonal set of electrocardiographic leads. Fig. 2 shows a vertical and lateral view of the tank with an indication of electrode positioning and lead polarity. Critical problems concerning constant temperature, oxygenation of the solution and absence of bubbles were overcome using special technical solutions.
The source localization was obtained using a new method proposed by our group and discussed in detail elsewhere (Gonnelli and Durin, 1989). Using this approach it is possible to determine, for every instantaneous field distribution, the source model which minimizes a so called Best Localization (BL) index and produces the best source localization from the statistical point of view (BL method).

RESULTS

Quite different results have been obtained in measurements on "in vivo" and on isolated rabbit hearts. In electric and magnetic signals of "in vivo" hearts waves P, QRS and T are always present and have the same polarity and field distribution observed in normal human subjects. At the peak of the R wave, usually, isofield maps of rabbit heart present a higher degree of dipolarity and an electric axis more vertical in comparison with humans.
In all the experiments with isolated rabbit hearts the existence of sinus rhythm during the whole measurement period was clearly indicated by the presence of P waves with normal atrium-ventricular conduction. Moreover, in all the cases, the frequency of the sinus node was reduced by the perfusion from 190-220 to 100-160 beats/min. An increase of the duration of the P-R interval (from 21 to 44 %) was observed in 3 out of the 5 cases. A prolonged QRS interval was also present in 3 cases with variations between 10 and 17 % in comparison with "in vivo" hearts. In Fig. 3 an example of the electric signals recorded inside the conductive bath and of the magnetic field distribution produced by an isolated rabbit heart and detected few millimetres over the conductive solution surface is shown. Until the onset of ventricular activation, electric signals and magnetic isofield maps of isolated rabbit hearts are regular and the current dipoles representative of the atrium and septal activation have the expected localization and direction. Then, during the QR phase, a new contribution appears which adds positive isofield lines in the upper right part of the map and negative ones in the lower left. In the 5 observed cases, this term, rapidly increasing, produces a left deviation of the electric axis and, at the R wave peak, the field polarity is completely reversed in comparison with maps at the same instant when the heart is inside the rabbit chest. The left deviation of the electric axis is well confirmed by electric signals recorded in the conductive bath by leads F1, F2, F3 and F4 as it is shown in fig. 3. The electric axis at the maximum of ventricular activation has always a direction close to -90 degrees. This anomalous behaviour has been consistently and repeatedly observed *in all the experiments with isolated hearts*. Some measurements were repeated with the heart rotated along its axis to present the left ventricle upward but the anomalous behaviour during R wave remained practically unchanged. Some alterations of the ventricular repolarization were observed in electric and magnetic signals of isolated rabbit hearts. In all the cases

a depression of signals during S-T interval was present and a prolonged Q-T duration (corrected for the heart rate) was observed in 2 out of the 5 hearts. In some isolated hearts low amplitude T waves were observed and, in 2 cases, a complete inversion of the T wave was present at the beginning of the perfusion only (see electric traces in fig.3).

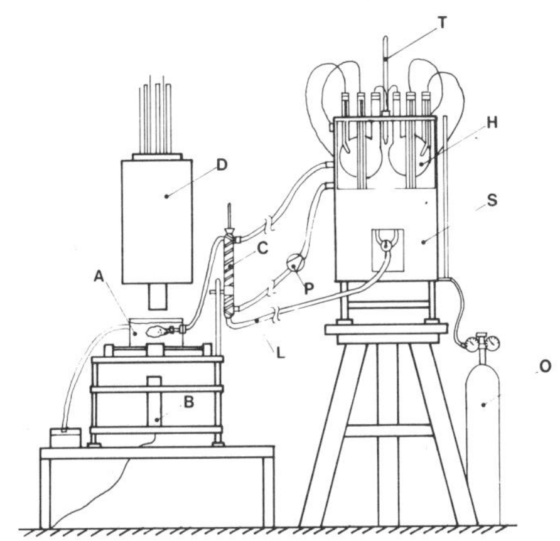

Fig. 1. Schematic representation of our experimental setup for measurement of the magnetic field of isolated hearts.
O. oxygen bottle S. perfus. set
H. Tyrode solut. T. thermostat
L. perfus. line P. plast. pump
C. warming coil D. dewar
A. conduc. solut. B. laser beam

Fig. 2. Lateral and vertical view of the tank for the experiments with isolated hearts in conductive solution. ECG electrodes position and lead polarities are shown.

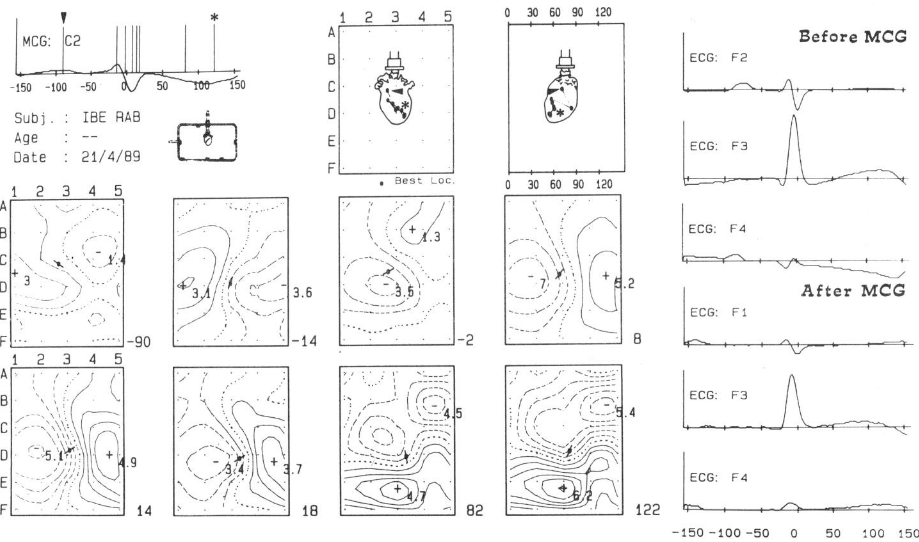

Fig. 3. Electric signals and magnetic field distributions produced by an isolated rabbit heart immersed in a homogeneous conducting bath during P, QRS and T waves. In the upper two maps source localizations using the Best Localization (BL) approach are shown in frontal and sagittal planes.

DISCUSSION

Electric and magnetic measurements on "in vivo" and on isolated perfused rabbit hearts should give different results due to the different contributions of volume currents. Nevertheless, the effect of volume currents is not able to explain the large anomalies observed in our data from isolated hearts. The presence of electrically silent sources could produce differences between electric and magnetic measurements which have not been observed at the present level of sensitivity. On the other hand, we simulated the magnetic field produced during ventricular activation using our three-dimensional model (Gonnelli and Agnello, 1988). Using values found in literature for anisotropy of fiber geometry and primary generators and simulating also the effect of the absence of the conductive medium inside the left ventricle, we obtained a surprising good accordance between experimental and calculated maps. However we believe that the electric and magnetic experimental findings can be more appropriately explained in the framework of conduction disturbances. Phenomena observed at least in some experiments like: Repolarization alterations, prolonged Q-T and P-R intervals and depressed S-T intervals can be consequences of an unbalanced electrolyte concentration in the perfusing solution. As reported in literature for isolated dog hearts (Butcher et al, 1952), these findings are typical of a situation of hypopotassemia which could has occurred in our experiments too. On the other hand the large left deviation of the electric axis during ventricle depolarization in absence of a large QRS prolongation could be produced by interventricular conduction disturbances like a left anterior bundle branch hemiblock. This hypothesis is partially confirmed by source localization during ventricular depolarization which indicates a motion of the equivalent source (obtained by the BL method above mentioned) from inferior heart positions to anterior ones (see Fig.3). General conditions of heart pain connected with the complex experimental setup necessary for magnetic measurements and with particular anatomical features of the rabbit heart (left branch less developed and reached only by left coronary artery ramifications) could be possible causes of this phenomenon, recently observed also with higher potassium concentrations in the solution.
In conclusion further experiments are necessary for the definitive assessment of the presence of electrically silent sources in mammalian hearts but these first measurements of the magnetic field of an isolated heart can probably prove, in "in vitro" pathological situation, the localization power of the biomagnetic technique and of the BL method.

ACKNOWLEDGEMENTS

We are indebted to M. Sicuro and V. Petrizzi for the design and realization of perfusion experimental setup, to Istituto Elettrotecnico "G. Ferraris" for hospitality and to R. Fenici for invaluable discussions and suggestions on data interpretation. This work was completely supported by Assessorato alla Sanita' della Regione Piemonte.

REFERENCES

Brusca, A. and Rosettani, E., 1973, Am. Heart J., 86, 1:79.
Butcher, W.A., Wakim, K.G., Essex, H.E., Pruitt, R.D. and Burchell, H.B., 1952, Am. Heart J., 41, 6:801.
Gonnelli, R.S. and Agnello, M., 1988, in: "Biomagnetism '87", K. Atsumi, M. Kotani, S. Ueno, T. Katila and S.J. Williamson, ed., Tokyo Denki Univ. Press, Tokyo, 318.
Gonnelli, R.S. and Durin, G.F., 1989, "A method for best localization assessment of biomagnetic sources", Submitted for publication.
Roth, B.J., Guo, W. and Wikswo, J.P., Jr., 1988, Math. Biosc., 88:191.
Wikswo, J.P., Jr. and Barach, J.P., 1982, J. Theor. Biol., 95:721.

WHAT DOES AN ELECTROCARDIOLOGIST EXPECT OF A MAGENETOCARDIOGRAM ?

Kenichi Harumi, Sabro Mashima, Hiroshi Tsunakawa,
Tohru Hashimoto, Kazuhiko Shimizu, Genyo Nishiyama
Cardiology Division, Fujigaoka Hospital, Showa University
Yokohama 227, Japan

Electric phenomena in the heart are of low frequency or even quasi-static, so that accompanying magnetic events are at quite low level in intensity. Nevertheless, recent development of magnetocardiography[1,2] enables us to expect a contribution to the solution of several problems in the field of electrocardiography. The latter has a longer history with accumulation of empirical knowledge and recently additional techniques such as the body surface potential mapping and signal averaging method. Limitations of the method are still apparent in certain clinical applications, because of the essential complexity of the phenomenon or of the technical problems. Several examples are selected here, which have been challenged by electrocardiographers with unsatisfactory results. They will hopefully be improved by the combination with magnetocardiography.

SURFACE POTENTIALS AS A MANIFESTATION OF INTRACARDIAC SOURCES.

Voltage measurement has long been a fundamental tool for the diagnosis of ventricular hypertrophy, based on the higher voltage representing increased myocardial mass. Although various criteria are available now, their performance seems to be not satisfactory, that is, their sensitivity and specificity move inversely, in general. For instance, Romhilt and Estes proposed criteria for LVH, which have been shown as associated with sensitivity of 60 % and specificity of 96.8 %.[3] Our own experience is shown in Table 1, where several voltage criteria were compared with LV mass index obtained on the echocardiogram in 170 young athletes. The correlation is by no means perfect. One of the reasons for difficulties in obtaining a high level of both sensitivity and specificity is that many factors contribute to the body surface potentials, including complex geometry of the heart and thorax as well as different conductivities of intrathoacic tissues. On certain conditions, the MCG may eliminate the effect of inhomogeneity of tissues and hopefully, give more direct information on the current sources in the heart.

THE ST DISPLACEMENT AND DC COMPONENT

The ST segment of the electrocardiogram is of utmost clinical significance because the ST displacement is known to indicate myocardial injury in ischemic heart disease. On the other hand, ST and T waves are the portion most susceptible to a number of various other conditions: secondary changes due to alteration in the activation process, sympathetic

Advances in Biomagnetism
Edited by S.J. Williamson *et al.*
Plenum Press, New York

influences and other mechanisms including those causing so-called giant negative T waves. Differentiation of these conditions is most important in clinical practice.

The stimulation of unilateral stellate ganglion has been known to induce marked ST depression, which was attributed to the change in the action potential caused by increased sympathetic tone.[4,5] These observations provide an explanation for the ST-T changes in patients with neurocirculatory asthenia and other conditions. We experienced a typical pattern of exercise-induced ischemic ST depression in young athletes, who showed normal coronary perfusion on the exercise scintigraphy. An example is shown in Fig.1., where a similar pattern is provoked by the standing position.

Table 1. Sensitivity, specificity and predictive value of electrocardiogaphic criteria for left ventricular hypertrophy (LV mass index 140g)

	Sensitivity (%)	Specificity (%)	P.P.V. (%)	N.P.V. (%)
max R $\geq$ 2.0 mV I, II, III or aVF	44	68	44	68
$RV_5 >$ 2.6 mV	79	39	43	77
$SV_1 + RV_5 \geq$ 3.5 mV	92	23	41	83
Greatest R + Greates S $>$ 4.0 mV	100	7	38	100
$RV_5 \geq$ 4.0 mV	24	85	48	66
$SV_1 + RV_5 \geq$ 5.0 mV	34	71	40	65
Greatest R + Greatest S $\geq$ 6.0 mV	53	53	39	66

The ST shift due to myocardial injury is usually associated with the baseline displacement of the ECG, which is caused by the diastolic current of injury. A conventional ECG machine, utilizing registor-coupled amplifiers, does not show the absolute baseline. The contribution of the diastolic current of injury is to be detected by a DC amplifier, which is, not practical because high and unstable DC voltages due to other origins exist in the recording system. The MCG is expected to be useful in the detection of DC current in the diastole and consequently, in the differentiation of the injury current from other causes of ST. depression.

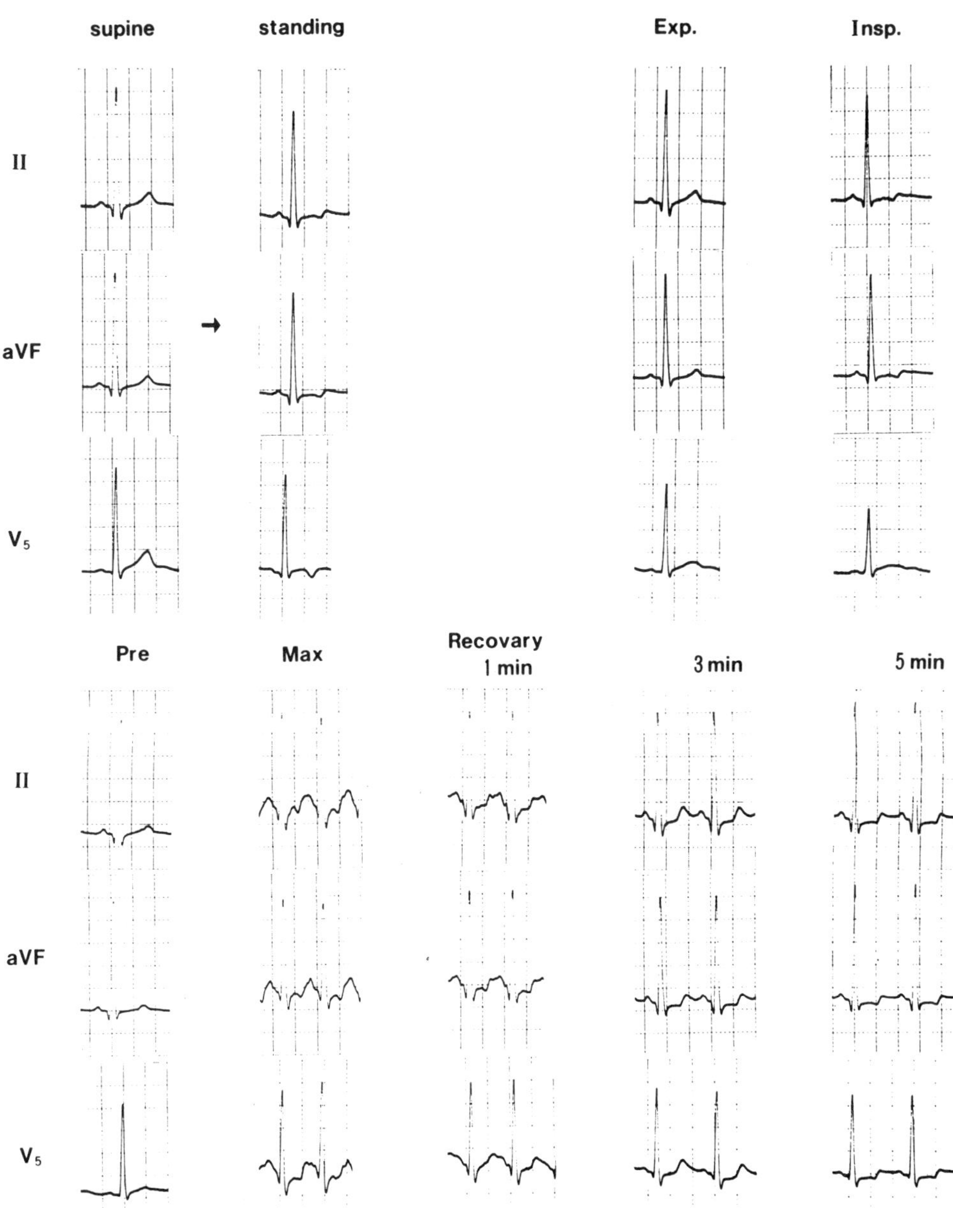

Fig.1. Positive exercise test in a young athletes

THE LOCATION OF THE DIPOLE

One of the purposes of ECG is to locate the equivalent dipole of the cardiac generator at an instant during a cardiac cycle, which leads to the estimation of the activation wave front, the site of Kent bundle, the origin of ventricular tachycardia, the location of myocardial infarction and so on. As long as the observed potential values are regarded as dipolar along with vectorcardiographers, the location of the dipole is not to be determined. Multiple body surface leads system makes it possible to locate a dipole from a body surface potential map containing nondipolar components in a certain degree of approximation. We developed a method to determine the location and moment of an instantaneous dipole from multiple body surface potential measurements, using the proximity function derived from minimizing the difference between measured potential values and those calculated with a single equivalent dipole.[6] The minimal value of the difference was called the residue, which was used as an index of the dipolarity of the surface potential.

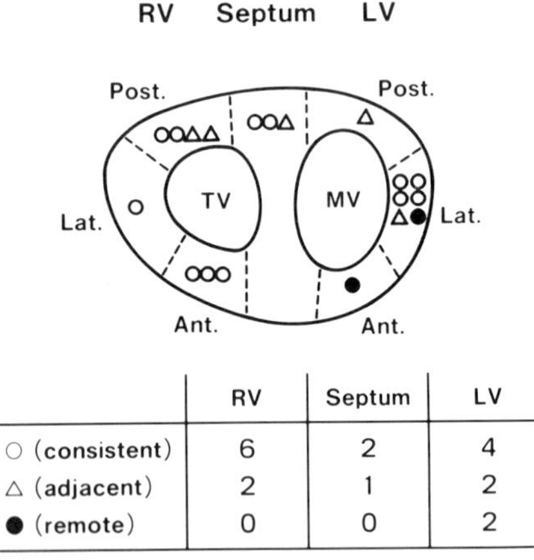

	RV	Septum	LV
○ (consistent)	6	2	4
△ (adjacent)	2	1	2
● (remote)	0	0	2

Fig.2. Determination of the location of Kent bundle from the measurement on the body surface.

The method was applied to locate an accessory A-V pathway in 19 patients with WPW syndrome, in which the site of Kent bundle was surgically confirmed. Results are shown in Fig.2. The section of the heart along the A-V ring was divided into 7 regions. Estimated and proved locations of Kent bundle were in the same region in 12 cases, in adjacent regions in 5 cases and other regions in the remaining 2 cases. The coincidence was relatively but not always satisfactory.

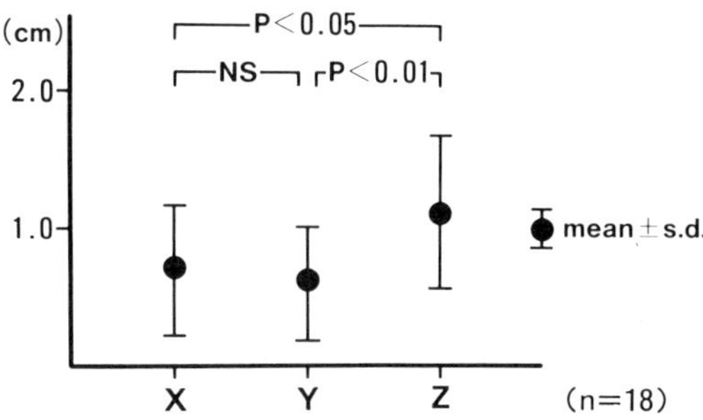

Fig.3. Distance between the site of stimulating electrodes and the calculated dipole location.

As an another application of the method, the location of bipolar stimulating electrodes attached to the dog heart was determined from the surface measurement of the initial QRS voltage of the stimulated beats. Calculated location of the dipole was about 1 cm away from the actual site of the electrodes on the average (Fig.3.). It was, however, sometimes over 1.5 cm. Similar results have been obtained in the estimation of the site of artificial pacemaker in human. The MCG might be of help for improving the accuracy of the inverse problem of this sort, if it would be relatively insensitive to complicated effects of tissue inhomogeneity and its individual variations.

MULTIPLE DIPOLES

It has been known that the excitation wave front of the heart is often separated into several parts. The large residue value obtained with the method above may indicate several dipolar generators in the heart. Multiple dipoles as an equivalent generator have been considered to explain multiple maxima and minima on the equipotential body surface mapping.[7] High residue values were also observed during the QRS interval in normal persons and the timing was similar to that of multiple maxima and minima on the potential mapping. In cases with anterior myocardial infarction, high residue values were obtained in the earlier portions of the QRS interval, which was found to be a diagnostic feature even in the presence of left bundle branch block.[8] High residue values were also observed in the later part of QRS in inferoposterior infarction. The presence of large residue in the earlier part of QRS in inferoposterior infarction was a good indicator of the extention of lesions to the anterior wall.

Our method for locating a dipole can be extended to 2 dipoles or even to 3 dipoles, which would be the limit within the present accuracy of potential measurement. We applied the method for the analysis of the T wave and found that a single dipole gave reasonable approximation in normal persons, while 2 separate dipoles were suitable for the potential field at the time of the negative T wave in anterior myocardial infarction,[9] the location of two dipoles during T wave was estimated (Fig.4.).

These results indicated that the body surface potential mapping and data processing of the measurements are a powerful tool in the inverse problem based on certain assumptions. MCG may be of help also in this field for reducing errors and simplifying the method.

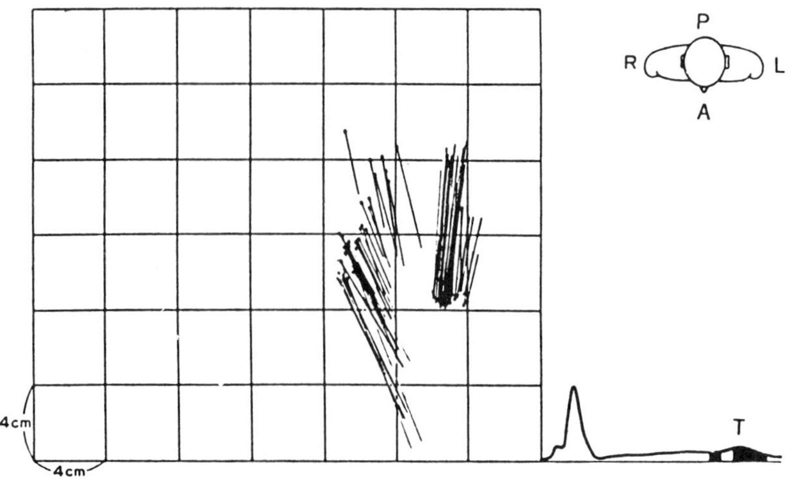

Fig.4. Movement of 2 dipoles during the T wave in cases of anterior myocardial infarction with negative T wave.

REFERENCES

1. Cohen PD, Lepeschkin E, Cuffin BN., et al (1983): Magnetic measurement of S-T and T-Q segment shifts in humans I & II Circ Res 53:264,274,
2. Nakaya Y, Sumi M, Saito K, et al (1984): Analysis of current source of the heart using isomagnetic and vector arrow maps. Jpn Heart J 25:701
3. Romhilt DW, Estes EH., (1968) : A point score system for the ECG diagnosis of left ventricular hypertrophy, Am heart J 75:752
4. Ueda H, Yanai Y, Murao S, et al (1974) : Electrocardiographic and vectorcardiographic changes produced by electrical stimulation of the cardiac nerves, Jpn Heart J 5:359
5. Murayama M, Harumi K, Mashima S, et al (1977) : Prolongation of ventricular action potential due to sympathetic stimulation, Jpn Heart J 18: 269
6. Okamoto Y, Teramachi Y, Musha T, et al (1977) : Moving multiple dipole model for cardiac activity, Jpn Heart J 23:293
7. Taccardi B.(1963) : Distribution of heart potentials on the thoracic surface of normal human subject, Circ Res 12:341
8. Tsunakawa H, Nishiyama G, Kanesaka S, et al, (1987) : Application of dipole analysis for the diagnosis of myocardial infarction in the presence of left bundle branch block, J Am Coll Cardiol 10:1015
9. Harumi K, Kanesaka S, Tsunakawa H, et al (1986) : Dipolarity of the T wave, Jpn Heart J 27:281

CLINICAL VALUE OF MAGNETOCARDIOGRAPHIC MAPPING

Y. Nakaya, H. Mori and M. Nomura

The Second Department of Internal Medicine, School of Medicine the University of Tokushima, Tokushima, Japan

Steady effort on research of the magnetocardiogram (MCG) has been made since the introduction of SQUID gradiometer to measure weak magnetic field of the heart.[1,2] The isomagnetic map was useful to study instantaneous magnetic field of each phase of cardiac cycle like the isopotential map. However, compared with the isopotential map, few studies on MCG mapping have been made, and previous studies on the MCG did not provide us with a clear answer about whether the MCG is a clinically useful tool. In order to obtain the answer, we should study the MCG more quantitatively in clinical setting. But most of the previous studies have been theoretical ones. Our studies on the MCG mapping in the clinical cases showed that in some conditions the MCG mapping was superior to the ECG mapping. These conditions were: (1) the detection of the opposing dipoles,[3,4] (2) detection of the current source close to the anterior chest wall,[5,6] and (3) source localization (inverse solution).[7-10] In this paper, we compared the two mapping methods based on our clinical cases, to fill a gap between the theoretical studies and clinical cardiology.

RECORDING OF THE MCG AND ISOMAGNETIC MAP

The MCGs were recorded with a second derivative SQUID gradiometer (SHE Corp. model BMP), and the magnetic components perpendicular to the frontal plane (normal component) were recorded. Recording sites are shown in Fig. 1. This area was smaller compared with those reported by Saarinen et al.[11] The isomagnetic map was constructed using the same methods as for construction of the isopotential map.[11] To deduce current source, we applied "Biot-Savart law", which shows the relation between the electric and magnetic fields.[12]

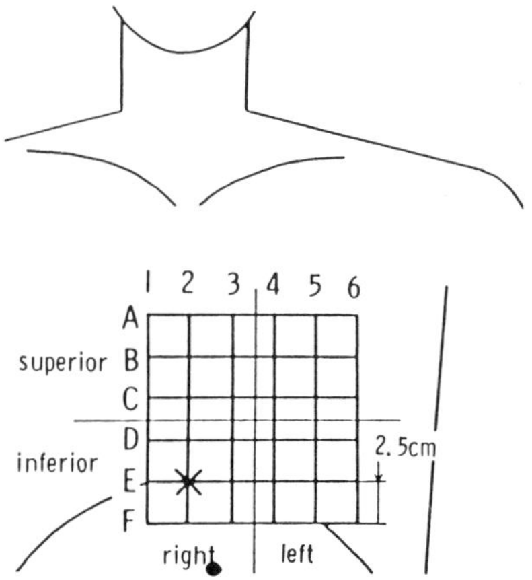

Fig. 1 Recording position of the MCG mapping

OPPOSING DIPOLES

Opposing pair of the dipoles produce the depressed potential but produced large magnetic field.[13] This dipole pair is expected to be detected more easily by the MCG mapping than by the ECG mapping.

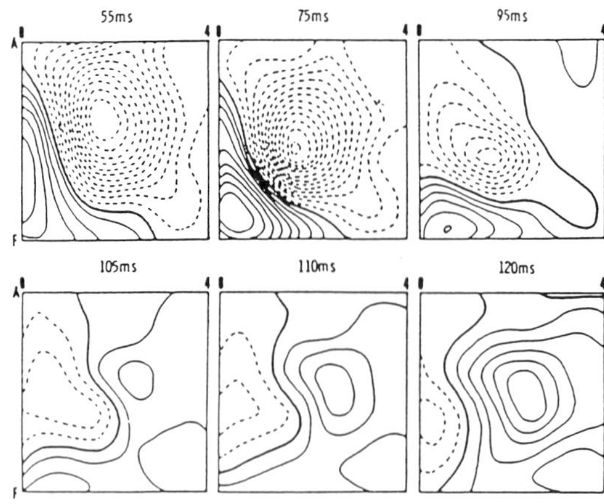

.069pT/L

Fig. 2 Isomagnetic map of the atrial depolarization in a patient with intraatrial conduction disturbance (cited from Ref.5)

1) Atrial depolarization

Fig. 2 shows the isomagnetic maps in a patient with biatrial overloading with intra-atrial conduction disturbance. The isomagnetic map at 55 ms shows a positive area in the right lower portion and a negative area in the left portion, suggesting a dipole directed inferiorly and to the left, which was similar to that of right atrial overloading. From 95 ms a negative area moved to the right, and a positive area appeared in the left superior portion, suggesting that two dipoles due to the right and left atrial depolarizations appeared at the same time. The isomagnetic map at 110 ms showed a negative area on the right and a positive area on the left. At 120 ms, a negative area is located in the right portion and a positive area in the left portion, suggesting a dipole directed superiorly and to the left.

It has been difficult in the isopotential mapping to find two maxima or minima, even epicardial mapping showed two excitation front by each atrium. In the present study, the isomagnetic map clearly showed the depolarizations of the right and left atria at the same time, respectively. Takeuchi et al.[14] found that the 50 % of the patients with left atrial dimension of more than 40mm showed two maxima in the isomagnetic map of the P wave at 40 or 60 msec, suggesting the presence of multiple dipoles. These results suggest that the MCG can add considerable information of electromotive force of the P wave in addition to the ECG.

2) Ventricular repolarization

Fig. 3 shows the ECG, isopotential and isomagnetic maps of a normal subjects at the peak of the T wave. The T wave in the ECG is upright in all lead except for aV_R. In the isopotential map, the negative area was located in the right upper portion and the positive area in the other portion, and the T vector was directed leftward and inferiorly. The isomagnetic shows the negative area in the left upper portion and the positive area in the right lower portion. The deduced current sources were directed leftward and inferiorly. In normal subjects, the direction of the T vector determined by the isomagnetic map and isopotential map were similar to each other.

Fig. 4 shows the ECG, and the isopotential and isomagnetic maps of the T wave in a patient with old inferior myocardial infarction. This patient showed typical ECG during the acute stage, but the Q wave and the coronary T wave became obscure with the progress of the recovery process. The isopotential map shows a single normal dipole directed inferiorly and to the left. From the isomagnetic map we can deduce two dipoles one located on the right and directed inferiorly, and the other located on the left and directed superiorly.

These opposing pair of dipoles detected only in the MCG has been reported in other pathological conditions[3,15,16] and help to detect localized abnormalities.

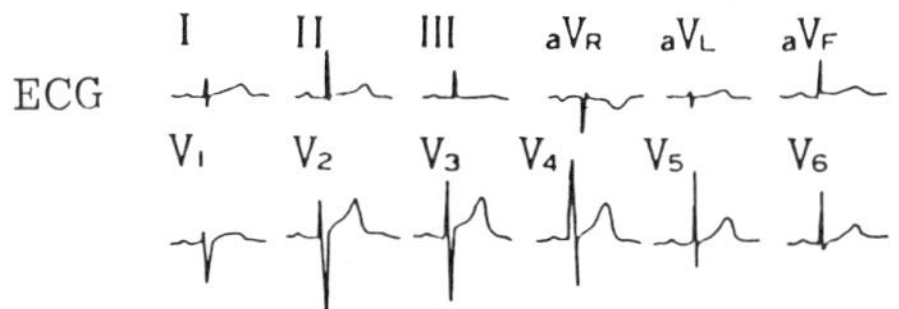

Isopotential map Isomagnetic map

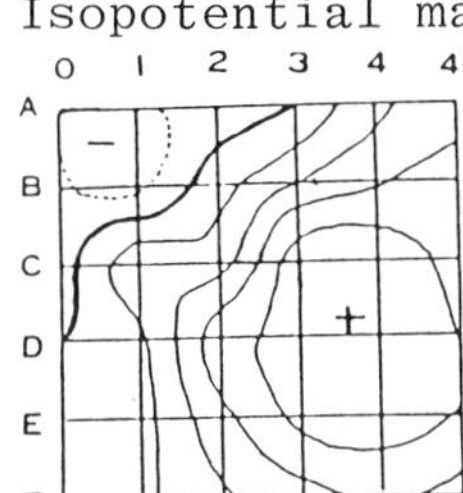

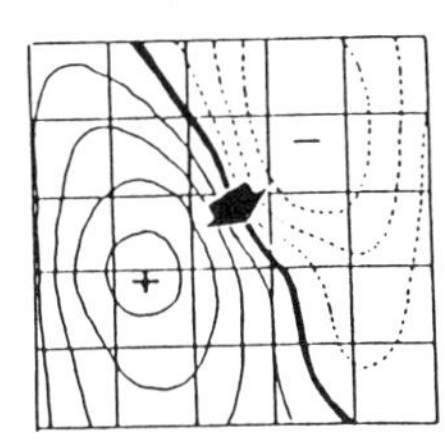

Fig. 3 ECG, isopotential and isomagnetic maps of a normal subject (cited from Ref.4)

DETECTION OF CURRENT SOURCE CLOSE TO THE DETECTOR

Fig. 5 shows the relationship between the amplitude of the signal detected by the gradiometer and the distance from the detector to the current source.[6] As this type of detector rejects both the uniform field and the uniform gradient of the magnetic field, there is a rapid fall-off rate with distance from the pickup coil. Therefore, in this system the current from remote portions is greatly decreased but the magnetic source close to the detector is decreased much less. The sensitivity of the ECG for detecting right ventricular or atrial overloading is low, especially in mild cases. In our previous studies, the isomagnetic map was found to have significantly higher diagnostic sensitivity for these conditions than the ECG.

1) Right atrial overloading

Table 1 shows the sensitivities and sepcificities of the MCG and ECG for the diagnosis of right atrial overloading.[5] Consistent with previous

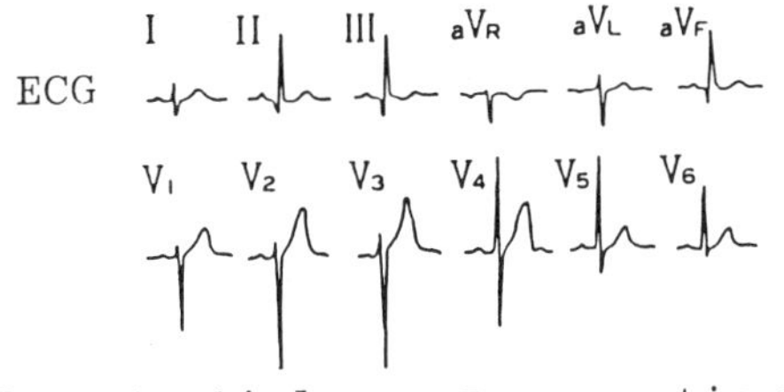

Isopotential map Isomagnetic map

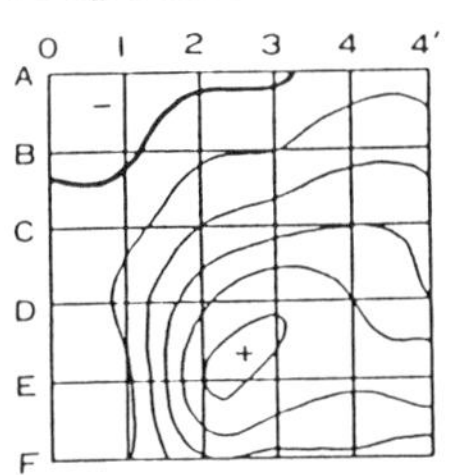

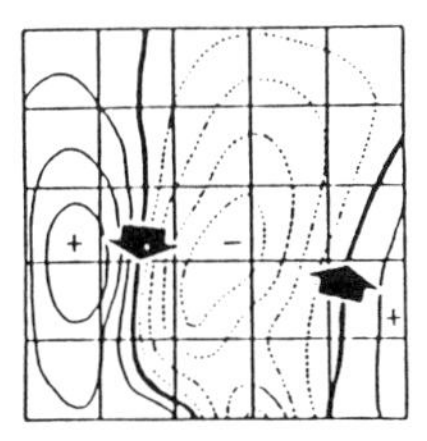

Fig. 4 ECG, isopotential and isomagnetic maps of a patient with inferior infarction (cited from Ref.4)

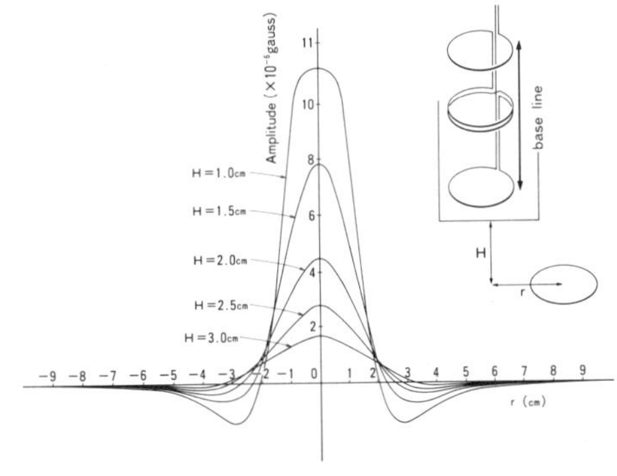

Fig. 5 Relation between the amplitude of the signal detected by the gradiometer and the distance from the detector (cited from Ref.6)

TABLE 1 The incidences of the Positivity of the ECG and MCG Criteria for right atrial overload

Right ventricular pressure(mmHg)	30-60 n=12	>60 n=13	Sensitivity n=25	Specificity n=69
-ECG criteria				
1.P amplitude in lead II>2mm	2	3	20%	96%
2.P intial force in V_1 0.06mm sec	1	4	20%	97%
-MCG criteria				
1. Nesative amplitude in C-2>2.3 10pT	5	9	56%	96%

studies, our study shows that the sensitivity of the ECG criteria for right atrial overloading was low. The diagnostic sensitivity of right atrial overloading was improved using the isomagnetic map, suggesting the possible usefulness of this method. This improved sensitivity was partly due to the recording system, which can easily detect the current sources close to the detector coil. The sensitivity of the MCG for diagnosis of left atrial overloading was not different from that of ECG. The left atrium was located behind the right atrium and it was difficult to detect the current source of the left atrium by the second derivative gradiometer, although the pattern of the isomagnetic map was useful for the diagnosis of left atrial overloading.

2)Right ventricular overloading (RVO),

Fig. 6 shows the location of the maxima and minima in the normal subjects and patients with RVO. Relative to values of the normal subjects, the maxima of the patients with RVO were displaced to the right and superiorly, especially in patients with pulmonary artery pressure of more than 40 mmHg. Table 2 shows that the minimum in the inferior portions was significantly greater in the patients with RVO than in the normal subjects, while the minimum in the superior portion was significantly less in the patients with RVO than in the normal subjects. We also found that in the morphological studies the MCG was more sensitive in diagnosis for RVO than the ECG, as in the isomagnetic map.

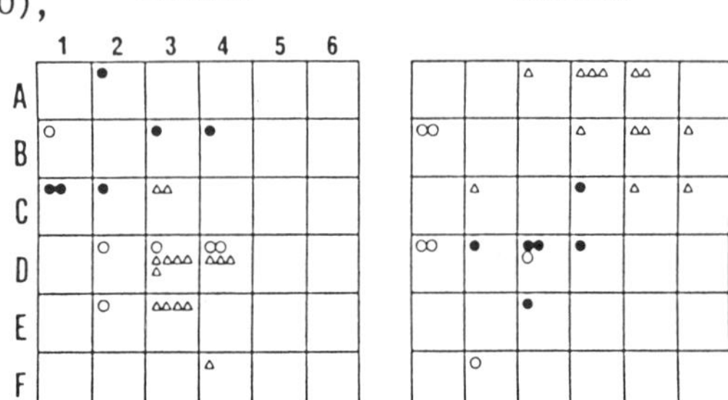

Fig. 6 Locations of the maxima and minima in normal subjects and patients with right ventricular overloading(RVO)

Δ, control group; O, ●, RVO group with the systolic pulmonary arterial pressure of ≤ 40 mmHg and > 40 mmHg

LOCALIZATION OF THE CURRENT SOURCE AND SOLUTION OF INVERSE PROBLEM

Initially, in the normal component of the MCG, the contribution of the volume current of the field of a current dipole was considered to be uninfluenced by the boundaries of semi-infinite

TABLE 2 Maximal and minimal values in each portion for control subjects and patient with right ventricular overioading

Group		Control(pT)	RVO(pT)	
Superior	Maximum	1.67±.72	1.74±1.43	
	Minimum	.97±.60	.59± .56	p<0.05
Inferior	Maximum	2.13±.56	1.80± .72	
	Minimum	.34±.40	.87± .78	p<0.05

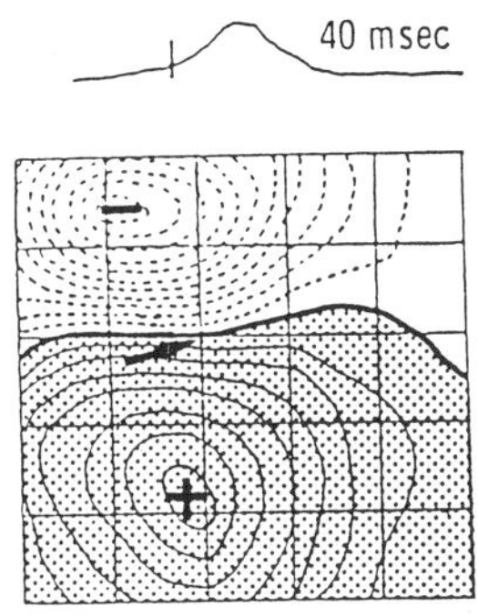

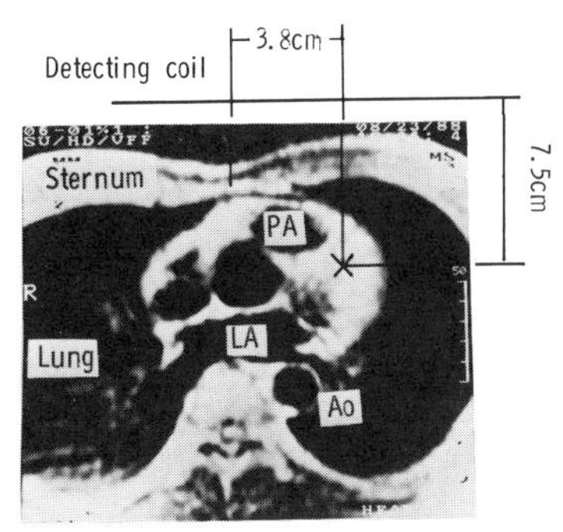

Fig. 7 Isomagnetic map and MRI in a patient with WPW syndrome

homogeneous medium. However, recent studies of the forward calculation of the MCG showed that the effect of the boundaries on the magnitude of the calculated signals is as large for the MCG as for the ECG.[17,18] Although these controversies, inverse solutions by the MCG mapping has been made successfully, e.g., localization of Kent bundle,[7,8] origin of ventricular arrhythmia[9,10] and late potential.[19] Equivalent current dipole algorithm (Williamson and Kaufman)[20] is used as the most elegant and simple solution to the inverse problem.

Fig. 7 shows an isomagnetic map of a patient with WPW syndrome the location of the deduced current dipole (site of the early excitation) by the isomagnetic map on the schematic picture of the MRI. The combination of the MCG mapping and MRI will help to catheter ablation of the accessory pathway in patients suffering resistant reciprocal tachycardia. Single channel SQUID system could detect the site of early excitation, while the introduction of higher order multichannel SQUID system is mandatory to detect the origin of the ventricular arrhythmias.

Hosaka et al. [21] and Nakaya et al.[22] reported that current sources deduced from the vector arrow map methods was in good agreement with the results of the experimental studies and simulation studies. This is most simple method for multiple dipole approximation, however, in the future more elegant method for inverse solution should be done as in those by the electrocardiogram.

CONCLUSION

Although the MCG and ECG signals are both from the same current source, the data deduced by the isopotential and isomagnetic map are not exactly same. Our previous studies and theoretic studies by others (Stroink et al.)[23,24] suggest that combination of the isopotential and isomagnetic maps will enhance our ability to locate the origin of cardiac sources responsible for the maps. Surgical interventions or catheter ablation procedures to eliminate arrhythmogenic tissue in life-threatening arrhythmias is one of the major concerns in the clinical cardiology. These results indicate that the MCG is expected to play an important role in determining the arrhythmogenic tissues in the future.

REFERENCES

1. Zimmerman JE, Thiene P, Harding JH : . J Appl Phys 41:1572,1970
2. Cohen D, Edelsack EA, Zimmerman JE: Appl Phys Letters 16:278,1970
3. Nomura M, Fujino K, Katayama M, Tekeuchi A, Fukuda Y, Sumi M, Murakami M, Nakaya Y , Mori H: J Electrocardiol 21:174,1988
4. Nomura M, Nakaya Y, Ishihara M, Katayama M, Tekeuchi A, Watanabe K, Hiasa Y, Aihara T, Mori H: Eur Heart J 10:8, 1989
5. Takeuchi A, Watanabe K, Nomura M, Ishihara S, Sumi M, Murakami M, Saito K, Nakaya Y , Mori H: J Electrocardiol 21:181,1988
6. Nakaya Y, Takeuchi A, Nii H, Katayama M, Nomura M, Fujino K, Saito K, Mori H: J Electrocardiol 21: 168, 1988
7. Katila T, Montonen J, Makijarvi M, Nenonen J, Raivio M, Siltanen P: Biomagnetism'87 Tokyo Denki University Press, p 274, 1987
8. Uchikawa Y, Erne SN: Biomagnetism'87, Tokyo Denki University Press, p 282, 1987
9. Fenichi RR, Masselli M, Lopez L, Melillo G: Biomagnetism'87, Tokyo Denki University Press, p 282, 1987
10. Schmitz L, Oeff M, Erne SN: Biomagnetism'87, Tokyo Denki University Press, p 286, 1987
11. Saarinen M, Karp PJ, Katila TE , Siltanen P: Cardiovasc Res 8:820, 1974
12. Sumi M, Takeuchi A, Katayama M, Fukuda Y, Nomura M, Fujino K, Murakami M, Nakaya Mori H: Jpn Heart J 27: 621, 1986
13. Cohen D , Hosaka H: J Electrocardiol 9:409, 1976
14 Takeuchi A, Katayama M, Watanabe K, Nomura M, Nakaya Y, Mori H: Medical Progress through Technology, (in press)
15. Fujino K, Sumi M, Saito K, Murakami M, Higuchi T, Nakaya Y , Mori H: J Electrocardiol 17:219, 1984
16. Mori H, Nakaya Y: CV World Report 1:78, 1988
17. Grynszpan F, Geselowits DB: Byophys. J13: 911, 1973
18. Cuffin BN, Cohen D: IEEE Trans Biomed Eng BME-24: 372, 1977
19. Erne SN, Fenici RR, Hahlbohm HD, Jaszczuk W, Lehmann HP, Masseli M: II Nuovo Cimento 2D:340, 1983
20. Williamson SJ, Kaufman L: Biomagnetism, Walter de Gruyter & Co., Berlin, p 353, 1981
21. Hosaka H, Cohen D: J Electrocardiol 9:426, 1976
22. Nakaya Y, Sumi M, Saito K, Fujino K, Murakami M , Mori H: Jpn Heart J 25: 701, 1984
23. Stroink G, Purcell C, Laothe R, Merritt R, Horacek BM, ten Voorde BJ: Biomagnetism'87, Tokyo Denki University Press, p. 74, 1987
24. ten Voorde B J, Stroink G, Montague TJ: Biomagnetism'87, Tokyo Denki University Press, p. 326, 1987

BIOMAGNETIC IMAGING IN THE CARDIAC CATHETERIZATION LABORATORY

Riccardo R. Fenici, Guido Melillo

Clinical Physiology, Cardiovascular Biomagnetism Unit, Catholic University, Rome, Italy

INTRODUCTION

At the beginning of the eighties still no demonstration had been given that magnetocardiography could be performed in a noisy unshielded hospital environment. Furthermore, when the first so called "high resolution MCG measurements" were reported (Farrel et al 1978; Fenici et al 1980), their interpretation and potential diagnostic utility were questionable. Tentative interpretation and validation of the experimental measurements on the basis of mathematical models (Leoni et al 1982; Erne' et al 1985; Lorenzana et al 1985), although clearcut and impressively coherent with what expected from the anatomy and physiology of the heart, were strongly criticized. Few experimental animal investigation had given counterdicting results (Leifer et al 1983). Both cardiac electrophysiologists and cardiologists asked for direct demonstration that magnetocardiography could really provide new information with respect to the less expensive and troubleless electric measurements and that the MCG could be easily recorded in an hospital setting. For this reason at the Clinical Physiology Laboratory of the Catholic University of Rome a perspective project was started in 1980 to set up a Cardiovascular Biomagnetism Unit in the hospital, which should feature both the characteristics of a Biomagnetism and Cardiac Catheterization laboratory, without the use of any electromagnetic shielding.

First high resolution MCG recordings in this hospital laboratory were carried out in 1982 (Fenici et al 1982), however only in 1985 first simultaneous magnetocardiographic and invasive electrophysiologic measurements were successful. This provided the first direct clinical validation for the interpretation of high resolution MCG recordings (Fenici et al 1985a). Furthermore the first demonstration was given of the MCG accuracy for the 3D localization of cardiac accessory pathways (Fenici et al 1985b) and of an artificial current dipole pacing the human heart (Fenici et al 1986). First MCG localization of ectopic atrial and ventricular tachycardias were reported by us in 1987 (Fenici et al 1987,89). Once demonstrated the possibility to use magnetocardiography as a routine diagnostic tool, the second step has been to start

Advances in Biomagnetism
Edited by S.J. Williamson *et al.*
Plenum Press, New York

perspective projects to apply the biomagnetic investigation potentiality on a large number of cardiac patients. In particular our attention has been devoted to the study of patients affected by cardiac arrhythmias, to attempt a non-invasive localization of the origin of life-threatening arrhythmias, evaluate the predictive value of MCG for the assessment of risk of sudden death and to establish the accuracy of arrhythmogenic tissue localization. The latter point is particularly relevant for the future application of the MCG functional imaging as an advanced monitoring tool during antiarrhythmic surgery or catheter ablation procedures.

In this view our development of an integrated system to perform MCG mapping during cardiac catheterization and pacing is of unquestionable relevance. However, although such pionieristic clinical work has been published since 1985, it is usually not quoted as relevant for the progress of SQUID-based measuring techniques, non even in the most recent review article on clinical applications of Biomagnetism (Hoke 1988). A possible explanation of this phenomenon could be a lack of communication capability or clarity in reporting our results. Thus, in order to fill this information gap, in this paper our experience, developed on the basis of in-hospital measurements will be briefly summarized, with special attention to magnetic studies carried out in the catheterization laboratory on patients affected by cardiac arrhythmias.

MATERIAL AND METHODS

A detailed description of the Cardiovascular Biomagnetism Unit at the Catholic University has been given in previous papers and recent review articles (Fenici et al 1985-89). Here we will only discuss some specific solutions developed to combine catheterization procedures with magnetocardiographic mapping. Apparently the two methods would have been incompatible. Both electronics and electrocatheters in fact may produce strong magnetic fields and induce artifacts impeding reliable MCG mapping procedures. On the other hand the wooden beds usually constructed for MCG measurements were absolutely not adequate for the use of the fluoroscopic equipment necessary for catheters positioning. Moreover looking perspectively at the MCG mapping as a dynamic procedure to be repeated during the catheterization, a quick and simple system had to be developed to wheel the patient from fluoroscopic to biomagnetic imaging and viceversa.

At first endocardial recordings and pacing were attempted with different kinds of commercial electrocatheters. All of them, including platinum ones, induced wide fluctuations of the baseline which impeded, or at the best strongly affected, the MCG recordings. Therefore custom non ferromagnetic electrocatheters were manufactured differently designed for intracardiac recordings, pacing and energy delivery (patented) (Fenici et al 1986-89, CNR/R. Fenici patent N.89830349).

During the last three years 150 MCG mappings have been performed in this catheterization laboratory in 102 patients affected by cardiac arrhythmias due to cardiac preexcitation, ischemic heart disease, and different kinds of cardiomyopaties.

The reproducibility of the measurements was tested in 45/102 patients. The effect of several antiarrhythmic drugs (verapamil, flecainide, ajmaline) was evaluated as well.

In 23 patients MCG mapping was performed during cardiac catheterization. In 10/23 MCG mapping was carried out during cardiac pacing, with different extension of the recording grid to test at what extent the accuracy of source localization could be affected by reducing the number of recording points. The minimum amount of averaged beats compatible with satisfactory source localization was also tested.

RESULTS

Wolff-Parkinson White Syndrome

MCG localization of the preexcitation area was satisfactory, provided that a sufficient degree of ventricular preexcitation was spontaneously present or pharmacologically obtained by intravenous infusion of verapamil during mapping.

Aside the results of Kent bundle localization reported elsewhere in this book (Fenici et al, this Conference), 19 patients with septal accessory pathways will be here discussed in more detail. A clear distinction was possible between two completely different magnetic field distribution patterns (fig. 1). A typical dipolar pattern was found in the majority of the patients (17/19) (fig. 1, right) which accounts for preexcitation of the right side of the interventricular septum (Fenici et al 1987- 89). In 9/17 (6/17 posteroseptal and 3/17 anteroseptal) the MCG localization was confirmed by catheter mapping. In 8/17, the MCG septal localization could not be validated, as an invasive study was not clinically necessary. In 2/19 patients a quadrupolar field distribution was found during the delta wave (fig. 1, left), very similar to the one generated by an intramural activation ellipsoidal wavefront, approaching a right breakthrough (Uchikawa et al 1988). As expected, while the Equivalent Current Dipole model failed, a left paraseptal localization of the preexcitation site was diagnosed with the Current Multipole inverse solution (Gonnelli et al 1988). In 1/2 of the latter patients invasive electrophysiology was carried out for clinical problems and MCG localization was validated with catheter mapping.

Life-threatening Ventricular arrhythmias

20 patients with ventricular arrhythmias were studied with two different end-points: 1) the localization of the site of onset of the arrhythmia (4 cases with sustained ventricular tachycardia); 2) the risk-analysis evaluation according to Schmitz (1988) (10/20 arrhythmogenic right ventricular disease, 4/20 congestive cardiomyopathy, 4/20 myocardial infarction, 2/20 hyperthophic cardiomyopathy).

The reproducibility and localization accuracy of ventricular tachycardia has been described in detail elsewhere in this book (Fenici et al, this Conference). In 1/4 cases, catheter mapping and pacemapping validated the MCG findings, giving an uncertainty range less than 2 cm. More recently in the same patient coronary artery by-pass surgery was necessary after a second acute myocardial infarction. Although it was not possible to map the ventricular tachycardia during surgery, as the arrhythmia was fully controlled by the pharmacological treatment, the anatomical finding were consistent with the previous electrophysiological and MCG localization.

In fact an area of pericardial adhesion was found, stretching the myocardium of the postero-inferior wall of the left ventricle, where the onset of the tachycardia had been localized (Fenici et al 1989). As concerns risk analysis, an abnormal field distribution during the S-T segment was found in only two of the first 20 investigated patients. One of these patients died suddenly four years after the MCG mapping had been carried out.

MCG mapping during cardiac catheterization

Since the prototypes of our custom electrocatheters were employed, magnetic mapping during intracardiac recording or pacing procedures was successfully attempted in 23 patients. The method, although somehow time-consuming at the moment, has provided useful information for the study and interpretation of the MCG patterns related to atrial repolarization and His-Purkinje system activation (Fenici et al 1986-89). Moreover it has been useful to calibrate the MCG localization accuracy of endocardial sources (Fenici et al 1989). A more detailed description of the results of this study has been given elsewhere in this book (Fenici et al, this Conference).

DISCUSSION

Wolff-Parkinson-White Syndrome

During the last ten years the development of surgical techniques for Kent bundle's ablation has provided a wider knowledge of the anatomy and electrophysiology of the WPW syndrome (Sealy et al 1978, Cox et al 1985). By combining, in a step-by step sequence, surgical manoeuvres and electrophysiological monitoring, Guiraudon and coworkers (1986) have given a "surgical insight" to cardiac preexcitation anatomy and a clear guide to avoid operative failure in patients with "atypical" or multiple pathways. In fact in the latter patients in order to decide the surgical route and the need for normothermic cardiopulmonary bypass when the epicardial technique is used, it can be important to distinguish preoperatively between true posteroseptal and left paraseptal pathways. In this view MCG "functional localization" is invaluable, as it can provide a clearcut image of the direction of septal depolarization (fig. 1) thus differentiating a right from left insertion of paraseptal accessory pathways. The former in fact generate a typically dipolar field pattern oriented from right to left (fig. 1, right). However at the moment it can be still difficult to interpret all the "septal" localization images found so far, in particular the complex quadrupolar fields (fig. 1, left), which are relatively rare. In one patient invasively studied, this pattern was correlated to a left paraseptal Kent bundle.

A further improvement of the preexcitation imaging could in theory permit in the future a pre-operative differentiation between epicardial, endocardial and true "atypical" intraseptal accessory pathways, which could be useful to screen patients candidates for catheter ablation. However for this purpose further experience ,on a larger number of patients, is needed with accurate surgical validation of the location of the accessory pathways (Guiraudon et al 1986).

Moreover the presentation of the localization figures should be given on 3D anatomical images of the heart. This is in our opinion a critical point. Indeed in our experience the major limitation so far encountered even in validating the MCG localization accuracy, has been the difficulty to transfer both magnetic and invasive data on a realistic representation of the patient's anatomy without errors related to uncontrolled variables. The heart position in respect of the recording grid significantly changes with respiration, with minor rotations of the body along its longitudinal axis and with the position of the arms. Intracardiac catheter position can be unstable and affected by respiration and heart beating. During surgery, even using the "epicardial approach" without cardio-pulmonary by-pass (Guiraudon et al 1986), is difficult to obtain a precise positioning of a radiopaque marker on the preexcitation area. In fact subsequent dissection and cryoprobe applications may significantly alter the original anatomy and prevent from quantitative three-dimensional estimate of the original source of interest within the desired accuracy range (in the order of millimeters).

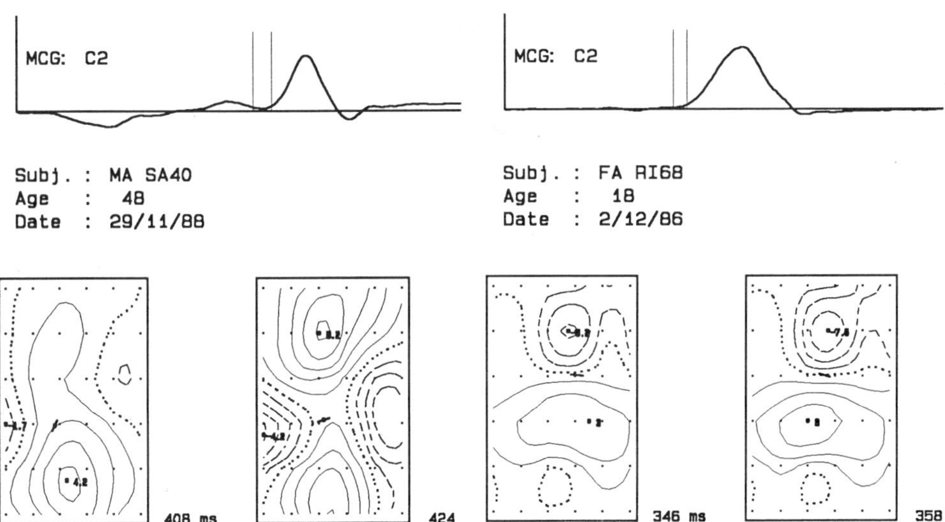

Fig. 1. Examples of dipolar (right) and quadrupolar (left) field patterns generated by paraseptal pathways.

Life threatening arrhythmias

The reproducibility of MCG localization of the site of origin of ventricular tachycardia has been found satisfactory in all the investigated patients (Fenici et al, this Conference). Moreover the localization accuracy, recently validated in one patient, both with catheter endocardial mapping and during surgery, has been in the order of 2 centimeters. The focal mechanism of the arrhythmia in this patient was pathophysiologically correlated to pericardial adhesion of an old infarcted area. In fact after resection of pericardial "adherences" no relapse of the VT was observed during withdrawal of previous antiarrhythmic therapy. By comparison with surgical results, the origin of VT had been properly magnetically localized at the border zone of the postero-inferior aspect of the infarction scar, adherent to the diaphragmatic pericardium.

MCG mapping during cardiac catheterization

This procedure, originally developed to calibrate the localization accuracy of magnetocardiography (Fenici et al 1986), has demonstrated that MCG mapping and catheterization are not incompatible. Moreover, as we have found that properly designed catheters can be accurately localized by the biomagnetic imaging, we have proposed (and recently patented) an integrated biomagnetic system to drive mapping and ablation catheters as close as possible to the arrhythmogenic target (Fenici 1987).

ACKNOWLEDGEMENTS

The authors are indebted to Dr. R. Gonnelli and Dr. G. Durin, who have recently provided our laboratory with their software for current multipole localization. A special thank is due to Prof. G. Romani, Dr. V. Pizzella e G. Torrioli for invaluable help in managing the cryogenic instrumentation. Partially supported by Grants : CNR N.85.00462.04, CNR N. 86.00062.04, CNR N. 88.00503.04, Contract Elettronica S.p.A/ IMI (Law n.46 17/02/82) and Italian Ministery of Education (60 %) 1986-88.

REFERENCES

Cox J.L., Gallagher J.J., Cain M.E. Experience with 118 consecutive patients undergoing operation for the Wolff-Parkinson -White syndrome, 1985. J. Thorac Cardiov Surg 90: 490.

Erne' S.N., Lehmann H.P., Masselli M., Uchikawa Y., 1985 Modelling of the His -Purkinje Heart conduction system. In Biomagnetism: Applications and theory, Pergamon Press, 127.

Farrel D.E., Tripp J.H., Nordgren R., 1978, Non-invasive information on the PR segment of the cardiac cycle: an assessment of the clinical potential of the electric and magnetic methods. In Proc. SPIE 167:173.

Fenici R.R., Romani G.L., Barbanera S., Zeppilli P;, Carelli P;, Modena I;, 1980, High resolution Magnetocardiography: Non-invasive investigation of His-Purkinje system activity in man. G. Ital. Cardiol. 10: 1366.

Fenici R.R., Romani G.L., Leoni R., Masselli M., Modena I.,1982, Magnetocardiographic recording of the His-Purkinje system activity in man. Japan. Heart J. Vol 23: 728.

Fenici R.R., Masselli M., Lopez L., Sabetta F.,1985a, First simultaneous magnetocardiographic and invasive recordings of the PR interval electrophysiological phenomena in Man. Med.& Biol. Eng. & Comp. 23, Suppl. Part 2: 1483.

Fenici R.R., Masselli M., Lopez L., 1985b, First simultaneous MCG and invasive Kent bundle localization in Man. New Trends in Arrhythmias 1: 455.

Fenici R.R., Masselli, M., Lopez L., Sabetta F., 1986, Simultaneous MCG mapping and invasive electrophysiology to evaluate the accuracy of the Equivalent Current Dipole inverse solution for the localization of human cardiac sources. New Trends in Arrhythmias 2: 357.

Fenici R.R., Masselli M., Lopez L., Melillo G., 1987, Catheter ablation of cardiac arrhythmias: MCG localization of electrocatheters and arrhythmogenic foci. New Trends in Arrhythmias Vol. III, 4: 723.

Fenici R.R., Masselli M., Lopez L., Melillo G., 1989, Clinical value of magnetocardiography. In : Electrocardiography and cardiac drug therapy. Hombach V., Hilger H.H. (eds), Kluwer Academic Publishers, Dordrecht/ Boston/ London: 239.

Gonnelli R.S., Sicuro M. 1988, Use of current multipole for the cardiac source localization in normal subjects. In Biomagnetism 87, Atsumi K, Katila T, Kotani M, Williamson SJ, Ueno S (eds). Tokyo Denki University Press: 314.

Guiraudon G.M., Klein G.J., Sharma A.D., Milstein S., McLellan D.G. 1986, Closed-heart technique for Wolff-Parkinson-White syndrome: further experience and potential limitations. Annals of thoracic surgery, vol. 42 / 6: 652.

Hoke M., 1988, SQUID-based measuring techniques - A challenge for the functional diagnostics in medicine. In : The art of measurement. VCH Weinheim 1988.

Lorenzana H.E., Pipes P.B., Zaitlin M.P. James D., 1985, A study of the p-r segment in the human magnetocardiogram. In Biomagnetism: applications and theory. Weinberg H., Stroink G., Katila T. (eds), Pergamon Press: 107.

Schmitz L., 1988, Magnetocardiography: the clinician's point of view. In Biomagnetism 87, Atsumi K., Katila T., Kotani M., Williamson S.J., Ueno S. (eds). Tokyo Denki University Press: 66.

Sealy W.C., Gallagher J.J., Pritchett E, 1978, The surgical anatomy of kent bundles based on electrophysiological mapping and surgical exploration. Journ. of thoracic and cardiovascular surgery, Vol. 76 / 6: 803.

Uchikawa Y., Erne' S.N., 1988 Modelling the Wolff-Parkinson-White syndrome for magnetocardiography. In Biomagnetism '87, Atsumi K., Katila T., Kotani M., Williamson S.J., Ueno S. (eds). Tokyo Denki University Press: 322.

DETECTION OF THE ABNORMAL REPOLARIZATION VECTOR IN DIABETES MELLITUS BY MEANS OF THE ISOMAGNETIC MAP

Masahiro Nomura, Katsusuke Watanabe,
Mariko Katayama, Akemi Takeuchi,
Kazuya Fujino, Yutaka Nakaya,
and Hiroyoshi Mori

The Second Department of Internal Medicine, School of Medicine, The University of Tokushima, Tokushima, Japan 770

INTRODUCTION

The magnetocardiogram (MCG) recorded with the second-derivative SQUID gradiometer may be more useful to detect the current source parallel to the anterior chest wall and multiple current dioples than the electrocardiogram (ECG). We have already reported that the abnormal repolarization vector could be detected more frequently by the MCG than ECG in patient with left ventricular overloading and myocardial infarction.[1,2] In the present study, we investigated the clinical usefulness of the isomagnetic map analysis for the diagnosis of repolarization abnormality in diabetic patients.

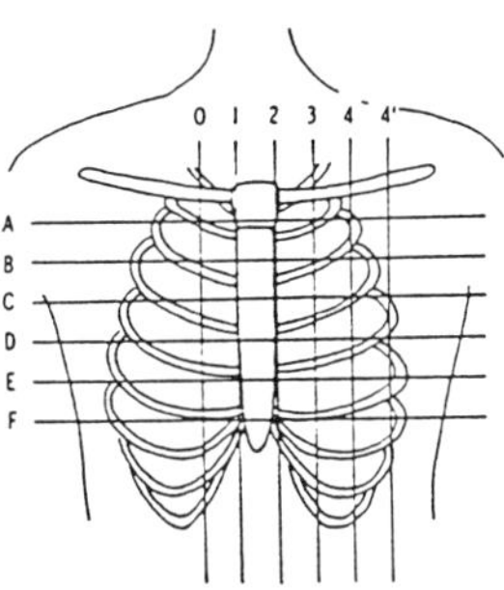

Fig. 1 Recording sites for MCG

SUBJECTS AND METHODS

We studied 50 normal subjects (N group) and 31 diabetic patients (DM group). The MCG was recorded with a second-derivative SQUID gradiometer. The patients laid on a wooden bed in supine position. The detector was placed close to the anterior chest wall and the magnetic field perpendicular to the anterior chest wall was recorded. The MCGs were recorded at the 36 points as shown in Fig. 1. Lead II of the standard ECG was used as a time reference. Body surface isopotential and isomagnetic maps were constructed at the peak of the T wave of lead II of the standard ECG. By simple observation of the isomagnetic map, the location and direction of the current source were deduced by applying "the Biot-Savart Law". To evaluate the repolarization abnormality in the DM group, departure maps of the isopotential and isomagnetic maps (ECG and MCG departure maps) were constructed following the method reported by Flowers at al.[3] Averaged normal isopotential and isomagnetic maps were drawn based on the mean values of the unipolar chest lead ECG and MCG. The ECG and MCG departure maps were drawn at intervals of every one standard deviation (SD) by substructing these normal isopotential and isomagnetic maps from those of patients with DM group, respectively.[2]

RESULTS

1) T wave of the ECG and MCG in the N group

In the ECG of the N group, negative T wave was observed in the middle and upper right portions of the anterior thorax and positive T wave in the

Advances in Biomagnetism
Edited by S.J. Williamson *et al.*
Plenum Press, New York

other portions in the N group. In the MCG, negative T wave was observed in the middle and left upper portions and positive T wave in the middle and right lower portions.

Fig. 2 a shows the isopotential and isomagnetic maps in a normal subject. In the isopotential map, the negative area was located in the right upper portion, the rest of the area being positive, and the T vector was directed leftward and inferiorly. In the isomagnetic map, the negative area was located in the left upper portion and the positive area in the right lower portion. According to "the Biot-Savart Law", the T vector was deduced to be directed leftward and inferiorly.

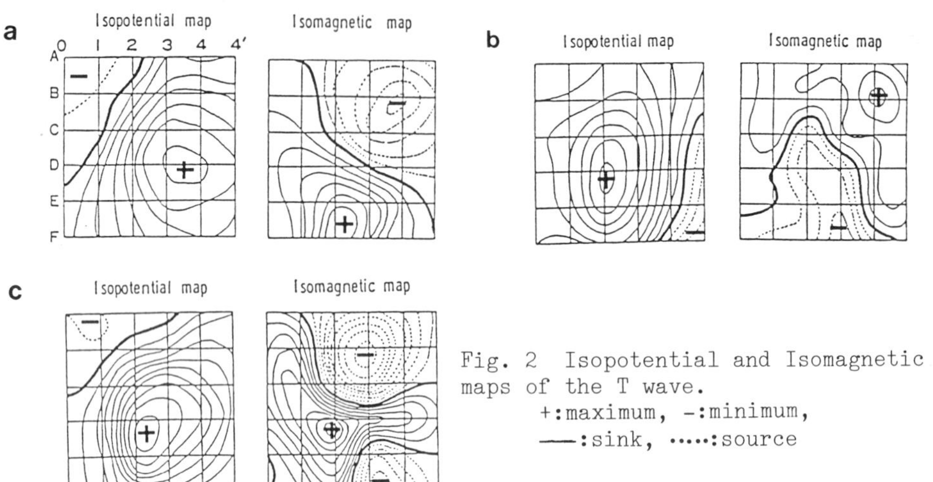

Fig. 2 Isopotential and Isomagnetic maps of the T wave.
+:maximum, -:minimum,
—:sink, ·····:source

2) T wave of the ECG and MCG in the DM group

In the ECG of the DM group, positive T waves were more frequently observed in the middle and right upper portions than in the N group. In the MCG, positive T waves were observed more frequently in the middle and left upper portions, and the negative T waves in the middle and left lower portions.

Fig. 2 b shows the isopotential and isomagnetic maps of a patient with DM which shows an abnormal T wave in the standard ECG. The isopotential map showed positive area in the right upper portion indicating a T vector directed rightward. The isomagnetic map showed a minimum in the lower portion and a maximum in the left upper portion indicating a T vector directed to the right.

Fig. 2 c shows the isopotential and isomagnetic maps of a patient with DM which shows normal T wave in standard lead ECG. In the isopotential map, T vector was directed leftward and inferiorly similarly to that of the normal subject. The isomagnetic map shows two minima at the left upper and lower portions, indicating two current dipoles, one of which directed rightwards.

3) Departure map and vectorcardiogram in the DM group

Fig. 3 a shows the ECG and MCG departure maps of the same patient as shown in Fig. 2 b. In the ECG departure map, the area greater than mean+2SD was observed in the middle and right upper portions and the area smaller than mean-2SD in the left portion, suggesting an increased repolarization vector directing to the right similarly to the isopotential map. In the MCG departure map, the area smaller than mean-2SD was observed in the lower portions of the anterior thorax and area greater than mean+2SD in the left upper portions, suggesting an increased rightward-directing current. In this patient, the T loop of the vectorcardiogram was directed to the right. Fig. 3 b shows the ECG and MCG departure maps of the same patient as shown in Fig. 2 c. The ECG departure map showed no area exceeding 2SD. On the other hand, an area smaller than mean-2SD was present near F-3 and an area greater than mean+2SD near D-4 in the MCG departure map, suggesting the presence of the T vector directed rightward. In this patient, the T loop of the vectorcardiogram was directed to the right. In this patient, the isopotential and ECG departure maps showed no repolarization abnormalities. But, the MCG departure map suggested an increased the rightward repolarization vector.

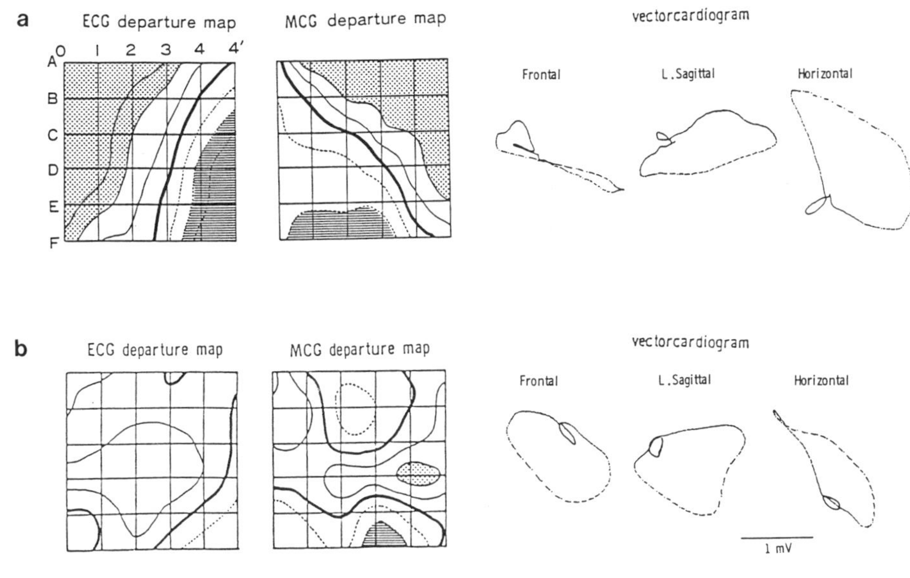

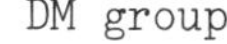

Fig. 3 ECG and MCG departure maps and vectorcardiogram. shaded area: the area where the amplitude of the T wave is smaller than mean-2SD, stipple area: where the amplitude of the T wave is greater than mean+2SD

4) Spatial velocity electrocardiogram in the DM group

Fig. 4 shows simultanous recording of the three scalar ECG (the Frank system) and spatial velocity ECG (SV-ECG) of the same patient as in Fig. 2 c. In this patient, the c/a ratio[4] was 1.63, showed normal T wave in the SV-ECG.

5) Comparison between isopotential and isomagnetic maps

Table 1 shows the incidences of the abnormal repolarization vector in the isopotential and isomagnetic maps. The isopotential and isomagnetic maps agreed in 24 cases (77.4%). An abnormal repolarization vector was recognized only in the isomagnetic map in 6 cases (19.4%), but no patients showed an abnormality only in the isopotential map. Multiple dipoles were recognized in 0 and 4 patients in isomagnetic maps, but were not recognized in isopotential maps.

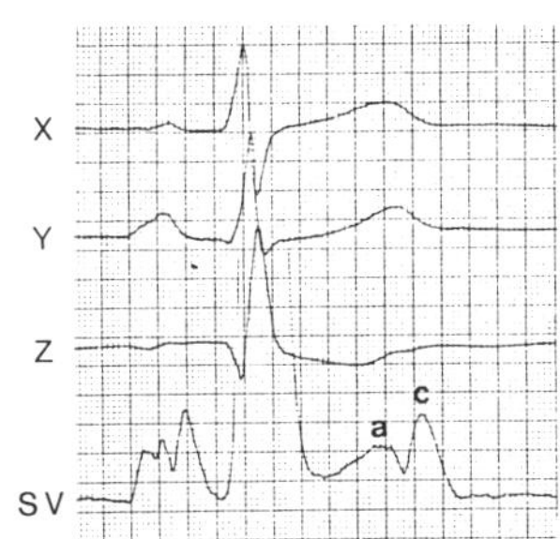

Fig. 4 Scalar ECG (Frank system) and spatial velocity ECG

DISCUSSION

Several investigators reported that the vectorcardiogram, SV-ECG[4] and body surface isopotential map[5] were useful for the early diagnosis of myocardial injury in diabetic patients even if their standard ECG were normal. Selvester, Riff and Zoneraich et al. reported that the QRS loop had a bit more frequently in vectorcardiogram of diabetic patient.[6-8] Atake et al. reported that Fourier analysis of the body surface isopoten-

Table 1. Relationship between abnormality in the isopotential and isomagnetic maps

Isopotential map	Isomagnetic map	Abnormal cases
+	+	1
+	-	0
-	+	6
-	-	24

tial map was of value in evaluating myocardial injury.[5] Furthermore, Shiraiwa et al. reported that the SV-ECG might show various abnormalities in diabetic patients.[4] But, in the case of Fig. 2 c, there was no abnormality in the QRS loop and the T wave of the SV-ECG. On the other hand, an abnormal local tangential current was detected only in the MCG.

Cohen et al. reported a case with angina pectoris in which T wave abnormality was detected by the MCG, but not by the ECG.[9] Therefore, we have further analyzed the T wave abnormality in the MCG of the diabetic patients. In the present study, we compared the incidence of an abnormal repolarization vector between isopotential and isomagnetic maps in normal subjects and diabetic patients. Repolarization abnormality was detected more frequently in the latter. Myocardial damage in diabetic patients might be caused by the macro- and/or micro-angiopathy. These myocardial changes may cause inhomgenity of action potential duration of the various portions of the heart. These inhomogeneity may result in multiple current dipoles during ventricular repolarization phase. As the MCG is more sensitive to localize the current source than the ECG, multiple dipoles, (especially, opposing dipoles) may easily be expressed on the isomagnetic map. Such kind of inhomogenity of the electromotive force may be difficult to detect by isopotential map. Usually one dipole can be deduced from isopotential map as a summation of these localized current.[2] In the present study, localized repolarization abnormalities could be detected only by the isomagnetic map in 19.4%. These results indicated that the MCG might show a repolarization abnormality in diabetic patients even if their standard ECG and isopotential map were normal. Thus, the MCG was considered to be useful for the early diagnosis of myocardial injury in diabetic patients.

CONCLUSION

The isomagnetic map was more useful than the isopotential map in detecting the multiple dipoles in the repolarization phase of the ventricle and also in the early diagnosis of the myocardial injury in diabetic patients.

REFERENCES

1. H.Mori and Y.Nakaya: CV World Report 1:78, 1988
2. M.Nomura et al: J Electrocardiol 21:174, 1988
3. NC.Flower et al: Circulation 54:906, 1976
4. H.Shiraiwa et al: Shikoku Acta Medica 36:49, 1980
5. Y.Atake et al: Jpn J Electrocardiol 4:157, 1984
6. R.Selvester et al: Am Heart J 75:335, 1968
7. ER.Riff et al: Diabetes 23:572, 1974
8. O.Zoneraich et al: J Electrocardiol 10:207, 1977
9. D.Cohen et al: J Electrocardiol 9:398, 1976

MAGNETOCARDIOGRAPHY IN PATIENTS WITH THE LONG QT-SYNDROME

K. Brockmeier, L. Schmitz, L. Trahms*, and S. N. Erné*

Department of Pediatric Cardiology, KAVH, Freie Universität Berlin
*Physikalisch- Technische Bundesanstalt (PTB), Institut Berlin D- 1000 Berlin, FRG

INTRODUCTION

Patients with Romano-Ward Syndrome show abnormal long QT-intervals in ECG and have a high risk of sudden cardiac death. The QT-syndrome is a pure electrophysiological disease in otherwise normal hearts. The underlying electrophysiological mechanism triggering ventricular flutter/fibrillation in these patients is an uneven depolarization and repolarization of the myocardium and the specialized conducting tissue (Schwartz et al., 1975). Like in other autosomal dominant inherited diseases expression of symptoms is variable among family members. Up to now a specific method for the discrimination of these high-risk patients does not exist.

The objectives of our investigations are as follows: 1. Is Magnetocardiography an appropriate diagnostical tool to identify the patient at risk for severe ventricular tachycardias, 2. does this method allow monitoring of the protective effect of drug treatment?

METHODS

The measurements were performed in the Berlin Magnetically Shielded Room using a superconducting SQUID magnetometer with an equivalent input white noise below 10 $fT/\sqrt{Hz}$ under measuring conditions (Erné et al., 1981). The magnetic field component normal to a plane tangential to the chest has been recorded in 36 positions defined according to the Finish standard grid. The recording bandpass for the signals was between 0.016 Hz and 250 Hz with a RC high pass filter (-3dB) of the first order and a Bessel low pass filter of the 8th order. The signals have been digitized with 12 bit resolution and 1000 Hz sampling rate. We examined the temporal fluctuation of magnetic fields distribution during the ST-segment by means of the "Relative Smoothness" (RS) parameter. This parameter is given by:

$$RS = \sum_{j=1}^{j=3} C_j$$

C_i denotes the correlation coefficients between two subsequent magnetic field maps of a series of maps taken at intervals of 25 ms, starting at the end of the QRS complex.

Standard 12 lead ECG, bicycle stress testing , 24-hour Holter monitoring and invasive electrophysiological study (1 patient) were performed as approved diagnostical procedures.

PATIENTS

Nine patients out of four families with Romano-Ward syndrome were studied. One additional patient had a symptomatic QT-prolongation after traumatic head injury. Symptoms, reaching from severe arrhythmias (6/10) to sudden cardiac arrest (1/10), occurred in six individuals of the study group.

RESULTS

The RS-score values ranged from 2.6 to 0.4 (Tab.1). In patients with Romano-Ward syndrom thev were out of the normal range (Schmitz, 1988). Even in the small number of patients studied up to now there is a correlation between severity of symptoms and RS-score values. Notably, the mean RS-score values of medically treated patients are higher than those of the non-symptomatic non-treated individuals (Fig 1). In one patient a correlation could be demonstrated between RS-score values and the inducibility of ventricular tachycardias during bicycle stress testing (Fig 2). Clearly lower score values were correlated with the occurrence of life threatening arrhythmias and inefficient treatment due to low drug levels.

Tab. 1. QT_c = QT interval corrected for heart frequency, upper limit of normal is 0.48. Maximal QT_c during stress testing is given. (+) indicating patients with normal QTc in standard ECG. (*) indicating that the mother died from Long QT-Syndrome. (#) indicating a patient without Romano-Ward Syndrome.

	Patient	Age	Events	Drugs	QT_c	RS
1	MAKE	38	syncopes	ß-blocker	0.51	1.9
2	CLKE	19	none	none	0.52+	1.0
3	GIMO	17	none *	none	0.51+	2.1
4	URMO	16	none *	none	0.55+	1.7
5	GEKL	44	syncopes	none	0.52	0.4
6	PEKL	14	syncopes	none	0.58	1.7
7	DESC	8	syncopes	ß-blocker	0.55	0.7
8	DEHA	16	syncopes	none	0.57+	0.5
		17	none	ß-blocker	0.52+	2.3
9	JAHA	12	none	none	0.57	1.6
10	PEOH#	13	arrhythmias	none	0.5	2.6

Standard ECG showing normal QT-intervals was non-diagnostical in four patients. ECG recordings during stress testing disclosed abnormal QT intervals in all tested patients (7/10). Even repeated 24-hour ECG recordings in 4 out of 10 patients and an invasive electrophysiological study in one patient did not contribute to the final diagnosis.

One patient (PEOH) measured after traumatic head injury had a QT-prolongation with a normal RS-score. 24-hour ECG recordings showed supraventricular premature beats and AV-block.

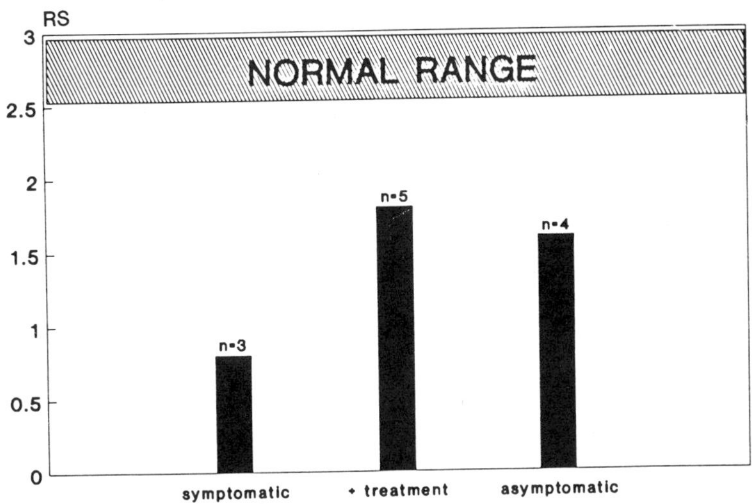

Fig.1 RS-score values in symptomatic QT patients before and after treatment are apparently different. Asymptomatic QT patients with intermediate RS-score values yet out of normal.

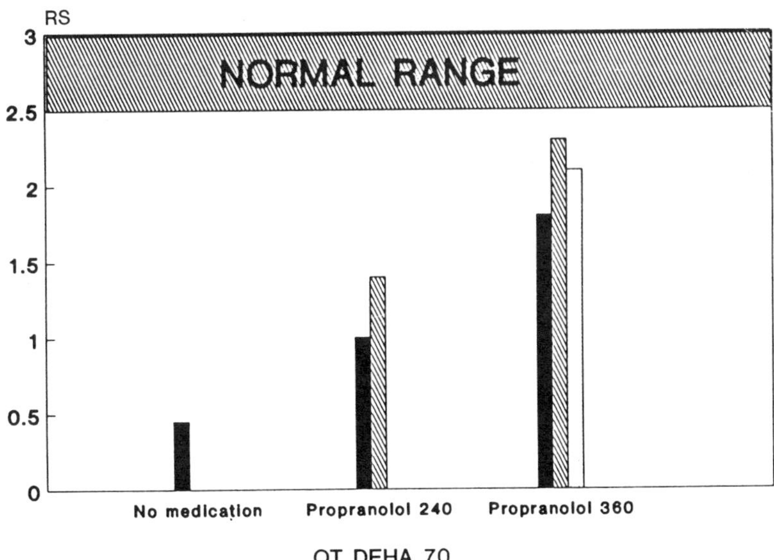

Fig.2 Influence of drug treatment on the RS-score for a patient suffering life threatening arrhythmias and sudden cardiac arrest due to QT-syndrome. Different bars indicate repeated measurements under identical medication.

DISCUSSION

In patients with functional disturbance of depolarization and repolarization of the myocardium we were able to demonstrate abnormal fluctuations of magnetic fields during the course of the ST-segment of the limb ECG used as time reference. These abnormal patterns exist even in patients without detectable abnormalities in the surface ECG. Concerning Romano-Ward patients our experience shows that among all applied methods magnetocardiography seems to be the most sensitive one in the detection of the patients at risk for life threatening arrhythmias. QT-prolongation in individuals not suffering from Romano-Ward Syndrome seem to have a normal RS-score in absence of ventricular arrhythmias. Similar results were obtained in comparable investigations in patients with ventricular tachycardias after myocardial infarctions (Erné et al., 1983) and in patients with cardiomyopathies and arrhythmias (Schmitz, this volume).

Due to the small number of patients this study cannot provide any statistical evaluation of the data.

Our preliminary results in one patient, repeatedly investigated during drug treatment with different doses of Propranolol, show a good correlation between the RS-score , drug dosage and efficacy of treatment. This might be a hint that MCG can be used as a monitoring tool during antiarrhythmic therapy.

REFERENCES

Erné, S.N., Fenici, R.R., Hahlbohm, H.-D., Jaszczuk, W., Lehmann, H.P., and Maselli, M. , 1983, High-Resolution Isofield Mapping in Magnetocardiography. Il Nuovo Cimento, 2D, 291-300

Erné, S.N., Hahlbohm, H.-D., Scheer, H.J., and Trontelj, Z., 1981, The Berlin Magnetic Shielded Room (BMSR): Section B - Performances. In: "Biomagnetism" S.N. Erné, H.-D. Hahlbohm and H. Lübbig eds., W. De Gruyter, Berlin, pp. 79-87

Schmitz, L., 1988, Magnetocardiography: The clinician's point of view. In: "Biomagnetism'87", Atsumi et al. eds. Tokyo Denki University Press, Tokyo, pp. 66-73

Schwartz, P.J., Periti, M., Malliani, A., 1975, The long QT syndrome. Am Heart J. 89, 378-390

MEASUREMENT OF CARDIAC MAGNETIC FIELD VECTOR

Y.Sakauchi, H.Kado*, N.Awano, N.Kasai*, M.Higuchi**, K.Chinone***, M.Nakanishi*, K.Ohwada, S.Kariyone

Fukushima Medical College, 1 Hikarigaoka, Fukushima 960-12 Japan
*Electrotechnical Laboratory, 1-1-4 Umezono, Tsukuba 305 Japan
**Tsukuba University, 1 Ten-nohdai, Tsukuba 305 Japan
***Seiko I Co. Tokyo, Japan

INTRODUCTION

The component of Magnetocardiogram(MCG) perpendicular to the anterior chest has been recorded in almost all the reports except a few of them. The conventional method is to detect the location of equivalent current dipole by using the iso-magnetic field mapping over the anterior chest. This method is unavailable when the order and/or number of poles increase. It is significant to carry out vector measurement of MCG to estimate the current elements associated with intracardiac electrical events more precisely. We carried out vector measurement of MCG by using vector SQUID system and tried to estimate the cardiac activities by the distribution of magnetic field vector over the anterior chest.

METHODS

We performed vector measurments of MCG at 36 points over the anterior chest in 5 healthy human subjects by using the SQUID system in a magnetically shielded room and the simultaneous ECG (II lead) was recorded as time reference. The SQUID system, developed by the Electrotechnical Laboratory, enable us to measure the three orthogonal components of MCG simultaneously. Fig.1 shows the schematic figure of the experimental set up. The configuration of the vector magnetometer system is shown in Fig. 2. The vector magnetometer consists of three integrated DC-SQUID magnetometers and these magnetometers are attached to adjacent surfaces of the corner cut from a cube in order to be located perpendiculer to each other to detect 3 orthogonal components of the magnetic field simultaneously. The diameter of each pickup coil is 8.0 x 8.0mm^2 and the resolution of the magnetic field is 11fT/Hz$^{1/2}$ in the white noise region(1).

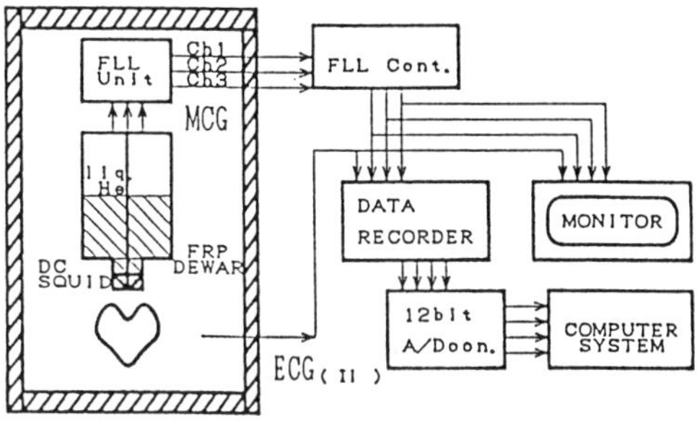

Fig.1 experimental set up

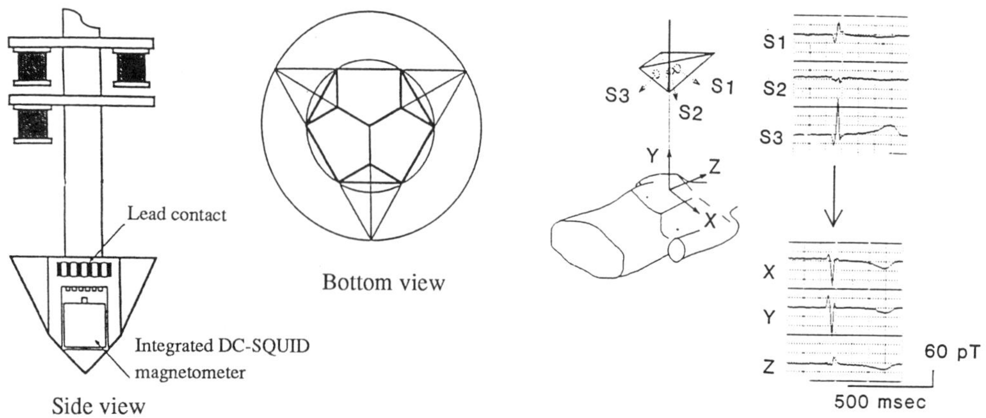

Fig. 2. Vector magnetometer system.

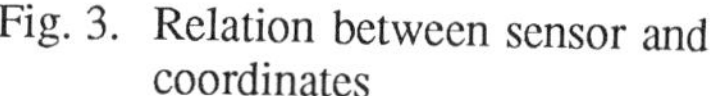

Fig. 3. Relation between sensor and coordinates

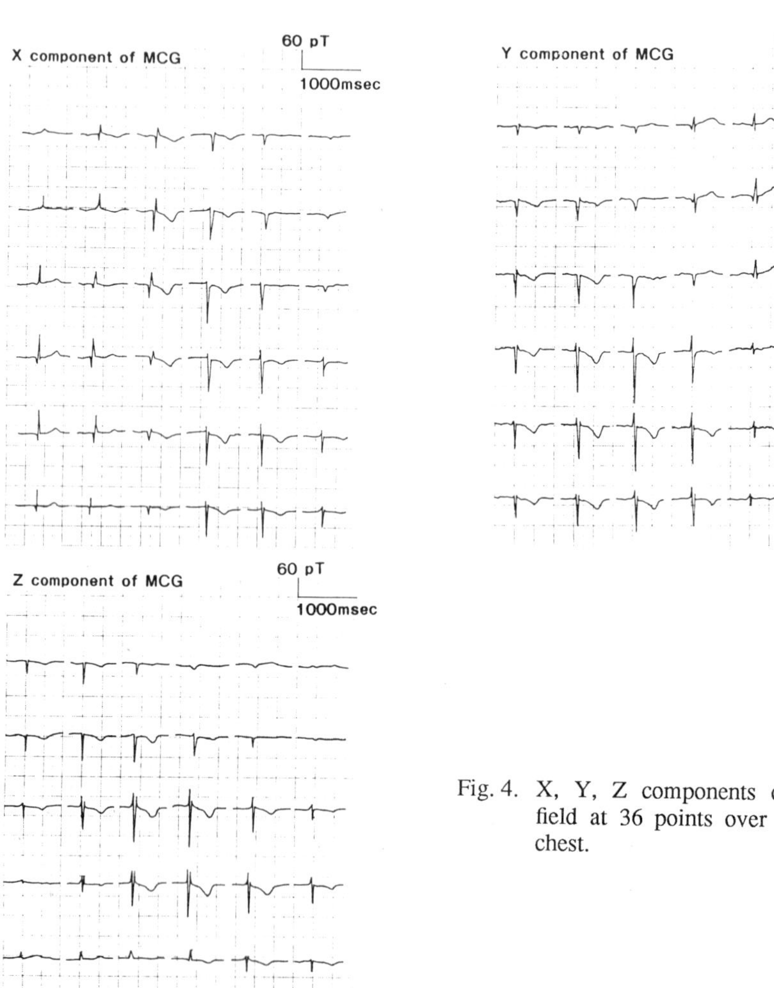

Fig. 4. X, Y, Z components of magnetic field at 36 points over the anterior chest.

The conventional X, Y, Z components of magnetic field were obtained from the S1, S2, S3 components detected by the vector magnetometer system by converting the coordinates (Fig. 3). Then, the spacial distribution maps of magnetic field vectors at each time instant during the ventricular depolarization were prepared.

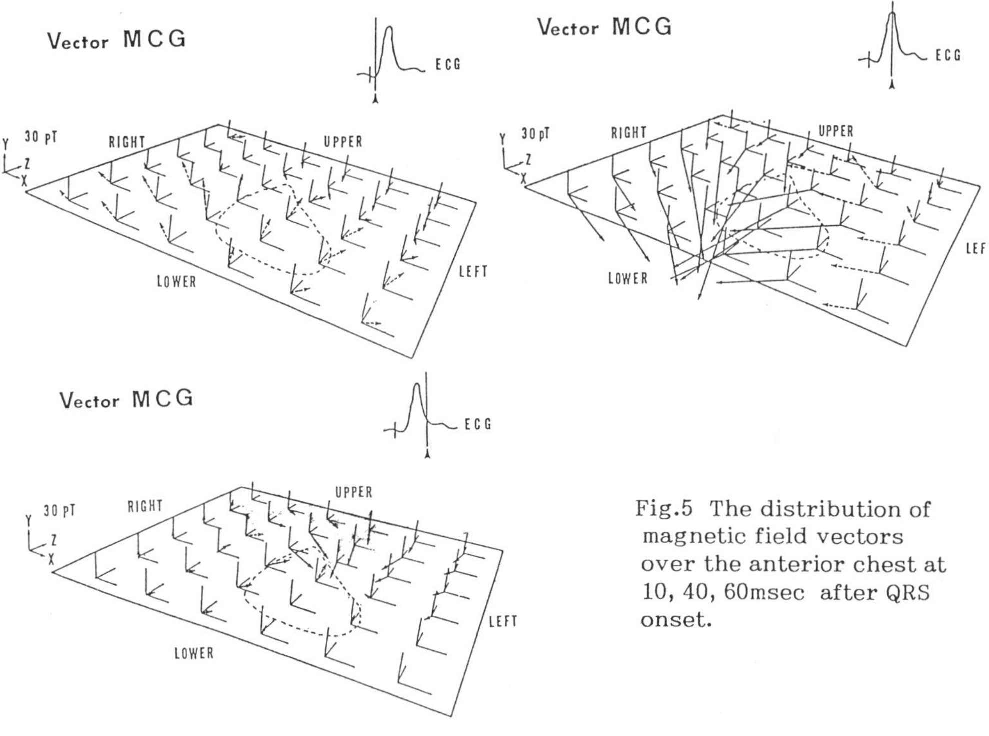

Fig.5 The distribution of magnetic field vectors over the anterior chest at 10, 40, 60msec after QRS onset.

RESULTS

Fig.4 shows the distribution of three components of magnetic fields over the anterior chest and Fig.5 shows the spatial distribution mapsof magnetic field vectors at 10, 40, 60msec. after the QRS onset, respectively. The sedistributions of spatial magnetic field vectors having different directions indicatedthe plural currents rather than single current throughout the ventricular depolarization.

DISCUSSION

To estimate the cardiac electric phenomena more precisely, we measured cardiac magnetic field vectors using a vector magnetometer system which enable us to record the three orthogonal components of MCG simultaneously. The iso-magnetic mapping method is conventionally used to detect the location of current dipole and certainly, the current from iso-magnetic map has been reported to be almost dipolar as from iso-potential map (2). We think these findings depends on that this method is limited to estimate the parallel electric component with body surface.

A few prior investigaters reported vector magnetocardiogram, for example Shirae et al. (3) developed a original SQUID system built in gradiometer type and estimated the current dipole movement using 2 or 3 dimensional displays. However, electric phenomena of the heart has spatial distribution and certainly is not dipolar in itself.

It was in this study, quite understandable to assume the plural currents during every phase of ventricular depolarization more than single one as cardiac current source for explaining the distribution of magnetic field vectors having different directions over the anterior chest.

Taking account of Durrer's excitation map[4], the magnetic field vectors over the anterior chest may yield information about "local currents" associated with cardiac electric activity during ventricular depolarization.

REFERENCE

1. Nakanishi,M., Kasai,N., et al: DC-SQUID MAGNETOMETER SYSTEM FOR DETECTING VECTOR VALUE OF MAGNETIC FIELD. IEEE TRANSACTION ON MAGNETICS, 25-2: 1162-1165, 1989
2. Taccardi,B.: Distribution of heart potential on the thoracic surface of normal human subjects. Circulation Res. 12: 341-352, 1963
3. Shirae,K., Furukawa,H., Katayama,M.: MEASUREMENT AND CHARACTERISTICS OF VECTOR MAGNETOCARDIOGRAPHY. 6th international conference on Biognetism, Tokyo: 294-297, 1987
4. Durrer,D., Van Dam,R.T., Freud,G.E., et al: Total excitation of the isolated human heart. Circulation, 26: 1050-1055, 1987

CLASSIFICATION OF INFARCTS

USING ELECTRIC AND MAGNETIC INVERSE SOLUTIONS

C. J. Purcell[1], G. Stroink[1,2] and T. J. Montague[2]

Department of Physics[1], and Physiology and Biophysics[2]
Dalhousie University
Halifax, N.S., Canada, B3H 3J5

INTRODUCTION

Single moving dipole inverse solutions provide a means of compressing the information content of body surface potential and magnetic maps into a few parameters which have a simple physical interpretation. The repolarization phase of the normal cardiac cycle is well fit by a single moving dipole, and is also sensitive to the changes caused by abnormalities such as infarction, as noted by Mirvis and Holbrook (1981). We have applied electric and magnetic single moving dipole inverse solutions to the T-wave of normal subjects and subjects with old myocardial infarction. Our purpose was to determine if inverse solutions provide a useful means of detecting the presence and perhaps location of old myocardial infarct scars and to compare the relative diagnostic sensitivities of electric and magnetic recording techniques.

METHODS

Simultaneous 120 channel body surface potential recordings and sequential 56 channel magnetocardiographic recordings were made of normal subjects and myocardial infarct patients using instrumentation and methods described by Stroink et al. (1987). Electric and magnetic inverse solution fits were made to these recordings, specifically to the T-waves of 10 normal male subjects of mean age 55 (s.d.± 6); and 15 myocardial infarct (MI) patients (13 male, 2 female) of mean age 57 (± 12), whose maps were recorded on average 77 (± 28) days following their first documented infarction.

Subjects are considered normal under our protocol if they have no personal history of high blood pressure, hypertension, or heart disease, and no evidence of heart disease apparent during a physical, 12 lead ECG and echocardiogram examination performed just prior to their mapping session. The diagnosis of myocardial infarction was based on clinical history of chest pain, enzyme elevation, and 12 lead ECG evidence. The MI study group included several non-Q infarct patients for whom there was no clinical evidence of diagnostically significant Q-waves in the 12 lead ECG. In addition to the echocardiogram, MI patients had a nuclear ventriculogram performed to assess wall motion abnormality and confirm the 12 lead ECG diagnosis.

Advances in Biomagnetism
Edited by S.J. Williamson *et al.*
Plenum Press, New York

The T-wave duration is taken to be 5/8 of the ST-T interval ending at T-wave offset as used by Montague et al. (1981), with the timing of intervals determined by the computer program used to align and average the cardiac complexes. In all subjects 32 maps were obtained from this interval at equal time increments. This time normalizes the T-waves of all subjects to the same duration. The inverse solutions were applied to each of these maps. The mean and mean ± s.d. of the subjects' dipole moment and location parameters as found by the inverse solutions and the error of fit were plotted against % of T-wave interval.

Our electric and magnetic inverse solutions utilize a volume conduction model shaped like a human torso, but with homogeneous conductivity. This form of inverse solution became technically feasible only after the development of a non-iterative solution of the integral equations for the potential described by Purcell and Stroink (1987, 1989). The potentials found using this method are then numerically integrated to give the magnetic fields following Horacek (1973). The non-linear least squares fitting algorithm used is a version of the Marquardt algorithm which computes finite differences of the residuals with respect to the dipole parameters to guide the search for the best fitting dipole.

RESULTS

Figure 1 shows plots of the means (and mean ± 2 s.d.) of the 6 dipole parameters (3 for location, and 3 for dipole moment) and error of fit of our 10 normal subjects as functions of % of T-wave as obtained from electric data. The error of fit (fractional residual) in Fig 1 has a mean value of 19 (±1) % for the first 80 % of the T-wave and rises afterwards, probably because the signal then decreases into the noise. It was found using this mean value for the error of fit that a single moving dipole estimated with the electric inverse solution on average could account for 98 % of the information in body surface potential maps of the first 80 % of the T-wave of the 10 normal subjects by using the definition of 'information' of Horan et al. (1972). Thus the electric single moving dipole inverse solution is an effective means of data compression for this portion of the normal T-wave. When the dipole parameter plots made by the electric inverse solution of the 15 members of the MI patient group were compared to the mean plots of the normals it was found that in all 15 cases they could be classified as abnormal, i.e., at least one of their 6 dipole parameters lay outside the mean of the normals by more than 2 s.d. at some time during the T-wave. An example of this is given in Fig 1 where the dipole parameters for a subject with inferior infarction are shown. This indicates good sensitivity for the detection of old infarct scars, but nothing can be claimed for the specificity because of the small number of subjects analyzed. It was possible to visually classify the 15 MI subjects into subgroups with similar parameter plots, which were retrospectively identified (from their clinical records) as containing subjects with inferior infarctions, with 8 of the 8 known cases so classified; anterior infarctions, with 4 of 4 known cases classified; non-Q infarctions, with 2 of 3 known cases classified; and with 1 non-Q subject being classified as different from the normals, inferiors, anteriors, or other 2 non-Q infarctions.

Figure 2 shows plots of the 6 dipole parameters of our 10 normal subjects as in Figure 1 except they are obtained from magnetic} data. It was found using Fig 2 that the mean error of fit of the magnetic inverse solutions for the first 80 % of T-wave was 37 (± 6) %. From this it can be estimated that a single moving dipole obtained from the magnetic inverse solution on average will account for 93 % of the information in magnetocardiographic maps of the first 80 % of the T-wave of 10 normal subjects. Thus there was only a small difference (5 ± 3) % in the information content of the electric and magnetic data of this portion of normal repolarization and this may be due to differences in the measurement methodology such as numbers of leads and signal to noise ratio. When the dipole parameter plots made by the magnetic inverse solution of the MI patient group were compared to the mean plots of the normals it was found that 10 of 15 MI subjects could be classified as abnormal as defined above. It was possible to retrospectively classify 5 of these 10 abnormal MI subjects into only one subgroup with similar parameter curves, and the other 5 were all visually distinct. The subgroup which was homogeneous enough to classify was identified as a group of inferior MI's.

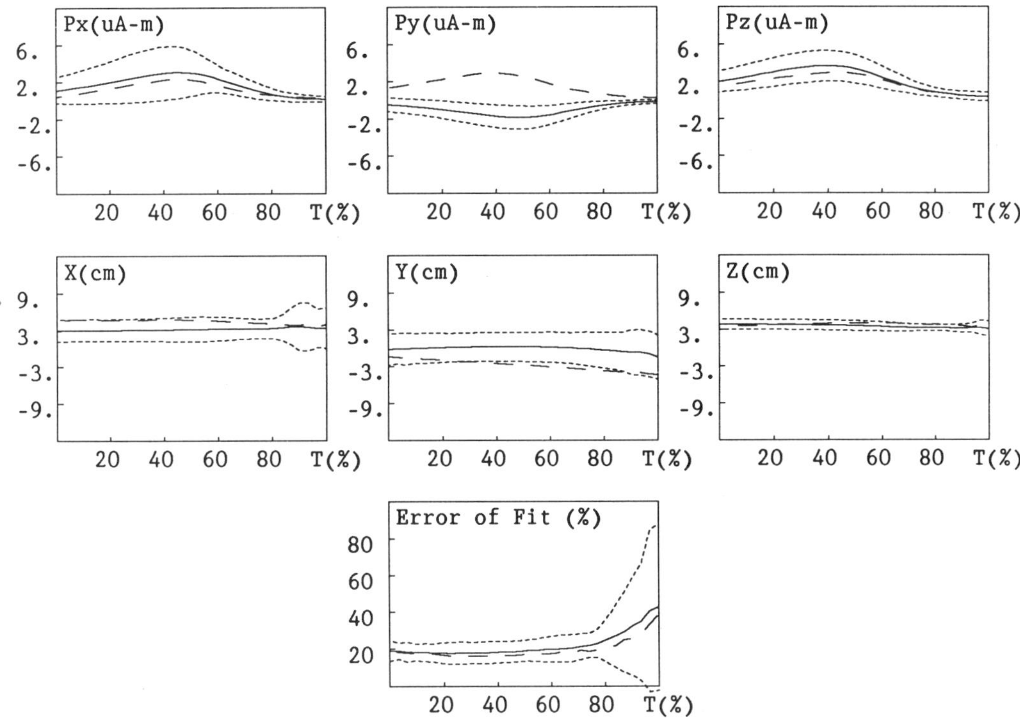

Figure 1. Solid lines indicate mean electric inverse solution parameters of 10 normal subjects: x,y,z components of dipole moment **P** and location **X**, and error of fit plotted against % of T-wave interval. The small dashed lines indicate the mean ± 2 s.d. The large dashed lines represent results from a subject with inferior infarction.

DISCUSSION

Our method of classification of these dipole parameter plots was purely visual, we intend to make this more quantitative, e.g., by fitting orthogonal polynomials to them. These preliminary results suggest that our electric and magnetic maps differ in their ability at detecting old myocardial infarction scars and predicting their location. It appeared possible to confirm the clinical diagnosis of the scarred segment of the myocardium more clearly using the body surface potential data than with the magnetocardiographic data. These results are preliminary due to the small sample sizes. We will extend this study to include larger sample sizes. Also changes to our methodology must be made so that the electric and magnetic recordings have a similar number of leads, coverage of the torso surface, and signal to noise ratio.

ACKNOWLEDGEMENTS

This work was funded through the support of the Medical Research Council of Canada (Program Grant No. PG-30), the Natural Sciences and Engineering Council of Canada, and the Nova Scotia Heart Foundation.

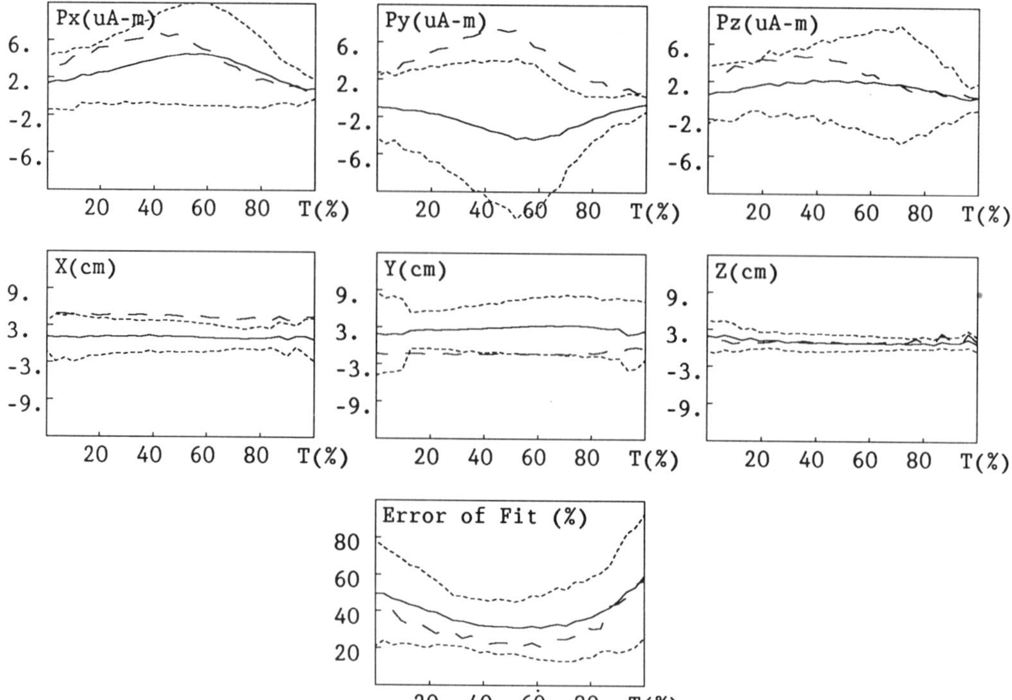

Figure 2. Solid lines indicate mean magnetic inverse solution parameters of 10 normal subjects, x,y,z components of dipole moment **P** and location **X**, and error of fit plotted against % of T-wave interval. The small dashed lines indicate the mean ± 2 s.d. The large dashed lines represent results from the same subject with inferior infarction as in Fig.1 .

REFERENCES

Mirvis, D. M., and Holbrook, M. A., Body surface distributions of repolarization potentials after acute myocardial infarction, 1981, J. Electrocardiology, 14:387.

Purcell, C. and Stroink G.,and Horacek, B.M., Magnetic inverse solution using a homogeneous torso model, 1987, Proc. 9th Ann. Conf. IEEE Eng. Med. Biol. Soc., 1:214.

Purcell C. and Stroink G., 1989, submitted to IEEE Trans. Biomed. Eng..

Montague T., Smith E. R., Cameron D. A. , Rautaharju P. M. , Klassen, G. A. , Felmington, C. S., and Horacek, B. M., 1981, Isointegral analysis of body surface maps, Circulation, 63(5):1166.

Horacek, B. M., 1974, Numerical model of an inhomogeneous human torso, Adv. Cardiology, , 10:51.

Horacek, B. M., 1973, Digital model for studies in magnetic cardiography, 1973, IEEE Trans. Magn., Mag-9(3):440.

Horan, L.G., Flowers, N.C., and Miller, C.B., A rapid assay of dipolar and extradipolar content in the human electrocardiogram, J. Electrocardiology, 5(3):211.

Stroink, G., Purcell, C., Lamothe, R., Merritt, R., Horacek, B.M., and ten Voorde, B., 1987, Body surface potential and magnetic mapping, in: "Biomagnetism '87", Astumi, K., Kotani, M., Ueno, S., Katila, T. and Williamson, S.J., Tokyo Denki Univ. Press, Tokyo, p.74.

DISCRIMINATION BETWEEN PATIENTS WITH MYOCARDIAL INFARCTION AND THOSE WITH VENTRICULAR TACHYCARDIA USING MAGNETIC AND POTENTIAL MAP EXTREMA AND TRAJECTORY PLOTS

J.Lant[1], G.Stroink[1,2], D.Vardy[1] and M.J.Gardner[2,3]

Departments of Physics[1], Physiology and Biophysics[2] and Medicine[3]
Dalhousie University
Halifax, Nova Scotia, Canada B3H 3J5

INTRODUCTION

The comparatively high mortality rate among patients surviving the acute phase of myocardial infarction (MI) has been attributed, in part, to their susceptibility to conduction arrhythmias such as ventricular tachycardia (VT) (Josephson, 1982). Hence there exists a pressing need for an efficient, non-invasive, discriminatory test with which to diagnose vulnerable patients. Spatial trajectory plots of signal extrema in body surface potential maps (BSPM) have been used to characterize normal subjects (Taccardi et al., 1976) and patients exhibiting cardiac arrhythmia (Gardner et al., 1986). We have used BSPM and magnetic field map (MFM) trajectory plots to facilitate inter-group separation of normal subjects (N), MI patients and VT patients.

METHODS

The study group of 45 subjects comprised three, 15 membered, sex (11 men, 4 women) and age matched groups. Ten patients in the MI group (mean age 57 ± 10 years) had previous inferior MI (IMI) and 5 had anterior MI (AMI). All patients were admitted to the coronary care unit with 1st acute MI. In the VT group (mean age 55 ± 8 years), 4 patients were diagnosed as idiopathic, 7 had previous AMI (VTA) and 4 had previous IMI (VTI). None of the 15 normal subjects (mean age 53 ± 14 years) had a history of cardiac disease and all had normal physical and echo-cardiographic examinations and 12-lead electrocardiograms.

56-lead magnetocardiographic (MCG) recordings, using a 2nd order asymmetric gradiometer (Stroink et al.,1986), and 120-lead BSPM recordings (Montague et al., 1986) were obtained in a eddy-current shielded room. All recordings were made with the patient in the supine position, in sinus rhythm, during tidal volume respiration. Patient recordings occurred within a 9 day to three week time span following release from hospital.

The data was averaged off-line and base-line corrected. Edited ECG limb leads were used to locate the onset/offset times of signal intervals within the averaged complexes. For both BSPM and MFM, the QRS and ST-T waveforms were separately time normalized and represented by 20 and 30 samples (maps) respectively. Thus the time interval between consecutive QRS maps is of the order of 5ms; between ST-T maps it is approximately 10ms. Amalgamation of all normal map sets, for a given time interval , defines the range/area of normal extrema trajectories for that interval. Group mean normal (QRS, ST-T) maps provide the group mean signal extrema trajectories

Advances in Biomagnetism
Edited by S.J. Williamson *et al.*
Plenum Press, New York

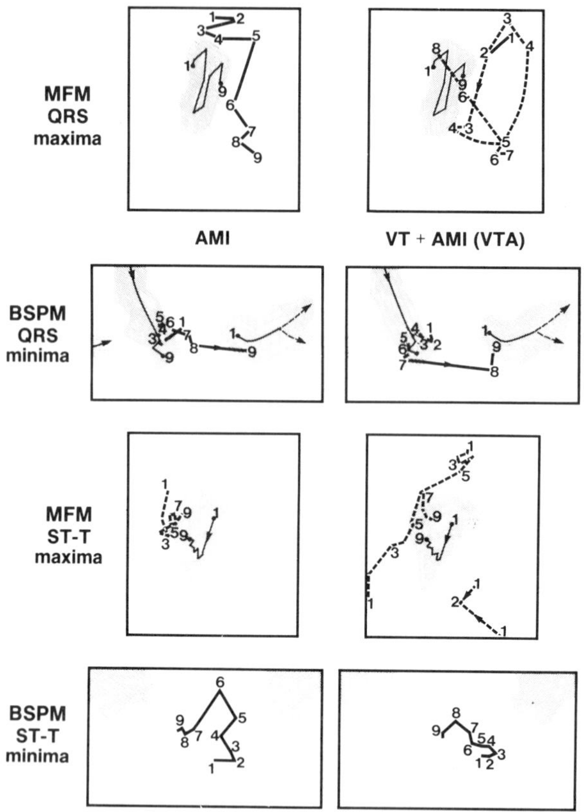

Figure 1. (top) MFM and BSPM trajectory plots of QRS extrema for a patient with AMI (left) and for a VT patient with previous AMI (right). Normal range is indicated by shaded area upon which the mean normal trajectory is superposed. The patient trajectories (heavy line) may display multiple tracks (dashed heavy line).
(bottom) MFM and BSPM trajectory plots of ST-T extrema for a AMI and a VTA patient. MFM multiple trajectories separate AMI and VTA patients; BSPM trajectories are similar for VTA and AMI patients.
The electrical potentials of the entire (front and back) torso is mapped in BSPM. The MFM depicts the magnetic field of the anterior torso only.

within the normal ranges. The trajectory plots, of signal maxima and minima, were constructed from each set (MFM and BSPM) of individual patient maps and compared with the corresponding group-mean normal trajectory plots.

RESULTS

Figure 1 shows typical MFM and BSPM QRS (top) and ST-T (bottom) extrema trajectory plots for, respectively, an AMI patient and for a VTA patient. The normal ranges in BSPM and MFM trajectories are indicated by the shaded regions. Within these regions are drawn the group-mean normal trajectories for 10 time-normalized instants. Normal BSPM trajectories, for both QRS and ST-T intervals, agree with previously published plots (Taccardi et al., 1976; Pham-Huy et al.,1981).

The MFM trajectory plots (Figure 1), for both QRS and ST-T intervals, clearly show AMI and VTA trajectories to be outside of the normal range and to share certain similarities. However, the VTA trajectory tends to be more widespread and fragmented than the AMI trajectory. The figure also shows the BSPM trajectories for the same two patients to be abnormal, but the distinction between the VTA and AMI patient is not as obvious as in the MFM plots. This is so because trajectory fragmentation is not as common in BSPM trajectory plots as it is in MFM trajectory plots. Trajectory fragmentation is affected by the appearance of an independent secondary extremum or of an additional pseudopodic extremum having signal strength comparable to , or exceeding that of the principal extremum.

In this study, trajectories falling outside the normal range for time periods exceeding 30ms in QRS and exceeding 90ms in ST-T were considered abnormal. Using this criterion, we found, for the QRS interval, MFM trajectory plots to be 100 % accurate in both MI/N and VT/N classification (all 30 patients exhibited abnormal MFM QRS trajectories); BSPM accuracy for the same bi-group separation is 86 % and 97 % respectively. Using ST-T time normalized maps, MFM trajectory plots are respectively 90% and 97 % accurate for MI/N and VT/N bi-group separation; BSPM trajectory plots are 100 % and 97 % accurate.

Table 1 Positive predictive values for MI and VT patient identification using MFM and BSPM trajectory plotting.

		QRS	ST-T
MI	MFM	73%	58%
	BSPM	100%	93%
VT	MFM	73%	86%
	BSPM	50%	21%

Using the trajectory plots previously identified as abnormal, the appearance of double-trajectories, of duration 30ms or longer during QRS and/or exceeding 60ms in ST-T, was then applied (to the plots) as a criteria for MI/VT separation. Employing

QRS trajectory plots, MFM correctly classified 11 of 15 VT's; BSPM correctly classified 7 of 14 VT's. When ST-T maps are employed, MFM correctly classified 13 of 15 VT patients but BSPM distinguished only 3 of 14 VT's. Table 1 indicates the relative success (positive predictive value) of MFM and BSPM in correctly classifying VT and MI patients.

DISCUSSION

Despite the fact that MCG interrogates a smaller torso area than BSPM (the MFM maps the anterior torso, the BSPM covers the entire torso), the results of this preliminary study indicates that MI/N, VT/N bi-group separation is as readily accomplished with MFM trajectory plots as with BSPM trajectory plots. MFM trajectory plots, for the QRS interval , show greater intragroup homogeneity than do BSPM plots. As well, the extended (spatial and temporal) fragmented trajectories of VT patients are more consistently obvious in MFM plots than in BSPM plots. As indicated in Table 1, MFM trajectory plots are a better (than BSPM) means of recognizing VT patients; BSPM plots provide a more reliable (than MFM) way of identifying MI patients. Moreover, the Tabled data shows that the accuracy of VT/MI classification using MFM (QRS, ST-T) trajectory plots is 73 % and 74 % respectively. By comparison, BSPM (QRS, ST-T) plots are 72% and 58 % respectively.

This study suggests that combined BSPM and MFM trajectory plotting may provide a means of localizing secondary sources associated with arrhythmic events and of identifying incipient VT patients in the at-risk MI population.

ACKNOWLEDGEMENTS

This work has been funded through the support of the Nova Scotia Heart Foundation, The Medical Research Council and the Natural Science and Engineering Research Council of Canada. Special thanks are extended to Reina Lamothe, Dorothy Marshall, Robert Merritt, Dr. B. M. Horacek, Paul Charlebois and to Dr. T. J. Montague.

REFERENCES

Gardner, M. J., Montague, T. J., Armstrong, C. S., Horacek, B. M. and Smith, E. R., 1986, Vulnerability to ventricular arrhythmia: Assessment by mapping of body surface potentials.Circulation 73: 684.

Josephson, M.E., 1982,Ventricular Tachycardia: Mechanisms and Management, Futura Publications, New York:10.

Montague, T .J., Johnston, D. E., Spencer, C. A., Lalonde, L. D., Gardner, M. J., O'Reilly, M. G.and Horacek, B. M., 1986, Non-Q wave Acute Myocardial Infarction: Body Surface Potential Mapping and Ventriculographic patterns, Am. J. Cardiol. 58:1173.

Pham-Huy, H., Gulrajani, R. M., Roberge, F. A., Nadeau, R. A., Mailloux, G. E. and Savard, P., 1981, A Comparative Evaluation of Three Different Approaches for Detecting Body Surface Isopotential Map Abnormalities in patients with Myocardial Infarction, J. Electrocardiology,14(1):43.

Stroink, G., ten Voorde, B., Horacek, B. M. and Montague, T .J., 1986, High Resolution Magnetocardiographic Field Mapping and Analysis,Proc. 8th Ann. Conf. IEEE Eng. Med. & Biol. Soc.1: 415.

Taccardi, B., DeAmbroggi, L. and Viganotti, C, 1976, Body Surface Mapping of Heart Potentials,in: Nelson,C. C. and Gesolowitz,D. B., eds, Theoretical Basis of Electrocardiography Clarendon Press, Oxford., p.436.

MAGNETOCARDIOGRAPHIC AND ELECTROCARDIOGRAPHIC RECORDINGS OF PATIENTS WITH VENTRICULAR TACHYCARDIA

G. Stroink[1,2], D. Vardy[1], R. Lamothe[1] and M. Gardner[2,3]

Department of Physics[1], Physiology and Biophysics[2] and Medicine[3]
Dalhousie University
Halifax, Canada B3H-3J5

INTRODUCTION

In recent years many researchers have shown the presence of low level, high frequency potentials in vector electrocardiograms of patients prone to ventricular tachycardia (VT) or fibrilation. These late potentials (LP) can be observed at the end of the QRS complex and last for a variable time into the ST segment. These signals have been associated with delayed or fragmented electrical activity in areas of damaged myocardium where reentry is assumed to occur. The LP are believed to be sensitive predictors of inducible sustained VT (Simson, 1981). Recently several groups (Erne et al, 1983; Montonen et al, 1988; Fenici et al., 1988; Merritt et al., 1988) have reported the existence of similar low level magnetic fields (LF) during the same time-period that the LP are recorded.

In this paper we report the measurements and analysis of both LP and LF in the electrocardiographic and magnetocardiographic records of three subject groups: 15 patients with inducible sustained VT, 11 of this group had previous myocardial infarction; 12 patients with previous myocardial infarction without VT and 14 normals. Our aim is to see if these LF 's can be used together with the LP's to formalize a sensitive and specific diagnostic marker for the presence of VT.

METHODS

The vector-electrocardiogram based upon the X, Y and Z Frank leads were recorded for each subject for 15 s and amplified using a high gain (2000x), low pass (125 Hz) amplifier. Using the method described by Simson (1981) the ECG averaged signals were then filtered bi-directionally using a 25 Hz four-pole high pass butterworth filter and combined to form a vector magnitude. The average rms noise level after filtering, over all subjects, during the ST segment was 2.5μV; the average Rmax/noise level was 413. The QRS onset and offset were set manually by displaying these segments of the vector ECG at high amplification. QRS offset was set at the end of any low-amplitude, high-frequency components exceeding the noise.

Twelve magnetocardiographic leads, forming a 3x4 grid with a spacing of 4 cm in the precordial area were recorded for 15 s with an asymmetric gradiometer (built by CTF Systems Inc., noise level 27 fT/$\sqrt{}$Hz) and processed in an equivalent manner. A composite MCG lead was formed for each subject by calculating the rms of the twelve bi-directionally filtered leads. The average rms noise level during the ST segment of each averaged and filtered lead was 46 fT; the average Rmax/noise level was 146. The data

Advances in Biomagnetism
Edited by S.J. Williamson *et al.*
Plenum Press, New York

was similarly analysed using, for each subject, the MCG lead with the largest amplitude. The average Rmax/noise level of this lead over all subjects is 349. MCG QRS on and offset were also set manually.

To quantify late ventricular activity the average signal strength during the 40 ms before QRS offset of the composite ECG or MCG rms signals was calculated. LP was defined as present if the activity during this time interval was less than 25 μV (Simson,1981); LF if this activity was less than 300 fT.

RESULTS & ANALYSIS

Fig. 1 shows the signal averaged ECG and MCG of a patient with MI and VT as well as the 25 Hz bi- directional signal (smaller signal). The low amplitude late activity in the filtered ECG and MCG is indicated by the darkened region. Generally the group of normals does not show late ventricular activity and the QRS complex ends abruptly. Such an abrupt change results in relatively large rms signals during the last 40 ms. The average rms voltage (field) during these last 40 ms is 60 ± 20 μV (.36 ± .15 pT) for the normals, 39 ± 31 μV (.38 ± .22 pT) for the MI patients and 30 ± 19 μV (.35 ± .25 pT) for the VT group.

In Table 1 we show for the ECG vector magnitude lead, the composite 12 lead MCG, and the largest MCG lead, the number of times LP and LF were found within the different subject groups. Comparing the ECG lead with the MCG composite lead (between brackets) we find late potentials (late fields) in 40% (53%) of the VT-group, 50% (42%) of the MI group and none (28%) in the group of normals, resulting in a diagnostic performance (the average of the sensitivity and specificity of this test) in detecting LP's (LF's) in the VT group and not in normals of 70% (62%). Separating the VT- from the MI- group is more challenging. Using LP's or LF's as criterion results in a diagnostic performance of 45% and 56% respectively. The number of times LF are detected in the MCG composite lead is not significantly different for the MCG largest lead.

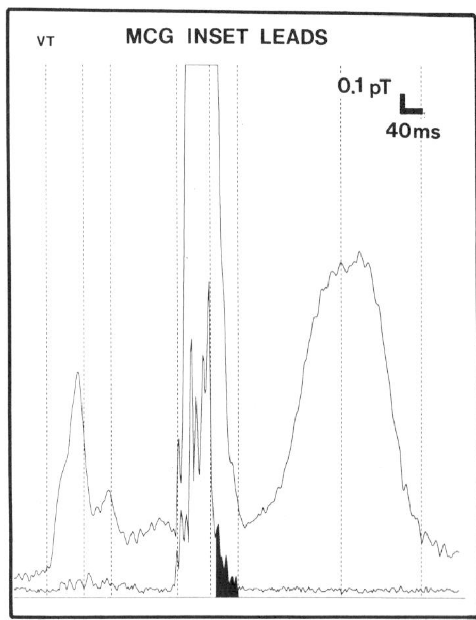

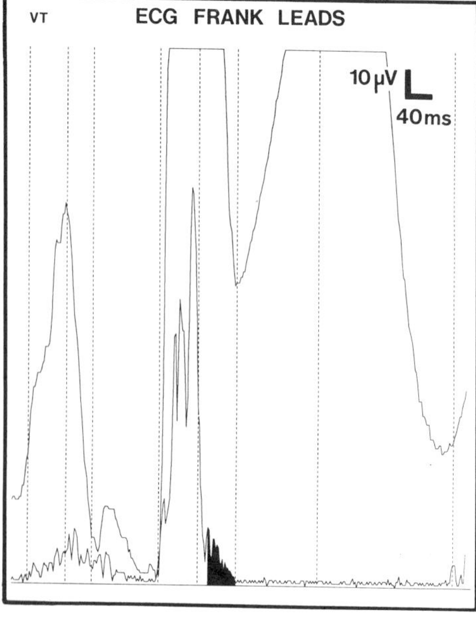

Fig 1. Signal averaged rms 12 lead composite MCG (left) and ECG vector magnitude (right) of the same patient with myocardial infarction and VT. The larger clipped signal is the unfiltered, the smaller signal the filtered signal. The dark area at the end of the MCG and ECG QRS indicates the LF and LP respectively.

Table 1. Number of subjects that show a late potential (LP) or late field (LF) during the last 40 ms of the QRS (top three rows). Number of subjects with a MCG or ECG for which the ratio of signal strength of the unfiltered signal at Rmax, over the average signal during the last 40 ms of the QRS, exceeds 23 (next 3 rows). The number of subjects for which the QRS duration is larger than 110 ms (last 2 rows). The subscript C refers to the 12 lead composite MCG, L refers to the largest MCG only.

	NM (14)	MI (12)	VT (15)
LP	0	6	6
LF_C	4	5	8
LF_L	4	2	4
$R_{max}/\overline{LP} > 23$	4	6	13
$R_{max}/\overline{LF_C} > 23$	3	4	10
$R_{max}/\overline{LF_L} > 23$	5	8	9
$ECG - QRS > 110\ ms$	0	1	6
$MCG_C - QRS > 110\ ms$	0	2	5

In identifying LP's or LF's we observed that a false positive finding can occur when the overall signal strength for the subject was low, resulting in small filtered signals during the last 40 ms of the late QRS. To account for this and to obtain a dimensionless quantity valid for both ECG and MCG we calculated the ratio of Rmax (unfiltered) to a computer calculated average rms signal during the last 40 ms of the QRS complex. Based on the average value obtained for the group of normals we estimated that a value larger than 23 indicates delayed QRS activity in both the ECG and MCG. The incidence of LP and LF based on this criterion is also included in Table 1. Using this ratio as a marker to identify VT patients we find a somewhat better diagnostic performance when compared with the normals: 79% for ECG and 72% for the 12- lead composite MCG. The average duration in the ECG vector magnitude lead of the QRS complex of the VT group is 105 ms, compared to 98 ms ($p < 0.2$) for the MI-patients and 86 ms ($p < 0.001$) for the normals. The average duration of the MCG composite rms signal is 101 ms for VT patients,

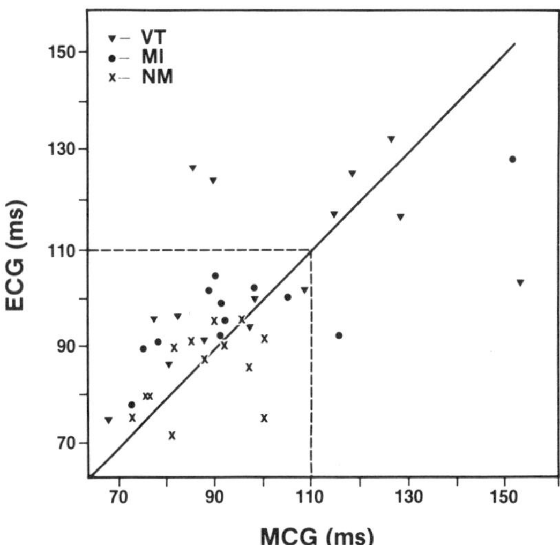

Fig.2. Duration of the rms ECG vs MCG (composite 12 lead) QRS time interval for each subject.

compared with 96 ms ($p < 0.6$) for the MI-patients and 86 ms ($p < 0.03$) for normals. Fig. 2 is a plot of the time duration of the ECG vs MCG QRS complex. It shows that 7 VT patients have either a ECG or a MCG QRS duration longer than 110 ms against 2 MI without VT and none of the normals (see also table 1).

DISCUSSION

The study demonstrates that LF can be identified in patients with VT as has been reported previously. Although the number of subjects used in each group is too small to draw firm conclusions, several trends are apparent and suggestions can be made for future studies. The overall better diagnostic performance and predictive value of the ECG leads as compared to the MCG composite leads, to detect late ventricular activity in VT patients and not in normals, agrees with similar observations by other researchers (Montonen et al, 1988). It is not clear from this study alone if this is due to the smaller signal/ noise ratio in the MCG lead as compared to the ECG lead or due to a lesser sensitivity of the MCG leads, studied here, to such activity.

Using the QRS duration of both the rms ECG and MCG signals shows some success in identifying VT patients and separating them from normal and MI subjects. It is interesting to note that, on average, the MCG duration is, on average, shorter (see Fig. 2) for all groups. This is even more apparent for the MCG largest lead which has a similar S/N ratio as the ECG vector magnitude lead. This confirms the observations made by Montonen et al. (1988) and probably reflects the different sensitivity of the two methods in detecting cardiac sources.

We conclude that longer MCG measuring times, MCG noise levels comparable to ECG noise levels and/or a more optimal MCG lead-system is required before conclusions can be drawn about the comparative sensitivity of temporal ECG and MCG recordings to low level late ventricular activity. In the meantime the analysis of magnetic field maps provides a more promising avenue to use MCG to obtain a sensitive marker for the presence of VT (Lant et al, 1990).

ACKNOWLEDGMENTS

This work has been funded through the support of the Nova Scotia Heart Foundation , The Medical Research Council and the Natural Science and Engineering Research Council of Canada. Special thanks are extended to Dorothy Marshall, Robert Merritt, John Lant, Paul Charlebois and to Dr. T. J. Montague.

REFERENCES

Erne, S. N., Fenici, R. R., Hahlmbohm, H. -D., Jaszczuk, W., Lehmann, H. P. and Masselli, M., 1983, High resolution magnetocardiographic recordings of the ST segment in patients with electrical late potentials, Il Nuovo Cimento, 2D: 340.

Fenici, R. R., Masselli, M., Lopez, L., and Melillo, G.,1988, Magnetocardiographic localization of arrythmogenic tissue, in: "Biomagnetism '87", Atsumi, K., Kotani, M., Ueno, S., Katila, T., and Williamson, S. J., eds., Tokyo Denki Univ. Press, Tokyo, pp. 282.

Lant, J., Stroink, G., Vardy, D. and Gardner, M.J., 1990, Discrimination between patients with with myocardial infarction and those with ventricular tachycardia using magnetic and potential map extrema trajectory plots, These proceedings.

Merritt, R., Stroink, G., Gardner, M. J. and Horacek, B. M., 1988, Cardiac potential and magnetic maps of V-T patients, Physics & Biology, 33, Suppl.1:60.

Montonen, J., Katila, T., Leinio, M., Madekivi, S., Makijarvi, M., Nenonen, J. and Siltanen, P., 1988, Time and frequency domain analysis of cardiac micropotentials, in: Biomagnetism '87 , Atsumi, K., Kotani, M., Ueno, S., Katila, T., and Williamson, S. J., Tokyo, Denki Univ. Press, Tokyo, pp.278.

Simson, M. B., 1981, Use of signals in the terminal QRS complex to identify patients with ventricular tachycardia after myocardial infarction, Circulation, 64: 235.

ATRIAL AND VENTRICULAR TACHYCARDIAS : INVASIVE VALIDATION AND REPRODUCIBILITY OF MAGNETOCARDIOGRAPHIC IMAGING

Riccardo Fenici, Guido Melillo, Alessandra Cappelli, Claudio De Luca, Mariella Masselli

Clinical Physiology - Cardiovascular Biomagnetism Unit, Catholic University, Rome, Italy

INTRODUCTION

Magnetic localization of the site of onset of cardiac arrhythmias both of atrial and ventricular origin was first reported in 1986 (Fenici et al, 1987-89). However the accuracy of such localization procedures had not been validated so far. In this paper the reproducibility of such measurements is reported in several patients. Moreover the validation of magnetic localisation of ventricular tachycardia with conventional invasive endocardial mapping is described in one patient with previous myocardial infarction (MI).

METHODS

8 patients were magnetically studied. 4/8 with permanent focal atrial tachycardia. 4/8 with episodes of sustained ventricular tachycardia (VT). 3/4 VT patients were affected by arrhythmogenic right ventricular dysplasia (ARVD), 1/4 had a post myocardial infarction ventricular aneurysm , complicated by sustained iterative ventricular tachycardia. In all patients the arrhythmias were hemodynamically well tolerated.

MCG mapping was performed with a RF-SQUID based single channel instrumentation and protocols previously described in detail (Fenici et al 1985-89). The measurements reproducibility was tested by repeating MCG mapping in different recording sessions (for 1 to 24 months apart). In particular in 2/4 VT patients, MCG mapping was also repeated during ventricular bigeminy, to test the localization reproducibility of the arrhythmogenic areas even when mapping single extrasystoles.

In the post-MI VT patient, apparently refractory to previous antiarrhythmic therapy, invasive electrophysiological study (EPS) was performed in order to identify the electrogenetic mechanism of the arrhythmia and to establish the appropriate pharmacological treatment. The MCG VT localization therefore was compared with that inferred by conventional catheter mapping (Josephson et al., 1978) and pacemapping (Waxman et al., 1982) (fig. 1). One year later coronary heart surgery was necessary in the latter patient, because of triple vessel disease with impending angina.

RESULTS

In 4/4 patients with focal atrial tachycardia, MCG mapping provided a reproducible three-dimensional localization of the site of origin of the arrhythmia, which was electrically classifiable in only 1/4. However only the measurements reproducibility accounted for their accuracy, as invasive EPS was not clinically required.

In the 3 patients with ARVD, the site of origin of the ventricular arrhythmia was reproducibly identified by MCG mapping during sustained ventricular tachycardia (avg. 3D uncertainty: 16 mm.). In all subjects the origin of VT was magnetically localized in correspondence with areas of the right ventricle, which appeared to be the most jeopardised at the echocardiogram (RV Inferior wall, 1 case and RV Outflow tract, 2 cases). Ventricular depolarization pattern during VT was reproducibly depicted by magnetic imaging, and provided a reasonable explanation of the ECG morphology of individual VTs. The 3D uncertainty of arrhythmogenic area's localization was as high as 45 mm. when comparing, in the same patient, MCG maps taken during sustained VT and bigeminal PVCs of apparently same morphology.

In the patient with post-MI VT, the onset of ventricular depolarization was magnetically localized in the postero-infero-lateral wall of the left ventricle, where catheter mapping recorded the site of earliest endocardial activation with fragmented countinous activity and endocardial pacemapping fairly reproduced the VT morphology (fig. 1).
This localization was in agreement with the scintigraphic imaging of the infarcted area. Moreover, although ventricular tachycardia, fully controlled by the antiarrhythmic therapy, was not inducible during the intervention,a large scar was found in the postero-inferior wall of the left ventricle, adherent to the diaphragmatic pericardium.

DISCUSSION

This is the first report describing the reproducibility of biomagnetic localization of focal cardiac arrhythmias. It was satisfactory for both atrial and ventricular tachycardias. Unfortunately the invasive validation of MCG localization accuracy in these patients is limited to a single case, because in 7/8 case the arrhythmias were well tolerated and there was no clinical indication for invasive electrophysiology. On the other hand sustained ventricular tachycardias, which requires invasive electrophysiological study, are rarely sufficiently tolerated for a period of time long enough to allow a safe MCG mapping. Notwithstanding the coincidence found, in the patient with previous myocardial infarction, between magnetocardiographic and catheter localization of the site of origin of ventricular tachycardia is striking and well in agreement with the anatomical lesion observed during surgery. This result strongly supports the MCG capability to provide a reliable "functional imaging" and localization of ventricular arrhythmias. Moreover, the antiarrhythmic effect of surgical excision of the myocardial scar from the diaphragmatic pericardium (Fenici and Melillo, this Conference) further confirms that the ventricular arrhythmia originated in that area.

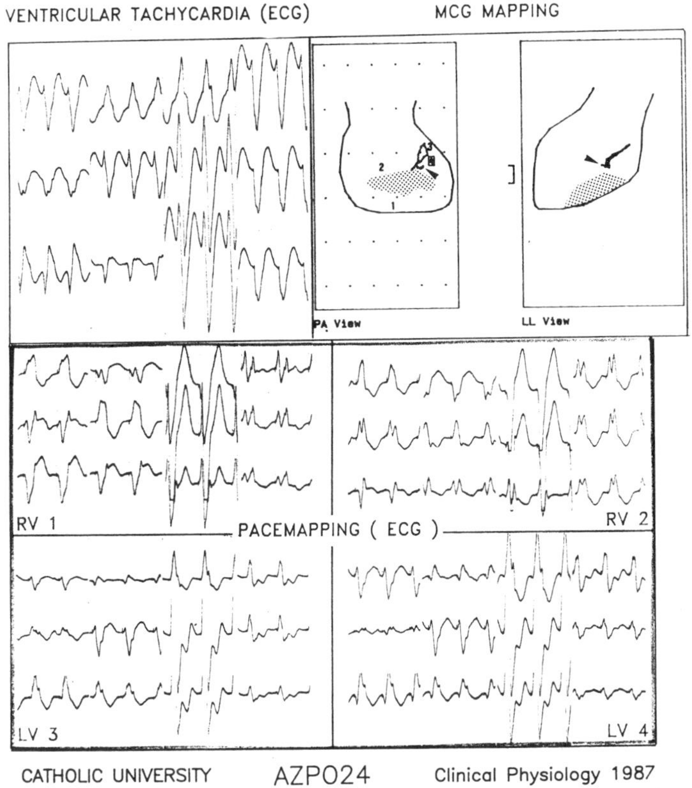

Fig. 1. Validation of MCG localization with pacemapping technique : Standard leads ECG morphology similar to spontaneous VT (top left) was obtained by pacing the Left Ventricle at site LV 4 (bottom right) (3D distance from MCG localization: 12 mm., top right).

Obviously only four investigated cases and one invasive validation are insufficient to extrapolate the reliability of the MCG method for the localization of all kinds of cardiac arrhythmias. In fact especially in patients with post-MI ventricular arrhythmias, pathologic anysotropy of myocardial tissue could generate more complicated field patterns of non-dipolar configuration. In such situations current multipole expansion could be a more appropriate model for source localization (Katila et al 1987, Gonnelli et al 1988, Erne' et al 1988, Fenici and Melillo, this conference).

ACKNOWLEDGEMENTS

Partially supported by grants: CNR N. 85.00462.04, CNR N.86.00062.04, CNR N. 88.00503.04, Contract Elettronica S.p.A./IMI (law n.46, 17/02/82) and Italian Ministery of Education (60%) 1986-88.

REFERENCES

Erne' S.N., Trahms L.,Trontelj Z., 1988, Current multipoles as sources of biomagnetic fields. In: Biomagnetism 1987. Atsumi K, Katila T, Kotani M, Williamson SJ, Ueno S (eds). Tokyo Denki University Press: 302.

Fenici R.R., Masselli M., Lopez L., Sabetta F., 1985, High resolution magnetocardiography: electrophysiological and clinical findings. In: Proc. of the XIV ICMBE and VII ICPM, Espoo, Finland: 1475.

Fenici R.R.,Masselli M., Lopez L., Melillo G., 1987, Catheter ablation of cardiac arrhythmias: MCG localization of electrocatheters and arrhythmogenic foci. New Trends in Arrhythmias, Vol. III, N.4: 723.

Fenici R.R., Masselli M, Lopez L., Melillo G., 1988, Magnetocardiographic localization of arrhythmogenic tissue. In: Biomagnetism '87. Atsumi K., Katila T., Kotani M., Williamson S.J., Ueno S. (eds). Tokyo Denki University Press: 282.

Fenici R.R., Masselli M., Lopez L., Melillo G., 1989a, Clinical value of magnetocardiography. In: Electrocardiography and cardiac drug Therapy. Hombach V., Hilger H.H. (eds), Kluwer Academic Publishers, Dordrect/ Boston/ London: 239.

Fenici R.R., Masselli M., Lopez L., Melillo G., 1989b, Clinical magnetocardiography. Localization of arrhythmogenic structures. In: Advances in Biomagnetism; Functional localization: a challenge for biomagnetism. I.S.I., Erne' S.N., Romani G.L., (eds), World Scientific: 102.

Fenici R.R., Masselli M., Lopez L., Melillo G., 1989c, High resolution electrocardiography and magnetocardiography. In: "High resolution electrocardiography", El Sherif N., Hombach V., Futura Publishing Company (in press).

Fenici R.R., Melillo G., Biomagnetic imaging in the cardiac catheterization laboratory. (this conference).

Gonnelli R.S., Sicuro M., 1988, Use of current multipole for the cardiac source localization in normal subjects. In: Biomagnetism '87, Atsumi K., Katila T., Kotani M., Williamson S.J., Ueno S. (eds). Tokyo Denki University Press: 314.

Katila T., Maniewski R., Markijarvi M., Nenonen J., Siltanen P., 1987, On the accuracy of source localization in cardiac measurements. Phys. Med. Biol., Vol 32 N.1: 125.

Josephson M.E., Horowitz L.N. et al., 1978, Recurrent sustained ventricular tachycardia: 2. Endocardial mapping. Circulation, Vol.57 N.3, 440.

Waxman H. L., Josephson M. E., 1982, Ventricular activation during ventricular endocardial pacing: I. Electrocardiographic patterns related to the sites of pacing. Am. J. Cardiol., Vol.50 N.1, 1.

THE INFLUENCE OF HEART MOTION ON MAGNETIC FIELDS

U. Tachinardi, S.S. Furuie,
S. Sirota and C.P. Melo

Coordenadoria de Informática - INCOR
C.P. 11.450 - Sao Paulo - SP
Brazil

INTRODUCTION

The identification and comprehension of the many factors that influence the cardiac magnetic fields, is fundamental for a better understanding of the MCG signals. Cardiac anisotropy and volume conductor seem to be two of those factors. The former was studied in a previous report (Campos et al, 1988). In that study, a multiple dipole model taking into account the orientation of the depolarization wavefront was proposed and tested . The MCG calculated using that method revealed some features similar to those found in experimental measurements. Those findings were also observed by others (Roth et al, 1988; Gonelli and Agnello, 1987), who used different approaches to show the effects of cardiac anisotropy on the MCG. Those models however, did not consider some other factors such as cardiac motion that could also influence the MCG. The present study is a first approach to analyze the possible effects of the heart dynamics on the MCG.

Although motion is a well known characteristic of the heart, its measurement is made difficult because of the complex three-dimensional deformation that occurs during contraction and relaxation (Walley et al, 1982). Left ventricular contraction in humans were analyzed by Hood and Rolett (Hood and Rolett, 1969), showing that shortening was about 20% along the major axis (base-to-apex) and 36% along the minor axis (transverse). Using biplane radiographic markers, Ingels and co-workers (Ingels et al, 1982), showed that the heart contracts in an assymmetric and inhomogeneous manner, with little rotation of the center of the mass and little rotation of the long axis (about 1 ^{o}). They also showed that the minor axis twists transversely to the long axis some 0 to 7 degrees, depending on the region. These findings were attributed to the complex geometry of myofibrils in the ventricular wall.

METHODS

A multiple dipole model described elsewhere was used (Campos et al, 1988). Two models of ventricular depolarization were adopted (fig. 1): (1) isochronic potentials obtained from a human isolated heart (Durrer et al, 1970), and (2) a theoretical line model of depolarization, represented by 7 consecutive rectangular isochrones. A uniform density of dipoles, oriented normally to the wavefront (homogeneous hypothesis), were placed along the midline between two consecutive isochronic curves. The magnetic fields (Bz) were obtained using the Biot-Savart equation, for an ideal detector positioned at the center of each cell of the grid. The distance from the detector to the grid plane was 4 cm. The isofield maps were calculated for a 6 X 6 position grid (35 cm X 28 cm).

The simulation of the heart swinging motion consisted of fixing one point of the model (fig. 1), and displacing the model a variable number of degrees (Θ) counterclockwise, with a constant angular velocity. For each consecutive isochronic curve, the model was rotated the corresponding fraction of Θ (Θ/number of isochrones).

Advances in Biomagnetism
Edited by S.J. Williamson *et al.*
Plenum Press, New York

The isofield map sequences (one map for each isochronic curve) were analyzed by means of their principal maps. Details of this technique are found elsewhere (Tachinardi et al, 1988).

(a)

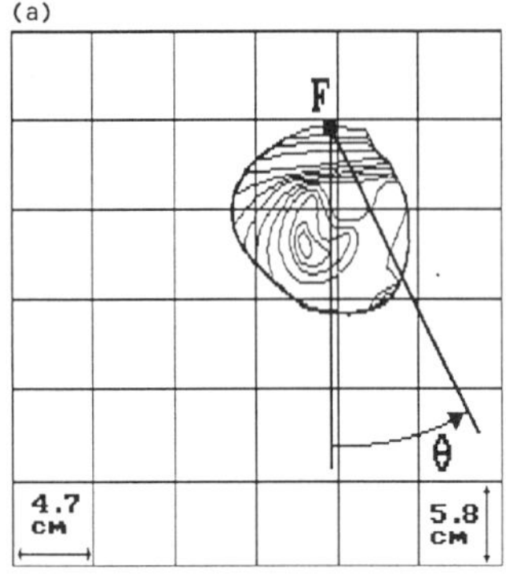

(c)

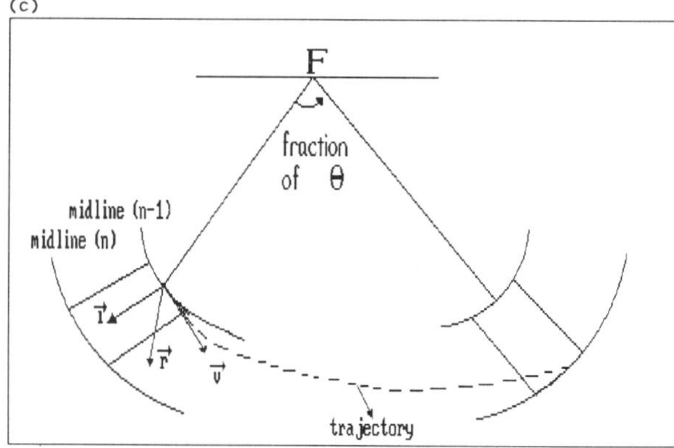

(b)

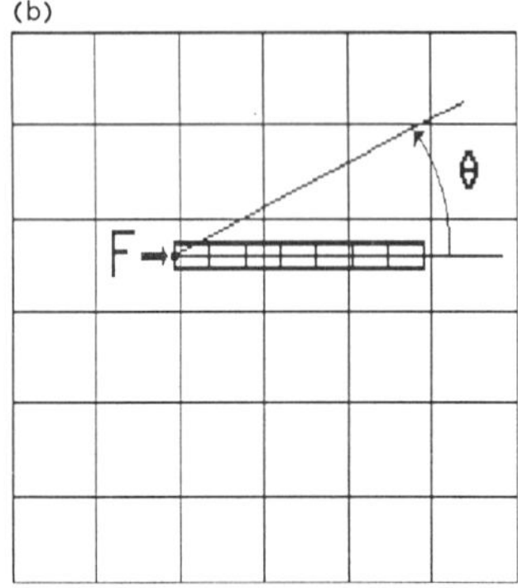

Fig. 1.
Two depolarization models used in the simulation: (a) isochronic potentials of an isolated human heart, (b) theoretical isochronic potentials. "F" indicates the fixed point, and θ is the angle by which the model is rotated. (c) diagram showing the current dipole element $\vec{i}$, moving between two consecutive isochrones (n-1 to n). $\vec{v}$ represents the motion component, and $\vec{r}$ the resulting vector. The model and the grid are shown at the same position and scaling as used for calculations. The distance between the model and the grid plane is 4 cm.

RESULTS

Figure 2 shows the principal maps of some sequences of isofield maps obtained with both the static and the dynamic heart models. A minor effect on the magnetic field configuration can be observed. Figure 2d shows the differences between the maximum and minimum field values obtained for different values of Θ. An increased value between the maxima values can be observed for the calculations with motion. The calculations made using the line model, showed that motion affects the isofield maps configuration (fig. 3).

DISCUSSION

The maps calculated for the line model have shown a variation in the isofield map patterns for different values of Θ. The MCG calculated with the heart model however, revealed to be little influenced by motion, except for a small increase in the unbalance between the maxima values. These results suggest that the complex configuration of the isochronic curves of that model, formed mostly by closed curves, results in cancelation of most of the effect of the simulated motion. It should be noted that severe limitations are assumed for the models and the motion simulation. The homogeneous medium was adopted to enable the analysis of heart motion as an isolated factor. Unpublished results obtained with anisotropic models have shown comparable results.

The results observed for both models, show that only very high degrees of motion are needed to elicit a visible effect on the maps. Since this amount of rotation is not observed in the real case, even when the whole cycle is considered, it seems that heart motion has little effect on the MCG. However,

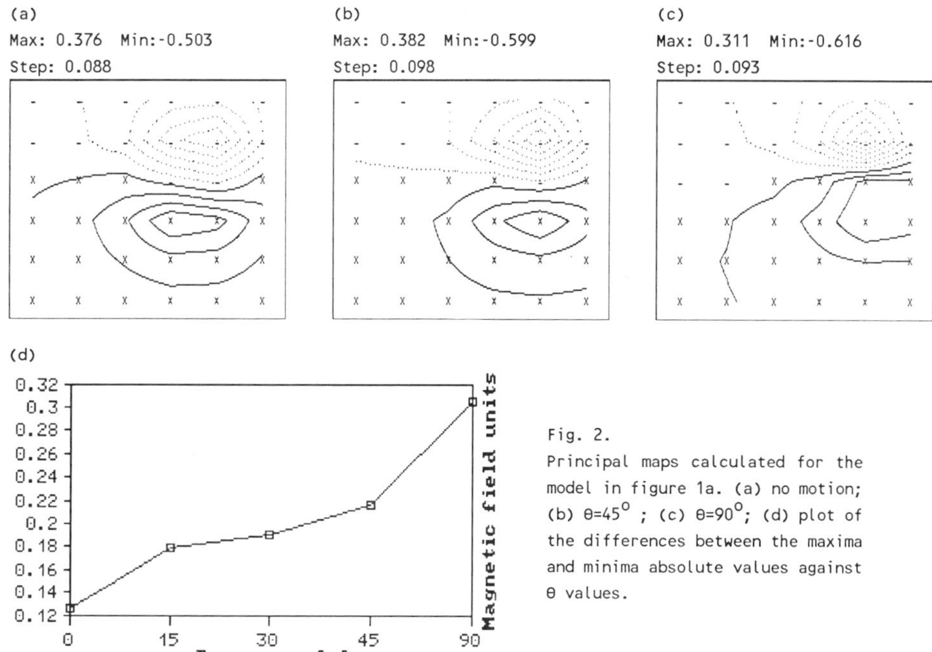

Fig. 2.
Principal maps calculated for the model in figure 1a. (a) no motion; (b) $\theta=45^{o}$; (c) $\theta=90^{o}$; (d) plot of the differences between the maxima and minima absolute values against θ values.

in diseases that alter the heart mobility (i.e. pericardial effusion), this effect should be more relevant. It is important to note that electrical and mechanical systole do not occur simultaneously. The left ventricular contraction starts about 20 ms after the onset of the QRS, whereas the left ventricular pressure almost reaches its maximum value within the QRS limits. That means that the heart movement is not constant along the systole. The segment contraction varies for different regions of the heart, suggesting that magnetic fields produced by some regions can be more sensitive to motion than others. More detailed studies are needed to analyze the regional influence of motion on the MCG.

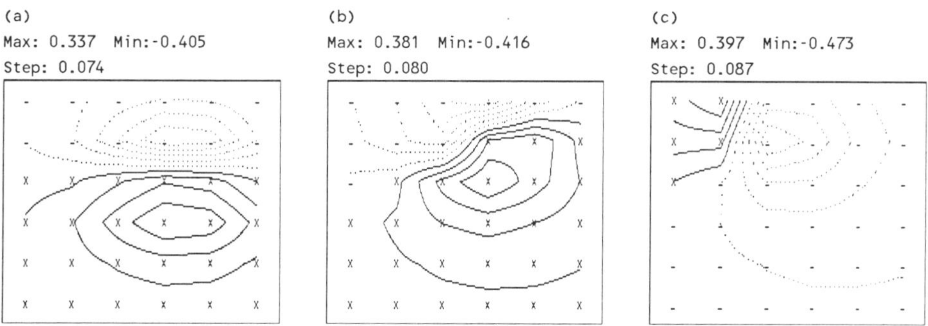

Fig. 3. Principal maps calculated using figure 1b model. (a) no motion; (b) $\theta=45^{o}$; (c) $\theta=90^{o}$.

ACKNOWLEDGEMENTS

The authors are grateful to Dr. Moffa and Prof. Costa Ribeiro for many helpful discussions. This project is supported by FINEP.

REFERENCES

Campos, J. C., Tachinardi, U., Melo, C. P. and Costa Ribeiro, P. C., 1988, Depolarization orientation in a multiple dipole model for the direct problem in magnetocardiography, in: Biomagnetism'87 - Proceedings of the 6th International Conference on Biomagnetism, K. Atsumi, M. Kotani, S. Ueno, T. Katila and S.J. Williamson, eds., Tokyo Denki University Press, Tokyo.

Durrer, D., Van Dam, R. Th., Freud, G. E., Janse, M. J., Meijler, F. L. and Arzbaicher, R. C., 1970, Total excitation of the isolated human heart, Circulation, 41:899-912.

Gonelli, R. S. and Agnello, M., 1987, Inverse problem solution in cardiomagnetism using a current multipole expansion of the primary sources, Phys. Med. Biol., 32:133-142.

Hood Jr., W. P. and Rollet, E. L., 1969, Patterns of contraction in the human left ventricle, Circulation, 39-40(Suppl.3):109.

Ingels Jr., N. B., Daughters II, G. T., Stinson, E. B. and Alderman, E. L., 1982, Left ventricular midwall dynamics from surgically implanted markers in intact unanesthetized man, in: Cardiovascular system dynamics - Models and measurements, T. Kenner, R. Busse and H. Hinghofer-Szalkay, eds., Plenum Press, New York.

Roth, B. J., Guo, W. and Wikswo Jr, J. P., 1988, The effects of spiral anisotropy on the electric potential and the magnetic field at the apex of the heart, Math. Biosci., 88:191-221.

Tachinardi, U., Furuie, S. S., Campos, J. C. and Melo, C. P., 1988, The use of singular value decomposition in the analysis of the QRS complex isofield maps, in: Biomagnetism'87 - Proceedings of the 6th International Conference on Biomagnetism, K. Atsumi, M. Kotani, S. Ueno, T. Katila and S.J. Williamson, eds., Tokyo Denki University Press, Tokyo.

Walley, K. R., Grover, M., Raff, G. L., Benge, J. W., Hannaford, B. and Glantz, S. A., 1982, Left ventricular dynamic geometry in the intact and open chest dog, Circ. Res., 50:573-589.

EFFECT OF CONSTITUTIONAL VARIABLES ON MAGNETOCARDIOGRAM

J. Nousiainen, O.S. Oja and J. Malmivuo

Tampere University of Technology,
Institute of Biomedical Engineering
P.O. Box 527, SF-33101 Tampere, FINLAND

INTRODUCTION

Many non-cardiac factors like age, sex and constitutional variables of the body have an effect on the electrocardiogram (ECG) (Pipberger et al., 1967; Ishikawa, 1976; Nemati et al., 1977). Several criteria for normal ECG have been established separately for men and women. The correlation of constitutional variables and MCG parameters has not been studied so far. In this study we present with normal material the effect of sex, age, height and weigh of the body and dimensions of the chest on the amplitude and direction of the QRS vector in MCG.

MATERIAL AND METHODS

The material of the study consisted of 188 normal, healthy subjects without history of cardiac disorders. The age of 105 male and 83 female subjects ranged from 20 to 79 years.

The MCGs were recorded with the first order vector gradiometer using the corrected unipositional lead system (Eskola, 1987). The equivalent magnetic dipole located in the geometrical center of the heart was calculated from the three orthogonal components of the magnetic field. As an approximation for the location of the equivalent dipole was used the depth of one third of the thickness of the chest. The thickness and width of the chest were measured at the level of the fourth intercostal space.

The joint effect and the relative importance of the constitutional variables on 50 MCG parameters was examined by means of multiple regression analysis. The simple regression analysis was also performed to calculate the coefficients of correlation by using the Pearson's product-moment method and to determine the regression line between the dependent and independent variables. Student's t-statistics was used to determine the significance of the correlation and regression.

RESULTS

The multiple regression analysis showed that the most important explanatory factors of MCG amplitudes were age as well as in men the height

Advances in Biomagnetism
Edited by S.J. Williamson *et al.*
Plenum Press, New York

and in women the weight and to a minor extent the width of the chest. The highest correlation was in the maximum spatial QRS amplitude (R = 0.65).

Sex: Table 1. shows that the most prominent effect of the sex on MCG was that the MCG amplitudes were in female subjects on an average about 40 % smaller than in male subjects. However, in the age over about 50 years this difference became equalized.

The only statistically significant difference in the orientation of the QRS vectors between men and women was in the angle of the maximum QRS vector in frontal plane that was more cranial in men.

Age: Table 2. shows that the main effect of the age on MCG was the decrease of the MCG amplitudes with advancing age. The correlation of MCG amplitudes with age was pronounced in men in which the differencies in the calculated MCG amplitudes between the youngest and the oldest subgroups were statistically significant. The only notable change in women was the decrease of the Y amplitude. According to the regression line the spatial maximum QRS amplitude decreased 0.15 μAm^2 per a decade in male subjects.

The fact that only the Y amplitude in women correlated with age gave rise to the shift of the maximum QRS vector to the right which can be seen in the frontal and transverse planes.

Body height: The height of the body was the most important single constitutional factor of the body affecting almost all MCG amplitude measurements in men. Table 3. shows the mean maximum QRS amplitudes in three height categories. According to the regression line, the maximum spatial QRS amplitude increased about 0.35 μAm^2 when the height increased 10 cm.

Body weight: Many MCG amplitude measurements of female subjects correlated with the weight. The greatest correlation coefficient was observed with the maximum spatial QRS magnitude ($r = 0.28$). The slope of the regression line was in the maximum amplitude of the spatial QRS vector only 0.01 $\mu Am^2/kg$ so that the effect of the weight was not tabulated.

Chest dimensions: Many amplitude measurements of the Y component had a weak negative correlation with the width of the chest especially in men. In women also some measurements of the Z amplitude and the spatial QRS amplitude correlated with the chest width. The separate tabulation of the effect of chest dimensions was omitted because of its minor importance.

Table 1. Mean values and standard deviations (SD) of some MCG parameters in three groups and the statistical significance of difference between the mean values of male and female subgroups.

MCG parameter	All n = 188 Mean	SD	Men n = 105 Mean	SD	Women n = 83 Mean	SD	p-value
X_max (μAm^2)	0.88	0.47	1.07	0.46	0.64	0.39	<0.0001
Y_max (μAm^2)	0.43	0.23	0.52	0.24	0.32	0.17	<0.0001
Z_max (μAm^2)	0.86	0.47	1.07	0.48	0.60	0.25	<0.0001
M_max (μAm^2)	1.06	0.51	1.29	0.51	0.74	0.27	<0.0001
QRS_Sag. (degr.)	-43	21	-42	21	-44	21	(ns)
QRS_Fro. (degr.)	76	30	81	35	68	18	<0.005
QRS_Tra. (degr.)	177	34	174	32	179	30	(ns)

X_max, Y_max, Z_max: maximum peak-to-peak QRS amplitudes in X, Y and Z leads;
M_max: maximum magnitude of spatial QRS vector;
QRS_Sag., QRS_Fro., QRS_Tra.: angles of maximum vector in sagittal, frontal and transverse planes; n: number of cases; ns: not significant

Table 2. Mean values and standard deviations of some MCG parameters in three age groups of male and female subjects and the statistical significance of the difference between the youngest and oldest subgroups.

MCG parameter	Sex	20-35 years 34 men 15 women Mean SD	36-50 years 31 men 20 women Mean SD	51-78 years 49 men 47 women Mean SD	p-value sub-groups 1 vs. 3	Correlation coeffient
X_max (μAm^2)	m	1.22 0.46	1.22 0.39	0.81 0.39	<0.0001	-0.43
	f	0.61 0.30	0.61 0.48	0.67 0.33	(ns)	(ns)
Y_max (μAm^2)	m	0.62 0.24	0.52 0.22	0.42 0.21	<0.0005	-0.39
	f	0.42 0.09	0.34 0.16	0.28 0.15	<0.005	-0.49
Z_max (μAm^2)	m	1.16 0.46	1.16 0.54	0.92 0.42	<0.05	-0.28
	f	0.62 0.29	0.59 0.27	0.60 0.25	(ns)	(ns)
M_max (μAm^2)	m	1.47 0.48	1.47 0.50	1.02 0.42	<0.0001	-0.42
	f	0.78 0.16	0.75 0.30	0.74 0.27	(ns)	(ns)
QRS_Sag. (degr.)	m	-41 18	-37 15	-47 25	(ns)	(ns)
	f	-33 10	-49 28	-46 18	<0.05	(ns)
QRS_Fro. (degr.)	m	75 27	83 36	84 41	(ns)	(ns)
	f	60 20	61 13	74 16	<0.005	0.51
QRS_Tra. (degr.)	m	183 38	188 15	182 38	(ns)	(ns)
	f	206 12	200 36	186 37	<0.1	-0.26

<u>Effect on the variation in MCG amplitudes:</u> Table 4. summarizes the effect of sex and constitutional variables on the variation of some MCG amplitudes. The change in the coefficient of variation (CV) describes the influence of the sex on the variation: for instance the CV in the maximum spatial QRS magnitude decreased from the value 48 % in the whole group to the values 40 % and 36 % when the population was divided into male and female subgroups, respectively. The coefficient of multiple determination (R^2) describes, what fraction of variation in the amplitudes can be explained by the joint effect of constitutional variables. Table 4. shows that in case of the whole population up to 42 % of the variation in the maximum spatial QRS magnitude could be explained by the joint effect of constitutional variables. When the effect of sex was eliminated the proportion of variance due to the regression was 25 %.

Table 3. Mean values and standard deviations of MCG parameters in three height subgroups of men and the statistical significance of the difference between the shortest and tallest subgroups.

MCG parameter	≤ 175 cm 34 men Mean SD	176 - 181 cm 39 men Mean SD	≥ 182 cm 32 men Mean SD	p-value subgroups 1 vs. 3	Correlation coeffient
X_max (μAm^2)	0.93 0.56	1.05 0.40	1.18 0.40	<0.05	0.20
Y_max (μAm^2)	0.49 0.31	0.50 0.23	0.53 0.27	(ns)	(ns)
Z_max (μAm^2)	0.86 0.41	1.06 0.48	1.22 0.58	<0.005	0.34
M_max (μAm^2)	1.08 0.50	1.25 0.46	1.62 0.46	<0.0001	0.42

Table 4. Coefficients of variation (CV) and coefficients of multiple determination (R^2) of MCG amplitude measurements in the whole material and in male and female subgroups.

MCG parameter	CV			R^2		
	All	Men	Women	All	Men	Women
X_max	0.53	0.43	0.57	0.22	0.17	0.09
Y_max	0.53	0.46	0.51	0.24	0.14	0.24
Z_max	0.55	0.45	0.36	0.27	0.13	0.15
M_max	0.48	0.40	0.36	0.42	0.25	0.24

DISCUSSION

The effects of the constitutional variables on MCG parameters observed in the present study were very consistent with the corresponding effects on ECG reported in the literature. Some correlation coefficients were observed to be higher in MCG than in ECG. The difference in amplitudes between male and female subjects was steeper in MCG than in ECG.

The MCG measurements were affected in different ways by many constitutional variables and the effects were not always parallel in men and women. It is very difficult to conclude which variables were primary factors because of their intercorrelation. In men the diminishing of MCG amplitudes with the advancing age was strengthened by the correlation of the MCG amplitudes with the body height that decreased with age. In women the situation was different. The body weight was clearly more important factor than the height. The decrease of the amplitude with the increasing age was partially eliminated by the increase of the amplitude with the increasing weight which was characteristic for the female group.

The results showed that the sex and the age were so prominent factors affecting MCG that they must be considered when assessing the clinical value of MCG in heart diseases where the diagnosis is based mainly on the amplitude criteria. This kind of heart disorder is e.g. ventricular hypertrophy (Oja et al., 1988) in which the diagnostic sensitivity of MCG was improved in female subjects and in male subjects over 50 years old when the age and the sex were accounted for in the normal reference group.

ACKNOWLEDGEMENTS

This work was supported by the Academy of Finland.

REFERENCES

Pipberger, H.V., Goldman, M.J., Littmann, D., Murphy, G.P., Cosma, J., and Snyder, J.R., 1967, Correlations of the Orthogonal Electrocardiogram and Vectorcardiogram with Constitutional Variables in 518 Normal Men, Circ., 35:536

Ishikawa, K., 1976, Correlation coefficients for electrocardiographic and constitutional variables, Am. Heart J., 92:152.

Nemati, M., McCaughan, D., Doyle, J.T., and Pipberger, H.V., 1977, The Influence of Constitutional Variables on Orthogonal Electrocardiogram of Normal Women, Circ., 56:989,

Eskola, H.J., Malmivuo, J.A.V., Nousiainen, J.J.O. and Lekkala, J.O., 1987, Corrected Unipositional Lead system for Vector Magnetocardiography, IEEE Trans. on Biomed. Eng., **BME-34**:81.

Oja, O.S., Nousiainen, J. and Malmivuo, J., 1988, Magnetocardiogram in Left Ventricular Hypertrophy, in: "Biomagnetism '87," Atsumi, K., Kotani, M., Ueno, S., Katila, T. and Williamson, S. eds. Tokyo Denki University Press, Tokyo

MAGNETOCARDIOGRAPHY IN PATIENTS WITH CARDIOMYOPATHY AND OPERATED CONGENITAL HEART DISEASE

L. Schmitz, K. Brockmeier, L. Trahms* and S. N. Erné*

Department of Pediatric Cardiology, KAVH, Freie Universität, Berlin
*Physikalisch- Technische Bundesanstalt (PTB), Institut Berlin D-1000 Berlin, FRG

INTRODUCTION

Patients with dilated and hypertrophic cardiomyopathies represent a high risk group for sudden cardiac death (Griffin et al.,1988 and McKenna et al.,1988). Usually they die from ventricular fibrillation as a result of micro-reentry mechanisms in the severely compromised myocardium (Swerdlow et al.,1983). Most often the left ventricular myocardium is involved. These cardiomyopathies are either acquired as the result of viral infections or they are the result of an inborn error of metabolism. A comparable anatomical and functional state of the heart can be seen after surgical correction of Tetrade of Fallot (TOF). These hearts offer a suitable model of abnormal pressure and/or volume load of the right ventricular myocardium. The significant mortality and morbidity in this patient group is also related to severe ventricular arrhythmias. Because mortality in both groups of patients depends on pathological electrophysiological phenomena, which usually can only be studied by invasive catheter procedures, the possibility of a non-invasive assessment of these changes by magnetocardiography is an intriguing idea.

This study was conducted to describe the diagnostic power of the MCG in the detection of electrophysiological disturbances of the right or left ventricle.

METHODS

Using the biomagnetic facilities of the PTB, described elsewhere (Erné et al.,1981), we examined the fluctuations of magnetic fields within the ST-segment. The measurements were performed normal to the anterior chest wall according to the Finnish standard grid. The data evaluation procedure was standardized following ref. (Erné et al.,1983): 1. Data reduction algorithm were applied to obtain a noise reduced set of 36 averaged MCG corresponding to the 36 positions (Erné et al.,1988). 2. Four instantaneous field distributions were selected during 75 ms starting at the end of the QRS-complex with a time gap of 25 ms each, 3. For each subsequent pair of field distributions, the correlation coefficient was calculated. The sum of the three coefficients called "relative smoothness" (RS) reaches a maximum value of 3, if no fluctuations occur and moves towards 0 if rapid and profound changes occur. Standardized methods for routine follow-up as Holter monitoring, stress-testing and echocardiography were done at the same time and compared with the MCG-data.

Advances in Biomagnetism
Edited by S.J. Williamson *et al.*
Plenum Press, New York

PATIENTS

Cardiomyopathy. The study group of ten patients covers the entire spectrum of primary and secondary cardiomyopathies of the right and the left ventricle. Both symptomatic and asymptomatic patients were included. An Arrhythmogenic Right Ventricular Dysplasia (ARVD) was diagnosed in one patient, a dilated cardiomyopathy of the right ventricle (dil CMP RV) of unknown origin in another patient (SUKR), and dilatation after operation of atrial shunts in another two patients. In the two patients with dilated cardiomyopathy of the left ventricle (dil CMP LV), one was idiopathic inherited, the other due to severe aortic valve incompetence (AoI). Among the four patients with hypertrophic obstructive cardiomyopathy (HOCM) one patient had a secondary form due to severe valvular aortic stenosis.

Tetralogy of Fallot. Four patients with good results were compared with two patients with poor results (dilated cardiomyopathy of the right ventricle due to pulmonary valve incompetence) after surgical correction.

RESULTS

Cardiomyopathy. One of the lowest RS-scores within the whole study group was found in a patient (STSC) with ARVD and repeated life threatening arrhythmias completely resistant to drug treatment (Tab.1). This patient died during the course of the study as a result of ventricular fibrillation. The patient (ERVO) with an end stage dilated CMP of the LV is accepted for heart transplantation and suffers from recurrent ventricular flutter. For ethical reasons he could only be investigated under antiarrhythmic medication so that his relatively high RS-score of 1.8 might be influenced by an effective treatment. In three patients with dilated CMP of the RV RS-scores correlated with the presence (GEVO 1.1) and with the absence (MAGA 2.1; SUKR 2.6) of ventricular arrhythmias during Holter monitoring and load testing.

Tab. 1. Risk analysis in Cardiomyopathy

	Patient	Age	Diagnosis	Events	NYHA	SCORE	Medication
1	STSC	13	ARVD	VT,syncope	II	0.9	ß-blocker
		14	ARVD	VT	II	0.8	ß-blocker
2	SUKR	17	dil CMP RV	none	I	2.6	none
3	GEVO	14	dil CMP RV	VT	II	1.1	none
4	MAGA	15	dil CMP RV	none	I	2.1	none
5	ERVO	36	dil CMP LV	VT,syncope	II	1.8	ß-blocker
6	HUMS	16	AoI dil LV	none	II	2.8	digitalis
7	RARO	11	HOCM	none	I	2.7	none
8	DOKI	45	HOCM	none	II	1.8	ß-blocker
9	DAKI	16	HOCM	none	III	1.4	ß-blocker
10	HOHI	19	HOCM	syncope	II	0.8	none

The patient (HOHI) with a secondary form of HOCM due to a stenotic outgrown artificial aortic valve suffers from repeated cardiac syncopes due to ventricular tachycardias. In this patient for many years repeated investigations (Holter and load test) failed to demonstrate a high risk form of arrhythmia so that the low RS-score (0.8) was the only sign of a severe electrophysiological disease. Two months ago we succeeded in monitoring of nonsustained ventricular tachycardias in this young man. In the adolescent (HUMS) with dilated LV as a result of aortic regurgitation we could not find dangerous ventricular premature beats, and RS-score showed to be normal (2.8). In patients with primary HOCM, those without demonstrable ventricular arrhythmias (RARO and DOKI) had normal RS-scores (2.8 and 2.7) at least under medication. The worst clinical course in HOCM (DAKI) accordingly showed a depressed RS-score (1.4) even under drug treatment and after operation.

Tetralogy of Fallot. Seven magnetocardiograms in six patients showed the following results: in two patients with moderate pressure load of the right ventricle but without volume load the RS-scores were 2.9 and 2.7 (Tab.2). In these patients no risk criteria could be found in ECG, Holter monitoring and echo. All the other patients with combined pressure and volume load showed a score ranging between 2.4 and 1.4 dependent on the severity of the volume load. Accordingly in those patients we could demonstrate higher degrees of ventricular arrhythmias during Holter monitoring (3 pts) and load testing (4 pts). One of these patients (RS = 1.4) had three cardiac syncopes in his recent history. The incomplete right bundle branch block did not influence the score per se.

Tab. 2. Risk analysis in TOF

	Pts	Age	Events	RV	SCORE
1	KOSC	7	none	mild PS	2.9
2	MADA	11	none	mild PS	2.4
3	DEBO	9	none	mild PS	2.7
4	STWE	9	none	mild PS	2.1
5	ANBL	14	syncopes	dil CMP	1.4
6	CIAC	12	NYHA III + VT	severe PS	1.5
		13	NYHA II	dil CMP	2.1

DISCUSSION

Previous studies (Schmitz,1988) done in 62 healthy volunteers demonstrated the normal values of the RS-score to be in the range between 2.5 and 2.95. A significant difference in the RS-scores between normals and patients with known electrophysiological disturbances could be demonstrated. Furthermore, we could demonstrate that the depression in RS-score is obviously mainly dependent on the electrophysiological state of the myocardium, more than on its pure anatomical shape (Fig. 1).

Patients with the most advanced electrophysiological disturbances show the lowest RS-scores corresponding with their high risk of sudden cardiac death. Patients with low degree ventricular arrhythmias and patients under effective drug treatment show a less decreased RS-score according to their lower risk. In patients with TOF RS-scoring in the ST-segment showed results according well to clinical findings and to the results of approved diagnostical procedures so that a clear discrimination of the patient with electrophysiological disturbance was possible. MCG seems to react equally sensitive on the arrhythmogenic activities in both the left and right ventricle. Our findings demonstrate that magnetocardiography using the RS-score is an appropriate method to describe the individual risk for the development of life threatening arrhythmias in patients with different underlying cardiac diseases.

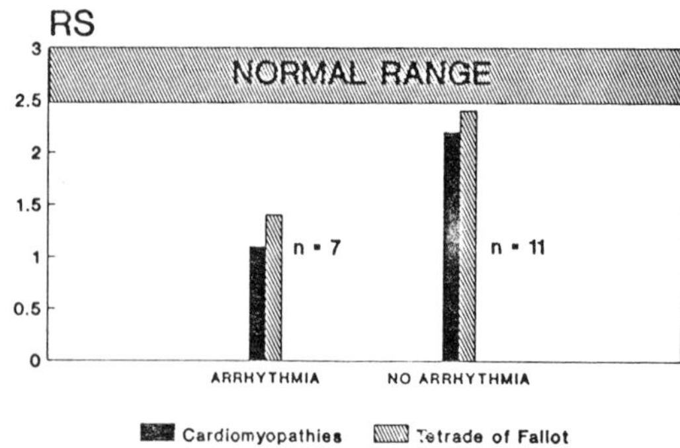

Fig.1. Dependence of the RS-score on the anatomical state and electrophysiologic situation.

REFERENCES

Griffin, M.L., Hernandez, A., Martin, T.C. et al. (1988). Dilated cardiomyopathy in infants and children. J Am Coll Cardiol 11, 145-146.m

McKenna, W.J., Franklin, R.C., Nihoyannopoulos, P. et al. (1988). Arrhythmia and prognosis in infants, children and adolescents with hypertrophic cardiomyopathy. J Am Coll Cardiol 11, 147-153.

Swerdlow, C.D., Winkle, R.A., Mason, J.W. (1983). Determinants of survival in patients with ventricular tachyarrhythmias, N Engl J Med 308, 1436-1442.

Erné, S.N., Hahlbohm, H.-D., Scheer, H.J. et al. (1981). The Berlin Magnetic Shielded Room (BMSR): Section B - Performances. In: Erné, S.N., Hahlbohm, H.-D., and Lübbig, H., Biomagnetism. W. De Gruyter, Berlin, pp. 80 - 87.

Erné, S.N., Fenici, R.R., Hahlbohm, H.-D. et al. (1983). High resolution isofield mapping in magnetocardiography. Il Nuovo Cim 2D, 291-300.

Erné, S.N., Trahms, L., Trontelj, Z. (1988). Clustering - a novel approach for selected averaging of biomagnetic signals. In: Atsumi et al.Biomagnetism'87. Tokyo Denki University Press, Tokyo, pp. 298 - 301.

Schmitz, L. (1988) Magnetocardiography: The clinician's point of view. In: Atsumi et al.Biomagnetism'87. Tokyo Denki University Press, Tokyo, pp. 66-73.

THE MAGNETOCARDIOGRAM IN PATIENTS WITH SYSTOLIC AND DIASTOLIC OVERLOAD OF THE RIGHT VENTRICLE

Mariko Katayama, Masahiro Nomura, Katsusuke Watanabe, Akemi Takeuchi, Kazuya Fujino, Yutaka Nakaya, and Hiroyoshi Mori

The Second Department of Internal Medicine
School of Medicine, The University of Tokushima
Tokushima, Japan

The second derivative gradiometer is expected to detect the current source from the right ventricle more specifically, where it is located close to the anterior chest wall because of its unique system. Therefore, we investigated the magnetocardiogram (MCG) in patients with right ventricular overload (RVO), and correlated the MCG findings with hemodynamic parameters. This study was also aimed to diagnose RVO in the presence of right bundle branch block (RBBB), which so far has been considered to be difficult to diagnose by the conventional electrocardiogram (ECG).

METHODS

The control group consisted of 35 healthy subjects (48.7 ± 16.7 years). The RVO group was divided into two groups; (1) RVO-s group: 37 patients with systolic overload of the right ventricle (44.9 ± 10.4 years). Of these patients, 25 mitral stenosis, 6 pulmonary stenosis, 4 primary pulmonary hypertention and 2 Tetralogy of Fallot. (2) RVO-d group: 14 patients with diastolic overload of the right ventricle (44.9 ± 16.6 years). All of these patients were atrial septal defect. All of the RVO group underwent right heart catheterization. In order to diagnose RVO in the presence of RBBB, we also studied the patients RBBB group (17 patients, 55.4 ± 17.3 years) with RBBB without any underlying diseases which cause RVO.

The MCG was recorded at the 36 points over the anterior chest wall (Fig.1) with a second-derivative SQUID gradiometer (BTi,model BMP), and the magnetic field perpendicular to the anterior chest wall was measured. The MCG was recorded at a paper speed of 25 mm/sec with the lead II ECG as a time reference.

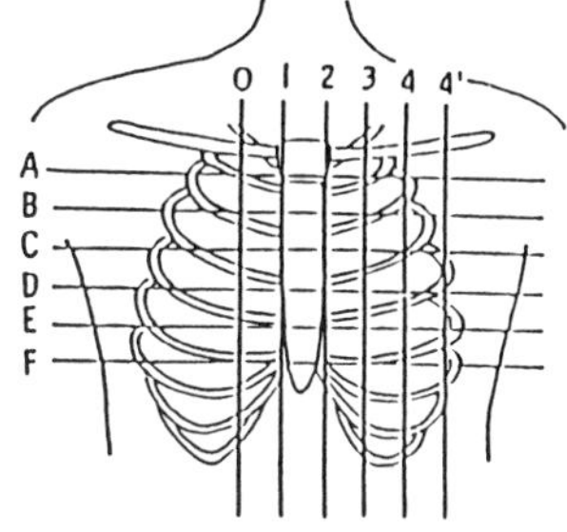

Fig. 1 Recording sites of MCG

RESULTS

The control group (Fig.2): The QRS wave of the MCG of normal subjects showed QS or Qr pattern in the upper portion, qR or R pattern in the lower portion of the anterior chest wall.

The RBBB group (Fig.3): The QRS wave of the MCG showed Qr pattern in the upper portion and Rs pattern in the lower portion.

The RVO group: (1)RVO-s group; Fig. 4 shows the standard ECG and MCG of a patient with primary pulmonary hypertention. The ECG showed a tall R wave in V_{1-2}, and a deep S wave in V_{2-6}, suggesting the presence of right ventricular systolic overload. The MCG showed a tall R wave at B-1,-2 and -3, and C-1,-2 and -3, and a deep S wave at E,F-1,-2 and -3, suggesting an increase in rightward force. (2) RVO-d group; Fig. 5 shows the standard ECG and MCG of a

Advances in Biomagnetism
Edited by S.J. Williamson *et al.*
Plenum Press, New York

patient with atrial septal defect. The ECG showed right axis deviation and right bundle branch block pattern. The MCG showed a tall R wave at B-1,-2,-3 and -4, and C-1,-2,-3 and -4, and a deep S wave at E-1,-2,-3 and -4, and F-1,-2,-3 and -4, suggesting increased rightward force.

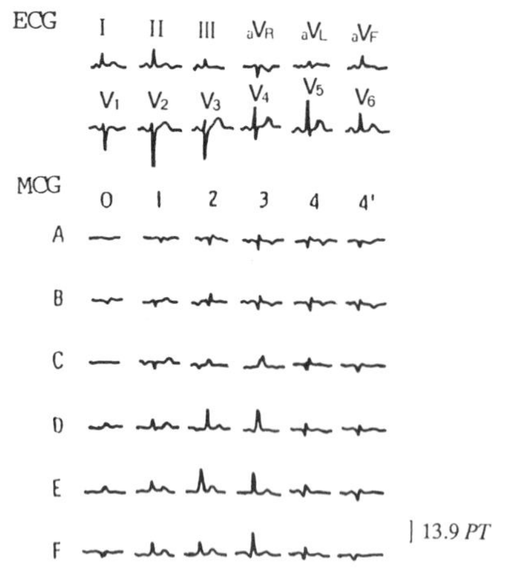

Fig.2 ECG and MCG of a normal subject (51 years, male)

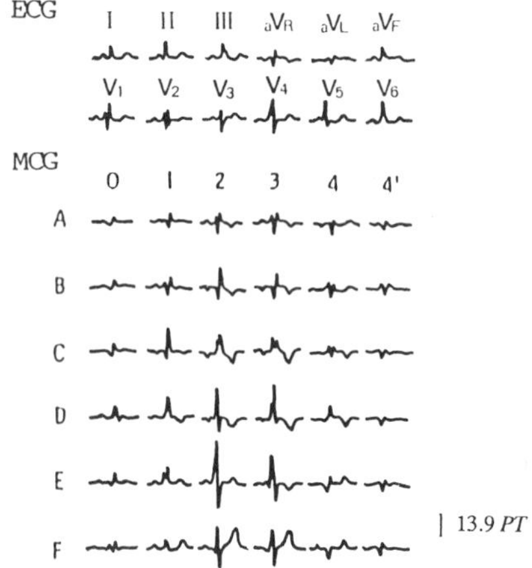

Fig.3 ECG and MCG of a RBBB patient (49 years, female)

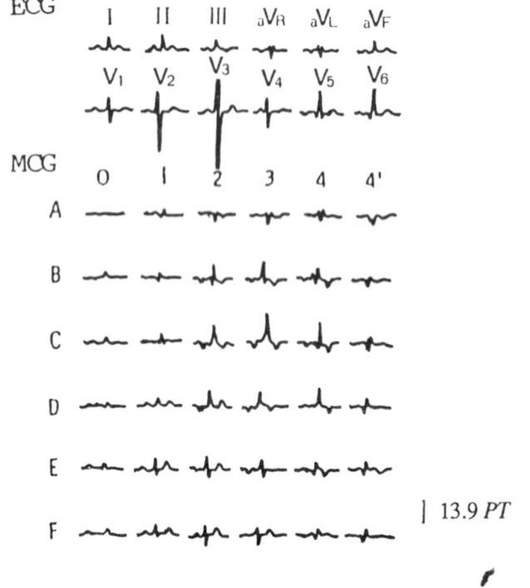

Fig.4 ECG and MCG of a patient with primary pulmonary hypertention (46 years, female)

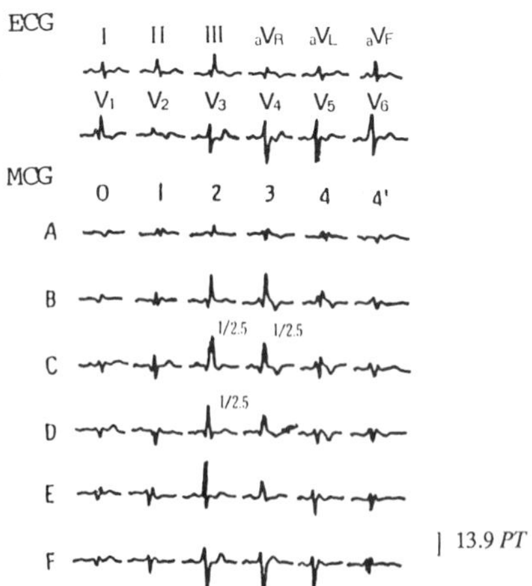

Fig.5 ECG and MCG of a patient with atrial septal defect (55 years, female)

Table 1 Sensitivity (%) of the MCG and ECG criteria

criteria		control (n=35)	RBBB (n=17)	RVO-s (n=37)	RVO-d (n=14)
ECG criteria (Roman et al.)		6%	65%	19%	64%
MCG criteria	$R_{B-2} \geq 13 \times 10^{-12}$ tesla	3%	12%	24%	43%
	$S_{F-3} \geq 3 \times 10^{-12}$ tesla	6%	77%	38%	86%
	$(R_{B-2}+S_{F-3})/(R_{F-3}+S_{B-2}) \geq 1.0$	9%	77%	30%	93%

Comparison between ECG and MCG: We have already reported that the typical MCG finding in RVO were an increase in amplitude of the R wave in the upper portion at the anterior chest, and of the S wave in the lower portion. MCG criteria for the diagnosis of RVO were set as follows on the basis of mean ± 2SD (SD = standard deviation) of the normal values. (1) R wave at B-2 (R_{B-2}) $\geq 13 \times 10^{-12}$ tesla, (2) S wave at F-3 (S_{F-3}) $\geq 3 \times 10^{-12}$ tesla, (3) $(R_{B-2} + S_{F-3})/(R_{F-3} + S_{B-2}) \geq 1.0$.

Table 1 shows the reliability of MCG and ECG criteria for the diagnosis of RVO. The criteria proposed by Roman et al. were used as ECG criteria in the RVO-s group. The positivities were 24-38% by the MCG criteria and 19% by the ECG criteria, and in the RVO-d group 43-93% by the MCG criteria and 64% by the ECG criteria, respectively. But the RBBB group showed higher false positivity. Therefore we set different MCG criteria for RVO-d group with RBBB based on the mean ± 2SD of the RBBB, i.e., (1) $R_{C-3} \geq 25 \times 10^{-12}$ tesla, (2) $S_{F-4} \geq 11 \times 10^{-12}$ tesla.

Table 2 shows the sensitivities and specificities of the ECG and MCG criteria in the systolic and diastolic overload. The RVO group was divided into three subgroups according to the right ventricular pressure. (1) RVO-s group: The MCG and ECG criteria showed similar specificities. In the patients with a right ventricular pressure of >30mmHg, the MCG criteria showed higher sensitivities than the ECG criteria ($p<0.05$). (2) RVO-d group: Sensitivity of the MCG criteria was slightly higher than that of the ECG, although the difference was not statistically significant. But the specificity of the MCG was significant higher than that of the ECG.

Table 2 Sensitivity and specificity of MCG and ECG criteria for the diagnosis of RVO

(1) RVO-s group (37 cases)

	right ventricular pressure (mmHg) 0-30	30-50	50-	specificity
ECG	0%	7%	38%	100%
MCG	0%	50%	85%	91%
	ns	p<0.05	p<0.05	ns

ns: not significant

(2) RVO-d group (14 cases)

	right ventricular pressure (mmHg) 0-30	30-50	50-	specificity
ECG	25%	33%	75%	35%
MCG	25%	33%	100%	94%
	ns	ns	ns	p<0.01

ns: not significant

Correlation of the MCG parameters and right ventricular pressure: Table 3 shows the coefficients of correlation of the MCG parameters and right ventricular systolic pressure. There was a significant correlation between the MCG parameters and right ventricular pressure.

Table 3 Coefficients of correlation (r) between MCG index and right ventricular systolic pressure

MCG index	r
R_{B-2}	0.58*
S_{F-3}	0.63*
$(R_{B-2}+S_{F-3})/(R_{F-3}+S_{B-2})$	0.45*
R_{C-3}	0.77*
S_{F-4}	0.40

*: $p<0.01$

DISCUSSION

Typical QRS pattern of the MCG in the MCG in the RVO group is an increase of the R wave in the upper portion, and of the S wave in the lower portion of the anterior chest wall, reflecting increased electromotive forces directed to the right. The MCG criteria for the diagnosis of RVO in this study showed significantly higher sensitivity or specificity than the ECG criteria in patients with RVO. In the patients with a right ventricular systolic pressure of more than 30mmHg, especially in those of more than 50mmHg, the sensitivity of the MCG criteria was much higher than that of the ECG criteria. Significant positive correlation was also found between MCG parameters and the right ventricular pressure. At the present time, ECG is widely used for the diagnosis of RVO, but its sensitivity and specificity are low. The higher sensitivity of the MCG criteria for the diagnosis of the RVO was considered to be due to the characteristics of the magnetic measurements which is different from that of the electric measurement, and the unique property of the second derivative gradiometer. The MCG gives better positional resolution and is more sensitive to detect a current source located closely to the anterior chest wall, such as the right ventricle. Therefore, the MCG seemed to be more useful for the diagnosis of RVO than the ECG, even in cases associated with RBBB.

MAGNETIC MICROPARTICLES CAN MEASURE WHOLE-BODY CLEARANCE, CELL ORGANELLE MOTIONS, AND PROTEIN POLYMER VISCOELASTICITY

Peter A. Valberg, Ken S. Zaner*

Respiratory Biology Program, Harvard University, School of Public Health
Boston, MA 02115
*Hematology-Oncology Section, Boston City Hospital, Boston, MA 02118

INTRODUCTION

Magnetic particles in the size range of 0.5 to 2 μm diameter can serve to quantify a number of disparate phenomena when these particles are enmeshed in tissues, cells, or polymer fluids. Proteins (including iron-containing proteins) and other tissue components are not ferromagnetic, but tiny ferromagnetic crystals can be introduced as probe particles. Such particles can be magnetically aligned by application of a strong magnetic field, after which they act in unison to produce a *remanent magnetic field* (RMF) measured at the body surface. The magnitude and time course of the RMF depend, respectively, on the quantity of magnetic material present and on the degree of particle motion. Magnetic particles can be used to examine clearance or dissolution of particulate material from the lungs, liver, or other organs. Particle rotation within the body or within cells causes the RMF to decay after magnetization, a phenomenon called *relaxation;* the initial magnitude of the RMF can be restored by remagnetization, and relaxation begins again. The decay rate of the RMF is related to the time constants of particle motions, and relaxation can noninvasively quantify cell organelle movement. A torque can be applied to magnetic particles by external fields, and the resulting rate of particle rotation depends on the viscoelasticity of the particle environment, e.g., airway mucus, lung surfactant, cytoplasm, or purified protein gels. When magnetic particles are ingested by cells, magnetic elutriation techniques can be used to separate cells into subpopulations according to the quantity of magnetic material they have internalized.

RETENTION AND CLEARANCE OF PARTICLES

Like *radioactivity, magnetism* can be used as a label for noninvasive quantification of particulate contaminants within body tissues. In occupational settings, some aerosols contain magnetic components which can serve as a tracer of lung retention [Cohen *et al,* 1981; Freedman *et al,* 1988; Kalliomäki *et al,* 1988]. Since magnetite is nearly insoluble at physiological pH, it makes an ideal test aerosol for investigating the fate of inhaled particles. The RMF outside the chest is related to lung content of magnetic material; measurements repeated over weeks or months, describe lung clearance curves [Valberg and Brain, 1979]. The iron in the magnetic particles can be neutron activated, and a comparison of RMF measurements with more traditional radiometric techniques has shown good agreement [Halpern *et al,* 1981].

CELL ORGANELLE MOTIONS AND CYTOPLASMIC CONSISTENCY

In humans and animals, RMF from lung-retained ferromagnetic particles drops rapidly over the first hour after magnetization, or *relaxes* [Cohen, 1973; Valberg and Brain, 1979]. The majority of this motion is due to particles which have become sequestered in lung cells, specifically, macrophages. These cells reside on lung surfaces and ingest the micrometer-sized magnetic particles into intracellular vesicles, and cytoplasmic streaming moves the phagocytized particles, causing decay of the RMF. Time-lapse video observation of the magnetization process and of the subsequent reorientation of γ-Fe_2O_3 particles has confirmed that relaxation is associated with motions of the macrophage cytoplasm; macrophages collected from lungs and studied in culture exhibit relaxation quantitatively similar to that seen in intact animals [Valberg, 1984; Valberg and Albertini, 1985]. The character of the relaxation curve can provide information about the intrapulmonary environment of particles and about cell health. Magnetometric studies of macrophages cultured *in vitro* have shown that relaxation is slowed by inhibitors of the metabolic enzymes involved in ATP production [Nemoto *et al,* 1989].

MOLECULAR DETERMINANTS OF CELL VISCOELASTICITY

Magnetometric viscoelastometry

Cytoplasm has the capacity to both generate force and resist deformation. However, little is known about the physical factors involved in cell spreading, locomotion, phagocytosis, organelle movement, and division. The properties of several mechanical and force-generating proteins in the cortical cytoplasm has been reviewed [Stossel, 1988]; the microfilament system is particularly important. It consists of filamentous actin (F-actin), a protein polymer that is ubiquitously present in motile cells. F-actin can be crosslinked by a 540 kD molecular weight protein known as actin binding protein (ABP) which gels F-actin by binding the filaments together into orthogonally-branched structures [Hartwig and Shevlin, 1986].

In order to interpret in more molecular terms the rheologic information being obtained from intact cells by the magnetic particle method [Valberg and Albertini, 1985], we used the same magnetic particle method to measure the viscoelastic properties of F-actin solutions and F-actin+ABP gels. The instrumental approach was to magnetically monitor the movement of tiny ferromagnetic particles enmeshed in F-actin. In contrast to conventional rheologic methods, which are "bulk" measurements not applicable to cytoplasm within individual cells, the magnetic particle method probes rheology at the "microscopic" level. Ferromagnetic particles can be magnetically aligned by application of a strong magnetic field, and the particle rotation can be followed magnetometrically by measuring the RMF. Since the fluxgate detectors are sensitive to the vector component of the RMF that is parallel to the initial direction of magnetization, any rotation of the particles decreases the net RMF sensed.

Magnetic microparticles were generated in aerosol form by controlled combustion of iron pentacarbonyl vapors [Valberg and Brain, 1979]. About 3 mg γ-Fe_2O_3 was collected on each of several filters for dispersion into test fluids. Particles were also sampled onto carbon-coated copper grids, and shadowed, for examination by electron microscopy. The appearance of the magnetic particles was crystalline, with individual units approximately 0.2μm diameter, and with agglomerates in chains about 0.5μm long. After viscous fluids or F-actin gels had been prepared with dispersed magnetic microparticles, the magnetic directions of particles were aligned using a pulsed magnetic field of 93 mT. The particles produced a weak RMF, which was measured in a magnetically-shielded apparatus with 4 fluxgate detectors [Valberg and Butler, 1987].

Magnetometric studies of viscosity standards

An RMF decrease for particles in test solutions results either from random, independent motion of each particle, driven by thermal energy (*relaxation*), or from the action of an externally-applied magnetic field (*twisting*). The direction of the twisting-field is set perpendicular to the direction of particle initial magnetization, and the magnetic torque created acts to rotate particles toward the direction of this applied field. Monitoring the RMF decrease can be used to quantify particle rotation in response to a known torque. The rate of particle rotation is related to the viscoelasticity of the medium trapping the particles [Valberg and Butler, 1987].

Both relaxation and twist were measured for particles suspended in Newtonian-viscosity standards (dimethylpolysiloxane fluids). The torque is proportional to the strength of the twisting field, but rotation of the particles is opposed by the viscosity of the medium. When the twisting field is first applied, it is perpendicular to the particle magnetic moments and torque is at a maximum. As particles begin to rotate toward the applied field, torque falls off; the maximum possible particle rotation is 90°. The RMF curve generated in this process (Fig. 1) provided a means of calculating the stress that the particles are applying to their environment as a function of particle magnetic orientation relative to the applied field.

Particle rotation in a 100 Pa-s viscosity standard is shown in Fig. 1. The vertical axis gives the magnitude of the measured RMF; additional vertical scales show the corresponding angle of particle rotation in degrees, and the stress being applied to the particles in dy/cm^2. In this inertialess situation, magnetic torque (τ) and shear stress ($\eta\omega V$) are always in balance; the mathematical form of this curve can be derived [Valberg and Butler, 1987]. If $B_r(t)$ is the RMF at time t and B_{r0} is the initial RMF, their relationship to θ and t is (if $\theta=\pi/2$ at $t=0$)

$$B_r(t) = B_{r0} \sin\theta \qquad \text{where } \theta \text{ is related to time by} \qquad \ln\tan(\theta/2) = -t\,c/\eta$$

η is the viscosity of the dispersing fluid and c is the magnitude of the stress applied by the twisting field at $t=0$. Linear regression of $[\ln\tan(\theta/2)]$ versus t, for the data on Fig. 1 yields $c = 10.9$ dy/cm^2. This analysis is independent of particle diameter. Relaxation due to Brownian motions of magnetic particles suspended in a viscous fluid is given by [Nemoto, 1982] :

$$B_r(t) = e^{-\lambda t} \qquad \text{where} \qquad \lambda = 2kT/\pi\eta d^3$$

The relaxation curve in Fig. 1 gives particle hydrodynamic diameter as 0.61μm.

Magnetometric studies of F-actin

G-actin was purified from an acetone powder of rabbit skeletal muscle. Actin-binding protein (ABP) was purified from rabbit lung macrophages. G-actin with or without ABP was allowed to polymerize after magnetic iron oxide particles (γ-Fe_2O_3) were added at a concentration of 50μg/ml. Magnetic particle volume was approximately 0.001% of gel volume. When ABP was used, the molar ratio of ABP:G-actin was 1:200. Light microscopy showed the particles to be

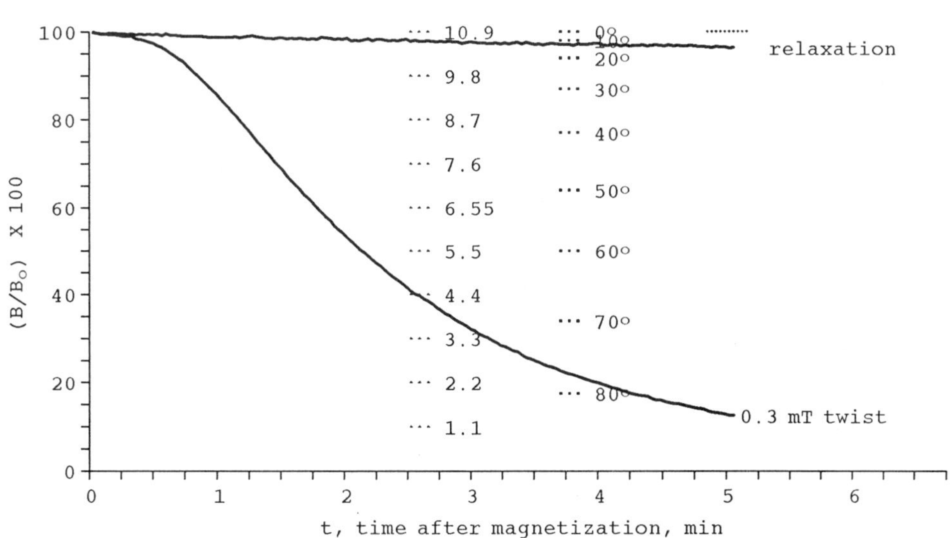

Fig. 1. Remanent magnetic field (RMF) as a function of time for particles suspended in 100 Pa-s dimethylpolysiloxane. Upper curve: relaxation. Lower curve: 0.3 mT twisting field perpendicular to the original magnetization (see text).

uniformly dispersed throughout the gel; over 24 hrs there was no indication of particle sedimentation. Particle entrapment was quite efficient; at an actin concentration of 6 mg/ml, the total length of F-actin is about 2×10^{10}cm of filament per ml of gel, and inter-filament separation is less than 0.1μm.

F-actin gels were maintained at 25°C, and we monitored the RMF from particles enmeshed in the F-actin gels while applying twisting magnetic fields from 0 to 3.0 mT. The F-actin gel opposed the particle rotation by viscous and elastic forces. The twisting field was turned on and off in one-minute intervals. The rate at which particles reoriented toward the twisting field and then recoiled, was recorded over 5 min via the RMF produced.

The mechanical response of F-actin (4 mg/ml) over a variety of strains is shown in Fig. 2. As the twisting force increased from 0.15 mT to 3.00 mT, there was a progressive increase in the rotation of the particles. In addition, the recovery of strain during 1 min intervals of stress-release progressively decreased. A subsequent sequence of progressively increasing twisting pulses yielded nearly superimposable results, suggesting that twisting of the particles was not irreversibly disrupting F-actin structure. This is further supported by the fact that a second relaxation measurement, made by remagnetizing the particles, was unchanged from relaxation measured prior to the particle twisting protocol; thus, particle diffusion in the F-actin was not being enhanced by particle twisting. Table I gives the "secant modulus" at 60 seconds, G_{60}, defined as the stress/strain ratio after 60 seconds of twisting. The modulus is nearly constant over the range of twisting strengths examined, and the second set of measurements is close to the first. The rigidities obtained by this technique are within a factor of two of previously-reported values using other, more conventional techniques [Zaner and Stossel, 1983]. The viscosity, η, can be calculated from the curves in Fig. 2, and for actin concentrations of 4 mg/ml was found to be 200 Pa-s at a shear rate of 0.0025 sec^{-1}. This value is also in reasonable agreement with previously reported values [Zaner and Stossel, 1983].

The effect of ABP on F-actin is shown in Fig. 3. The twisting field for both RMF curves is 3.0 mT, and equivalent concentrations of F-actin (4mg/ml) are shown. The upper curve is for F-actin plus ABP and the lower curve is without ABP. For F-actin+ABP, applying a stress of 3.0 mT results in an average particle rotation of 40° at the end of 1 min, but a complete recovery of

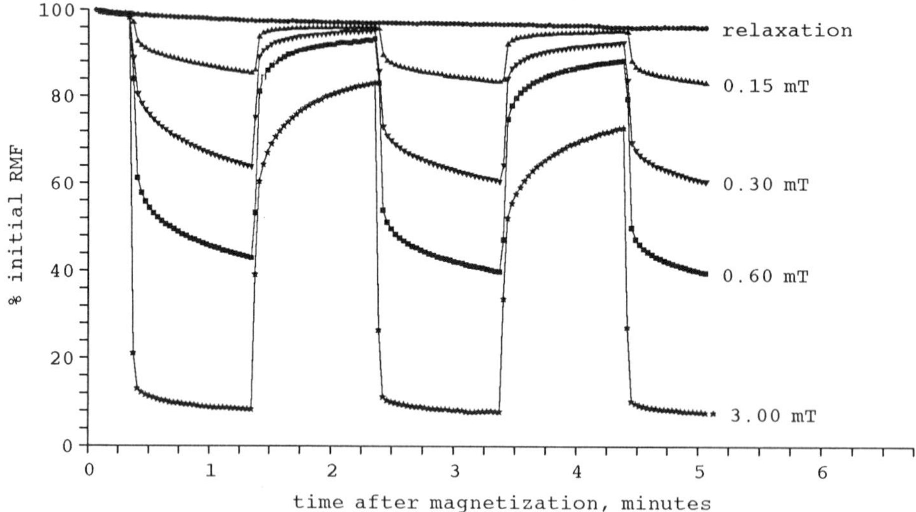

Fig. 2. Particles in F-actin show progressively larger rotations as the magnitude of the stress, i.e., the twisting field was increased from 0.15 to 3.00 mT.

Table 1

G_{60} = stress-strain ratio at 60 sec after stress application; F-actin concentration = 4 mg/ml

twisting field, mT	first trial (F-actin only) stress σ dy/cm^2	strain γ radians	G_{60} σ/γ dy/cm^2	second trial (F-actin only) stress σ dy/cm^2	strain γ radians	G_{60} σ/γ dy/cm^2
0.15	4.6	0.55	8.3	4.6	0.56	8.1
0.30	7.0	0.87	8.1	6.6	0.92	7.2
0.60	9.2	1.14	8.1	8.8	1.16	7.6
3.00	11.8	1.46	8.1	11.5	1.47	7.8
	first trial (F-actin + ABP)			second trial (F-actin + ABP)		
6.0	21.4	0.185	116	21.3	0.190	112
30.0	90.5	0.591	153	89.3	0.609	147

strain after stress release. At a twisting field of 0.6 mT, particle rotation is less than 10°. The G_{60} at 3.0 mT is about 153 dy/cm^2, somewhat higher than at 0.6 mT, where the G_{60} is 116 dy/cm^2 (Table 1). The compliance is time-independent over the course of the measurement, and is nearly 20-fold lower than the actin control. This apparent increase in rigidity (~20×) most likely represents the fact that when the filaments are physically crosslinked into a network, movement of the particles cannot occur by rotation of the filaments, but now requires bending of the filaments near the crosslink point.

Lung macrophages

Hamster lung macrophages were obtained by lung lavage from animals that had breathed magnetic iron oxide aerosol [Valberg and Albertini, 1985]. During magnetometry measurements,

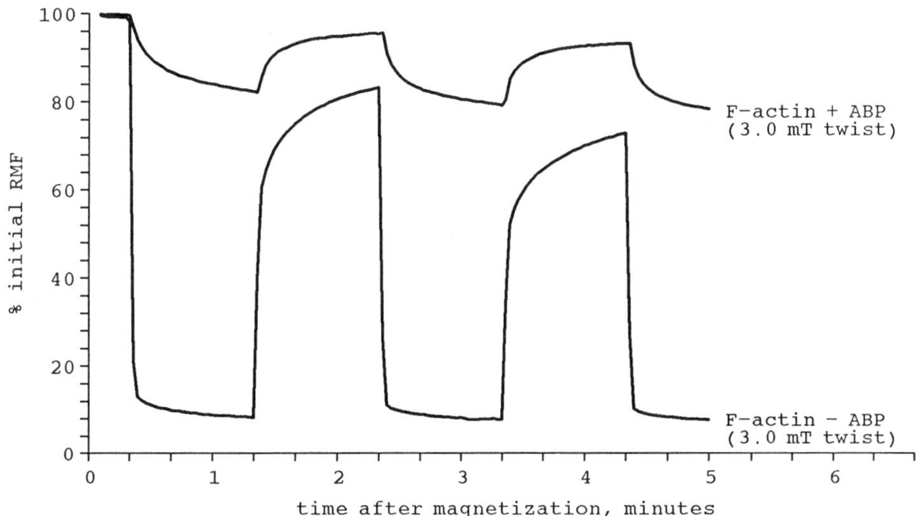

Fig. 3. ABP addition dramatically increases the rigidity of F-actin.

cells were maintained in culture medium, adherent to the bottom of glass vials, oxygenated, and at 37°C. The RMF curves were generated from ~10^5 adherent cells containing a total of about 7 μg of ingested γ-Fe_2O_3. Fig. 4 depicts both relaxation and twist response for particles within hamster lung macrophages. The upper curve shows that *relaxation* for particles in cell vesicles is quite rapid, reflecting active biochemical processes moving and rotating cell organelles [Valberg, 1984]. The lower curve shows the result of applying the same twist protocol (2.5 mT) to the macrophages as was used for F-actin gels. A comparison of this result to Fig. 3 shows that the elasticity of the cytoplasm is better approximated by an F-actin+ABP gel than an F-actin solution. Viscous losses appear to be greater, in that less of the particle orientation is recovered upon release of the twist. From the RMF curve, we can calculate that at a shear rate of 0.002 sec^{-1} the apparent viscosity of the cytoplasm is 2500 Pa-s, in agreement with other reports [Buxbaum *et al*, 1987]. [Valberg and Feldman, 1987].

Discussion

Measurements of cell mechanical properties help identify the mechanisms by which cells can maintain and alter their shape. Magnetometric tracking of cell-ingested ferric oxide particles is one of the few methods which can provide these data. By extending this method to model protein systems approximating the conditions present in cortical cytoplasm, we generated data for interpreting the *mechanical* properties of living cytoplasm in molecular terms. The behavior of actin-ABP gels, as measured by magnetometry, is qualitatively in good agreement with previous reports; the magnetic-particle approach gives a compliance for F-actin about a factor of two lower, and for F-actin+ABP about six-fold lower as compared to bulk viscoelastometry measurements [Zaner, 1986]. Traditional viscoelastometers utilize a single centrally-located "macroscopic" source of shear. Typically, the sample is placed between two surfaces, and the displacement or strain of the sample is observed in response to an applied force or stress. The validity of the measurement is based on the assumption that the sample is continuous and homogeneous in the region between the surfaces and that shear takes place uniformly in this region. Heterogeneity in the sample would bias the results toward the properties of those areas that sheared

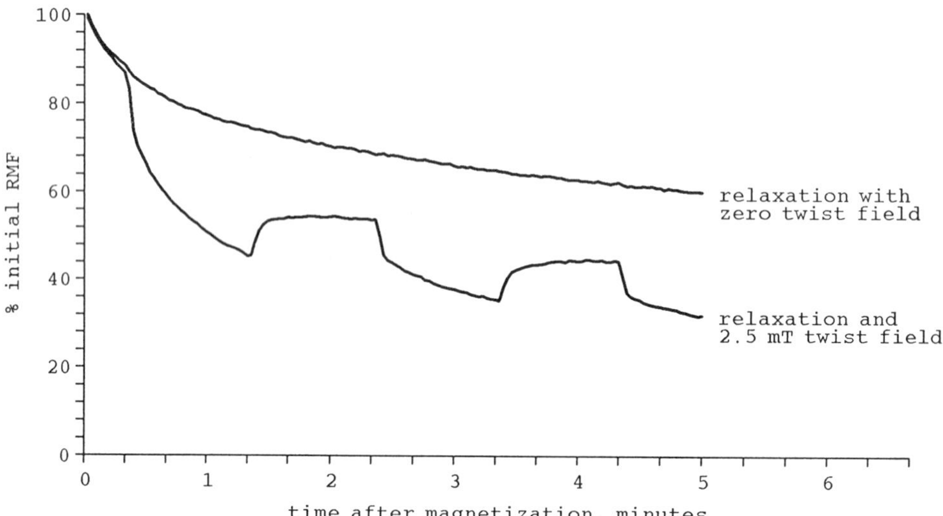

Fig. 4. RMF curves for particles within lung macrophages maintained in culture at 37°C. Upper curve: organelle motions cause rapid relaxation. Lower curve: 2.5 mT twisting causes additional decrement in the RMF, and indicates that the cell interior has high apparent viscosity (see text).

more readily. Magnetic particles provide "dispersed", microscopic shear locations, and the method produces a measurement which reflects the local environment or individual particles. Microscopic rheology would be less affected by long range heterogeneity or domain-like structure, and a lower compliance would be expected.

CONCLUSIONS

Magnetic particles can be either phagocytized by cells into intracytoplasmic vesicles or suspended in purified protein gels. Particle orientation and realignment can be carried out nonoptically *in vivo* and *in vitro*. Organelle motions, diffusion mobility, rigidity, and viscosity can be extracted from the RMF curves.

REFERENCES

Buxbaum, R.E., T. Dennerll, S. Weiss, and S.R. Heidemann, 1987, F-actin and microtubule suspensions as indeterminate fluids. *Science.* **235:** 1511.

Cohen, D., 1973, Ferromagnetic contaminants in the lungs and other organs of the body. *Science.* **180,** 745.

Cohen, D., T.S. Crowther, G.W. Gibbs, and M.R. Becklake., 1981, Magnetic lung measurements in relation to occupational exposure in asbestos miners and millers of Quebec. *Environ. Res.* **26,** 535.

Freedman, A.P., S.E. Robinson, and M.R. Street., 1988, Magnetopneumographic study of human alveolar clearance in health and disease. *J. occup. Hyg.* **32,** (Supp.1) 809.

Halpern, M., S.J. Williamson, D.M. Spektor, R.B. Schlesinger, and M. Lippmann., 1981, Remanent magnetic fields for measuring particle retention and distribution in the lungs. *Expt. Lung Res.* **2,** 27.

Hartwig, J.H., and P. Shevlin, 1986, The architecture of actin filaments and the ultrastructural location of actin-binding protein in the periphery of lung macrophages. *J. Cell Biol.* **103:** 1007.

Kalliomäki, K., P.L. Kalliomäki, and M. Molianen, 1988, Relaxation studies among mild steel (MS) and stainless steel (SS) welders. *In:* Biomagnetism '87. K.Atsumi, M.Kotani, S.Ueno, T.Katila, S.J.Williamson, editors. Tokyo Denki University Press, Tokyo, pp. 382.

Nemoto, I., 1982, A model of magnetization and relaxation of ferrimagnetic particles in the lungs. *IEEE Trans. Biomed. Eng.* **BME-29:** 745.

Nemoto, I., K. Ogura, and H. Toyotama, 1989, Estimation of the energy of cytoplasmic movements by magnetometry: Effects of temperature and intracellular concentration of ATP. *IEEE Trans. Biomed. Eng.* (in press).

Stossel, T.P., 1988, The mechanical properties of white blood cells. *In:* Inflammation: Basic Principles and Clinical Correlates. J.I. Gallin, I.M. Goldstein and R. Snyderman, editors. Raven Press, New York 325.

Valberg, P.A., 1984, Magnetometry of ingested particles in pulmonary macrophages. *Science.* **224,** 513.

Valberg, P.A., and D.F. Albertini, 1985, Cytoplasmic motions, rheology, and structure probed by a novel magnetic particle method. *J. Cell Biol.* **101:** 130.

Valberg, P.A., and J.D. Brain, 1979, Generation and use of three types of iron-oxide aerosol. *Am. Rev. Respir. Dis.* **120:** 1013.

Valberg, P.A., and J.P. Butler, 1987, Magnetic particle motions within living cells: Physical theory and techniques. *Biophys. J.* **52:** 537.

Zaner, K.S., 1986, The effect of the 540-kilodalton actin cross-linking protein, actin binding protein, on the mechanical properties of F-actin. *J. Biol. Chem.* **261:** 7615.

Zaner, K.S., and T.P. Stossel, 1983, Physical basis of the rheologic properties of F-actin. *J. Biol. Chem.* **258:** 11004.

ESTIMATION OF ENERGY OF INTRACELLULAR MOVEMENT AND APPARENT VISCOSITY BY MAGNETOMETRY

Iku Nemoto, Kazuhito Ogura* and Hiroyuki Waki
Department of Methematical Sciences,
Tokyo Denki University, Hatoyama, Saitama, Japan
*Stanley Electric Company
Tokodai, Tsukuba, Ibaragi, Japan

INTRODUCTION

Magnetometry has been employed to investigate intracellular movements by several researchers [1-6]. The principle is quite simple: Ferrimagnetic particles are introduced into pulmonary macrophages through phagocytosis. The particles are magnetized by a strong external magnetic field so that the magnetic moments of the phagosomes and secondary lysosomes containing the particles (hereafter referred to as phagosomes for simplicity) get aligned in the direction of the magnetizing field. The remanent magnetic field produced by the particles (RMF) can be measured by a flux-gate magnetometer and is a measure of the intracellular movements of the phagosomes. The magnetized particles can be manipulated by a weak field, and the measurement of the cellular field yields information about the energy E_r responsible for randomization of the orientations of the phagosomes and the apparent viscosity η of the medium surrounding the phagosomes.

We estimated the apparent viscosity by two methods. The first method combines the relaxation measurement and what we call 'secondary magnetization'. The other method measures the dynamic behavior of phagosomes under an external field of medium strength. The estimates of the apparent viscosity by the two methods gave contradicting results when their dependencies on intracellular ATP concentration were investigated. The purpose of the present paper is to present a model which explains these contradicting results.

THE MODEL

First we briefly review the Brownian-motion model[1] of the motion of the phagosomes. By Brownian Motion, we do not necessarily imply thermal energy, but use the term in the mathematical sense. We assume that phagosomes undergo rotational Brownian motions (RBM) due to active movements of the surrounding structures. Let r, η, H, and μ denote the radius of the phagosome, the apparent viscosity of the surrounding medium, the intensity of the external magnetic field and the magnetic moment of the phagosome (due of course to the magnetized particles), respectively. The probability density $p(\theta, t)$ of the orientation of the moment of the phagosome, where t is the time and θ the angle shown in Fig. 1, is governed by the following partial differential equation:

Advances in Biomagnetism
Edited by S.J. Williamson *et al.*
Plenum Press, New York

$$\frac{\partial p}{\partial t} = \frac{1}{\sin\theta}\frac{\partial}{\partial\theta}\left[\sin\theta\left(D\frac{\partial p}{\partial\theta} + \frac{\mu H\sin\theta}{\zeta}p\right)\right] \tag{1}$$

where the diffusion constant D is given by $E_r/8\pi r^3\eta$. In the equilibrium state under H, the field produced by the particle-containing cells is proportional to

$$B_H = \coth a - 1/a \ , \ a = \mu H/E_r \ . \tag{2}$$

Therefore, one can estimate E_r by the measurement of B_H. When the external field is removed, the cell field decays (relaxation) according to

$$B(t) = B_H \exp\left\{-\frac{E_r t}{4\pi r^3\eta}\right\} . \tag{3}$$

Therefore, combining this relaxation measurement with the equilibrium measurement, one can also estimate η. We denote the apparent viscosity thus estimated by η_s.

EFFECTS OF ATP CONCENTRATION

Effects of intracellular ATP concentration on E_r and on η_s were investigated. The results reported in [4] show that E_r heavily depends on ATP concentration whereas η_s was constant over the range of the ATP concentration employed in the experiments. This result is interesting but somewhat intriguing, considering that the deficiency of ATP causes the state of rigor in the muscle. The apparent viscosity can be measured *directly* by applying a magnetic field of an appropriate intensity such that the field does not change the magnetization of each particle and yet its magnetic potential energy on the particle is much stronger than E_r. We denote by η_t the apparent viscosity estimated by this way. (For this purpose, Valberg [5] used a field perpendicular to the original magnetization. He called this method 'twisting'.) Fig. 2 shows the result. The cells were first strongly magnetized and then incubated for $\simeq$1 hour. During the incubation period, relaxation took place and the cell field decreased to 10-15% of the saturation value. KCN was then added to the cells to lower the ATP concentration. After another 30 minutes, we applied a field of $\simeq$6mT for 12s and the RMF was measured. The figure shows that when ATP concentration was lowered, the cell field did not go back up so much as the control, indicating that the apprent viscosity η_t was larger than the control. To estimate the increase in η_s, the theoretical magnetization curve[1] was used which is shown in the right portion of Fig. 2. This curve is expressed by

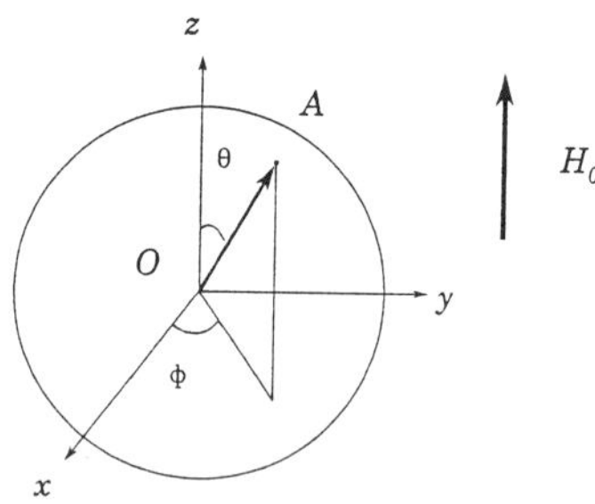

Fig. 1 The polar coordinates.

$$B(t) = -1 + \frac{2}{1-e^{-\gamma t}} - \frac{2e^{-\gamma t}\gamma t}{(1-e^{-\gamma t})^2}, \qquad \gamma = \frac{\mu H}{4\pi r^3 \eta_t} \tag{4}$$

Comaparison of l_1 with l_2 in the figure shows that in the ATP deficiency condition η_t was about 40% of the control value.

We thus have a situation where the two estimates η_s and η_t for apparent viscosity behave differently. The following model for the random motion of the phagosomes can explain the difference.

A MODEL OF THE INTERACTION OF PHAGOSOMES WITH FILAMENTS

It is widely conjectured that intracellular movements involve acto-mysin systems as in the movement of muscle. The model shown in Fig. 3 is an analogy to muscle contraction. A random impulse is given to a phagosome when some point of its surface touches a point in a fiber and gets a rotational kick when the two points of contact are pushed apart (possibly by the hydrolysis of ATP). We assume that the association of the phagosome with a filament is the Poisson process with the average rate of association a. Assume also that their

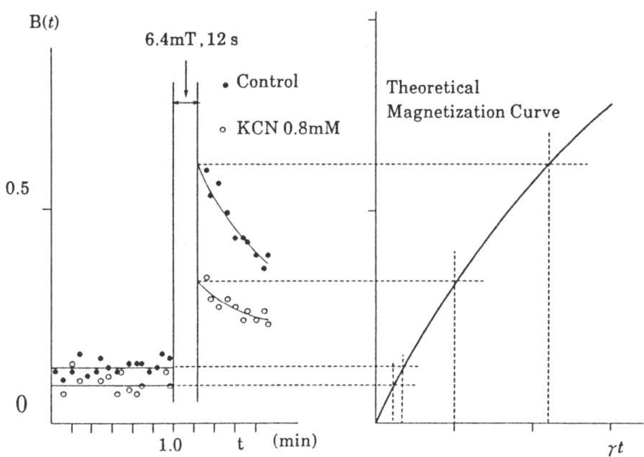

Fig. 2 Realignment of phagosomes by an external field of 6.4 mT after ≃1hour of relaxation period. The curve in the right is the theoetical curve which is used to estimate the increase in η_t.

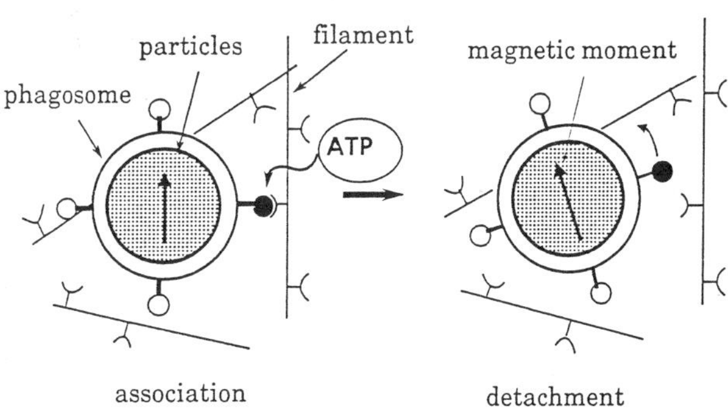

Fig. 3 Interaction of a phagosome and filaments.

detachments are independent and the 'locked' period is exponentially distributed according to $f(t) = \beta e^{-\beta t}$. Then it is shown that the free period per unit time period tends to $e^{-\alpha/\beta}$ as the observation period tends to infinity. If the medium surrounding the phagosome has a constant viscosity, η_t would be proportional to $e^{\alpha/\beta}$ because time comes into eq. (4) in the form of γt where γ is proportional to η_t^{-1}. Therefore, if β decreases with decreasing ATP concentration, η_t would increase accordingly. However, η_s would not change for the following reason. It is shown that the ratio of the number of 'effective' impulses to the total number of impulses is proportional to $e^{-\alpha/\beta}$. E_r is proportional to the ratio according to the RBM model. The rate of relaxation should also be proportional to $e^{-\alpha/\beta}$. Therefore, the apparent viscosity η_s would be estimated to be constant.

The contradicting results of the viscosity measurement can be thus explained by a simple model of phagosome motion. It is not known what causes the phagosomes and other organelles to move within cells, but their association with the surrounding filamentous strucures is considered to be a candidate. Magnetometry may be a probe for infestigation of the intracellular motility further in this direction

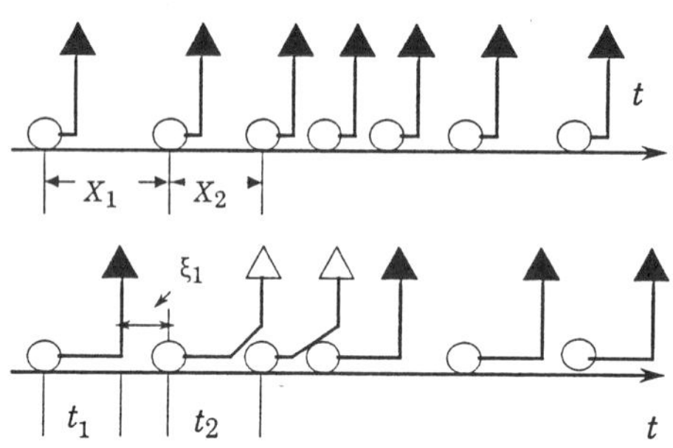

Fig. 4 Association and detachment of phagosome and a filament.

REFERENCES

[1] I. Nemoto,"A model of magnetization and relaxation of ferrimagnetic particles in the lung," *IEEE Trans. Biomed. Eng.*, vol. BME-29, pp. 745-752, 1981.

[2] P. Gehr, J.D. Brain, I. Nemoto and S.B. Bloom,"Behavior of magnetic particles in hamster lungs: Estimates of clearance and cytoplasmic motility", *J. Appl. Physiol.:Respir. Environ. Exercise Physiol.*, vol. 55, pp. 1196-1202, 1983.

[3] I. Nemoto, H. Toyotama, J.D. Brain and P. Gehr,"In vivo and in vitro measurements of magnetic relaxation in hamster pulmonary macrophages", in *Biomagnetism: Application and Theory*, eds. H. Weinberg et al., pp. 401-405, Pergamon Press, 1985.

[4] I. Nemoto, K. Ogura, and H. Toyotama, " Estimation of the energy of cytoplasmic movements by magnetometry, *IEEE Trans. Biomed. Eng.*, vol. 36, pp.598-607, 1989.

[5] P.A. Valberg and J.P. Butler, "Magnetic particle motions within living cells: Physical theory and techniques", *Biophys. J.* vol. 52, pp. 537-550, 1987.

[6] P.A. Valberg and H.A. Feldman, "Magnetic particle motions within living cells: Measurement of cytoplasmic viscosity and motile activity", *Biophys. J.*, vol. 52, pp.551-561, 1987.

INTRACELLULAR MOTILITY OF PULMONARY MACROPHAGES FROM SMOKERS AND NONSMOKERS

Peter Gehr, Markus Klauser* and Vinzenz Im Hof**

*Division of Histology, Department of Anatomy and **Division of Pneumology, Inselspital, University of Berne, Berne, Switzerland

INTRODUCTION

The pulmonary macrophages (PM) with their locomotory, phagocytic and lytic potentials are an essential line of defence in the lungs, keeping the airway and alveolar surfaces clean and sterile (Bowden, 1987). Stimulating collagen producing fibroblasts and secreting lysosomal proteolytic enzymes (collagenase, elastase), the same cells, however, also participate in the pathogenesis of lung diseases, such as fibrosis (Leibovich et al., 1986) and emphysema (Brain, 1988). An increased inhalation of particles causes the number of PM to increase. In chronic smokers (S) the number of PM has been found to be manifold increased as compared to nonsmokers (NS) (Crapo et al., 1982). Moreover, the PM from S have more and larger phagosomes and secondary lysosomes (organelles), containing indigestible material (Pratt. et al., 1971). Thus, we expected the PM of S to exhibit a more extensive phagocytic activity and organelle motion than PM from NS. To test this hypothesis, we harvested PM from human S and NS by bronchoalveolar lavage (BAL) and analysed the cells by magnetometric means (cytomagnetometry). This technique consists of the measurement of the remanent magnetic field, that emanates from macrophages which have phagocytized ferromagnetic particles (Fe_3O_4), after magnetization by an external magnetic field. This non-invasive technique allows the estimation of the phagocytic activity and the motion of organelles (Gehr, 1983; Gehr, 1985; Valberg, 1984).

MATERIALS AND METHODS

PM from 11 S (5 pack-years) and 9 NS (never smoked) were collected by BAL (6 washes of 50 ml saline per subject). The subjects of both groups were between 22 and 32 years old and included both females and males. For each subject the total volume and cell recovery, the volume and cell recovery per wash, the viability of the cells (trypan blue test) and the fraction of PM of the recovered cells were determined. The pooled cells of each subject were then incubated at 37 °C and 5% CO_2. After 60 min the non-adherent cells were rinsed off and the remaining monolayer of macrophages was reincubated with submicrometric Fe_3O_4-particles for 1 hour. Non-phagocytized particles were rinsed off. Afterwards the culture

Advances in Biomagnetism
Edited by S.J. Williamson *et al.*
Plenum Press, New York

dishes were placed in a pulse magnetic field of 0.5 - 1 T for 1 - 2 msec. The remanent field strength, produced by the phagocytized magnetite particles, was measured with a fluxgate magnetometer probe and recorded every second by a PDP-11 computer. It decays with time due to random progressive rotations of the particles (relaxation). The initial field strength, B_0, i.e. the field strength at the time the magnetizing field is turned off, and the initial relaxation rate, λ_0, i.e. the exponential decay coefficient calculated from the values within the first 60 sec after magnetization, were determined according to the equation $B_{(t)} = B_0 \times e^{-\lambda o(t)}$ where $B_{(t)}$ is the field strength measured at time t after magnetization (Nemoto, 1982). B_0 is an estimate for the amount of magnetite the macrophages have phagocytized and λ_0 is an estimate for the organelle motility (Gehr, 1983; Valberg, 1984).

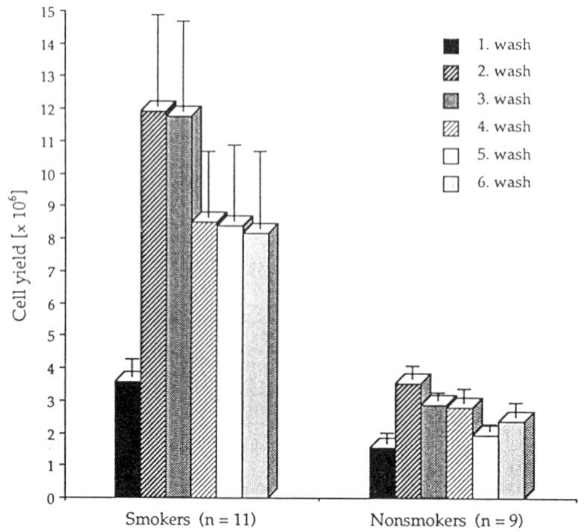

Figure 1. BAL data. Cell yields per wash (mean values, SE)

RESULTS

Our BAL data are in accordance with the data given in literature (Davis, 1982; Ettensohn, 1988). As expected, the cell yield per wash, as well as the one per lavage both were larger in S than in NS (figure 1).
B_0 of PM from S was not significantly different from B_0 of NS, the values being 13.24 nT (SE 0.79 nT) and 11.74 nT (SE 1.39 nT), respectively (table 1). Figure 2A shows all 20 normalized relaxation curves of the 11 S and the 9 NS. It is obvious that the remanent magnetic field of PM from both S and NS decayed in a very similar manner (fig. 2B), and, the relaxation rates (λ_0) of the two groups were found to be the same. These were calculated as 3.14 x 10^{-3} sec^{-1} (SE 0.18 x 10^{-3} sec^{-1}) in S and 3.17 x 10^{-3} sec^{-1} (SE 0.22 x 10^{-3} sec^{-1}) in NS, respectively (table 1).

Table 1. Magnetometric data.

Smokers

Subject No.	B_0 [nT]	B_{60} [nT]	λ_0 [$\times 10^{-3}\cdot sec^{-1}$]
1	14.13	12.56	2.35
2	16.89	14.28	3.15
3	14.84	12.72	2.88
4	8.79	7.10	3.87
5	10.29	8.16	4.13
6	9.23	7.93	2.89
7	15.13	12.20	3.96
8	14.13	12.21	2.81
9	14.61	12.62	2.75
10	13.58	11.58	2.90
11	13.98	11.95	2.85
Mean	13.24	11.21	3.14
SE	0.79	0.71	0.18

Nonsmokers

Subject No.	B_0 [nT]	B_{60} [nT]	λ_0 [$\times 10^{-3}\cdot sec^{-1}$]
12	12.89	10.96	2.95
13	10.80	9.31	2.79
14	18.00	15.30	3.07
15	8.48	7.64	2.08
16	6.02	4.98	3.76
17	8.34	5.74	4.42
18	11.18	9.39	3.46
19	18.31	15.47	3.13
20	11.64	9.94	2.89
Mean	11.74	9.86	3.17
SE	1.39	1.23	0.22

DISCUSSION

The macrophages of both S and NS had phagocytized the same amount of magnetite, and hence, demonstrated the same phagocytic activity. This is in agreement with earlier observations (Ando, 1984; Cohen 1971). The relaxation phenomenon is caused by misalignment of the magnetic particles due to random progressive rotations of the particle containing phagosomes and secondary lysosomes. The rotations are attributed to contractile forces exerted on these organelles, mainly due to actin-myosin interactions (Gehr, 1983, 1985; Valberg, 1984; Valberg and Albertini, 1985). Despite the burden of phagosomes and secondary lysosomes which were increased in number and volume due to the increased amount of foreign material phagocytized in situ, PM of S were still able to continue

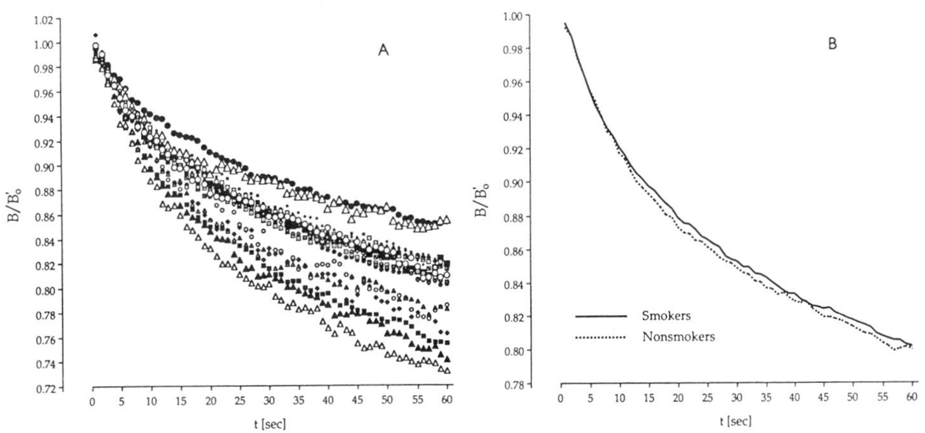

Figure 2. Relaxation curves
A) All subjects, 11 S (closed symbols) and 9 NS (open symbols)
B) S versus NS (mean values)

phagocytosis in vitro at the same rate as PM from NS. The relaxation of S and NS was found to be the same, hence the macrophages of both groups exhibited the same organelle motility. The increase in number, size and density of the phagosomes in PM from S obviously does not impair the movements of the organelles caused by the contractile elements of the cytoskeleton. The relaxation rate, λ_0, of PM from NS was found to be the same as the one recently reported in an abstract by Valberg et al. (1988). There exists some disagreement, however, as far as the findings of PM from S are concerned: λ_0 of PM from S was found to be 8.5 x 10^{-3} sec^{-1} (SE 1.3 x 10^{-3} sec^{-1}) by Valberg et al. as compared to 3.1 x 10^{-3} sec^{-1} (SE 0.18 x 10^{-3} sec^{-1}) in our study. In order to compare the results of the two studies the following considerations have to be made: 1) The characteristics of the lavaged subjects in the study of Valberg et al. have not been specified, 2) their cytomagnetometric measurements were performed with the cells in suspension, and 3), may be most important, Valberg et al. incubated their harvested PM with magnetite "over night", i.e. many hours longer than we did. Our findings give strong evidence that the PM of young S and NS have the same phagocytic properties and the same organelle motility.

ACKNOWLEDGEMENTS

We thank Ch. Furter, K. Babl and Ch. Lehmann for their assistance. This work was supported by the Swiss NSF.

REFERENCES

(1) M. Ando, M. Sugimoto, R. Nishi, M. Suga, S. Horio, K. Kohrogo, K. Shimazu, S. Araki: Thorax, 39, 850-856, 1984.
(2) D. H. Bowden: Exp. Lung Res., 12, 89-107, 1987.
(3) J. D. Brain: In: Handbook of Physiology, The Respiratory system, I. chapter 14, ... Press, pp. 447-471, 1988.
(4) A. B. Cohen, M. J. Cline: J. Clin. Invest., 50, 1390-1398, 1971.
(5) E. D. Crapo, B. E. Barry, P. Gehr, M. Bachofen, E. R. Weibel: Am. Rev. Respir. Dis., 125, 332-337, 1982.
(6) G. S. Davis, M. S. Giancola, M. C. Constanza, R. Low: Am. Rev. Respir. Dis., 126, 611-616, 1982.
(7) D. B. Ettensohn, M. J. Jankowski, P. G. Duncan, P. A. Lalor: Chest, 94, 275-280, 1988.
(8) P. Gehr, J. D. Brain, S. D. Bloom, P. A. Valberg: Nature, 302, 336-338, 1983.
(9) P. Gehr, J. D. Brain, I. Nemoto, S. B. Bloom: In:Biomagnetism: Applications and Theory. Pergamon Press, NY, pp. 395-400, 1985.
(10) S. J. Leibovich, R. Ross: Am. J. Pathol., 84, 501-514, 1976.
(11) I. Nemoto: IEEE Trans. Biomed. Eng., 29, 745-752, 1982.
(12) S. A. Pratt, M. H. Smith, A. J. Ladman, T. N. Finley: Lab. Invest., 24, 331-338, 1971.
(13) P. A. Valberg: Science, 224, 513-516, 1984.
(14) P. A. Valberg, D. F. Albertini: J. Cell Biol., 101, 130-140, 1985.
(15) P. A. Valberg, W. A. Jensen, R. M. Rose: Am. Rev. Respir. Dis. (abstract), 137 (2/2), 316, 1988.

WELDING FUME RETENTION IN LUNGS OF PREVIOUSLY UNEXPOSED SUBJECTS

Mikael Forsman[1] and Per Högstedt[1,2]

[1]Department of Applied Electronics, Chalmers University of Technology
S-412 96 Göteborg, Sweden

[2]Projekt Lindholmen IDC, P.O. Box 8714
S-402 75 Göteborg, Sweden

INTRODUCTION

Previous studies of long-term exposed arc welders revealed gross differences in lung dust retention among arc welders. Explanations to this observation were sought e.g. in the time the welder had been exposed to arc welding fumes and the concentration of welding fume in the workshops. Even though these variables did explain some of the variability in the data, the remaining ratio between the welders having the highest retention to those having the lowest was over 50. Variables other than duration and intensity of the exposure could be responsible for this observation. Inter individual differences in retention pattern and clearance may explain some of the remaining variability. In this paper we describe a study addressing this question by measuring the rate of increase of retention in previously unexposed subjects being exposed to relatively homogeneous dust concentrations. The changes in retention is compared to the estimated individual exposure. A novel model for estimating individual retention and clearance is used.

METHODS

A group of eight trainees in welding school, aged 16-49, 4 smokers, and with no previous exposure to arc welding fumes, was followed during the first few months of their MMA mild steel welding training. Magnetopneumography (MPG) was used to estimate the subjects' magnetizable lung dust retention before and during the training period. MPG measurements was taken at least three times per subject during the experiment. The day-to-day working schedule for each individual was examined to account for variations in exposure level. Exposure was stratified into three levels assigned weighting factors based on previous experience of the average dust concentration in different situations. The days the subject was welding were assigned a weight factor of 3, days when he was present in the training workshop but not welding were assigned an exposure level of 1, whereas days of total absence from welding fume exposure were given zero weight. The MPG instrument used in this experiment (Kalliomäki, 1981; Högstedt, 1987) is equipped with first order fluxgate gradiometers having a noise level of approximately 45 $pT/\sqrt{Hz}$. Post measurement signal processing was necessary in order to detect the weak magnetic fields obtained from the minute amounts of magnetizable

Advances in Biomagnetism
Edited by S.J. Williamson *et al.*
Plenum Press, New York

dust particles in the lungs of these subjects. The retention, B_o, was estimated from repeated transversal scans (>25) taken at the dorsal side of the thorax along a line located at the xiphoids. A 5 second magnetization pulse was used. The distance between the near probe and the back of the subject was 59±2 mm. Scans were taken starting approximately 3.5 seconds post magnetization, up to 500 seconds. Each scan consisted of 40 samples, separated 15 mm along the scanning line. Using a weighted mean of the outer 9 samples of each scan to estimate a baseline, the 18 central samples were used to calculate the mean flux density of the scan, $B_c(t)$. Due to the low signal to noise ratio, normal relaxation analysis could not be applied to the data (Högstedt, 1983). The relaxation model applied in the analysis was an exponential, $B(t)= B_o e^{-t/\tau}$. The two free parameters of this model were estimated using the Marquardt algorithm. Asymptotic confidence intervals for the estimates were also calculated. The retention estimate, B_o, was plotted versus the number of days since onset of exposure for each individual. In these plots, the discrete exposure weighting factor, W_i, for each day

$$R_n = \sum_{i=1}^{n} W_i \, a_r \, e^{-(n-i)/\tau_c} \qquad \text{(Eq. 1)}$$

was also plotted. Using B_o and W_i, the parameters of a simple retention-clearance model (Eq. 1) could be estimated. In this model, R_n refers to the total amount of magnetizable dust remaining in the lungs of a subject on a given day, n, since onset of exposure. The parameter a_r is the retention per exposure weight unit and day, and τ_c the clearance time constant. Finally, the result of this model was plotted for each individual.

RESULTS

In Figure 1, a representative example of the measured $B_c(t)$ is shown (subject JD at day 33). Also the relaxation curve, resulting from fitting the model to the data, is illustrated. The

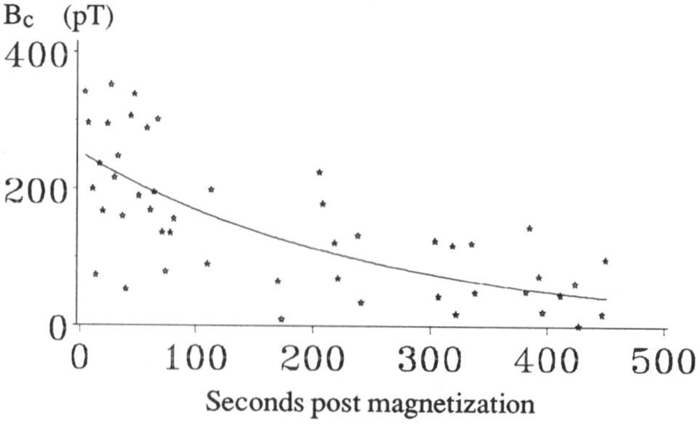

Figure 1.
Relaxation in subject JD, at 33 days after onset of exposure. Stars indicate measured data taken at the dorsal side at a distance of approximately 60 mm from the skin. The curve is the flux density predicted by the single exponential relaxation model.

width of the 95 % confidence interval for B_o is less than ±50 pT. In Figure 2, the retention as a function of time since onset of exposure is illustrated for all subjects. The vertical bars mark the 95 per cent confidence interval for B_o. The exposure weights W_i (0,1,or 3) assigned to each day is inserted in the diagram on the x axis. Here, the height of the fat bars represents the estimated relative dust concentration to which the subject is exposed. The curve predicts retention by the simple retention-clearance model previously described.

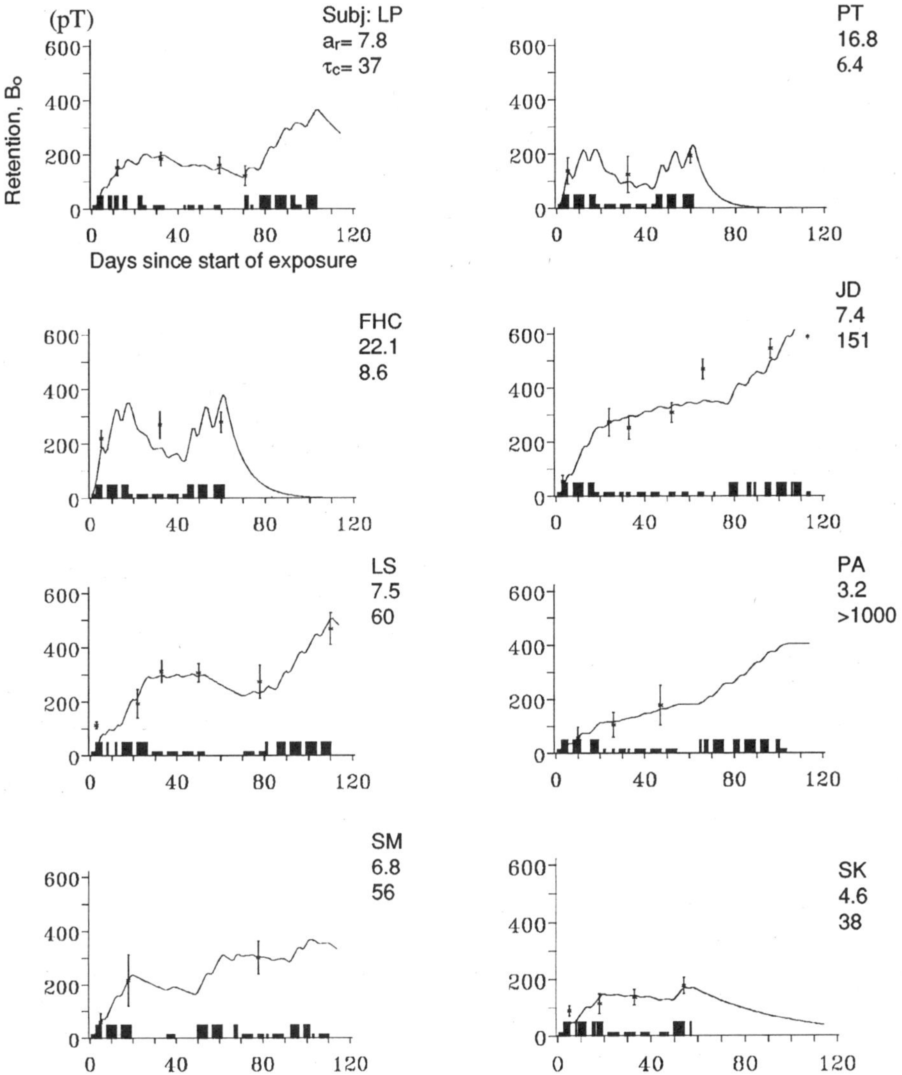

Figure 2. Retention as measured in MPG, with 95 % confidence intervals for B_o marked by thin bars, versus days since start of the arc welding training programme. The exposure weights, W_i, are indicated by fat bars on the x axis. The upper number in the insert in each figure is the retention parameter, a_r, from the retention model in Equation 1. The lower number is the clearance time constant, τ_c. The curves illustrate retention predicted by the model. In subject JD on day 114, loss of raw data impaired post measurement data processing.

DISCUSSION

The study described in this paper was designed to address the hypothesis of a possible influence of inter individual retention and clearance differences on the long-term ackumulation of arc welding dust in the lungs of welders. The design aimed at estimating individual retention and clearance rate using data from previuosly unexposed subjects, not having the confounding background retention found in professional arc welders. Data were presented on retention of magnetizable dusts in lungs of the subjects from the point when they started their training up to 114 days of exposure. These data were compared to the exposure time and to a novel estimate of intensity of exposure. Unfortunately, some of the subjects in this study did not participate in both parts of the training programme, hence most of the MPG data covers only 60 days of exposure history. It is obvious from Figure 1, that in order to be able to arrive at a high quality estimate of the relaxation time constant, τ , and to be able to utilize more elaborate relaxation models, an increase in signal-to-noise ratio is necessary. The parameter of primary interest to this study, B_0, was however possible to estimate with an acceptable degree of confidence. The exposure weighting technique used here is the result of a careful penetration of each individuals tasks during the training. The weights assigned to different situations are based on previous dust samplings in other workshops, and can only be expected to resemble the real dust concentration to which the subjects are exposed. Analysis of measurements of the actual dust concentration by personal and stationary dust samplers are under way. During periods of intense welding (high bars, Figure 2), the retention increases. When the subject is not welding but exposed to the ambient workshop air (low bars), the retention appears to level off. Absence of exposure results in a decrease in retention. There appears to be an inter individual difference in the slope of the retention, Figure 2, but the dust concentration measurements will also have to be considered. Also, the possibility of translocation of the dust within the lungs could be a confounding factor. This could however be accounted for by measuring over the entire lung, which is the standard procedure in our MPG measurements. Some subjects were not available for MPG measurements after some period of time (60 days). Since exposure data was available, the retention-clearance model was used to predict the retention up to day 114. The retention-clearance model used is a first order model that does not account for other than the very basics of this complex process. Nevertheless, it is able to fit the observed data reasonably well. Furthermore, the predictions made by the model outside the period of time where MPG data is available appears to be consistent with what could be expected. Some of the instances where the model fail (see subject FHC, Figure 2) probably depends on the model being forced by the fitting procedure to assume R= 0 at day 0. This will be changed in the near future.

These preliminary results indicate that combining MPG measurements with careful monitoring of dust concentration levels on the subject and in the workshops and keeping day-to-day records of work tasks and presence, will supply valuable information on the role of the individual retention and clearance for long-term buildup of dusts in the lung. Current plans include an extended study, where MPG measurements will be taken at more regular intervals and where periods of zero exposure will be used for estimation of the individual clearance.

This work was supported in part by the Swedish Work Environment Fund, under grant 86-0563.

REFERENCES

Högstedt, P., Kadefors, R., and Näslund P.-E., 1983, Magnetopneumography in welders: observations on relaxation and clearance, Il Nuovo Cimento, 2D:608.

Högstedt, P., Kadefors, R., and Näslund P.-E., 1987, Magnetopneumography: methodological aspects of non invasive measurements of iron oxide retained in lungs, Technical report, Dept. Appl. Electronics, Chalmers UoT, ISBN 91-7546-048-3.

Kalliomäki, K., Aittoniemi, K., Kalliomäki, P.-L., Moilanen, M., 1981, Measurement of lung retained contaminants in vivo among workers exposed to metal aerosols, Amer. Ind. Hyg. Assoc. J., 42:234.

IN VIVO SQUID MEASUREMENTS OF THE MAGNETISED HUMAN THORAX

D Rassi[*], B H Blott[+], H Al-Sewaidan[*], S Davies[*] and C Ni[+]

[*] Physics Department, Univ. Coll. of Swansea, SA2 8PP, U.K.

[+] Physics Department, Univ. of Southampton, SO9 5NH, U.K.

INTRODUCTION

We have been investigating for some time the possibility of obtaining diagnostically useful information from the magnetic field distributions observed over the human thorax magnetised in a uniform applied field. The aim is to correlate the measured field distribution with the highly inhomogeneous structure of the thorax which contains a diversity of organs (heart, lungs, liver) and tissues (muscle, fat, bone, blood). Although generally quite small, the differences in the diamagnetic susceptibilities of these tissues and organs produce measurable field variations (of the order of nanoteslas in an applied field of milliteslas) on the surface of the thorax. There are, of course, other contributions from physiological processes (heart activity, blood flow etc.) and volume changes which occur during the cardiac and respiratory cycles. This latter problem has been discussed in some detail by Maniewski et al. (1988). *In vivo* susceptometry has also been used by Farrell et al. (1983) and by Bastuscheck and Williamson (1985) to study hepatic iron levels. In contrast to these and other similar studies, which have been mainly concerned with measuring changes in the susceptibility signal at specific points over the thorax, in the present work susceptibility "images" of the entire thorax are constructed by recording the magnetic signal at several hundred points.

Computer simulation of a magnetised human thorax, using anatomically accurate data, was discussed by Khenia et al. (1986) and the computational procedure was subsequently improved by Hoare et al. (1988) who made use of the reciprocity theorem. Phantom studies comparing the predictions of the computer model with SQUID measurements (Rassi et al. 1988) indicated the feasibility of this method and we now present further evidence of the ability of *in vivo* susceptometry to provide information on structure (and possibly pathology) of thorax components.

METHODS

Thoracic magnetic field distributions were measured with a commercial SQUID magnetometer (BTi 601) equipped with a second-order gradiometer detection coil of diameter 19.8 mm and baseline 50.4 mm. The subject, lying on his back on a wooden platform, was moved in two orthogonal directions in the horizontal (x-y) plane under the fixed SQUID cryostat.

Taking the long axis of the body as the y-axis with the sternal notch corresponding to y=0, the subject was scanned along the x-axis (across the thorax) whilst the SQUID output was recorded at 10 mm intervals by the computerised data-logging system. Three such scans were taken consecutively and averaged at each y-coordinate. The subject was then moved 20 mm along the y-axis and the above procedure was repeated at 12 to 17 y-coordinates, depending on the length of the thorax being imaged.

A container consisting of a strong, thin, elastic membrane sealed to a 0.6 m x 0.6 m flat perspex sheet was placed over the subject in all measurements. This was supported on a wooden frame the height of which could be adjusted for each subject such that the highest point of the thorax just touched the underside of the perspex sheet. The distance between the bottom of the SQUID cryostat and the surface of the thorax varied between 15 and 25 mm in the *in vivo* measurements. When filled with approximately 50 l of distilled water, the water-bag completely engulfed the thorax, while for measurements in air the bag was evacuated. The magnetic signal due to the perspex sheet and plastic membrane was measured separately and found to be negligible.

The applied magnetic field was produced by a pair of square coils of 2.5 m side and separation, each wound with 27 turns of 12 A-rated wire, having their axis in the vertical (z) direction. The non-uniformity at the centre of this coil system was corrected with a third coil of the same dimensions having 18 turns in the same sense as the first pair, connected in series with and positioned midway between them. In this way a central field uniformity of 1 ppm was achieved and with the centre of the pick-up gradiometer fixed at the centre of the coil system, the gradiometer was balanced to better than 10 ppm. Fields of up to 0.25 mT (including the vertical component of the geomagnetic field) could be applied during measurements by passing currents of up to 8 A through the coil system.

RESULTS

In order to quantify the effects on the signal-to-noise ratio of applied field strength and detector-to-source distance, a series of measurements was carried out on a plastic bottle containing a liquid of known magnetic susceptibility. The bottle, which produced negligible signal when empty, was in the shape of a long cylinder of cross-sectional diameter 58 mm. With its axis along the y direction, the centre of the bottle was scanned along the x-axis under the SQUID magnetometer. The results of four such measurements at two different detector-to-source distances, and with two values of applied field, are shown in Fig. 1. Each curve is an average of ten scans with standard deviation represented by error bars. The conclusions concerning signal-to-noise deduced from this series of measurements will be discussed in the following section.

Figures 2 and 3 are three-dimensional plots of thoracic magnetic field distributions of two normal male subjects, obtained by the method described in the previous section. For the measurements shown in Fig. 2 the water-bag was evacuated so that a diamagnetic signal corresponding to the air-thorax interface is observed. The results in Fig. 3, obtained when the water-bag was filled with distilled water, show the (relative) paramagnetic signal due to the tissue-lung interface. In these figures the measured fields are displayed in units of the SQUID magnetometer's output; 1 V corresponds to a field of 0.24 nT normal to, and passing only through, the bottom coil of the gradiometer . This is an idealised case of a point source located very close to the bottom (pick-up) coil; it can therefore be expected that the actual fields associated with a magnetised thorax are somewhat larger than suggested by Figs. 2 and 3.

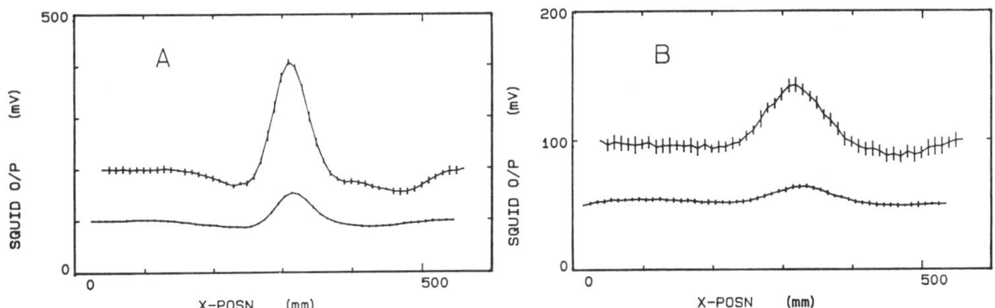

Fig. 1. Signal-to-noise studies on a 58 mm diameter cylindrical object having the same magnetic susceptibility as the human lung (i.e. $-4x10^{-6}$ SI units), showing the effect of increasing the applied field from 0.05 to 0.25 mT. The detector-object distances were (A) 38 mm, and (B) 79 mm. For clarity the traces are displaced by an arbitrary zero shift on the vertical axis.

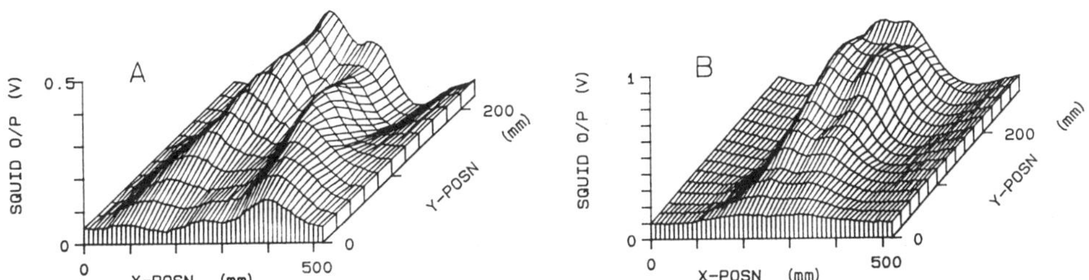

Fig. 2. Thoracic magnetic field distributions of two normal male subjects in an applied DC magnetic field of 0.25 mT. The medium external to the chest wall was air (susceptibility $+0.34x10^{-6}$ SI units)

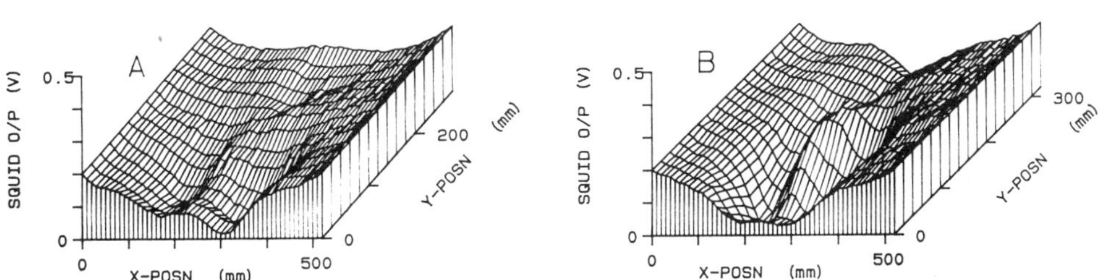

Fig. 3. As Fig. 2 but with the chest wall completely surrounded by 50 l of distilled water of susceptibility $-9x10^{-6}$ SI units.

DISCUSSION

The measured standard deviations in the data showed considerable improvement with increased magnetising field in regions where time-varying signals (e.g. from the electrical currents in the heart) were significant. The signal showed a strong dependency on the detector-object separation as expected from the previously determined instrument function of the gradiometer (Blott et al 1988). The signal-to-noise ratio, however, showed little variation with this separation, suggesting that the noise is not coupled to the gradiometer via the sample. The main advantage of increasing the applied field is therefore to enhance the susceptibility signal, thus reducing the interference from the physiology-related time-varying magnetic fields.

In the course of our investigations a total of twelve human subjects (seven male and five female) were studied. Thoracic maps measured in air, as shown in Fig. 2, reveal significant inter-individual differences which are clearly related to the surface morphology of the body. These were highly reproducible between successive measurements on the same person, and indicate the sensitivity of the technique to interfaces between two regions of different susceptibility. For imaging internal organs this external shape effect must be effectively removed by using a water-bag to match the susceptibility of the chest wall tissue. Fig. 3 illustrates the success of this technique; thoracic maps measured using the water-bag exhibit features common to all our subjects, both male and female. A diamagnetic signal is seen over the centre of the chest while the lungs, and to some extent the liver, give rise to minima corresponding to relative paramagnetism.

In conclusion, these experiments show that magnetisation measurements of the thorax are sensitive enough to detect internal magnetic anomalies in the body and may possibly have applications in the diagnosis of certain pathologies. Further research is in progress to refine the mapping of the thorax by incorporating reciprocity methods.

REFERENCES

Bastuscheck C.M. and Williamson S.J., 1985, Techniques for measuring the ac susceptibility of portions of the human body or other large objects, J. Appl. Phys., 58:3896.

Blott B.H., Janday B.S., Melville D., Hoare A., Rassi D. and Samadian V. 1988, Design and assessment of SQUID magnetometers using reciprocity methods, J. de Physique, 49-C8:2061

Farrell D.E., Tripp J.H., Brittenham G.M., Danish E.H., Harris J.W. and Tracht A.E., 1983, A clinical system for accurate assessment of tissue iron concentration, Il Nuovo Cimento, 2:582.

Hoare A., Melville D., Rassi D. and Samadian V., 1988, Rapid methods for the calculation of the magnetic field associated with the human thorax, IEEE Trans. Magn., 24:1978.

Khenia S., Melville D. and Rassi D., Magnetic mapping of the human thorax using a SQUID magnetometer, <u>in</u>: "Biophysical Effects of Steady Magnetic Fields", G. Maret, N. Boccara and J. Kiepenheuer, ed, Springer-Verlag, Berlin (1986).

Maniewski R., Katila T., Poutanen T., Siltanen P., Varpula T. and Wikswo J.P., 1988, Magnetic measurements of cardiac mechanical activity, IEEE Trans. Biomed. Eng., 35:662.

Rassi D., Hoare A., Samadian V. and Melville D., SQUID measurements and computational modelling of a simple thorax phantom, <u>in</u>: "Biomagnetism '87", K. Atsumi, M. Kotani, S. Ueno, T. Katila and S.J. Williamson, ed., Tokyo Denki University Press, (1988).

A STUDY OF MAGNETIC CONTAMINANTS IN *POST MORTEM* LUNG SAMPLES FROM ASBESTOS MINERS

D. Rassi[*], V. Timbrell[+], H. Al-Sewaidan[*], S. Davies[*], O. Taikina-aho[#] and P. Paakko[#]

[*] Physics Department, Univ. Coll. of Swansea, SA2 8PP, U.K.

[+] MRC Epidemiological Unit, Cardiff, U.K.

[#] University of Oulu, Oulu, Finland

INTRODUCTION

Over the past decade magnetopneumography has been successfully used in *in vivo* studies of the contamination levels of the human lung with inhaled dust. However, before this information can be used to assess the health hazard of a given dust, dose-response relationships for the various dust-related pulmonary diseases will have to be established. This involves detailed analysis of large numbers of *post mortem* lung samples containing different amounts of contamination and exhibiting various degrees of pathology. Such analysis, inevitably involving electron microscopy, is extremely time-consuming and expensive since a large spread in the contamination levels will have to be obtained for meaningful dose-response correlations.

An area of intense current interest is the disease-producing effects of inhaled asbestos dust. These include asbestosis (an interstitial pulmonary fibrosis), mesothelioma (a cancer of the pleura and peritoneum) and lung cancer. Significant progress has been made in the understanding of the relative importance of the various measurable dust parameters such as mass concentration, fibre length, diameter, surface area etc. (Lippmann 1988, Timbrell et al., 1989).

In this paper we demonstrate how remanent magnetisation measurements on *post mortem* lung samples can be used to preselect samples for electron microscopic and other analytical investigation. This leads to much more rapid data-processing in large-scale epidemiological studies aimed at establishing dose-response relationships.

METHODS

The *post mortem* lung specimens were collected from a large sample population of asbestos miners from Wittenoom (Western Australia), North Western Cape Province (South Africa), Transvaal (South Africa) and Paakkila (Finland). In order to extract the mineral content of the partially dried lung samples, these were first soaked in filtered and

Advances in Biomagnetism
Edited by S.J. Williamson *et al.*
Plenum Press, New York

de-ionised water for 10 to 30 days. They were then ashed in a low-temperature asher (BIO-RAD Plasma Asher E2000) for 48 hours at temperatures of 100 to 120 ^{o}C and the ash was placed in test tubes which were heated for a further 48 hours at 80 ^{o}C.

The magnetic studies on these ash residues were performed using a SQUID magnetometer (BTi 601) equipped with a second-order gradiometer detection coil of diameter 19.8 mm and baseline 50.4 mm. The samples were magnetised in fields of 0.05, 0.1 and 0.2 Tesla for 5 seconds after which the remanent magnetisation was measured for each magnetising field. The results were calibrated against known quantities of magnetite powder embedded in polyurethane foam magnetised in the same field as the samples.

RESULTS

Over eighty lung specimens from more than twenty individuals were examined by the methods described above. Total dust, and magnetite concentrations in the lung tissue samples of ex-employees of the Wittenoom crocidolite-asbestos mine are shown in Fig. 1. Data points associated with lung samples from the same person are linked; the presence of many such sets of linked points indicating our aim to take account of intra- and inter-subject variability. The magnitude of intra- and inter-subject variations in ash (and magnetite) concentration necessitates the use of logarithmic scales in Fig. 1.

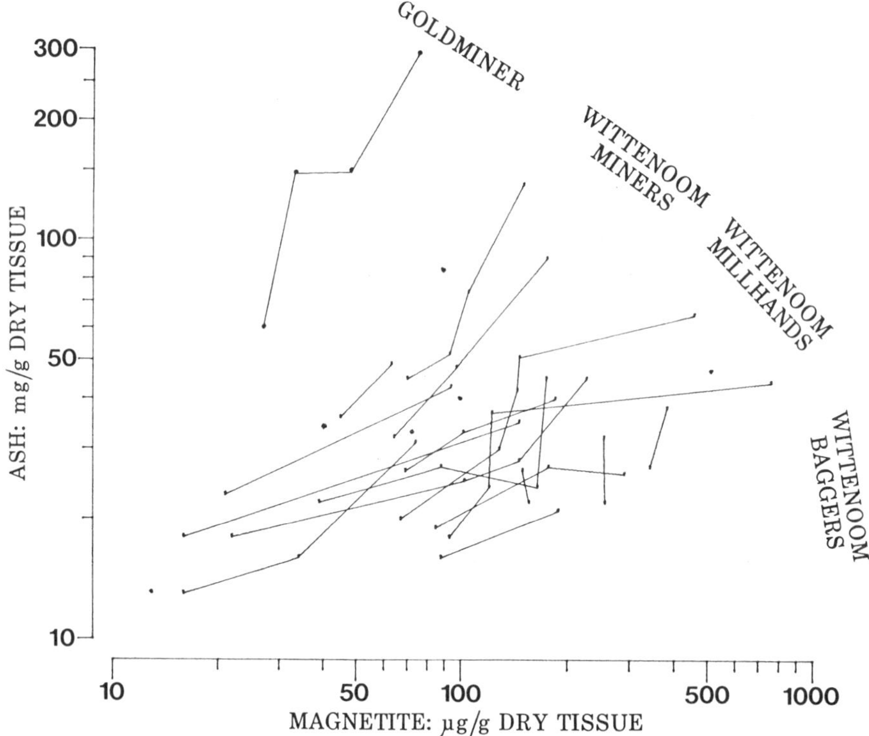

Fig. 1. Concentrations of ash and magnetite in the *post mortem* lung tissue samples. Linked data points relate to specimens from the same person.

A striking feature of the results shown in Fig. 1 is the tendency of data points to occur in bands relating to the various occupations within the mine. This reflects the multi-stage nature of the production of asbestos. In principle, the asbestos ore is extracted intact so that the mine dust clouds are poor in magnetite-containing asbestos. Dust clouds subsequently become richer in magnetite, reaching peak magnetite concentration in the bagging department where the purity of the asbestos has to meet given specifications. The results in Fig. 1 illustrate the need to determine the relationship between magnetite and ash for each of the major occupations. Fortunately, all the main asbestos mines have kept accurate job-records virtually since they started operations decades ago, making it possible to determine the specific relationships for any mine. The goldminer, exhibiting high ash concentrations, had worked for a few months as a miner at Wittenoom and for several years as a miner at a gold mine. The relevance of these data will be discussed below.

DISCUSSION AND FURTHER APPLICATIONS

The magnetite concentration of asbestos-bearing rocks varies with the geographical location of the deposit. Within each mining area, however, the magnetite concentration is fairly constant and determinable. Typical results of EDAX compositional analysis carried out on ashed lung samples similar to those used in the present study are shown in Fig. 2. Many such analyses were performed by Timbrell et al (1989) who found that often the predominant mineral type in a specimen was not the nominal work material. Nevertheless, in most mines there is good consistency in the relative proportions of the various minerals. Thus, the results shown in Fig. 1 for the goldminer would resemble satisfactorily the results obtained from other employees of the same mine.In the case of asbestos, as mentioned before, the relative concentration of magnetite is expected to vary according to the stage of production. However, the relationships between magnetite concentration, ash concentration and occupation can be established by means of graphs such as Fig. 1. Combining this information with corresponding sets of measurements relating pulmonary pathology (e.g. fibrosis) to dust concentration (Timbrell et al., 1988), leads to quantitative dose-response relationships.

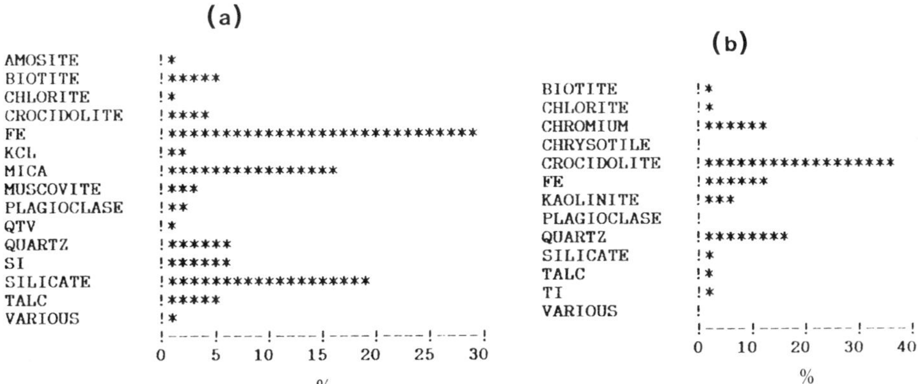

Fig. 2. Mineral composition determined by EDAX of ashed tissue specimen from a lung exposed (a) at a platinum mine in South Africa, and (b) at the Wittenoom crocidolite mine in Australia.

The main advantages of the magnetic technique presented here are its great speed and sensitivity. The method can therefore be used to preselect realistic numbers of samples for detailed (and time-consuming) microscopic investigations (Timbrell 1982). This leads to a major reduction in the effort required to achieve a given accuracy in the results of epidemiological studies on large numbers of *post mortem* tissue samples.

Finally, the method described here has the sensitivity required for the detection of magnetite in tissues of brain, kidney and other organs. This facility is valuable in investigations of possible translocation of asbestos fibres from the lungs to various parts of the body. The rapidity with which measurements can be made allows the accurate mapping of the distribution of asbestos in the lung by examination of large numbers of small samples excised from whole-lung sections.

REFERENCES

Lippmann M., 1988, Asbestos exposure indices, Environ. Res., 46:86.

Timbrell V., 1982, Deposition and retention of fibres in the human lung, Ann. Occup. Hyg., 26:347.

Timbrell V., Ashcroft T., Goldstein B., Heyworth F., Meurman L.O., Rendall R.E.G., Reynolds J.A.,Shilkin K.B. and Whitaker D., 1988, Relationships between retained amphibole fibres and fibrosis in human lung tissue specimens, Ann. Occup. Hyg., 52:323.

Timbrell V., Taikina-aho O., Paakko P., Ashcroft T., Meurman L.O. and Shilkin K.B., 1989, Similarities in the fibrogenicity of asbestos fibres and other mineral particles retained in human lungs, 1989, to be published in: "Proc. VIIth Int. Pneumoconiosis Conf." Pittsburgh, U.S.A., August 23-26, 1988.

EFFECTS OF LATEX AND DIFFERENT DOSES OF SILICA ON BEHAVIOR OF IRON PARTICLES IN RABBIT LUNGS

Yoshiharu Aizawa, Tsutomu Takata, Kiichiro Hashimoto, Mamoru Tominaga, Hiroshi Tatsumi, Makoto Kotani* and Keizo Chiyotani**

Department of Preventive Medicine and Public Health, School of Medicine, Kitasato University, Kanagawa, Japan
* Electronics, Tokyo Denki University, Tokyo, Japan
** Rosai Hospital for Silicosis, Tochigi, Japan

INTRODUCTION

Silica is known to have a fibrogenic effect on pulmonary tissue and give rise to silicosis. Frequent complications of pulmonary infection suggest the disturbed clearance in the silicotic lung. Early studies on the pathogenesis of silicosis suggested that the basic lesion was to macrophages. Silica has been shown to be toxic for macrophages.

Magnetopneumographic studies have revealed that remanent magnetic fields generated by an external magnetization of ferrimagnetic particles in the lung decreased gradually with time(1,2). This phenomenon called relaxation is considered attributable to the rotation of phagocytized ferrimagnetic particles in macrophages. The clearance of deposited particles in the alveolar spaces is carried out by macrophages. Brain et al. observed delayed clearance and fast relaxation in hamster lungs by the intratracheal administration of various doses of silica(3). Authors previously observed delayed clearance and relaxation in rabbit lungs exposed to high dose of silica(4).

The present study was designed to evaluate the effect of exposure of high and low doses of silica on the relaxation and clearance of ferrimagnetic particles in the rabbit lungs. The other object of this study is to examine the effect of intratracheal injection of inert particle as latex on these phenomena.

MATERIALS AND METHODS

Fe_3O_4 particles (0.4 micron diameter) suspended in saline were intratracheally instilled into 20 male white rabbits weighing 3-4 kg. The suspension prepared by dispersing 20 mg of Fe_3O_4 particles into 1 ml of saline was instilled into the trachea using silicon rubber catheter. One of the suspension of silica 300mg, silica 30mg or latex 2.2×10^6 in 2 ml of saline was instilled into the trachea of 5 rabbits in each group, while 2 ml of saline was instilled into 5 control rabbits. The silica particles (2.16 micron diameter, with range of 0.3-4.0 micron) were obtained as a generous gift from Dr. K. Homma, National Institutes of Industrial Health. Solid-latex, Polybead-polystyrene Microspheres, with nominal diameter 1.0 micrometer was obtained from Polyscience, Inc., U.S.A.

After instillation, a 50 mT field was applied to the chest of the rabbit placed between a pair of coils of enameled copper wire driven by a DC power

Advances in Biomagnetism
Edited by S.J. Williamson *et al.*
Plenum Press, New York

supply. The rabbits were exposed to this field for periods of 15 seconds to magnetize.

Upon removal from the external magnetic field, the remanent field from the lungs was measured by a flux-gate magnetometer for at least 40 minutes. The magnetization and measurement of magnetic field of the lungs were repeated as long as the presence of remanent magnetic field detected in the control rabbits.

The first five minutes of relaxation was fitted to the exponential function, $B = B_0 exp(-\lambda t)$, where B is the field strength at time t, B_0 is the field strength at time t=0, λ is the relaxation rate (decay constant) for the first 5 minutes. Linear regression of the natural logarithms of the field strengths on t by the least-squares method was used to fit the line. B_0 was estimated by extrapolating the function back to time zero. Because initial remanent magnetic fields were not always constant in each experiment, percent magnetic field strength was calculated with a formula of $B/B_0 \times 100$ as in Fig. 1 and Fig. 2.

The data for clearance were calculated with a formula of (B_0 of a rabbit at each day) / (B_0 of the same rabbit immediately after instillation) x 100. The mean percent of magnetic fields were obtained from 5 rabbits.

Microscopical and ultrastructural examinations of the lungs were performed 6 and 12 weeks after instillation. The lung tissue from experimental animals was prepared for study by a transmission electron microscope, a scanning electron microscope, the energy dispersible X-ray microanalysis. Portions of the each lobe were fixed and stained with hematoxylin and eosin, Berlin blue and examined by a polarizing microscope to localized the silica particles.

RESULTS AND DISCUSSION

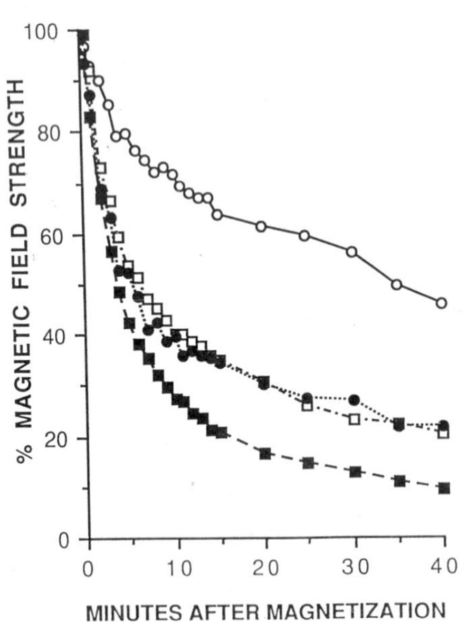

Fig. 1 Relaxation curves 3 days after exposure. Means of normalized data of rabbits exposed to saline (—•—), latex(-▪-), SiO2 30mg(··□··) and SiO2 300mg(—○—)are plotted.

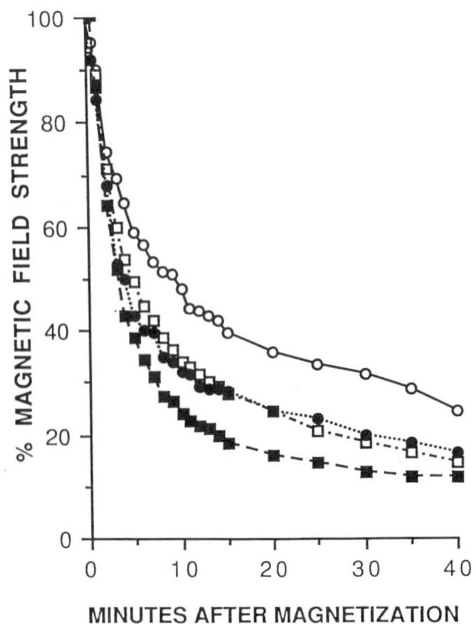

Fig. 2 Relaxation curves 7 days after exposure. Means of normalized data of rabbits exposed to saline (—•—), latex(-▪-), SiO2 30mg(··□··) and SiO2 300mg(—○—)are plotted.

Relaxation

The mean percent of magnetic fields calculated from five rabbits at one minute intervals until 15 minutes and at five minutes intervals until 40 minutes after magnetization are plotted. The relaxation curve obtained three days after instillation of ferrimagnetic particles and silica 300mg was remarkably delayed compared with those of silica 30mg, latex and controls as shown in Fig. 1. The difference of relaxation curves between silica 300mg group and those of other three groups became obscure at the 7th day following instillation as shown in Fig. 2. The same finding was obtained at the 14th day. Four relaxation curves appeared essentially same 21 days after instillation.

Because the delayed relaxation curves of exposed rabbits are considered attributable to a decreased initial relaxation, decay constants for first five minutes were calculated as in Table. The mean decay constants of the exposed group were significantly lower than those of controls at one, two, three and four ($p<0.05$), and six days ($p<0.01$) after exposure.

The delay of relaxation in exposed rabbits was considered attributable to the functional disturbance of alveolar macrophages due to phagocytized silica. This cytological dysfunction appeared recovered 7 days after instillation.

Clearance

The mean maximum percent magnetic field strengths at each day after instillation are plotted in Fig. 3. The clearance curves of ferrimagnetic particles from lungs exposed to higher dose as well as lower dose were delayed after 7 days of exposure. The clearance of the lungs exposed to latex was not disturbed.

Histological examination

Microscopic examinations of grossly consolidated areas of lungs exposed to silica showed extensive cellular infiltrates. Granulomatous lesions were occasionally found. These granulomatous areas contained silica particles identified by their typical appearance and ability to polarize light. The alveolar air spaces in regions of diffuse infiltration contained large mono-

Table Decay Constant for the first five minutes after magnetization

		decay constant[α]		
time	Saline	Latex	$SiO_2$30mg	$SiO_2$300mg
0 day	2.20±3.00	1.24±0.60	0.94±0.40	0.73±0.65
1 day	2.23±0.84	1.78±0.10	1.38±0.41	0.55±0.14*
2 days	2.08±0.82	2.41±0.17	1.52±0.41	0.83±0.45*
3 days	2.86±1.14	2.98±0.15	2.17±0.39	0.89±0.28*
4 days	2.39±0.39	3.28±0.12*	2.39±0.41	1.66±0.42*
5 days	3.77±2.41	3.51±0.54	2.52±0.58	——
6 days	4.88±1.22	3.55±0.35	2.56±0.47*	1.71±0.55**
7 days	3.07±1.64	3.46±0.53	2.63±0.52	2.25±0.80
14 days	2.73±1.38	3.51±0.36	2.33±0.42	1.75±0.68
28 days	3.00±1.41	2.82±0.51	1.73±0.22	2.49±1.00

α All values represent $(M \pm SD) \times 10^{-3}$ per second. Decay constant is the initial decay rate calculated with the equation of $B=B_0\exp(-\lambda t)$.
* $p<0.05$, ** $p<0.01$.

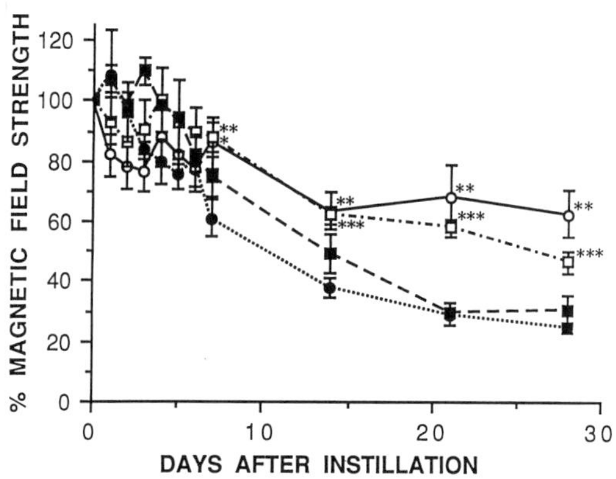

Fig. 3 Clearance curves. Means of normalized B_0 of rabbits exposed to saline(—•—), latex(-▪-), SiO_2 30mg(··□··) and SiO_2 300mg(—○—) are plotted. * $p<0.05$, ** $p<0.01$, *** $p<0.001$.

nuclear cells that were probably macrophages. The ferrimagnetic particles stained with Berlin blue coexisted with silica in some areas.

The coexistence of iron oxide particles either with silica or latex was observed in the phagocytized cells by an transmission electron microscope.

CONCLUSIONS

The intratracheal instillation of high dose of silica into rabbits disturbed relaxation during first 6 days, and it impaired clearance of ferrimagnetic particles later. The exposure of low dose of silica did not disturb relaxation but caused delayed clearance. Because the exposure of latex did not affect either relaxation or clearance, the effects of silica are considered specific to phagocytic cells in lungs.

ACKNOWLEDGMENTS. Histological examinations offered by Professor T. Kameya and technical assistance of Ms. Y. Sugiura, Ms. K. Yajima and staffs in Electron Microscopy Laboratory Center are gratefully acknowledged.

REFERENCES

1) Gehr, P., Brain, J.D., Nemoto, I. & Bloom, S.B.: Behavior of magnetic particles in hamster lungs: estimates of clearance and cytoplasmic motility. J Appl Physiol Respirat Environ Exercise Physiol 55:1196-1202, 1983.
2) Brain, J.D., Bloom, S.B., Valberg, P.A. & Gehr, P.: Correlation between the behavior of magnetic iron oxide particles in the lungs of rabbits and phago-cytosis. Exper Lung Res 6:115-131, 1984.
3) Brain, J.D., Hu, T., and Bloom, S.B.: Effects of SiO_2 and Fe_2O_3 on macrophage motility and on clearance of magnetic particles from hamster lungs. 5th World Conference on Biomagnetism, 1984.
4) Aizawa, Y., Kurihara, M., Hashimoto, K., Maeda, A., Takata, T., Kotani, M., Chiyotani, K. and Yagami, T.:Effect of silica on relaxation and clearance of iron particles in rabbit lungs. Biomagnetism'87 p.374-377, Tokyo Denki University Press, Tokyo, 1988.

RESEARCH ON BIOMAGNETIC TECHNIQUE USED FOR TRACING PNEUMOCONIOSIS OF METALLURGICAL WORKERS

Yu Baigang*, Xiang Ke*, Hu Peilie**, Li Lian**

*Beijing University of Science and Technology, Beijing, China
**Industrial Hygiene Institute of Ben Xi Iron and Steel Corporation
Ben Xi, China

INTRODUCTION

There are many workers in metallurgical factories suffering from silicosis. So far there is not a diagnostic method which may be able to examine the patients' conditions exactly. Luckily, iron oxide always in the dusts of metallurgical factories and can be considered to serve as a natural tracer; it gives an opportunity to apply the biomagnetic technique to tracing silicosis. Baigang et al.(1987a, b) reported that the silicosis of animals caused the mean relaxation parameter Q (defined in Fig. 1) to decrease and clearance caused Q to increase; the parameter Q was more sensitive to the animals' silicosis than relaxation rate. Aming to determine the relationship between relaxation parameters and pneumoconiosis state, we studied 36 workers of an iron-ore sintering workshop in the Ben Xi Iron and Steel Corporation.

SUBJECTS

The exposure period of subjects working in an iron-ore sintering workshop varied from 8 to 39 years, and the mean exposure period was 30.6 ± 0.5 years. They were examined with a x-ray and a magnetopneumographic instrument; their pneumonographs and relaxation curves were measured. It is recognized that the pneumonograph is the only direct way to examine the clinical state of pneumoconiosis, although it is not so accurate as using pathological sections of cadaver lungs. The pneumoconiosis states of the subjects were divided into 12 grades on the basis of the pneumonography.

METHODS

The subjects were magnetized with a mobile magnetizing bed for 10 min, and then they were measured with a mobile testing bed. The magnetizing bed consisted of a mobile bed and a pair of magneto-poles with an area of 45×35 cm. The magnetic induction of the field at the face of magneto-poles was 20 mT, and at the center of the magnetic field space was about 10 mT. The testing bed was made up of a mobile bed and a fluxgate gradiometer, with a microcomputer used to collect and treat the measuring data. The fluxgate sensing a single z-component of the field was placed at the center between the mamillies of each subject. The relaxation curves of the subjects' remanent field $B_r(t)$ were measured from 1 to 11 min after the magnetization process. In this paper three characteristic parameters are used as follows: mean relaxation quantity $Q(2)$, characteristic time T_i, characteristic time T_n, where T_i, T_n are the characteristic time for the relaxation curves when $B_r(t)$ is plotted against $\ln(t)$. T_i represents the time at an inflection point, and T_n shows the time at an intersection point of two tangents; one is the tangent at the inflection point, and the other is at t=1 min. The characteristic parameters are diagramed in Figs. 1 and 2.

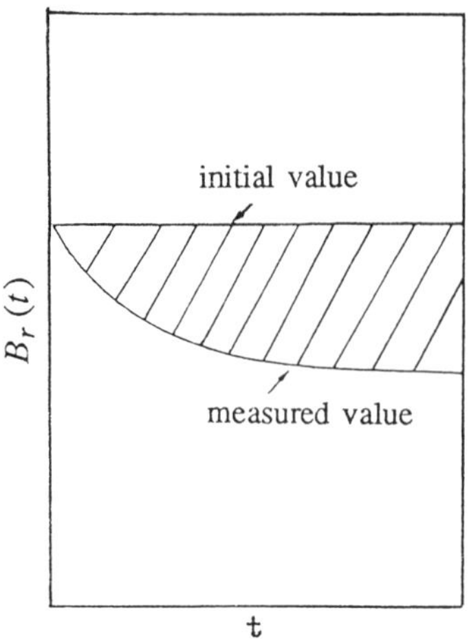

Fig. 1. Relaxation parameter Q is defined as the cross hatched area between the initial value and the measured value lines.

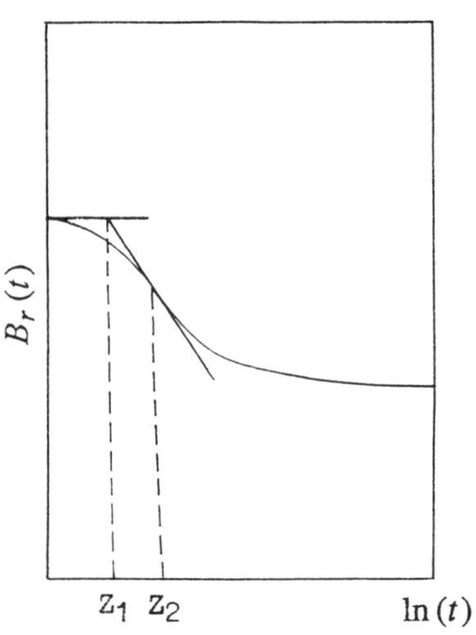

Fig. 2. T_i, T_n are the time values corresponding to the point Z_1, Z_2 expressed in ln (t) coordinate.

Then correlations was made between the measured values of each relaxation parameter and graded data of pneumoconiosis states according to the pneumonographs. Data of 36 subjects were fit by the following empirical formula:

$$Y = a + bX \quad (1)$$

Where Y is the measured values of each relaxation parameters, X is the graded data of pneumoconiosis state, and a,b are the fitted constants.

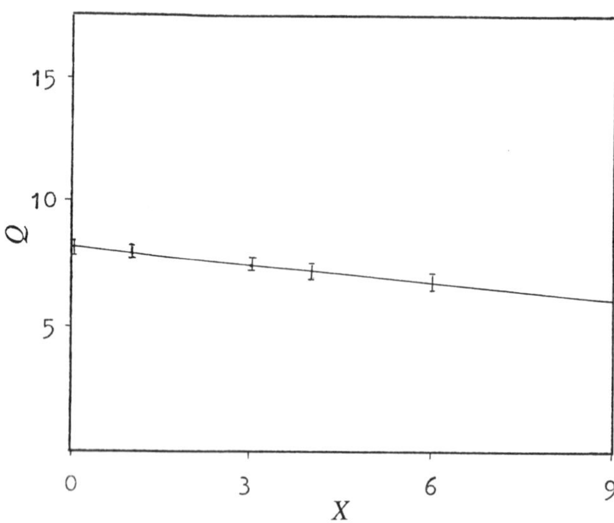

Fig. 3. The best-fitting line relating the relaxation parameter Q to pneumonographs state X.

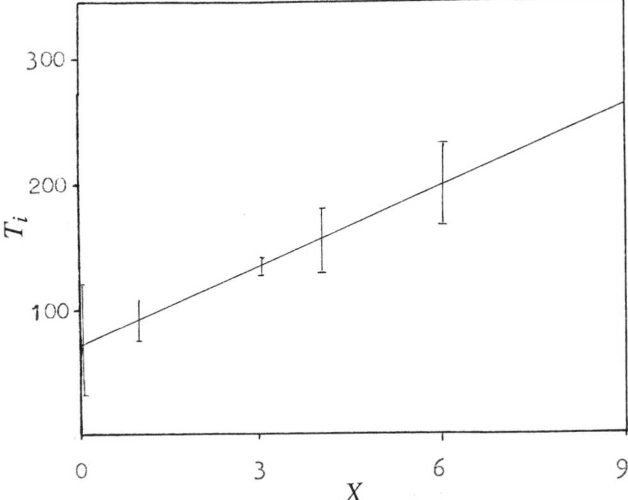

Fig. 4. The best-fitting line for the empirical values of T_i

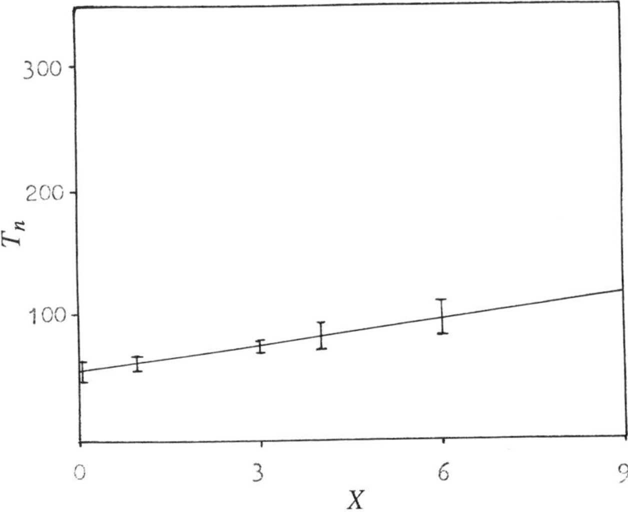

Fig. 5. The best fitting line for the empirical values of T_n

RESULTS

The results of these experiments and their fitting lines are shown in Figs. 3, 4, 5. The regression coefficient of the lines in Figs. 3, 4, 5 are calculated respectively, and the goodness of fitting of each line, p, is made as Table 1.

Table 1

Parameters	a	b	p
Q	8.4	-0.1	0.1
T_i	72.0	21.3	0.05
T_n	58.4	7.1	0.01

DISCUSSION

This study provides new evidence of that relaxation parameters Q, T_i, T_n may be able to give us some information about the pneumoconiosis states. It is clear that the goodness of fit of Q is less than for T_i, T_n , because the initial time of the relaxation measured curves is fairly late. The constant b is the slope for Eq. 1. The constant b is greater, the greater the difference of values for Y among the grades of pneumoconiosis states. If the constant b is bigger, the patients' conditions determined with magnetopneumography are more accurate. Obviously, the measured values of Y are not strictly to the values of X: there are some deviation from Eq. 1. It has been found that the x-ray technique is not be able to examine the patient condition exactly, and there exist some errors in magnetopneumographic method.

REFERENCES

Yu Baigang , Shi Fan , Hu Peilie, Yang Guixin, Li Na, Li Lian, Wang Yanghou, 1987a, Research on biomagnetic technique used for tracing silicosis -Relaxation and clearance in process of pathologic chance of hamsters, in: *Biomagnetism '87*, K. Atsumi, M. Kotani, S. Ueno, T. Katila, and S. J. Williamson, Eds., Tokyo Denki University Press, pp. 288-289.

Yu Baigang, Dong Qingfei, 1987b, Research on biomagnetic technique used for tracing silicosis(3) -Characteristic parameters of relaxation curves of animals in: *Biomagnetism '87*, K. Atsumi, M. Kotani, S. Ueno, T. Katila, and S. J. Williamson, Eds., Tokyo Denki University Press, pp. 292-293.

THE HAMBURG BIOSUSCEPTOMETER FOR LIVER IRON QUANTIFICATION

D.N. Paulson*, R. Engelhardt, R. Fischer, and H.C. Heinrich

Division of Medical Biochemistry, University Hospital Eppendorf, 2000 Hamburg 20, Germany
*Biomagnetic Technologies, Inc., San Diego, CA 92121, U.S.A.

INTRODUCTION

SQUID biosusceptometric studies for the non-invasive in vivo quantification of paramagnetic iron in the liver started in 1978 (Harris et al., 1978; Farrell et al., 1980, 1983; Bastuschek et al., 1981, 1985). This technique has been further developed into a commercial prototype instrument with the sensitivity necessary for the detection of iron overload .

INSTRUMENTATION AND METHODS

The main system components (Figure 1.) with peripheral equipment are installed in a newly constructed magnetically clean building placed in a calm corner of the hospital area.
The sensor assembly comprises two 2nd order gradiometers of different radii (3.4 and 1.4 cm) rf SQUIDS, and two persistent-current superconducting magnetic field coils wound as 1st order gradiometers of different radii (1.6 and 3.6 cm) of 780 turns 2 cm long at each end of the coil forms. The magnetic field coils can be energized in single or combined mode with maximum magnetic field strength of 20 mT and 50 mT, respectively, at the skin surface. The different magnetic field profiles may be used to provide better definition of the liver and overlying tissue. The detection coils and the SQUIDs have been mounted in the vacuum space of the dewar and thermally connected to the liquid helium bath. The dewar has a holding time of max. 7 days (boil off rate 3 liters/day). The water bag is filled from a reservoir on the side of the gantry and the pressure monitored. The bed, made from carefully selected materials (wood, brass, plastics), is motorized with pancake DC motors which are linked with pulleys to 4 jack screws. This enables the bed to handle safely 200 kg at speeds to 1 cm/sec. Locator loops are used to position the subject under the sensor assembly (x, y direction) and to measure the distance to the lowest gradiometer coil (z) as the bed is lowered during measurement. The bed distance is registered separately by a position transducer assembly and may be used favorably in phantom measurements. The locator loops are a single turn of 1.5 cm diameter copper wire for distance determination and a crossed "double D" coil set used with 2 frequencies and lock-in amplifiers to provide x-y positioning aid. All three coils were encapsulated in magnetically clean epoxy.

For measurements, the motor driven bed is raised until the patient is in contact with the dewar tail and then lowered smoothly about 6 cm in 10 seconds while data from the SQUID channels, the pressure sensor of

Advances in Biomagnetism
Edited by S.J. Williamson *et al.*
Plenum Press, New York

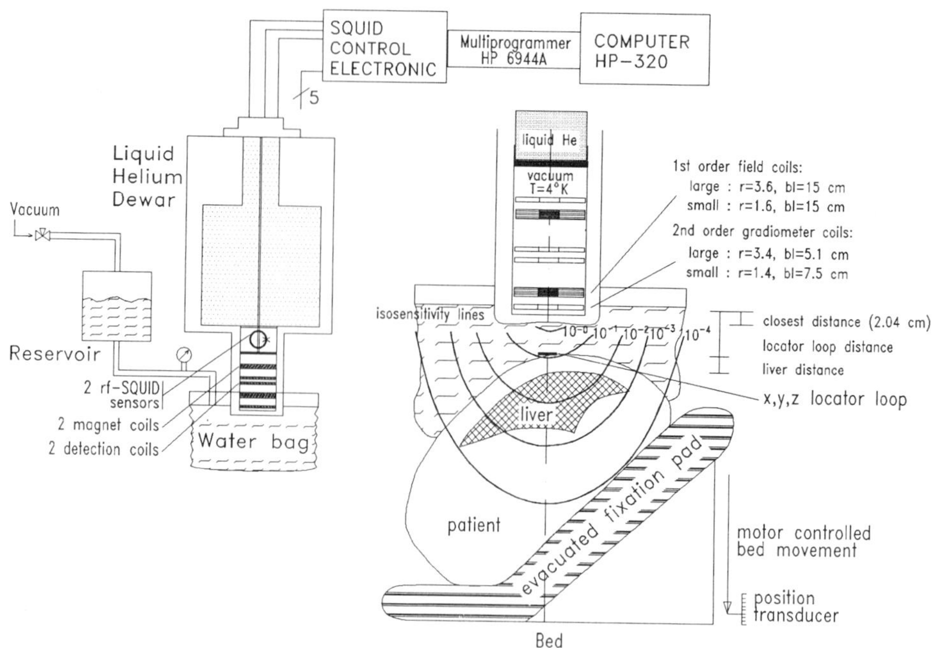

Fig. 1. Schematic illustration of the Ferritometer.

the water coupling membrane, the locator loop and the position transducer are sampled at a rate of 50 Hz. The patient is supported on the bed in a stabilized and reproducible position by an evacuated plastic cushion containing polysterol microspheres. The measuring position above the patient's liver has to be selected with respect to maximum liver volume and minimum skin-liver distance, maximum distance to lung tissue and intestine (air!), enough area for the water coupling membrane, flatness of the torso and capability of withstanding the water bag (false distance measurements!). Normally, the resulting compromise is a more lateral position on the chest and patients are measured in an exhaled state. A water bag pressure equivalent to 6-9 kg avoids any air contribution between body and latex membrane if its positioning on the skin is done carefully. Geometrical information used in the analysis (the liver-skin distance, the torso and liver shape, regions of lung tissue) is extracted from ultrasound images and contour mapping.

The equivalent iron concentration is determined according to equation (1) by a linear fit of the actual Ferritometer system response at a certain depth, $\Delta V(z)$, versus the calculated response of the system to a model volume (flux integral) at the same depth.

$$(1) \quad \Delta V(z) = \text{const} \cdot \Delta\Phi(z) = \text{const} \cdot \frac{\Delta\chi}{\mu_o I_d} \cdot \int \mathbf{B}_f(\mathbf{r}) \cdot \mathbf{B}_d(\mathbf{r})\, d^3r$$

The slope of the linear fit between system response and the calculated response (flux integral) yields the volume susceptibility which is assumed homogeneous over the whole volume and which corresponds with the ferritin-hemosiderin equivalent iron concentration, C_{Fe}, via the Weidemann relation, $\Delta\chi = \chi - \chi_o \approx \chi_{Ftn} \cdot C_{Fe}$, with a mean ferritin-hemosiderin susceptibility of $\chi_{Ftn} = 1600 \cdot 10^{-6}$ [SI] (Shoden and Sturgeon, 1960).

A straight forward calculation (eq. 1.) is performed rapidly by linear correlation of SQUID voltage output versus tabulated standard volume flux integrals during run time. An analytical model with two homogeneous layers (liver and overlaying tissue) with correction terms for the system background (water bag, locator loop) was developed to analyze the system output (Fischer et al., 1989).

SYSTEM PERFORMANCE, NOISE, AND CALIBRATION

The major sources of noise have been identified as vibration, bubbling liquid helium, rf shielding, and moving magnetic objects. By minimizing the contributions from these sources, the low frequency instrumentation noise has been reduced by at least a factor of 30 in relation to an earlier instrument. An rf stripping transformer was installed in the input to reduce the system reponse to rf signals above 1 kHz. The coil region has an approximate 2 hour response time to pressure or temperature changes which were $< 10\,V/K^o$ or $< 0.02\,V/mHg$ at gain 10 on the SQUID control unit (BTi, model 330X) and the system drift is $< 5 \cdot 10^{-4}\,V/h$. There is a long time constant (0.5 day) associated with stability after a major field change in the magnets. Several heaters were installed in the flux loops to minimize this effect.

The SQUID detection coils were balanced with respect to the magnets to <1% and to external fields by <700 ppm. Most of the moving potentially magnetic system components (especially in the bed assembly) have been modified to reduce their noise contribution. Instrumental noise spectra have been taken at the site of the new building. At frequencies below 3 Hz, the total noise is equivalent to 0.016 mg Fe/g liver ($< 1\,pT/\sqrt{Hz}$ at 0.1 Hz) during normal hospital daytime and ten times smaller at midnight. Background signals from different parts of the system (water bag, locator loop, bed) have been investigated and were found to be small but not negligible (equivalent to 0.4 mg Fe/g at typical liver depth of 20 mm below the skin). This background, causing a systematic error, is removed by a correction term in the iron calculation software.

The calibration was first calculated and corrections were made by susceptibility measurements with a SHE VTS-905 susceptometer on an hemispherical epoxy model. A better calibration was then performed with spherical DURAN glass flasks of diameter 159 mm and walls 2.3 mm filled with aqueous solutions of iron(III)-hydroxide-polymaltose ($\chi/\rho = 769 \cdot 10^{-9}\,m^3/kg$) and ferric chloride, $FeCl_3 \cdot 6H_2O$ (pH=2, $\chi/\rho = 3467 \cdot 10^{-9}\,m^3/kg$) in the concentration range of 0.05 -4.0 mg ferritin equivalent iron per ml. The glass balls were installed inside a water-filled cylindrical lucite torso phantom at a realistic depth of 15 mm. A linear correlation of the Ferritometer results versus ferritin equivalent iron concentrations calculated from susceptibilty measurements on aliquots with a Gouy balance (Evans method) is shown in Figure 2.

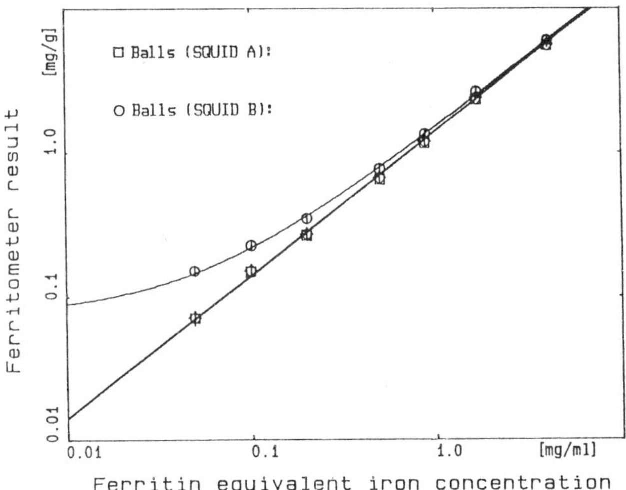

Fig. 2. Calibration of the system for the two SQUID channels (large A and small B gradiometer coils) in a water-filled torso phantom at 15 mm depth. Linear regression fits of Ferritometer estimations to concentrations of ferric iron solutions inside spherical DURAN glass flasks.

The data show excellent linear relationship ($r=0.9998$, $\chi^2<2$) for both SQUID gradiometer channels with instrumental in vitro detection limits of 0.02 and 0.03 mg Fe/ml for the large and small coils, respectively. The slope represents the calibration factor whereas the intercept describes the mean backgound from the lucite torso phantom and the glass spheres.
A fast and more elegant method which may be used for monitoring purposes, especially, is a difference measurement of a geometrical well defined object versus water and air. According to equation (1), this results in a relation for the SQUID output voltage difference, $\Delta V_{water}-\Delta V_{air}$, with the susceptibility difference of $\chi_{air}-\chi_{water}=9.396\cdot 10^{-6}$ [SI]. This relation may be fitted exclusively for the calibration constant, const, or an effective geometry, $\int ...\, d^3r$.

FUTURE ASPECTS

The analysis algorithms will be improved in order to extract the susceptibilities of liver and overlying tissue, simultaneously, as described here elsewhere (Fischer et al., 1989). Also minor experimental magnetic field deviations from theoretical calculations have to be investigated in order to reduce small errors in flux integral calculations. Since there is a strong correlation between tissue and liver susceptibility, noise from bed movement, the most important source left, and errors from unprecise geometry determination have to be minimized.
The weak point of this method is the relative poor spatial resolution of gradiometer coil configurations for tissue and liver susceptibility. In order to extend the clinical application of the instrument also to normal and even reduced liver iron concentrations, this problem has to be solved. Since magnetic resonance imaging with its localization capacity but severely limited quantification range is the only competitor for the non-invasive quantification of liver iron, biomagnetometry will be the method of choice if the discrimination between magnetic susceptibilities of the liver and and the overlaying tissue has been improved.

ACKNOWLEDGEMENTS

This work is supported by grant 01 VF 8603 of the Bundesministerium für Forschung und Technologie, Federal Republic of Germany, and supported in part by National Institutes of Health grant, No. 2R44AM33424, U.S.A.

REFERENCES

Bastuscheck C.M., and Williamson S.J. (1985). Technique for measuring th ac susceptibility of portions of the human body or other large objects. J. Appl. Phys., 58: 3896-3906.

Farrell D.E., Tripp J.H., Zanzucchi P.E., Harris J.W., Brittenham G.M., Muir W.A. (1980). Magnetic measurement of human iron stores. IEEE Transactions on Magnetism, MAG-16, 818-823.

Farrell D.E., Tripp J.H., Brittenham G.M., Danish E.H., Harris J.W., Tracht A.E. (1983). A clinical system for accurate assessment of tissue iron concentration. In: Romani G.L., Williamson S.J., Proc. 4th Int. Workshop Biomagnetism, Nuovo Cimento 2D, Rome, pp. 582-593.

Fischer R., Eich E., Engelhardt R., Heinrich H.C., Kessler M., and Nielsen P., 1989. The calibration problem in liver iron susceptometry - comparison of magnetical and chemical liver iron quantification. In: Williamson S.J., Proc. 7th Int. Conf. Biomagnetism, Plenum Press, New York.

Harris J.W., Farrell D.E., Messer M.J., Tripp J.H., Brittenham G.M., Danish E.H., and Muir W.A., 1978. Assessment of human iron stores by magnetic susceptibility measurements (in vivo and in vitro studies), Clin. Res., 26: 504A abstract.

Shoden A., and Sturgeon P., 1960. Hemosiderin - a physico-chemical study, Acta Haematol., 23: 376-392.

THE CALIBRATION PROBLEM IN LIVER IRON SUSCEPTOMETRY

COMPARISON OF MAGNETICAL AND CHEMICAL LIVER IRON QUANTIFICATION

R. Fischer, E. Eich*, R. Engelhardt, H.C. Heinrich,
M. Kessler, and P. Nielsen

Division of Medical Biochemistry, University Hospital Eppendorf
2000 Hamburg 20, Germany
* S.H.E. GmbH, 5100 Aachen 1, Germany

INTRODUCTION

The concentration of non-heme storage iron in human liver ranges from 0.02-0.1 mg/g (wet weight) in iron deficient to 0.1-0.5 mg/g with normal iron stores and from 1 to 30 mg/g in different stages of iron overload. The reference standard for all non-invasive in vivo methods of liver iron quantification (Computer Tomography, Biosusceptometry, Magnetic Resonance Imaging) is the direct in vitro determination of non-heme iron in liver biopsies by colorimetry or atomic absorption spectrometry. Susceptometry of the paramagnetic iron in the liver with a SQUID biomagnetometer was introduced at CWRU in Cleveland (Harris et al., 1978; Brittenham et al., 1982; Farrell et al., 1983) for iron overloaded patients using prototype instrumentation.
If the magnetic structure of the human body around the liver in the presence of an external magnetic field is known in detail a resulting magnetic field distribution can be calculated at any point in the space. Although the geometrical information is obtained satisfactorily by ultrasound imaging and contour mapping, the inverse problem of determining the magnetization of the liver from magnetic flux change measurements outside the body gets unsolvable with the degree of complexity in the magnetic properties of the human body. For particular models of the liver and the surrounding tissue, e.g. torso models with magnetically homogeneous layers, this problem can be solved numerically, but in practice the solutions lack from the poor spatial resolution of present day pick-up coil configurations.

ANALYSIS METHODS

The Hamburg biosusceptometer with 2 rf SQUID channels as 2nd order gradiometers different in diameter, and 2 different field magnets of similar size was used and is described here elsewhere (Paulson et al., 1989). Almost all measurements were performed with the small size magnet which was energized to generate a field strength of 20 mT at the patient's skin surface. Iron in the liver biopsies was estimated by atomic absorption spectroscopy.
The analysis of simulated data show a fairly high correlation between liver and tissue susceptibility for the single gradiometer channels as well as for both channels considered simultaneously. It also turned out that tiny system background and noise contributions are another serious problem which causes susceptibility deviations due to an altered voltage characteristic.

Advances in Biomagnetism
Edited by S.J. Williamson *et al.*
Plenum Press, New York

At the moment, analysis of the SQUID output voltages is done for a 2-layer model consisting of a hemispherical liver and the overlaying torso tissue with cylindrical or hemispherical shape. The magnetic susceptibility of the liver is determined primarily by the hemosiderin/ferritin susceptibility of the liver iron. The non-iron contribution from the liver tissue itself is assumed to be small and constant for all individuals.

The data from the two SQUID channels, are fitted with distance, z, for the voltage intercept, V_o, the difference susceptibilities, $\Delta\chi = \chi - \chi^{ref}$, and a ramp parameter, α. Normally, the reference medium is water with $\chi^{ref} = -9.032 \cdot 10^{-6}$ [SI], since the patient is displaced by a water bag. According to equation (1) these parameters are estimated separately or simultaneously for the two gradiometer configurations by a non-linear Marquardt algorithm in flux integral space.

$$(1)\quad V_{net}(z) = V_o + c\left[\Delta\chi^{liv}\int \mathbf{B}_f(r)\cdot\mathbf{B}_d(r)\,dV_{liv} + \Delta\chi^{tis}\int \mathbf{B}_f(r)\cdot\mathbf{B}_d(r)\,dV_{tis}\right] + \mathcal{O}(\alpha\cdot z)$$

Background contributions from the locator loop, water bag and bed were measured very carefully and are subtracted from the raw voltage in advance. Nevertheless, there is a small, significant error term, $\mathcal{O}(z)$, of different sources which is assumed linear with distance. Recently, the influence of this error term could be reduced by eliminating a considerable background contribution in the patient's bed which depended on the bed distance and the patient's position. The ramp parameter was typically 6 and 12 mV/cm for the small and large SQUID, respectively.

The present analysis procedure is to fix the ramp parameter, α, of the error term, first, by fitting the data according to equation (1) with a reasonable but constant tissue susceptibility for both the SQUIDs. Then the data from both SQUID channels are fitted independently and/or simultaneously for the susceptibilities and the intercept. The final result is achieved from a linear regression fit (1st approximation of equation (1)) with constant tissue term from the multiple fit procedure. Figure 1 shows the remaining experimental net voltage together with simulated contributions of tissue ($-8.68 \cdot 10^{-6}$ [SI]) and liver, exemplarily, for an obese patient with 0.36 mg Fe/g liver which was established by the measurement of liver biopsy iron. Because of the relative small distance of the overlaying tissue this signal results in the predominant contribution to the total signal in fig. 1.

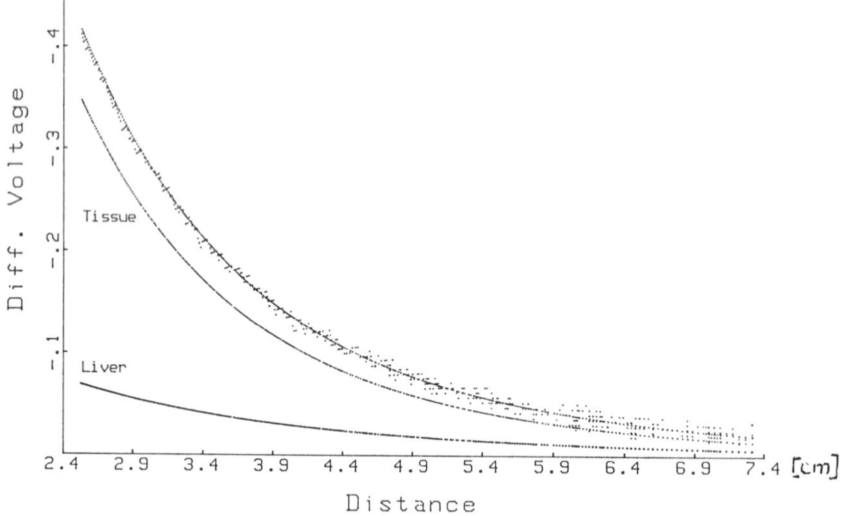

Fig. 1. SQUID output net voltage of large 2nd order gradiometer (raw voltage - system background) for a patient of 97 kg with liver iron concentration of 0.36 mg/$g_{w.w.}$ and simulated liver and tissue contribution and the sum of both.

RESULTS AND DISCUSSION

Various analysis strategies have been derived as approximations from equation (1) and their results were correlated with iron concentrations from liver biopsies in figure 2.

Mean tissue susceptibility model

The relatively simple and fast straight forward model of a representative tissue background for all individuals (i.e. intercept of the linear mean tissue susceptibility model curve in fig. 2) as used by Brittenham et al. (1982) results in a poor correlation ($r = 0.5$) and large quantification errors of 1.2 mg/g below 2 mg $Fe/g_{w.w.}$ ($\chi^2 = 260$!). Also, the approach of extracting a mean tissue susceptibility from iron deficient patients failed, since the interindividual tissue susceptibilities varied by far more than 1% (Farrel et al., 1983). In fact, a liver susceptibility variation of 1% ($\Delta\chi = 0.1 \cdot 10^{-6}$ [SI]) will correspond to a subject noise of 0.05 mg Fe/g liver, but the same variation in the overlaying tissue will cause already a change in liver iron concentration between 0.3 and 0.5 mg Fe/g liver. Therefore, major changes in tissue susceptibilities may mislead to false iron concentrations of 1-2 mg Fe/g liver, even in iron deficiency anemia as shown in fig. 2 (analysis model o).
Another approach was to find other body regions like the thigh with its simple and stable geometry which could represent individual tissue susceptibilities. But the quantification became sometimes even worse and it seems to be, that d. c. magnetic fields due to ionic currents in the leg superpose the magnetization from the field coils of the instrument (Grimes et al., 1985).

Individual tissue susceptibility (2-layer) model

In a more sophisticated model (2-layer model curve in fig. 2) tissue and liver susceptibilities were fitted simultaneously for both the SQUID channels. The correlation could be improved ($r = 0.96$) as well as the estimation errors ($\chi^2 = 8$) at least beyond normal iron concentrations of ≥ 0.3 mg/g. The slope coefficient of $1.05 \pm .09$ indicates that the calibration derived originally from phantom measurements is also valid for in vivo liver susceptometry. The intercept indicates a vanishing or at least a small non-ferric susceptibility of liver tissue. This

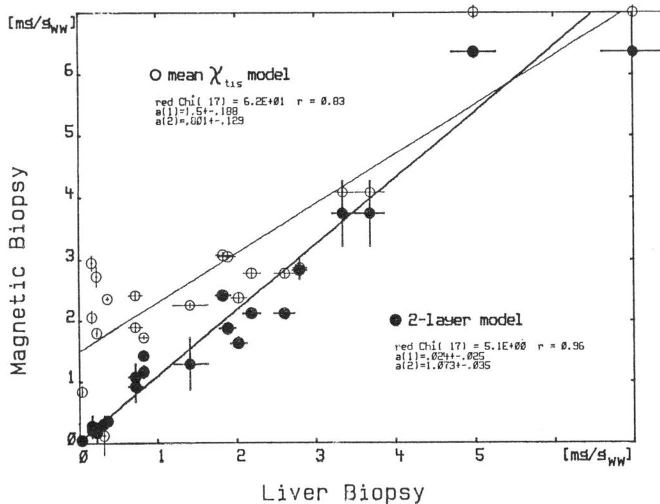

Fig. 2. Liver iron concentrations from biomagnetometer measurements versus chemical estimation of total iron in hepatic biopsies for mean tissue susceptibility model (o) and 2-layer model (●).

could be expected from estimations of the susceptibility contribution from the blood content of the liver. Considering only the blood in the small-capacitance vessels with less than 15 - 18 ml/100g liver tissue (Campra and Reynolds, 1988), the corresponding iron concentration is less than 0.078 - 0.094 mg Fe/g liver. This is in agreement with the intercept of 0.058 mg Fe/g due to the hemoglobine susceptibility, which was found to be $1543 \pm 50 \cdot 10^{-9} m^3/kg$ iron.

Especially, in obese patients we found relative paramagnetic tissue susceptibilities of $-8.8 \cdot 10^{-6}$ to $-8.6 \cdot 10^{-6}$ [SI] by the 2-layer model analysis, and a slight correlation with weight.

From the linear regression analysis in fig 2. (model ●) and a mean standard deviation of 0.1 mg Fe/g for the "magnetic biopsy" a lower detection limit of 0.23 mg Fe/g is derived, whereas, the quantification range is unlimited for high iron concentrations in contrast to magnetic resonance imaging. There are possibly systematic differences due to the fact that magnetic and liver biopsy originate from different parts of the liver.

In simulations on calculated data without noise the correct liver iron concentration, e. g. a liver iron concentration of 1.0 mg Fe/g with a tissue susceptibility difference of 1% relative to water, is reproduced within a 1σ confidence range from 0.875 to 1.125 mg/g. If, however, the noise component is increased to experimental values, it becomes more difficult to retain the input values for the susceptibilities, e. g. the 1σ confidence range extends from 0.750 to 1.250 mg Fe/g liver. Imposing a side condition of positive equal liver iron concentrations for both SQUID channels on the fitting procedure of the data restricts liver iron concentrations not only to the χ^2 minimum, which is highly sensitive to any perturbation, but to more realistic and stable values. This has been done in figure 2 for the 2-layer model analysis and seems to reflect the fact, that inhomogeneities in the overlaying tissue (ribs and minor tissue deformations!) will cause different effective tissue susceptibilities for both the SQUID channels due to different sensitivity areas.

The main difficulties arise from the relative poor spatial resolution of both the gradiometer configurations. So, a ferritometer with a significantly improved resolution characteristic may solve some of these calibration problems.

ACKNOWLEDGEMENTS

This work is supported by grant 01 VF 8603 of the Bundesministerium für Forschung und Technologie, Federal Republic of Germany.

REFERENCES

Brittenham G.M., Farrell D.E., Harris J.W., Feldman E.S., Danish E.H., Muir W.A., Tripp J.H., and Bellon E.M., 1982. Magnetic-susceptibility measurement of human iron stores, N. Eng. J. Med., 307: 1671-1675.

Campra J.L. and Reynolds T.B., 1988. The hepatic Circulation. In: Arias I.M., Jakoby W.B., Popper H.P., Schachter D., and Shafritz D.A., The Liver: Biology and Pathobiology, Raven Press, New York, pp. 911-930.

Farrell D.E., Tripp J.H., Brittenham G.M., Danish E.H., Harris J.W., Tracht A.E., 1983. A clinical system for accurate assessment of tissue iron concentration. In: Romani G.L., Williamson S.J., Proc. 4th Int. Workshop Biomagnetism, Nuovo Cimento 2D, Rome, pp. 582-593.

Grimes D.I.F., Lennard R.F., and Swithenby S.J., 1985. Macroscopic ionic currents within the human leg, Phys. Med. Biol., 30: 1101-1112.

Harris J.W., Farrell D.E., Messer M.J., Tripp J.H., Brittenham G.M., Danish E.H., and Muir W.A., 1978. Assessment of human iron stores by magnetic susceptibility measurements, Clin. Res., 26: 504A

Paulson D.N., Engelhardt R., Fischer R., and Heinrich H.C., 1989. The Hamburg biosusceptometer for liver iron quantification. In: Williamson S.J., Proc. 7th Int. Conf. Biomagnetism, Plenum Press, New York.

MAGNETIC MAPPING OF DC FIELDS RELATED TO TISSUE SUSCEPTIBILITY IN THE HUMAN BODY

S. Di Luzio, G. Obletter*, S. Comani, C. Del Gratta**, and G.L. Romani

Istituto di Fisica Medica, and *Istituto di Semeiotica Medica
Universita' "G. D'Annunzio", 66100 Chieti, ITALY
**Supported by grant by CITEC S.p.A., Roma, ITALY

INTRODUCTION

Several studies on dc magnetic fields outside the human body have been performed in the past (Kalliomaki, 1983; Farrell, 1983; Cohen, 1983; Swithenby, 1983; Varpula, 1983; Maniewski et al., 1988). As the major constituent of tissues in the body is water, it has usually been assumed that most tissues actually exhibit diamagnetic properties with the magnetic susceptibility of pure water, $\chi = -9 \times 10^{-6}$ SI (Varpula, 1983). However, this is no longer true if a quantitative analysis is carried out to evaluate the magnetization in the earth field of a specific portion of the body as, for instance, the upper or the lower leg. Significant differences from a "water-like" diamagnetic behaviour are observed, which may provide interesting information on diverse contributions to the overall magnetization. These may originate from small amounts of paramagnetic components in specific tissues, or from slight differences in the susceptibility value of various constituents of the body itself. For example, it has been recently estimated (Maniewski et al., 1988) that the susceptibility of the lungs may be assumed as $\chi \sim -4 \times 10^{-6}$ SI, due to the "sponge-like" structure of this organ. Similarly, estimated values for the magnetic susceptibility of the arterial ($\chi \sim -9.3 \times 10^{-6}$ SI) and veneous blood ($\chi \sim -7.8 \times 10^{-6}$ SI), the bone ($\chi \sim -10.0 \times 10^{-6}$ SI), the muscle ($\chi \sim -9.0 \times 10^{-6}$ SI), and other tissues have been recently reported (Rassi et al., 1988). Such estimates, however, were based on *in vitro* measurements of the magnetic behaviour of oxi- and deoxihemoglobin in red cells, whereas no susceptibility value was available from *in vivo* measurements. In this paper we present the preliminary results of a detailed mapping of dc magnetic signals originating from body tissues in the earth field.

MODELING

In order to take account of different contributions to the magnetic induction from different parts of the body, we have represented these parts, with a simplified geometry, in a very crude model. For instance, we can assume that the upper leg is homogeneous from a magnetic point of view and can be regarded as a cylinder of constant radius and isotropic susceptibility χ, immersed in a uniform magnetic field $\mathbf{B}_0$ (i.e. the earth field). In the case of a cylinder with a horizontal axis, two extreme cases may be figured: the horizontal component of the earth field $\mathbf{B}^h_0$ lies either on the same plane as the cylinder axis, or on a plane orthogonal to it. In the former configuration, the contribution of $\mathbf{B}^h_0$ to the vertical component $\mathbf{B}^V$ of the magnetic induction outside the cylinder is negligible unless the measurement is performed in proximity of a transverse boundary (cylinder edge). In the latter configuration, $\mathbf{B}^h_0$ always produces a magnetization that contributes to the measured field. For this reason the following analysis will account only for the first case. The experimental measurements have been performed according to the same configuration. In the case of the sphere, due to the different symmetry conditions, the horizontal component of the earth field always contributes appreciably to the body field, and has been taken into account in the following analysis.

The evaluation of the magnetic induction $\mathbf{B}$ outside the cylinder, at a point P at a distance x from the vertical plane containing the cylinder axis (see Fig. 1), is then straightforward. The vertical component $\mathbf{B}^V$ of this field is given by the following expression:

$$B^V = \{ [B^V_0 R^2 \chi] / [2 (h + R)^2] \} [(1 - u) / (1 + u^2)^2] \quad (1)$$

where R is the cylinder radius, h is the distance between the cylinder surface and a horizontal plane where the field is measured, and $u = x / (R + h)$. In order to represent specific organs it may be useful to consider also the very simple case of a uniformly magnetized sphere. In the case of a sphere with its center lying on the vertical passing through the origin of the plane of measurement, the vertical component of the magnetic induction at a point P of coordinates (x,y) is :

$$B^V = \{ [\chi R^3] / [3 (h + R)^3] \} \{ [B^V_0 (2 - u^2 - v^2) + B^h_0 v] / (1 + u^2 + v^2)^{5/2} \} \quad (2)$$

where R is the radius of the sphere , h is the distance between the sphere and the horizontal plane where the field is measured, $u = x / (R + h)$, and $v = y / (R + h)$.

More complex configurations - i.e. a sphere inside a cylinder, or two coaxial cylinders, etc. - can be represented by a combination of the previous formulas, and the spatial distribution of the resulting $\mathbf{B}^V$ can be calculated.

METHODS AND RESULTS

Relation (1) was checked on a model consisting of a plastic cylinder, 9 cm in diameter and 30 cm in length, filled with isotonic solution (0.9% NaCl). The measurement was carried out using a single channel biomagnetic system (Romani et al., 1982), consisting of a 7 cm baseline, 1.5 cm pickup coil diameter second order gradiometer coupled to a rfSQUID, with a noise figure of about 40 $fT \times (Hz)^{-1/2}$ above 0.5 Hz. The same system was used to perform *in vivo* measurements, and in all cases the recording bandwidth was dc-1 Hz. For the model study the measurement was performed with the cylinder axis parallel to the horizontal component of the earth field. The vertical component of the field was scanned in a transverse direction with respect to the cylinder axis, along a plane such that the minimum vertical distance between the pickup coil and the upper edge of the cylinder was about 2.5 cm. The measured field value $\mathbf{B}^V = 61.5 \pm 2.0$ pT was in good agreement with the theoretical prediction $\mathbf{B}^V_{theor} \sim 63$ pT, obtained using the measured value $\mathbf{B}^V_0 = 3.4 \times 10^{-5}$ T for the vertical component of the earth field. The relatively large error is due to the contribution from 1/f noise in the recording bandwidth.

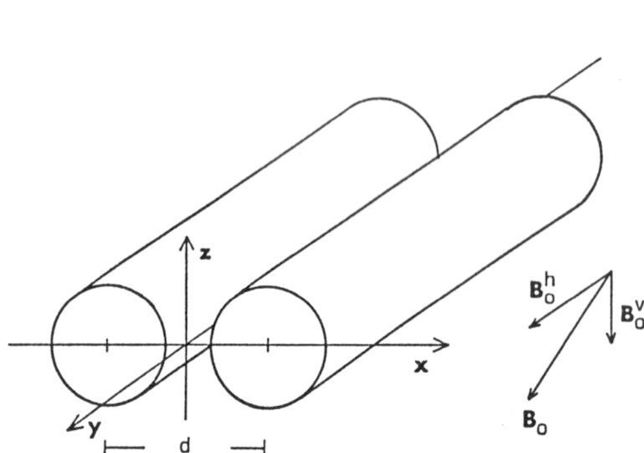

Fig. 1. Perspective view of the model used to compute the values of $\mathbf{B}^V$ on a plane at a distance h for the upper edge of the cylinders with radius R. Both cylinders have an isotropic susceptibility χ and are immersed in an external field $\mathbf{B}^V_0$.

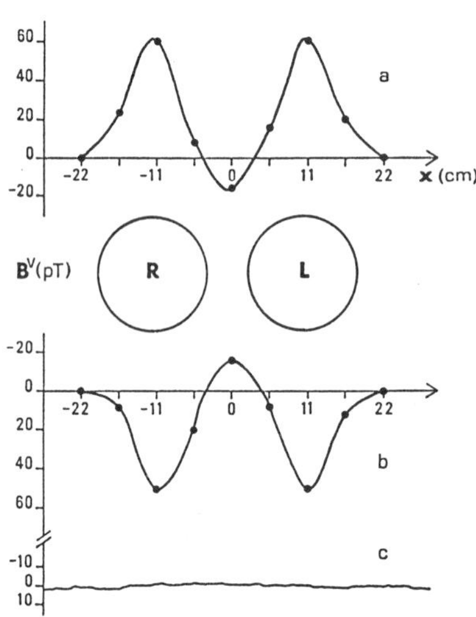

Fig. 2. Measured $\mathbf{B}^V$ over the thighs of subj. AT (a, front; b, back), at the level shown in Fig. 3, c, d). The zero line was arbitrarily chosen at $x = \pm 22$ cm. The solid curves reproduce continuously recorded data, and the dots identify the grid points. c) Typical noise during a scan period.

Magnetic field mapping was performed on thirteen normal volunteers (eleven males, two females) by scanning the body along transverse lines, in the East-West direction. The subjects were carefully demagnetized and their skin was cleaned before each session, to reduce or, possibly, eliminate undesired contribution from contaminating particles in the skin and in the lungs. The subjects laid on a plastic mattress over a wooden bed, oriented in the North-South direction, and the bed itself was moved under the gradiometer in a transverse (East-West) direction. In order to find out whether any contribution to the measured field was due to magnetization of the mattress or the bed, these were thoroughly checked through complete scans. The overall contribution turned out to be lower than 2 pT, i.e. the "overall" noise of the instrument mentioned above. Subject scanning was performed according to a 9×21 point grid normalized to the subject's dimensions. The chosen step for the anterior grid was 1/8 of the distance between the two acromians for the transverse coordinate , and 1/10 of the distance between the cricoid cartilage and the perineum for the longitudinal coordinate. For the posterior side, the field was measured at a similar grid. In this way the whole body was scanned, from the neck to the ankle, on both the anterior and posterior sides. Typically, two sequential, transverse scans were performed at each longitudinal grid position, to check signal reproducibility. All subjects were mapped at least twice in different days, and two (LC and SD) were studied three times, the last one being at a month distance from the previous two for both subjects.

Two typical traces of the measured component $\mathbf{B}^V$ are shown in Fig. 2. They have been recorded over middle thighs of subject AT. The anterior and posterior traces have been combined in a unique figure for clarity. A typical noise trace within a time interval corresponding to that of a scan is also reported at the bottom.

Two examples of whole-body isofield maps are shown in Fig. 3 (a: subject SD, front; b: subject SD, back; c: subject AT, front; d: subject AT, back). The isofield step is 10 pT. The shaded areas represent negative field values, i.e. a polarity coinciding with the orientation of the normal component of the earth field. The unshaded areas therefore identify diamagnetic magnetization of tissues. The longitudinal frames are slightly different for the two subjects, due to the difference in their respective heights.

DISCUSSION

The maps clearly show that several parts of the body do not behave according to the assumption that tissue susceptibility is that of pure water, the major deviations from that assumption being related to the torso area. Minor discrepancies are however observed also in the leg district. This discrepancy may be reduced by considering the actual anatomy of the upper leg, where the femoral bone occupies a non symmetric position with respect to the rest of the muscular mass. Taking into account the data inferable from

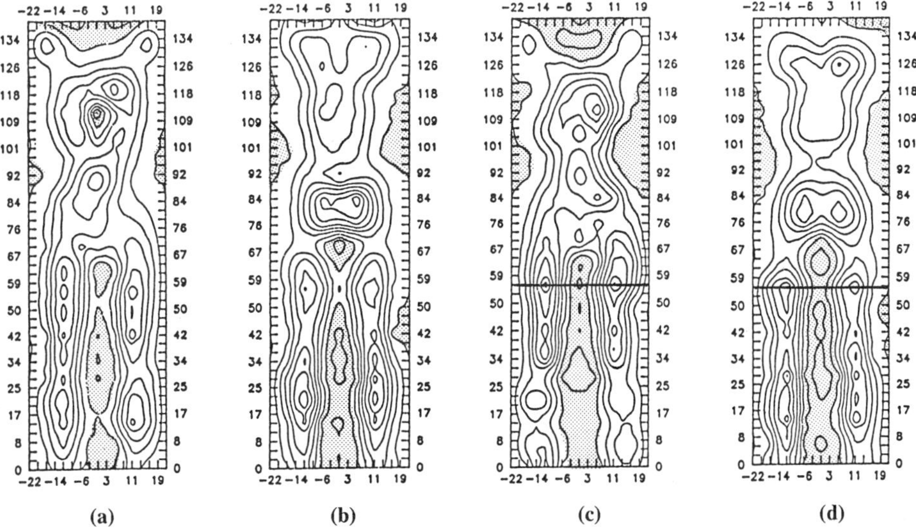

Fig. 3. Isofield maps showing the distribution of $\mathbf{B}^V$ over front and rear body sides (subj. SD, a: front, b: back; subj. AT, c: front, d: back). The isofield step is 10 pT and the shaded areas identify negative field polarities. Units are in cm. The dashed lines in c), d) identify the cross sections used in Fig. 2. and 4.

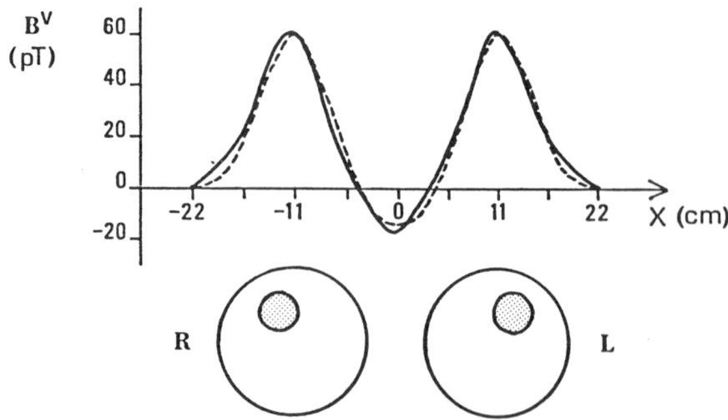

Fig. 4. Fit (dashed line) of the experimental data (solid line) reported in Fig. 2,a using a model which includes the femoral bone (bottom).

a standard anatomy textbook for the bone-muscle relative dimensions and positions typical of a cross section of the upper leg at the level indicated in Fig. 3, it is possible to perform a simple fit of the measured data shown in Fig. 2. This fit also accounts for the actual geometry of the detection coil, in that the measurement has been performed by means of a 7 cm baseline gradiometer, whereas the magnetic "source" has larger physical dimensions and, consequently, the effect of the baseline must be included. The results are shown in Fig. 4, and satisfactorily agree with the measured behaviour. However, a value $\chi = -11 \times 10^{-6}$ SI for the bone susceptibility is obtained from the fit. This figure is slightly larger than that cited at the beginning as estimated by Rassi and coworkers (1988).

The purpose of the present work was to investigate the possibility of achieving a low-resolution magnetic imaging by dc measurements of the body magnetization in the earth field. Indeed this magnetization reflects differences in tissue susceptibility, which so far have been mainly estimated from *in vitro* measurements. Our results demonstrate that it is possible to evaluate susceptibility values for different tissues by *in vivo* measurements, with the use of simple, but realistic models. At present, this analysis has been limited to the leg district, with satisfactory results. More complex modeling is required to investigate other areas (such as the torso) where major deviations are observed.

REFERENCES

Cohen, D., 1983, Steady fields of the body, in: "Biomagnetism: An Interdisciplinary Approach", S. J. Williamson, G. L. Romani, L. Kaufman, and I. Modena, Plenum Press, New York and London.

Farrell, D. E., 1983, Assessment of iron in human tissue: the magnetic biopsy, in: "Biomagnetism: An Interdisciplinary Approach", S. J. Williamson, G. L. Romani, L. Kaufman, and I. Modena, Plenum Press, New York and London.

Grimes, D., Lennard, R., and Swithenby, S., 1983, DC magnetic fields of the human leg as a function of position and relaxation, Il Nuovo Cimento, 2D:650.

Kalliomaki, K., Kalliomaki, P. L., Aittoniemi, K., Moilanen, M., 1983, Magnetic technique for measuring lung contamination, in: "Biomagnetism: An Interdisciplinary Approach", S. J. Williamson, G. L. Romani, L. Kaufman, and I. Modena, Plenum Press, New York and London.

Maniewski, R., Katila, T., Poutanen, T., Siltanen, P., Varpula, T., Wikswo, J. P. Jr., 1988, Magnetic measurements of cardiac mechanical activity, IEEE Transactions on Biomedical Engineering, 35:662

Rassi, D., Hoare, A., Samadian, V., and Melville, D., 1987, SQUID measurement and computational modeling of a simple thorax phantom, in: "Biomagnetism87", K. Atsumi, M. Kotani, S. Ueno, T. Katila, and S.J. Williamson eds., Tokyo Denki University Press, Tokyo, 402-405.

Romani, G. L., Williamson, S. J., and Kaufman, L., 1982, Biomagnetic instrumentation, Rev. Sci. Instr., 53:1815.

Varpula, T., 1983, Magnetic susceptibility plethysmography, Il Nuovo Cimento, 2D:624.

IONIC CURRENTS WITHIN DEVELOPING CHICK EGGS

S.M.Freake, B.S.Janday[1], S.J.Swithenby and I.M.Thomas

Physics Department, Open University, Milton Keynes MK7 6AA, U.K.
[1]Department of Vision Sciences, Aston University
Birmingham B4 7ET, U.K.

INTRODUCTION

DC ionic currents that change slowly over the time scale of development have been measured in many different organisms using vibrating-probe electrometers (Jaffe, 1974). Other recent work described in a multi-author review in *Experientia* (1988) has emphasised the relevance of the electrochemical environment in the development of biological structures, and it has been suggested that the ionic currents may play a significant role in this morphogenetic process. We have investigated the development of the chick embryo *Gallus domesticus* by making mainly non-invasive *in ovo* measurements of the associated magnetic fields with SQUID magnetometers. Our initial aim was to identify the dominant dc ionic current flows and to relate these to the embryo development. During early incubation, we observed consistent simple field patterns. The amplitude of the patterns increased during the first three days, but the patterns then became unpredictable. In this paper we describe the data taken during early incubation stages, discuss possible source models and postulate the biophysical processes that give rise to the signals.

EXPERIMENTAL METHODS

The eggs were incubated at 38°C and 65% relative humidity (40% in later experiments) in a fixed orientation with their long axes horizontal. To prevent adhesion of the embryo to the shell membranes, the eggs were turned every six hours through 90°. By following this protocol, healthy chicks were hatched after 21 days. Magnetic field measurements were made variously at three, six or twelve hour intervals for the first five days of incubation. For a few eggs, the measurement period was extended until the completion of incubation.

The measurements were made with each egg positioned reproducibly (to within ± 5° about each axis) on a non-magnetic support beneath the dewar. The ambient field was nulled to less than 10^{-8} tesla, and each egg was tested for magnetic contamination. The distance between the top of the egg and the bottom of the dewar was 1–2 mm, and was measured to ± 0.2 mm in each case. The magnetic field was recorded by moving the egg beneath the detector along a series of equally spaced scan lines perpendicular to the egg's long axis. A full mapping took approximately 4 minutes, during which time the field did not change significantly, and the egg was then returned to the incubator.

Our initial studies (described briefly in Swithenby, 1988) utilized a commercial rf SQUID and second-order gradiometer with 23 mm diameter coils, with the lowest coil about 11 mm from the outside of the dewar. With this system, the fields above 60 eggs were recorded along six scan lines separated by 14 mm. The data for each scan was averaged into 5mm wide bins.

In order to improve the spatial resolution of the field maps, subsequent measurements were made on 32 eggs using a dc SQUID with a miniature asymmetric second-order gradiometer (Freake, 1988),

Advances in Biomagnetism
Edited by S.J. Williamson *et al.*
Plenum Press, New York

in which the lowest pick-up coil had a diameter of 4 mm and was separated from the outside of the dewar by 6.7 mm, (now reduced to 5.5 mm). The field was measured along 20 scan lines separated by 5 mm and, within each scan line, the data was averaged into 3 mm wide bins.

There are two significant problems associated with the interpretation of these measurements. First, the stage of development of the embryo at a particular time is uncertain; there can be up to 10 hours variation in the laboratory incubation time at which the embryo reaches any specified developmental stage. Second, the orientation of the embryo within the egg is variable; in the majority of cases the embryo's body axis is roughly perpendicular to the long axis of the egg, but in 25 per cent of eggs the body orientation differs by more than 45° from this direction.

To overcome these problems, further experiments with both systems were carried out on 15 eggs that had been windowed by carefully scoring through the shell and removing a rectangular piece of shell together with the underlying shell membrane. The window was covered with a piece of transparent film to guard against airborne infection and desiccation. In this way, it was possible to record the developmental stage and orientation of the embryo for comparison with the magnetic field maps. In addition, a limited series of invasive experiments were carried out on dissected systems.

RESULTS

We have measured the magnetic fields produced by 92 eggs *in ovo*. We first describe the broad pattern of the results from this entire batch, omitting only the 25 per cent of the eggs which proved to be infertile or failed to develop through the stages appropriate to the period of the experiment.

From about 24 hours after the start of incubation, the eggs generated magnetic fields that were detectable above the system noise level. The magnitudes of the fields increased for the next two days. The maximum peak-to-peak signals recorded were very variable, corresponding to magnetic fields of between 10 pT and 80 pT at the lowest gradiometer coil. Figure 1 shows a typical set of scans and a

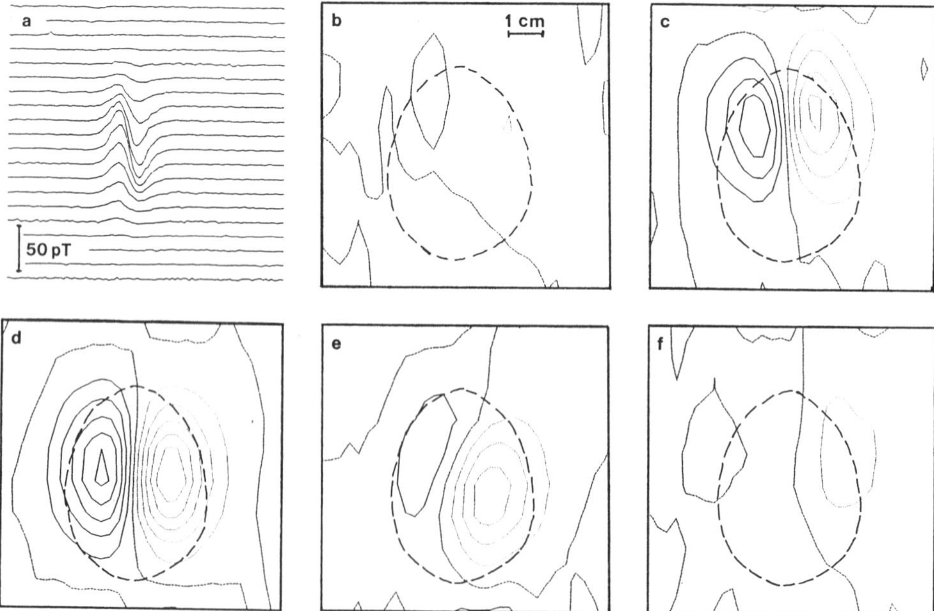

Fig. 1. (a) The signals produced by a set of scans in the horizontal plane 8 mm above an egg at 56 hours incubation time; scan length 300 mm, scan separation 5 mm.
(b)-(f) Contour maps showing the equivalent field in the plane as a function of incubation time: (b) 28 hr, (c) 42 hr, (d) 56 hr, (e) 66 hr, (f) 75 hr. Solid contours indicate that the vertical component of the field is upwards, dotted contours indicate that the field is downwards, and the dashed contour indicates zero vertical field. The contour separation is 2.7 pT in b, c, e and f, and 5.4 pT in d. The broken line indicates the position of the egg. Note that the peak field produced by this egg occurred earlier than normal.

typical series of equivalent field contour maps, both obtained using the miniature gradiometer. After the three days of growing signals, the observed fields tended to diminish and to change in magnitude in a more complex manner without any simple egg to egg consistency. During the initial period of increasing signal magnitude, 90 per cent of the eggs produced contour maps that were superficially consistent with having been produced by a single current dipole. In two-thirds of these eggs, the equivalent dipole was oriented during this period within 45 degrees of the longitudinal blunt-sharp egg axis. However, at approximately 75 hours, the orientation of the pattern became highly unpredictable: for example, the polarity was sometimes completely reversed during a twelve hour period.

These gross statistics are dominated by the measurements made with the 23 mm coil system. Recent data taken with the miniature system show the same trends but also suggest some more complex sources. A few eggs have produced contour maps that are not simple dipolar patterns (Figure 2).

DISCUSSION

In those cases where the field contours appear to be dipolar, we have used a dipole-in-a-conducting-sphere model to determine the position, orientation and strength of the equivalent source dipole. Our results show that throughout the first three days the equivalent dipole is located at a depth corresponding to the centre of the yolk, and has a strength of about 3×10^{-7} A m. This depth localisation is highly consistent from egg to egg; the variability is $\pm$ 3 mm. There is some variability in embryo location, but in all cases it is found on the surface of the yolk near the top. Clearly these results indicate that the active (dipolar) source is *not* the embryo itself.

In those eggs that were windowed and where development was normal, we looked for correlations between the position and orientation of the field contours and the position and orientation of the embryo. These observations confirm that the embryo itself is not the source: the effective current dipole in these eggs is located to the side of the embryo, at a horizontal displacement of approximately 1 cm. However, more measurements with windowed eggs are needed to confirm this tentative result.

Is there an alternative localised source? There is no obvious structure to act as such a source at the centre of the yolk. In addition, the strength of the calculated dipole is large in comparison with localised sources in other biological systems. It appears, therefore, that a localised dipole model is inappropriate for this system.

The existence of a superficially dipolar pattern does not necessarily imply a simple dipolar source. It is well understood that the fields produced by an extended source region or by a collection of dipole sources will tend to a dipolar form as the separation from the source increases. Okada (1985)

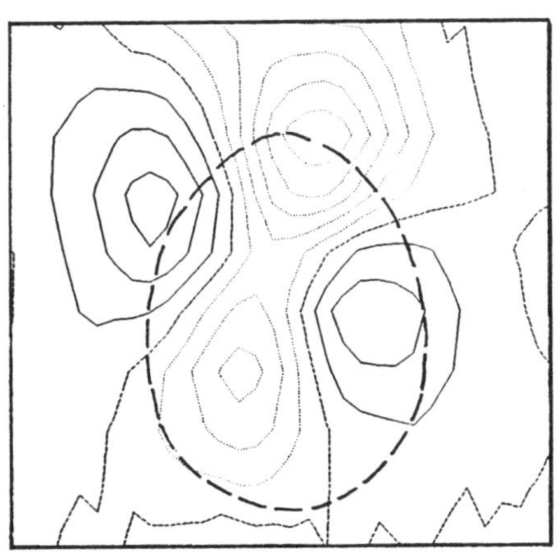

Fig. 2. Contour map showing a distinctly non-dipolar field in a horizontal plane 8 mm above a developing chick egg (contour separation = 2 pT).

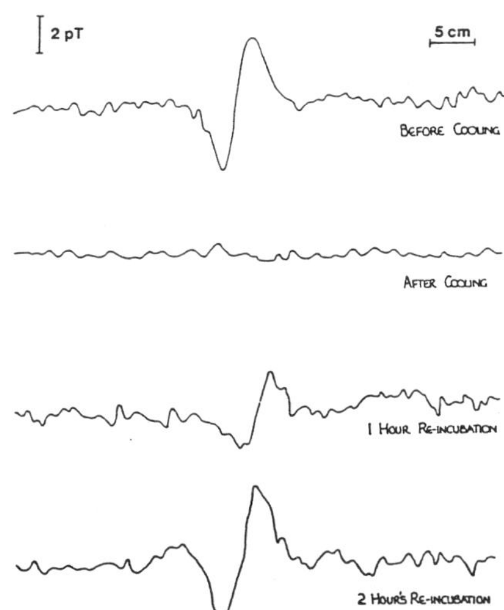

Fig. 3. The effect of cooling an incubating egg. Note that occasional drops in temperature are a regular part of normal egg incubation.

has shown that an extended region of current dipoles with a common orientation can produce a field similar to that from a deeper localised source. In our case this tendency to the adoption of a dipolar form will be enhanced by the smearing of the signal by the inappropriately large coil system (23 mm diameter, about half the diameter of a typical egg) used for part of this study.

We have performed several invasive tests to help to elucidate the source of the fields that we have measured. When 4 of the eggs were refrigerated after incubation had started, the signals disappeared, only to reappear when the eggs were warmed again to incubation temperature (Figure 3). This is evidence that the source is associated with a metabolic process, and not with the presence of biogenic magnetite. This conclusion is supported by evidence from magnetisation and susceptibility experiments: in each case any signals induced with magnetic fields could be accounted for by the diamagnetic susceptibility of the egg and its contents.

No signals were produced by empty shells, but signals were observed from the embryo plus yolk plus associated membranes when they were floated out of the shell into a saline bath. Very pertinently, in three cases we have dissected away the embryo from its underlying membranes and found little change in the signal for about 20 minutes. However, in two cases, breaking or mixing the upper region of the yolk membrane did cause the signal to disappear immediately.

We cannot unambiguously identify the source of our signals. However the data are consistent with the existence of an extended source distribution in the extra-embryonic membranes. These membranes are highly active electrophysiologically. Recent vibrating electrode measurements (Kucera, 1989) suggest the existence of sodium ion currents in the peripheral regions of the yolk sac membrane and establish that these currents are inhomogeneously distributed. Deeming et al (1987) suggest that active pumping of sodium ions in the periphery of the developing yolk sac is responsible for the formation of the sub-embryonic fluid. In addition, measurements of the extracellular embryonic pH (Gillespie, 1987) show that an active pH gradient is maintained in the region between the ectoderm and endoderm in this period of development. This gradient is believed to be created by epithelial activity: its function may be to modulate cell development, possibly by modifying the mechanical properties of the membrane surfaces. Unfortunately there is limited information available about the expected quasi dc current flows due to these and other possible mechanisms deeper within the egg, partly because the use of vibrating probe techniques is essentially limited to superficial regions. This makes it difficult to distinguish between the possible source mechanisms.

Analytical methods of identifying 3-d current density distributions from external magnetic field data have recently been developed (Clarke, 1989) and we believe that these will help us to more definitively identify the source and relevance of the signals we observe. Further information will come from more careful perturbative experiments. Through such techniques we hope to be able to determine the relationship between the ionic currents and the biological development of the chick.

REFERENCES

Clarke, C.J.S., Ioannides, A.A. and Bolton, J.P.R., 1989, Localised and distributed source solutions for the biomagnetic inverse problem, in these proceedings.

Deeming, D.C., Rowlett, K. and Simkiss, K., 1987, Physical influences on embryo development, *J. Exp. Zool. supp.*, 1:341.

Freake, S.M., Swithenby, S.J. and Thomas, I.M., 1988, A miniature SQUID magnetometer for the detection of quasi-dc ionic current flow in developing organisms, *in*: "Biomagnetism '87" (Proceedings of the Sixth International Conference on Biomagnetism), Tokyo Denki University Press.

Gillespie, J.I., 1987, Measurement of intra-embryonic pH during the early stages of development in the chick embryo, *Cell Tissue Res.*, 247:445.

Jaffe, L.F. and Nuccitelli, R., 1974, An ultrasensitive vibrating probe for measuring steady extracellular fields, *J. Cell Biol.*, 63:614.

Kucera, P., Katz, D.C. and de Ribaupierre, Y., 1989, Ionic pathways in the early chick embryogenesis, *Proc. 31st Int. Cong. of Physiological Sciences*, Helsinki.

Multi-author review, 1988, New perspectives in morphogenesis, O'Shea, P.S., ed., *Experientia* 44:631

Okada, Y., 1985, Discrimination of localised and distributed current dipole sources and localised single and multiple sources, *in*: "Biomagnetism: Applications and theory", Weinberg, H., Stroink, G. and Katila, T., ed., 266-72, Pergamon, New York.

Swithenby, S.J., 1988, Non-invasive monitoring of ionic currents during development by SQUID magnetometry, *Experientia*, 44:673.

MAGNETIC FIELD MEASUREMENTS OF THE ELECTRIC ORGAN OF *GYMNOTUS CARAPÓ*

O. Baffa, S. Lopes Côrrea, C. A. Pelá and A. Tannus*

Fac. Filosofia Ciências e Letras de Ribeirão Preto–USP, 14049–Ribeirão Preto, SP, Brazil
*Instituto de Física e Química de São Carlos–USP, 13560–São Carlos, SP, Brazil

INTRODUCTION

The measurement of the magnetic field associated with the spontaneous activity of the electric organ (EO) of the fish *Gymnotus Carapó* is described. Its low voltage EO gives a steady, pulsed electric signal with frequencies in the range 30–70 Hz and amplitude 200mV . The frequency can vary depending on the water temperature and to avoid signal jamming by other fish nearby (Bullock et al, 1979). This fish has poor eyesight and usually lives in turbid waters. It is thought that the EO creates an electric field pattern in its surroundings that can be recognized by the fish through its electroreceptors. When obstacles, prey or other objects are close, a distortion of the electric field pattern is sensed by the electroreceptors allowing the fish to react. This electric signal has been extensively exploited to study either electric location, the fish's behaviour, and to detect the fish's presence in ecological studies (Scheich, 1983).

METHODS

a) Magnetic Field Measurements

The electric and magnetic signals were detected using the arrangement shown in figure 1a. The fish was restrained in water on a small plywood board using a fine net. Two copper electrodes 1 cm appart were in contact with the tail of the fish to pick up the electric signal. The magnetic signal was detected using a ferrite toroidal probe with 80 turns and external diameter 16 mm, internal diameter 9 mm and thickness 7.4 mm (Wikswo, 1983 and Gielen, 1986) inserted around the tail. The inductance of the sensor was measured with a General Radio LC bridge, operating at 1 KHz giving 11.5 mH. The magnetic probe was connected to a Tektronix 7904 oscilloscpe equipped with a 7A22 differential preamplifier.

b) Probe Calibration

To calibrate the probe the amplified electric signal produced by the fish was fed to a resistor placed on the axis of the probe. This procedure assures that the same Fourier components present in the actual magnetic signal will be present in the calibration signal.

Advances in Biomagnetism
Edited by S.J. Williamson *et al.*
Plenum Press, New York

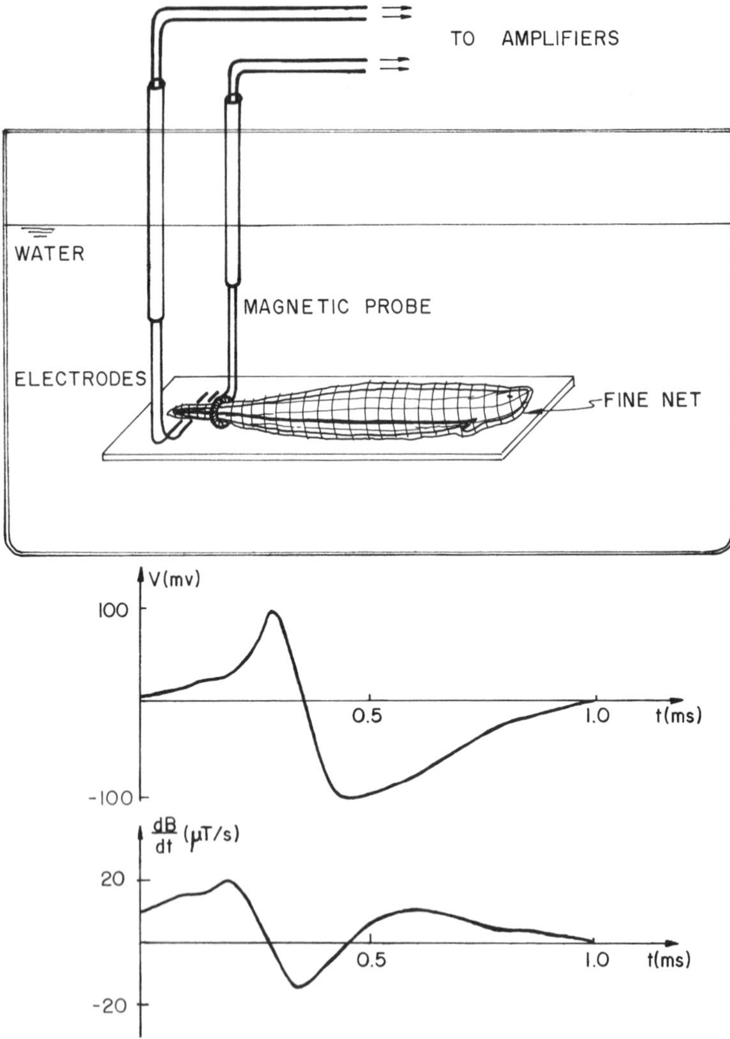

Figure 1. (a): Experimental arrangement used to detect the magnetic field from the electric fish *Gymnotus Carapó*. The continuous line along the fish's side indicates the location of the electric organ. (b): The electric and magnetic (first time derivative) signals are also shown.

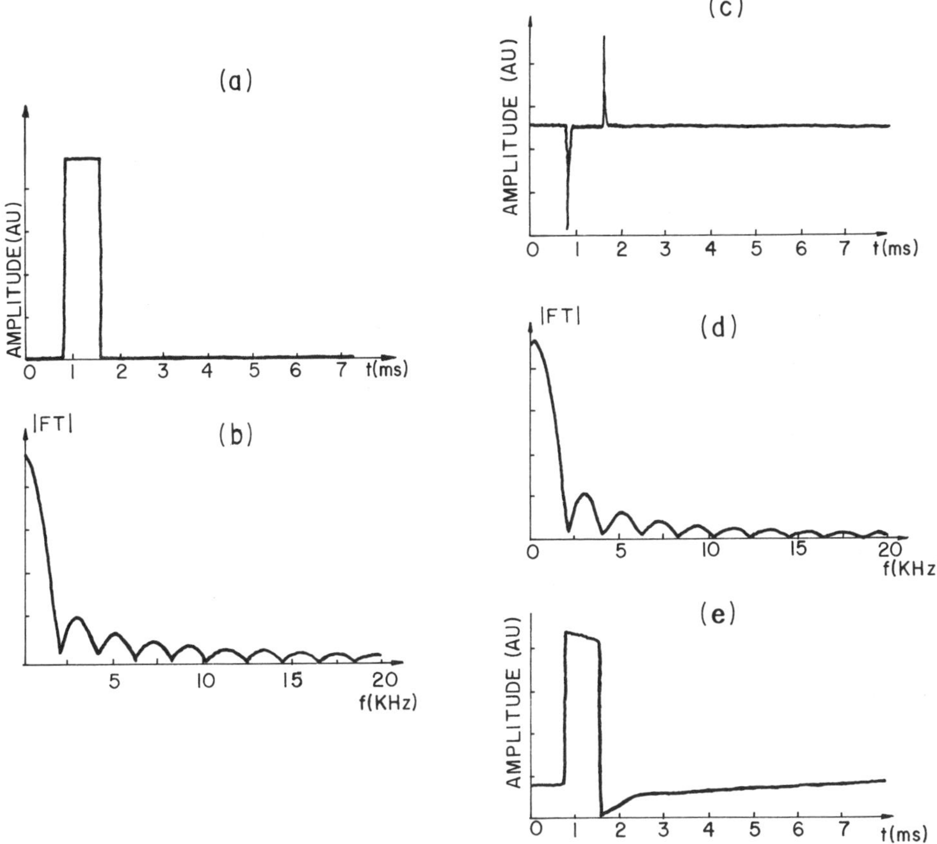

Figure 2. Fourier analysis of the frequency response of the sensor (see text for details).

To check for the frequency response of the probe, a square current pulse of 1 mA with 1 ms duration was applied to a wire threading the toroid. Figure 2 shows the input pulse (a) and the modulus of its Fourier Transform–FT (b). The response of the probe to the input pulse (2a) is shown in 2c. Instead of integrating pulse 2c in the direct space and then FT it to compare with the input signal, an alternative approach was used. The signal 2c was transformed and the real and imaginary parts of its FT were divided by $i\omega$, the resulting functions were combined to give the FT modulus of the integral of signal 2c. This procedure saves the step of integration of signal 2c in the real space, and base line corrections that are almost always present, are intrinsically corrected by the algorithm. The reverse FT of signal d is displayed in 2e. Except for a small base line drift the response of the probe is very good as can be seen from the steepness of the rise and fall of the signal 2e. Furthermore, the expected power spectrum of the fish's signal does not extend beyond 1kHz, so the measured transfer function can be considered flat over that region.

RESULTS AND DISCUSSION

Figure 1b shows the electric signal and the first derivative of the magnetic signal detected. Inversion of the probe relative to the tail inverts the polarity of the magnetic signal, as would be expected according to Ampere's law. When the tail is positioned just outside the probe no signal is detected, indicating no capacitive coupling. The magnetic and electric signals are being analysed to estimate the electric current produced by the low voltage electric organ in *G. Carapó* and to better characterize this EO. The experiments done so far indicate that the EO behaves like a current source. Measurements made at the tail dried with paper towels, with the fish placed outside the water, gave a voltage as high as 2V between its head and tail, and no magnetic field was detected by our system. However when the fish was placed in the water the electric signal decreased and the magnetic signal was then easily detected, indicating an increase in the electric current. The fact that the tail was dry ruled out the hypothesis that no signal was detected due to a resulting null current passing through the toroid. A first calculation of the electric current gives a peak value of $500\mu A$ in the portion of the tail where the measurements were made. This value agrees with the fact that the low voltage EO is obtained through the parallel association of the electroplates. A previous study was published regarding the detection of the magnetic fields produced by electric fish (Costa Monteiro, 1987), but as far as we know, this is the first experiment reporting the value of the electric current produced by the EO of the electric fish. Due to the relatively simple experimental arrangement used to obtain the electric and magnetic signals, with no biological preparation and employing standard electronic equipment, the present experiment could be used in a teaching laboratory. Experiments are under way to better characterize the current source properties of the EO.

ACKNOWLEDGEMENTS

The authors are grateful to the financial support of the Brazilian agencies: Coordenação de Aperfeiçoamento de Pessoal de Nível Superior (CAPES) and Conselho Nacional de Desenvolvimento Científico Tecnológico (CNPq). The discussions with R.L. Zimmerman are also appreciated.

REFERENCES

Bullock, T.H., Fernandes-Souza, L., Graf, W., Helligenberg, W., Langner, G., Meyer, D.L.,Pimentel-Souza, F., Scheich, H. and Viancour, T.A., 1979, Aspectos do Uso da Descarga do Orgão Eletrico e Eletrorecepção nos Gymnotoidei e Outros Peixes Amazonicos. Acta Amaz. 9(3):549.

Costa Monteiro, E.,Bruno, A.C., Louro, S.R.W., Costa Ribeiro, P. and Fonseca Costa, A. (1987) Study of Magnetic Field of Electrophorus Electricus. In "Biomagnetism'87", Tokyo Denki University, Tokyo (1987).

Gielen, F.L.H., Roth, B.J. and Wikswo, J.P., 1986, Capabilities of a Toroid-Amplifier System for Magnetic Measurement of Current in Biological Tissue. IEEE Trans. Biomed. Eng. BME 33(10):910.

Scheich, H. Biophysics of Electroreceptors In "Biophysics", Hoppe, W., Lohmann, W., Marki, H. and Ziegler, H. (Editors), Springer Verlag, New York (1983).

MEASUREMENT OF MAGNETIC FIELD NEAR AN ACUTE SURGICAL INJURY ON THE RABBIT'S THIGH

Z. Trontelj, J. Pirnat, J. Lužnik, V. Jazbinšek

Physics Department and Institute of Mathematics, Physics and Mechanics, University E. Kardelj of Ljubljana, Jadranska 19, 61000 Ljubljana, Yugoslavia

V. Valenčič, D. Križaj, L. Vodovnik, A. Jerčinović

Faculty of Electrical and Computer Engineering, University E. Kardelj of Ljubljana, Tržaška 25, 61000 Ljubljana, Yugoslavia

INTRODUCTION

The relation between the injuries in skin, muscles and bones in humans or animals and the increased electrophysiological activity in the injured area is a subject of research since 19th century[1,2]. However, it seems that this research has become especially acute (and necessary) in the last years with the accelerated use of external electric and magnetic fields in different clinical applications, like the promotion of healing of wounds or fractured bones. In order to understand the healing processes and the role which have the external electromagnetic fields during the process of healing it is necessary to explore at the beginning the inner electrophysiological processes which take place in the injured area. That means, we have to find out more about the sources of endogeneous electric activity in injured limbs. In last years several authors have measured electric potentials and currents, called endogeneous potentials and currents, which accompany injuries in skin muscels and bones[3,4,5,6,7,8]. There was also an attempt to detect injury currents magnetically.[9]

Since the measurements of small endogeneous dc voltages and currents of the order of few mV and nA on the skin and/or within injuries requires special techniques[3,4,10] it is not easy to detect them. Moreover, the experimental results of different groups are not always consistent[8]. Therefore it is worthwhile to extend the present methods by the measurements of magnetical field caused by the endogeneous current(s). This way we might get an additional independent information on the endogeneous current(s). We will report here on preliminary results of magnetic measurements above the surgical injury on the rabbit's thigh.

EXPERIMENTAL RESULTS

The measurements were performed on 5 rabbits; one of them was measured repeatedly after 6 months with a good reproducibility of the measured results. Each animal was under general anaesthesia. The hair was removed from the lateral part of the hind leg and the hairless area was cleaned with etanol before the incision was made. Subsequently the skin incision was enlarged in steps and surgical injury in the upper layer of the thigh's muscle tissue was the final step. The final injury was approximately 5 cm long and 2 cm broad.

Advances in Biomagnetism
Edited by S.J. Williamson *et al.*
Plenum Press, New York

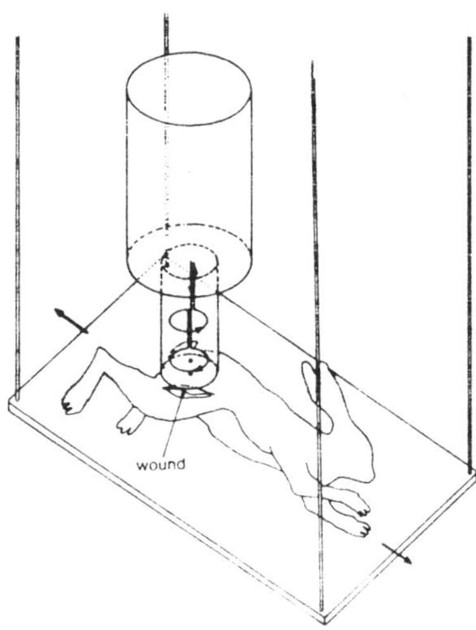

Figure 1. The measuring set-up

The first magnetic measurements had been carried out just before the incision was made through the upper layer (stratum corneum) of the skin. Later-on the magnetic field was measured above the injury at each intermediate step. After the measurement was completed, the injury was properly treated.

The magnetic field above the wound was measured with the SQUID magnetogradiometer of 1st order. The pickup coil had 2 cm diameter and the base line was 10 cm. At the beginning the measurements were carried out in the magnetically quiet part of Physics Department and later with considerably better s/n ratio in the biomagnetic laboratory in the rural area. The Hewlett-Packard microcomputer system HP-200 was used for data processing and analysis. Because of dc character of the measured magnetic field the rabbit was laid on a small wooden table swinging with frequency about 0.3 Hz under the cryostat with SQUID senzor. The schematic drawing of the measuring set-up is seen on Fig. 1.

The main sequences in the magnetic field measurements were the same for all test animals:

a) after receiving anaesthetic

b) after the incision in the stratum corneum

c) after the physiological solution was added

d) after the incision through all skin layers was completed

e) after the injury in the upper layer of muscle tissue was made.

Some typical results obtained in the biomagnetic laboratory corresponding to the sequences a) and e) are shown on Figs. 2a and 2b. These figures show single sequences without averaging because the s/n ratio is considerably better in the biomagnetic laboratory in comparison to

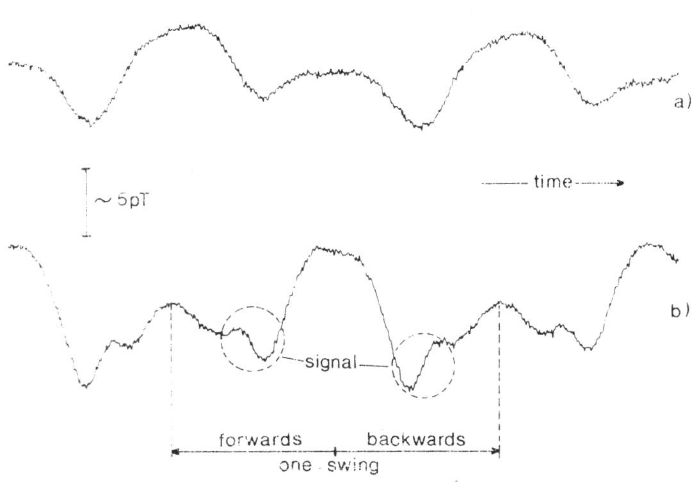

Figure 2. Typical records a) after receiving anaesthetic and b) after the injury in the upper layer of muscle tissue was made.

the measurements done at the Physics Department. The measurements on each animal were completed in about 2 hours.

DISCUSSION

Studying magnetic fields we want to learn something about the current which causes the measured magnetic field. The research of skin electric activity by Barker et al.[4] showed that driving force for the ionic currents comes from the "battery" located in the living epidermis (the skin layer under the stratum corneum). The experiments of Chakkalakal et al.[3] and of Lokietek et al.[5] which involve also the muscle injury and the bone injury confirm the existance of the epidermal battery and suggest an additional battery in the bone area - the endosteal battery in order to explain the injury currents in the bone area.

With the electric measurements one cannot avoid the influence of the measuring electrodes. However, with the magnetic measurements the current loops are closed only inside the body, i.e. within the skin, through the liquids in the wound (the physiological solution applied to the injury is also included) and through the conducting tissue.

We have observed the first magnetic signals which can be related to the endogeneous injury current during the measuring sequence following the complete incision through all skin layers with the physiological solution added to the the injury. The signals were contaminated with the rather strong background dc signal. The magnetic signals appeared at each passing of the edge of the injury under the pickup coil of SQUID system, see Fig. 2b. It has to be mentioned that at this point of measurement the incision became already broader. We expect that the short circuit currents at the edge of the injury contribute the main part to the measured magnetic signal. Magnetic signals increase by a factor 3 to 5 and reach the maximum value 1 to 2 pT during the mesuring sequence following the injury in the upper layer muscle. The same increase, but in the voltage measurements, has also been noticed by Lokietek[5]. It is expected that the muscle injury brings additional possibilities for the short circuit currents. The polarity change in the measured magnetic signal speaks in favour to our explanation of the measured signal. The same can be said for the time evolution of the measured magnetic signals during each oscillation of the table with rabbit on it.

The background dc signals were quite strong for some animals. It is very likely that they are caused by the magnetical contamination of rabbit's digestive organs. Some animals were not suitable for measurements due to clearly magnetically contaminated rests of food in their digestive organs.

We can say in the conclusion that it is possible to measure magnetic signals related to the injury current. However, we have to admit that there are still many open questions and it is necessary to continue with these experiments before more decisive statements can be made.

ACKNOWLEDGEMENT

We express our sincere appreciation to V. Cotič, M.D. for the anaesthesia of rabbits.

REFERENCES

1. E. Du Bois-Reymond, *Ann. Phys. Chem.* (Leipzig), 58:1 (1843).
2. E. Du Bois-Reymond, "Untersuchungen ueber tierische Elektrizitaet," Vol.2, p.2., Reimer, Berlin (1860).
3. D.A. Chakkalakal, R.F. Wilson and J.F. Connolly, Epidermal sources of endogeneous electricity in injured canine limbs, *IEEE Trans. on Biomed. Eng.* 35:19 (1988).
4. A.T. Barker, L.F. Jaffe and J.W. Vanable, The glabrous epidermis of cavies contains a powerful battery, *Amer. J. Physiol.*, vol. 242, *Regulatory Integ. Comp. Physiol.*, vol. 11, pp R358-R366 (1982).
5. W. Lokietek, R.J. Pawluk and C.A.L. Bassett, Muscle injury potentials: A source of voltage in the undeformed rabbit tibia, *J. Bone Joint Surg.* 56B:361 (1974).
6. Z.B. Friedenberg and C.T. Brighton, Bioelectric potentials in bone, *J. Bone Joint Surg.* 48A:915 (1966).
7. A. Herlitzka, Ein Beitrag zur Physiologie der Regeneration, *Wilhelm Roux Arch. Entwicklungsmech. Org.* 10:126 (1910).
8. R.B. Borgens, Natural voltage gradients and the generation and regeneration of limbs, *in:* "Regulation of vertebrate limb generation", 2. pp.6-31 (1985).
9. D. Cohen and L.A. Kaufman, Magnetic determination of the relationship between the S-T segment shift and the injury current produced by coronary artery occlusion, *Circulation Research* 36:414 (1975).
10. L.F. Jaffe and R. Nuccitelli, An ultrasensitive vibrating probe for measuring steady extracellular currents, *J. of Cell Biology*, 63:614 (1974).

BIOCHEMICAL MAGNETITE FORMATION AND ITS APPLICATION

T. Hamaya and K. Horikoshi

Bio Science Laboratories, Meiji Seika Kaisha Ltd., Chiyoda, Sakado-shi, Saitama, Japan. and Department of Bioengineering, The Tokyo Institute of Technology, Meguro-ku, Tokyo Japan

INTRODUCTION

Magnetic particles have important applications in biochemistry and in medicine, for example, in magnetoliposomes for cell sorting[1] and for magnetic separation techniques[2]. Particles from magnetotactic bacteria are most suitable for such applications by virtue of their size[3], but cannot be recovered in sufficient quantities for commercial purpose, because the growth of magnetotactic bacteria in culture is limited. This study was designed to gain an understanding of the mechanisms of magnetite formation in living organisms, and to synthesize magnetite particles for industrial applications.

The distribution of magnetite among living organisms is unexpectedly diverse. Examples include polyplacophora (marine chiton), honey bees, and magnetotactic bacteria[4], suggesting that magnetite can be formed under widely differing conditions. It is believed that magnetite in sediments is produced authigenically, or with the contribution of magnetotactic bacteria[5], although the mechanism of biogenic formation are unknown. In the case of magnetotactic bacteria, assimilatory nitrate reduction seems likely to participate in the magnetite forming reaction, but the precise role remains unclear[6]. We propose that the formation of both intra- and extracellular magnetite can result from enzymatic reactions which affect the balance of pH and ORP (oxidation-reduction potential). This study was undertaken to gain more understanding of the mechanisms of magnetite formation and to establish a method for *in vitro* synthesis of magnetite for use in investigations of its applications.

In addition to magnetite, other iron substances, including goethite (α-FeOOH) and lepidocrocite (γ-FeOOH), have been found in the ANIMALIA kingdom, and maghemite (γ-Fe_2O_3) might exist in the MONERA kingdom[7]. Although the distribution of these bio-iron materials is diverse, the mechanisms of biomineralization are almost completely unknown. Each of the bio-iron materials described above can be formed through the same enzyme reaction as the magnetite forming one, under different pH and ORP conditions, suggesting that the composition of bio-iron materials depends on the reaction conditions.

METHODS

Enzyme

Jack bean urease (Type IX) was purchased from Sigma Chemical Co. Other chemicals were of analytical grade.

Assay of Urease Activity

Urease solution (100 μl) and 2.0% urea solution (1.9 ml) in 0.2M

Na_2HPO_4-KH_2PO_4 buffer (pH 6.5) was incubated at 37 °C for 5 min., and produced ammonia was measured with Ammonia-Test Wako (Wako Pure Chemical Industries, LTD.).

X-ray analysis

The sample was examined by means of X-ray diffraction using CuKα radiation and its chemical formulas were identified using data files.

Electron microscopy

For scanning electron microscopy, the solids were coated on aluminium stubs with the aid of silver paste.

Moessbauer analysis

Moessbauer measurement was performed using conventional constant acceleration spectrometer.

RESULTS AND DISCUSSION

Urease hydrolyzes urea to ammonia and CO_2, with a concomitant increase in pH. One hundred ml of substrate mixture containing 2.0g of potassium nitrate, 50 mg of urea and 80 mg of ferrous chloride, 4-hydrate was prepared in a glass bottle (200ml). Oxygen was removed by degassing with nitrogen and the bottle was sealed with a rubber cap. Jack bean urease, 1000U, was injected through the cap and the reaction mixture incubated at 37 °C without shaking.

From an initial turbid yellowish-white, the reaction mixture slowly turned green; 30-60 min later, the solution had cleared and dark green precipitates formed at the bottom of the bottle. This suggested that the enzyme hydrolyzes the urea, precipitating Fe^{2+} and OH^- ions to form an insoluble ferrous hydroxide gel. After 20-40 hr incubation, the precipitates had darkened and become slightly magnetosensitive. A further 20-40 hr of incubation resulted in complete oxidation of the precipitates to black magnetic crystalline particles. The oxidation is presumably a caused by nitrate, with a trace amount of oxygen probably a catalyst in initiating and maintaining the redox potential. On the other hand, the reaction was performed without urease, no precipitate was formed. The pH of the solution changed from 4.8 before injection of urease solution to 8.6 after formation of black precipitates. The crystallization was considered to be syneresis taking place with water being removed from the gel as the components condensed to form a hydrophobic matrix.

The X-ray diffraction pattern of the black magnetic solids was obtained and is presented in Fig. 1. These data agree with those of magnetite[8]. The Moessbauer spectrum of the product is shown in Fig. 2, and is in agreement with that for magnetite.

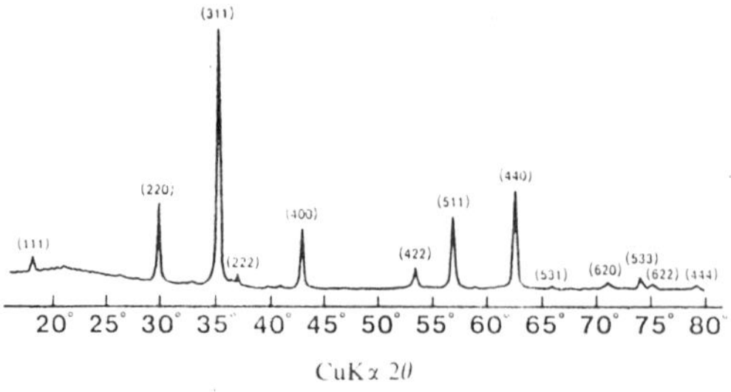

Fig. 1. X-ray Diffraction Pattern of the Black Magnetic Precipitates.

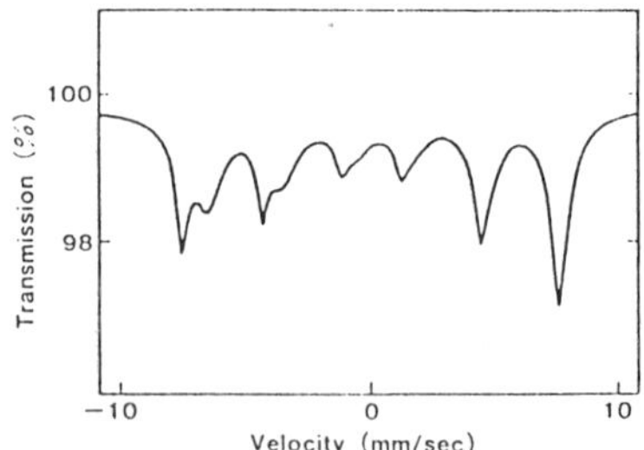

Fig. 2. The Moessbauer Spectrum of the Products at Room Temperature.

Table 1. Reaction Conditions and Products.

Conditions	$FeCl_2$ (mM)	Urea (mM)	Atmosphere	Temp. (°C)	Final pH	Product
A	4.2	8.0	N_2	30	7.8	Magnetite(M)
B	4.2	2.0	N_2	30	6.5	Lepidocrocite(L)
C	1.4	2.7	N_2	30	8.3	M and Goethite(G)
D	4.2	8.0	aeration	30	3.7	L and Akaganeite
E	4.2	8.0	N_2	37	8.6	M
F	4.2	8.0	liq.paraffin	37	9.2	Maghemite and G

Magnetite particles found in sediments are heterogeneous in size and shape. In this work, roughly spherical particles 150-250 nm diameter were observed. When magnetite is formed intracellularly, the size and shape of particles vary between different organisms. In polyplacophora, for example, magnetite particles are not uniform either in size or shape[5]. In magnetotactic bacteria, however, particles are usually 40-120 nm in size[3] and can be hexagonal, cuboid, or tear-shaped. It has been suggested that[5] the maximum size of these particles is constrained by the magnetosome envelope[3], but there is no evidence for a specific biological control. We propose a general mechanism by which some enzymatic reactions can create the appropriate conditions to catalyze the formation of magnetite.

As described, urease is not directly involved in magnetite formation, but create an appropriate balance of pH and ORP during the hydrolysis of urea. This implies that magnetite particles can be formed from ferrous iron during any enzymatic reactions which create the appropriate conditions of pH and ORP. Other such enzymes may include nitrate and nitrite reductases, which act together to produce ammonia from nitrate. This reaction also increases pH and decreases ORP, creating similar conditions to those in the urea-urease reaction.

It has been suggested that nitrate reduction is necessary for synthesis of magnetite in magnetotactic bacteria. Blakemore and co-workers noted that magnetotactic bacteria living under microaerobic conditions could reduce nitrate and form magnetite, but when grown on ammonium, no magnetite was formed[6]. This observation is consisted with our work.

Reaction conditions effected the products. The condition of the enzymatic reaction and the identities of the precipitated products are summarized in Table 1. The products changed when the ratio of urea/$FeCl_2$ was changed. When the ratio was higher than 1, the solution became alkaline because of ammonia production through hydrolysis of urea. On the other hand, a lower ratio resulted in acidic conditions, under neutral to alkaline conditions, only magnetite was formed (A), but under acidic conditions only lepidocrocite was formed (B). When the concentration of both $FeCl_2$ and urea were reduced to a third those in the case of A by dilution (C), without changing the urea/$FeCl_2$ ratio, a small amount of goethite was formed in addition to magnetite. The reason for the formation of goethite, which is more highly oxidized than magnetite, may be as follows. In C, the ratio of dissolved oxygen/$FeCl_2$ was higher than that in A, so a part of the formed ferrous hydroxide is expected to be oxidized to goethite under neutral to alkaline conditions. When the reaction mixture was aerated (D), oxidative and acidic conditions were created because of evaporation of the ammonia formed from the urea. As a result, lepidocrocite and a small amount of akaganeite (β-FeOOH) were formed. Lepidocrocite is expected to be formed for the same reason as in the case of B. It is known that akaganeite can be formed from ferric chloride through a chemical reaction, so in D, some ferrous iron might be oxidized to ferric iron through aeration and akaganeite would be formed from ferric iron under acidic conditions. The reaction temperature had no effect on the nature of the products formed (A,E). Maghemite and a little goethite were formed when the reaction mixture was covered with 1 cm of liquid paraffin (F). Under these conditions, a small amount of oxygen could be supplied constantly to the reaction mixture. In this case, most of the formed ferrous hydroxide was oxidized to magnetite and the remainder was much more oxidized. Then the formed magnetite might be oxidized slowly into maghemite and goethite might be formed for the same reason as in the case of C. We believe that the ratio of maghemite/goethite might be changed by the rate of oxygen supplementation.

Our results indicate that the pH and ORP conditions are very important as to the chemical nature of the reaction products. Furthermore, the data imply that the variation observed in the nature of the iron materials formed in living organisms may not depend upon the sort of metabolic enzyme system, but mainly upon the enzymatic reaction conditions. The urease activity itself was significant for the magnetite formation only in its creation of the required pH and ORP conditions. Various other enzymes which influence pH and ORP may be useful also for producing magnetite *in vitro*. From our results, we could not identify the enzymatic reaction which results in the formation of bio-iron materials in living organisms. But, in any case, these enzymes apparently function to create the necessary pH and ORP conditions.

REFERENCES

1. L. B. Margolis, V. A. Namiot and L. M. Kljukin, Magnetoliposomes : Another Principle of Cell Sorting,. *Biophys. Acta* 735 : 193 (1983).
2. J. T. Kemshead and J. Ugelstad, Magnetic Separation Techniques : Their Application to Medicine, *Molecular and Cellular Biochem.* 67 : 11 (1985).
3. R. P. Blakemore and R. B. Frankel, Magnetic Navigation in Bacteria, *Sci. Am.* 245 : 42 (1981).
4. R. B. Frankel, Magnetic Guidance of Organisms, *Ann. Rev. Biophys. Bioeng.* 13 : 85 (1984).
5. R. Karlin, M. Lyle and G. R. Heath, Authigenic Magnetite Formation in Suboxic Marine Sediments, *Nature* 326 : 490 (1987).
6. D. A. Brazylinski and R. P. Blakemore, Denitrification and Assimilatory Nitrate reduction in *Aquaspirillum magnetotacticum*, *Appl. Environment. Microbiol.* 46 : 1118 (1983).
7. H. A. Lowenstam, Minerals Formed by Organisms, *Science* 211 : 1126 (1981)
8. International Centre for Diffraction Data, Powder Diffraction File (1986)

IMMUNOSENSOR USING BACTERIAL MAGNETITES

Noriyuki Nakamura and Tadashi Matsunaga

Department of Biotechnology
Tokyo University of Agriculture and Technology
Koganei, Tokyo 184, Japan

INTRODUCTION

Magnetotactic bacteria contain magnetic particles which consist of magnetite (Fe_3O_4). They are 500-1000 Å in size, covered with organic thin films, and do not aggregate. It is therefore possible to immobilize larger quantities of bioactive substances. Moreover, such immobilized bioactive substances can be moved by a magnetic field. Recently, the author's group has succeeded in culturing magnetotactic bacteria in a large amount. Bacterial magnetites were separated from these cells using several methods such as ultrasonication, lysozyme treatment, etc.. Separated bacterial magnetites have been employed for enzyme immobilization[1]. Glucose oxidase and uricase were immobilized on bacterial magnetites. Enzyme immobilized on bacterial magnetites showed higher activities than those immobilized on artificial magnetic particles and retained initial activities when they were reused. Furthermore, bacterial magnetites were also introduced into erythrocytes and leucocytes. Blood cells containing bacterial magnetites were separated with a magnet[2,3]. This article describes the immobilization of antibody on bacterial magnetites. The immunosensor system using these bacterial magnetites and the fluorescence spectrophotometer was constructed for the detection of mouse IgG.

MATERIALS AND METHODS

The cells of magnetotactic bacteria were cultured in a chemically defined growth medium (MSGM) containing 10 ml of Wolfe's vitamin solution, 5 ml Wolfe's mineral solution, 2 ml 10 mM ferric quinate, 0.45 ml 0.1% resazurin, 0.68 g KH_2PO_4, 0.12 g $NaNO_3$, 0.05 g sodium thioglycollate, 0.37 g tartaric acid, 0.37 g succinic acid, 0.05 g sodium acetate, and distilled water to make a volume of 1 l[4]. The pH of the medium was adjusted to 6.75 before sterilization. The cells were cultured in 5 l of medium under microaerobic condition at 25 °C for 5-7 days. Magnetotactic bacteria were centrifuged at 5000 x g for 10 min. The collected cells were washed with 10 mM HEPES (N-2-hydroxyethyl-piperazine-N'-2-ethanesulfonic acid) buffer (pH 7.4) and suspended in 20 ml of same buffer. Magnetotactic bacteria were disrupted by the ultrasonic disrupter (TOMY Seiko Co. LTD., UR-200P) operated for 5 min at 0 °C over 10 times. Magnetotactic bacteria were observed with a light microscope (OLYMPUS, BH-2) and a transmission electron microscope (HITACHI, H-700H). For electron microscopy, the cells were placed on the surface of carbon-coated collodion-covered copper mesh grids and air-dried. Bacterial magnetites were separated from a cellular disrupted fraction with samarium-cobalt (Sm-Co) magnet. Bacterial magnetites were washed with distilled water, and incubated with 2.5% glutaraldehyde solution in 1 ml of phosphate buffered saline (PBS; pH 7.4) for 1 h at 25 °C. The treated bacterial magnetites were washed with PBS, dispersed, and incubated with FITC-conjugated anti-mouse IgG for 12 h at 4 °C. The amounts of antibodies in the solution were determined by Lowry method[5] before and after immobilization and the quantities of antibody immobilized on bacterial magnetites were calculated.

IgG samples were diluted in gelatin veronal buffer (GVB; pH 8.3) containing Tween 20 (0.16% v/v). 100 µg of immunomagnetic particles and 100 µl of each diluted standard sample were mixed and incubated at 37 °C for 15 min. The aggregation reaction of FITC-conjugated anti-mouse IgG bacterial magnetites was enhanced by applying a magnetic field, when the immunomagnetic particles reacted with mouse IgG. Then 2 ml of GVB containing Tween 20 was added to the mixture. Fluoroscence intensity of FITC-conjugated immunomagnetic particles decreased because of aggregation. Fluorescence intensity of FITC-labeled magnetic particles aggregation was determined using the fluorescence spectrophotometer (HITACHI, F-1200) with the excitation wavelength set at 490 nm and the emission wavelength at 520 nm using 10 x 10 mm glass cuvette at 25 °C (Fig. 1). The value was estimated after 15 min when the fluorescence intensity became stable.

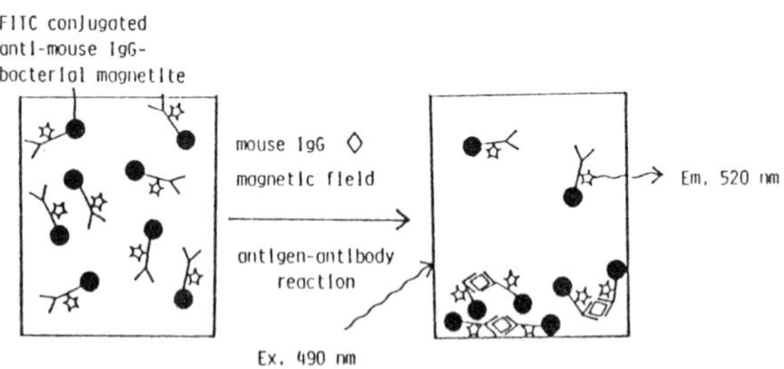

Fig. 1 LgG seneor using FITC conjugated anti-mouse IgG bacterial magnetite.

RESULTS AND DISCUSSION

Bacterial magnetites separated by ultrasonication were only slightly aggregated and well dispersed in HEPES buffer. They were covered with organic thin films and thickness of film was about 40 Å. When these magnetites were treated with chloroform- methanol (2:1 v/v) for 1 h, electron microscopic observations showed that bacterial magnetites were not covered with organic thin films. Bacterial magnetites without organic thin films formed aggregations. The quantity of antibody coupling with bacterial magnetites extracted by ultrasonication was 263 µg/mg particles, while that coupling with artificial magnetites was 68 μg/mg particles. There was slight aggregation in each particle by its own magnetic property. Bacterial magnetites were superior in dispersion and immobilization as compared with artificial magnetites in the same size in aqueous solution. Thus the quantity of antibody coupling with bacterial magnetites was about 4 times that which coupled with artificial magnetites.

Immunomagnetic particles were efficiently aggregated in an inhomogeneous magnetic field (0.4 T and 20 T/m in average) using Sm-Co magnet. Figure 2 shows the effect of magnetic field on aggregation of immunomagnetic particles. The reaction of aggregation proceeded on slightly without magnetic field. After 45 min incubation, the relative fluorescence intensity decreased to 50%. When the antigen-antibody reaction of immunomagnetic particles was carried out in the magnetic field, aggregation reached constant after 10 min incubation. Relative fluorescence intensity decreased to 67%, 52% and 20% in the magnetic fields of 400 G, 2000 G and 3000 G respectively. Therefore, the aggregation of immunomagnetic particles reacted with the antigen was enhanced by applying the magnetic field during incubation. Immunomagnetic particles were also easily separated. Gelatin was employed in order to clarify the difference between the decrease of fluorescence intensity based on specific-aggregation. Low gelatin concentration (0.1%) and high concentration (2%) in GVB were not suitable to

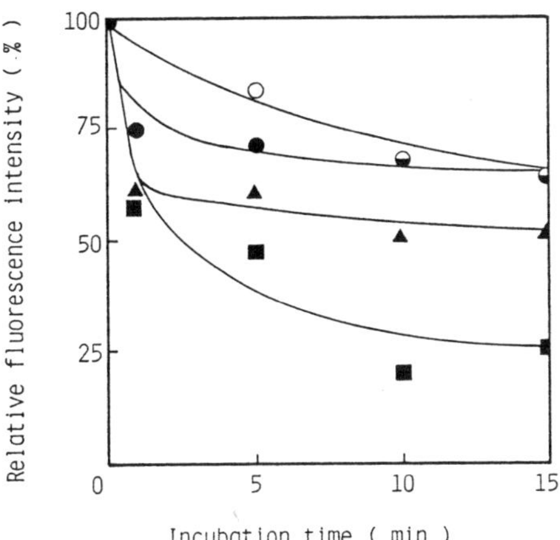

Fig. 2 Effect of magnetic field on antigen-antibody reaction using bacterial magnetites.

○: No magnetic field, ●: 400 G
▲: 2000 G, ■: 3000 G

Bacterial magnetites : 100 μg
Mouse IgG conc. : 100 ng/ml

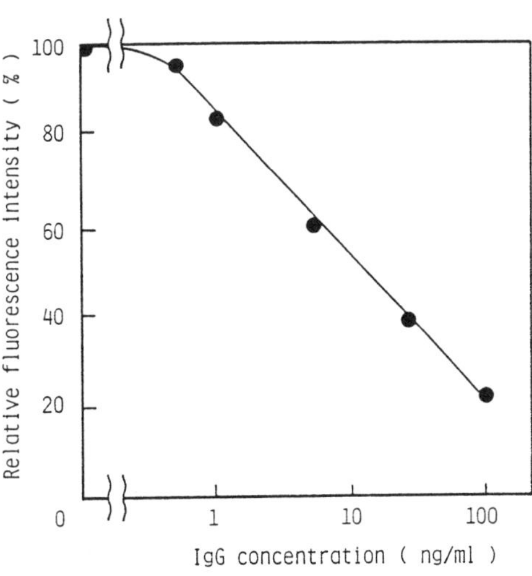

Fig. 3 Calibration curve of mouse IgG using FITC conjugated anti-mouse IgG immobilized on biogenic magnetic particles.

Temp. : 37°C
pH : 8.3
Incubation time : 15 min
Magnetic particles : 100 μg

clarify the differences because of quick or slow sedimentation of immunomagnetic particles caused by the viscosity of gelatin. The relative fluorescence intensity was most decreased at 1% gelatin.

Figure 3 shows the relationship between the relative fluorescence intensity and mouse IgG concentration. The relative fluorescence intensity decreased with increasing mouse IgG concentration. A linear relationship was obtained between the relative fluorescence intensity and mouse IgG concentration in the range of 0.5-100 ng/ml. Above 100 ng/ml, the relative fluorescence intensity was constant. The relative fluorescence intensity did not decrease when other proteins such as mouse IgE or human albumin were added in the range of 1-100 ng/ml. The minimum detectable concentration of mouse IgG was 0.5 ng/ml. Fluoroimmunoassay of mouse IgG using bacterial magnetites could be measured in the wider concentration range than that using artificial immunomagnetic particles.

There are some immunoassays based on aggregation of the latex particles by the particle counting, but the aggregation reaction still requires time consuming and has low sensitivity. In the present method based on the aggregation of bacterial magnetites covalently coated with FITC-conjugated anti-mouse IgG and decrease of the fluorescence intensity of immunomagnetic particles caused by aggregation, the magnetic field enhanced the aggregation reaction and shortened the measurement time. This sensor system provides rapid and easy technique and good accuracy for assay.

ACKNOWLEDGEMENTS

This work was partially supported by grant-in-aid for scientific research on priority areas no. 63604525 from the Ministry of Science and Culture.

REFERENCES

1. T. Matsunaga and S. Kamiya, Use of magnetic particles isolated from magnetotactic bacteria for enzyme immobilization, Appl. Microbiol. Biotechnol., 26: 328 (1987).
2. T. Matsunaga and S. Kamiya, Introduction of bacterial magnetic particles into red blood cells with cell fusion, in: "Biomagnetism '87," K. Atsumi, ed., Tokyo Denki Univ. Press, Tokyo (1988).
3. T. Matsunaga, K. Hashimoto, N. Nakamura, K. Nakamura, and S. Hashimoto, Phagocytosis of bacterial magnetite by leucocytes, Appl. Microbiol. Biotechnol., (in press).
4. R.P. Blakemore, D. Maratea, and R.S. Wolfe, Isolation and pure culture of a freshwater magnetic spirilllum in chemically defined medium, J. Bacteriol., 140: 720 (1979).
5. O.H. Lowry, N.J. Rosebrough, A.L. Farr, and R.J. Randall, Protein measurement with the folin phenol reagent, J. Biol. Chem., 193: 265 (1951).

LOCALIZED STIMULATION OF THE HUMAN CORTEX BY OPPOSING MAGNETIC FIELDS

S.Ueno*, T.Matsuda*, and M.Fujiki**

*Department of Electronics, Kyushu University, Fukuoka, 812, Japan

**Department of Neurosurgery, Medical College of Oita, 879-56, Japan

INTRODUCTION

A method of transcranial pulsed magnetic stimulation of the brain has been proposed by Barker et al (1985,1986). Parameters of muscular action potentials, such as conduction velocity, latency and amplitudes have been studied by the electromyographic (EMG) responses to the stimulation of the motor cortex (Barker et al,1986,1987; Hess et al,1987; Day et al, 1987; Rothwell et al,1987). Single coils are used for these studies. By the previously reported method, however, it is unable to stimulate localized area in the brain, as it causes broad area of the brain to be stimulated simultaneously.

We have proposed a new method of magnetic brain stimulation which alleviates this shortcoming (Ueno et al,1988a,1988b). In the present report, we apply our method to the stimulation of the human motor cortex. The results show that magnetic brain stimulation can be realized within a 5 mm resolution.

METHOD

The basic idea of localized stimulation is to concentrate induced eddy currents in a targeted area by a pair of time-varying magnetic fields (Ueno et al.1985,1987). As shown in Fig.1, a pair of coils are positioned outside the head so that time-varying magnetic fields pass through the head in the opposite directions around a target which should be stimulated.

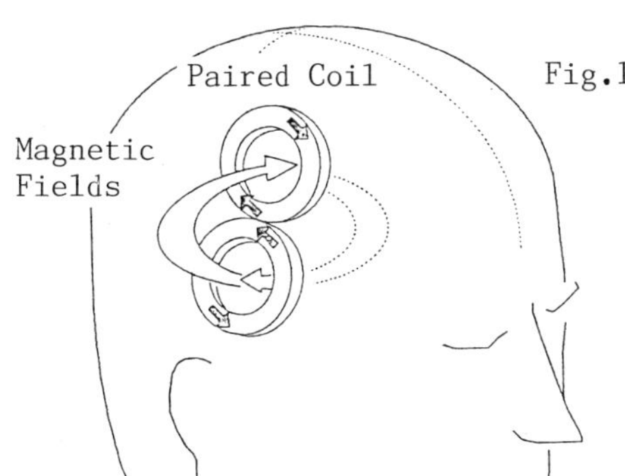

Fig.1 Principle of localized stimulation of the brain. A pair of coils are positioned outside the head so that magnetic fields path through the head in the opposite directions around a target which is located beneath the cross point of the paired coil.

Advances in Biomagnetism
Edited by S.J. Williamson *et al.*
Plenum Press, New York

Eddy currents can be induced in the head in a manner that the current flows make themselves two vortexes which flow together at the target between coils, thereby eddy currents are concentrated in the target. A computer simulation shows that the current density at the target makes a peak which is higher by 2-3 times than current densities at non target regions (Ueno et al. 1988a,1988b). A pair of coils with a winding of 5 turns of 5 mm wide by 2 mm thick copper wire were used. The coil size was 65 mm in inside diameter and 85 mm in outside diameter. Magnetic stimulation of the human brain were delivered by discharge currents (4,000-7,500 A) which passed through the paired-coil from a capacitor bank 600-900 V. The discharged currents produced time-varying magnetic fields which gave rise to concentrated eddy currents of 50 A/m^2 for 0.1 ms duration at a point 10 mm below the cross point of the paired-coil. The various parts in the motor cortex were stimulated, and the corresponding muscular action potentials were recorded by the electromyograms (EMGs) from the thenar, hypothenar and brachioradial muscles.

RESULTS AND DISCUSSION

Let us define the co-ordinates on the surface of the head. The Y-axis is chosen so as to coincide with the line along the central sulcus. The Y-axis passes a point 20 mm posterior to Cz of the 10-20 system and reaches to the center of the zygomatic arch. The X-axis orients to the direction perpendicular to the Y-axis, and crosses the Y-axis at 40 % lateral from the point 20 mm posterior to Cz (The distance between the point 20 mm posterior to Cz and the center of the zygomatic arch is 100 %).

Definite EMG responses to magnetic brain stimulation were obtained. Fig.2 and Fig.3 show the results in the case of thenar muscle. The paired coil was placed at a point(X = 15.0 mm, Y = 0.0 mm), called "thenar point". Definite EMG response was obtained at the thenar point. No thenar muscle responses were obtained at a point 5 mm anterior or posterior to the thenar point. No thenar muscle responses were obtained at a point 5 mm upper or lower to the thenar point. In other words, the selective stimulation of the human motor cortex was realized within a 5 mm resolution. The maximal EMG response was obtained from hypothenar muscle when the brain was stimulated at a point (X = 10.0 mm, Y = 10.0 mm). whereas, the maximal EMG response was obtained from brachioradial muscle when the brain was stimulated at a point (X = 15.0 mm, Y = 20.0 mm).

It is important to know whether or not an optimal axis exists in the cortex for brain stimulation.

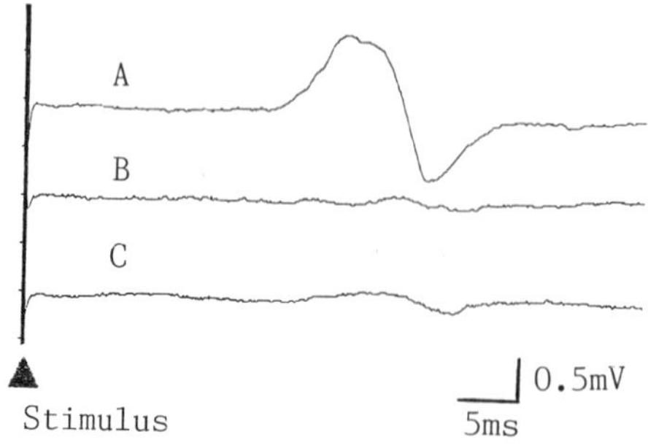

Fig.2 EMG responses to magnetic brain stimulation. A: Thenar point stimulation. B: Stimulation at a point 5 mm posterior to the thenar point. C: Stimulation at a point 5 mm anterior to the thenar point.

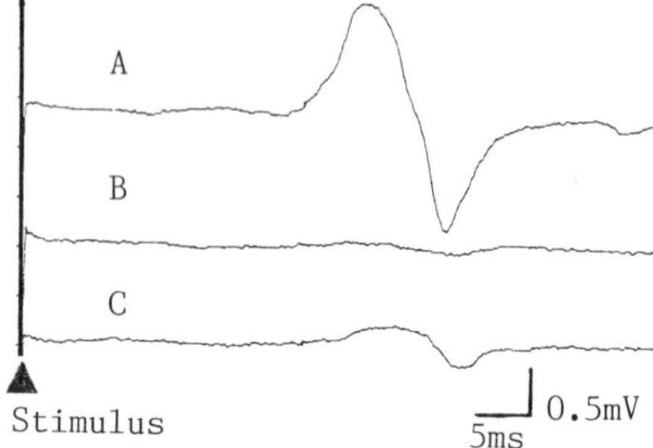

Fig.3 EMG responses to magnetic brain stimulation. A: Thenar point stimulation. B: Stimulation at a point 5 mm upper from the thenar point. C: Stimulation at a point 5 mm lower from the thenar point.

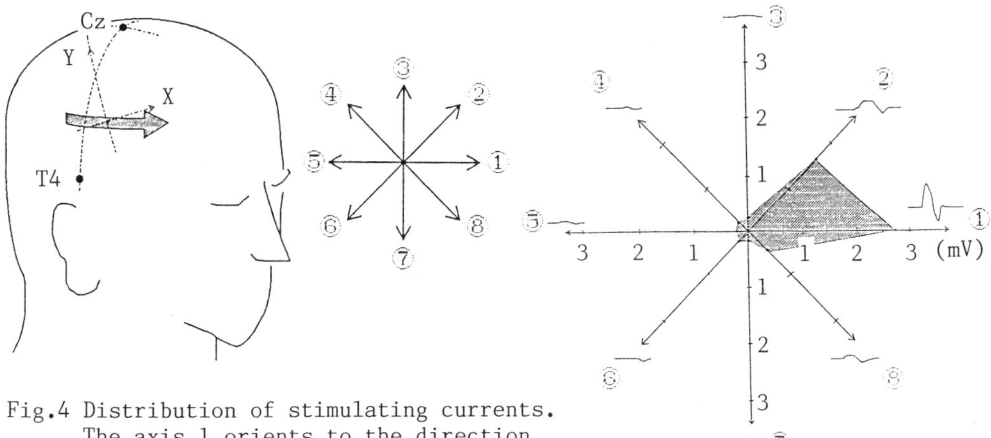

Fig.4 Distribution of stimulating currents. The axis 1 orients to the direction perpendicular to the midline which passes Cz and T4 of the 10-20 system.

Fig.5 Change of EMG responses to brain stimulation with the direction of stimulating currents.

Let us define that the axis 1 orients to the direction perpendicular to the midline which passes Cz and T4 of the 10-20 system as shown in Fig.4. Rotating the paired coil at the cross point of the coil, the thenar point in the motor cortex was stimulated. The peak-to-peak values of EMG signals which responded to the oriented brain stimulation were plotted on each axis as shown in Fig.5.

The maximum EMG responses was obtained in the direction 1, whereas, no EMG signals were obtained in the directions 3, 4, 5, 6 and 7.

The functional mapping of the human motor cortex related to the hand area was obtained as shown in Fig.6. Magnetic brain stimulation was carried out at all grid points on the meshed region in Fig.6. The distance between grid point is 5 mm each. The arrows show current directions for neural excitation. The circular, triangle and square points show the thenar, hypothenar and brachioradial muscle area, respectively. These marked points on the mesh indicate each functional area of which magnetic stimulation produced maximum EMG responses. Each functional area in the cortex corresponding to each muscle contraction in the hand area is localized in the region posterior to the Y-axis, and an optimal direction of stimulating currents for neural excitation exists in each functional area in the cortex.

Selective stimulation of each finger was also realized. Shifting the paired coil carefully from the thenar point to hypothenar point, we observed the movement of sum, index, middle finger, ring finger and little finger, separately.

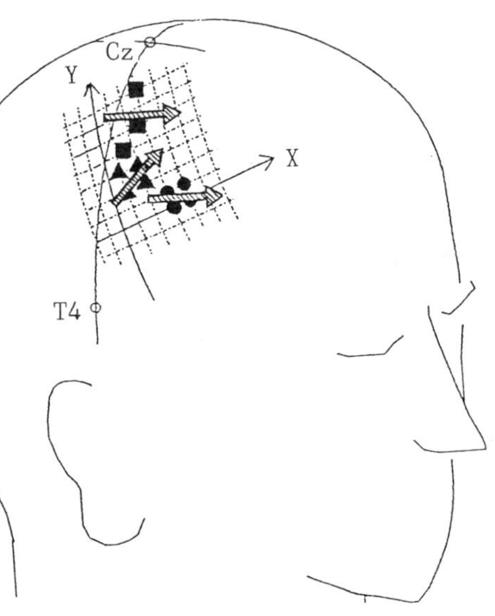

Fig.6 Functional map of the human motor cortex. The arrows show optimal current directions for neural excitation.
● Thenar muscle
▲ Hypothenar muscle
■ Brachioradial muscle

It is noted here that the localized functional area on the motor cortex diffuses relatively in a more wide regions if smaller EMG signals are taken into account in plotting the functional distributions of neural population which produces the EMG signals.

Fig.7 shows the functional localization of the motor cortex related to the thenar muscle in a subject of his hand muscles were totally relaxed. The effect of muscular tension on spatial distributions of functional organization of the cortex was also investigated.

Fig.8 shows the distribution of functional organization of the cortex related to the thenar muscle in the same subject maintained a 10 % maximum contraction of the muscle. Compared with the results in Fig.7, the area of the activated neural population in the cortex is spreaded, and a part of the region is shifted into the somatosensory area. It has been reported that both latency and amplitude of the EMG responses to magnetic stimulation of the motor cortex are depended on voluntary preactivation of the muscle (Rothwell et al.1987, Hess et al.1987). However it has been difficult to study the spatial properties of activated neural population in the cortex using a single coil technique. The magnetic brain stimulation introduced in the present study has enabled us to get fine distributions of functional organization in the human cortex within 5 mm resolution. This work was supported in part by the grants 63460113 and 63850090 from the Ministry of Education, Science and Culture in Japan.

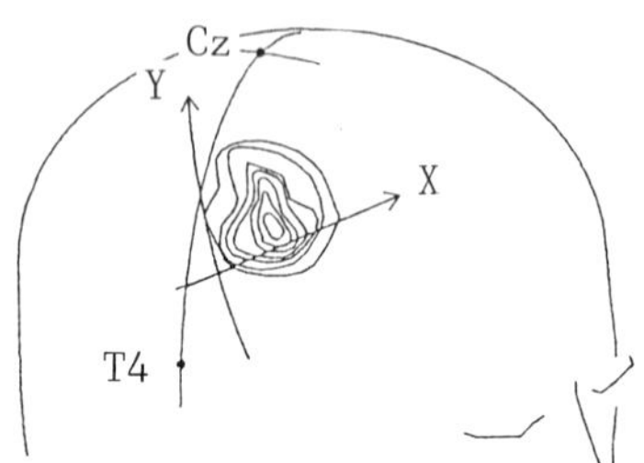

Fig.7 Functional localization of the human motor cortex related to the thenar muscle in one subject with the muscle totally relaxed. The equipotential lines which show peak-to-peak values of EMG responses to magnetic brain stimulation are quantized by 0.4 mV from 0 to 3.2 mV.

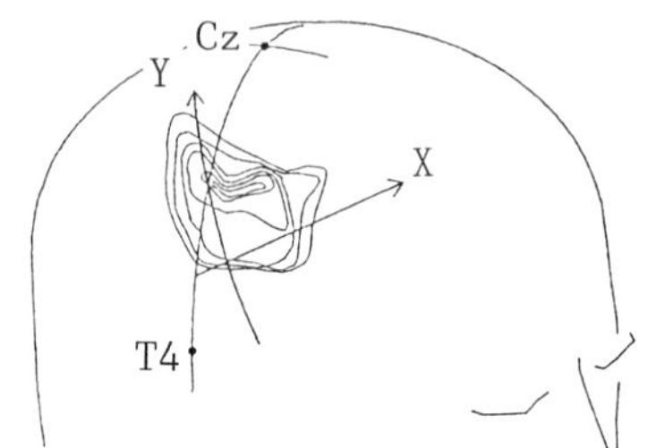

Fig.8 Functional localization of the human motor cortex related to the thenar muscle in the subject maintaining a 10 % maximum contraction of the muscle. The equipotential lines which show peak-to-peak values of EMG responses to magnetic brain stimulation are quantized by 2.0mV from 0 to 12.0 mV.

REFERENCES

Barker,A.T., Jalinous.R., and Freeston,I.L, May 1985, Lancet i, 1106-1107.

Barker,A.T., Freeston.I.L, Jalinous.R., and Jarratt,A.J., June 1986, Lancet i,1325

Barker,A.T., Freeston,I.L., Jalinous,R., and Jarratt,J.A., 1987, Neurosurgery 20,100

Hess,C.W., Mills,K.R., and Murray,N.M.F., 1987, J.Physiol.388,397

Day,B.L., Thompson,P.D., Dick,J.P., Nakashima,K., and Marsden,C.D., 1987, Neuroscience Lett.75,101

Rothwell,J.C., Day,B.L., Thompson,P.D., Dick,J.P.R., and Marsden,C.D.,1987, Neurosurgery 20,156

Ueno,S., Tashiro,T., Kamise,S., Osako,T., and Harada,K., April 1985 Digests of the Intermag Conference,BD-3,St.Paul,MN

Ueno,S., Tashiro,T., Kamise,S., and Harada,K., 1987 IEEE Trans.Magn,MAG-23, 2437

Ueno,S., Tashiro,T., and Harada,K., 1988, MMM-Intermag Conf.GR-13,Vancouver, Canada

Ueno,S., Tashiro,T., and Harada,K., 1988, J.Appl.Phys.,64,5862-5864

VOLUME CURRENT EFFECTS ON MEG AND MODELING

Eduardo Ducla-Soares*

Medical Neurology Branch
National Institute of Neurological Disorders and Stroke
National Institutes of Health
Bethesda, Md.

INTRODUCTION

Initial work on MEG assumed that the head is a sphere, either homogeneous or a set of successive concentric layers, and emphasized that if the magnetic field from the spherical head is recorded radially only the impressed current, the cellular current associated with some neural event like an epileptiform spike or an evoked response, needs to be taken into account (Williamson and Kaufman, 1982). The volume currents, those generated far from the excited cells, over the whole volume of the electrically conducting brain, CSF, skull, and scalp, and due to the electrical potentials generated by the impressed current, give no contribution if the sensors are oriented radially. The magnetic field can then be calculated from the current in a small region of space with Biot Savart's Law (Williamson and Kaufman, 1982). For this approximation, scanning around the head should give a symmetric map with two extrema of opposite signs. Recording from the occipital area, for example, offers support of this picture.

However, the head is not a sphere. It is a complex structure consisting of the brain, CSF, skull, and scalp. The skull, especially its cortical bone, is a good insulator compared with the other structures. It strongly limits the electrical currents issuing through the skull from electrical sources inside. In simulating the head for MEG studies, as a first approximation, it is appropriate to concentrate on the electrical currents inside the skull, which can be taken as an insulator, and neglect the scalp. In simulating the intracranial cavity, therefore, the spherical approximation is not very good in the low temporal and frontal areas. Also, near the jaw, if the neuromagnetometer is kept as close as possible to the outer surface of the head in order to get the

*On sabbatical leave from the Department of Physics, University of Lisbon, Lisbon, Portugal.

Advances in Biomagnetism
Edited by S.J. Williamson *et al.*
Plenum Press, New York

highest signal-to-noise ratio, it will not be perpendicular to the inner skull surface. This condition is especially difficult to satisfy with multichannel neuromagnetometers.

With recording of anterotemporal sharp waves, the MEG maps are in general very asymmetric (Rose et al., 1987) when scanning is done in the usual way, almost parallel to the face. Over the face, the sensors are tilted relative to the inner surface of the skull, and volume current effects should play a role through the tangential component of the magnetic field. In processing data from this area of the head, if the volume current effects are to be taken into account in the spherical approximation, it is necessary to use the equations for a dipole in a sphere (Stok, 1986; Hari and Ilmoniemi, 1987; Sarvas, 1987), which are available in analytic form. The main concepts emerging from these formulas are as follows:

1. The magnetic field generated by a radial dipole in a sphere (homogeneous or a succession of concentric layers with different conductivities) is zero. This is true for both the radial component and the tangential component of the magnetic field.

2. Even if the head is simulated as a set of concentric spheres, each layer with its own conductivity, the volume current contribution to the magnetic field does not depend on the conductivities of the different layers or on their radius. This statement is valid for any component of the magnetic field. The only head parameter that must be specified for this spherical approximation is the coordinates of its center. These coordinates, together with the position, orientation, and magnitude of the dipole, are all that are needed to calculate the magnetic field outside the head for any orientation of the sensors, with inclusion of volume current effects. Neither the radius nor the conductivities are needed for the calculation of the magnetic field for any direction in space. This is a very important point that deserves to be stressed.

It is important to determine how much the inclusion of volume current effects can improve the localization and quality of the calculated maps for the dipole that best fits the data, as compared with the experimental ones. This can be accomplished through correct handling of the tangential component of the magnetic field rather than just considering the field from the impressed current and depends on the area of the head under consideration, the importance of departures from sphericity, and the tilt of the sensors relative to the normal to the skull surface. Since in the National Institute of Neurological Disorders and Stroke (NINDS) an important area of research is temporal lobe epilepsy, we attempted to answer this question by concentrating first on the temporal area.

DIPOLES IMPLANTED IN A SKULL MODEL

A good way of separating the complexities due to geometry from other complexities such as multiple sources, inhomogeneities, or anisotropies in the head is to study dipoles implanted in a skull filled with gel. We studied six dipoles implanted in the temporal area of a plastic, gel-filled skull and scanned the neuromagnetometer rigorously in a plane almost parallel to the face, with the sensors nearly perpendicular to that surface (Rose et al., 1989a). For this geometry, a single current dipole (just the impressed current) should give a symmetric map with two extrema approximately identical and opposite in sign.

In the contour maps from the experimental data for the first of these six dipoles, the zero line is quite complex, and the map, with the minima near the jaw, is very asymmetric with the extrema differing by a factor of 4 (Fig. 1A). In the calculated maps for the dipole that best fits the data, which take into account only the impressed current, both the zero line and the relative amplitude of the extrema are very poorly represented (Fig. 1B). The calculated maps for a dipole in a sphere, with inclusion of volume current effects and with a reasonable position for the center of the inner skull surface, show a marked improvement in the quality of the maps for both the zero line and the relative amplitude of the extrema (Fig. 1C). The maps for the other five dipoles gave identical results (Rose et al., 1989a), with average errors in localization of 0.9 cm as compared with 2.5 cm when volume currents were not included. In the frontal area, the errors were of the same order.

Varying the position of the center of the sphere influences the accuracy of localization. Moving it in arbitrary directions by 2 cm from a reasonable estimate for the center of the intracranial cavity may introduce an extra error in localization of 1 to 1.5 cm. But if one tries to match a sphere to the local intracranial surface near the region where the measurements are being made, and chooses the center of the sphere accordingly, there is some improvement. For a dipole in the temporal region, for example, the accuracy improved from 8 mm to 5 mm.

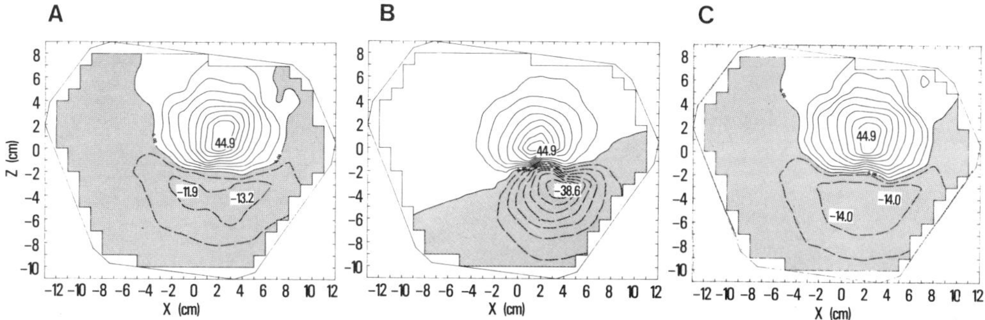

Fig. 1. Maps for a dipole in a skull model. Scanning was done in a plane almost parallel to the face.

DIPOLES IN A PATIENT

How much of this accuracy is related to the fact that the skull model is a homogeneous medium? At NINDS, candidates for surgical therapy of medically intractable seizures have subdural electrodes implanted in the surface of the brain as part of the presurgical work-up. These subdural electrodes record directly the origin of the epileptic spikes and seizures and also are used for stimulation of the brain to verify that the areas proposed for excision are not involved in motor control, somatosensory functions, or speech and memory. NINDS also has a research protocol to study the magnetic field generated by passing a current through the subdural electrodes to test the MEG models. The currents used in the MEG studies are approximately 100 times smaller then the ones used to stimulate the patient's brain (Smith et al., 1985). Figure 2 shows data from dipoles (subdural electrodes) implanted in the temporal lobe of a patient who subsequently had a temporal lobectomy (Rose et al., 1989b). The calculated maps (D-F) do not match the experimental ones as perfectly as in the skull, because we did not have as much control over every step of the procedure as we did for dipoles implanted in the skull model. Also, the presence of staples in the head from the craniotomy could be a source of error. In areas where the magnetic field varies quickly, as at the zero line, the calculated data closely reproduce the experimental results. The errors in location are 1 mm, 3 mm, and 4 mm. Even if the skull studies suggest that we could expect to have higher errors for other positions of the dipoles, these results seem to indicate that the influence of the real medium, although not a homogeneous gel, is not very large.

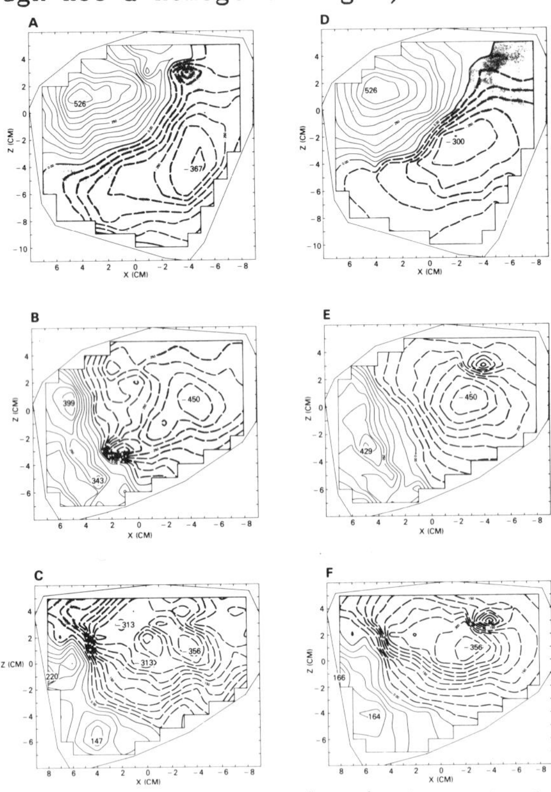

Fig. 2. Experimental maps (A-C) and calculated maps (D-F) for dipoles (subdural electrodes) implanted in the temporal lobe of a patient with epilepsy. Scanning was done as close as possible to the head surface.

HOMOGENEOUS, REALISTICALLY SHAPED HEAD MODEL

The results from the spherical models (skull and patient) are quite good, but we thought it would be interesting to push the model as hard as we can to improve accuracy and to avoid the somewhat arbitrary choice of the center of the head. We, therefore, processed the same data from the above studies in a homogeneous, realistically shaped head model limited by the inner surface of the skull (Ducla-Soares et al., 1988). Digitizing the inner surface with 640 points generated 1,216 triangles that approximate closely the inner surface of the skull (Fig. 3). A system of 1,216 equations allowed us to get the electrical potential in that surface. For each trial position of the dipole, we calculated the magnetic field from the impressed current with Biot Savart's Law. From the potential distribution at the surface of the skull, we calculated the effect of volume currents. The maps were very similar to those obtained before, but, as expected, the accuracy was better. For the four dipoles we tested, it was approximately 3 to 4 mm instead of 9 mm with the spherical models. The experimental error in position was approximately 2 mm.

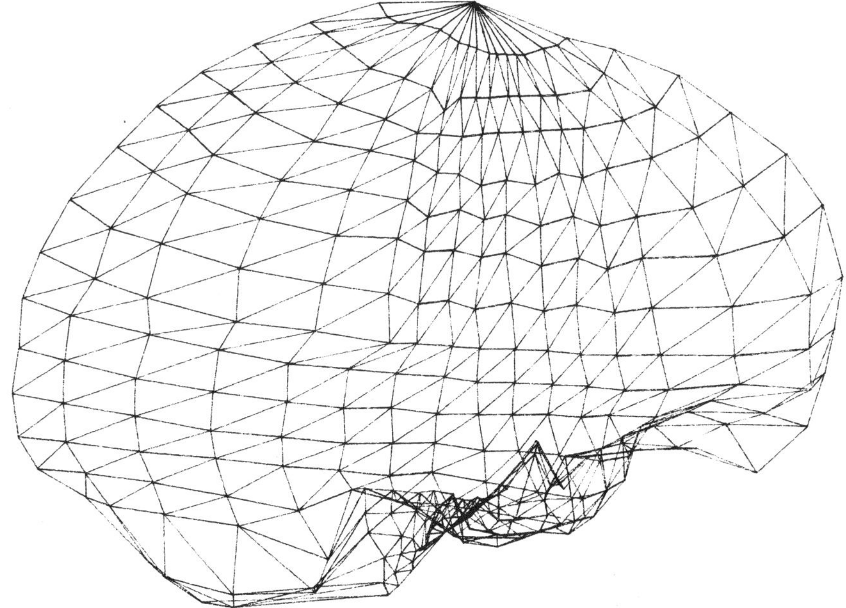

Fig. 3. Approximation of the inner surface of the skull by a set of small triangles.

FUTURE DEVELOPMENTS

Is it necessary to go beyond this approximation? Certainly it would be interesting to measure scalp currents to see if they really contribute less than 5% to the magnetic field maps (Hamalainen and Sarvas, 1987). It also would be desirable to have a clear picture of the conductivity of the brain, skull, and scalp in vivo. These new data might suggest some improvements in the models used to process MEG data, but both the spherical and the homogeneous, realistically shaped head models seem to give good results even now.

In the next 2 years, however, the most important modeling problem for MEG is to go beyond the single dipole approximation and handle extended as well as multiple sources. For this, it would be desirable to process, together with MEG, information obtained from EEG, which is more sensitive to radial dipoles. Unfortunately, spherical models for EEG are not as good as for MEG; in a four-sphere approximation, for example, it is necessary to specify the radius and the conductivities of the four spheres involved. Mixing together data from MEG and EEG in the spherical approximation is mixing models of different quality, and important errors will be introduced through the EEG data. It is, therefore, necessary to develop a sophisticated model to handle EEG correctly, which means considering explicitly the skull and the scalp. This kind of modeling, together with the new generation of multichannel neuromagnetometers now available, will open new possibilities that will clarify, in the near future, how far MEG and EEG can go as functional brain localization techniques.

REFERENCES

Ducla-Soares, E., Rose, D., and Sato, S, 1988, Volume current effects in magnetoencephalography, Phys. Med. Biol., 33(suppl. 1):33.

Hamalainen, M.S., and Sarvas, J., 1987, Feasibility of the homogeneous head model in the interpretation of neuromagnetic fields, Phys. Med. Biol., 32:91-97.

Hari, R., and Ilmoniemi, R.J., 1987, Cerebral magnetic fields, CRC Crit. Rev. Biomed. Eng., 14:93-126.

Rose, D.F., Sato, S., Smith, P.D., and White, J., 1987, Modeling the temporal region in patients with temporal lobe epilepsy, Phys. Med. Biol., 32:59-63.

Rose, D.F., Ducla-Soares, E., and Sato, S., 1989a, Improved accuracy of MEG localization in the temporal region with inclusion of volume current effects, Brain Topography, 1 (in press).

Rose, D.F., Sato, S., Ducla-Soares, E., and Kufta, C., 1989b, Magnetoencephalographic localization of dipoles implanted in an epileptic patient, submitted for publication.

Sarvas, J., 1987, Basic mathematical and electromagnetic concepts of the biomagnetic inverse problem, Phys. Med. Biol., 32:11-22.

Smith D.B., Sidman, R.D., Flanigin, H., Menke, J., and Labiner, D., 1985, A reliable method for localizing deep intracranial sources of the EEG, Neurology, 35:1702-1707.

Stok, C.J., 1986, The inverse problem in EEG and MEG with application to visual evoked responses. PhD thesis, Leiden University.

Williamson, S.J., and Kaufman L., 1982, Biomagnetism, J. Magnetism Magn. Materials, 22:129-201.

IMPACT OF DIFFERENT NOISE SOURCES ON DIPOLE LOCALIZATION IN THE SPHERICAL MODEL: A SIMULATION

D. S. Buchanan

Biomagnetic Technologies Inc.
San Diego, CA 92121

INTRODUCTION

In an effort to understand the impact of the different noise sources present in current multi-channel Neuromagnetometers® we have developed a set of modeling routines which allow us to independently add noise corresponding to these different sources to the forward solution for a current dipole in a homogeneous spherical conductor (Sarvas 1987). The resulting perturbed forward solution is then inverted using the non-linear least squares fitting routine in the Biomagnetic Technologies Inc. (BTi) Neuromagnetometer software. Unlike several previous analysis of noise effects (Ribeiro et al. 1988, Kaukoranta et al. 1986) we were interested in simulating a number of different sources to look at each contribution independently and together. We have included field noise, relative gain error of a multi-channel system, translational error in placement of the system, and rotational error in placement of the system. We have measured the statistics of the resulting fits as an estimate of the noise introduced into the localization.

METHOD

Sensor Array

Simulation of the impact of these noise sources required the ability to create and manipulate sensor arrays in software. Software was developed which could create circular arrays of sensors placed on either spherical or ellipsoidal surfaces. The individual sensors could be constructed of any configuration of loops including first and second order coaxial gradiometers of any baseline. Once created these sensor arrays (or probes) were placed in software, about the dipole source. The software could also manipulate 'realistic probes;' probes that had been generated by measurements of real sensor arrays (Buchanan 1989).

Results presented here are for a probe which was the image of a real seven channel system. This probe was placed on a 12 cm radius sphere at seven locations about the simulated dipole. One placement was radically above the dipole while the six others were equally spaced about a circle formed by the intersection of a cone of .802 rad. included angle and the sphere, the cone's vertex being placed at the center of the sphere and axis passing through the dipole. All probe placements were initially oriented radially before being perturbed (see below). The sensors were constructed of 12 loops of 0.0064 cm dia wire each loop having a radius of 0.9 cm and arranged as a 3-6-3 second order gradiometer of 4 cm baseline.

Forward Solution

The forward solution was calculated for each loop of each sensor for a homogeneous sphere model and then summed to give the sensor output. This solution was then perturbed according to the type of noise or noises being simulated.

For field noise a random number having a gaussian distribution of standard deviation σ_n was added to each calculated field points.

For translational and rotational noise the forward solution was calculated for each sensor in a given probe placement. The entire probe location or orientation was then perturbed. The inverse solution was then calculated using the perturbed probe locations. The translational perturbation consisted of adding a random number having a gaussian distribution of standard deviation σ_t to each of the x, y and z coordinates of the probe locations. The probe is moved as a rigid structure. The rotational perturbation consisted of adding a random number having a gaussian distribution of standard deviation σ_a to each of the orientation angles of the probe.

For noise introduced by relative gain errors (i.e. calibration errors) each sensor in the probe was assigned a gain of 1.0 ± g where g was a random number having a gaussian distribution of standard deviation σ_g These relative gains were then fixed for all seven probe placements. The calculated field values were multiplied by these gain values.

Any subset, or all of the above noise sources could be applied to a given simulation.

Inverse Solution

The inverse solution was calculated using the BTi Neuromagnetometer® Dipole Fit routine. The routine performs a non-linear least squares approximation to find the dipole location and size. The forward solution used in the least squares algorithm is for a homogeneous spherical model.

Analysis

For each set of input noise parameters simulations were run. A simulation consists of a forward calculation with perturbation followed by inverse solution for that perturbed data. A standard deviation was then calculated for each of the dipole parameters in the resulting sixty four fits. The results are presented in Figs. 1-4 for a variety of input parameters. Fig 3 represents an estimate for the errors in the current BTi Neuromagnetometer system.

RESULTS

Simulation results are plotted in the following figures. In each of the legends 'Perp. to Dipole' and 'Par to dipole' refer to tangential directions where the former is perpendicular to the direction of the dipole while the latter parallel to the dipole. 'Radial' refers to the radial direction. These coordinates are the natural ones for a tangential dipole and are independent of the dipole's location in the sphere. The vertical axis represents the standard deviation of the population of fits for each of these directions as indicated. The distances in the legends are the distance of the dipole from the origin of the sphere.

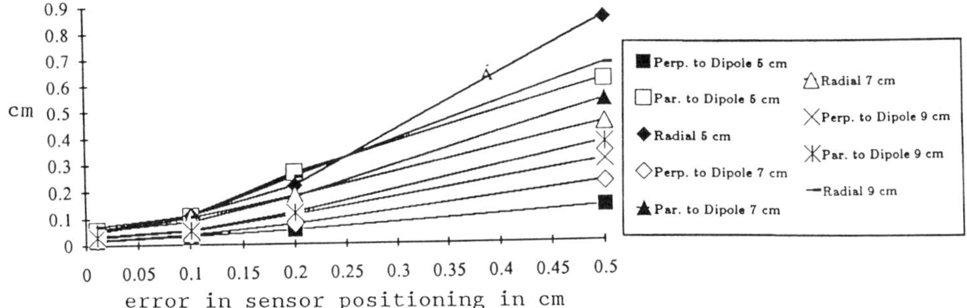

Fig. 1. Localization error as a function of translational error. The x, y and z coordinates of the probe position measurements are equally perturbed. The standard deviation of the perturbation is plotted along the horizontal axis.

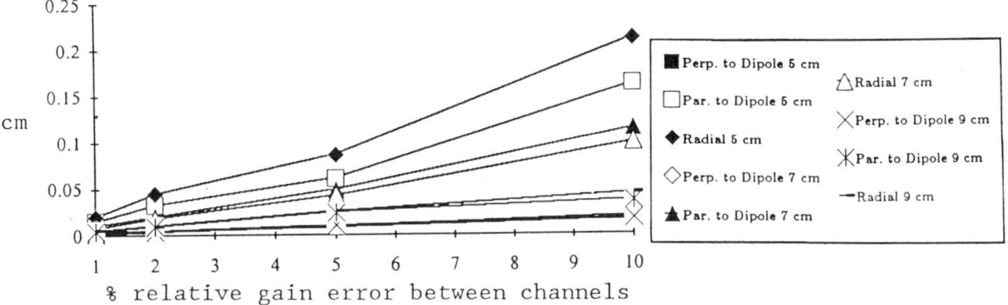

Fig. 2. Localization error as a function of relative gain error for a 7 channel sensor. The standard deviation of the gain perturbation is plotted along the horizontal axis in %.

DISCUSSION

Figs. 1-4 show the effects of various noise sources on dipole localization. Measurements on spherical phantoms have given a localization error of about 3 mm for large signal to noise sources (Paulson 1989). From Fig. 2 it is apparent that calibration errors are not limiting the system. This is different than the results of Ribeiro et al. (1988) because in this case there are 49 measurement points as opposed to their 5-14 measurement points. Because field noise was small this leaves probe positioning errors as the limiting source. This can be seen in Fig. 1 which shows that errors of about 2-5 mm could account for most the 3 mm error associated with the phantom measurement. This is consistent with measurements of the probe position measurement system which is used. It can easily give 2 mm errors.

Fig. 4 is very interesting in that it shows that for dipole localization where measurements positions are picked optimally, that is along the line connecting the extrema, only 2 probes resulting in 14 measurement locations are required even for realistic source sizes.

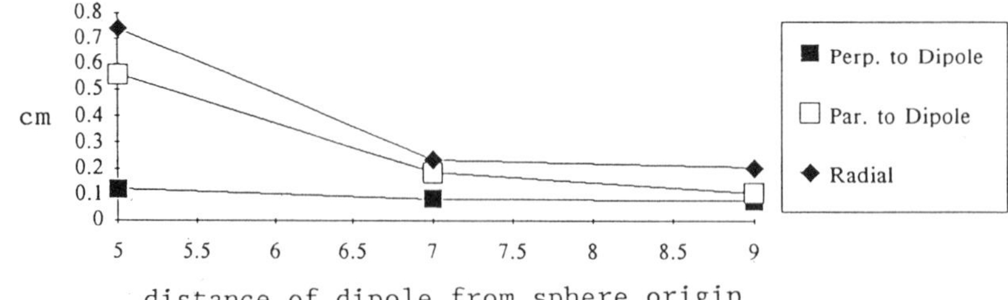

Fig. 3. Localization error as a function of dipole depth using the combined errors of a typical system for a 10 nAm source. The calculation is for a field noise of 20 fT, sensor positioning error of 1.5 mm, sensor angular positioning error of 2 degrees and a relative gain error of 1.5%. The distance of the dipole from the sphere origin is plotted along the horizontal axis.

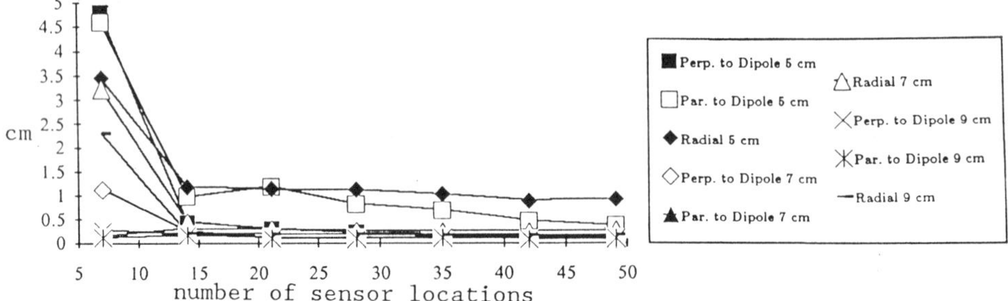

Fig. 4. Localization error as a function of the number of probe placements. The noise parameter were set as in Fig. 3. The single probe was placed radially above the dipole. The probes in the 2 probe position were placed on either side of the 1 probe placement along the line connecting the field extreme. The 3 probe placement filled the 1 probe position back in while 4-7 continued to fill around the circle described earlier.

ACKNOWLEDGEMENTS

This work was supported in part by NINCDS Grants 2 R44 NS 24098 and 1 R43 NS 24484 under the SBIR program. I would like to thank Steve Robinson for providing the forward calculation. I would also like to thank Richard Greenblatt and Doug Paulson for any helpful discussions.

REFERENCES

Sarvas, J. (1987). Basis Mathematical and Electromagnetic Concepts of the Biomagnetic Inverse Problem. UPhys. Med. Biol.32:11-22

Ribeiro,P. C., Williamson, S. J., and Kaufman L. (1988). SQUID Arrays for Simultaneous Magnetic Measurements: Calibration and Source Localization Performance. IEEE Trans. Biomed. Eng. 35n7:551.

Kaukoranta, E., Hamalainin, M. Sarvas, J. and Hari, R. (1986). Mixed ans sensory nerve simulations activate different cytoarchitectonic areas in the human primary somatosensory cortex SI. Exp. Brain Res. 63:60.

Buchanan, D. S. and Paulson, D. N. (1989) Neuromagnetometer Calibration Using an Array of Small Coils. This Proceedings.

Paulson, D. N., and Buchanan, D. S. (1989). Experimental Accuracy of Localization of Current Dipoles in a Spherical Phantom. This Proceedings.

MONTE CARLO ANALYSIS OF LOCALIZATION ERRORS IN MAGNETOENCEPHALOGRAPHY

Patricia A. Medvick, Paul S. Lewis, Cheryl Aine, and Edward R. Flynn

Neuromagnetism Laboratory, Los Alamos National Laboratory
Mail Stop M715, Los Alamos, NM 87545, U.S.A.

INTRODUCTION

In magnetoencephalography (MEG), the magnetic fields created by electrical activity in the brain are measured on the surface of the skull. To determine the location of the activity, the measured field is fit to a parameterized source generator model by minimizing chi-square. In the case of a current dipole model, the parameters computed by the fitting procedure are the location and orientation of the dipole. For current dipoles and other nonlinear source models, the fit is performed by an iterative least squares procedure such as the Levenberg-Marquardt algorithm (Press 1986). Once the fit has been computed, analysis of the resulting value of chi-square can determine whether the assumed source model is adequate to account for the measurements. If the source model is adequate, then the effect of measurement error on the fitted model parameters must be analyzed.

Several computer modeling studies have explored the effects of measurement errors on fitting simulated MEG data to dipole models in conducting spheres. Cuffin (1985, 1986) analyzed the effects of additive error by computing individual parameter variances from 10-run Monte Carlo simulations. Two-parameter confidence regions were computed by Hari et al. (1988) by making a number of simplifying assumptions. Stok (1987) compared estimates of parameter variances computed via analytic model linearization with estimates computed by Monte Carlo simulations of 100 runs and found that the linearization approach could underestimate the variances by a factor of up to 25.

Although these kinds of simulation studies can provide a rough idea of the effect that measurement error can be expected to have on source localization, they cannot provide detailed enough information to determine the effects that the errors in a particular measurement situation will produce. In this work, we introduce and describe the use of Monte Carlo-based techniques to analyze model fitting errors for real data. Given the details of the measurement setup and a statistical description of the measurement errors, these techniques determine the effects the errors have on the fitted model parameters.

METHODS

The effect of measurement error on fitted model parameters is usually analyzed statistically by computing covariances and/or multidimensional confidence regions of the parameters. These statistics can be computed by traditional analytic methods if the measurement errors are additive and normally distributed, and if the model is linear (Press et al. 1986). When these conditions do not hold, analytic computation requires either 1) a detailed analysis of the statistics for the particular case, or 2) approximation, such as model linearization.

Most MEG source models are nonlinear in some of their parameters. The current dipole model, for example, has a nonlinear dependence on its location parameters. MEG measurement errors contain both additive components, such as unrelated brain activity, intrinsic sensor noise, and environmental interference, and nonadditive components, such as sensor location errors. Furthermore, the distribution of some of these errors may not be normal. Because of these conditions, analytic approximations may provide incorrect results, as evidenced by Stok (1987) in the calculation of parameter variances.

To provide an alternative to the analytic-approximation approach, we have developed MEG localization error analysis techniques based on Monte Carlo simulation (Press et al. 1986). These techniques are not limited to computer simulation studies of the general effect of measurement errors. Instead, they are intended to provide an error analysis tool for real data, tailored to the specifics of the particular measurement situation.

The basic approach of Monte Carlo error analysis can be summarized as follows. The measurements we use to compute the source model parameters correspond to one particular experimental realization. Because of the random nature of the measurement errors, repetition of the experiment would result in a slightly different set of measurements. Fitting the model to this different set of measurements would result in slightly different values for the model parameters. The most robust method of analyzing the effect of measurement errors on the fitted parameters is to repeat the experiment many times and fit the model to each set of the resulting measurements. This would provide a sample of the parameter population that could be directly analyzed.

Since repetition of the experiment is usually impractical, the approach of Monte Carlo error analysis is to simulate the measurements that would have been obtained if the experiment had been repeated. Using the parameters found by fitting the model to the real measurement data as surrogates for the unknown "true" parameters, multiple copies of the "ideal" field measurements produced by the model are generated. Each of these ideal fields is then perturbed by a different set of simulated errors. These sets of simulated errors are randomly generated on a computer with distributions that mimic those of the errors in the measuring process. The simulated errors can be used to perturb the ideal field additively, as when one simulates the error caused by noise sources, or nonadditively, as when one simulates the error (shift) caused by imprecise location of the sensors. The result is a number of simulated measurement sets. The source model is then fit to each measurement set, providing an ensemble of model parameters. This ensemble approximates the joint distribution of the parameters, and from it any statistics describing the parameter error can be directly estimated (e.g. variances, confidence regions).

Like all procedures for analyzing the effect of measurement error on fitted model parameters, Monte Carlo analysis depends on statistical knowledge of the error processes. As a consequence, the validity of the final results are dependent on the accuracy of this knowledge. Unlike most alternate procedures however, this is the only requirement for the Monte Carlo approach. Error processes do not have to be normal and additive, linear approximations are not required for the source model, and detailed statistical analyses are unnecessary.

APPLICATION EXAMPLES

Monte Carlo simulations have been used to analyze parameter uncertainty in a variety of MEG experiments at Los Alamos. In a recent auditory attention study (Arthur et al. 1989), we used Monte Carlo error analyses to demonstrate that the closely spaced sources of the N1m and Ndm activity are spatially different and can be distinguished from one another. In a visual attention study (Aine et al. 1989), Monte Carlo analyses have indicated that, for the particular paradigm, the source locations of the attend and not-attend responses could not be distinguished. In another visual study (George et al. 1989), we employed Monte Carlo analyses to demonstrate distinct sources at differing latencies.

In this section we present two examples to illustrate the use of Monte Carlo error analysis. The data used in these examples are drawn from the third study cited above. For graphical clarity, the ensembles from 100 point Monte Carlo simulations are presented. Detailed statistical analyses will generally require larger ensembles. For these examples, we employed a simple five-parameter "dipole in a sphere" model. The forward field computations for this model took into account both the second-order gradiometer configuration and finite coil areas of the SQUID sensors.

In the first example, Monte Carlo analysis is used to compare dipolar fits of visually evoked fields at latencies of 90 and 110 ms. The evoked field was a response to a sinusoidal grating displayed in the lower right quadrant of the visual field. Field measurements were taken at 56 points on the head and each measurement is the average of 75 trials. This is an example of a relative analysis in which the objective is to determine if the sources of the two fields can be distinguished by the MEG measurements. Since the sensor location errors are the same for both fields, only measurement noise errors were incorporated into the analysis. For this example, the noise was assumed to be independent from channel-to-channel and normally distributed. A standard deviation of 21.1 fT for the noise was computed by averaging the standard deviations of the prestimulus intervals for the measurements at each location.

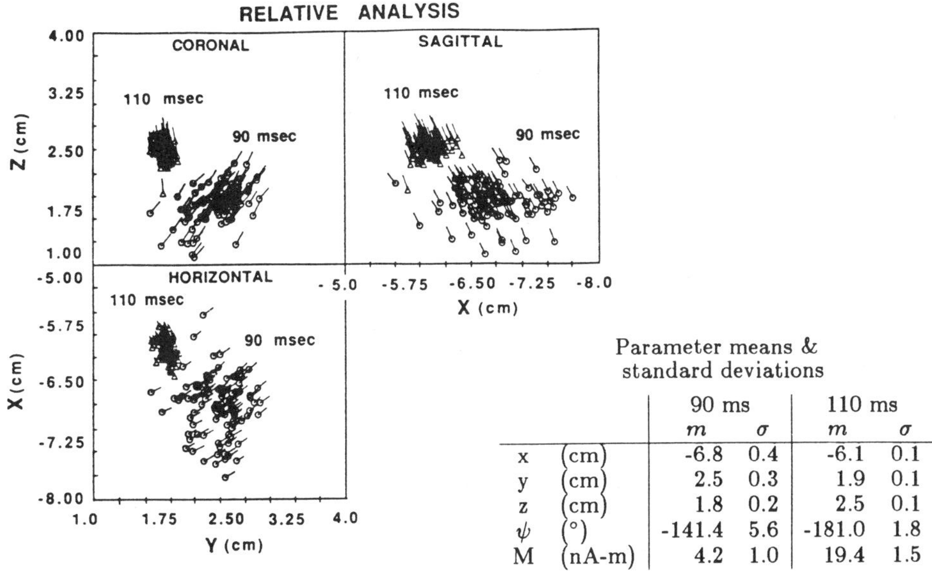

Parameter means & standard deviations

		90 ms		110 ms	
		m	σ	m	σ
x	(cm)	-6.8	0.4	-6.1	0.1
y	(cm)	2.5	0.3	1.9	0.1
z	(cm)	1.8	0.2	2.5	0.1
ψ	(°)	-141.4	5.6	-181.0	1.8
M	(nA-m)	4.2	1.0	19.4	1.5

Fig. 1. Monte Carlo-generated ensembles for visually evoked fields at 90 ms and 110 ms latencies using additive noise with a standard deviation of 21.2 fT.

The parameter ensembles generated by a 100-point Monte Carlo analysis are shown in Fig. 1. The three frames show the ensemble dipoles from three orthogonal views, with the symbols marking the locations and the tails indicating the moment and orientation. The accompanying table lists the standard deviations of the dipole parameters for both cases. In this example, the sources for the two evoked fields are clearly distinguishable.

In the second example, Monte Carlo error analysis is used to examine absolute localization accuracy. The visually evoked field used in this example is a response at a latency of 90 ms to a sinusoidal grating in the central visual field. The evoked field was sampled at 42 points on the head and each field measurement is the average of 100 trials. Measurement errors caused by both

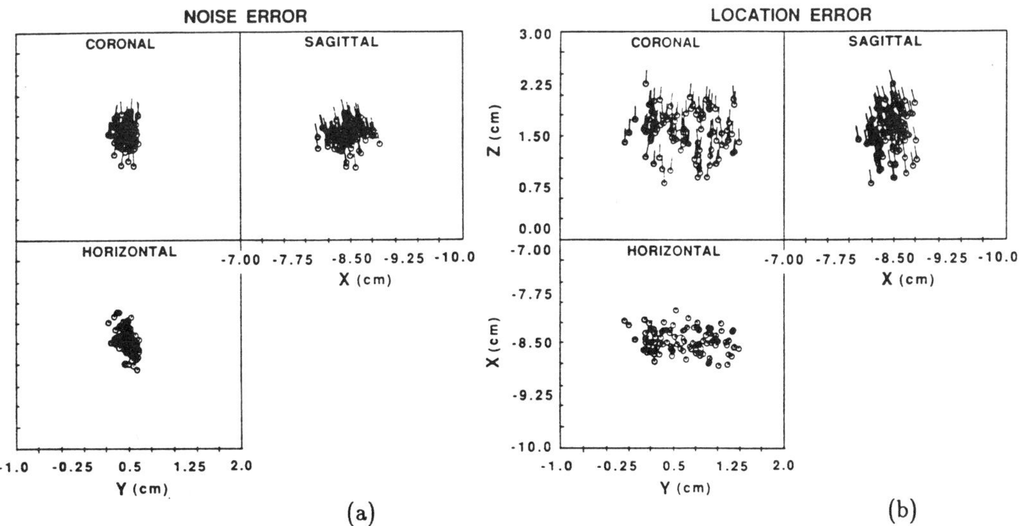

Fig. 2. Monte Carlo-generated ensembles for a visually evoked field at a 90 ms latency. (a) Additive noise error only, using a standard deviation of 12.4 fT. (b) Nonadditive location error only of ± 1 cm.

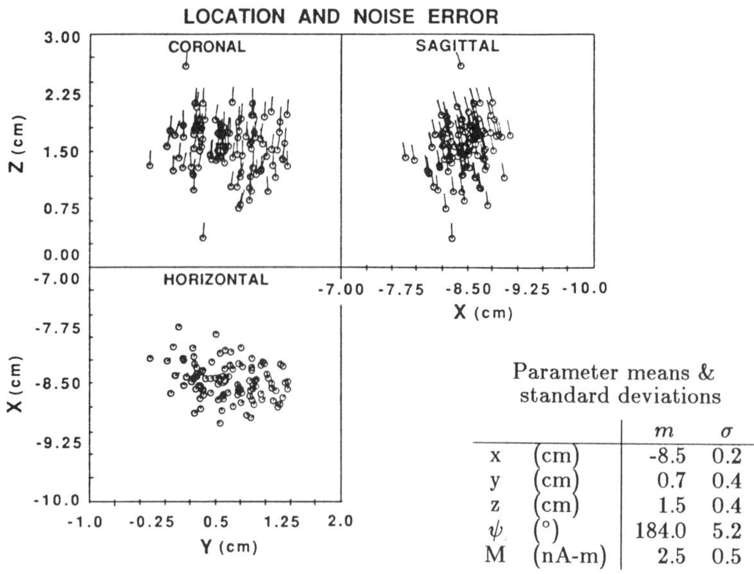

		m	σ
x	(cm)	-8.5	0.2
y	(cm)	0.7	0.4
z	(cm)	1.5	0.4
ψ	(°)	184.0	5.2
M	(nA-m)	2.5	0.5

Fig. 3: Monte Carlo-generated ensemble incorporating both noise and location error.

additive noise and sensor location uncertainty were incorporated into this analysis. The noise was again assumed to be independent and normally distributed. Analysis of the prestimulus intervals for this data set yielded a noise standard deviation of 12.4 fT. Fig. 2(a) shows a 100-point Monte Carlo ensemble generated using only noise error.

The sensor location error was modeled by random shifts of the sensor locations along the surface of the measurement sphere. These shift errors are used to perturb the ideal field by using the field values at the actual or shifted sensor locations in place of the values at their nominal locations. In this example, the shift error was modeled by independent shift errors in the north-south and east-west directions. The shift errors were generated from a uniform distribution of $\pm$ 1 cm. Since our measurements were taken with a seven-sensor SQUID, the shift errors were not independent from channel-to-channel. To incorporate this into our error model, we randomly shifted the blocks of seven sensors rather than the individual sensors. Fig. 2(b) shows a 100-point Monte Carlo ensemble generated using location error only. Fig. 3 shows a 100-point Monte Carlo ensemble incorporating both noise and location error. In this particular example, it can be seen that the parameter uncertainty caused by sensor location error is significant and must be taken into account for a realistic error analysis.

REFERENCES

Aine, C.J., George, J.S., Medvick, P.A., Oakley, M.T., Davis, L., and Flynn, E.R. (1989). Effects of spatial attention on the visual-evoked neuromagnetic response. Submitted to *Jour. Cognitive Neuroscience*

Arthur, D.L., Lewis, P.S., Medvick, P.A., and Flynn, E.R. (1989). A neuromagnetic study of selective auditory attention. Submitted to *EEG.*

Cuffin, B.N. (1985). A comparison of moving dipole inverse solutions using EEG's and MEG's. *IEEE Trans. Biomed. Eng.* BME-32, 905–910.

Cuffin, B.N. (1986). Effects of measurement errors and noise on MEG moving dipole inverse solutions. *IEEE Trans. Biomed. Eng.* BME-33, 854–861.

George, J.S., Aine, C.J., Medvick, P.A., and Flynn, E.R. (1989). Spatial/temporal resolution of multiple sources: paths of activation in the human visual cortex. *Proc. Seventh Int. Conf. Biomagnetism.* New York, NY.

Hari, R., Joutsiniemi, S.-L., and Sarvas, J. (1988). Spatial resolution of neuromagnetic records: theoretical calculations in a spherical model. *EEG* 71, 64–72.

Press, W.H., Flannery, B.P., Teukolsky, S.A., and Vetterling, W.T. (1986) *Numerical Recipes.* Cambridge University Press, New York.

Stok, C.J. (1987). The influence of model parameters on EEG/MEG single dipole source estimation. *IEEE Trans. Biomed. Eng.* BME-34, 289–296.

VARIATIONAL PRINCIPLES FOR THE RETURN CURRENT

IN ENCEPHALOGRAPHY

Leon Heller

Theoretical Division
Los Alamos National Laboratory
Los Alamos, New Mexico 87545

INTRODUCTION

The total electric current within the brain has been written as a sum of two terms of distinctly different nature (Geselowitz, 1967; Barnard, 1967). The first, $\vec{J}^{i}$, is the 'primary' or 'impressed' intracellular current that flows within the neurons, and is the quantity of interest in neuroscience. This current leaks across the cell membrane, however, and since the cells are embedded in an electrically conducting medium the extracellular ('return') current flows through a large volume of this medium before returning to the cell. With the return current written as the product of the conductivity σ and the electric field intensity $\vec{E} = -\nabla V$, at low frequencies the electric potential V is determined by the continuity equation (Geselowitz, 1967).

$$\nabla\cdot(\vec{J}^{i} - \sigma\nabla V) = 0. \tag{1}$$

Although the three-dimensional partial differential equation (1) can be solved numerically for the potential V for any assumed functions $\vec{J}^{i}$ and σ, it is instructive to consider other mathematical formulations of the problem that are equivalent to Eq. (1). Some of these reformulations may provide some practical advantages, such as greater efficiency of the numerical solution. In addition, as will be shown below, some exact properties of the solution are exposed, which are not obvious by looking at Eq. (1).

One such reformulation of Eq. (1) that has been used recently in encephalography (Meijs, 1987; Hämäläinen, 1989) makes use of the assumption that the conductivity σ can be treated as a different constant in different regions, e.g., brain, skull, and scalp. With this assumption the three-dimensional partial differential equation (1) can be converted to a two-dimensional integral equation, where the integration runs over all the surfaces of discontinuity of σ (Geselowitz, 1967; Barnard, 1967).

We now consider some other reformulations of Eq. (1) based upon a variational principle (Heller, 1989).

VARIATIONAL PRINCIPLE

The variational principle states that the correct potential function $V(\vec{r})$ is the one that makes P[V] a maximum, where

$$P[V] = -\int d^3r[2V\,\nabla\cdot\vec{J}^{i} + \sigma(\nabla V)^2] \ . \tag{2}$$

A straightforward calculation of the first order variation δP produced by a change δV shows that if $\delta P = 0$ for arbitrary δV then (i) V satisfies Eq. (1) at every interior point, and (ii)

$$\vec{n} \cdot \sigma \nabla V = 0 \tag{3}$$

at every point on the surface. Equation (3) states that no current crosses the surface, and is the appropriate boundary condition provided the conductivity vanishes outside the surface.

It can also be shown that an extremum of P is actually a maximum; and furthermore, the solution for ∇V is unique (Heller, 1989). This is also important for numerical work since any change in V that increases P is a step in the right direction.

CONSERVATION OF ENERGY

One special variation of V about its correct value consists of multiplying the entire function by a constant. When this is done it leads to the result that at the correct solution P[V] has the value

$$P_0 = - \int d^3r \; V \; \nabla \cdot \vec{J}^{\ell} = \int d^3r \; \sigma (\nabla V)^2 \quad . \tag{4}$$

We shall now show that the first integral in Eq. (4) represents the rate at which the neurons do work in creating the current $\vec{J}^{\ell}$, and the second integral in Eq. (4) represents the rate at which electrical energy is dissipated (ohmic heating) in the extracellular medium. Consequently, Eq. (4) represents the *conservation of energy*. To see this recall that for any current $\vec{J}$, $\int d^3r \; \vec{J} \cdot \vec{E}$ represents the rate at which the electric field does work *on* the current. Since $\vec{E} = - \nabla V$, it takes only an integration by parts on the first integral in Eq. (4) to prove the two statements made above.

It is true, of course, that the conservation of energy, as embodied in Eq. (4), could have been written down *ab initio* without any reference to the variational principle, Eq. (2). But the variational principle leads naturally to this result, and that is one of the benefits of formulating the return current problem in this way. Eq. (4) can serve as a check on any numerical solution for V, no matter from what equation that solution was obtained.

POINT SOURCES

Equation (2) is not suitable for numerical work if the divergence of the primary current is concentrated at individual points, which is the case, for example, with a current dipole, because near such a point $\int (\nabla V)^2$ diverges. To overcome this problem write V as a sum of a known term V^{ℓ} and an unknown term ϕ, $V = V^{\ell} + \phi$, where

$$V^{\ell}(\vec{r}) = - \frac{1}{4\pi} \int d^3r' \; \frac{\nabla' \cdot \vec{J}^{\ell}(\vec{r}\,')}{\sigma(\vec{r}\,') \, |\vec{r} - \vec{r}\,'|} \quad , \tag{5}$$

and consequently $\nabla^2 V^{\ell} = \nabla \cdot \vec{J}^{\ell} / \sigma$.

With this decomposition, $P[V] = P^{\ell} + p[\phi]$, where P^{ℓ} is known (in terms of $\vec{J}^{\ell}$ and V^{ℓ}) and $p[\phi]$ contains all the dependence on the unknown function ϕ,

$$p[\phi] = \int d^3r \; [2\phi \nabla\sigma \cdot \nabla V^{\ell} - \sigma (\nabla\phi)^2] \quad . \tag{6}$$

The return current problem has now been reduced to finding the function ϕ that makes $p[\phi]$ a maximum.

REGIONS OF CONSTANT CONDUCTIVITY

If it can be assumed that the conductivity is a different constant in different regions, e.g., brain, skull, and scalp, then the only places where $\nabla\sigma$ does not vanish are on the surfaces where σ jumps in value, including the outermost surface. Furthermore, $\nabla\sigma$ is normal to these surfaces, and Eq. (6) can be rewritten as

$$p[\phi] = -\sum_j \int dS\vec{n}\cdot[2(\sigma_j'-\sigma_j'')\nabla V^{\iota} + (\sigma_j'\nabla'\phi-\sigma_j''\nabla''\phi)]\phi + \sum_j \sigma_j\int d^3r\phi\nabla^2\phi \quad ,(7)$$

where we have followed the convention that the unit normal vector $\vec{n}$ points outward from the region designated with single primes, and into the region designated with double primes. The summation in Eq. (7) runs over all the surfaces of discontinuity of σ.

In trying to maximize $p[\phi]$ in either Eq. (6) or Eq. (7) there are no restrictions on the trial function ϕ. We know, however, from Eqs. (1) and (5) that the correct function ϕ satisfies $\nabla^2\phi = 0$ *inside* every region of constant σ, and consequently the sources of ϕ are all located on the surfaces separating regions having different values of σ. It makes sense, therefore, to parameterize the variational function ϕ in terms of a surface charge density τ,

$$\phi(\vec{r}) = \frac{1}{4\pi\epsilon_0}\sum_j \int dS'\frac{\tau(\vec{r}')}{|\vec{r}-\vec{r}'|} \quad . \tag{8}$$

Since Eq. (8) satisfies $\nabla^2\phi = 0$ inside every region for any choice of τ, the final term in Eq. (7) can now be set equal to zero. The return current problem has now been reformulated into finding the surface charge density τ that makes $p[\phi]$ a maximum.

NUMERICAL METHODS

The original differential equation (1) for V can be solved directly, by a finite difference scheme, for example. If it is desired to model the primary current $\vec{J}^{\iota}$ with fine spatial resolution then this would require a very large number of grid points and lead, therefore, to a very large system of linear equations to be solved. The two-dimensional integral equation for the potential also leads to a system of linear equations (Meijs, 1987; Hämäläinen, 1989), which would become large if more and more regions having different conductivity values are considered.

The variational principle can also be converted to a set of linear equations, by the method of finite elements, for example. Such a procedure has been used in electrocardiography (Yamashita, 1984; Pilkington, 1985), but which differs from Eqs. (2) or (6) in two important respects. In the ECG problem one tries to relate the potential on the surface of the heart to that measured on the body surface, and it is assumed that there are no current sources in the volume between these surfaces. The term linear in V in those equations is not present, therefore. A second difference between ECG and encephalography is that the boundary condition on the heart surface is not given by Eq. (3) since current can flow across that surface. Instead, the values of the potential there are taken as a constraint upon the allowed functions V.

There is another way to treat the variational principle, Eq. (7), that does not lead to a system of linear equations. It is based upon the integral equation for the surface charge density τ (Gelernter, 1964; Barnard, 1967), which can be written

$$\frac{1}{2\epsilon_0}\frac{\sigma'+\sigma''}{\sigma'-\sigma''}\tau(\vec{r}) = -\vec{n}\cdot\nabla V^{\iota}(\vec{r}) + \frac{1}{4\pi\epsilon_0}\vec{n}\cdot\int dS'\tau(\vec{r}')\frac{\vec{r}-\vec{r}'}{|\vec{r}-\vec{r}'|^3} \quad , \tag{9}$$

where $\vec{r}$ is a point on any of the surfaces of discontinuity of σ, and the integration runs over all the surfaces. One can, of course, try to solve Eq. (9) directly, in a manner analogous to solving the integral equation for V.

It is also possible to attempt a solution by iteration (Gelernter, 1964), but it is not clear whether this procedure will always converge. On the other hand, by combining Eqs. (7), (8), and (9), an iteration-variation procedure can be used, which systematically approaches the correct solution (Heller, 1989). Analysis of a homogeneous sphere shows that (barring accidental cancellations) a *single* iteration-variation step comes within 4% of the correct solution, even for very shallow primary currents. For deep currents the accuracy is much greater.

We intend to study the relative merits of a number of these techniques for finding the potential V that is produced by a variety of assumed primary currents $\vec{J}^{i}$ and conductivity functions σ.

ACKNOWLEDGMENTS

I am grateful to the members of the MEG group at Los Alamos for introducing me to this problem, and especially want to thank E. R. Flynn, D. Van Hulsteyn, J. Lewine, and C. C. Wood for many informative discussions. This work was supported by the U. S. Departments of Energy and Defense.

REFERENCES

Barnard, A. C. L., Duck, I. M., and Lynn, M. S. (1967). The application of electromagnetic theory to cardiology I. Derivation of the integral equations. Biophys. J. 7, 443-462.

Gelernter, H. L., and Swihart, J. C. (1964). A mathematical-physical model of the genesis of the electrocardiogram. Biophys. J. 4, 285-301.

Geselowitz, D. B. (1967). On bioelectric potentials in an inhomogeneous volume conductor. Biophys. J. 7, 1-11.

Hämäläinen, M. S., and Sarvas, J. (1989). Realistic conductivity geometry model of the human head for interpretation of neuromagnetic data. IEEE Trans. Biomed. Eng. BME-36, 165-171.

Heller, L. (1989). The return current in encephalography: variational principles. Submitted for publication.

Meijs, J. W. H., Bosch, F. G. C., Peters, M. J., and Lopes da Silva, F. H. (1987). On the magnetic field distribution generated by a dipolar current source situated in a realistically shaped compartment model of the head. Electroenceph. Clin. Neurophysiol. 66, 286-298.

Pilkington, T. C., Morrow, M. N., and Stanley, P. C. (1985). A comparison of finite element and integral equation formulations for the calculation of electrocardiographic potentials. IEEE Trans. Biomed. Eng. BME-32, 166-173.

Yamashita, Y., and Takahashi, T. (1984). Use of the finite element method to determine epicardial from body surface potentials under a realistic torso model. IEEE Trans. Biomed. Eng. BME-31, 611-621.

MAGNETOENCEPHALOGRAPHIC LOCALIZATION OF SIMULATED EVOKED RESPONSE SOURCES AFFIRMS THE IMPORTANCE OF ADEQUATE MODELLING

Capt Paul J. De Rego and Capt Albert F. Badeau

Human Engineering Division
Armstrong Aerospace Medical Research Laboratory
Wright-Patterson AFB, Ohio 45433

INTRODUCTION

A popular claim of magnetoencephalography (MEG) is it's ability to precisely estimate the location, orientation, and strength of the neural current sources responsible for the observed fields outside the head (Hari et. al., 1988). The estimation procedure usually involves a least squares fit between the observed magnetic field and a modelled magnetic field.

Our research group measures auditory and visual evoked responses to study the behavior of components under various workload conditions. An evoked field will have several latency components occurring after stimulus onset, each with inverse solutions typically localizing to a unique location (Hari et. al., 1988). The response can not be modelled as a single generator reversing polarity, but rather two or more activated regions summing to form the observed components. Colleagues and visitors often ask how accurate our position and strength estimates are for the sources of these components. In this paper, Gaussian waves were used to simulate regions of many closely packed neurons, and localization was evaluated.

METHODS

A soft sponge wrapped in chamois cloth and soaked in conductive fluid was placed within a human skull. Four current dipoles were constructed from 36 AWG single conductor shielded cable with two each placed in the temporal and occipital regions of the head/brain model. The anode and cathode ends of the dipoles were exposed so the return currents would freely flow through the surrounding conductive medium. Variations in conductivity due to compressed portions of the sponge were assumed negligible.

With the skull mounted in a plexiglass mount, an x-ray image was taken parallel to each axis of a designated "head reference" coordinate system. The x-axis exited just above the right ear canal, the y-axis passed between the nasal bones, and the z-axis exited superiorly. Since the x-ray procedure produced expanded images as a function of object position, a computer program corrected dipole image position to true "head reference" coordinates. The program also computed actual dipole length, tangential component, and orientation. The tangential component was defined as the projection of the dipole vector normal to the intersecting radius of the

Advances in Biomagnetism
Edited by S.J. Williamson *et al.*
Plenum Press, New York

best local sphere (described later). Orientation was computed as the ccw angle between the tangential component and the N-to-S meridian of the best local sphere. The scaling parameter "cosine", computed by dividing the tangential component into the dipole length, was used to predict the dipole strength visible to the homogeneous conducting sphere model.

Auditory and visual evoked responses (AER and VER) were simulated by activating appropriate dipoles with Gaussian shaped current waveforms. Four stimulus conditions were performed in each of the two cranial regions. In the first condition, one dipole was activated with a Gaussian mean of 100 millisecond (ms) and the other dipole with a Gaussian mean of 200 ms. In the second condition, the 100 ms dipole was unchanged but the 200 ms dipole's polarity was reversed, and in the third and fourth conditions each dipole was activated solely. The peak dipole currents were 40 and 50 micro-Ampere in the auditory and visual simulations respectively.

The magnetic field normal to the skull surface was measured with a DC-SQUID 2nd order gradiometer (50 mm baseline). Thirty sweeps for each of the four stimulus conditions, filtered 0.3-30 Hz, were averaged at fifty locations above each of the cranial regions. Stimulus conditions were performed sequentially before moving the gradiometer to the next measurement location. Measurement locations in "head reference" coordinates were determined using an instrumented articulating apparatus. The apparatus converted potentiometer positions to Cartesian coordinates with about 3 mm accuracy, then transformed the coordinates to the "head reference" system using the ear canals and nasal bones as axes landmarks.

Least squares fit by gradient-expansion (Marquardt, 1963, Bevington, 1969) was used in three steps in the analysis. The first step, only performed when two sources were activated, estimated source contributions to each recorded waveform using a model of two independent Gaussian waves. The estimated parameters were amplitude, mean latency, and standard deviation for each Gaussian. The second step determined the best local sphere by fitting a spherical surface to the field measurement positions on the external skull surface in each experimental condition. The fit parameters were origin position and radius. The third step estimated parameters for the best fit equivalent dipoles. The forward solution employed the Biot-Savart law for magnetic flux density propagating through free space. The equation was written in spherical coordinates, operated in the best local sphere, considered only the radial component of magnetic flux density from tangential dipoles, and modelled the 2nd order gradiometer used in the measurements. Dipole fit input data were peak waveform amplitudes in all conditions, and estimated Gaussian amplitudes in conditions with two active dipoles. The output parameters in spherical coordinates were dipole moment, range, orientation, meridian position, and elevation position. Upon fit completion, the equivalent dipole positions were transformed to the "head reference" Cartesian coordinate system.

RESULTS

The actual strengths, locations, and orientations were not known until after the skull was sealed and the x-ray images evaluated. The strengths for dipoles V100, V200, A100, and A200 were 80, 120, 250, and 200 nAmp-meters respectively. The dipole parameters are given in the IMAGE rows of Table 1, where the moments were scaled to reflect only the tangential strength. The equivalent dipoles' parameters are in rows titled by the appropriate condition.

When solely active, V100 was localized within 7 mm and it's strength estimated with 15% error. However, solely active V200's localization was 35 mm in error, estimated strength 23% in error, and fit correlation rather low. Solely active A100, deep but entirely tangential, localized 4 mm from the actual, and the strength was estimated with only 3% error. Similar to V200, solely active A200 had a large localization error of 20 mm and the strength was grossly over estimated by 163%.

With two dipoles active, the fits using peakpicker data underestimated and overestimated V100 strength by greater than 20% in conditions 1 and 2 respectively. The peakpicker method does not consider the effects of the contributing fields from the early activation of the V200 source. When the simulated evoked components were modelled with their known shape (in this case Gaussian), the percent error in V100 strength was reduced to half or better. The accuracy in localization remained very good.

Peakpicker analysis of A100 with both auditory sources active produced small strength errors with localization within 6 mm. However, the estimated component fits for A100 grossly overestimated strengths, and despite A100's 100% tangential orientation, localization was in error by more than 1 cm. This might be explained by the unmodelled filter characteristics of the Gaussian fits. The highpass filter response causes the first component to overshoot, interfering with the second component. The unmodelled overshoot is misinterpreted by a model which considers only the summation of two undisturbed Gaussians. The error is more pronounced in the auditory simulation due to the large A100 moment (250 nA-M).

DISCUSSION

Because each model surface was fit to the local external surface, the measured radial vector (normal to the external skull surface) would be equal to the desired radial vector (normal to the internal skull surface) in regions where the internal and external surfaces are parallel. However, in other regions, an unmodelled flux component tangent to the internal volume conductor surface would have been measured. Because dipoles V100 and A100 were localized well, this modelling error apparently causes only slight inaccuracy in the occipital and temporal regions.

A larger error deserving discussion is evident when a radial dipole component is present. The assumption of spherical symmetry must specify no contribution from radially oriented sources (many MEG references). With only local spherical symmetry, unmodelled magnetic flux was measured when radially oriented sources were active. The results from dipoles V200 and A200 indicate that this error is very large in both cranial regions.

The inverse solution was slightly improved by modelling the dynamics of interfering dipoles in the V100 case, where the unmodelled filter overshoot was not a major factor. The spherical model fit to the local external surface yielded good results for tangential dipoles in both the occipital and the auditory regions, where one dipole was 2 cm and the other was 4 cm in depth. Non-tangential dipole components produced significant fields normal to the skull surface and should not be considered negligible. The methods used by this laboratory produce sufficient results in the occipital and temporal regions, but only if the evoked sources are tangential. Because many contributing neural sources are non-tangential and the evoked response contains interfering components, better volume conductor models (Hamalainen and Sarvas, 1989) and source dynamics models should be further developed to reap the full potential of magnetoencephalography.

Table 1. Dipole parameters computed from the x-ray images and estimated from the MEG data. The stimulation conditions for the MEG fits are given in parentheses. The method of determining peak dipole stimulation is indicated by "PP" (Peak Picker) or "EC" (Estimated Components). Coordinates "X,Y,Z" are head coordinates (mm) with error being the distance from the "IMAGE" position. Parameter "P" is peak dipole moment (nA-M) multiplied by the parameter "cosine" in the IMAGE rows, and best fit moment in all other rows. Orientation "Or" is degrees ccw between the tangential component and the N-->S meridian of the best local sphere. Dipole depth (mm) is from the skull surface and "Corr" is fit correlation.

	X	Y	Z	err	cosine	P	%err	Or	err	depth	Corr
V100											
IMAGE	-17	-53	26		1.0	80		99			
(V1)PP	-14	-46	25	7		92	+15	87	12	24	.95
(V1+V2)PP	-15	-50	25	4		59	-26	95	4	20	.96
(V1-V2)PP	-13	-45	24	9		99	+23	86	14	25	.96
(V1+V2)EC	-16	-48	25	5		91	+13	94	5	21	.97
(V1-V2)EC	-19	-49	23	5		82	+3	92	7	20	.95
V200											
IMAGE	-10	-35	44		0.36	43		47			
(V2)PP	6	-4	44	35		53	+23	45	2	57	.65
(V1+V2)PP	-9	-22	35	17		559	+1200	182	135	49	.90
(V1-V2)PP	15	19	42	60		477	+1009	197	150	67	.88
(V1+V2)EC	3	-17	24	29		362	+742	-46	93	45	.92
(V1-V2)EC	14	19	42	59		495	+1051	196	149	68	.90
A100											
IMAGE	-24	0	43		1.0	250		-72			
(A1)PP	-22	1	40	4		257	+3	-52	20	40	.98
(A1+A2)PP	-22	2	38	6		230	-8	-53	19	39	.99
(A1-A2)PP	-22	2	38	6		243	-3	-54	18	40	.99
(A1+A2)EC	-14	3	34	15		578	+131	-53	19	47	.97
(A1-A2)EC	-18	6	33	13		433	+73	-55	17	43	.97
A200											
IMAGE	-29	-15	59		0.30	60		112			
(A2)PP	-19	-6	44	20		158	+163	129	17	42	.89
(A1+A2)PP	-30	-2	44	20		97	+62	129	17	32	.98
(A1-A2)PP	50	5	-30	121		206	+243	-48	177	105	.28
(A1+A2)EC	-27	-3	43	12		149	+143	133	21	35	.98
(A1-A2)EC	-37	24	24	53		29	-52	114	2	23	.55

REFERENCES

Bevington, P., 1969, "Data Reduction and Error Analysis," McGraw-Hill, New York.

Hamalainen, M. S., and Sarvas, J., 1989, Realistic Conductivity Geometry Model of the Human Head for Interpretation of Neuromagnetic Data, IEEE Trans. Biomed. Engr., 36:165-171.

Hari, R., Joutsiniemi, S. L., and Sarvas, J., 1988, Spatial Resolution of Neuromagnetic Records: Theoretical Calculations in a Spherical Model, EEG and Clin. Neurophys., 71:64-72.

Marquardt, D. W., 1963, An Algorithm for Least-Squares Estimation of Non-Linear Parameters, J. Soc. Ind. Appl. Math., 11:431-441.

MONTE CARLO STUDY OF CONFIDENCE REGION ACCURACY FOR MEG INVERSE DIPOLE SOLUTIONS

L. Goldstein, P. Teale and M. Reite

Department of Psychiatry
University of Colorado Health Sciences Center
Denver, CO 80282, USA

INTRODUCTION

Localization and characterization of neuromagnetic sources is often attempted assuming the model of a dipole current source in a spherical homogeneous conductor volume and solving the inverse problem for a given measured external field (Tanday (1987)). Evaluation of experimental results and clinical procedures also requires accurate confidence regions. Statistical methods exist for defining these regions by analyzing the fit of the data to the best fit model prediction without independent estimates of the measurement noise. We have empirically evaluated three of these methods in a Monte Carlo study.

METHODS

We describe the three tested methods for defining confidence regions and the Monte Carlo study itself. The most common method of defining a confidence region in nonlinear inverse parametric estimation is linearization (Dennis, et.al. (1983) and Donaldson (1985)).

Linearization

Let $\mathbf{x}$ be the 1 x 5 matrix of the five unknown dipole parameters. Let $\mathbf{x}_*$ represent the optimum dipole in the least squares sense. Let there be n measurements B_i of the radial B field amplitude at locations external to the conducting sphere, and let $M_i(\mathbf{x})$ be the n predicted radial B field amplitudes at these same n locations for dipole $\mathbf{x}$. Then define

$$R_i = B_i - M_i(\mathbf{x})$$

$$\text{(I)} \qquad f(\mathbf{x}) = \sum_{i=1}^{n} R_i^2$$

We have $f(\mathbf{x}_*) \leq f(\mathbf{x})$ for all dipoles $\mathbf{x}$ since $\mathbf{x}_*$ is optimum in the least squares sense of minimizing $f(\mathbf{x})$. Now let

$$g_i(\mathbf{x}_o) = \left.\frac{\partial f(\mathbf{x})}{\partial \mathbf{x}_i}\right|_{\mathbf{x}_o}, \quad i = 1 \,..\, 5$$

$$\mathbf{H}_{ij}(\mathbf{x}_o) = \left.\frac{\partial^2 f(\mathbf{x})}{\partial \mathbf{x}_i \, \partial \mathbf{x}_j}\right|_{\mathbf{x}_o}, \quad i = 1 \,..\, 5, \; j = 1 \,..\, 5$$

That is, $\mathbf{g}$ is a vector of first partial derivatives of f and $\mathbf{H}$ is a matrix of second partial derivatives of F. The affine model $\hat{f}$ of f around $\mathbf{x}_*$ may then be written

Advances in Biomagnetism
Edited by S.J. Williamson *et al.*
Plenum Press, New York

(II) $\bar{f}(x) = f(x_*) + g(x_*)\,(x - x_*) + \frac{1}{2}(x - x_*)^T\, H\,(x - x_*)$

or since $g(x_*)$ is 0 for the optimum dipole x_*

(III) $\bar{f}(x) = f(x_*) + \frac{1}{2}(x - x_*)^T\, H\,(x - x_*)$

We define the confidence region using $\bar{f}(x)$ rather than f(x) to simplify the task of constructing the region. The criterion is then

$$\text{(IV)} \quad \frac{\bar{f}(x) - f(x_*)}{f(x_*)} \leq \frac{p}{n - p} F_{p;\, n - p;\, 1 - \alpha}$$

Where p is the number of fit parameters and n the number of measured field points. F is the Snedecor's F distribution with degrees of freedom p and n-p at the confidence level $1 - \alpha$. The Snedecor's F distribution describes the ratio of the two independent Chi-Square random variables on the left hand side of (II).

Maximum Likelihood Criterion

The second method uses the maximum likelihood criterion

$$\text{(V)} \quad \frac{f(x) - f(x_*)}{f(x_*)} \leq \frac{p}{n - p} F_{p;\, n - p;\, 1 - \alpha}$$

The difference between this and (IV) is that the true nonlinear function f(x) is used rather than the affine approximation $\bar{f}(x)$. While much more difficult to compute, regions based on (V) will be exact for some class of nonlinear functions, while (IV) is only exact for linear functions.

Lack-of-fit Method

The lack-of-fit method (Donaldson (1985), Halperin (1963), Hartley (1964), Williams (1962)) provides an exact statistic for determining confidence regions for any nonlinear function. The existence of such an exact statistic is an argument for the validity of constructing confidence regions without relying on independent estimates of all possible noise sources. Although there are different versions of this statistic we chose a version that reduces to (IV) for linear functions.

The basic idea of this method is to linearize f(x) around x, the dipole parameter set which is being tested for inclusion in the 100 $(1 - \alpha)$ confidence region. We then determine the optimum dipole x_0 for the linearized version $\bar{f}(x)$ of f(x). The criterion is then

$$\text{(VI)} \quad \frac{f(x) - \bar{f}(x_0)}{\bar{f}(x_0)} \leq \frac{p}{n - p} F_{p;\, n - p;\, 1 - \alpha}$$

The formula we used is

$$\text{(VII)} \quad \frac{R(x)^T\, P(x)\, R(x)}{R(x)^T\, (I - P(x))\, R(x)} \leq \frac{p}{n - p} F_{p;\, n - p;\, 1 - \alpha}$$

where R is the vector with components R_i defined in [I] above, **I** is the identity matrix, and

$$\text{(VIII)} \quad P(x) = J(x)\,(J(x)^T J(x))^{-1}\, J(x)^T$$

$$J_{ij}(x) = \frac{\partial M_i(x)}{\partial x_j}, \quad i = 1 \,..\, n,\ j = 1 \,..\, p$$

Monte Carlo Study

The Monte Carlo study was performed as follows. A set of radial B field values was computed for a transverse dipole in a homogenous conducting sphere as they would be measured by a third order finite-coil gradiometer. The values were computed for a grid of points spaced over a region 100° wide in both longitude and latitude centered over the current dipole. For the maximum likelihood test statistic, the distance of the dipole from the center of the sphere was varied from 0.50 to 7.5 cm, the noise to signal ratio (N/S) was varied from .1 to .4, and the number of field points computed was varied between 35 and 121. For each data set, the Monte Carlo study consisted of repeatedly adding independent Gaussian noise to the measurements, solving for the optimum dipole using a hookstep modified Newton's method (Dennis (1983)), and computing the various confidence region test statistics for the known true solution to determine whether it would have been included in the confidence regions (Donaldson (1985)). At least 500 trials were run for each data set. The observed coverages could be computed for each statistic's nominal 100 $(1 - \alpha)$ percent confidence region. The final computed coverages are point estimates. The following method was applied to compute 95% confidence tests for the accuracy of these point estimates. For a 100p percent confidence interval, the true solution should be included with a probability p, and excluded with a probability $q = (1 - p)$, for each of the n individual trials. This series obeys a binomial distribution, which has a known mean and standard deviation. For very large n such as we have here, we may accurately apply the normal distribution to find the $1 - \alpha$ confidence interval

$$\text{(IX)} \quad \left[\, p - z_{\alpha/2}\sqrt{\frac{pq}{n}}\,,\; p + z_{\alpha/2}\sqrt{\frac{pq}{n}}\,\right]$$

The lack-of-fit method was used to check the accuracy of the simulations. Its coverage was within the 95% confidence interval for an exact statistic 29 times out of the total of 30 tests, consistent with the exactness of this statistic.

In addition, a smaller confidence interval was computed for the linearization and maximum likelihood methods by comparing them to the exact lack-of-fit method. For each study of n trials, a sequence y_i, $i = 1 \ldots n$ was created by comparing the test statistic to the lack-of-fit statistic. If in the ith trial, the test statistic and the lack-of-fit statistic both included or both excluded the true solution, then $y_i = 0$. If the test statistic included the true solution, but the lack-of-fit method excluded it, then $y_i = 1$. If the test statistic excluded the true solution but the lack-of-fit method included it, then $y_i = -1$. Hence, the difference in the coverage of the test statistic and the lack-of-fit method was the mean value of the y_i. Although we don't know the true distribution function for the y_i, for the large values of n encountered here we may apply the Student's t distribution (Maksoudian (1969)) giving us a confidence interval for the difference between the test statistic and the exact lack-of-fit method

$$\text{(X)} \quad \left[\, \bar{y} - t_{\alpha/2}\frac{s_y}{\sqrt{n}}\,,\; \bar{y} + t_{\alpha/2}\frac{s_y}{\sqrt{n}}\,\right]$$

where $\bar{y}$ is the mean value of the y_i, n is the number of trials, $t_{\alpha/2}$ is the Student's t distribution value for the $1 - \alpha$ confidence level and $n - 1$ degrees of freedom, and s_y is the variance of the y_i.

For the 99% confidence intervals, the number of non-zero y_i (≈ 5) was too small to accurately apply the Student's t distribution.

RESULTS

The 5 studies on the maximum likelihood method show that it is exact to within the resolution of these tests. In the 25 confidence regions evaluated, all of them passed the

95% confidence test for having the appropriate coverage using the binomial intervals. In the 20 comparisons to the lack-of-fit method, the largest error was 1.2% ± 1.24% for the 50% confidence interval. The 95% maximum likelihood confidence interval had a largest error of .35% ± .49%. In order to obtain these accuracies without paired comparison to the lack-of-fit method, n would have to have been from 4 to 16 times larger, which would have been computationally prohibitive.

The one study on the linearization method (for a dipole 3.5 cm from the center of the sphere) showed coverage from 3.3 to 15.2 standard deviations away from the correct values using the binomial confidence intervals, and similar results for the paired comparison to the lack-of-fit statistic. The 95% linear confidence interval had a coverage 7.8% ± 2.5% less than the exact lack-of-fit interval. Only the 10% confidence interval passed the tests for exactness, consistent with the smaller linearization error associated with a smaller confidence region.

DISCUSSION

Further tests are being done on the linearization method at different dipole depths and signal to noise ratios, as well as with alternate linearization methods. However, alternate linearization methods have been found to give similar results (Donaldson (1985)) in other nonlinear problems. These results suggest that it would be worthwhile to develop efficient methods of constructing confidence regions using the maximum likelihood statistic. We are currently testing several ways of doing this.

This research was supported by USPHS Grants No. RR03259, MH41396, and MH46335.

REFERENCES

Dennis, Jr, J.E. and Schnabel, Robert B. (1983). Numerical Methods for Unconstrained Optimization and Nonlinear Equations. Prentice-Hall Inc., Englewood Cliffs N.J.

Donaldson, Janet R., (1985), Computation Experience with Confidence Regions, Thesis, Univ. of Colorado at Boulder.

Halperin, M. (1963) "Confidence Interval Estimation in Nonlinear Regression", Journal of the Royal Statistical Society (B), 25(2), pp 330-333.

Hartley, H.O. (1964). "Exact Confidence Regions for the parameters in Nonlinear Regression Laws", Biometrika, 51(3,4) pp. 347-353.

Maksoudian, Y. Leon (1969). Probability and Statistics, with Applications. International Textbook Co., Scranton, PA. Pg. 188.

Tanday, B.S. and Swithenby, S.J. (1987). "Analysis of Magnetoencephalographic data using the homogeneous sphere model: empirical tests", Physics in Medicine and Biology, 32(1), pp. 105-413.

Williams, E.J. (1962). "Exact Fiducial Limits in Nonlinear Estimation", Journal of the Royal Statistical Society (B), 24(1), pp.125-139.

INFLUENCE OF THE FINITE PICKUP COIL SIZE ON THE LOCALIZATION OF CURRENT SOURCES WITH QUADRUPOLAR COMPONENTS

V. Jazbinšek, Z. Trontelj

Physics Department and Institute of Mathematics, Physics and Mechanics, University E. Kardelj of Ljubljana. Jadranska 19, 61000 Ljubljana, Yugoslavia

S.N. Erné, L. Trahms

Physikalisch-Technische Bundesanstalt (PTB), Institut Berlin
Abbestr.2-12, D-1000 Berlin, Germany

INTRODUCTION

Geselowitz and Grynszpan have considered the current dipole as a source of the biomagnetic field[1]. This is a natural and successful first approximation in many electrophysiological cases. Williamson and Kaufman have introduced the concept of a current dipole as an equivalent current source (E.C.S.) of biomagnetic field in some aspects of brain research. They have also emphasized the influence of the finite magnetometer pickup coil size and calculated the correction factor[2] which is needed when estimating the spatial position of an equivalent current dipole source from the extrema of the measured magnetic field distribution.

Later, several authors (T.Katila[3,4], J.Wikswo[5], Erné et al.[6]) have included the quadrupolar term in the E.C.S. description, i.e. the first two terms in the current multipole expansion are considered.

Here we present an analytical expression for the average magnetic field due to a quadrupolar source taking into account the finite pickup coil size.

CALCULATION

We usually select the plane of isofield lines perpendicular to the geometrical axis of the pickup coil which means that we have to consider only one component (B_z) of the magnetic field. The magnetic flux can be calculated by contour integration of the magnetic vector potential around the pickup coil

$$\Phi = \oint \vec{A} \cdot \vec{dl} \tag{1}$$

The vector potential can be described by a multipole expansion of a source. Considering the first two terms, this expansion takes the form[7]

$$\vec{A}(\vec{R}) = \frac{\mu_0}{4\pi R}\vec{p} + \frac{\mu_0}{4\pi R^3}\vec{R}\underline{Q} \tag{2}$$

$\vec{p}$ is the current dipole vector and $\underline{Q}$ is the current quadrupole tensor[3] consisting of 9 components q_{ij}.

Advances in Biomagnetism
Edited by S.J. Williamson *et al.*
Plenum Press, New York

Using $\vec{B} = \text{curl}\,\vec{A}$ all components of magnetic field can be obtained. Assuming the source is embedded in a homogeneous conducting half space, the normal component of magnetic field B_z is given by

$$\begin{aligned} B_z &= B_z^{(1)} + B_z^{(2)} = \frac{\mu_0}{4\pi R^3}(yp_x - xp_y) + \\ &+ \frac{\mu_0}{4\pi R^5}[3xyQ_{dd} + 3(y^2 - x^2)Q_{od} + (3z^2 - R^2)Q_{mz} + 3z(yQ_{zx} - xQ_{zy})] \,, \end{aligned} \qquad (3)$$

where x,y,z are the observation point coordinates with regard to the source position, R is the distance between the source and the observation point, μ_0 is the induction constant, p_x and p_y are components of the current dipole, $Q_{dd} = q_{xx} - q_{yy}$, $Q_{od} = (q_{xy} + q_{yx})/2$, $Q_{mz} = (q_{xy} - q_{yx})/2$, $Q_{zx} = q_{zx}$, $Q_{zy} = q_{zy}$.

From Eqs. (1) and (2) an average magnetic field $\overline{B}_z^{(2)} = \Phi^{(2)}/\pi a^2$ through the pickup coil of radius a is found. The contribution $\overline{B}_z^{(1)}$ of the first term is the well known dipolar field[2]. For the quadrupolar term $\overline{B}_z^{(2)}$ we have obtained

$$\begin{aligned} \overline{B}_z^{(2)} = \frac{\mu_0}{\pi^2 a r^2}\frac{1}{(R^2 + a^2 - 2ar)\sqrt{R^2 + a^2 + 2ar}}\{[xyQ_{dd} + (y^2 - x^2)Q_{od}][af(k) + rg(k)] \\ + Q_{mz}[aE - rg(k)]r^2 + z[yQ_{zx} - xQ_{zy}]rg(k)\} \end{aligned} \qquad (4)$$

with $k^2 = 4ar/[z^2 + (a+r)^2]$, $f(k) = \{8(1-k^2)(2-k^2)K(k^2) - [k^4 + 16(1-k^2)]E(k^2)\}/k^4$,
$g(k) = [(2-k^2)E(k^2) - 2(1-k^2)K(k^2)]/k^2$ and $r^2 = x^2 + y^2$.

Here $K(k^2)$ and $E(k^2)$ are complete elliptic integrals of the first and the second kind, respectively. The first test for the calculated average magnetic field is the evaluation in the limit of $a/z \ll 1$. We obtain $k^2 \approx 4ar/R^2$, $\lim_{a\to 0} af(k) = 0$, $\lim_{a\to 0} aE = \pi a/2$, $\lim_{a\to 0} rg(k) = 3\pi ar^2/4R^2$, $\lim_{a\to 0}[aE - rg(k)] = \pi a(3z^2 - R^2)/4R^2$. Considering these values , the average measured magnetic field, $\overline{B}_z^{(2)}|_{a\to 0}$ has exactly the same form as $B_z^{(2)}$ in expression (3) at a constant depth z. That means the average magnetic field measured with a pickup coil of infinitely small diameter is the same as the magnetic field calculated at the center of the magnetometer pickup coil.

DISCUSSION

It is characteristic for the current dipole that its isofield line distribution in the plane above the current dipole clearly shows two extrema. The depth, d, of the current dipole can be estimated by using the distance between the extrema. Similarly, the depth for the quadrupolar terms Q_{dd}; Q_{od}; Q_{zx}, Q_{zy}; which clearly show the extrema, can be calculated. The corresponding formulae are

$$d = \begin{cases} \frac{\Delta}{\sqrt{2}} & \text{for the current dipole} \quad (5a) \\ \sqrt{\frac{3}{4}}\Delta & \text{for } Q_{dd} \text{ or } Q_{od} \text{ terms} \quad (5b) \\ \Delta & \text{for } Q_{zx} \text{ or } Q_{zy} \text{ terms} \quad (5c) \end{cases}$$

where Δ is the distance between minimum and maximum.

We have to be careful with the term Q_{mz} because in this case, B_z has the maximum value in the center of the circular isofield pattern and the minimum value at a rather larger radius $r = 2d$. Therefore, it is more suitable to choose the radius where $B_z = B_{max}/2$, which is within 0.2% of the radius $r = d/2$, as the second value for the estimation of the E.C.S. depth.

We now consider the influence of the pickup coil size on the detected field. For the sake of simplicity only the Q_{od} and Q_{zy} terms of the quadrupolar E.C.S. are taken into account, since these sources generate extrema on the x-axis. The position of the maximum value of the average field $\overline{B}_z$ is calculated for pickup coils with different radii. The results are shown on Figs. 1a and 1b. We see that as pickup coil radius increases, the position of the maximum of the detected average magnetic field shifts farther away from the center of the coordinate system, below which the E.C.S. is located.

Using the separation of extrema obtained simply from the isofield distribution (only the maximum is shown on Fig.1), it is clear that the depth of the E.C.S. determined from (5b,c) would be too large. The necessary correction factors, calculated from the results used to compute Figs. 1a,b, are displayed on Figs. 2: $d/\overline{d}$ vs. $2a/\overline{\Delta}$ is shown on Fig. 2a and $d/\overline{d}$ vs. a/d on Fig. 2b. For comparison, the correction factors for the dipolar E.C.S. published in ref.2 are added in Fig. 2a.

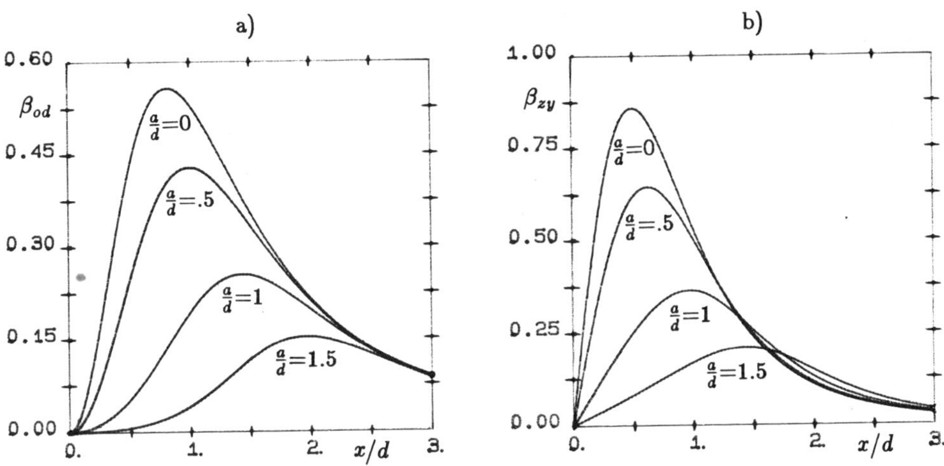

Figure 1. Dependence of the normalized average magnetic field $\overline{B}_z$ on the pickup coil position along the x-axis: a) $\beta_{od} = \frac{4\pi d^3 \overline{B}_z}{\mu_0 Q_{od}}$, b) $\beta_{zy} = \frac{4\pi d^3 \overline{B}_z}{\mu_0 Q_{zy}}$ for a set of parameters a/d.

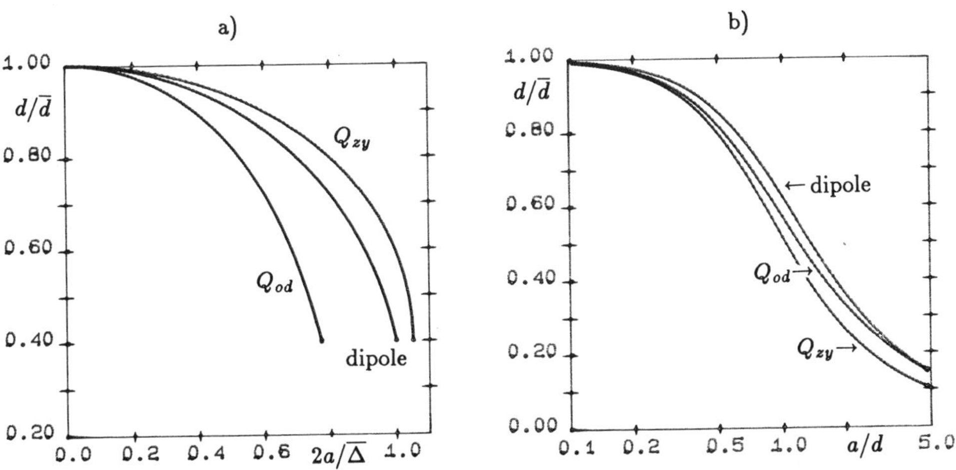

Figure 2. The correction factors $d/\overline{d}$ as a function of the pickup coil radius.

REFERENCES

1. F. Grynszpan and D.B. Geselowitz, Model studies of the magnetocardiogram, *Biophys. J.* 13:9 11 (1973).
2. S.J. Williamson and L.Kaufman, Magnetic fields of the cerebral cortex, *in*: "Biomagnetism," S.N. Erné, H.D. Hahlbohm and H. Lübbig, eds., Walter de Gruyter, Berlin, New York (1981).
3. T. Katila and P. Karp, Magnetocardiology: Morphology and multipole representation, *in*: "Biomagnetism - An Interdisciplinary Approach", S.J. Williamson, G.L. Romani, L. Kaufman and I. Modena, eds., Plenum Press, New York and London (1983).
4. T. Katila, R. Maniewski, M. Mäkijärvi, J. Nenonen and P. Siltanen, On the accuracy of source localization in cardiac measurements, *Phys. Med. Biol.* 32:125 (1987).
5. J.P. Wikswo Jr., Theoretical aspects of the ECG-MCG relationship, *in*: "Biomagnetism - An Interdisciplinary Approach", S.J. Williamson, G.L. Romani, L. Kaufman and I. Modena, eds., Plenum Press, New York and London (1983).
6. S.N. Erné, L. Trahms and Z. Trontelj, (1988). Current multipoles as sources of biomagnetic fields. *in*: "Biomagnetism '87", K. Atsumi, M. Kotani, S. Ueno, T. Katila and S.J. Williamson, eds., Tokyo Denki University Press, Tokyo (1987).
7. J.A. Stratton, "Electromagnetic Theory," McGraw-Hill Book Company,Inc., New York and London (1941).

CONSIDERATIONS ON A SPATIO-TEMPORAL TWO-DIPOLE MODEL

K. Lehnertz, B. Lütkenhöner, M. Hoke and C. Pantev

Institute of Experimental Audiology
University of Münster, Münster
Federal Republic of Germany

INTRODUCTION

Dipole localization methods (DLM) for estimating the source locations of sensory evoked magnetic fields (EF) are usually based upon the assumption that the observed field pattern at a given instant of time can be approximated by that of a single equivalent current dipole (ECD). To account for the temporal variation of the observed field pattern each ECD parameter is allowed to vary in time. Such a model, however, is often inappropriate since complex neuronal excitation processes generate multiple, spatially separated sources whose activation may overlap temporarily. In these cases, DLM based on a single-ECD assumption may yield virtual source locations being far off the actual ones (e.g., Nunez, 1986).

In order to reduce the ambiguity inherent in the single-ECD model, Scherg (1984) and Scherg and von Cramon (1985) introduced a spatio-temporal dipole model (STDM) for locating, from the electric potential distribution on the surface of the head, the sources of different deflections of the auditory evoked potential. The basic concept underlying Scherg's STDM is that the surface distribution due to each generator population can be approximated by that of an ECD with fixed location whose moment varies with time. Achim et al. (1988) employed the STDM approach in simulation studies of evoked magnetic fields, but did not consider the influence of superimposed noise on the resulting estimates. The present investigation was undertaken to study the biomagnetic inverse problem inherent in a spatio-temporal two-dipole model in the presence of superimposed noise.

METHODS

Model

It is assumed that two dipoles having fixed locations and temporarily overlapping Gaussian-shaped activation functions (Fig. 1a) are immersed in a semi-infinite volume conductor. Three different situations will be compared (the depth of the first dipole was set to 3 cm):

(1) Locations of the two dipoles being 1.41 cm apart (1 cm each in one horizontal dimension and depth), second activation function with opposite polarity and delayed by 60 ms.
(2) Same locations and activation functions as in (1), but delay of 100 ms.
(3) Same activation functions as in (1), but locations 2.60 cm apart (1.5 cm in all three dimensions of a Cartesian coordinate system).

To approximate realistic physiological conditions, the model parameters were chosen such that the largest deflection of the magnetic field component normal to the surface of the volume conductor amounted to 600 fT, while the superimposed noise had a standard deviation of 50 fT.

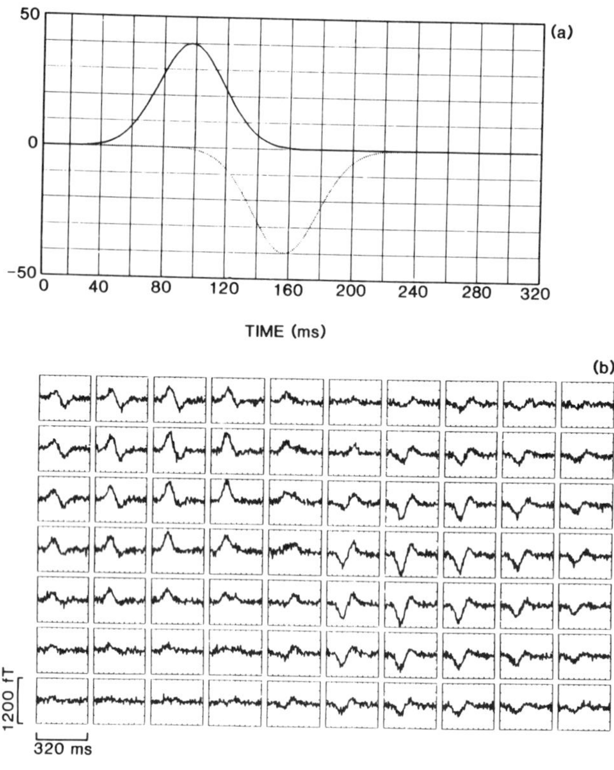

Fig. 1. (a) Gaussian-shaped activation functions for the two-dipole model. (b) EF waveforms for situation (1).

Forward calculation

If the component of the magnetic field perpendicular to the surface of the volume conductor is denoted by B, the time-dependent activation functions of the two dipoles are denoted by $P_i(t)$ and the location and orientation of the two dipoles by $\mathbf{R}_i$ and Θ_i [i=1,2], then the model field distribution as recorded by an arbitrary gradiometer configuration at a given point $\mathbf{r}$ can be written as

$$B(t,\mathbf{r}) = P_1(t)\, D(\mathbf{r};\mathbf{R}_1,\Theta_1) + P_2(t)\, D(\mathbf{r};\mathbf{R}_2,\Theta_2) + \epsilon(t,\mathbf{r}) \tag{1}$$

where D is the magnetic field produced by a dipole having a dipole moment of magnitude 1, and ϵ is the superimposed noise. The magnetic field was assumed to be measured with a second order gradiometer (coil diameter: 2.0 cm; baseline: 5.0 cm) at 7 x 10 equidistantly spaced (1.5 cm) measurement positions. The waveforms obtained for situation (1) are presented in Fig. 1b.

Inverse calculation

If B_{mk} denotes the field measured at measurement position $\mathbf{r}_m$ at time instant t_k, then the function to be minimized can be written as

$$Q = \sum_{m=1}^{M}\sum_{k=1}^{K}\{B_{mk} - B(\mathbf{r}_m, t_k)\}^2 \tag{2}$$

Given the parameter values $\mathbf{R}_i$ and Θ_i of the two dipoles [i=1,2], the least-squares estimates for the function values $P_i(t_k)$ can be obtained as a solution of a system of 2K linear equations. Inserting these estimates into Eq. (2) results in a function $\bar{Q}$ which depends only on the position and the orientation of the two dipoles and on the values of B_{mk}. The function $\bar{Q}$ was minimized using an iterative downhill simplex method in multidimensions (Press et al., 1986), which requires only the evaluation of the function values, but not of the derivatives. The initial simplex required for starting the minimization procedure was defined by selecting, for each ECD parameter, random numbers having a uniform distribution centered at the respective theoretical parameter value (range of ± 2 cm for coordinate values and ± 90° for angles). The procedure was terminated if the minimization program claimed to have found the minimum of the function $\bar{Q}$ (i.e., if an iteration step resulted in a relative decrease of $\bar{Q}$ less than 10^{-5}) or if the maximum number of iteration steps (1000) was exceeded.

RESULTS

In agreement with Achim et al. (1988), the minimization procedure supplied the correct values for all model parameters in the absence of noise. However, when noise was added, the estimated parameter values were found to depend on the starting simplex. In Fig. 2a an attempt was undertaken to visualize the multidimensional results obtained for situation (1) in a two-dimensional representation: The distance between the estimated locations of the two dipoles is plotted versus the residual variance $\bar{Q}$. For pragmatical reasons, a classification of the results into three categories was undertaken:
(A) All estimated parameter values are close to the values used for the forward calculation.
(B) The estimated locations of the two dipoles are almost identical ("quasi one-dipole solution").
(C) Neither (A) nor (B).
For N=76 randomly selected starting conditions the three categories were found to have nearly the same frequency (34% for (A), 37% for (B) and 29% for (C)). Figs. 2b-d show retrieved activation functions for typical members of the three categories. Only in the case of (A) are the activation functions similar to those of the model. In case of (B) the two activation functions are nearly identical except for the sign, whereas in (C) the retrieved activation function is a superposition of the two model activation functions.

In the case of situation (2) the relative frequencies of the three categories were about the same as in case of situation (1). However, if the spatial separation of the two dipoles is increased (situation (3)), solutions belonging to (A) become dominant (Fig. 3): They were found in 69% of N=51 cases.

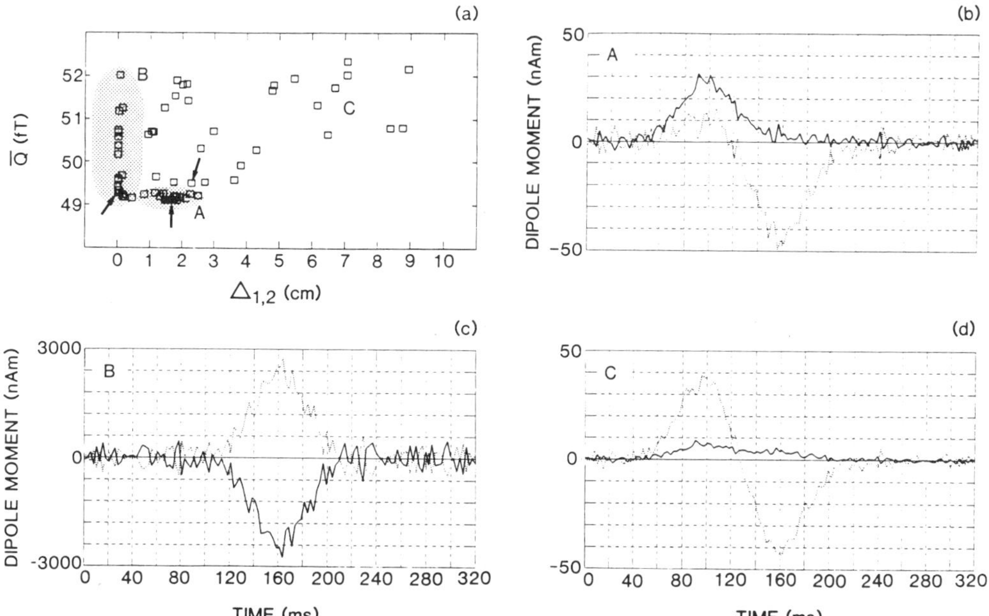

Fig. 2. (a) Dependence of the residual variance $\bar{Q}$ on the distance between estimated locations of the two dipoles for situation (1). For pragmatical reasons, the simulation results shown in the figure were subdivided into three categories. (b-d) Activation functions obtained for typical members, marked with arrows in panel (a), of the three categories.

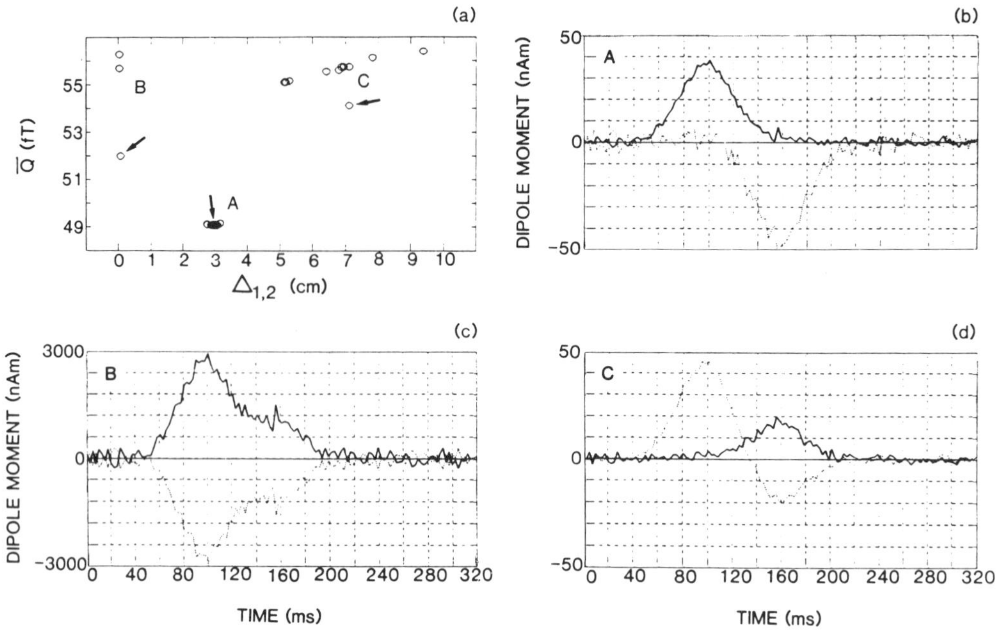

Fig. 3. same as Fig. 2, but for situation (3).

DISCUSSION

The model studies presented in this paper show that in the case of a spatio-temporal two-dipole model the solution of the inverse problem is a rather delicate task, if the two dipoles are arranged in close, but physiologically reasonable proximity (1.41 cm): If noise is added to such an extent that favourable physiological conditions are simulated, the downhill simplex minimization procedure, which is commonly regarded as a very robust method (Press et al., 1986), may yield for different starting conditions totally different dipole solutions with nearly the same residual variance $\bar{Q}$. This suggests that when solving the inverse problem always a certain number of repetitions with different starting conditions should be carried out in order to reduce the risk of arriving at a non-optimum solution. However, one must be aware that even this solution might not be consistent with the underlying physiology, especially when the model is not detailed enough to account for the actual anatomical and physiological conditions. More consistent results might be obtained if the number of degrees of freedom of the model is reduced by limiting the possible coarses of the activation functions (e.g., Scherg and von Cramon, 1985). In this case, however, an extensive a priori knowledge about the activation pattern is required, which is not always available.

REFERENCES

Achim, A. Richter, F., Saint-Hilaire, J.M., 1988, Methods for separating temporally overlapping sources of neuroelectric data, Brain Topography, 1:22-28.

Nunez, P., 1986, The brain's magnetic field: Some effects of multiple sources on the localization methods, Electroencephalogr. clin. Neurophysiol., 63:75-82.

Press, W.H., Flannery, B.P., Teukolsky, S.A., Vetterling, W.T., 1986, "Numerical Recipes. The art of scientific programming", Cambridge University Press, Cambridge.

Scherg, M., 1984, Spatio-temporal modelling of early auditory evoked potentials, Rev. Larnyg. (Bordeaux), 105:163-170.

Scherg, M. and von Cramon, D., 1985, Two bilateral sources of the late AEP as identified by a spatio-temporal dipole model, Electroencephalogr. clin. Neurophysiol., 62: 34-44.

RULE–BASED LOCATION OF MULTIPLE CURRENT–DIPOLE SOURCES FROM BIOMAGNETIC DATA

N.M.Palfreyman, K.D.Singh and S.J.Swithenby

Physics Department,
Open University, Walton Hall,
Milton Keynes MK7 6AA, U.K.

Introduction

The biomagnetic inverse problem is concerned with the derivation of the current distribution in a biological organism from measurements of the magnetic field outside the organism. This problem is characteristic of many inverse problems in being ill-posed and poorly convergent, yet in the past considerable success has been achieved in its solution by using human intervention to control otherwise blind numerical algorithms [4]. We have investigated the possibility of replacing this intervention by an expert system. In this paper we describe the resulting implementation which we have named ABIS (A Biomagnetic Inference System), and report on the success we have had in identifying multiple current dipole sources in a spherical volume conductor from a knowledge of the magnetic field over a discrete set of measurement points.

ABIS

ABIS is a rule–based system implemented in Prolog on a VAX cluster. It integrates a number of different inverse–problem tools into a single framework suitable for use in an everyday research setting. Its aim is not to provide a universal inverse–problem solver, but rather an environment within which a biomagnetic researcher can experiment with newly developed tools and combine them to build more complex problem–solving tools.

ABIS was written in response to two basic design requirements:

- The problem should be described in high–level, problem–oriented terms.
- The knowledge of biomagnetism available to the system should be represented in the form of modular rules which can be modified, removed or added without having to take into account their effect on each other.

The first of these requirements is fully satisfied by the current system; the second has been compromised to some extent, as we shall see in the following section.

The resulting system forms a convenient environment for investigating and reasoning about the biomagnetic problem in both its forward and inverse forms. Within this environment, using simple commands, the user can define, manipulate and graphically display datasets of magnetic field values which we term *maps*. For example the ABIS command "map1 equals grad1(distrn1) over patch1." defines the map *map1* to be the result of measuring the field of a source distribution *distrn1* using the gradiometer *grad1* over an orthogonal coordinate patch *patch1*. Graphical representations of the map such as those in Figure 1 can then be displayed with a command of the form "contour map1.". While such facilities belong properly to the forward, rather than inverse, problem, they are tools which are necessary to the inverse (dipole location) process, and also provide a convenient means of exploring new configurations and models — for example one of the authors (K.D.S.) is using the system in the exploration of novel gradiometer designs. In addition, and most relevantly for this paper, all of these facilities can be orchestrated and manipulated from rulebases written in an extended Prolog-style syntax which can be loaded and unloaded from the system. The dipole location process (DLP) to be described in the following section is such a rulebase containing at present 17 rules.

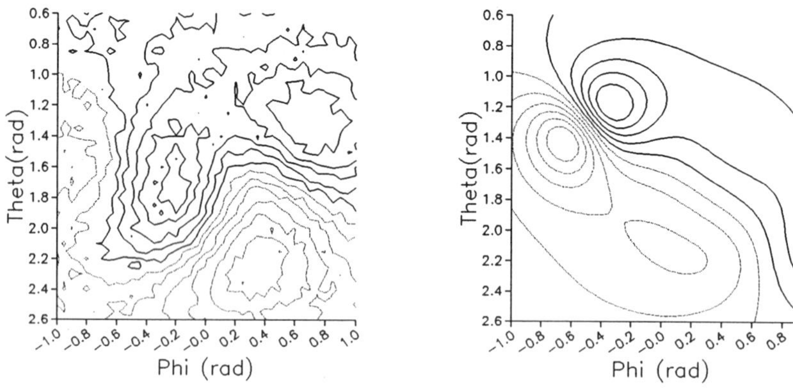

Figure 1. Two typical contour maps corresponding to second-order gradiometer measurements of the radial field over the surface of a uniformly conducting sphere of radius 15cm, with sources shown. (a) includes 10% noise; (b) does not. Solid and dotted lines indicate respectively positive and negative field values.

The Dipole Location Process

Our primary interest has so far been in the identification of current dipoles in a sphere from gradiometer measurements of the type shown in Figure 1. By *current dipole* we mean a current element of vanishing length which feeds current into and out of a conducting volume.

At first sight this seems like a standard problem in syntactic pattern recognition — much work [1] has for instance been done on the analysis of EEG data. However the heavy overlap of signals from different sources is inherent to the biomagnetic inverse problem and takes it well outside the essentially context-free domain of standard pattern recognition techniques. In particular overlap makes it impossible to establish a straightforward 1:1 correspondence between map features and source parameters. The unravelling of this overlap dictates the presence of a procedural element to the solution process which in turn leads to coupling between rules and the breakdown in modularity of the DLP rulebase mentioned above. While much can be done to minimise this coupling, a procedural element nevertheless remains intrinsic to the biomagnetic inverse problem.

DLP was constructed to mimic the way in which an expert operator views a map. This expert view provides an initial picture of the underlying source distribution but is insufficient to extract all the available information. Because of this DLP incorporates a procedural means for refining this estimate. We now present an account of the way in which DLP arrives at and then refines its estimate of the locations of the dipoles underlying a map.

The first point to note is that Prolog is essentially a symbol-manipulation language, and as such is incapable of dealing with arrays of data of the type produced by magnetic field measurements. Consequently our first step is to convert all features of a map which are relevant to reasoning concerning the underlying sources into a symbolic form capable of manipulation by DLP within Prolog. We interpolate the data onto a regular, orthogonal grid representing equal steps in the spherical polar coordinates (θ, ϕ) — this is the form in which maps are stored for manipulation by ABIS. A procedural program then converts this numerical array into a set of features which form DLP's view of the data. These features fall into three types:

Edges are vectors positioned at local gradient maxima of the map and oriented at an angle of $-\frac{\pi}{2}$ to the local gradient. Cohen *et al.* [2] first proposed the use of these features as a heuristic guide to the locations and orientations of underlying dipoles, and Ioannides [3] has shown that these estimates are correct to first order.

Dots are local extrema of curvature of the map, and may be either positive or negative. In many cases the position of a dot approximates closely to the position of a signal extremum. The importance of using dots rather than signal extrema lies in the fact that they are tied more closely to sources, so that for instance the single large minimum on the bottom–right of Figure 1(a) can be resolved into two separate dots corresponding to different dipoles.

Weights elaborate the relationship between each edge–dot pair. They contain information on the *separation* between the two, a measure of the *relevance* of the dot to the edge — the likelihood that both are caused by the same dipole, and the *contribution* which the edge makes to the magnitude of the dot.

Once this symbolic view of the map has been obtained DLP derives an approximate source set as follows. The only edge which definitely corresponds to a current dipole is the most prominent edge of the map, so the (θ, ϕ) coordinates and orientation of this edge are used as the position and orientation of the corresponding dipole. Next the most relevant dot to this edge is found and the separation between them is used to calculate the radial location of the dipole. A dipole with this position and orientation is then postulated and assigned the strength required to give the appropriate contribution to the dot. In this way the first dipole has been obtained and its effect can be subtracted from the map; the process is then repeated with the residue until it falls below a threshold value.

At this stage the dipoles collected so far are investigated to see whether any are close enough together to be combined into a single source, and the result constitutes the preliminary assessment of the underlying sources. A drastic refinement of this initial set can now be achieved by recalculating each dipole (including the most prominent) in the light of knowledge of the others in the set.

Results

It is important to realise that the DLP rulebase is completely automatic in its operation — the entire analysis of the map *map1* is initiated by the simple command "workset1 underlies map1", which places the dipole solution set into the set *workset1*.

The rulebase described in the previous section has so far proven successful with a number of source configurations. In particular, given maps of the type shown in Figure 1, resulting from several heavily overlapping dipole sources, DLP has proven successful in a variety of test situations. It has been tested trivially on 1–dipole maps and in six 3–dipole situations. In each accuracies of better than 5mm have been obtained for the radial location and better than 0.03 radians for the angular location of the sources. To our knowledge DLP is the first system capable of dealing with source distributions of this complexity, although a more general system which can handle a wider range of models and instrument types is currently being developed at the Open University (Ioannides, in preparation).

Because of the wide variety of possible source configurations it is impossible to give an exhaustive assessment of the system's capability. Clearly it must fail when the dipoles are either too weak or too close together. However we can illustrate its performance in the far from trivial situation of Figure 1(b). Here it is not immediately obvious that three dipoles are involved, due to the heavy overlap between them. Using arbitrary units for the dipole strength P, the source specifications are:

dipole	x_r/cm	x_θ/rad	x_ϕ/rad	P_r	P_θ	P_ϕ
1	11.00	1.27	-0.50	0.00	1.60	1.20
2	9.00	2.17	0.70	0.00	2.00	0.00
3	7.00	1.67	0.20	0.00	4.00	3.00

The solution set to this problem obtained by DLP was:

dipole	x_r/cm	x_θ/rad	x_ϕ/rad	P_r	P_θ	P_ϕ
1	11.09	1.27	-0.50	0.00	1.38	1.11
2	9.45	2.18	0.70	0.00	1.19	0.09
3	7.45	1.68	0.22	0.00	2.29	2.14

This solution is remarkably accurate considering the overlap of the sources. However, as can be seen the magnitudes are quite low — this occurs solely as a consequence of the fact that DLP has consistently overestimated the radial position. In fact, the calculation of depth on the basis of edge–dot separation is the most fragile part of the process at present.

When presented with a problem DLP has no knowledge of the number of dipoles in the source set. While it has in this case found the correct number, it will sometimes find an additional deep source which mops up the residue left from inaccuracies in the estimation of the others. This "additional" dipole can be eliminated by demanding a solution containing a specific number of sources, but there are obvious dangers in such a strategy when deep sources may be present. Further work is needed to clarify the status of individual dipoles within a solution set. A first step towards this goal is provided by a confidence measure which DLP assigns to a given solution set (92% in the above example). However more work is required to relate this parameter to modelling errors and noise.

Restrictions and future prospects

There are three main restrictions on the existing DLP rulebase. One is the depth calculation, which has already been mentioned. The other two are calculation time and noise tolerance. Bench tests show that DLP requires about 6.5 minutes to solve a three dipole problem at present. This length of time has two causes. One is that we currently use an interpreted version of Prolog; the Prolog code can be speeded up by a factor of 10 by using a compiled version. A more significant contribution to the time taken comes from the inability of our version of Prolog to communicate with procedural code written in other languages. Consequently, each call to procedural code requires two files to be both written and read, in order to pass parameters between the two. Given a compiled version of Prolog which permits parameter passing to and from procedural code, we foresee such problems taking about 30 seconds to solve.

The present system is not as noise–tolerant as we should like. When presented with the map shown in Figure 1(a), containing 10% noise, DLP finds the correct solution, yet does not recognise it as such and continues processing, thereafter diverging from the solution without terminating. We are quite clear as to why this is happening and how to rectify the situation. However, we are currently considering an alternative representation of maps in terms of cubic splines, and it may be that the preprocessing necessary for this representation obviates the need for further work on noise rejection.

References

[1] J.R.Bourne, V.Jagannathan, B.Giese & J.W.Ward (1980): "A software system for syntactic analysis of the EEG", *Computer Programs in Biomedicine, 11,* 190.

[2] D.Cohen, Y.Palti, B.N.Cuffin & S.J.Schmid (1980): "Magnetic fields produced by steady currents in the body", *Proc. Nat. Acad. Sci. USA, 77,* 1447.

[3] A.A.Ioannides (1986): "Graphical representation of biomagnetic signals", Proceedings of the Workshop on Interdisciplinary Inverse Problems, Dec.1986, Montpellier, France.

[4] A.A.Ioannides & D.I.F.Grimes (1986): "A method for reconstructing line current sources from magnetic field data", *Inverse Problems, 2,* 331.

A LINEAR ESTIMATION APPROACH TO BIOMAGNETIC IMAGING

W.H. Kullmann, K.D. Jandt, K. Rehm*, H.A. Schlitt*, W.J. Dallas*, W.E. Smith+

Philips GmbH, Forschungslaboratorium Hamburg, 2000 Hamburg 54, FRG
*University of Arizona, Department of Radiology and Optical Sciences Center, Tucson, Arizona 85724, U.S.A.
+University of Rochester, Institute of Optics, Rochester, New York 14627, U.S.A.

INTRODUCTION

A reconstruction algorithm based on linear estimation theory in combination with Moore-Penrose pseudoinverse techniques is presented in order to image complex current distributions. Phantom experiments with current dipoles immersed in saline solution inside a glass phantom head and computer simulations demonstrate the applicability to biomagnetic imaging.

METHOD

The inversion of the discretized Biot-Savart law

$$\vec{B} = A \cdot \vec{j} + \vec{n}$$

($\vec{B}$: measured magnetic field, A: Biot-Savart matrix, $\vec{j}$: current density, $\vec{n}$: experimental noise) will be carried out by using pseudoinverse techniques and statistical second order a-priori information of the current density and the experimental noise (Dallas et al. 1987, Kullmann 1988). For an ensemble of the current density, where $\vec{j}$ is one sample object, the covariance matrix can be constructed

$$K_{\vec{j}} = \langle(\vec{j}-\langle\vec{j}\rangle)\cdot(\vec{j}-\langle\vec{j}\rangle)^T\rangle = \sum_{\vec{j}} p(\vec{j})(\vec{j}-\langle\vec{j}\rangle)\cdot(\vec{j}-\langle\vec{j}\rangle)^T$$

(< > indicates ensemble averages, $p(\vec{j})$: probability of occurence of $\vec{j}$, T indicates the transpose). In analogy the covariance matrix for the noise is given by

$$K_{\vec{n}} = \langle\vec{n}\cdot\vec{n}^T\rangle = \sum_{\vec{j}} \sum_{\vec{n}} p(\vec{n}|\vec{j})\vec{n}\cdot\vec{n}^T$$

($p(\vec{n}|\vec{j})$: conditional probability for the of occurrence of the noise $\vec{n}$ with given object $\vec{j}$). The reconstruction procedure searches for an optimal linear estimator, which minimizes the mean square error MSE between the object class $\vec{j}$ and the reconstruction class $\hat{\vec{j}}$

Advances in Biomagnetism
Edited by S.J. Williamson *et al.*
Plenum Press, New York

$$MSE = \mathrm{Trace} \sum_{\vec{j}} \sum_{\vec{n}} p(\vec{n}|\vec{j})\,p(\vec{j})\,(\vec{j}-\hat{\vec{j}})\cdot(\vec{j}-\hat{\vec{j}})^T .$$

Such a linear estimator is given by (Pratt, 1978)

$$\hat{\vec{j}} = [A^T K_{\vec{n}}^{-1} A + K_{\vec{j}}^{-1}]^{-1} A^T K_{\vec{n}}^{-1} (\vec{B}-\langle\vec{B}\rangle) + \langle\vec{j}\rangle.$$

In this method the measurement region of the magnetic field as well as the interesting region of current density can be chosen arbitrarily.

The reconstruction method was tested by computer simulations and phantom experiments. In the experiment current dipoles (two 5 mm long parallel alligned platinum wires with drilled leads) were immersed in a saline solution inside a glass head phantom (mannequin head). The current generators were fed by a 10 Hz ac current (I=50 μA) and the SQUID output signal was measured by lock-in technique. The magnetic field was measured with a second order one-channel SQUID gradiometer (BTI, baseline 50.4 mm, diameter 19.8 mm) in a plane (proximal coil 1.5 cm above the vertex) of equidistantly spaced (2.0 cm) detection points. In the reconstructions a planar area or a volume of interest was defined, where the current distribution was considered. The a-priori information of the current density was confined to the fact, that the individual current elements are independent of each other. The ensemble averages of the current density and the magnetic field are assumed to be zero.

RESULTS

Phantom experiments and computer simulations often show a similar bipolar behavior of the magnetic field arising from multiple electrical sources and widely spreaded current generators (compare Figs 1,2,4). For example, Figure 1a shows the experimentally measured magnetic field of two current dipoles, symmetrically located in y-direction 3.0 cm apart from the origin (below vertex) and directing into negative x-direction (anterior-posterior). Both dipoles are located in the same depth. The z-component of the magnetic field is measured in a plane 4.4 cm above the dipoles. The occurring fields asymmetry results from small asymmetries of the dipoles. The conventional reconstrction, using the equivalent current dipole model, would suggest one dipole next to the origin, as indicated in Fig. 1b. Fig. 1c shows the reconstruction based on the linear estimation algorithm. The arrows indicate the strength and the direction of the current elements. The "return currents" around the areas of the original currents (largest arrows) originate predominantly from filtering effects

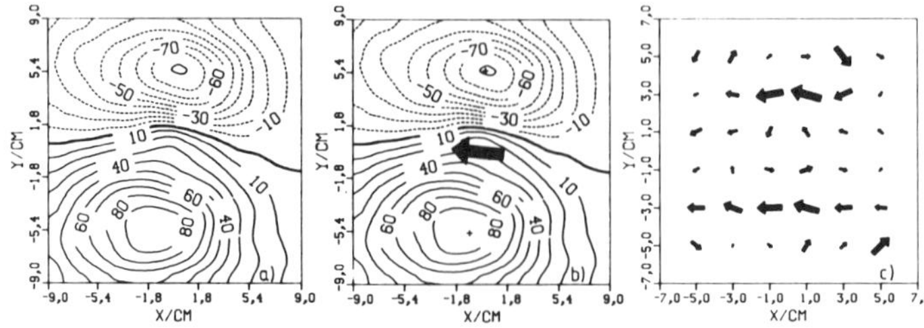

Fig. 1. Magnetic field and current density reconstruction of two experimental current dipoles in a glass phantom head: a) measured magnetic field B_Z (relative units) b) projection of the equivalent current dipole, c) reconstructed current density in the original current plane (arrows indicate the relative strength and direction of the current density).

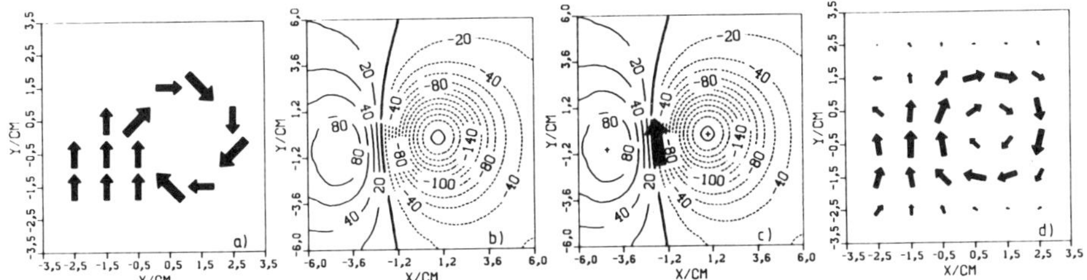

Fig. 2. Computer simulation of a complex planar current density distribution: a) input current density, b) calculated magnetic field (B_Z) in a plane 3.0 cm above the current, c) projection of the equivalent current dipole, d) reconstruction with linear estimation theory.

of the method. The reconstruction only uses the z-component of the field in the measurement plane.

Computer simulations demonstrate the ability of imaging of lateral components of more complex current arrangements. Fig. 2a indicates a planar current density distribution composed of 14 current elements. Figs. 2b,c represent the z-component of the magnetic field 3.0 cm above the current and the projection of the equivalent current dipole. In contrast to the current dipole model the linear estimation reconstruction, based only on B_Z, reconstructs the intrinsic structure as well as the extension of the source, if the reconstruction plane is located in the right depth of the current (Fig. 2d). If the reconstruction plane is located deeper than the original current source, the image shows a similar character, but increased smearing effects occur (Fig. 3a,b). In the case of a reconstruction above the original depth a disturbed image, inconsistent with the images from deeper planes, appears (Fig. 3d).

The above results are based on planar current arrangements and planar reconstructions. Now a computer simulation of two current generators in different depths is discussed in combination with a volume reconstruction. One current element is located at (+0.5,-1.5,-2.0) cm, the second at (-0.5,+1.5,-1.0) cm. The orientation of both dipoles of equal strengths is parallel to the y-axis (projection in Fig. 4a). The z-component of the corresponding magnetic field is illustrated in Fig. 4b. Now the reconstruction region is a volume, composed of two planes in z-direction at z= -1.0 cm and z= -2.0 cm. The reconstructed images, based on B_X, B_y, B_Z, show in both planes the right locations and directions of the current sources (Figs. 4c, d). However the intensity of the deeper current element is reduced. Planar reconstructions only show a projection of both sources in the upper original plane. Reconstructions of multiple current generators at deeper locations yield only projections of the generator elements in the upper face of the reconstruction volume.

DISCUSSION

The biomagnetic reconstruction method based on linear estimation theory in combination with Moore-Penrose pseudoinverse techniques allows the imaging of the lateral components of complex current arrangements. The location, strength, direction, and the spatial extension of planar current density distributions can be determined if the depth is known by a-priori information. Shallow sources in different depths can be distinguished, also in depth, by reconstructions using threedimensional current volume regions and all three components of the magnetic field in one measurement plane. For deep lying multiple sources in different depths only the projection of the lateral current distribution can be resolved because of the

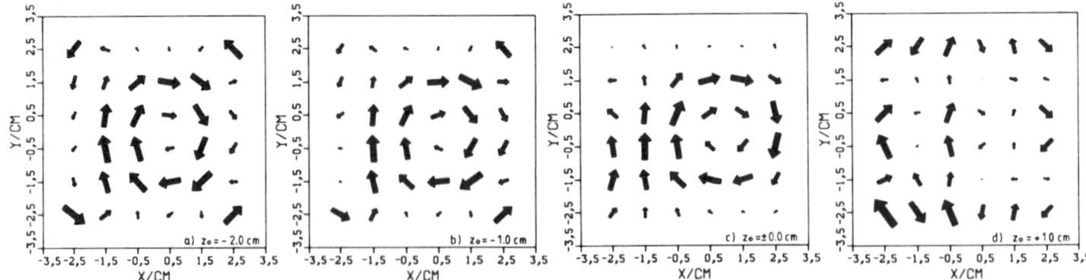

Fig. 3. Computer simulated reconstruction of the current denstiy (Fig. 2a) in different depths: a) z_0=-2.0 cm, b) z_0=-1.0 cm, c) z_0= ±0.0 cm, d) z_0=+1.0 cm. The original current depth is z_0=±0.0 cm.

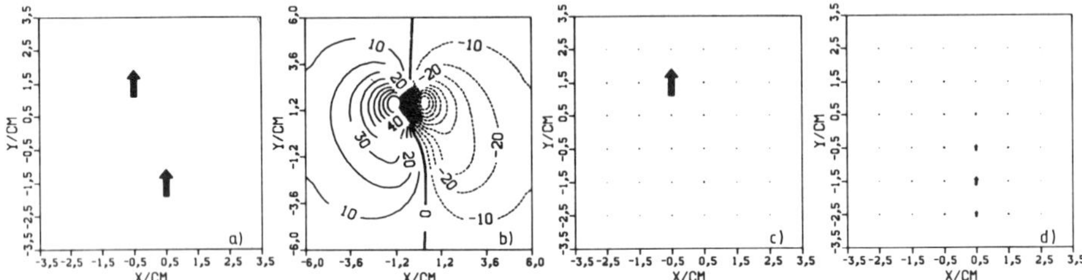

Fig. 4. Computer simulated reconstruction of two shallow current elements in different depths: a) projection of the current elements located at (+0.5,-1.5,-2.0) cm and (-0.5,+1.5,-1.0) cm into the xy-plane, b) magnetic field (B_Z) in the xy-plane at z=0.0 cm, c) reconstructed image in the plane of the upper dipole (z=-1.0 cm), d) reconstructed image in the plane of the deeper dipole (z=-2.0 cm).

smoothing properties of the Biot-Savart law. For planar deep lying sources the depth may be determined by moving a reconstruction plane through the volume conductor. While with increasing depth, starting from the original current plane, blurring effects dominate the reconstructions, just above the right location a discontinuity in the imaged current density occurs. This discontinuity of the imaged current elements can be used as a rough estimation of the depth. The method may not give an exact positioning with millimeter accuracy, but it is able to image the internal structure of complex current distributions within centimeter resolution. Volume conductor dependent magnetically silent sources of course cannot be visualized.

ACKNOWLEDGEMENTS

We gratefully thank Dr. O. Doessel for stimulating and helpful discussions throughout the whole work. This work was financially supported in part by the German Government, Bundesministerium für Forschung und Technologie, grant number 13 N 5377 0.

REFERENCES

Dallas, W.J., Smith, W.E., Schlitt, H.A. and Kullmann, W. (1987). Bioelectric current image reconstruction from measurement of the generated magnetic fields. In: Schneider, R.H. and Dwyer III, S.J. (Eds.), Medical Imaging, Proc. SPIE 767, 2-10.

Kullmann, W.H. (1988). Biomagnetic Imaging. In: Harris, G. and Walker, C. (Eds.), Proc Annual International Conference of the IEEE Engineering in Medicine and Biology Society, New Orleans, Vol. 10, Part 1/4: Cardiology and Imaging, 439-440.

Pratt, W.K. (1978). Digital image processing. John Wiley, New York.

DISCUSSION OF BIOMAGNETIC IMAGING SYSTEM AND RECONSTRUCTION ALGORITHM

H. Haneishi, N. Ohyama and K. Sekihara*

Imaging Science & Engineering Lab., Tokyo Inst. of Tech.
4259 Nagatsuta Midoriku, Yokohama 227 Japan
*Central Research Laboratory, Hitachi Ltd.
PO Box 2, Kokubunji, Tokyo 185 Japan

INTRODUCTION

The reconstruction of electric current distribution in a human brain from measured magnetic fields has been studied by many researchers. Most of these studies model the human head as a sphere casing filled with a homogeneous conductive medium in which only one electric current dipole exists. In case of complex current distribution, however, single dipole model is a poor match, and thus the current distribution should be modeled as multiple current dipoles.

In this paper, a method of estimating of the location and vector components of multiple dipoles is discussed. In this estimation, the least squares fitting is used, and this fitting causes nonlinear optimization problem. Conventional algorithms to solve this optimization problem involve the steepest descent method, the conjugate gradient method and the Newton method. These methods, however, cannot prevent their solution from being trapped at local minima and the solution can be incorrect when the minimized function contains many local minima. Estimating multiple current dipole parameters is just this case. This paper proposes to apply simulated annealing to this optimization problem. Simulated annealing is an algorithm which can provide the globally optimum solution beyond some local minima.

In this paper, first formulation of the problem and the simulated annealing procedure are reviewed. Next, results from the computer simulation are presented; these results clearly show the superiority of simulated annealing over the conventional methods. Finally, the annealing schedule is also discussed.

FORMULATION OF THE PROBLEM

Let us define N as the number of current dipoles, $\hat{\mathbf{r}}_n$ as the estimated position vector of n-th dipole and $\hat{\mathbf{q}}_n$ as its estimated current vector. Let $\mathbf{r}_m$ be the position vector of m-th measured point. The magnetic field $\mathbf{B}(\mathbf{r}_m)$ given by the current dipoles is calculated by Biot-Savart's low:

$$B(\mathbf{r}_m)=\sum_{n=1}^{N}\frac{\mu_0}{4\pi}\frac{\hat{\mathbf{q}}_n\times(\mathbf{r}_m-\hat{\mathbf{r}}_n)}{||\mathbf{r}_m-\hat{\mathbf{r}}_n||^3}\ . \tag{1}$$

Since the external magnetic field normal to the surface is measured on the hemispherical surface, the measured component $B_d(\mathbf{r}_m)$ is scalar, and given by

$$B_d(\mathbf{r}_m)=\sum_{n=1}^{N}\frac{\mu_0}{4\pi}\cdot\frac{\hat{\mathbf{q}}_n\cdot(\mathbf{r}_m \times \hat{\mathbf{r}}_n)}{\|\mathbf{r}_m-\hat{\mathbf{r}}_n\|^3\,\|\mathbf{r}_m\|}. \tag{2}$$

Consequently, letting $B_t(\mathbf{r}_m)$ be the actually measured magnetic component, the cost function, which is minimized through the optimization process, is given by the square error as:

$$E(\hat{\mathbf{r}}_1,\hat{\mathbf{q}}_1;,.,;\hat{\mathbf{r}}_N,\hat{\mathbf{q}}_N)=\sum_{m=1}^{M}\{\sum_{n=1}^{N}\frac{\mu_0}{4\pi}\frac{\hat{\mathbf{q}}_n\cdot(\mathbf{r}_m \times \hat{\mathbf{r}}_n)}{\|\mathbf{r}_m-\hat{\mathbf{r}}_n\|^3\,\|\mathbf{r}_m\|}-B_t(\mathbf{r}_m)\}^2. \tag{3}$$

Here, M is the total number of measured points. Our goal is to find the solution which globally minimizes this function. In this paper, it is proposed that simulated annealing is applied to this optimization problem.

SIMULATED ANNEALING

Simulated annealing has been originally proposed by Kirkpatrick et al.(1983) to solve the optimization problems using the analogy of thermodynamics. One of most important characteristics of the algorithm is the possibility that its estimates reach the globally optimum solution beyond some local minima. For the sake of this advantage, we propose to apply this algorithm to reconstructing the electric current distribution. The procedure of simulated annealing is described as follows.

First the initial estimate of current dipoles are arbitrarily given. If some a priori knowledge about dipole position and/or orientation are given, the knowledges might be taken into account to set appropriate initial estimates. Next, a perturbation is introduced to those estimates by adding or subtracting a small value called a grain. Then, the change of this cost function due to the introduction of the perturbation, ΔE, is calculated. If $\Delta E<0$, the grain is accepted as a favorable change decreasing the energy and the value of the parameter is updated. If $\Delta E>0$, the grain is accepted subject to the Boltzmann probability statistics $p(\Delta E)=\exp(-\Delta E/T)$, where T is a factor that can be associated with the thermodynamic temperature.

This stochastic acceptance is essential to avoid trapping at local minima. These trials and updates over all parameters are repeated until the thermal equilibrium is established; the thermal equilibrium is equal to the condition that the number of accepted grains that raise the energy is equal to that of accepted grains that decrease the energy. When the thermal equilibrium is established, the temperature is decreased according to a predetermined schedule. The same procedure is repeated until next thermal equilibrium is obtained. The whole process described here enables the estimates to reach the global minimum of the cost function. It should be noted that the cost function is often called the energy because of the analogy of simulated annealing with the thermodynamics.

COMPUTER SIMULATION

In our simulation, the head surface is modeled by a sphere with a radius of 60 (arbitrary unit), and the external magnetic field normal to the surface is measured at 64 sampling points on the hemispherical surface. In this measurement scheme, the current vector component aligned with the sphere's radii produce no measurable magnetic field. Therefore we can neglect this component. Consequently, the parameters to be estimated are three components of the position and two components of the current vector per one current dipole.

(A) COMPARISON BETWEEN SIMULATED ANNEALING AND STEEPEST DESCENT

First we show a comparison between a performance of simulated annealing and of conventional optimization algorithms. Here, the steepest descent method is used as a typical method of those conventional algorithms.

The number of the current dipoles is assumed to be known in the simulation, and ranges from one to four. Table 1 lists the final energy for each number of dipoles. In one or two dipole cases, both methods provide good estimates. In three or four dipole cases, however, the steepest descent method provides incorrect estimates compared to simulated annealing. This is because the estimate is trapped at a local minimum in the steepest descent case. Table 2 shows the final estimates obtained by both methods in four dipole case. This result clearly shows the superiority of simulated annealing over the steepest descent method and verifies the use of simulated annealing in this optimization problem.

Table 1 final energy

the number of dipoles	1	2	3	4
simulated annealing	0.32	0.06	1.91	5.14
steepest descent	0.01	0.04	83.50	2262.59

Table 2 final estimates in four dipole case (arbitrary unit) p_x, p_y, p_z are x,y,z components of the position vector, respectively, and q_u, q_v are two tangential components of the current vector.

parameter		position vector component			current vector component	
		p_x	p_y	p_z	q_u	q_v
original	#1	0.00	20.00	40.00	-20.00	-8.94
	#2	0.00	40.00	0.00	20.00	-20.00
	#3	0.00	0.00	20.00	0.00	50.00
	#4	-25.00	-25.00	25.00	-28.28	-16.33
estimate by simulated annealing	#1	-0.38	19.37	38.52	-24.13	-11.41
	#2	0.55	38.61	-0.95	19.71	-24.60
	#3	-5.06	0.99	20.00	21.49	-49.77
	#4	-24.89	-25.08	25.11	-28.24	-15.92
estimate by steepest descent	#1	-8.03	13.04	25.43	-90.73	57.32
	#2	23.67	19.42	0.94	-37.16	33.90
	#3	-22.44	-30.77	-3.28	63.06	-9.52
	#4	40.27	-8.65	-37.23	-21.70	55.64

(B)ANNEALING SCHEDULE

Although simulated annealing provides better estimates than the steepest descent method, we found through the computer simulation that the scheduling of the temperature reduction is a crucial factor to obtain the good solution. We tested two kinds of scheduling;

$$T_k = aT_{k-1} \quad (\text{e.g. } a=0.95) \tag{4-a}$$

$$T_k = T_0/(1+k) \ , \tag{4-b}$$

where T_k denotes k-th value of the temperature. Figure 1 shows the results of the comparison between the two kinds of scheduling. These results indicate that the scheduling shown in Eq. (4b) should be used to estimate the current dipole parameters.

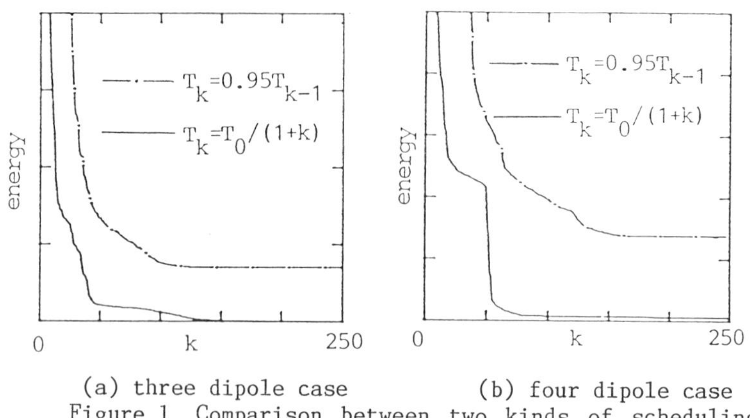

(a) three dipole case (b) four dipole case

Figure 1 Comparison between two kinds of scheduling

CONCLUSIONS

In order to estimate the parameters of multiple current dipoles, we have proposed to use simulated annealing as an optimization algorithm. According to the computer simulation results, when one or two dipole model is assumed, no difference can be observed between the performances of the conventional algorithm and simulated annealing. On the other hand, when three or four dipole model is assumed, only simulated annealing can provide the correct solution.

We have also found that the scheduling in the temperature reduction is very important to obtain the correct estimate. Two kinds of scheduling were tested in our computer simulation. According to the results of the simulation, only the scheduling shown in Eq.(4-b) can provide correct solution for three and four dipole cases.

We have also tried the five current dipole case. In this case, the estimates are trapped at a local minimum even by simulated annealing. A slower schedule, $T_k=T_0/\log(1+k)$, will be tested for this case. Moreover, we consider that some technique, for example, re-heating and cooling down, can lead the estimate to the global minimum.

REFERENCES

Jeffs,B., Leahy,R. and Singh,M.(1987). An evaluation of methods for neuromagnetic image reconstruction. IEEE Transaction on Biomedical Engineering, Vol.BME-34, No.9

Kirkpatrick,S., Gellatt,C.D.,Jr, and Vecci,M.P.(1983). Optimization by the simulated annealing. Science 220, 670-680

DIRECT APPROACH TO AN INVERSE PROBLEM: A TRIAL TO DESCRIBE SIGNAL SOURCES BY CURRENT ELEMENTS DISTRIBUTION

H. Kado, S. Kashiwaya, M. Higuchi*, H. Miura

Electrotechnical Laboratory,
1-1-4 Umezono, Tsukuba 305 JAPAN

*Tsukuba University,
1 Ten-nohdai, Tsukuba 305 JAPAN

INTRODUCTION

The conventional procedures for analyzing the magnetic field source in biomagnetism are to estimate the location, the direction and the intensity of an equivalent current dipole which is assumed as a representative of biological activity. The iso-magnetic field mapping is mostly used to determine the location of the dipole by finding the two extrema of magnetic field on the surface of observation. The dipole is estimated directly from the extrema or calculated by some mathematical procedures such as least square fitting of dipole model.

To estimate a single dipole, the mathematical operation comes to an unique solution in the solution space which consists of six coordinate corresponding with the parameter of dipole. A dipole is described with parameters of three components of position, two of direction and one of intensity. If we have magnetic field signals without any noise, these unknown parameters are estimated with at least six independent observations. In this case, the model is evaluated by the value of residue between observed data and magnetic field generated by model. If we expand the model being more complex system[1,2,3] like current multiple expansion (CME), multi source model (MSM) and distributed current model, there is no unique solution any more. We encounter a kind of combinatorial optimization problem and the mathematical approach should introduce a novel evaluation concept. To assume the MSM like multi current dipoles, even two or three current dipoles, we should observe twelve or eighteen signal which should be strongly independent each others and be without noise. Furthermore, on the way of parameter estimation there will be many local minimum. Simulated annealing[4] is one of the method to escape from local minimum. There is, however, still no concrete strategy for a model of large number signal sources.

To consider more general aspect of inverse problem, first we think a model of a system (like cardiac or central nervous system in biomagnetism). There is no practical idea which teach us to adopt a particular model. The CME is to reduce the residue such as ℓ_2 norm[4] between measured data and magnetic field generated by the model. We still have no rational idea to select a model, even incidentally the location of estimated poles are equal to the exited portion of biological system.

Advances in Biomagnetism
Edited by S.J. Williamson *et al.*
Plenum Press, New York

MODEL

In this study, we tried to establish an approach to describe magnetic sources by distribution of current elements which converge to a specific distribution of source. We think every observable magnetic field signal consists of summation of magnetic fields each of which is generated by each current element. The model of the signal source consists of large number current elements. Each element is described as a current dipole. Each element has same intensity. Position and direction of each element are not specified. The inverse problem on this model is that , by using an algorithm mentioned below, the distribution of the elements is expected to converge to a signal source current pattern.

ALGORITHM

To assume N number of current elements $I_{i\ ,\ i=1,...,N}$. The position of I_i is $\mathbf{r}_i$, the direction of I_i is $\mathbf{n}_i$.

Step 1: To distribute the elements randomly into the volume which is subject of biological function being in active. Then, to calculate the magnetic field $\mathbf{B}_{model}$ generated by distributed current elements $(I_1,..,I_N)$ at measurement positions $(\mathbf{R}_j,..,\mathbf{R}_M)$.

$$\mathbf{B}_{j,model} = \Sigma\ \mathbf{B}_i\ , \qquad j=1,...,M,$$

where $\mathbf{B}_i = \mathbf{B}(\mathbf{r}_i\ , \mathbf{n}_i)$ is magnetic field generated by current element I_i at position $\mathbf{r}_i$ and direction $\mathbf{n}_i$.

Step2: To calculate an evaluation value L of model fitting by norm between model field $\mathbf{B}_{j,model}$ and measured magnetic field $\mathbf{B}_{j,measured}$ at position of measurement $\mathbf{R}_j$.

$$L = \Sigma\ \text{norm}\ (\ \mathbf{B}_{j,model}, \mathbf{B}_{j,measured})\ ,$$

where, norm is ℓ_2 criterion of two vectors.

Step3: To select an arbitrary current element. The element moves to the vicinity of its original position in the solution space $\mathfrak{S}_i$ to reduce L. The element motion is limited within value as an algorithm parameter. There are N number of solution space, each of which belongs to each current element I_i.

$$\mathfrak{S}_i = \mathfrak{S}_i(\ \mathbf{r}_i\ , \mathbf{n}_i\ )$$

Solution space is specified by coordinate of position and direction vector of each current element.

Step4: In the case of L being reduced the element has new position. In the case of L being not reduced the element stay at it's original position. The algorithm operation return to Step3 and the algorithm select next arbitrary element.

The algorithm is not clarified its mathematical characteristics. It might be quite difficult to analyze the characteristics by means of analytical method but by the empirical and heuristic way. The major purpose of this study is to verify the algorithm could make the distribution of current elements to describe magnetic source within practical cpu time.

A SIMULATION

As the first step of mathematical clarification of the algorithm, the following simulation has been carried out. The circle current was assumed as a magnetic source which is located in a cube volume. Magnetic field vectors at several positions of surface of a cube generated by a circle current was adopted as a measured magnetic field vectors $\mathbf{B}_{measured}$. Magnetic field vectors at measurement positions generated by elements are calculated. The algorithm was carried by main frame computer (CRAY XMP-216) with using the vectors of measured magnetic field and of distributed current elements.

In the initial stage of the simulation, we should decide the every parameters which specify the signal source, the model and the algorithm. The parameters of the signal source which are not essential but practical for this method are size of cube, diameter of circle current, position and direction of circle and current intensity. The intensity of element, the number of elements and distribution are model parameters. The algorithm is specified by rule of element motion and termination rule of iteration.

In steps of algorithm, an arbitrary selected element moves it's vicinity in the solution space $\mathfrak{S}_i$ where is five dimensional space specified by position and direction of the element I_i. Fig.1 shows the signal source (circle current in the cube). Fig.2 shows a successive results of current elements converge from random distribution to signal source pattern. The cpu time of 3600 iteration is about 40 second.

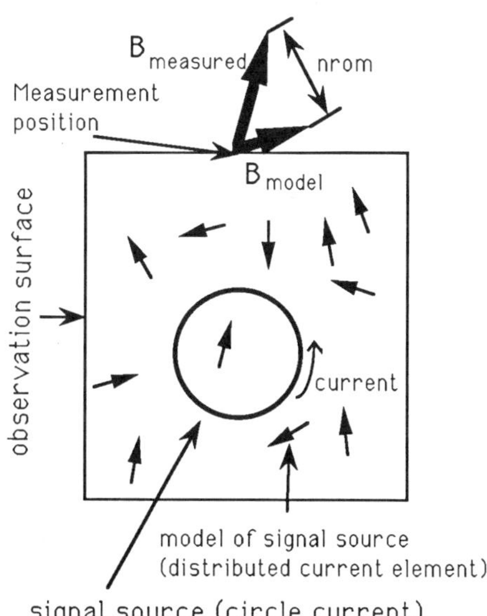

Fig.1 The circle current which is source of magnetic field in a cube. The model is evaluated by a value of summation of norm between model field $\mathbf{B}_{model}$ and measured field $\mathbf{B}_{measured}$.

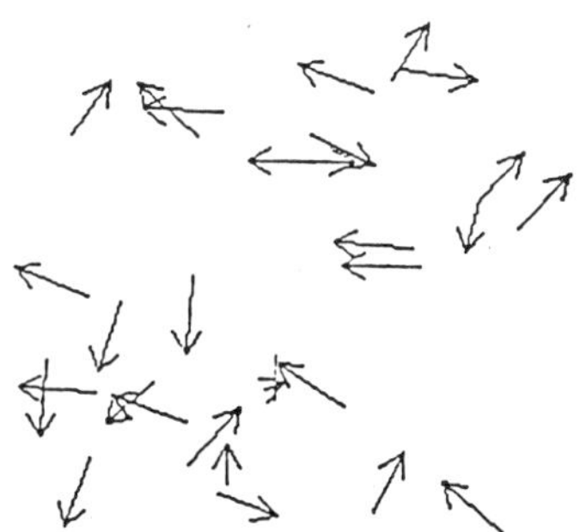

Fig.2(a) Initial distribution of current elements in the algorithm. 28 current elements were distributed randomly as a starting situation of the inverse problem.

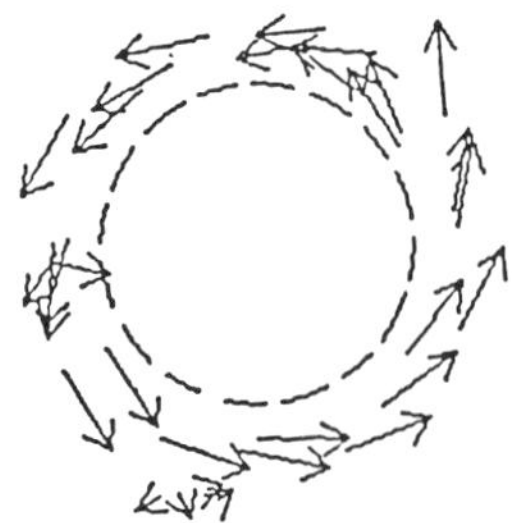

Fig.2(b) The distribution of current elements after 2400 iteration. They seems to be going to converge to the pattern of magnetic source.

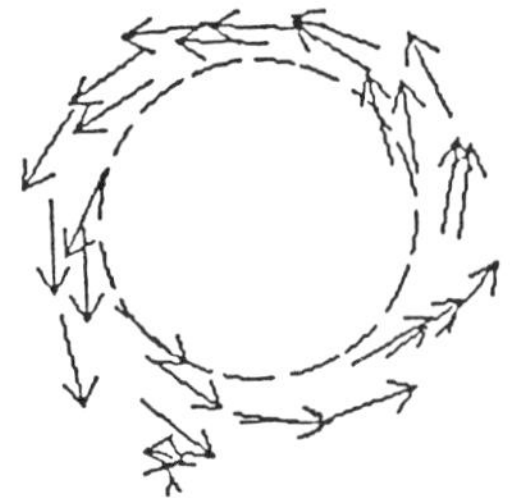

Fig.2(c) The distribution of current elements after 3600 iteration.They converged to the pattern of magnetic source which is a solution of this inverse problem.

DISCUSSION

The result is quite well posed to the signal source, even though it is not sure the algorithm may be effective for arbitrary ill posed situation. In the practical application, we should introduce many heuristics and the a-priori knowledge on the measurement in order to restrict the solution space and to avoid the local minimum solution.

Returning to the specification of this simulation, number and intensity of elements are decided arbitrary. It is, however, necessary to select concrete values of the parameters. It is proposed that, before the algorithm, intensity of an equivalent current dipole is estimated and, from the histological and physiological knowledge, the number of elements are decided. Then, the current intensity of element is decided from the energy value of the equivalent dipole divided by the number. As increasing the iteration number, element come to be a pair of elements. The pair of elements which face to each other make very small magnetic field and it effects small contribution for norm. It is a kind of local minimum.

There might be many of the pair when the number of elements is large. The appearance of the elements pair is a sign to terminate the iteration of algorithm. This algorithm is quite heuristic. It was examined to apply a inverse problem of describing circle current signal source. We could not have a perspective of possibility of the algorithm for applying general inverse problem. We, however, would like to insist that elements could figure out the three dimensional pattern of electric current which hides in a volume without any strict parametric model like CME. If we introduce a strategy like CME, we have to measure more and more data as the unknown parameters increase.

ACKNOWLEDGEMENT

Authors thank Dr. Koyanagi and Dr. Nemoto for supporting this research work. Kado thanks Dr. Oshima for supporting computer facilities.

REFERENCES

T. Katila and P. Karp, 1983, Magnetocardiology: Morphology and Multipole Presentations, in: *Biomagnetism: An Interdisciplinary Approach* , S. J. Williamson, GL. Onmani, L. Kaufman and I. Modena, Eds., Plenaum Press, New York and London.

S. J. Williamson and L. Kaufman, 1981, in: *Biomagnetism, Journal of Magnetism and Magnetic Materials*, **22**, 129-201.

S. Kirkpatrick, C. D. Gelatt Jr. and M. P. Vecchi, 1983, Optimization by simulated annealing, in: *Science*, **220**, 671-680

R. S. Gonnelli and M. Sicuro, 1987, Use of the current multipole model for the cardiac source localization in normal subjects, in: *Biomagnetism'87*, 314-317.

A. Tarantola, 1987, *Inverse Problem Theory*, Elseiver, New York.

MAGNETIC FIELDS OF CURRENT MONOPOLES

A. Stewart Ferguson and Dominique Durand

Applied Neural Control Laboratory, Dept. of Biomedical Engineering
Case Western Reserve University
Cleveland, OH 44106, U.S.A.

INTRODUCTION

Neuronal current sources are usually modelled as dipole or higher-order current terms. The assumption of dipolar behaviour is valid when the observation distance is many times greater than the source size and the sensing device (eg. SQUID coil) tends to low-pass filter the magnetic field characteristics. As smaller sensors become available, assumptions implicit in dipole sources may not be satisified and more accurate source models would be required (Wikswo and Roth, 1988). In addition, the common practice of neglecting fields arising from volume currents may not be desirable if the volume current fields can provide additional information to aid in source localization (Ilmoniemi et al., 1985).

A more accurate model of the extracellular current of a neuron is possible if a patch of membrane is modelled as a current monopole (literally a point in space from which current radiates equally in all directions) with a strength equal to the transmembrane current. We have developed the equations describing the magnetic field produced by the volume currents of monopoles in both semi-infinite and spherical volume conductors. Using these equations, the magnetic field of the extracellular current can be computed from a weighted summation of the magnetic field of each membrane patch or monopole. Using superposition, the magnetic field due to intracellular currents can be added to this to obtain the total magnetic field of the neuron.

DERIVATION OF MONOPOLE EQUATIONS

It is important to understand that a monopole of current, while not a closed circuit, is capable of generating a magnetic field in the same manner as the volume current of a dipole generates a magnetic field (which also is not a closed circuit until the dipole current itself is included). Similar to the dipole volume current, a monopole generates no magnetic field when the surrounding conductive medium is infinite because the current flows directly away from the source. In any bounded medium, the magnetic field results from the secondary current sources or boundary effects.

Semi-Infinite Volume Conductor.

A monopole situated at a position (0,0,-d) in an infinite conducting region generates a current density vector given by

$$\mathbf{J}^{m} = \frac{I_0}{4\pi\,|R|^2}\,\mathbf{a}_R \qquad \text{where } \mathbf{R} = x\,\mathbf{a}_x + y\,\mathbf{a}_y + (z+d)\,\mathbf{a}_z \tag{1}$$

at a distance R from the monopole and oriented away from the monopole. The magnetic field associated with this current flow in an infinite region is zero. If the region $z > 0$ now becomes non-conducting, the boundary condition requires the application of an applied current density using the method of images, given by

$$\mathbf{J}_{\text{applied}} = \frac{-I_0}{4\pi\,|R|^2}\,\mathbf{a}_R \;(z>0) \quad = \frac{+I_0}{4\pi\,|R'|^2}\,\mathbf{a}_{R'} \;(z<0) \qquad \text{where } \mathbf{R}' = x\,\mathbf{a}_x + y\,\mathbf{a}_y + (z-d)\,\mathbf{a}_z \tag{2}$$

The magnetic field associated with this applied current density only has a B_ϕ component (using cylindrical coordinates) and can be derived for any (r,z) observation point using Ampere's Law

$$B_\phi = \frac{\mu I_0}{4\pi r}\left(\frac{|z|+d}{\sqrt{r^2+(|z|+d)^2}} - 1\right) \tag{3}$$

and represents the magnetic field generated in both the conducting and non-conducting regions by a current monopole in a semi-infinite medium. More generally, the magnetic field at any point (x,y,z) in space generated by a monopole located at (x_0,y_0,z_0) in a conducting medium extending below z=0 is

$$B_x^m(x_0,y_0,z_0)=-(y-y_0)\zeta; \quad B_y^m(x_0,y_0,z_0)=(x-x_0)\zeta; \quad \text{where } \zeta=\frac{\mu I_0}{4\pi[(x-x_0)^2+(y-y_0)^2]}\left[\frac{|z|-z_0}{\sqrt{(x-x_0)^2+(y-y_0)^2+(|z|-z_0)^2}}-1\right] \tag{4}$$

The magnetic field of a monopole can be compared to that of a line segment of current. The magnetic field line of current extending along the z-axis, in the +z direction from $z = z_1$ to $z = z_2$ is

$$B_\phi = \frac{\mu I}{4\pi\sqrt{x^2+y^2}}\left[\frac{z-z_1}{\sqrt{x^2+y^2+(z-z_1)^2}} - \frac{z-z_2}{\sqrt{x^2+y^2+(z-z_2)^2}}\right] \tag{5}$$

A comparison of (3) and (5) indicates that the magnetic field in the non-conducting medium (z>0) due to the current monopole is identical to that of a line of current extending along the z-axis from z=-d to z=-∞. In the conducting region, the field is equivalent to that generated by a line of current running from z=+∞ to z=d.

From these results it is possible to obtain the magnetic field for the volume currents of a dipole, $\mathbf{B}^d$, in the same conductor. A dipole with finite length $2y_0$ (actually a bipole), centered at (0,0,-d), oriented in the +y direction with current strength I_0 generates the same volume current as two monopoles - situated at $(0,+y_0,-d)$ and $(0,-y_0,-d)$ with strengths $+I_0$ and $-I_0$ respectively. As y_0 approaches zero, the bipole approaches a dipole of differential length 2dy and the magnetic fields are related as

$$\mathbf{B}^d = \lim_{2y_0\to 0}[\mathbf{B}^m(0,+y_0,-d)-\mathbf{B}^m(0,-y_0,-d)] = 2\,dy\left(\frac{\partial \mathbf{B}^m(0,y_0,-d)}{\partial y_0}\right)_{y_0=0} \tag{6}$$

where $\mathbf{B}^m$ is the magnetic field of a monopole. When (6) is applied to each of the components in (4), the results previously published for dipole volume currents (Cuffin and Cohen, 1977a) can be obtained identically.

Spherical Volume Conductor

In a sphere, the dipole volume current is equivalent to that of two oppositely signed monopoles rotated in opposite directions from an axis by some angle θ_0 (see Fig 1). As the angle of rotation approaches zero (and current approaches ∞), the magnetic field of the monopole $\mathbf{B}^m$ is related to that of the dipole $\mathbf{B}^d$ as

$$\mathbf{B}^d = \lim_{\theta_0\to 0}[\mathbf{B}^m(+\theta_0)-\mathbf{B}^m(-\theta_0)] = 2\,d\theta_0\left(\frac{\partial \mathbf{B}^m}{\partial \theta_0}\right)_{\theta_0=0} \tag{7}$$

Without loss of generality, the monopole can be located on the z-axis at the position (0,0,a) within a spherical conductor centered at the origin. Using symmetry, it is clear that the magnetic field must only have a B_ϕ component that precesses around the z-axis. Therefore, (7) can be expanded for each of the spherical components of the B field to get the identities

$$B_\theta^d = \frac{-1}{a}\,dL\,\frac{y\sqrt{x^2+y^2+z^2}}{(x^2+y^2)}B_\phi^m; \quad B_\phi^d = \frac{1}{a}\,dL\left[-z\frac{\partial B_\phi^m}{\partial x}+x\frac{\partial B_\phi^m}{\partial z}\right]; \quad \text{where } dL = \text{dipole length} \tag{8}$$

The results for $\mathbf{B}^d$ have previously been published (Cuffin and Cohen, 1977a) for a dipole located at (0,0,a) oriented in the +x direction. The first part of (8) can be applied to these results to yield the final result for the magnetic field of a monopole located at (0,0,a) in a conducting sphere

$$B_\phi^m = \frac{\mu I}{4\pi\sqrt{x^2+y^2}}\left[\frac{z-a}{\sqrt{x^2+y^2+(z-a)^2}} - \frac{z}{\sqrt{x^2+y^2+z^2}}\right] \tag{9}$$

This solution can be shown to satisfy the second part of (8), although the details are omitted here. The magnetic field of the monopole, given in (9), can be compared to that of a line of current given in (5). The field of the positive current monopole is identical to that of a line segment of current extending from the position of the monopole source ($z_1 = a$) to the center of the sphere ($z_2 = 0$). Likewise, a negative current monopole (or a sink) generates a magnetic field identical to that of a line segment of current extending from the center of the sphere to the position of the monopole.

APPLICATION OF MONOPOLE SOURCES

Although the monopole equations can be used to accurately calculate the magnetic field of any neural source that generates volume currents, it is still unclear under what conditions a simple dipole model may also be "sufficiently accurate". The relative error in computing the magnetic field of a neural source using both monopoles and dipoles is shown here to quantify the range over which a dipole approximation is valid.

The neural source being modelled consists of a cell body and an equivalent dendrite with distributed current sources (Fig 2). The source contains a strong monopole sink (cell body) connected to a chain of weak monopole sources (membrane patches). Intracellular current flows from the cell body to each membrane patch and drops with increasing distance from the cell body. The magnetic field is generated by both the intracellular current and the volume currents of the 51 monopoles. The distributed source has unit length, extending from $x = -0.3367$ to $x = +0.6633$ The source is positioned in this manner so the equivalent dipole is located at $x=0$ and has a dipole moment of 0.51 Both the distributed and dipole sources are oriented parallel to the x-axis, at $y=0$, and at varying depths in a semi-infinite conducting medium which extends below the plane $z=0$. Arbitrary units are used for distance and subsequently magnetic field because only a relative error is being computed.

The magnetic field was computed in each plane (z=constant) above the conducting medium for an x-y grid of points. The greatest discrepancy between the magnetic fields generated by the dipole and monopoles was found in B_y (the y component of $\mathbf{B}$). This is understandable since this is the only component which both the intracellular and volume currents generate (B_z is generated by intracellular currents and B_x by volume currents alone). On each observation plane, the magnetic field from both sources was normalized to the largest magnetic field generated by the distributed source (shown in Fig 3). The difference between the two field maps, after normalization, provides a "relative" error between the fields produced by the two sources. The largest such error in B_y is shown in Fig 4 for different observation heights above the conducting medium and for different source depths in the medium. The largest errors occur close to the conducting medium regardless of source depth. However, the maximum error does not exceed 1% whenever the observation height or the source depth exceeded 2.0 Since the distributed source length was 1.0, a dipole approximation appears to be valid whenever the observation point is approximately two source lengths above the medium or the source depth is at least twice the source length.

DISCUSSION

The solutions to the magnetic field generated by a current monopole in these volume conductors are considerably simpler than those published for dipole volume currents although many of the field characteristics are preserved. The monopole and dipole solutions share some similar characteristics: (1) the field at the surface of the conductor is parallel to the conducting boundary and contains no perpendicular

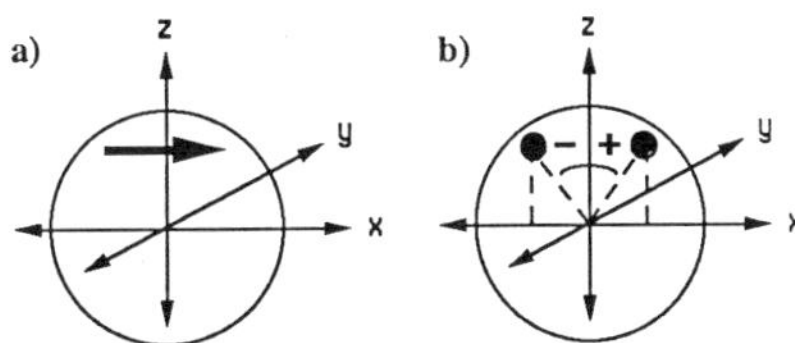

FIGURE 1. *The volume current of two oppositely signed monopoles (b) rotated away from each other is equivalent to the volume current of a dipole (a).*

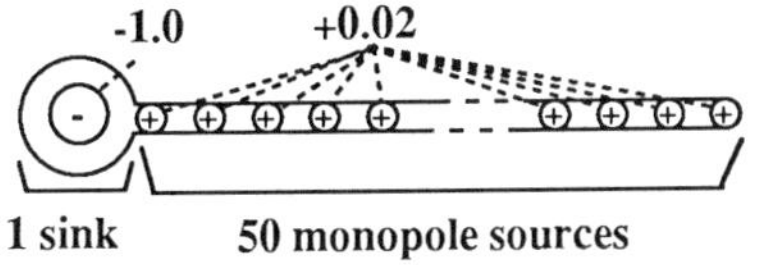

FIGURE 2. *The distributed current source consists of a single monopole sink of strength -1.0 connected to a chain of 50 monopole sources each with strength +0.02 spaced at equal intervals (see text).*

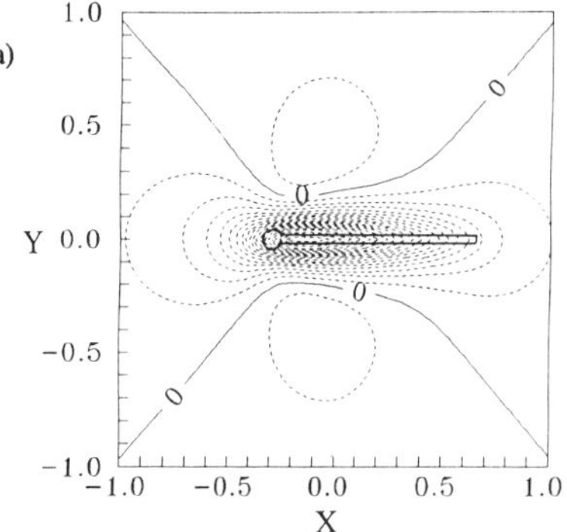

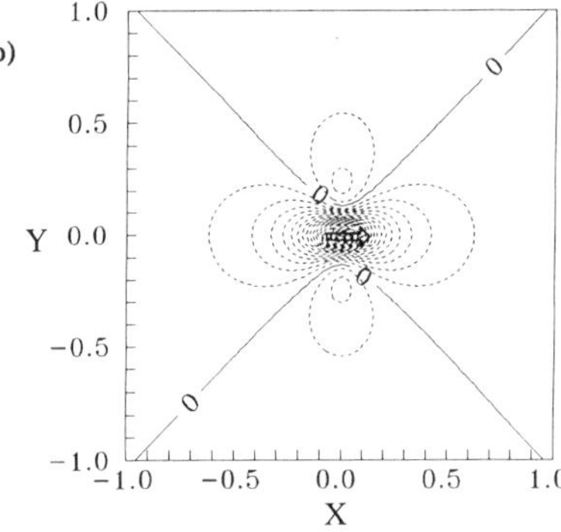

FIGURE 3. *Contour maps of B_y generated by "intracellular" and volume currents of the distributed (a) and dipole (b) source. The sources are located at a depth of 0.1 below the interface and maps show B_y on the interface (z=0). The values shown were normalized to the largest value of B generated by the distributed source. Contour intervals represent 0.05 (a) and 0.1 (b) of this value.*

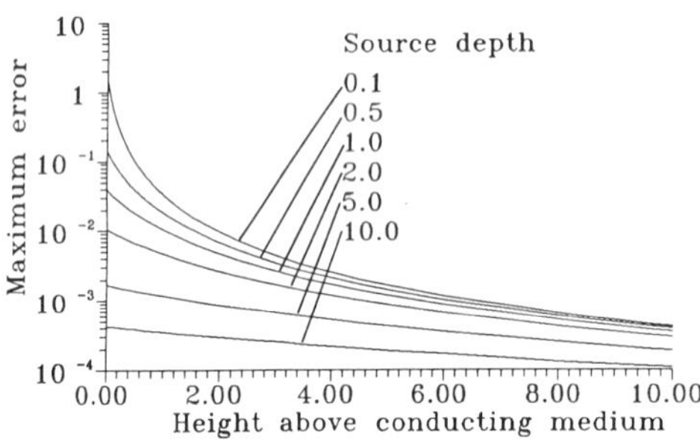

FIGURE 4. *The maximum error in B_y using the dipole approximation compared to the distributed source. Maximum error is defined as the largest difference between the magnetic field generated by the dipole source and that generated by the distributed source normalized to the largest magnetic field generated by the distributed source. Errors were computed at different plane heights above the conducting medium for different source depths (different lines in plot).*

component, (2) in a homogeneous conductor, conductivity does not affect the magnetic field, and (3) inhomogeneities, where the boundary of the inhomogeneity lies parallel to the conductor surface, do not affect the magnetic field (thus planar and concentric spherical inhomogeneities do not effect the semi-infinite and spherical models respectively).

Monopole current sources would be expected to be of greatest use in describing distributed current sources such as would occur in brain slices or myelinated axons. Attempts to model such sources using dipoles essentially involve integrating the field of a dipole (Cuffin and Cohen, 1977b). Since we have shown the field of a monopole to be the integral of the dipole field, one might expect the monopole to be the more sensible source model. The simple example presented in this paper indicates that the validity of a simple dipole approximation can be checked by using a more accurate monopole model for volume currents of neural sources. We are currently investigating the use of monopoles in modelling the fields produced by neurons in an attempt to determine the limits at which neural sources can truly be considered dipole current generators.

REFERENCES

Cuffin, B.N. and Cohen, D., 1977a, Magnetic fields of a dipole in special volume conductor shapes, IEEE Trans. Biomed. Eng., BME-24,:372-381.

Cuffin, B.N. and Cohen, D., 1977b, Magnetic fields produced by models of biological current sources, J. Appl. Phys, 48:3971-3980.

Ilmoniemi, R.J., Hamalainen, M.S., and Knuutila, J., 1985, The forward and inverse problems in the spherical mode, in: Biomagnetism: Applications and Theory, H. Weinberg, G. Stroink, and T. Katila, eds., Pergamon Press, New York.

Wikswo Jr., J.P. and Roth, B.J., 1988, Magnetic determination of the spatial extent of a single cortical current source: a theoretical analysis, EEG. Cl. Neur., 69: 266-276.

This work was supported by an NSF Presidential Young Investigator Award to D. Durand.

LOCALISED AND DISTRIBUTED SOURCE SOLUTIONS

FOR THE BIOMAGNETIC INVERSE PROBLEM I

C. J. S. Clarke
Faculty of Mathematical Studies, University of Southampton, Southampton, UK

A. A. Ioannides and J. P. R. Bolton
Physics Department, The Open University, Milton Keynes, MK7 6AA, UK

INTRODUCTION

Until recently, equivalent current dipole sources have been used almost universally to describe the biomagnetic signals generated by ionic currents in conducting body tissues but, as the performance of multichannel systems improves, clinical applications will emerge which require PET-like pictures demonstrating increased activity (or the absence of activity) in relation to normal background levels. A vital step in this direction is the development of a reliable, efficient and mathematically well-founded method of studying continuous source densities. A number of attempts to treat biomagnetic data in a model-independent way have been reported [1,2,3,4]. Starting from maximum entropy arguments [5] we have developed a very general method of inversion. In a certain limit, our method reduces to that of reference [1] but, in general, it is more powerful in its ability to take account of prior information about the source space and the noise spectrum of the magnetometers. It is implemented within a comprehensive computing environment that can deal with a wide range of experimental geometries and accommodate discrete or continuous sources, including both ionic flows and magnetic dipoles. In this paper we provide an outline of the method and computing environment and we discuss two simple examples. A more detailed description of the method will be given elsewhere, but its application to 3D inversions and the analysis of real MEG data is given in the next paper [6].

PHILOSOPHY AND MATHEMATICAL FOUNDATION

What appears to be the simplest method of source estimation – namely, varying the source within a chosen space of model sources so as to get the best least-squares fit to the data – suffers from many disadvantages. For example, the method is unstable unless the model space excludes "magnetically quiet" sources; but there is no natural way to split a given source into a quiet part and a remainder. Also, the best fit approach leads to an optimisation problem which is numerically tractable only for discrete sources or for very coarse discrete approximations to continuous sources.

To achieve a better method one requires the probability theory ideas that were introduced into the subject by Hämäläinen [7], and had earlier been introduced into other inverse problems by Daniell and Gull. One recognises that the magnetometer readings, subject to noise whose magnitude is usually roughly known, together with possible physiological data, gives one *partial information* about the source, which can be represented by a *probability distribution* over the space of possible sources (whether continuous or discrete). One can then choose to either (i) calculate the *expectation* of the source, in the probability theory sense; or (ii) find the *most likely* source, that is, the mode (provided the probability distribution can be expressed as a density); or (iii) extract other statistical information about different possible sources. Option (ii) involves an optimisation problem which can suffer from drawbacks analogous to those for the least-squares method. We have concentrated on option (i), calculating the expected current density, since it yields efficient and mathematically natural algorithms [5].

Advances in Biomagnetism
Edited by S.J. Williamson *et al.*
Plenum Press, New York

In the case of continuous current sources (in the ideal mathematical sense) with prior probability distribution $w(\mathbf{r})$ over a region Q the expected current density emerges as a linear combination of vector-valued basis functions $\boldsymbol{\phi}_k$, one for each of the field detectors:

$$\mathbf{j}(\mathbf{r}) = \sum_k A_k \boldsymbol{\phi}_k(\mathbf{r}) w(\mathbf{r}) \tag{1}$$

The basis function $\boldsymbol{\phi}_i(\mathbf{r})$ is defined by writing the general solution of the forward problem as

$$m_i = \int_Q \boldsymbol{\phi}_i(\mathbf{r}) \cdot \mathbf{j}(\mathbf{r}) d^3r \tag{2}$$

where m_i is the predicted measurement at the ith detector due to the current density distribution $\mathbf{j}(\mathbf{r})$. By solving the forward problem for an arbitrary delta function source we can evaluate $\boldsymbol{\phi}_i(\mathbf{r})$ throughout Q. Combining Equations 1 and 2, we obtain the linear set of equations

$$m_i = \sum_k P_{ik} A_k \tag{3}$$

$$P_{ik} = \int_Q \boldsymbol{\phi}_i(\mathbf{r}) \cdot \boldsymbol{\phi}_k(\mathbf{r})\, w(\mathbf{r})\, d^3r \tag{4}$$

The coefficients A_k, and hence the expected current density $\mathbf{j}(\mathbf{r})$, can then be obtained by inverting Equation 3, provided the matrix P is non-singular (the case where P is singular is treated in the next section). The method is both efficient and elegant. The vector function $\boldsymbol{\phi}_i(\mathbf{r})$ contains just the right amount of information that can be associated with the detailed nature, position and orientation of the ith detector and the specific assumptions made about the source space; note in particular that the contribution of silent sources to the basis functions vanishes by construction. In the case of a uniform weight (i.e. $w(\mathbf{r}) = 1$ throughout the allowed space Q) the solution reduces to that of reference [1]; amongst all the solutions that fit the given data this is the one of minimum power dissipation.

IMPLEMENTATION AND EXTENSIONS

The basic method described above has been implemented within a comprehensive biomagnetism computer program developed by one of us (AAI) at the Open University. This system deals with both the forward and inverse problems for a wide variety of source spaces, detectors and experimental geometries. In the current context, the first step is to calculate the $\boldsymbol{\phi}$ functions by solving the forward problem for the assumed source space and numerically integrating over the response functions of the detectors. Our program is able to do this for current and magnetic sources and for any given collection of detectors, in any orientation or spatial arrangement.

When a large number of $\boldsymbol{\phi}$ functions are used as basis for the expansion of the current density, many of them are close to linear combinations of the others and the matrix P is nearly singular. The inversion procedure described above then runs into numerical difficulty; however, precisely because the $\boldsymbol{\phi}$ functions are so similar, we can afford to expand $\mathbf{j}$ in terms of a smaller subset of these functions. We wish to do this in a way that does not ignore hard-won and potentially valuable measurements. The simplest method is to restrict the number of expansion terms but to include all the data so that Equation 3 becomes an overdetermined system whose least-square solution gives an estimate of the A_k. A more satisfactory procedure admits from the outset that very large currents are physiologically implausible and restricts their likelihood by requiring the *a priori* probability distribution of current density to have a finite standard deviation β. This limits our ability to fit the data exactly – but this turns out to be an advantage in the presence of noise as there is no point in fitting the data more accurately than its own standard deviation, σ. Using these ideas and taking s data values and $t \le s$ expansion terms, Equation 3 is replaced by the square system

$$\tilde{m}_i = \sum_{k=1}^{t} \tilde{P}_{ik} A_k \qquad (i = 1 \ldots t) \tag{5}$$

where the "dressed" quantities $\tilde{m}_i$ and $\tilde{P}_{ik}$ are defined by

$$\tilde{m}_i = \sum_{j=1}^{s} P_{ij} m_j \qquad \text{and} \qquad \tilde{P}_{ik} = \sum_{j=1}^{s} P_{ij} P_{jk} + \zeta P_{ik} \tag{6}$$

where $\zeta = \sigma^2/\beta^2$. For convenience we also introduce the dimensionless quantity $\tilde{\zeta} = \zeta s/\mathrm{Tr}P$, where this normalisation makes unity a rough divide between large and small values. For $\tilde{\zeta} > 0$, numerical problems are avoided because the matrix $\tilde{P}$ is positive definite. In the limit $\tilde{\zeta} \to 0$ the method reduces to the least-squares approach mentioned above.

TEST CASES

In the first test case (Figure 1) the target field is generated by two current dipoles (heavy arrows) located in the x-y plane. Measurements are made with a standard symmetric second-order gradiometer with symmetry axis along the z-direction. The entire measurement set consists of 121 readings in a plane 10 cm above the sources. The assumed source space Q is a disk of radius 13 cm in the x-y plane, with a uniform *a priori* probability distribution for the current density vector field. Figure 1a shows a continuous solution of the inverse problem, sampled at evenly spaced points in Q (light arrows). This solution is based on Equations 1 - 4 using only 5 of the gradiometers (dots) and the corresponding 5 ϕ functions. The results are reasonably good, bearing in mind the paucity of data and the lack of a priori assumptions made about the distribution of currents over the plane. The solution is, however, unsafe: if we compare signals from the initial sources and our estimated current distribution we find perfect agreement at the 5 chosen detectors (as expected) but a standard error of 35% over the whole array of detectors. Figure 1b shows the solution when 25 detectors and their corresponding ϕ functions are retained. The unsatisfactory nature of this solution reflects the numerical problems that arise when some of the ϕ functions are close to linear combinations of others. The problem can be resolved by using the "dressed" quantities of Equations 5 and 6, with the same 25 expansion functions and all 121 data values. For small values of $\tilde{\zeta}$ the solution is indistinguishable from that of Figure 1b but as $\tilde{\zeta}$ is increased the solution is stabilized: once stability has been achieved the solution is rather insensitive to $\tilde{\zeta}$. Figures 1c and 1d illustrate the solution for $\tilde{\zeta} = 0.1$ and $\tilde{\zeta} = 0.3$. In Figure 1d we also show a contour plot of the square of the current density. Although Figures 1a, 1c and 1d may seem similar it is important to note that Figures 1c and 1d represent much safer solutions since they have standard errors over the whole array of detectors of only 11% and 14% respectively.

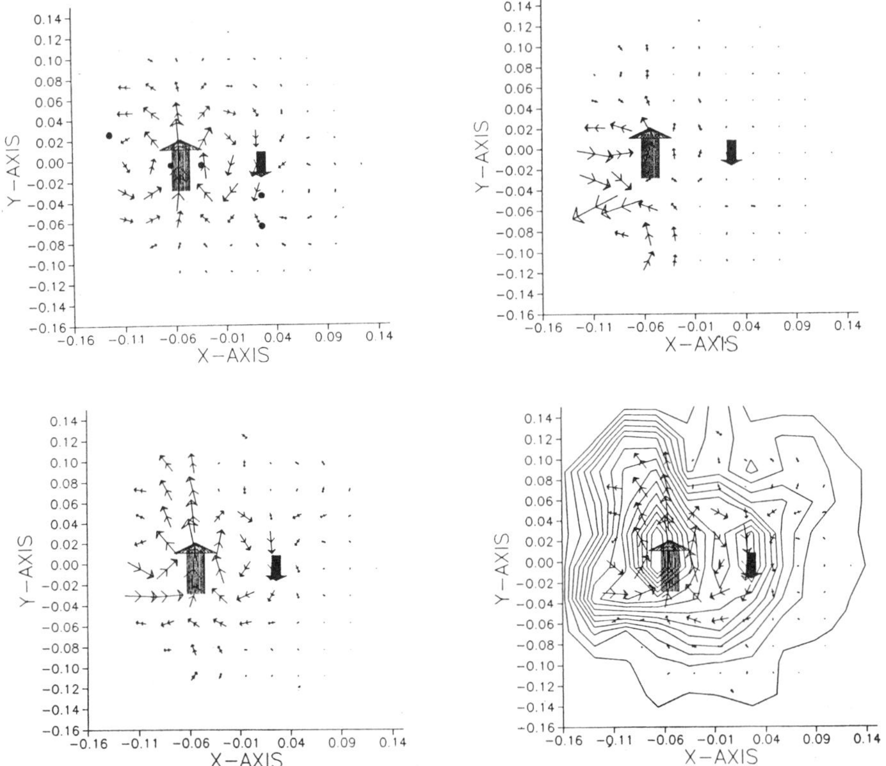

Figure 1. Solutions for two point sources in a homogeneous disk. Light arrows represent our continuous solution sampled at regular intervals. Heavy arrows indicate the target source.

Solving the inverse problem for a field generated by two point sources provides a severe test for our method which is designed to deal with continuous current densities. The next example uses the same measurement geometry and a target field produced by a set of 11 current dipoles. These dipoles extend along the x-axis from -10 cm to $+10$ cm at a fixed depth of 7 cm below the plane of measurements; they point along the y-axis and their strength varies smoothly. This source distribution is a good approximation to a 1D continuous current density. The source space Q is taken to be the x-axis with uniform probability from -13 cm to $+13$ cm and zero elsewhere; all components of the current density are allowed. Figure 2a shows the result of inverting using Equations 1 - 4 with just 5 data points and their ϕ functions. Using our improved method based on Equations 5 and 6 a much more satisfactory solution can be achieved. Our best result (Figure 2b) was obtained by using all 121 data, 20 expansion functions and $\tilde{\zeta} = 0.1$. The target field considered here approximates that of a single current dipole and standard inversion methods, based on fitting to point sources, would give the misleading impression that the source was indeed localised. Our method is able to give a more realistic picture of the true current density.

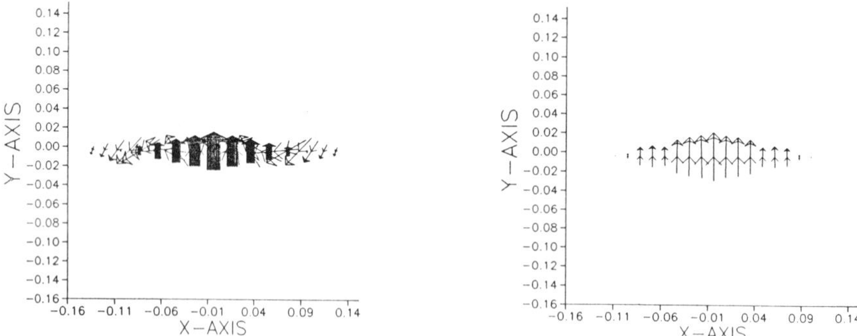

Figure 2. Solutions for a quasi-continuous 1D distribution of current density. The heavy arrows representing the target source have been omitted from Fig. 2b so as not to obscure our solution.

The results in this paper illustrate the potential of our method to resolve distinct regions of activity as well as provide reasonable estimates for distributed sources through simple examples. A more detailed description of our method, including a comprehensive range examples with different types of sources and experimental arrangements will be given elsewhere. In the next paper [6] we describe full 3D inversions and animations of the reconstructed current density at the level of the visual cortex, as a function of latency, from visually evoked field measurements following the reversal of a checkerboard pattern.

References

[1] M. S. Hämäläinen and R. S. Ilmoniemi. Preprint TKK-F-A559, Helsinki University of Technology (1984).

[2] A. A. Ioannides, In: Advances in Electronics and Electron Physics Supplement 19, Inverse Problems: An Interdisciplinary Study,pp 205-216, P. C. Sabatier ed, Academic Press, Orlando (1987).

[3] L. Narici, I. Modena, M. Peresson, V. Pizzella, G. L. Romani and G. Torrioli, In: Biomagnetism 1987, pp 134-137 K. Atsumi, M. Kotani, S. Ueno, T. Katila and S. J. Williamson eds,Tokyo Denki University Press, Tokyo 1988.

[4] R. J. Ilmoniemi, S. J. Williamson and W. E. Hostetler, In: Biomagnetism 1987, pp 182-185 K. Atsumi, M. Kotani, S. Ueno, T. Katila and S. J. Williamson eds,Tokyo Denki University Press, Tokyo 1988.

[5] C. J. S. Clarke and B. S. Janday, In Inverse Problems 5 (1989) 483-500.

[6] A. A. Ioannides, J. P. R. Bolton R. Hasson and C. J. S. Clarke ; Localised and distributed source solutions for the biomagnetic inverse problem II. In this volume.

[7] M. S. Hämäläinen, H Haario and M S Lehtinen. Preprint TKK-F-A620, Helsinki University of Technology (1987).

LOCALISED AND DISTRIBUTED SOURCE SOLUTIONS FOR THE BIOMAGNETIC INVERSE PROBLEM II

A. A. Ioannides, J. P. R. Bolton and R. Hasson
Physics Department, The Open University, Milton Keynes, MK7 6AA, UK.

C. J. S. Clarke
Faculty of Mathematical Studies, University of Southampton, Southampton, UK.

INTRODUCTION

The previous paper [1] has described powerful techniques for solving the biomagnetic inverse problem and contained model inversions confined to one and two-dimensional trial source space. The basic formalism allows the use of prior knowledge about the sources through a probability weight fuction and regularisation parameter. A more detailed description of the method, its sensitivity to noise and detector position and some extensions, including a comprehensive set of examples with both current densities and magnetic dipoles will be given elsewhere.

Attempts to extend our calculations to fully three-dimensional reconstructions or to analyse time-varying MEG data lead to a serious difficulty: the computation time required on a standard university computer becomes prohibitively large. Some of our tests with two-dimensional reconstrunctions required ten hours of CPU time. To overcome this obstacle we exploited the natural way in which the biomagnetic inverse problem lends itself to parallelism [2]. One of us (RH) translated the bulk of our FORTRAN programs into an efficient OCCAM code running on our SERC funded transputer array; in this paper we report the first applications of this work.

PARALLEL PROCESSING

We are using an INMOS parallel processor, which has thirty separate T800 transputers, each with an integral floating point unit. The topology of our parallel processing array is dynamically variable, but since our algorithms are dominated by heavy computation, rather than by communication, we have chosen to arrange the transputers in a linear array; this simplifies some of the coding and leads to practically no loss in performance. We used the OCCAM2 programming language, which we have found to be both convenient and powerful enough for our needs.

Two of the transputers are allocated to specific tasks, namely input/output and graphics, while the remaining 28 constitute the main task force for number crunching. The problem can be divided between them in several ways. The way that we found to be most efficient was to divide space into 28 regions and allocate a transputer to each region (geometric parallelism).

THREE-DIMENSIONAL SOURCE RECONSTRUCTION

In general terms, it is harder to localise sources in three dimensions than in two. The use of data from more than one plane of measurement can help, as does a number of refinements of the basic technique — notably, the use of regularisation, weight functions [1] and iteration. Details of our comprehensive tests and model studies will be published elsewhere. Perhaps the most surprising discovery has been that it is possible to recover some depth information, particularly regarding the direction of the local current density, from data collected in a *single* plane of measurement. We show here just one example of a 3D reconstruction from an $x - y$ plane of measurements. The signal is gen-

Advances in Biomagnetism
Edited by S.J. Williamson *et al.*
Plenum Press, New York

erated by two current dipoles directly below the plane of measurement at depths of 4 and 8 cm below the bottom coil of the gradiometer, and pointing in opposite directions. The source space is taken to be a cylinder with top and bottom faces at the level of the two sources. The radius of the cylinder is 4.5 cm and the a priori probability is weighted to favour deep sources. Note that, although our continuous solution has difficulty reproducing the magnitude of the lower source, it does successfully predict a reversal in the direction of the current density, as the cylinder is traversed from top to bottom.

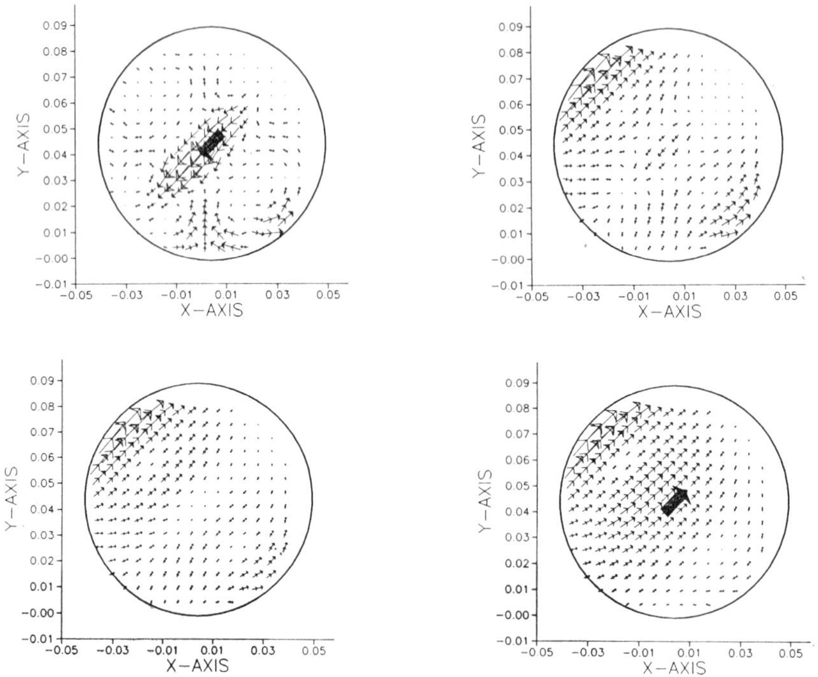

Figure 1. Three-dimensional inversion from computer generated data in a single $x - y$ plane; our continuous solution is shown at four slices through the cylindrical source space beginning at the level of the top source (Figure 1a) and successively increasing the depth until we reach the level of the bottom source (Figure 1d). Heavy arrows in Figures 1a and 1d represent the position and direction of the two point sources. Light arrows represent our continuous current density sampled at regular intervals. Note that the normalisation varies between figures; the maximum current density in Figure 1a is about 50 times greater than in Figure 1d.

ANALYSIS OF VISUALLY EVOKED RESPONSES

The problems we have examined so far all involved computer generated signals with added random noise of the order typically encountered in biomagnetic measurements. We now present our first attempt to analyse real MEG signals. These data were obtained at the Open University with a standard single-channel second order symmetric gradiometer [3]. They comprise sequences of evoked field measurements, on a single subject, following the reversal of a checkerboard pattern. Three sequences were generated, one in which the pattern occupied the right-bottom-quarter visual field (exp-B), one for top-quarter visual field (exp-T) and one for the half-right visual field (exp-H). Each data sequence consisted of 68 maps separated by 6 ms, with each map containing the z-component of the magnetic field, sampled at 42 points on an $x - y$ rectangular grid, tangential to the head at Cz (10-20 system). The minimum lower-coil scalp separation was 13 mm. In order to increase the signal-to-noise ratio all data sets were averaged over hundreds of repeated runs.

We have analysed these measurements in a variety of ways, restricting the source space to be a two dimensional disk as well as a full three dimensional region of space. For each case we have both allowed for return currents (within the conducting sphere model) and performed inversions in which the return currents were ignored. In all cases the results were quite similar, reflecting the fact that the experimental arrangement is preferentially sensitive to superficial sources. We will present results for just one analysis in which the middle coil of the gradiometer is at $z = 0.0$ and the source space is taken to be an $x - y$ disk of primary current density, with uniform a priori probability, embedded in a conducting sphere. The centre of the disk is at (0.0 0.04 −0.07)m while the centre of the sphere is at (0.0 0.04 −0.13)m. We have applied our regularised method using all 42 data, 42 expansion terms and $\zeta = 1.0$. Animated sequences, 68 frames long, clearly show the arrival of a signal at the visual cortex at a latency of about 84 ms with peak activity at about 100 ms. These animations [4] constitute the first example of truly functional imaging of biomagnetic signals: ***the source activity itself*** can be seen developing in space and time in both magnitude and direction! A number of different animations were constructed involving either the current density or its rate of change, the latter being particularly useful in pinpointing the onset of a new activity or the decay of a process. Of course, it is not feasible to show our animations here but Figure 2 shows some sample frames.

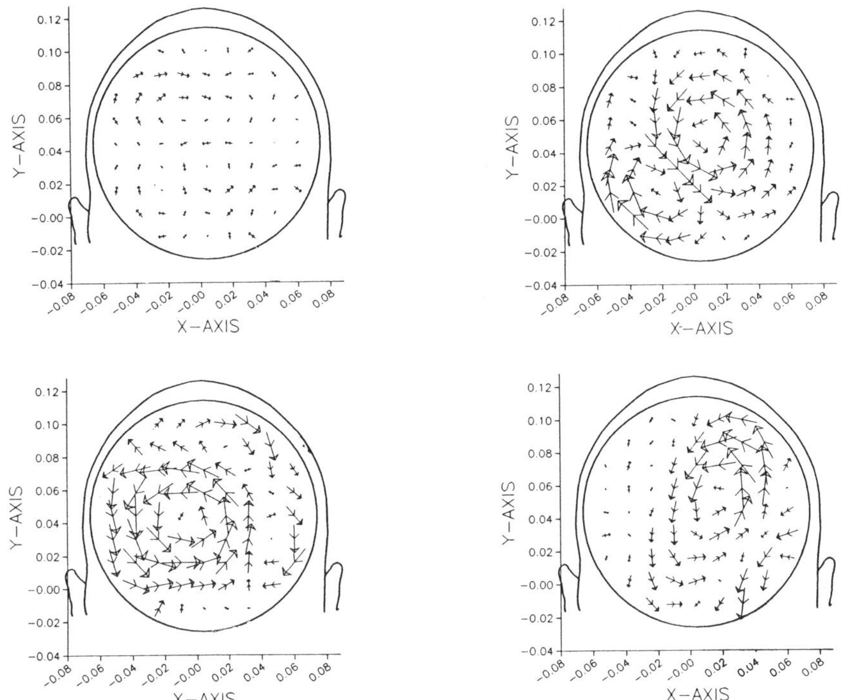

Figure 2. Figure 2a shows our solution at an early latency (36 ms) for exp-B while the rest show the solution at 102 ms latency (corresponding to maximum effective source power) for exp-B (2b), exp-T (2c) and exp-H (2d). The arrows represent the projection of the current density vector on the $x - y$ plane. For ease of comparison the arrows in each graph are normalised in an identical manner.

Our experience with model sources has shown that our method provides a very reliable guide to the *direction* of the true current density (cf. Figure 1). It is therefore interesting to note that our animations yield current density patterns that rotate as time progresses, consistent with models of the propagation of spiral waves in excitable media [5]. The suggestion that such a mode of propagation might exist in the brain was first made in connection with epileptic attack [6] but, so far as we are aware, this is the first time that evidence for spiral wave propagation has been associated with normal brain activity.

Further insight into our results can be obtained by following the time evolution of the square of the current density integrated over a region of source space and so finding the power output emanating from that region as a function of time. Figure 3 shows the results obtained from exp-B and exp-T by integrating the square of the current density over the entire (disk-shaped) source space. As expected, the most obvious feature is the peak at about 100 ms corresponding to the maximal activity at the visual cortex but other significant features are also discernible. A careful analysis of the frequency spectrum [7] reveals a strikingly consistent pattern in all three experiments and in particular a clear peak in source activity at a latency of 40 ms, much earlier than the arrival of the first signal at the visual cortex. This suggests that our method may be able to identify activity from deep within the brain. We believe that new and exciting results will be produced by applying our method to measurements taken with state of the art multi-channel systems.

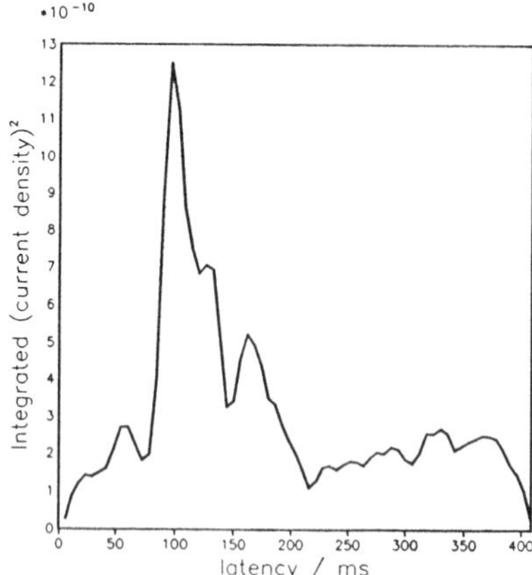

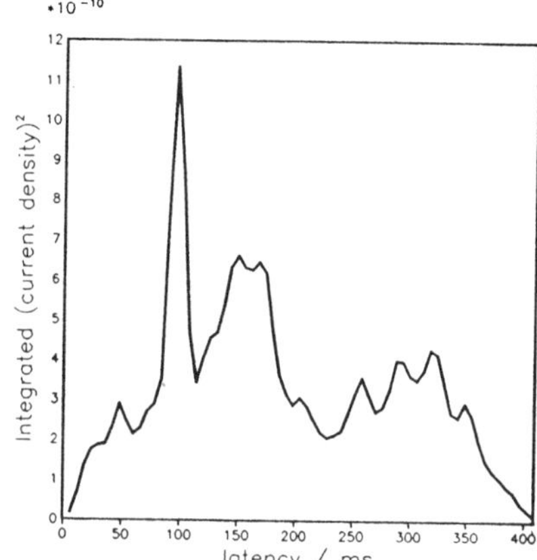

Figure 3. Plots of the square of the current density, integrated over the source space, as a function of latency, derived from MEG measurements for bottom-quarter-field (Figure 3a) and top-quarter-field (Figure 3b) pattern reversal stimulation.

CONCLUSION

In this paper we have outlined a small part of what can be done with the powerful methods and computational systems we have developed. In addition to obvious clinical applications, we believe that these results, and others obtained in a similar way, will contribute substantially to an understanding of the functional organization of the brain.

ACKNOWLEDGEMENTS

The work on parallel processing was supported by an SERC grant, under the Computational Science Initiative.

References

[1] C. J. S. Clarke, A. A. Ioannides and J. P. R. Bolton ; Localised and distributed source solutions for the biomagnetic inverse problem I. In this volume.

[2] A. A. Ioannides ; Trends in computational tools for biomagnetism: from procedural codes to intelligent scientific models in Phys. Med. Biol. 32 (1987) 77-83

[3] B. S. Janday, S. J. Swithenby and I. M. Thomas; Combined Magnetic Field and Electrical Potential Investigation of the Visual Pattern Reversal Response In: Biomagnetism 1987, pp 134-137 K. Atsumi, M. Kotani, S. Ueno, T. Katila and S. J. Williamson eds,Tokyo Denki University Press, Tokyo 1988.

[4] A. A. Ioannides, R. Hasson and J. P. R. Bolton ; Spatial and Temporal Evolution of Brain Activity; Open University video July 1989.

[5] John Tyson and J. D. Murray ; Cyclic AMP waves during aggregation Dictyostelium amoeba; In Development 106(3) (1989) 421-426

[6] H. Petche, O. Prohaska, P. Rappelsberger, R. Volmer and A. Kaiser; Cortical seizure patterns in multidimensional view: information content of equipotential maps; In Epilepsia 15 (1974) 439-463

[7] G. J. Miseldine and A. A. Ioannides; Cleaning up biomagnetic signals and biomagnetic inverse problem solutions; work in progress.

RANDOM DIPOLES AS A MODEL FOR SPONTANEOUS EEG- AND MEG- ACTIVITY

J.C. De Munck, P.C.M. Vijn, and H. Spekreijse

The Netherlands Ophthalmic Research Institute
and the Laboratory of Medical Physics
P.O.Box 12141, 1100 AC, Amsterdam ZO, The Netherlands

INTRODUCTION

A serious obstacle for the interpretation of evoked electromagnetic fields is the presence of noise in the data. The background EEG is considered as the major origin of noise for evoked potentials. Also for evoked magnetic fields (EMF) the spontaneous brain activity is an important factor (Knuutila and Hämäläinen, 1987). When the statistical properties of this noise are known, confidence limits of estimated (dipole) parameters can be calculated (Sarvas, 1987) and noise filters can be designed to improve the signal to noise ratio. For this purpose we studied the spontaneous brain activity and formulated a mathematical model, which predicts the statistics of the electromagnetic field of the brain. Since the model gives the spatial covariance matrix in analytic form, this matrix needs not to be estimated every time an EMF is recorded.

THEORY

Since the EEG reflects activity of many neurons the appearance of the EEG is chaotic. Our model assumes that the physical mechanisms responsible for the background EEG and EPs are similar. Contrary to the EPs, which are deterministic, the scalp EEG will be described with stochastic source parameters $\underline{\vec{P}}(t)$. These parameters give rise to a stochastic potential distribution, and a stochastic magnetic induction:

$$\underline{\chi}(\vec{x},\vec{P}(t)) = \psi(\vec{x},\underline{\vec{P}}(t)) \qquad ; \qquad \underline{\vec{B}}(\vec{x},\vec{P}(t)) = \vec{B}(\vec{x},\underline{\vec{P}}(t)) \qquad , \qquad (1)$$

where $\vec{x}$ is the recording site. These two equations form the basis of our theory. They imply that when an EEG or a MEG is recorded, a finite number of sources is active at randomly distributed positions and orientations. The source parameters result from stochastic processes. The stochastic signals, caused by the instantaneous source strengths are transmitted through the volume conductor, according to the laws of Maxwell. This transmission is determined by the volume conductor used, i.e. by the dependence of ψ and $\vec{B}$ on $\vec{P}$.

The statistics of the electromagnetic fields can be expressed in terms of the probability density function $f(\vec{P};\ t)$ of the sources. Assumptions about $f(\vec{P};\ t)$ can be

Advances in Biomagnetism
Edited by S.J. Williamson *et al.*
Plenum Press, New York

tested experimentally by estimating the covariance of the background activity and comparing the results with the theory. For simple volume conductor geometries and simple current source distributions, an analytic expression can be derived for the covariance of the EM-field. Estimation of the mean of the potential is not useful, since EEG-amplifiers are AC-coupled. Also MEG-signals are usually band-pass filtered. In both cases the means are zero. The expression for the covariance of the potential,

$$\begin{aligned} \mathrm{Cov}(\chi_1,\chi_2) &\equiv E\{\chi(\vec{x}_1,t_1),\chi(\vec{x}_2,t_2)\} \\ &= \int d\vec{P}_1 \int d\vec{P}_2\, f_{PP}(\vec{P}_1,\vec{P}_2;\, t_1,t_2)\; \psi(\vec{x}_1,\vec{P}_1)\; \psi(\vec{x}_2,\vec{P}_2) \end{aligned} \tag{2}$$

is not easy to handle in its general form. Therefore, assumptions are needed to obtain easier expressions, yet maintaining physiological significance.

First, it is assumed that the EEG is caused by a finite number N of statistically independent sources. Then the covariance can be expressed as the sums of the covariances of the single sources. Second, it is assumed that only the source strengths depend on time, and that the (random) geometry parameters of the sources are statistically independent of strength. In a formula these two assumptions can be represented as follows:

$$\mathrm{Cov}(\chi_1,\chi_2) = \sum_{n=1}^{N} \mathrm{Cov}(\chi_1^{(n)},\chi_2^{(n)}) = \sum_{n=1}^{N} S_n(t_1,t_2)\, X_n(\vec{x}_1,\vec{x}_2) \quad , \tag{3}$$

where S_n is the autocovariance of the n-th source, and $X_n(\vec{x}_1,\vec{x}_2)$ is the spatial covariance between the potential measured at $\vec{x}_1$ and $\vec{x}_2$. For the magnetic induction similar simplifications can be obtained.

To simplify this expression further, it will be assumed that the sources are dipoles, that are randomly distributed without preference for the ϑ- and φ- directions in a spherical volume conductor. With these assumptions the covariance depends only on the distance between the electrode pair. In the following this distance is expressed as the angle ω_{12} [degrees] with respect to the center of the head.

We found the following expansion of X_n in Legendre polynomials:

$$X_n(\vec{x}_1,\vec{x}_2) = \sum_{k=1}^{\infty} f_k^2\, r_0^{2k-2}\, \frac{2k^2 M_{rad}^2 + k(k+1)M_{tan}^2}{2k+1}\, P_k(\cos\omega_{12}) \quad , \tag{4}$$

where f_k describes the conductivities and radii of the volume conductor (De Munck, 1988). If the magnetic induction is measured with a first order gradiometer, normally oriented with respect to the head, the covariance between two such measurements is

$$\Sigma_n(\vec{x}_1,\vec{x}_2) = M_{tan}^2\, \mu_0^2 \sum_{k=1}^{\infty} \frac{k(k+1)^3}{2k+1}\, \frac{r_0^{2k-2}}{r^{2k+4}}\, P_k(\cos\omega_{12}) \quad . \tag{5}$$

The full derivation of Eqs. (4) and (5) can be found in De Munck (1989).

MODEL PREDICTIONS

To circumvent complications due to the reference electrode we will consider only the variance of potential differences, instead of the covariances themselves. This approach does not limit the generality, since the covariance between two differentially measured potentials can be expressed in terms of the variances:

$$\mathrm{Cov}(\chi_1\text{-}\chi_3,\chi_2\text{-}\chi_4) = \frac{1}{2}\Big\{ \mathrm{Var}(\chi_1\text{-}\chi_4)+\mathrm{Var}(\chi_2\text{-}\chi_3)-\mathrm{Var}(\chi_1\text{-}\chi_2)-\mathrm{Var}(\chi_3\text{-}\chi_4) \Big\} . \tag{6}$$

For magnetic recordings this complication does not exist.

In order to study the variance function of a rotationally symmetric model, we have plotted in fig. 1 the variance against the electrode distance ω_{12} for several depths r_0 of the sources. Fig. 2 gives similarly the covariance function for a first order gradiometer. It can be seen that the variance function is insensitive for depth. For small r_0 the function approaches $2\text{-}2\cos\omega_{12}$ which is the first term in the Legendre polynomial expansion. The mathematical reason for the depth invariance is that the smoothing effect of the skull appears quadratically in Eq. (4). For magnetic measurements, the covariance is more sensitive for source depth. If the random dipoles are at a spherical shell of radius *.7*, then the MEG-recordings which are separated more than about 50^0, become uncorrelated. For the electric potential such a correlation distance can not be given, since it depends on the location of the reference electrode.

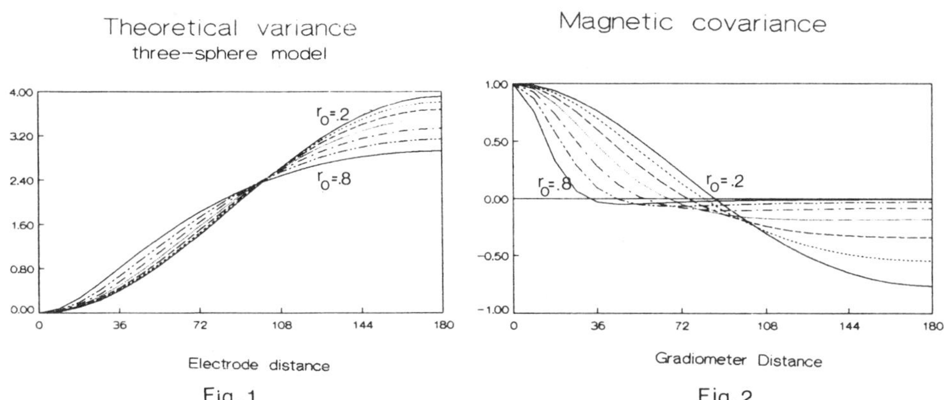

Fig.1

Fig.2

EXPERIMENTS

To test experimentally whether in some frequency bands the electric variance function is rotationally symmetric, as assumed in Eq. (4) we recorded segments of EEG of a subject watching random textures. The variances of these samples are plotted as a function of the electrode distance in figs. 3 (*0* - *8* Hz) and 4 (*12* - *30* Hz). The figures show that in the frequency bands chosen, the variance is mainly a function of electrode distance. For the α-band, (not shown), the variance changed less systematically with electrode distance.

To test the magnetic part of the theory, we used the magnetic covariance matrix estimated by Knuutila and Hämäläinen. These data are plotted in fig. 5 as a function of magnetometer distance. It can be seen that the spatial correlation decreases with distance, in accordance to the predictions of fig. 2. Since, however, the maximum magnetometer distance was only 42^0, further experiments are needed to test the theory more generally.

DISCUSSION

The agreement between theory and experiment suggests that the model predictions can be used for statistical analysis of evoked magnetic and electric fields. In particular, confidence limits and significance levels of (dipole) parameter estimations can be calculated.

Since the random dipole model used is based on physiologically meaningful assumptions, the estimated (co)-variance functions say something about the condition of the brain. Our data show that the generators of the EEG are in some frequency bands rotationally symmetric distributed, not so, however, for the α-band.

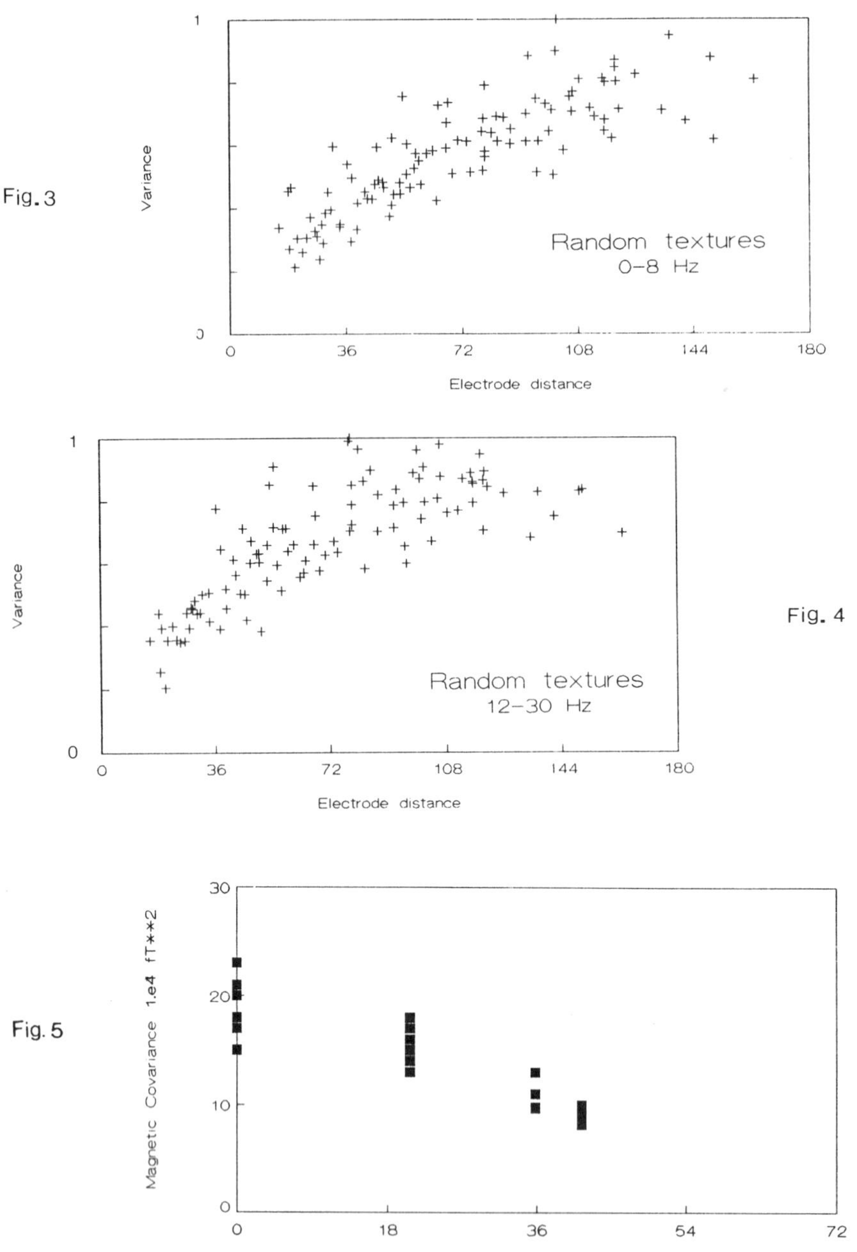

REFERENCES

J.C. De Munck, 1988, *The potential distribution in a layered anisotropic spheroidal volume conductor*, J. Appl. Phys. 64(2), pp. 464-470.

J.C. De Munck, 1989, *A mathematical and physical interpretation of the electromagnetic field of the brain*, PhD-thesis University of Amsterdam, Amsterdam.

J. Knuutila and M.S. Hämäläinen, 1987, *Characterization of brain noise using a high sensitivity 7-channel magnetometer*, Biomagnetism '87, Tokyo University Press, pp. 186-189.

J. Sarvas, 1987, *Basic mathematical and electromagnetic concepts of the biomagnetic inverse problem*, Phys. Med. Biol. 32(1), pp. 11-22.

THEORY AND PROPERTIES OF LEAD FIELD SYNTHESIS ANALYSIS

Stephen E. Robinson

Technology Department
Biomagnetic Technologies, Inc.
San Diego, CA 92121

INTRODUCTION

Background brain activity that is unrelated to that of the brain centers under study is often referred to as *brain noise*. This brain noise has posed a barrier to the measurement of brain activity arising from specific sites of interest within the brain. Signal averaging, which attenuates brain noise, is limited in use to measurement of brain activity evoked by repetitive stimuli. With present MEG and EEG technology it is brain noise, not sensor noise, that limits the ability of individual MEG and EEG sensors to discriminate spontaneous neural activity. For many studies, the ideal MEG or EEG sensor required should respond to one specific region of the brain, only, as do invasive depth electrodes. To address this need, we have developed a signal analysis process for combining simultaneous measurements made from multiple physical sensors into a synthetic *virtual sensor* having spatially selective and directional properties. This technique, termed *lead field synthesis* (LFS), was verified by computer model and with actual evoked field MEG measurements.

THEORETICAL BASIS

In the three-dimensional space of the brain (termed *source space*), each current source has a specific location and orientation[1]. Each current source in source space maps to a location in a multidimensional *signal space*[2] (Ilmoniemi, *et al*, 1987). A linear spatially-selective filter can be derived for a given current source $\vec{q}(\vec{r})$ as a projection operation in signal space -- that is, the dot-product of the signal vector $\vec{S}(t)$ with some weighting vector $\vec{W}(\vec{q},\vec{r})$:

$$\Lambda(\vec{q},\vec{r},t) = \vec{S}(t)\cdot\vec{W}(\vec{q},\vec{r}) \tag{1}$$

where $\Lambda(\vec{q},\vec{r},t)$ is the spatially-filtered time-series for the specified source. The term *target source* will be used here to distinguish the source to be measured from the brain-noise sources. The signal measured by the virtual sensor can be thought of as meaning *how much of the measured signals from all physical sensors could be attributed to the modeled target source*. The spatial filter is designated by parameters for the target source model -- for example, a current dipole, as used in the preceding example -- and the source's location and orientation, which may be specified using measurements from MRI or CT scans, from a brain atlas, or, where feasible, from a trial determination such as a dipole fit from averaged signals.

---

1 For the purpose of this discussion we assume that a given source is point-like, e.g.: a current dipole. Spatial filters may be designated for any realizable source model, including extended current sources.

2 An instrument simultaneously measuring 14 MEG channels and 6 EEG channels is said to possess a 20-dimensional signal space.

Advances in Biomagnetism
Edited by S.J. Williamson *et al.*
Plenum Press, New York

It is the weighting vector that determines the spatial and angular selectivity as well as the instrument noise level of the virtual sensor, given the sensor geometry, conductive model for the head and primary current source. The target source is represented by a signal space vector, as are all the brain-noise sources. Intuitively, one expects that the spatial filter weighting vector should be directed at the target source in signal space because the target signal projection on this vector will be maximal for this vector.

A simple spatial filter can be generated by normalizing the forward solution for the response B of each of M sensors to a unit (1 Ampere-meter) target source $\vec{q}(\vec{r})$. Each element of the weighting vector is:

$$W_i(\vec{q},\vec{r}) = \frac{B_i(\vec{q},\vec{r})}{\sum_{j=1}^{M} B_j^2(\vec{q},\vec{r})} \qquad i = 1 \cdots M \tag{2}$$

One observes that, since this $\vec{W}(\vec{q},\vec{r})$ has the maximal projection of $\vec{q}(\vec{r})$, it must therefore be the quietest virtual sensor in terms of equivalent instrumental noise (but not brain noise). In fact, the instrumental noise of any virtual sensor N_Λ is simply:

$$N_\Lambda = \sqrt{\sum_{i=1}^{M} (N_i W_i)^2} \tag{3}$$

where N_i is the noise of ith physical sensor.

More selective spatial filters may be generated by accounting for the rest of the source space, as well as the target source. As spatial selectivity is increased, brain noise decreases, because the spatial transfer function tends to attenuate these sources. However, an increase in spatial selectivity implies that $\vec{W}$ is being directed orthogonal to the projection of the brain noise sources. Since the signal-space representation of the brain noise sources are not necessarily orthogonal to that of the target source, a coefficient vector attenuating brain noise may also result in a smaller projection of the target signal. Maintenance of the target signal projection in source-strength units requires that the magnitude of the coefficient vector increase as $\vec{W}$ is rotated away from $\vec{q}(\vec{r})$. From equation (3) one sees that the virtual sensor instrumental noise increases in proportion to the magnitude of $\vec{W}$.

Some methods identified for generating coefficients for spatially selective filters are: spectral decomposition of the generalized inverse solution, optimal fitting (by minimization) of a coefficient vector to a specified modeled spatial transfer function, and adaptive signal processing, using measurements of signal and brain noise to generate the coefficients (for which the spatial transfer function is unknown and must be solved for *after* the adaptation process).

The tradeoff between the deltaness and variance of inverse solutions was first described by Backus and Gilbert; solutions to this tradeoff were reviewed by Parker (1977). As applied to spatial filtering, Backus-Gilbert theory (BGT) describes the tradeoff between spatial selectivity (deltaness) and error due to sensor noise (variance). To illustrate this tradeoff, a computer simulation of an array of sources in a two-dimensional space was performed. A family of spatial filter coefficients were calculated by varying the emphasis assigned to either a function of selectivity (the integral of the transfer function over the source region) and a function of sensor noise (the sum of squares of the coefficients). The resulting BGT tradeoff curve is shown in Figure 1. All realizable LFS weighting coefficients lie within the bounds of the tradeoff curve. The optimal LFS coefficients lie on the boundary of the tradeoff curve between minimum deltaness and minimum variance.

EXPERIMENTAL METHODS

An auditory evoked response measurement was made using two 7-channel Neuromagnetometers. Stimulus consisted of a 1 kHz tone bursts, repeated at 2 second intervals. The tone was delivered monaurally to the contralateral ear, using an etymotic earphone. Each run consisted of 100 trials. The evoked response was characterized by multiple runs with different sensor placements. Subsequently, a dipole fit was performed to the signal-averaged responses, in order to obtain the target parameters. From all the runs, one was selected in which both seven-channel sensors had been placed in the proximity of the radial field extrema for the evoked response. The spatial filter coefficients were computed by spectral decomposition, using the dipole fit parameters to describe the target, and an array of modeled sources to describe the brain noise. The coefficients were then used together with the *unaveraged* MEG data to generate a virtual sensor channel. The virtual sensor time-series for each individual trial was plotted and viewed.

RESULTS

An evoked response was not visible in every trial when viewing either the virtual or physical sensor time-series. When a response was detectable, it was always difficult to discern in any of the physical MEG channels (Figure 2a) and was well-characterized by the virtual sensor (Figure 2b). That is to say, brain noise was suppressed and the signal-to-noise ratio for the desired auditory evoked response was improved by the virtual sensor.

DISCUSSION

The following properties were observed using both computer simulations and actual MEG data:

1. LFS exhibits spatial and orientation selectivity; the virtual sensor responds maximally to the region of interest in the brain, attenuating signals from other regions of the brain, or signals from regions differing in source current direction.
2. LFS transforms the units of measurement (magnetic flux density and/or electrical potential) into a source strength estimate (such as Ampere-meters, for a dipolar source model). Measurement units are dependent on location of the measurement and the geometry of the measuring device, whereas source strength is independent of the measuring system.
4. LFS permits estimation of source activity using simultaneous MEG and EEG sensor information.
5. LFS can reduce the effective sensor instrumental (SQUID) noise level by spatial signal averaging.
6. LFS can be applied to any source model -- not merely the current dipole model.

ACKNOWLEDGEMENTS

This work was supported in part by the U.S. Air Force Armstrong Aerospace Medical Research Laboratory under SBIR contract F33615-87-C-0537. The author gratefully acknowledges assistance from C. Crowley in providing a two-dimensional simulation of the Backus-Gilbert tradeoff.

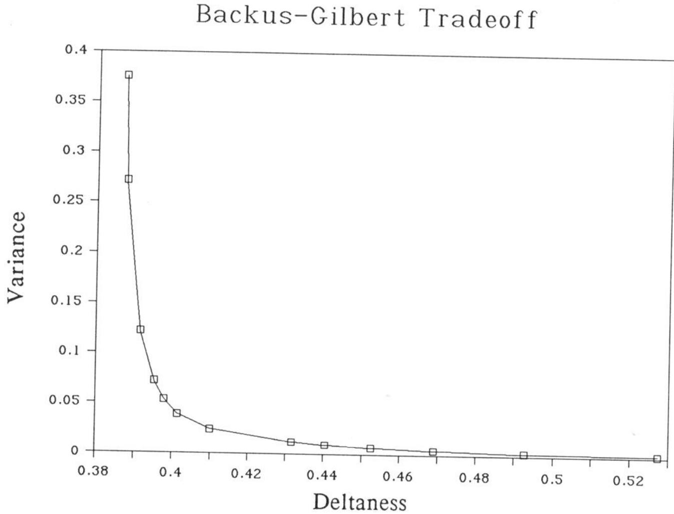

Figure 1. Backus-Gilbert tradeoff curve for two-dimensional simulation. Units of deltaness and variance are arbitrary. Deltaness is a measure of a virtual sensor's spatial selectivity; variance is a measure of a virtual sensor's noise level.

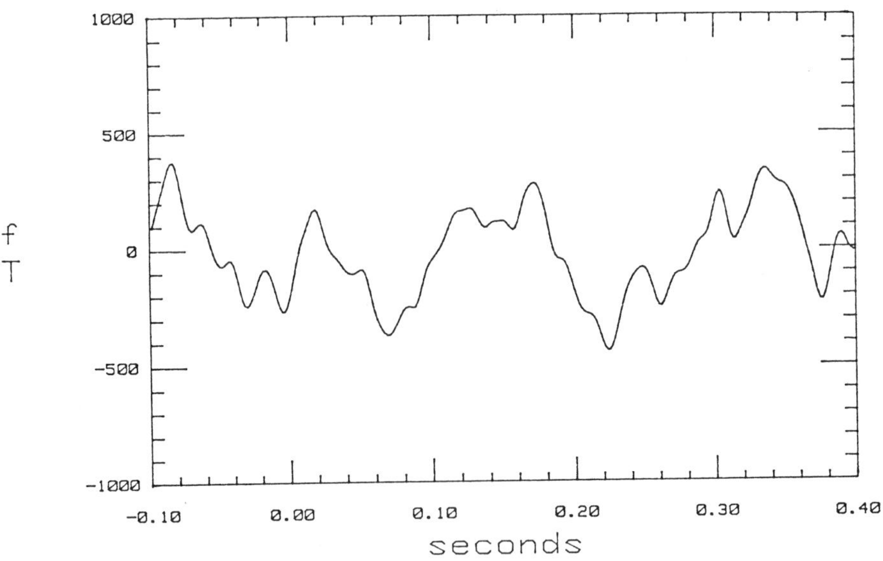

Figure 2a. Physical MEG sensor single-epoch (unaveraged) auditory evoked response. The stimulus onset is at 0.0 seconds. This sensor was near to a field extremum and has the best signal-to-noise ratio of the fourteen channels.

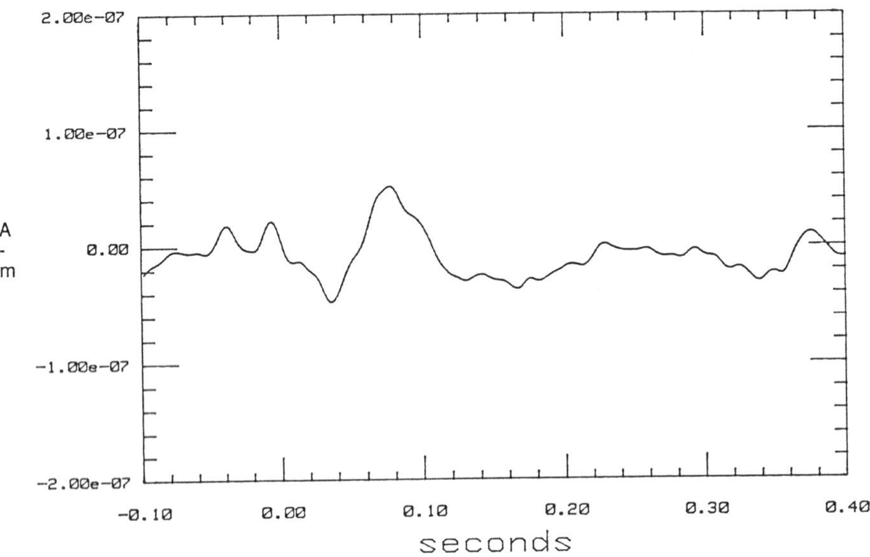

Figure 2b. Virtual sensor single-epoch (unaveraged) auditory evoked response. The data is for the same epoch as in Figure 2a. The response to the auditory stimulus is visible because brain noise has been suppressed. This virtual sensor is the linear combination of fourteen MEG channels.

REFERENCES

Parker, R.L. (1977). Understanding inverse theory. Ann Rev Earth Planet Sci 5, 35-64.

Ilmoniemi, R.J., Williamson, S.J., and Hostetler, W.E. (1987). New method for the study of spontaneous brain activity. In: Atsumi, K., Kotani, M., Ueno, S., Katila, T., and Williamson, S.J. (Eds.) "Biomagnetism '87". Tokyo Denki University Press, pp. 182-185.

MINIMUM NORM ESTIMATION OF CURRENT DISTRIBUTIONS IN REALISTIC GEOMETRIES

Christopher W. Crowley, Richard E. Greenblatt, Ismail Khalil
Biomagnetic Technologies Inc.
4174 Sorrento Valley Blvd.
San Diego, CA 92121 USA

INTRODUCTION

The inverse problem in biomagnetism is solved conventionally by representing the primary current distribution as a single equivalent current dipole via a non-linear iterative technique (Cuffin and Cohen, 1977). Such estimates may be unrealistic in some circumstances, however, such as with a distributed primary current. Linear estimation of the minimum norm current distribution (Sarvas, 1987) provides an alternative in cases where there is no *a priori* justification for assuming that the source activity is dipolar. Techniques for obtaining linear estimates of total current densities are described by Jeffs *et al.* (1987). Linear estimates of primary current density have been explored by several researchers for planar geometries (Hamalainen and Ilmoniemi, 1984; Dallas, 1985; Singh *et al.*, 1985). In this paper, we outline a technique that combines linear estimation theory with finite element analysis to construct primary current distributions in brain and heart models. The use of minimum norm estimation is motivated by mathematical rather than physiological or anatomical considerations, and one goal of our work is to investigate the feasibility of the method through experimental measurements.

THEORETICAL BASIS

The primary current distribution, $\vec{J}_p(\vec{r})$, is confined to some region, Ω, which may represent the brain or the heart. We consider $\vec{J}_p(\vec{r})$ to be an element of an infinite dimensional Hilbert space, $H(\Omega)$. Each primary current in $H(\Omega)$ is mapped to a field measurement, e_i, by

$$e_i = \int_\Omega \vec{J}_p(\vec{r}) \cdot \vec{G}_i(\vec{r}) \; d\vec{r} \tag{1}$$

The function $\vec{G}_i(\vec{r})$, which is often called the "lead field", depends on the location and orientation of the ith detector. Note that the lead field in Eq. (1) must account for the effects of volume currents and therefore the $\vec{G}_i(\vec{r})$ cannot be obtained directly from the Biot-Savart law. As Hamalainen and Ilmoneimi (1984) point out, from a set of n detector measurements, it is possible to determine the projection of the primary currents onto the span of the lead fields. Provided the lead fields are linearly independent, this projection represents the minimum norm estimate of $\vec{J}_p(\vec{r})$, in $H(\Omega)$. Note that the nonuniqueness of the inverse problem implies that no component of primary current orthogonal to the lead fields can be determined from any of the detector measurements.

In practice, minimum norm estimates are unstable with respect to measurement and modeling error. However, as described by Parker (1977), robust minimum norm estimates may be obtained by a spectral expansion that allows elimination of combinations of lead fields that are too sensitive. In realistic geometries, generally we do not have an explicit expression for the lead fields in Eq. (1), so our technique does not directly follow the methodology described by Parker. The basis of our method is to represent the primary current distribution parametrically by using a volumetric finite element discretization of the source region $H(\Omega)$ (Zinkiewicz, 1977). Using the finite element model, the continuous primary current distribution is represented

Advances in Biomagnetism
Edited by S.J. Williamson *et al.*
Plenum Press, New York

in terms of samples of J_p at discrete points $\vec{r}_j$, together with continuous finite element interpolation functions, $f_j(\vec{r})$:

$$\vec{J}_p(\vec{r}) = \sum_{j=1}^{j=n} \vec{J}_p(\vec{r}_j) f_j(\vec{r}) \tag{2}$$

Now by considering each of the polynomial functions in the source region as individual sources, we define a matrix D where $(\mathbf{D})_{ij}$ represents the measurement of the jth source polynomial at the ith detector. The norm of any current distribution in the finite element source region can be expressed as

$$\int_\Omega |\vec{J}_p|^2 = \mathbf{j}^T \mathbf{A} \mathbf{j}, \quad \text{where} \quad (\mathbf{A})_{ij} = \int_\Omega f_i(\vec{r}) f_j(\vec{r}) d\Omega \tag{3}$$

and $\mathbf{j}$ is the vector containing the samples of J_p at the discrete points $\vec{r}_j$.

Equipped with these definitions, our minimum norm estimation problem can be written as a standard optimization problem:

$$\textit{Minimize} \quad \mathbf{j}^T \mathbf{A} \mathbf{j} \qquad \textit{subject to} \qquad \mathbf{D}\mathbf{j} = \mathbf{e} \tag{4}$$

where $\mathbf{e}$ is the vector containing the actual measurements e_i in Eq. (1). The solution to Eq. (4) may be obtained by introducing a change of variables:

$$\mathbf{j}' = \mathbf{G}^T \mathbf{j} \qquad \textit{where} \qquad \mathbf{G}\mathbf{G}^T = \mathbf{A} \tag{5}$$

Eq. (4) then becomes

$$\textit{Minimize} \quad \mathbf{j}'^T \mathbf{j}' \quad \textit{subject to} \quad \mathbf{D}'\mathbf{j}' = \mathbf{e} \qquad \textit{where} \qquad \mathbf{D}' = \mathbf{D}\mathbf{G}^{-T} \tag{6}$$

It is well known that Eq. (6) can be solved for $\mathbf{j}'$ by computing the generalized inverse of $\mathbf{D}'$ using the singular value decomposition (Strang, 1986). Our method is similar to that proposed by Jeffs *et al.* (1987), except that we use minimum norm estimation to find a continuous **primary** current distribution, while Jeffs *et al.* obtained a constrained multiple dipole estimate of the **total** current.

EXPERIMENTAL RESULTS

Phantom Verification. The robust minimum norm technique was applied to magnetic field recordings taken at 84 sites around a plastic phantom (Paulson, 1989). Figure 1a displays a wire frame representation of the spherical phantom with contour lines indicating the recorded magnetic fields. For reference, a best fit dipole is displayed as a cone inside the phantom. The shaded surface inside the wire frame represents the source region used for this study. Figure 1b displays a gray scale plot of the magnitude of the minimum norm source activity. The light area near the top of the source region indicates that the minimum norm estimate is consistent with the conventional dipole fit.

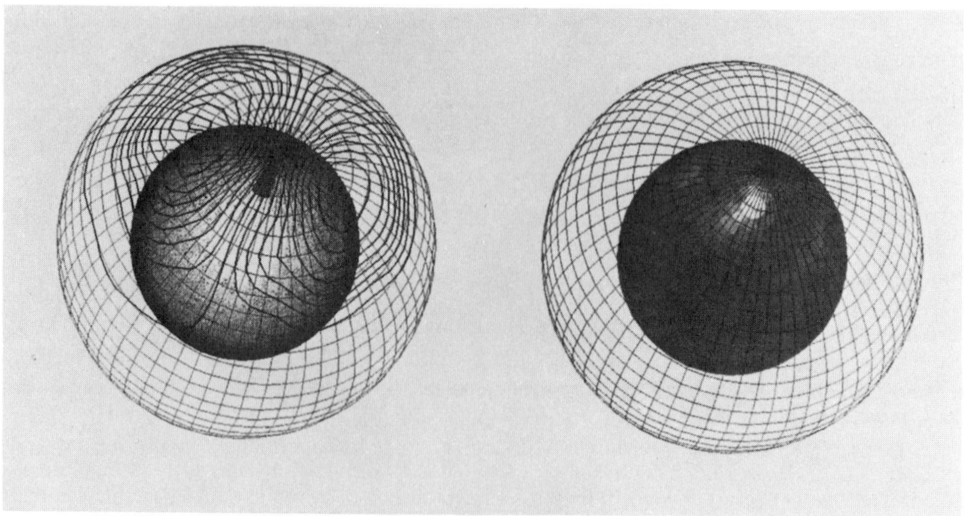

Figure 1. a) Wire frame representation of spherical phantom showing magnetic field contour lines, best fit dipole and source region Ω. b) Gray scale map shows magnitude of current density obtained by minimum norm estimation for the spherical phantom dipole.

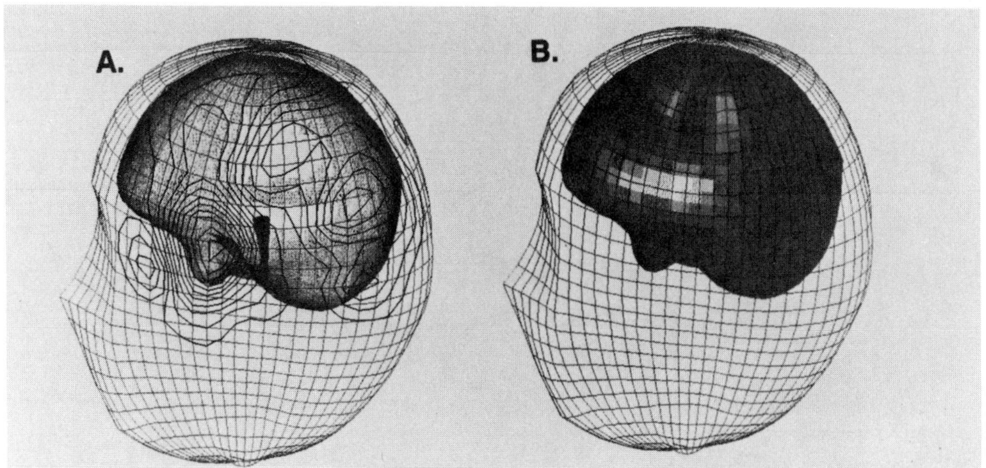

Figure 2. a) Field distribution and dipole location of the auditory evoked field 110 msec after the onset of a tone burst (average of 64 ipsilateral 500Hz tone bursts, 500 msec duration, 0 msec rise and fall time, recorded at 84 locations on the head with a BTi Model 607 second order 4 cm baseline Neuromagnetometer). The data was sampled at 200 Hz after analog filtering from 0.1-50 Hz. A mean interstimulus interval of 4 seconds randomized with a uniform distribution of ± 1 sec was used. Shaded brain shaped source region was modeled with 50 second order curvilinear finite elements. b) Gray scale activity map displays magnitude of the estimated primary current distribution (minimum norm estimate) for same latency.

Physiological measurements. Auditory evoked response measurements were obtained on two subjects using conventional techniques (e.g. Yamamoto *et al.*, 1988)as described in the legend to figure 2. Cardiac measurements for 1 subject were made as described in the legend to figure 3. In both cases, the inverse operator was computed for a parametric representation of primary current density using a local sphere polynomial representation for the forward solution for the individual current density elements (Sarvas, 1987), and this operator was then used to calculate the source activity maps at chosen latencies.

DISCUSSION

An auditory evoked field experiment for one subject is shown in figure 1. For both subjects tested, the m100 component, an apparently dipolar physiological source, produced a source map with much of the activity in the expected region. The mapped activity appeared to be somewhat more anterior and distributed than would be expected from the equivalent dipole solution. In addition, there appeared to be secondary sources of activity located caudal to the equivalent dipole. Figure 3 shows source activity maps for three phases of the cardiac cycle. Note in particular that activity appears in the right atrial region during the p-wave, and then moves to the ventricles during the rising phase of the r-wave.

Preliminary results indicate that linear source estimation techniques may be a useful complement to the conventional equivalent dipole representation for the MEG source localization problem. For the heart in particular, where equivalent dipole representations may be poor models of the underlying activity (Katila *et al.*, 1987), source activity mapping provides a physiologically plausible image of the pattern of electrical excitation. Our analysis of the data from the measurements shown here, as well as others not shown, indicate however, that the maps obtained from minimum norm estimation depend to a significant degree upon the sampling strategy employed. Unlike equivalent dipole solutions, which are fairly robust, minimum norm estimation will produce error if magnetic field extrema within the area used for the reconstruction are not sampled. As magnetometers with more channels become available, this problem may be reduced. In all cases, however, the minimum norm estimates appear to be somewhat superficial and delocalized.

ACKNOWLEDGEMENTS

Portions of this work were funded by HHS PHS grant 1R43NS24505. We thank S.E. Robinson and D.S. Buchanan for valuable suggestions and comments.

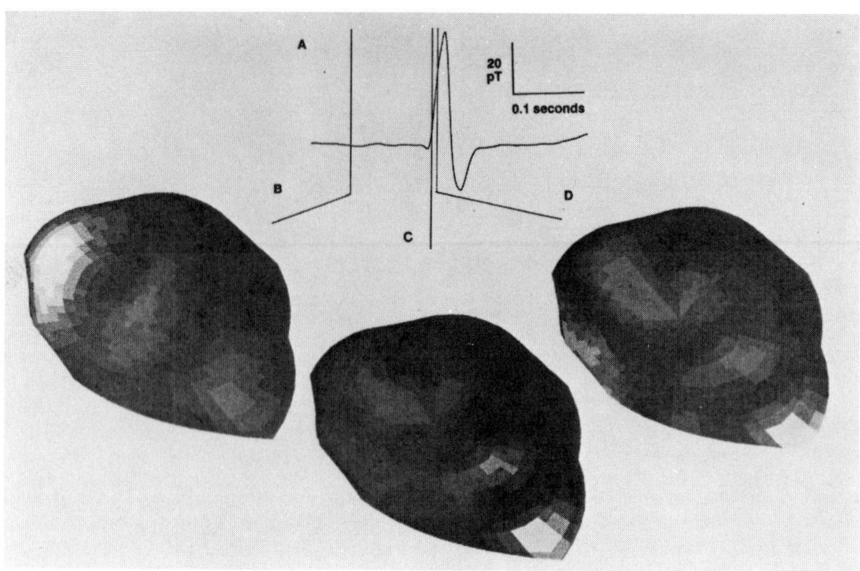

Figure 3. Source activity map for 3 time samples of the cardiac cycle. 3a illustrates an MCG lead from a normal adult male subject (average of 48 repetitions, aligned by maximizing ECG cross correlation). Data was acquired at a 512 Hz sampling rate after analog filtering from 0.1-100 Hz. The vertical lines (b, c, and d) indicate the time samples chosen for source activity mapping by linear estimation in figures 3b, 3c and 3d. Magnetic data were acquired on grid of 84 points on the torso with a BTi Model 607 magnetometer (7 channel, 1st order gradiometer detectors, 5 cm baseline). ECG data were acquired simultaneously using Ag/AgCl electrodes and a PAR Model 113 preamplifier. Electrical and magnetic data were digitized simultaneously, and the ECG data used to phase align magnetic data from differing sensor placements by maximizing cross correlation. 48-55 cycles were averaged at each location. For each time sample shown in figure 3a, source activity maps were constructed by linear estimation. Activity scales in b-d are normalized with respect to peak activity. Heart shaped source region was modeled with 50 second order curvilinear finite elements. Heart position, orientation, and size were determined from xray films.

REFERENCES

Cuffin, D.N. and Cohen, D. (1977) Magnetic fields of a dipole in special volume conductor shapes. **IEEE Trans. BME24**:372-381

Dallas, W.J, (1985) Fourier space solution to the magnetostatic imaging problem. **Appl. Optics** 24:4543-4546

Hamalainen M.S., and Ilmoneimi, R.J. (1984) Interpreting measured magnetic fields of the brain: estimates of current distributions. **Helsinki Univ. Tech. Report** TKK-F-A559.

Jeffs, B., Leahy, R. and Singh, M. (1987) An evaluation of methods for neuromagnetic image reconstruction. **IEEE Trans. BME-34**:713-723.

Katila, T., Montonen, J., Makijarvi, M., Nenonen, J., Raivio, M., and Siltanen, P. (1987) Localization of the accessory cardiac conduction pathway. In **Biomagnetism '87** (ed. Atsumi, K., Kotani, M., Ueno, S., Katila, T., and Williamson, S.J.) pp 274-277.

Parker, R.L. (1977) Understanding inverse theory. **Ann. Rev. Earth Planet. Sci. 5**:35-64.

Paulson, D.N., and Buchanan, D.S. (1989) Experimental accuracy of localization of current dipoles in a spherical phantom. (These **Proceedings**).

Sarvas, J. (1987) Basic mathematical and electromagnetic concepts of the biomagnetic inverse problem. **Phys. Med. Biol. 32**:11-22.

Singh, M., Doria, D., Henderson, V.W., Huth, G.C. and Beatty, J. (1984) Reconstruction of images from neuromagnetic fields. **IEEE Trans. Nucl. Sci. NS-31**:585-589.

Strang, G.S, **An Introduction to Applied Mathematics**, Wellesley, Mass.: Wellesley-Cambridge Press, 1986.

Yamamoto, T., Williamson, S.J., Kaufman, L., Nicholson, C., and Llinas, R. (1988) Magnetic localization of neuronal activity in the human brain. **Proc. Natl. Acad. Sci. 85**:8732-8736.

Zinkiewicz, O.C. (1977) **The Finite Element Method**. New York:McGraw-Hill.

LOCALIZING ABNORMALITIES IN MAPPING

S.S. Furuie, U. Tachinardi, S. Sirota, C.P. Melo

Coordenadoria de Informática-INCOR/ HC.FMUSP
Av. Dr. Enéas de Carvalho Aguiar, 44, 2. andar
Cx.Postal 11450 São Paulo - SP Brazil

INTRODUCTION

This work describes and analyzes a method for localizing abnormalities in temporal mapping, by applying the SVD (Singular Value Decomposition) technique over error signals. The error signals are obtained by subtracting original from estimated signals, which are calculated using orthonormal time vectors of a "normal" pattern. The method is unaffected by structure shift or rotation. It can be applied to Magnetocardiography (MCG) mapping. Some simulation results are given.

MODEL

The model, depicted in figure 1, is characterized by a source "S" which generates space-dependent temporal signals. These signals are detected by sensors positioned at the center of each cell of a square grid. It is assumed that the signal detected by any given sensor depends only on the intensity and direction of elements of "S" and the distance from them to the sensor. It is also assumed that the grid is large enough, so that signal energy near the grid boundaries is negligible.

For each row "r" and column "c" of the grid (figure 1) with "m" cells, the temporal quantized signal can be described by a vector $\vec{a}'_{rc} = \{a_{rc}(1), a_{rc}(2), ..., a_{rc}(n)\}$ in an n-dimensional space, where "n" is the number of temporal samples, and the symbol $'$ stands for transpose. Grouping these vectors together, we can form a data matrix $[A]_{mxn}$ consisting of "m" rows (signals) and "n" columns (temporal samples). $[A]_{mxn}$ contains all temporal signals and keeps spatial information . This matrix can be decomposed (Golub et al, 1970) using Singular Value Decomposition:

$$[A] = [U]\,[Q]\,[V]' = \begin{bmatrix} \vec{a}'_1 \\ \vec{a}'_2 \\ \vdots \\ \vec{a}'_m \end{bmatrix} \tag{1}$$

where $m \geq n$
$[Q]$: diagonal matrix
$[U],[V]$: orthonormal matrices

Equation (1) can be written (Andrews et al, 1976) as

$$[A] = \sum_{i=1}^{R} q_i\, \vec{u}_i\, \vec{v}'_i \tag{2}$$

where $R =$ rank ([A])
$\vec{u}_i, \vec{v}_i$ are the i-th column (vector) of [U] and [V] respectively.

The sets $\{\vec{u}_i\}$ and $\{\vec{v}_i\}$ contain, respectively, spatial and temporal information on the mapping data, and are the eigenvectors of [AA'] and [A'A]. These vectors can be denoted as orthonormal positional and time vectors, respectively (Groenewegen et al, 1985).

Advances in Biomagnetism
Edited by S.J. Williamson *et al.*
Plenum Press, New York

METHOD

The orthonormal set $\{\vec{v}_i\}$, i=1,2,...,R spans a linear vector space H that contains all rows of [A] ($\vec{a}'_j$, j=1,m). From eq.(2) it follows that:

$$\vec{a}'_j = \sum_{i=1}^{R} q_i \cdot u_{ji} \cdot \vec{v}'_i \qquad \text{where } u_{ji} \text{ is the j-th component of } \vec{u}_i. \tag{3}$$

If "S" is shifted and rotated parallel to the grid, there will be only an exchange between rows in matrix [A]. Since the set of signals is the same and [V] is related only to temporal information, [V] remains unchanged, i.e, it is invariant in relation to parallel shift and rotation of "S". These movements only affect [U].

Let [A] be data related to a "normal" source.

[B] be data corresponding to an "abnormal" structure which is formed by a "normal" component plus some noise. It is allowed that this structure be shifted and rotated (parallel to the grid) in relation to the case of [A].

Using the same notation for vectors in [B] , and assuming that the vectors ($\vec{b}_j$) in [B] belong to an equal or higher dimensional space than H, we can obtain an approximation of each $\vec{b}_j$ in H ,given by a linear combination of basis vectors:

$$\hat{\vec{b}}'_j = \sum_{i=1}^{R} c_{ji} \vec{v}'_i \qquad j=1,2,\ldots,m \tag{4}$$

From the orthogonality principle (least square error criterion), we have for each error vector(Giordano et al, 1985):

$$<\vec{b}_j - \hat{\vec{b}}_j , \vec{v}_i> = 0 \qquad \text{for all } i=1,2,\ldots,R \tag{5}$$

where

$$<\vec{x}, \vec{y}> = \sum_{i=1}^{m} x_i \cdot y_i = \vec{y}' . \vec{x} \qquad \text{denotes inner product in H} \tag{6}$$

Hence,

$$< \hat{\vec{b}}_j , \vec{v}_i> = < \vec{b}_j , \vec{v}_i> \tag{7}$$

Considering eq. (4) and orthogonality, yields:

$$c_{ji} = < \vec{b}_j , \vec{v}_i> \tag{8}$$

$$\hat{\vec{b}}'_j = \sum_{i=1}^{R} < \vec{b}_j , \vec{v}_i> \vec{v}'_i \qquad j=1,2,\ldots,m \tag{9}$$

The above approximation can be rewritten in a more compact and simpler form, using matrix notation:

$$[\hat{B}] = [C]\,[V]', \text{ where } [C] = [B]\,[V] \tag{10}$$

Therefore the error signals, [D] = [B] − [$\hat{B}$] will show those parts of [B] that cannot be explained by basis [V]. Applying SVD in [D], we have [D] = [T] [P] [W]', where [P] is a diagonal matrix and [T] and [W] are orthonormal matrices. By displaying the first positional vector (Stroink et al, 1985) of [D] (first column of [T]) on the grid it is possible to localize the abnormal source, because the components of vector $\vec{t}_1$ are projections of each error vector onto the most dominant error pattern ($\vec{w}_1$) (Furuie et al, 1989). In fact, as in equation (2), we have:

$$[D] = \sum_{i=1} p_i \cdot \vec{t}_i \, \vec{w}'_i \tag{11}$$

Multiplying both sides by $\vec{w}_1$ and using orthonormality of $\{\vec{w}_i\}$, we have:

$$\vec{t}_1 = [D]\,\vec{w}_1 / p_1 \tag{12}$$

Thus the k-th component of $\vec{t}_1$ is a measure of correlation between the k-th error signal and $\vec{w}_1$.

RESULTS AND DISCUSSION

This technique was applied to simulated mapping. We assumed a straight-line source "S" in vertical position (figure 1) that depolarizes along its structure in 12 instants of time, starting at its bottom. The grid of 6x6 sensors was positioned 3 cm away from "S" and only the orthogonal magnetic component to the grid was calculated. Figure 1 shows the "normal" temporal signals generated by "S", that forms matrix [A] containing 36 signals (rows) and 12 temporal samples (columns).

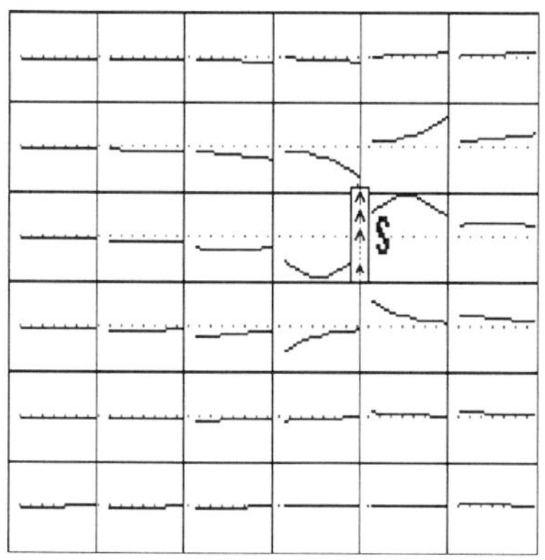

Figure 1. Temporal signals [A] generated by a "normal" structure "S" (depolarizaton in 12 instants)

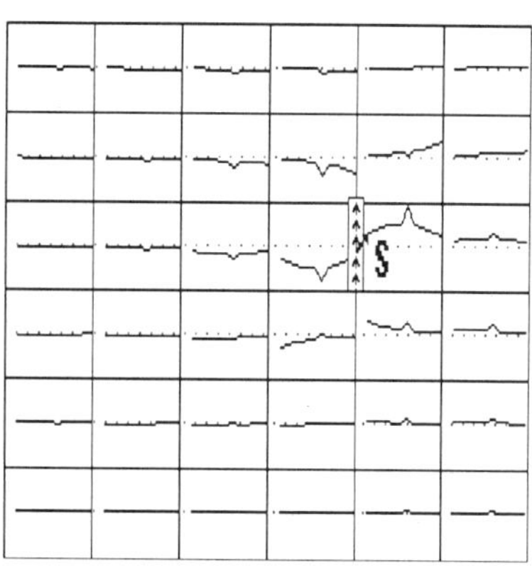

Figure 2.Temporal signals [B] of an 'abnormal' structure (noise at 7th instant)

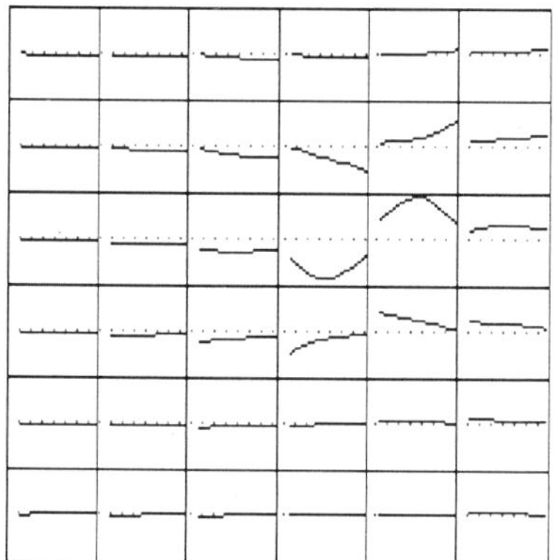

Figure 3. Estimated $[\hat{B}]$ temporal signals

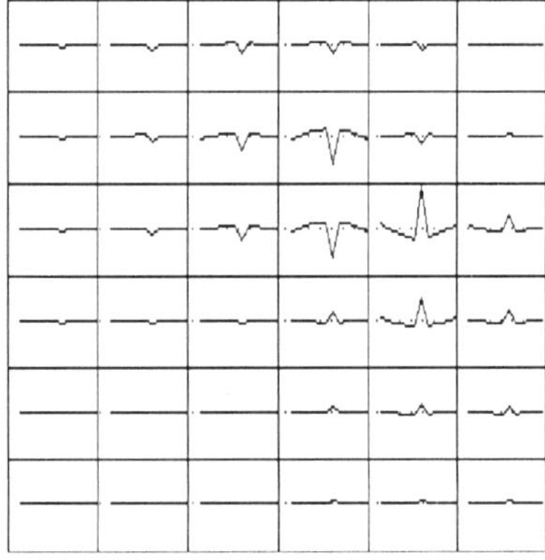

Figure 4. $[B - \hat{B}]$ temporal signals

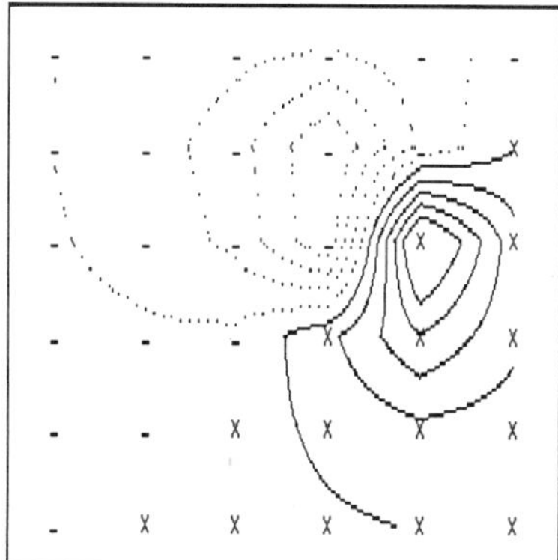

Figure 5. First orthonormal positional vector $(\vec{t}_1)$ of $[B-\hat{B}]$, and localization of 'noise' (singular value=0.263 , min=-0.399,max=0.593 ,step=0.090).

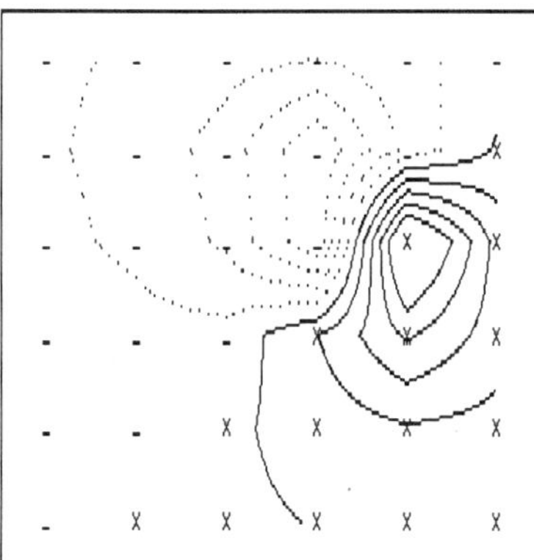

Figure 6.Positional vector of the "abnormal" component (fig.2) at 7th instant. (min=-0.117 , max=0.174 ,step=0.025)

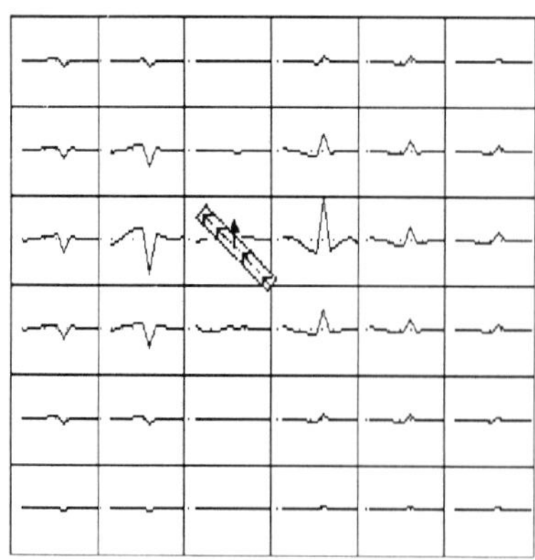

Figure 7. Temporal signals [B] of an "abnormal" structure after shift and rotation.

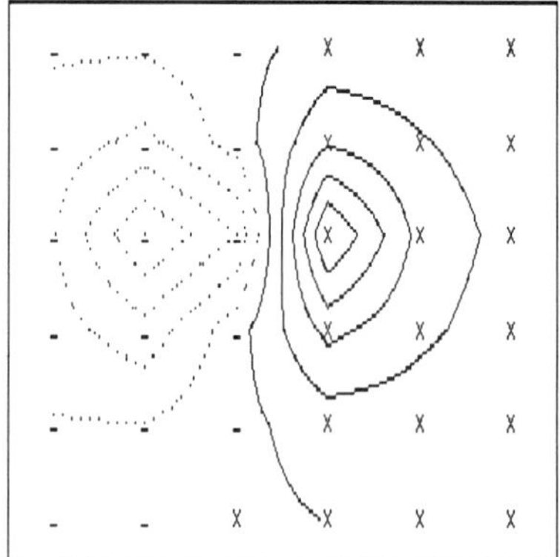

Figure 8. Localization of abnormality after shift and rotation.

In this example, the set of singular values is $\{q_i,\ i=1,12\}=\{1.058\ ,0.272\ ,0.141\ ,0.007\ ,0.004\ ,0.002,\ 0.002\ ,0.002\ ,0.001\ ,0.001\ ,0.001\ ,0.001\ \}$. In figure 2, an "abnormal" structure was created by adding some noise (dipole of same intensity, but oriented 45 degrees apart, at the 7th instant). Figure 3 shows on each cell the estimated temporal signal $[\hat{B}]$ using the first 4 orthonormal time vectors of [A], and figure 4 shows error signals $[B - \hat{B}]$. Applying SVD on $[B - \hat{B}]$, and displaying the first (normalized) positional vector $(\vec{t}_1)$ (figure 5), it is possible, by visual inspection, to localize the source of noise. Figure 6 shows isocurves generated by the 'abnormal' component alone, at the 7th instant. Figure 7 illustrates results obtained for another "abnormal" structure (noise dipole at the 7th instant) but after shift and rotation. The same procedure and time vectors [V] previously described were used in this case. Figure 8 confirms that using this technique it is possible to localize "abnormalities" even after shift and rotation. Examples in magnetocardiography involving more complex structures, such as cardiac depolarization in a plane, have been presented elsewhere (Furuie et al,1989).

If the rank of a testing data [B] is greater than the rank of a "normal" pattern [A] we can use $[A-\hat{A}]$, where $[\hat{A}]$ is estimated using basis of [B]. It should be pointed out that this method detects only those "abnormalities" that generate signals which are not fully a linear combination of $\{\vec{v}_i\}$. This technique also assumes simultaneous acquisition and that events in the "normal" pattern occur at the same temporal position in the testing mapping.

ACKNOWLEDGEMENTS

This work was supported by FINEP, Ministry of Science and Technology, Brazil. We gladly acknowledge the helpful comments and suggestions from Prof. P.C. Ribeiro (PUC-RJ), Prof. T. Tomitani (NIRS/Japan) and Dr L Moura (InCor).

REFERENCES

Andrews, H.C., Patterson, C.L.,1976, Singular Value Decomposition and digital image processing, IEEE Transactions on Acoustic, Speech and Signal Processing, ASSP-24 (1): 26-53.

Furuie, S.S , Tachinardi, U ,1989 A method to localize myocardial infarction using magnetocardiography: simulation studies, Med.&Biol. Eng. & Comp., 27:307-313.

Giordano, A.A and Hsu F.M ,1985 "Least square estimation with applications to digital signal processing", John Wiley & Sons Inc, New York.

Golub, G.H., Reinsch, C. ,1970, Singular Value decomposition and least square solutions, Numer. Math., 14: 403-420.

Groenewegen A.S, Spekhorst H.H.M, Reek E.J ,1985, A quantitative method for the localization of the ventricular pre-excitation area in the Wolff-Parkinson-White syndrome using Singular Value Decomposition of body surface potentials, J.Electrocardiology 18(2):157-168.

Stroink, G., Mac Aulay C. ,1985 Normal and abnormal Components in magnetocardiographic maps of a subject with myocardial infarction, Med. & Biol. Eng. & Comput., 23(1): 61-62.

PRELIMINARY TESTS OF MEG AND EEG LOCALIZATION

IN A HOMOGENEOUS SALINE HEAD

R. Maniewski, D. Cohen, B.N. Cuffin, K. Yunokuchi, C. Purcell

Francis Bitter National Magnet Laboratory
Massachusetts Institute of Technology
Cambridge, MA, 02139, USA

INTRODUCTION

As part of a larger project, to measure MEG and EEG localization due to an implanted dipole *in vivo* in the actual human head, it was important to first test the entire method *in vitro*. The purpose of this paper is to describe various aspects of this *in vitro* test. The head in this test consisted of a glass sphere filled with saline, hence was an idealized homogeneous spherical head. This head model is described here, including some features of the dipole electronics. Preliminary results are presented of MEG and EEG localization tests in this model. A serious problem was encountered in the EEG measurements of this test. It was temporarily circumvented so that the EEG localization results presented here are useful and valid. However, it must be dealt with before this project can proceed to the actual *in vivo* measurements, and is described because it will appear whenever this type of experiment is performed by others, using the same parameters.

METHOD

The saline head consisted of a spherical Pyrex flask of 9 cm radius. This was first cut in half, then teflon-insulated silver wire leads with 4-mm curled, stripped ends were cemented inside; the stripped ends of the wire served as the EEG electrodes. The locations were chosen to approximate those of the standard 10-20 system, as well as some extra half-way points. The two hemispheres were then cemented back together and mounted in an plastic frame. This frame allowed the sphere to be rotated in two ways about its center, similar to a globe of the earth, so that MEG locations on the sphere surface could readily be varied without moving the MEG dewar. Next, the sphere was filled with standard saline solution. Finally, the same string of electrodes (four or six) as to be implanted in the human head was suspended inside, on an accurate mounting, permitting any position or orientation of the current dipole made by any two electrodes. The general arrangement is shown in Fig. 1.

The design of the dipole electronics was dominated by two main constraints. First, that in the human subjects the current in each pulse be limited to 4 microamperes (set by the human-subject committee); this is considerably less than the current used in other studies on human subjects with implanted sources (Smith et al., 1985; Rose et al., 1989), which were already considered to be below neural stimulation level. However, in some tests in the saline head the current was raised to 10 microamperes, although most tests were made at 1-3 microamperes. Further, each current pulse must always occur as a plus-minus pair, to insure that there be no net chemical effect.

Advances in Biomagnetism
Edited by S.J. Williamson *et al.*
Plenum Press, New York

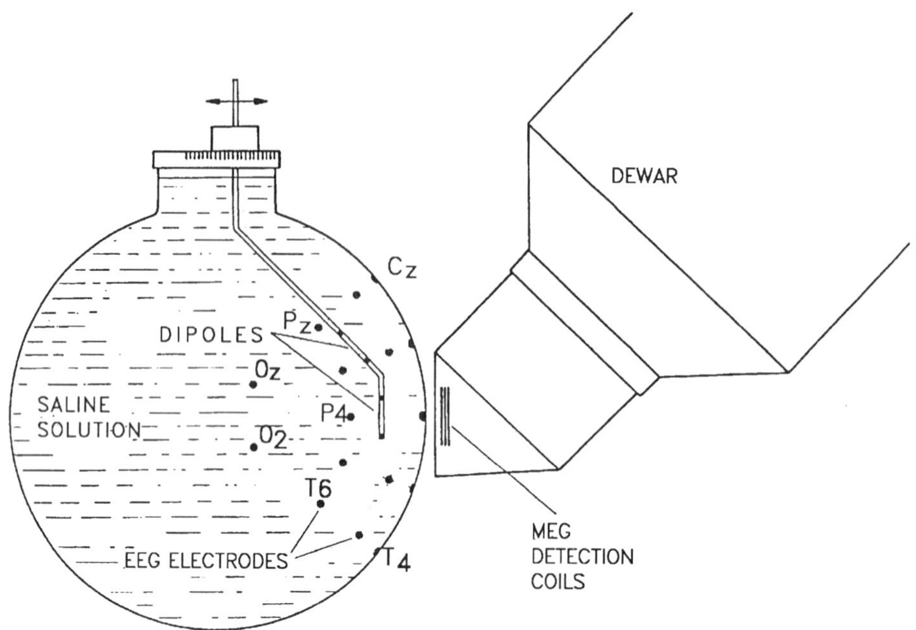

Fig. 1. Sketch of saline head, with MEG dewar in position for measurement.

The second constraint was that there be no possibility of leakage currents or unwanted currents of any kind, because of both patient safety and accuracy of measurement.

The current was produced by a computer-controlled Grass pulse generator which in turn fed an optically-isolated constant current source (the Grass SIU7 stimulator). This was followed by a passive current divider equipped with zener diode limiters, and capacitor coupling at two different stages to prevent any dc from ever flowing to the head electrodes. The initial choice of pulse shape was rectangular, of 1-msec duration, always occurring as a plus-minus pair. In testing, the pulse current was monitored using an optical isolation amplifier across a shunt resistor; for extra safety, this was not used in a human subject. The current stimuli were switched manually to various pairs of the electrodes (dipoles) in the head; as many as six separate dipoles, or combination of two dipoles, can be used in any recording session. In Fig. 1 the electrodes are seen as dark bands on the thin rod structure.

The measurements were made in the MIT magnetically-shielded room (Melcher and Cohen, 1988). The EEG signals were fed to 16 Grass 5P11J amplifiers via separate cables, to eliminate crosstalk; the Grass filters were set at 0.1 Hz to 3 KHz. The MEG measurements were made with the standard MIT dewar containing three SQUID channels, previously described (Melcher and Cohen, 1988). In brief review, two are each a planar 2-D bipolar gradiometer feeding a dc SQUID, and the third is a conventional Bz channel rf SQUID. One of the two bipolar gradiometers measures the change of Bz in the x-direction, while the other does so in the y-direction. The Bz channel is an in-line first-order gradiometer with 6.3 cm baseline; the error in localization due to the rear coil is of the order of 1 mm unless the source is very deep in the head, hence it usually need not be taken into account when doing localization calculations. The two planar gradiometers and the front Bz coil were almost coincident and are seen in Fig. 1, in side view, about 7 mm from the leftmost front face of the dewar tail. The MEG outputs were filtered similarly to the EEG channels, using band-pass filters adjusted to the falloff shapes of the Grass EEG amplifiers. Twenty-three locations over the sphere surface sequentially received MEG

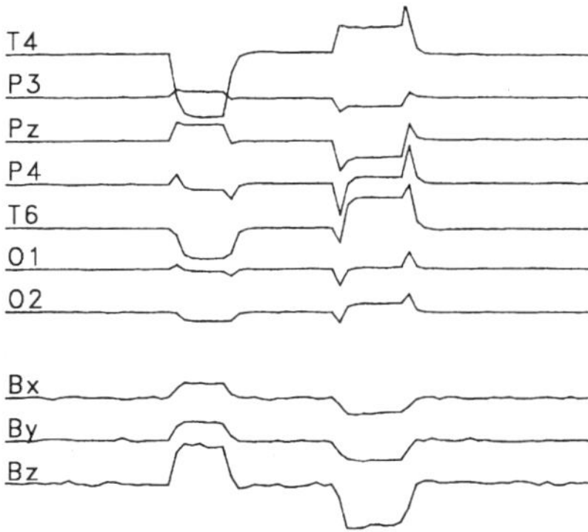

Fig. 2. Some raw traces of averaged EEG and MEG signals, showing typical spikes in the EEG.

measurements, somewhat more than the 16 MEG (and 16 EEG) locations planned for actual human measurement.

The MEG and EEG outputs were displayed on oscilloscopes, and were recorded by a DEC MicroVax II via a fast A/D converter. Because of the low dipole currents hence low EEG-MEG signals, signal-averaging was used, to improve the signal-to-noise ratio. Although the noise here was only SQUID and amplifier noise in the MEG and EEG noise, the actual human study would contain spontaneous brain signals, which would then dominate the noise. A study was therefore made of how many averaging sweeps were necessary for each expected spontaneous signal level, so that we would later be prepared; it was found that 500 sweeps should suffice for extreme cases of paroxismal EEG signals. For the MEG, the averaged waveform was an exact replica of the dipole rectangular current pulse pair, to within the accuracy allowed with the 3 KHz bandwidth. However, EEG test traces showed an unexpected problem. The averaged waveforms were no longer replicas of the dipole current pulse, but instead displayed a spike of varying amplitude and polarity at the leading and trailing edges of many of the pulses. This is seen in the example of raw traces shown in Fig. 2.

The upper seven traces are due to the EEG, and are part of the set of 16 traces obtained for each dipole position. The lower three traces are the three MEG channels at the location D8 (10-20 between point), where Bx and By are the planar 2-D gradiometer channels, and Bz is the conventional MEG monopolar channel. These are one MEG group out of the set of 23. The one-msec +/-pulses are separated by about two msec. The dipole is here tangential, of depth 1.6 cm, is 1.5 cm in length, with a current amplitude of 10 microamps. The spikes are clearly seen. Many efforts were then made to eliminate this artifact. For example, the system was shielded and grounded in the belief that the spike was due to radiation pick-up originating in the source circuit; these efforts reduced but did not eliminate the spikes. The reduced spikes were of an amplitude corresponding to a source of 1-3 microamperes, somewhat reduced from Fig. 2. They were quite independent of rectangular pulse current, hence are a major problem at the low pulse currents to which we are confined; this is because they showed an unusual EEG spatial distribution, hence produced large error in the EEG inverse solution if they were included. However, we temporarily excluded the problem by simply "working around them", that is, digitizing the signal amplitudes in periods where the spike was absent and did not spill into. This was not a final solution to the spikes, but at least allowed us to proceed with the remainder of the testing and did not degrade the localization accuracy. Certainly further work was necessary to eliminate the artifact before human implant experiments could be confidently performed.

After MEG and EEG measurements (or maps) were collected due to a variety of dipole strengths , moving-dipole inverse solutions (Cuffin, 1985) using a homogeneous spherical volume conductor model were performed to fit the measured maps and determine the MEG and EEG source locations. These computed solutions consisted of the dipole location in the three dimensions, and the two dipole angles of rotation (only one for the MEG), as well as the dipole strength. Further, they indicated how well the recorded data matched perfect dipole data.

RESULTS AND DISCUSSION

All the results of tests performed to date were very good, and showed that the MEG and EEG were both capable of accurate localization, in this ideal experimental model. For a tangential dipole in a depth range of 1.5 to 5.0 cm, both MEG and EEG localized the source to better than 4 or 5 mm, depending on the dipole depth; the deeper the dipole, the less accurate the solution. For example, for a depth of 2.5 cm the MEG accuracy was 2 mm. In the case of the EEG, the accuracy at first was not good for small depth if only the 10-20 locations were used; however, when the half-way electrodes were included in the dipole region (they had been too far apart compared with the depth hence only a few electrodes showed much signal) then the EEG solutions improved greatly. Thus, the accuracy of localization was about one mm for a dipole in the depth range of 1.5 to 4.0 cm. Radial dipoles have not been measured so far, but we would expect no new problems.

To our knowledge, this is the first report of localization measurements of both MEG and EEG, made *in vitro*. Some previous measurements of this general type have been reported, but using only MEG (Barth et al., 1986; Yamamoto et al., 1988), and show MEG localization accuracy similar to that reported here. Our results indicate that the MEG and EEG are *both* intrinsically capable of very good resolution, essentially as good as the spatial measuring system and grid system will allow. If the spatial locations and measurements in this type of ideal model are known to an accuracy of one mm, for example, then our results suggest that the localization accuracy of both MEG and EEG will be of this order, say to within 2 or 3 mm. However, the accuracy will certainly be degraded in the actual human head both because of spontaneous brain signals and modelling errors (non-sphericity and inhomogeneity); just how much MEG and EEG will lose in accuracy remains to be seen in actual human experiment, of the type planned here. In any case, it should be noted that under ideal conditions both MEG and EEG yield similar and good localization accuracy, as perhaps they should.

ACKNOWLEDGEMENTS

This work is supported by grants no. RO1NS26433 and no. RO1NS19558 to MIT (D. Cohen is PI), from the National Institutes of Health.

REFERENCES

Barth, D. S., Sutherling, W., Broffman, J., and Beatty, J., Magnetic localization of a dipolar current source implanted in a sphere and a human cranium, 1986, Electroenceph. clin. Neurophysiol., 63:260.

Cuffin, B. N., 1985, A comparison of moving dipole inverse solutions using EEGs and MEGs, IEEE Trans. Biomed. Engr., BME-32:905.

Melcher, J. R. and Cohen, D., 1988, Dependence of the Meg on dipole orientation in the rabbit head, Electroenceph. clin. Neurophysiol., 70:460.

Rose, D. F., Sato, S., Smith, P. D., Friauf, W., and Ducla-Soares, E., 1989, Subdural electrode as a dipole source for magnetoencephalography, Electroenceph. clin. Neurophysiol., 72:86.

Smith, D. B., Sidman, R. D., Flanigan, H., Henke, J. and Labiner, D., 1985, A reliable method for localizing deep intracranial sources of the EEG, Neurology, 35:1702.

Yamamoto, T., Williamson, S. J., Kaufman, L., Nicholson, C., and Llinas, R., 1988, Magnetic localization of neuronal activity in the human brain, Proc. Nat. Acad. Sci. USA, 85:8732.

PROJECTIVE METHODS FOR THE MAGNETIC DIRECT PROBLEM

S. Gonzalez[1], R. Grave de Peralta[1], R. Biscay[1], J.C. Jimenez[1], R.D. Pascual[1], J. Lemagne[2], P.A. Valdes[1]

[1]National Center for Scientific Research, POB 6880, [2]Havana University, Havana, Cuba

INTRODUCTION

The prediction of magnetic fields due to prescribed current sources in realistically shaped body models is usually approached by approximating the body as a set of piecewise homogeneous conductors with arbitrary geometry, separated by surfaces $S_l(l = 1, \ldots, M)$. One of the regions contains the primary current sources $\vec{j}(\vec{r})$ and S_1 encloses all other surfaces; $\vec{r}$ is a arbitrary position vector.

The resulting magnetic field vector $\vec{B}$ is (Geselowitz, 1970)

$$\vec{B}(\vec{r}) = \vec{B}_\infty(\vec{r}) + \sum_{l=1}^{M} \gamma_l \int_{S_l} V(\vec{r}_l)\vec{K}(\vec{r}, \vec{r}_l) \otimes d\vec{S}_l \tag{1}$$

where $\vec{r}_l \in S_l$ and $\vec{B}_\infty$ is the magnetic field produced by $\vec{j}(\vec{r})$ in an infinite homogeneous medium. The constants γ_l and the vector kernel $\vec{K}(\vec{r}, \vec{s})$ are defined in Table I, as are other special symbols used in this paper. The second term in (1) represents the contribution of secondary currents which explicitly involve the electric potentials $\vec{V}(\vec{r}_l)$ over each interface. Thus it is necessary to solve the electric direct problem (Barnard et al., 1967):

$$\alpha_k V_\infty(\vec{r}_k) = V(\vec{r}_k) + \sum_{l=1}^{M} \beta_l \int_{S_l} V(\vec{r}_l)\vec{K}(\vec{r}_l, \vec{r}_k) \circ d\vec{S}_l \tag{2}$$

where V_∞ is the potential distribution in an infinite homgeneneous medium due to the current sources and $k = 1, \ldots, M$.

Table I
Definitions of Symbols used in this paper

Symbol	Definition	Symbol	Definition
γ_l	$\frac{\mu_o}{4\pi}\Delta\sigma_l$	β_l	$\frac{\Delta\sigma_l}{4\pi\bar{\sigma}_k}$
α_k	$\frac{\sigma_s}{\bar{\sigma}_k}$	μ_o	magnetic permeability
$\Delta\sigma_l$	conductivity just inside S_l minus that just outside	σ_s	conductivity of region containing primary current sources
$\bar{\sigma}_k$	Average of electrical conductivities on both sides of S_k	$\vec{K}(\vec{r}, \vec{t})$	$\frac{\vec{r}-(\vec{t})}{\lvert\vec{r}-\vec{t}\rvert^3}$
$\vec{J}_l(u,v)$	$\frac{\partial\vec{r}_l}{\partial u} \otimes \frac{\partial\vec{r}_l}{\partial v}$	$d\vec{S}_l$	infinitessimal directed surface element

To date (1) and (2) have been solved numerically by the boundary element method (BEM), described by Barnard et. al. (1967). The computational burden is quite large, precluding its use in real time applications such as source localization (Fender, 1987; Williamson and Kaufman, 1987). A projective approch is an alternative.

PROJECTIVE SOLUTION

The unknown $V(\vec{r}_k)$ be expanded in terms of a set of known basis functions $\phi^j(\vec{r}_k)$†

$$V(\vec{r}_k) = \sum_{j=1}^{P} c_k^j \phi^j(\vec{r}_k) \tag{3}$$

Substitution into (2) yields a set of linear equations in the unknowns c_k^j. To determine these coefficients the method of collocation (Prenter, 1975, Goldberg, 1979) evaluates all terms at the "collocation points" $\vec{r}_k^i$ (where $i = 1, \ldots, N_k$, and $\sum N_k = N$), where the set of equations (2) is converted to: $\alpha_k V_\infty(\vec{r}_k^i) = \sum_{l=1}^{M} \sum_{j=1}^{P} d_{kl}^{ij} c_l^j$ where $d_{kl}^{ij} = \phi^j(\vec{r}_k^i)\delta_{lk} + \beta_l I_{lk}^{ij}$ (δ_{lk} is the Kronecker delta), and

$$I_{kl}^{ij} = \int_{S_l} \phi^j(\vec{r}_l) \vec{K}(\vec{r}_k^i, \vec{r}_l) \circ d\vec{S}_l \tag{4}$$

Let $\vec{C} = [c_1^1, \ldots, c_1^P, \ldots, c_M^1, \ldots, c_M^P]^T$ be an $M \times P$ vector;
$\vec{V}_\infty = [\alpha_1 V(\vec{r}_1^1), \ldots, \alpha_1 V(\vec{r}_1^{N_1}), \ldots, \alpha_M V(\vec{r}_M^1), \ldots, \alpha_M V(\vec{r}_M^{N_M})]^T$ an $M \times N$ vector;
$D_l^j = [d_{kl}^{ij}]_{k=1,M}^{i=1,N_k}$; and $\mathcal{D} = [D_l^j]_{l=1,M}^{j=1,P}$ is an $(M \times N)$ by $(M \times P)$ matrix.
The linear equation may now be stated as:

$$\vec{V}_\infty = \mathcal{D}\vec{C} \tag{5}$$

which may be easily solved by inverting $\mathcal{D}^T\mathcal{D}$ ($\mathcal{D}$ is usually rectangular).

It remains to evaluate the I_{lk}^{ij}. A solution to this problem depends on the representation of the surfaces S_l which has been usually based upon triangulation. An alternative is a parametric representation (Park and Lee, 1987; Evans et al., 1989). Let such a representation for each surface be: $S_l = (\vec{r}_l(u,v) | (u,v) \in T)$, where $\vec{r}_l(u,v)$ is a triplet of functions $[x(u,v), y(u,v), z(u,v)]$ and T is a rectangular domain. The surface integrals (4) may be transformed to the following double integrals (Biscay et al.,1989):

$$I_{kl}^{ij} = \int\int_T \phi^j(u,v)[\vec{K}[\vec{r}_k^i, \vec{r}_l(u,v)] \circ \vec{J}_l(u,v)]dudv$$

It is convenient to use the following type of parametric representation:

$$\vec{r}_l(u,v) = \sum_i \sum_j a_l^{ij} \vec{F}^{ij}(u,v) \tag{6}$$

where the a_l^{ij} are the coefficients and the $F^{ij}(u,v)$ are basis functions chosen to fulfill adequate regularity conditions in order to facilitate the calculations of the Jacobians.

As pointed out by Barnard et al. (1967), the BEM representation of equations (2) is ill-posed since there is a zero eigenvalue, corresponding to the non-uniqueness of potential references. Lynn and Timlake (1968), eliminate this problem by means of a Wielandt deflation. In the projective approach, the reference value for potentials in representation (3) corresponds to a constant function $\phi_o(\vec{r})$. Elimination of this term determines the reference and obviates the need for deflation.

Equation (2) may present other eigenvalues near zero when certain conductivity ratios are large. This produces instability and slow convergence for numerical solutions, a situation that becomes critical in the BEM due to the large size of the system. Multiple deflations have been proposed by Lynn and Timlake (1968) in order to reduce the spectral radius of the iterative

†The following convention will be used: subscripts refer to surface,m superscripts to basis

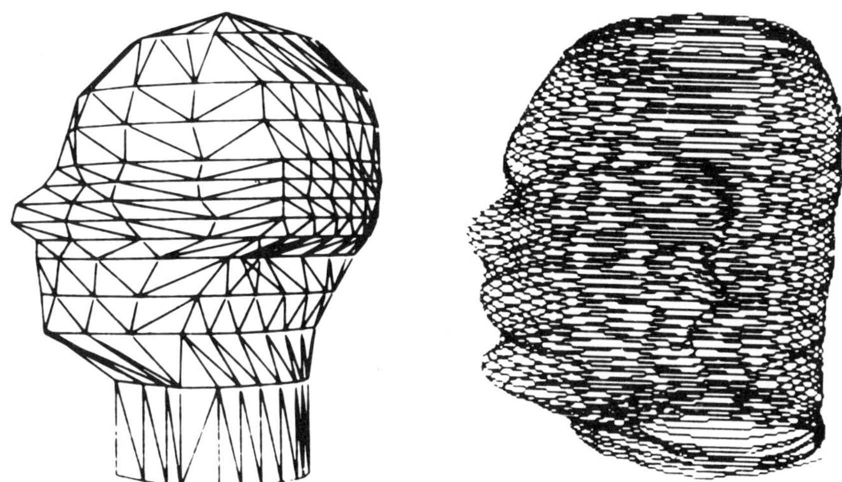

Figure 1. Representation of head skin by triangulation (left) and by 3-D Fourier Descriptors (right).

number and particular positions
schemes. However, in certain situations, such as a model of the head, in which conductivity of bone is much larger than that of brain, convergence is still too slow (Meijs, 1987).

Hämäläinen (1987) has introduced what Meijs has called the "Isolated Problem Approach" (Meijs et al., 1988), which puts $V(\vec{r}) = W(\vec{r}) = W_o(\vec{r})$, where $W_o(\vec{r})$ corresponds to the solution for a homogeneous conductor and $W(\vec{r})$ is a correction term. Solving a BEM formulation for both W and W_o obviates the need for multiple deflation.

This analysis carries over for the projective appproach of this paper. The eigenvalue analysis apparently applies to (2), not only for its BEM formulation. The "Isolated Problem" approach has therefore been used below when necessary.

If the magnetic field must be evaluated at point e then:

$$\vec{B}(\vec{r}_e) = \vec{B}_\infty(\vec{r}_e) + \sum_{l=1}^{M} \gamma_l \sum_{j=1}^{P} c_l^j J_l^{ej} \tag{7}$$

where $J_l^{ej} = \int\int_T \phi^j(u,v)[\vec{K}[\vec{r}_e, \vec{r}_l(u,v)] \otimes \vec{J}_l(u,v)]dudv$

The parametrric surface representation used in this paper is based upon Three Dimensional Fourier Descriptors (FD3) introduced by Park and Lee (1987), although the use of splines is currently being explored for the same purpose. As an illustration with actual head data, Figure 1 permits comparison of descriptions based upon FD3 (64 coefficients) and the plane element methods used in BEM (320 triangles). The FD3 description lends itself to simple surface data processing such as smoothing of noisy contours and the statistical analysis of body shape variations (Biscay et al., 1988).

The algorithm proposed in this paper consists of two different stages:

A)Calculation of Geometry Dependent Quantitites.

1) From X-Rays or MRI scans obtain the parametric representation (6) of the relevant body surfaces. Determine the $\vec{r}_e$ for which $\vec{B}$ will be evaluated and the collocation point $\vec{r}_k^i$ for each surface.

2) Choose the Basis functions ϕ^j. To date tensor products of algebraic and trigonometric polynomials have been explored.
3) On the basis of this representation evaluate the integrals I_{kl}^{ij} and J_l^{ej} which contain all the relevant geometrical information.
4) Form the matrix $\mathcal{D}$ for the system (5) which may be solved either by obtaining the inverse of $\mathcal{D}^T\mathcal{D}$ or its LU factorization.

B) Solution of Particular Electric and Magnetic Direct Problems

1) From a given current source configuration $\vec{\jmath}(\vec{r})$ calculate $\vec{V}_\infty$. Form $\vec{C} = (\mathcal{D}^T\mathcal{D})^{-1}\vec{V}_\infty$.
2) from $\vec{\jmath}(\vec{r})$ obtain $\vec{B}_\infty$ then use (7) to find $\vec{B}$.
3) additionally, values of V_l may be interpolated at arbitrary points r by using (3).

To prove the feasibility of the new method the simple model formed by two concentric spheres S_2 and S_1 was studied. The FD3 description in this case is particularly simple, only one coefficient being necessary for each sphere. In contrast, using BEM, as great number of triangles are necessary for a correct representation.

Since numerical problems are more acute for the electric direct problem only simulations for this case are presented. Dipole and sphere data are as reported by Meijs (1987). Error (with respect to the maximum theoretical V) of the estimated values at the collocation points and at 900 additional interpolated points was less than 3.4

The burden of computational time consists in forming the matrix $\mathcal{D}$ which is equivalent to calculating the solid angles matrix in BEM. Computation times are reasonably small for the new method: 5 hours with a basis of 63 Chebyshev polynomials and 64 collocation points on each surface, on an IBM PC AT compatible computer. Increasing the accuracy of the solution by including more collocation points does not change the time required to do the calculations.

REFERENCES

arnard, A. C. L., Duck , I. M., Lynn, M. S., 1967, The application of electromagnetic theory to electrocardiology, *I, Biophys. J.* 7:443-462.

Barnard, A. C. L., Duck , I. M., Lynn, M. S., Timlake, W. P., 1967, The application of electromagnetic theory to electrocardiology, *II, Biophys. J.* 7:463-491.

Biscay T., Aubert E. and Valdes P. A., 1988, Morphometric Analysis of contours and surfaces applied to biomegical images, *Revista CNIC Ciencias Biologicas*, 19:101-105.

Biscay, R. Jimenez, J.C., Valdes P. A., 1989, Numerical solutions of integral equations using parametric surface approximations, *Compilaciones sobre Electronica y Computaion*, 1:25-34.

Evans, A. R., and Sutherland Computer Corp., 1987, A generalized scanning technique for display of parametrically defined surfaces, *IEEE CG and A.*, Aug:15-26.

Fender, D. H., 1987, Source localization of brain electrical activity *in: Methods of Analysis of Brain Electrical and Magnetic Signals*, A. S. Gevins and A. Remond, Eds., Elsevier, Amsterdam-New York-Oxford.

Geselowitz, D. B., 1970, On the magnetic field generated outside and inhomogeneous volume conductor by internal sources, *IEEE Trans. Mag.*, 6:346-347.

Goldberg, M. A., 1979, A survery of Numerical Methods for Integral Equations. *in: Numerical Methods for Integral Equations*, Ed. Goldberg M. A., Pergamon Press.

Hamalainen, M.S., Sarvas, J., 1987, Realistic conductivity geometry model of the human head for interpretation of neuromagnetic data, *Report TKK-F-A614*, Helsinki University of Technology.

Lynn, M. S., Timlake, W. P., 1968, The use of multiple deflations in the numerical solution of singular systems of equations with applications to potential theory, *SIAM J. Numer. Anal.*, 5:303-322.

Meijs, J. W. H., Boom, H. B. K., Peters, M. J., Van Oosterom, A., 1987, Application of the Richardson extrapolation in simulation studies of EEGs, *Med. Biol. Eng. Comput.*, 25:222-226.

Meijs, J. W. H., Weier, O. W., Peters, M. J., Van Oosterom, A., 1988, On the numerical accuracy of the Boundary Element Method, *Ph. D. Thesis.*

Park, K. S., Lee, N. S., 1987, A three dimensional Fourier descriptor for human body representation/reconstruction from serial cross-sections, *Comput. Biomed. Res.*, 20:125-140. Prenter, P. M., 1975, *Splines and Variational Methods*, John Wiley and Sons, New York.

Williamson, S.J., and Kaufman, L., 1987, Analysis of neuromagnetic signals, *in: Methods of Analysis of Brain Electrical and Magnetic Signals*, Gevins, A.S., and Rémond, A., Eds., Elsevier, Amsterdam, 1987, pp. 405-448.

MECHANISM OF FLUX REVERSAL PHENOMENA IN SPATIAL DISTRIBUTIONS OF THE MAGNETOENCEPHALOGRAMS

K. Iramina and S. Ueno

Department of Electronics
Kyushu University
Fukuoka, 812, Japan

INTRODUCTION

It is difficult to solve the inverse problem in magnetoencephalography because of complexity of electrical sources and inhomogeneities of electrical conductivities in the head. The head consists of different materials with different electrical conductivities such as brain tissues, skull and ventricles. We have investigated the influence of small inhomogeneous regions in the head on spatial patterns of surface magnetic fields, and we have demonstrated that the flux reversal phenomena can be observed in special cases where conductivities of the inhomogeneous regions change with pathological situations (Ueno et al. 1985). A current dipole which orients radially in a homogeneous sphere produces no magnetic fields outside the sphere (Baule et al. 1965). We have also reported that radially oriented dipoles produce magnetic fields outside the sphere when inhomogeneous regions exist inside the sphere (Ueno et al. 1987, Iramina et al. 1988). The present study is focused on the mechanism of flux reversal phenomena which can be observed in spatial distributions of the magnetoencephalograms (MEGs). Computer simulation shows that the flux reversal can be caused by the change of flow patterns of currents which flow on the surface of boundary between different inhomogeneous regions in the head.

MODEL AND METHOD

The head is assumed to be a spherical volume conductor (radius R=0.1m) with a uniform electrical conductivity σ_1, in which small sphere (radius r=0.02m) with conductivity σ_2 is located in the left frontal region as shown in Fig.1. The small sphere is assumed to be brain lesions such as brain tumors and cerebrovascular lesions. The electrical conductivity of brain lesions can be vary with pathological situation such as edema and calcification.

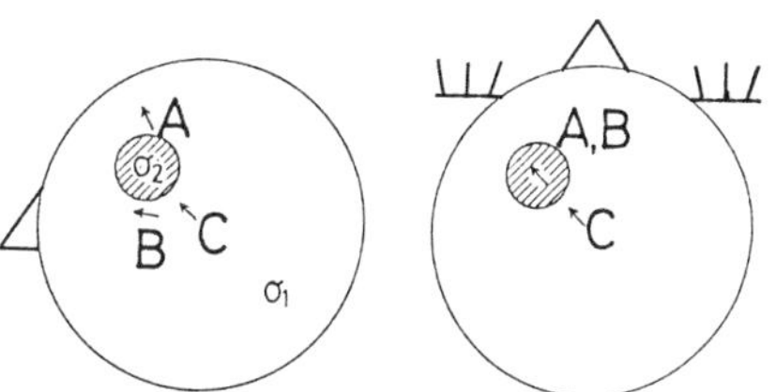

Fig.1. Head model and current dipoles.

In order to investigate the effect of inhomogeneities on surface magnetic fields, radial dipoles are used here as electrical sources of neural population. Magnetic fields on the surface of

Advances in Biomagnetism
Edited by S.J. Williamson *et al.*
Plenum Press, New York

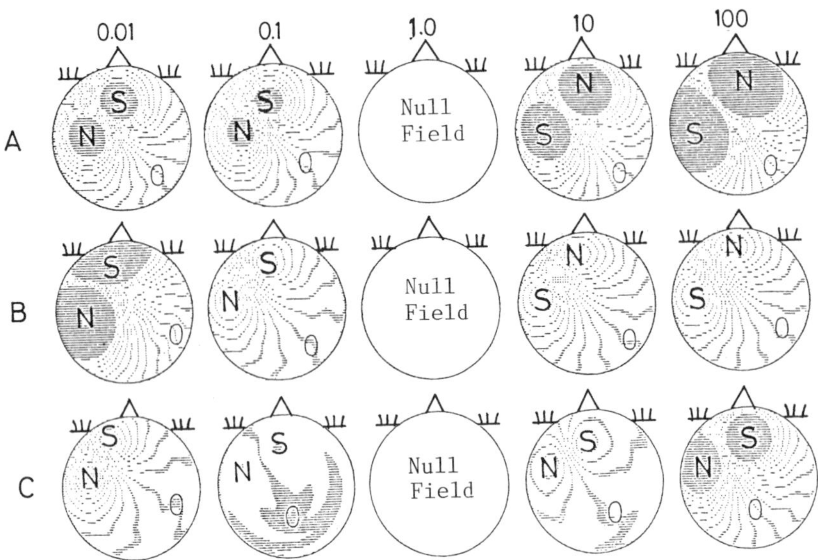

Fig.2. Spatial distributions of normal component of magnetic fields over the surface of the sphere generated by radial dipoles.

inhomogeneous volume conductor can be obtained as the sum of magnetic fields produced by current dipole and magnetic fields produced by the effect of inhomogeneities. Since radially oriented dipoles produce no magnetic fields outside the sphere, surface magnetic fields are generated only by the effect of inhomogeneities in the sphere. This simplified condition is useful in understanding the relationship between the surface magnetic fields and the inhomogeneities inside the sphere.

Radially oriented dipoles are located around the small sphere 0.01m apart from the boundary. The dipoles A, B and C are located at (x,y,z)= (0.025m,0.025m,0.0654m),(0.025m,0.025m,0.0054m) and (0.01m,0.01m,0.01414m), respectively, where X-axis is directed in parallel to the Inion-Anion axis. The dipole C orients radially to the small sphere, too.

Magnetic fields generated outside an inhomogeneous volume conductor by internal current sources can be calculated by an equation derived by Geselowitz(1970). Electrical potentials on the surfaces of both outer and inner small sphere are needed to solve the Geselowitz equation. The potentials are obtained by solving a simultaneous equation developed by Barr et al.(1966), where a solid-angle technique is used. We apply their methods to simulation of the MEG and EEG studies.

In field mapping, the surface of the upper hemisphere is projected into the unit circle. The calculated magnetic fields are interpolated and quantized, and finally isofield contour maps over the upper hemisphere are obtained.

RESULT AND DISCUSSION

Figure 2 shows change of spatial patterns of magnetic fields when a conductivity ratio σ_2/σ_1 varies from 0.01 to 100. In cases A and B, the North pole and the South pole are reversed when the conductivity ratio is changed from 0.1 to 10. In contrast, in case C, no flux reversal appears.

Figure 3 shows potential distributions over the surface of outer sphere. These maps are "subtracted potential distributions". The surface potentials produced by current dipoles which are located in the inhomogeneous sphere including small inhomogeneous region are subtracted by the potentials produced by the same dipoles which are located in the homoge-

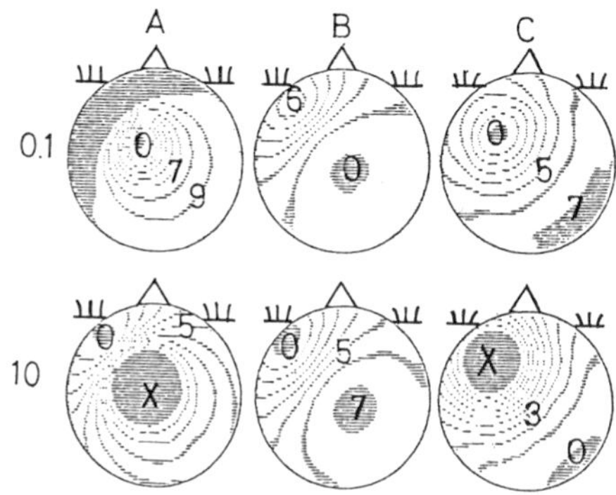

Fig.3. Spatial distributions of electrical potential produced by surface currents which flow on the surface of the sphere.

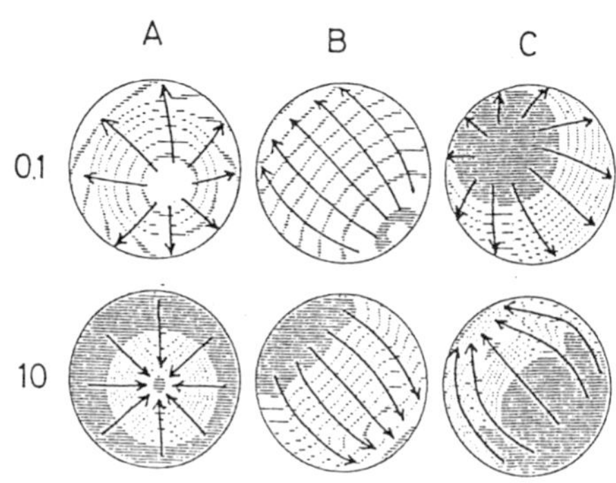

Fig.4. Spatial distributions of electrical potential on the surface of the inner small sphere. The arrows show the currents which flow on the surface of the sphere.

neous sphere excluding the small inhomogeneous region. In other words, these subtracted potentials are determined only by the effect of inhomogeneity of the small sphere inside the outer sphere. The spatial relation between peak value region and 0 level region is reversed when the conductivity ratio is changed from 0.1 to 10. Compared with spatial patterns of magnetic fields in Fig.2, potential distributions and magnetic field patterns are complementary. Phase reversal in potential distributions appears for all cases A, B and C, whereas flux reversal in magnetic distributions appears for A and B, but no flux reversal appears for C.

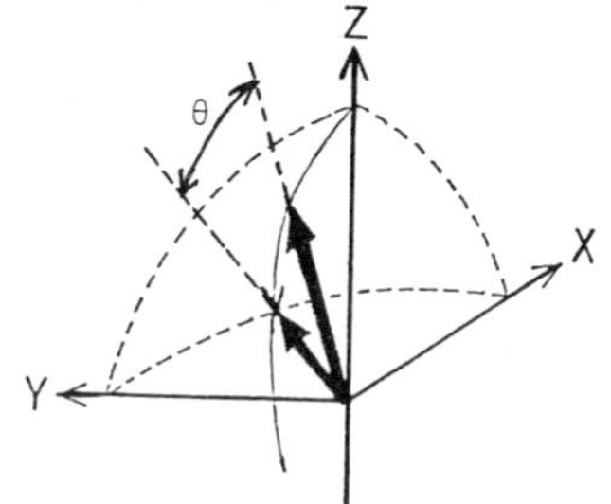

Fig.5. Direction of dipole orientation.

The mechanism for these effects is explained by obtaining current flow patterns on the surface of inner small sphere as shown in Fig.4. The surface currents are marked by arrows which flow in the direction perpendicular to the equipotential lines on the surface of the small sphere. These surface currents on the small sphere generate magnetic fields outside the outer sphere.

Directions of current flows on the small sphere are reversed with the change of conductivity ratio, thereby flux reversal in the outer sphere is brought in cases A and B. In case C, although current flows are reversed, the reversed currents cause no flux reversal because the current flows in the region which is located near the surface of the outer hemisphere contribute to generation of magnetic field outside the outer hemisphere.

It is important to determine the region in which flux reversal of magnetic fields can appear.

Rotating dipoles A, B and C as shown in Fig.5, magnetic field components perpendicular to the surface of the sphere at Fp2 in the 10-20 system are calculated as shown in Fig.6. In Fig.6, curves in column (a) show the change of magnetic fields produced by current dipole. Curves in column (b) show the change of magnetic fields produced by surface currents which flow on the surface of inner small sphere. Curves in column (c) show the sum of (a) and (b). In column (a), i.e., in the case of homogeneous sphere, the amplitudes in magnetic fields are strongly influenced by the direction of dipole orientation and distance between dipole and measured point. However, in column (b), i.e., in the case of inhomogeneous sphere, amplitude of magnetic fields are not so influenced by the dipole direction and the

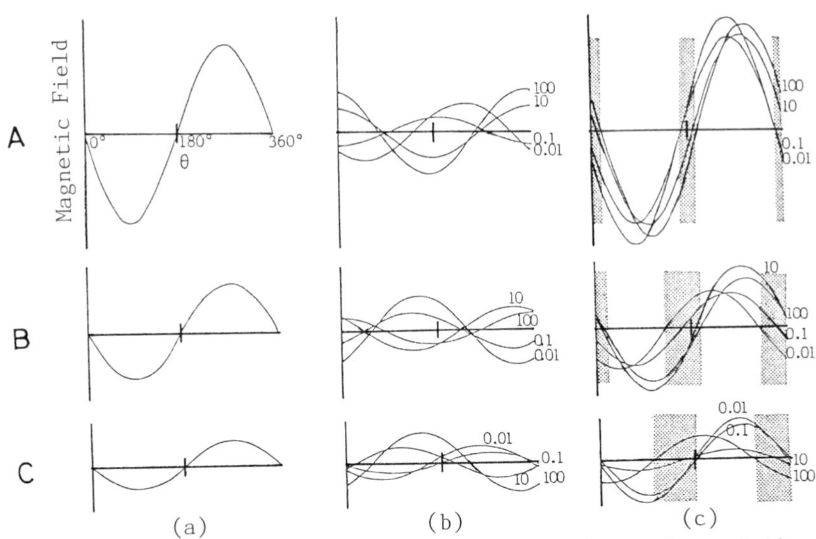

Fig.6. Magnetic field components perpendicular to the surface of the sphere at Fp2 in the 10-20 system produced by rotating dipoles. (a) Change of magnetic fields produced by current dipole. (b) Change of magnetic fields produced by surface currents which flow on the surface of inner sphere. (c) Sum of (a) and (b). Shadow patterns are regions in which flux reversal occurs.

distance between the dipole and the measured point. Therefore, in column (c) the effects of inhomogeneities on the change of magnetic fields show complicated patterns. Flux reversal occurs in the region marked with shadow. In case A, the range of flux reversal is narrow, because the rotation of dipole itself affects on the formation of magnetic fields. In contrast, in cases B and C, the range of flux reversal is wide because the change of dipole orientation and the change of inhomogeneities contribute in producing magnetic fields in a comparable order.

This study was supported in part by the Grant-63850090 from the Ministry of Education Science and Culture, Japan. Computation was carried out by a computer FACOM M 780 in computer center of Kyushu University.

REFERENCES

Barr R.C and Pilkington T.C., 1966, Determining surface potentials from current dipoles, with application to electrocardiography. IEEE Trans. Biomed. Eng., BME-13, 88-92

Baule G. and McFee R., 1965, Theory of magnetic detection of the hearts electrically activities. J. Appl. Phys. 2066-2073

Geselowitz D.B., 1970, On the magnetic field generated outside an inhomogeneous volume conductor by internal current sources. IEEE Trans. Mag-6, 346-347

Iramina K. and Ueno S., 1988, Spatial properties of magnetic fields produced by radially oriented dipole in inhomogeneous sphere. BIOMAGNETISM'87 (K.Atsumi, M.Kotani, S.Ueno, T.Katila and S.J.Williamson Eds.) Tokyo Denki University Press, 106-109

Ueno S., Wakisako H. and Harada K., 1985, Flux reversal phenomena in spatial distributions of the magnetoencephalograms. BIOMAGNETISM Applications & Theory (H.Weinberg, G.Stroink and T.Katila Eds.), Pergamon Press, New York, 289-293

Ueno S., Iramina K. and Harada K., 1987, Effects of inhomogeneities in cerebral modeling for magnetoencephalography. IEEE Trans. Mag-23, 3753-3755

CONSTRUCTING A REALISTICALLY SHAPED MODEL OF THE HUMAN HEAD

V. A. Konyshev, R. A. Maragey, Yu. A. Kholodov, V. M. Verkhlutov,
A. M. Gorbach

Laboratory of Electromagnetic Neurophysiology, Institute of Higher
Nervous Activity and Neurophysiology, Academy of Sciences
Moscow, USSR

INTRODUCTION

To increase the precision of measurements of the magnetic and electric fields of the human brain (in accordance with external and internal brain coordinates of the EEG and MEG grid points) and the precision of the solution of the inverse problem as well, a construction of the individual model of the head is required (Meijs et al., 1987; Meijs and Peters, 1987). It was shown (Witwer et al., 1972) that in order to diminish the dipole localization errors during the solution of the inverse problem in the EEG taking into account the head shape is more significant than inhomogeneouties of its conductivity. We developed a rather inexpensive technique of constructing a model of the human head, considering its individual shape.

METHODS

A patient was sitting in arm-chair set up in front of a TV-camera connected with the image processing and analysis system (Pericolor 2001, Numelec, France). The chair was rotated by engine or hand. A special rubber cap was used to press hair to head. The patient's head was softly fixed, with the vertical axis of rotation going through the vertex of his head and chair pivot. The plane passed through the inion and nasion was perpendicular to axis of rotation (Fig. 1). The series of the 18 images of the head were obtained by the sequential turning of the chair, each time by 10 degrees. After recognition, the contours were combined within a 3-D head model. So, by means of 36 meridians, arranging across 10 degrees, and latitudes, with distance between them being equal 1 cm, we described the surface of head. To calibrate all distance a image of ruler was used. The complete procedure took about 5 minutes.

The finite element method is used for solving the forward problem of EEG and MEG for realistically shaped model of the head (Witwer et al., 1972). For this purpose the nodes coordinates must be defined in internal areas of different cross-sections of the head, which coincide with areas outlined by contours at the corresponding latitudes. A full set of such 2-D nets forms the 3-D net.

Advances in Biomagnetism
Edited by S.J. Williamson *et al.*
Plenum Press, New York

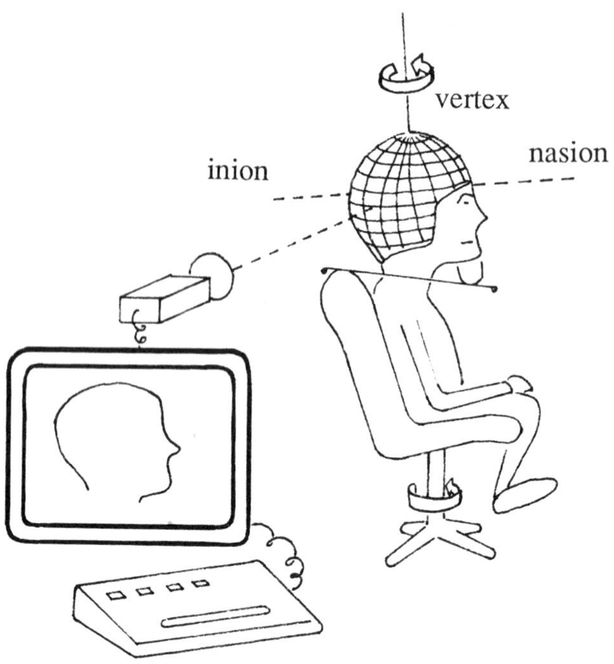

Fig.1. A patient was sitting in rotating arm-chair. His head was softly fixed by means of a special rubber cap and a support for the chin so that an axis of rotation passed through the vertex and had been perpendicular to inion-nasion line (IN-line). An immobile TV-camera was situated 2 m apart from the head and was aimed to a point of intersection of IN-line and axis of rotation.

RESULTS

Models of the head constructed for 4 patients were compared with those reconstructed from NMR-tomograms of these patients. The errors were negligible.

The realistically shaped model of the human head allowed:

1. To calculate the local curvature of the head in any point.
2. To estimate 3-D coordinates of EEG and MEG grid points.
3. To solve the direct and inverse problems of the EEG and MEG by the finite element method (Fig. 2).
4. To print the pattern of the individual helmet of the patient which can be used in routin EEG and MEG measurements. The external brain coordinates and MEG and EEG grid points were plotted on the helmet. The visualization of the fissures and girus reconstructed from NMR-slices on the helmet was also probed.

DISCUSSION

The proposed technique of constructing the realistically shaped model of the human head as compared to that using the NMR-slices does not allow to estimate the thickness of the skull. This may be compensated, however, by taking additional measurements of the thickness of the bone by ultrasound in each EEG and MEG grid point.

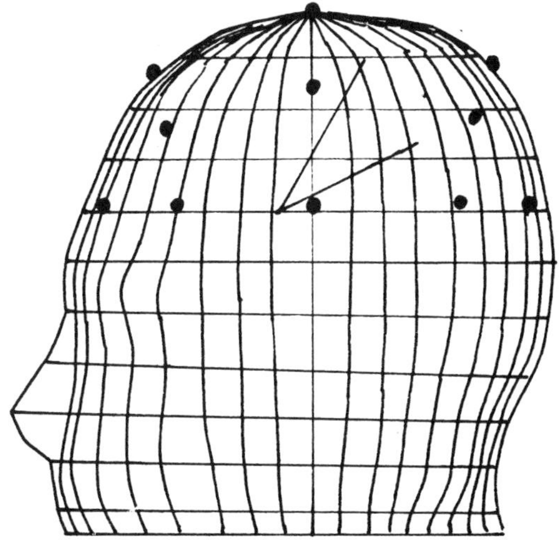

Fig.2. The model of head is formed by 36 meridians, and latitudes with distance between them 1 cm (at this figure they are drawn with a 2 cm interval). The proections of Rolandic and Sylvian fissures and EEG grid points, situated according to international system 10-20, was shown. MEG grid points corresponds to the crossing of meridians and latitudes.

We hope that such a technique of constructing a 3-D model of a real head and visualization of projections of the main fissures and gyric on the surface of the helmet may be used for MEG and EEG mapping and for solving the inverse problems of EEGs.

REFERENCES

Meijs, J. W. H., Bosch, F. G. C., Peters, M. J., Lopes da Silva F.H., 1987, On the magnetic field distribution generated by a dipolar current source situated in a realistically shaped compartment model of the head, EEG & Clin. Neurophys, 66:286-298.

Meijs, J. W. H., and Peters, M. J., 1987, The EEG and MEG, using a model of eccentric spheres to describe the head, Trans.Biomed.Engin., BME-34:913-220.

Witwer, J. G., Trezek, G. J., and Jewett, D. L., 1972 , The effect of media inhomogeneities upon intracranial electric fields, Trans. Biomed. Engin., BME-19:352-362.

COMPRESSION OF BIOMAGNETIC DATA BY COMBINING LINEAR PREDICTIVE AND VARIABLE-LENGTH CODING

B. Lütkenhöner, C. Pantev, M. Hoke, K. Lehnertz

Institute of Experimental Audiology
University of Münster
Münster, Federal Republic of Germany

INTRODUCTION

In consideration of the fact that with a multichannel magnetometer a huge amount of data can be acquired within a very short time, compression of biomagnetic data gains increasing importance. Two major classes of compression operations have to be distinguished: Entropy-reducing transformations, which result in a reduction in fidelity and are irreversible, and information-preserving (redundancy-removal) transformations (Blåsbalg and van Blerkom, 1962). Only the latter class will be considered in this paper.

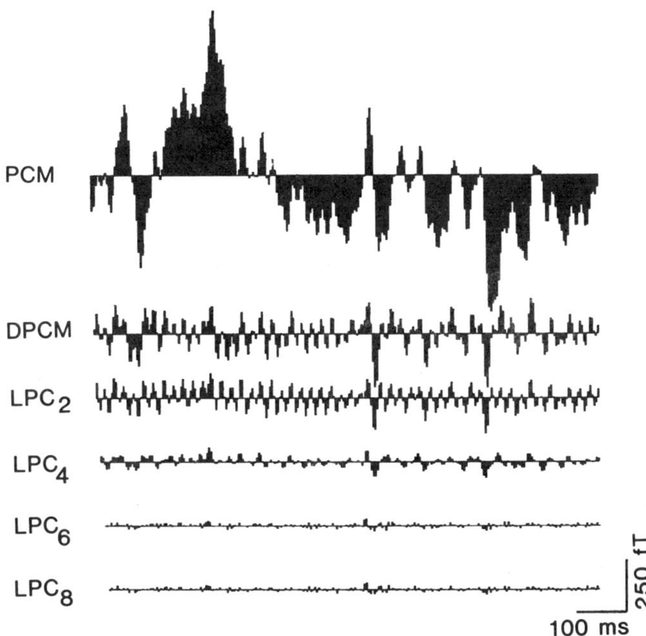

Fig. 1. Different representations of a typical MEG epoch.

Advances in Biomagnetism
Edited by S.J. Williamson *et al.*
Plenum Press, New York

Table 1. Frequency distribution of the lengths of the code-word kernels in case of suboptimum variable-length encoding (based upon 257 epochs, including the one considered in Fig. 1)

length	PCM	DPCM	LPC_2	LPC_4	LPC_6	LPC_8
1	387	1663	4171	9275	14324	15977
2	772	3374	5671	11715	17453	18681
3	1447	6683	10884	19177	22249	21533
4	2935	12689	18177	18986	9561	7023
5	5713	19754	19163	5148	572	438
6	11203	17315	6425	415	87	79
7	18771	3598	682	46	4	5
8	19024	407	103	2	0	0
9	5271	52	2	0	0	0
10	246	0	0	0	0	0
11	23	0	0	0	0	0

Table 2. Huffman codes for the lengths of the code-word kernels

length	PCM	DPCM	LPC_2	LPC_4	LPC_6	LPC_8
1	1011110	100010	10010	100	10	10
2	101110	10000	1000	11	01	01
3	10110	101	11	00	00	00
4	1010	11	01	01	110	110
5	1000	00	00	1010	1110	1110
6	11	01	101	10110	11110	11110
7	01	1001	100110	101110	11111	11111
8	00	1000110	1001110	101111	-	-
9	1001	1000111	1001111	-	-	-
10	10111110	-	-	-	-	-
11	10111111	-	-	-	-	-

BIOMAGNETIC MEASUREMENTS

By recording the magnetoencephalogram (MEG) in 3 subjects at 10 randomly distributed positions, 30 data sets have been acquired, each comprising 257 epochs (256 samples, 4 ms sampling interval). The measurements were carried out in an electrically (but not magnetically) shielded room using a second-order gradiometer (BTi model 601). Before digitization (12 bit A/D converter, full scale corresponding to $\pm$8921 fT), the signals were band-pass filtered (low-pass: Butterworth, cut-off frequency 40 Hz, 48 dB/oct; high-pass: Bessel, cut-off frequency 0.1 Hz, 12 db/oct). The overall noise decreased in the frequency range between 1 and 3 Hz from about 200 to about 40 fT/$\sqrt{}$Hz and remained more or less constant between 3 and 40 Hz.

ENCODING PROCEDURES

The simplest form of encoding is pulse-code modulation (PCM). In this approach, the amplitude values generated by the A/D converter are stored directly, without further manipulations (Davis, 1986). In the present paper the term *PCM representation* will be used for the amplitude values obtained after carrying out a digital de-meaning for each individual epoch. Subtracting from each sample of an epoch (except for the first sample) the value of the previous sample results in the DPCM (differential PCM) representation, whereas subtracting from each sample (except for the first n samples) the value predicted by an n-th order autoregressive (AR) model results in the LPC_n (linear predictive coding) representation (e.g. Press et al., 1986). Fig. 1 exemplifies for one typical epoch the differences between PCM, DPCM, and LPC_n (n=2,4,6,8) representation. It is obvious that in case of LPC_6 and LPC_8 the signal amplitude is highly reduced as compared to PCM.

All the above data representations were encoded using both Huffman's optimum variable-length encoding procedure (Huffman, 1952) and a suboptimum procedure (Lütkenhöner, 1989). Whereas in the first case Huffman's procedure is used for constructing a variable-length code word for each quantization level, in the second case each code word is composed of a kernel and a prefix specifying the length of the kernel, and Huffman's procedure is used only for constructing the codes of the prefixes. The kernels are formed according to the following principle: Non-negative integers (0,1,2,...) are represented by the codes **0**, **00**, **01**, **000**, **001**, **010**, **011**, **0000**, etc, whereas negative integers (-1,-2,-3,...) are represented by the codes **1**, **11**, **10**, **111**, **110**, **101**, **100**, **1111**, etc. Typical frequency distributions of the kernel lengths are shown in table 1. Huffman's procedure converts these frequency distributions into the variable-length codes presented in table 2. It is obvious that high frequencies result in short codes and vice versa.

COMPARISONS BETWEEN THE DIFFERENT ENCODING PROCEDURES

For comparing the performance of the different encoding procedures the mean code-word lengths have been determined for each of the different representations of the 30 data sets. The results are shown in Fig. 2, where

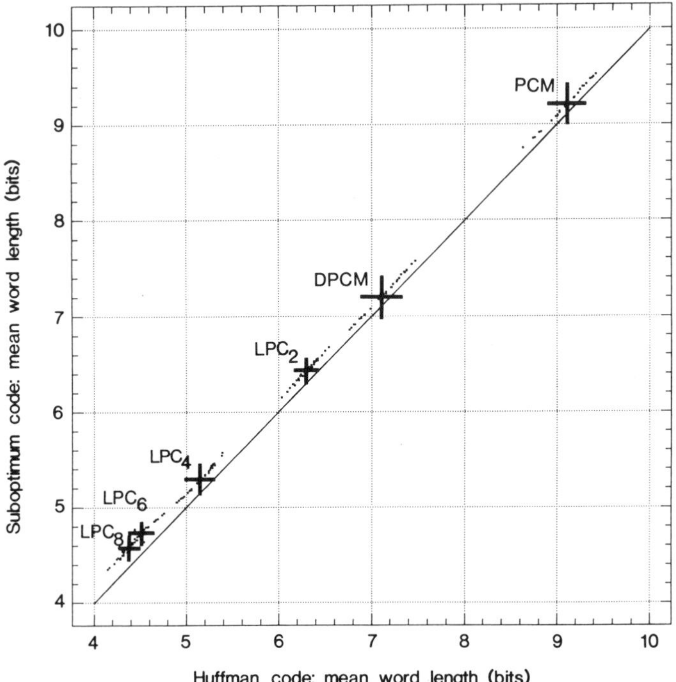

Fig. 2. Comparisons between the mean code-word lengths for the different encoding procedures

the mean code-word lengths in case of Huffman and suboptimum coding, respectively, are plotted versus each other (tiny dots). The fact that the dots form a line running parallel to the diagonal (distance only 0.1 to 0.2 bits) indicates that the suboptimum code is almost as effective as the more complicated Huffman code. Besides that, Fig. 2 shows the respective means and standard deviations. Obviously, LPC_6 combined with Huffman coding requires only half the storage capacity of PCM combined with Huffman coding, and the saving compared to the original 12 bit representation is even greater.

SOME REMARKS UPON THE REQUISITE COMPUTATION TIME

The computation time required for the different methods depends highly upon the available hardware and the degree of software optimization. Anyhow, it seems to be important to give at least a rough orientation: A straightforward FORTRAN 77 program running on a Motorola MVME147-1 microcomputer (68030 CPU with coprocessor 68882) needs about 130 ms to encode an epoch of 256 samples by means of a combination of LPC_6 and suboptimum variable-length encoding. Most of the time is used for evaluating the coefficients of the AR model (subroutine MEMCOF published by Press et al., 1986) and for packing the variable-length codes into fixed-length data blocks, which requires 66% and 14% of the total execution time, respectively.

DISCUSSION

The above results suggest that a combination of linear predictive and variable-length coding is capable of compressing biomagnetic data by more than factor of two. It must be emphasized that this compression factor is achieved without loosing a single bit of information, in contrast to the entropy-reducing transformations as commonly used e.g. for storing the electrocardiogram. LPC_6 combined with suboptimum variable-length coding seems to represent a reasonable compromise because it can be implemented quite easily, and with respect to the mean code-word length the method is nearly as efficient as linear predictive coding of higher order combined with Huffman coding. The method can be employed not only for off-line applications (e.g. for archiving of data), but also on-line applications are feasible: Since it can be expected that, after optimizing the software (e.g. Lütkenhöner and Ross, 1989), the computation time reported above will be reduced by a factor of 2 to 3, customary microcomputers are easily capable of on-line encoding the data provided by a 7-channel magnetometer, sampled at a rate of 250 Hz. Provided that a digital signal processor is available, on-line encoding of 32 or even 64 channels should be no insuperable problem.

REFERENCES

Blasbalg, H., and van Blerkom, R., 1962, Message compression, IRE. Trans. Space Electron. Telemetry, 8:228

Davis, R.O., 1986, Digital signal processing in studies of animal acoustical communication, including human speech, Comput. Methods Programs Biomed., 23:171

Huffman, D.A., 1952, A method for the construction of minimum redundancy codes, Proc. IRE, 40:1098

Lütkenhöner, B., and Ross, B., 1989, Software manipulations to speed up a real-valued fast Fourier transform algorithm, Comput. Methods Programs Biomed., 29:129

Lütkenhöner, B., 1989, A suboptimum variable-length encoding procedure for discrete quantized data (submitted for publication)

Press, W.H., Flannery, B.P., Teukolsky, S.A., and Vetterling, W.T., 1986, "Numerical recipes," Cambridge University Press, Cambridge

INTERACTIVE CONTROL AND DATA PROCESSING IN MULTICHANNEL SQUID INSTRUMENTATION SYSTEMS

J.H. Voskamp, R.M.H. Niessen and A.J. van der Wal

Department of Physics
Eindhoven University of Technology
P.O. Box 513, NL–5600 MB Eindhoven, The Netherlands

ABSTRACT

In the present article the architecture of a computer–controlled system for the acquisition and processing of signals and the simultaneous display of results is described for use in multichannel magneto–encephalography (MEG) experiments. It is shown that by selecting this architecture, that includes both state–of–the–art hardware concepts and interactive real–time software, a system has been developed that offers the combination of high performance and easy modifiability to the experiment.

The paper especially emphasizes the importance of modularity and flexibility in hardware and in software design, since both determine the (im)possibilities of future MEG experiments. The present architecture offers a contribution to defining the necessary standards for data acquisition and processing in magneto–encephalography. Finally we report on some preliminary performance results obtained from a system built and implemented according to this architecture.

INTRODUCTION

One of the problems that researchers in the field of experimental neurophysiology are faced with, is the problem of dealing with large volumes of data in real–time. The large data sets that are produced by even a relatively simple MEG experiment, have to be filtered, averaged, displayed and stored concurrently. The real–time constraints ask for a careful design in computer architecture.

Modern trends in neurophysiological research enhance the real–time constraints even more. First, the investigation of millisecond phenomena in MEG and EEG spectra calls for higher sampling rates, and produces proportionally more data. Secondly, multichannel systems enable the researcher to measure many signals simultaneously. The introduction of explicit hardware parallelism provides an obvious solution, although the costs involved may quickly become prohibitive. The alternative then is to share expensive hardware among the various channels, thereby transforming the economic problem into a real–time system design problem. The situation is further complicated by demanding that the data acquisition system should be extremely flexible, thereby precluding extremely dedicated hardware solutions.

In multichannel SQUID experiments a great variety of experimental set–ups exists. Under such circumstances a turnkey hardware configuration as well as a single sequential control–program, as generally applied in commercial, clinical equipment are of limited use. The lack of flexibility thus renders most commercial equipment unsuitable as instrumentation option for experimental neurophysiology.

Advances in Biomagnetism
Edited by S.J. Williamson *et al.*
Plenum Press, New York

During recent years software engineers and implementers of computer–based real–time systems have grown aware that real–time computer control involves many more features than can be incorporated in a single sequential computer–program under a single tasking operating system (Ref. 1,2). Apart from correctness and timeliness, an important design goal for a real–time computer system is the ability to adapt this hardware and software in an easy way to different configurations.

For the data acquisition and data processing in a typical multichannel MEG experiment, it should be possible to modify the number of channels, the digital filter coefficients, the way averaging is done and the way artefact rejection is done, in a user–friendly way. Generally the experimenter will adjust these parameters before running the experiment, although a flexible system would allow the experimenter to alter the organisation of the experiment interactively, i.e. during runtime. The latter can be achieved by means of subdividing the software controlling the experiment, in suitable concurrent processes and by providing the user with advanced facilities to interact with these processes.

This paper presents a description of the architecture of such a system, designed for use in the data acquisition and data processing in a 64–channel MEG and EEG experimental set–up. We will focus on the user aspects and the advantages offered by this architecture. Implementation details of the underlying system software can be found elsewhere (Ref. 1,3).

SOFTWARE ARCHITECTURE

The software architecture of the MEG data acquisition system is based on recent developments in software engineering. The most important of these is the concept of object–oriented programming, that is extensively used in languages such as Smalltalk, cf. Ref. 2. The same techniques have been applied in a number of other system implementations (Ref. 4).

Object–oriented programming offers an excellent tool for the implementation of a flexible and interactive real–time software package for experiment control and data acquisition. Here we will give only a short outline of the ideas. A more complete review can be found in Ref. 2.

An object consists of a data structure combined with a set of operations that can operate on that data structure. Each object is associated with a name, its identifier. All data relevant to the real–time system, as well as the operations pertaining to the experiment are assigned to objects. Various types of objects ("classes") exist in a system. The flexibility introduced by using object–oriented programming results mainly from the mechanism of <u>inheritance</u>, by means of which subclasses can inherit properties from already existing classes. The private data fields of objects are accessed in a protected way by the set of class–dependent generic operations.

An application implemented in such an environment may be considered as a relational database, containing both the instantaneous state of the experiment, as well as all operations that are allowed on the objects defining the experiment. The binding of the entities in the database is achieved during run–time by the user application, the experiment program. Without that program the separate entities exist, but they form a loosely coupled set. By using this <u>dynamic binding</u> (Ref. 2) mechanism the system is made more malleable at the cost of some processing power.

HARDWARE ARCHITECTURE AND IMPLEMENTATION

The hardware architecture employed to implement the multichannel MEG system is that of PHYDAS (Ref. 3). PHYDAS has originally been developed for the instrumentation and automation of medium and large scale experiments in physics. The main features of this system are a strongly real–time oriented design, high modularity and multiprocessor capabilities. This has been achieved by introducing a hierarchical triple–bus architecture (see Fig. 1), which reflects different real–time domains.

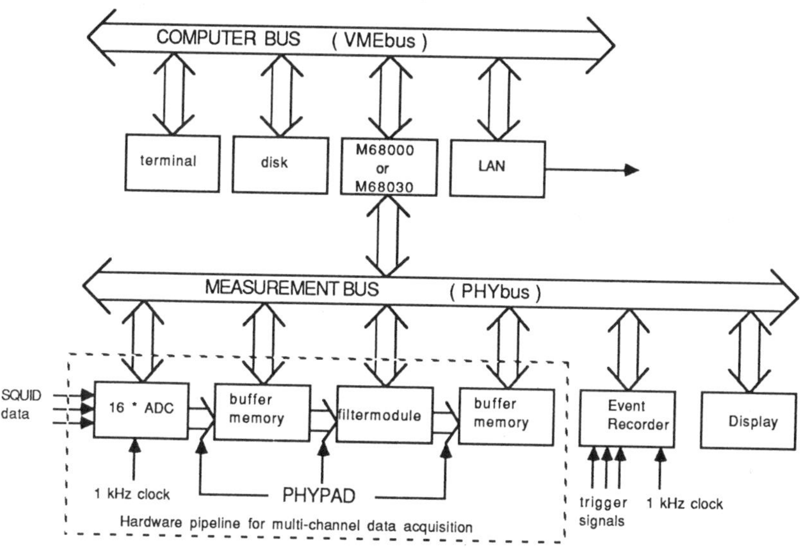

Fig. 1, An outline of the MEG hardware system.

The three busses consist of 1) the computer bus (standard VME–bus), 2) the asynchronous, processor independent measurement bus (PHYbus) and 3) the fast links, interconnecting elementary modules to form more advanced functional units (PHYPAD). Each bus has its specific functions and features which support the modularity of the system.

The VME–bus is used for the communication with standard I/O devices like terminal and a network controller. Here DMA actions may be used with cycle–stealing transfers, which are in time unpredictable. The asynchronous PHYbus deals with the communication between the CPU and all experiment–interfacing modules like the 16–channel ADC units, filter unit, local buffer memories and display unit. The transfers on the PHYbus (bandwidth 8 Mbyte/s, in blockmode 20 Mbyte/s) are completely controlled by the experimenter. The bus also contains control lines for multi–processor handling. The third bus, the PHYPAD, takes care of intermodule connections without support of the CPU.

In the MEG system data acquisition takes place at a maximum sample rate of 1kHz per channel. The data are filtered on–line, averaged and stored in memory. The data are subsequently transferred to harddisk, together with a time stamp and the classification of the event. At present a prototype system has been implemented for 3 MEG channels, using a Motorola 68000 CPU. The ultimate system will support 32 MEG and 32 EEG signal channels and will include a 68030 CPU.

It is worth noting that within the present architecture it is straightforward to incorporate future extensions, e.g. adding more processing power for computational intensive on–line data analyses. The triple–bus architecture facilitates the partitioning of a real–time system into independent functional parts. This in turn enables the experimenter to structure the system software as a number of concurrent tasks, for the MEG software:

- data acquisition and control of the ADC pipeline, including the digital signal processing.
- read–out of the eventrecorder, classifying the responses and stimuli.
- on–line averaging of the evoked response transients of the various types of events.
- display of transients.
- interactive intervention of the experimenter. By means of the user interface the operator is able to interact with the database describing the state of the experiment.

The hardware architecture provides the means to implement intelligent interfaces by interconnection of various modules. These interfaces operate autonomously without any risk to disturb the real–time actions of other interfaces. An example of an intelligent interface in the MEG system, is the pipeline (Fig. 1) formed by the multichannel AD converter, a local memory, the digital filter and a second local memory. CPU assistance is only required when a complete block of data (in the present implementation 4096 samples per channel) has been collected in the second memory. The process of reading the block of data from this second memory by the system processor is not time critical, because of the double buffered design of the memories.

The digital filter module in the ADC pipeline uses two cascadable IMS A100 digital signal processors (DSP) see Ref. 5. Each DSP can use up to 32 coefficients (16 bit, signed integers). The maximum throughput of the filter is $2.5 * 10^6$ samples/s. In the present implementation a throughput of $5 * 10^5$ samples/s has been used allowing for the filtering of more than 400 channels, each sampled with a sample rate of 1kHz. The intelligence of this pipeline is provided by a sophisticated dataflow controller, that has to switch each channel in turn to the filter, without loosing samples and without introducing artefacts due to the multiplexing and the internal DSP pipeline architecture. Output data from the filter are double buffered in blocks of 4096 samples at the end of the ADC pipeline, after which they are stored under CPU control.

RESULTS AND DISCUSSION

A three channel prototype of the MEG data acquisition system has been built and tested using experimental data, recorded on a multichannel analog recorder. Preliminary measurements show that the data acquisition pipeline, including A/D conversion at 1kHz, filtering, averaging and background storage, as well as the on–line visual display of the results for transients of 4 seconds duration, typically took 45 ms per channel. This performance has been achieved using a zero wait state M68030 computerboard running at 16 MHz and data compression techniques. From this figure it is evident that the present architecture will support the ultimate 64–channel MEG/EEG system.

In conclusion, it has been shown that by using a state–of–the–art real–time architecture, it is possible to design a powerful system for on–line data acquisition and analysis in multichannel neurophysiological experiments, that is flexible, user–friendly and affordable.

REFERENCES

1. P.W.E. Verhelst and N.F. Verster, "PEP, and interactive Programming system with an Algol–like programming language", Software practice and experience, 14(2), pp 119–133, 1984.

2. Brad J. Cox, "Object–oriented programming – An evolutionary appproach", Addison–Wesley Publishing Comp., Reading, 1986.

3. J.H. Voskamp, F.C. van Nijmweegen and A.J. van der Wal, "PHYDAS: a versatile architecture for data acquisition and control in physics experiments", submitted to Microprocessors and Microsystems.

4. L.J. Pinson, R.S. Wiener, "An introduction to object–oriented programming and Smalltalk, pp 29–30, Addison–Wesley Publishing Comp., Reading, 1988.

5. INMOS, Datasheet, 72TRN100 02, April 1987.

CHANNEL CAPACITY OF MULTICHANNEL MAGNETOMETERS

P. K. Kemppainen and R. J. Ilmoniemi

Low Temperature Laboratory
Helsinki University of Technology
02150 Espoo, Finland

INTRODUCTION

We have applied Shannon's theory of communication to develop a figure of merit for the comparison and optimization of multichannel magnetometers. This new measure is the channel capacity of the equipment in conveying information about cerebral currents. Like other figures of merit (Abraham-Fuchs et al., 1988; Carelli and Leoni, 1986; Erné 1985; Knuutila and Hämäläinen, 1989), it is a function of the SQUID noise level, the coil configuration, and the distance of the sensor array from the brain. Channel capacity as a cost function enables us to compare the marginal utility of different parameters, for example, of additional channels or a reduced brain-sensor distance, without specific source models.

METHODS

A magnetometer is a noisy channel conveying information from the sources of the field. Its output $v(t)$ is the sum of signal $b(t)$ and noise $u(t)$. When $b(t)$ and $u(t)$ are normally distributed and independent, the information gained through one sample of $v(t)$ is $I = \frac{1}{2}\log_2(P+1)$, where P is the power signal-to-noise ratio. If the same signal is transmitted N times and the received noisy signals are averaged, then the information per averaged sample is $I_N = \frac{1}{2}\log_2(NP+1)$ (Shannon and Weaver, 1949).

In order to reconstruct a band-limited signal of bandwidth Δf from samples recorded for a time interval Δt, the number of equally spaced samples required is $2\Delta t\Delta f$. If each sample has an information content I, the maximum information transfer rate of the channel, the channel capacity, is $C = 2I\Delta f$.

In addition to the noise level, the power signal-to-noise ratio of a single detector i depends on how well it is coupled to the source; this is described by the sensitivity pattern, i.e. by lead field L_i of the detector. As long as the conductivity is known, it is sufficient to formulate the lead field for the primary current J^p only. The sensor measures only the portion of J^p that is parallel to its lead field:

$$b_i = \vec{B}(\vec{r_i}) \cdot \vec{e_i} = \int_{V'} \vec{L_i}(\vec{r}\,') \cdot \vec{J^p}(\vec{r}\,')\, dv' \quad . \tag{1}$$

Here $\vec{B}(\vec{r_i})$ is the magnetic field at location $\vec{r_i}$ of the detector with sensitivity axis $\vec{e_i}$. The total current J is the sum of primary and volume currents, $J = J^p + J^v$,

Advances in Biomagnetism
Edited by S.J. Williamson *et al.*
Plenum Press, New York

where $\vec{J}^v(\vec{r}') = \sigma(\vec{r}')\vec{E}(\vec{r}')$; $\sigma(\vec{r}')$ is the conductivity and $\vec{E}(\vec{r}')$ the electric field. The definition of the primary current is identical to that of Plonsey for the impressed current but J^p refers to a macroscopic scale (Plonsey, 1969).

In our study, we modeled the conducting volume V' by a sphere. The results would be only marginally different for realistically-shaped head models. J^p was assumed to originate from a random process, which means that we have no specific prior knowledge about the nature of the sources. At each point in the sphere, the components of $\vec{J}^p$ are normally distributed: $J^p_\alpha(\vec{r}') \sim N(0, s^2)$, $\alpha = x, y, z$; they are also assumed uncorrelated with other components. Then, the signal-to-noise ratio is given by $P_i = \|L_i\|^2 s^2/\sigma_i^2$, where σ_i^2 is the variance of the noise u_i.

The total information of a multichannel magnetometer would be the sum of contributions from the single detectors, if the lead fields were orthogonal; the information from different channels would then be independent. With the orthogonalized set

$$\vec{L}'_i = \sum_j m_{ij}\vec{L}_j \ , \tag{2}$$

the transformed signal-to-noise ratios become $P'_i = \|L'_i\|^2 s^2/\sigma_i'^2$, where $\sigma_i'^2 = \sum_j (m_{ij}\sigma_j)^2$. The calculation of matrix $[\mathbf{M}]_{ij} = m_{ij}$ requires the inner-product matrix

$$[\mathbf{W}]_{ij} = \int_{V'} \vec{L}_i \cdot \vec{L}_j \, dv' \ . \tag{3}$$

As a normal matrix, $\mathbf{W}$ decomposes into $\mathbf{W} = \mathbf{U}\mathbf{\Lambda}\mathbf{U}^\mathbf{T}$, where $\mathbf{U}$ consists of the eigenvectors and the diagonal $\mathbf{\Lambda}$ of the eigenvalues of $\mathbf{W}$. We can choose $\mathbf{M} = \mathbf{U}^\mathbf{T}$, because then $\mathbf{W}' = \mathbf{U}^\mathbf{T}\mathbf{W}\mathbf{U} = (\mathbf{U}^\mathbf{T}\mathbf{U})\mathbf{\Lambda}(\mathbf{U}^\mathbf{T}\mathbf{U}) = \mathbf{\Lambda}$. The total information per sample is obtained from the signal-to-noise ratios $P'_i = s^2\lambda_i/\sum_j(u_{ij}\sigma_j)^2$ of the orthogonalized channels:

$$I_{tot} = \frac{1}{2}\sum_{i=1}^{N}\log_2(P'_i + 1) \ . \tag{4}$$

RESULTS

Figure 1 illustrates the first application of the proposed figure of merit. Magnetometer pickup coils were placed hexagonally on a spherical cap with 125-mm radius of curvature. The number of channels was increased by six at a time; the configuration was updated so that the centers of the outermost pickup coils were kept on a 73-mm circle. For the three densest configurations, the noise level was increased to account for the smaller coil size; when the energy sensitivity of a coil is constant, the magnetic field noise increases as $d^{3/2}$, where d is the diameter of the coil.

Because the area for the coils in the dewar is fixed, there is an optimal number of channels, after which the channel capacity decreases. This is due to the overlap of the lead fields and the increased noise level.

As a second application, the eight magnetometers listed in Table 1 were compared. BTI5, BTI7 and BTI37 refer to the commercial instruments of Biomagnetic Technologies Inc. The 7M and the planar gradiometer 24M are the magnetometers of our laboratory (Knuutila et al., 1987; Kajola et al., 1989). Dor22 is a two-dewar system of Dornier GmbH; it has 28 magnetometer channels, and the gradiometer output is calculated from the magnetometer outputs; typically 22 pickup channels are then used. S31M and S37M are the new flat-bottom magnetometers of Siemens Ag (Gudden et al., 1989).

Table 1. Eight magnetometers compared.

	BTI5	BTI7	7M	Dor22	24M	S31M	S37M	BTI37
Number of channels	5	7	7	22	24	31	37	37
Order of gradiometers	II	II	I	I	I	I	I	I
Baselength [mm]	40	40	60	133*	13	60	70	50
Noise level [$fT/\sqrt{Hz}$]	20	20	6	$15\sqrt{2}$	5	20	12	10
Array diameter [mm]	36	36	72	136	90	160	162	140
Coil diameter [mm]	15	15	20	20	30.5	30	25	20

* The smallest baselength. See text.

When calculating the conveyed information (4), each magnetometer was placed above a sphere of 95 mm radius so that its symmetry axis pointed to the center of the sphere. The distance between the spherical surface, which corresponds to the brain, and the center of the sensor grid was 30 mm in all setups, except with S31M and S37M where it was 40 mm because of the thick dewar bottom. The variance s of the source was set to correspond to an rms field amplitude of 100 fT.

The results are given in Fig. 2. The differences in information per channel can be explained mostly by variations in the noise levels. To find the effect of configuration only, information (4) was calculated with the equal flux noise level of 10 $fT/\sqrt{Hz}$ for each system (Fig. 2).

BTI5 conveys more information per channel than BTI7 because the area covered is the same. Adding channels to a fixed space results in larger overlap of lead fields, thus reducing the utility of additional sensors. The new channels would give maximum benefit if the gradiometers were constructed so that the lead fields were orthogonal.

The main reason for the difference between BTI7 and 7M is the larger area of the latter, but the baselength and the order of the gradiometers have small effects as well. Despite its large area, S31M had the lowest information per channel; this is due to the long distance from the source and the flat configuration. The gradiometers at the edges of the array are relatively distant from the conducting volume. Therefore the six additional channels in S37M do not increase the amount of total information essentially. However, 37 channels on a curved surface, as in BTI37, would give a much better result.

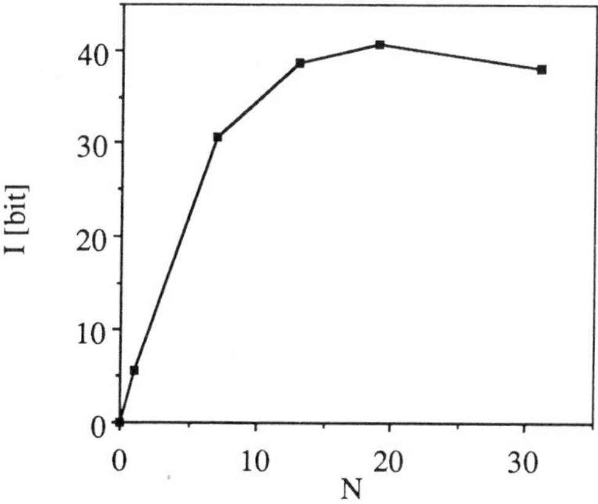

Fig. 1. Information per sampling time of a multichannel magnetometer.

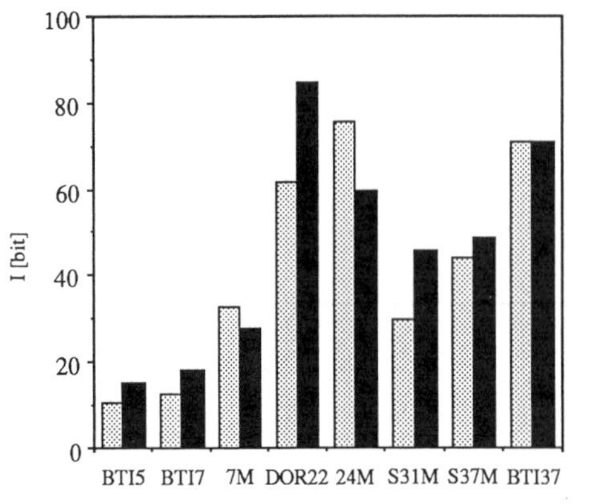

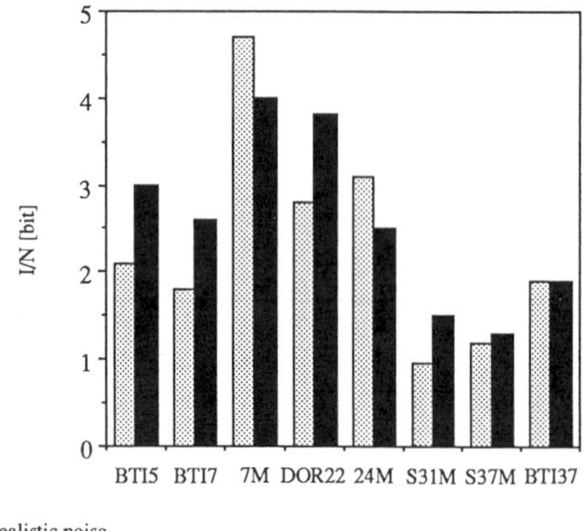

Fig. 2. a) Information I_{tot} (4) of different magnetometers. b) I_{tot} per channel.

DISCUSSION

Channel capacity as the figure of merit is applicable to any measurement setup; different conductivity and source distributions can be taken into account. For example, the sensitivity to deep sources can be evaluated by limiting the source volume for lead field calculations. Correlated noise, e.g., from the dewar, can be handled by a proper change of basis. The information-theoretical approach allows us to compare magnetometers without reference to a specific source model, such as the dipole model. Thus, we get results relevant for multi-purpose instruments.

REFERENCES

Abrahams-Fuchs, K., Schneider, S., Reichenberger, H., 1988, MCG inverse solution: Influence of coil size, grid size, number of coils, and SNR. *IEEE Trans. Biom. Eng.*, 35:573.

Carelli, P., Leoni, R., 1986, Localization of biological sources with arrays of superconducting gradiometers, *J. Appl. Phys.* 59:645.

Erné, S.N., 1985, SQUID measurement techniques in medical diagnosis, *in* "SQUID'85, Superconducting Quantum Interference Devices and their Applications", H.D. Hahlbohm, H. Lübbig, eds., Walter de Gruyter, Berlin.

Gudden, F., Hoenig, E., Reichenberger, H., Schittenhelm, R., Schneider, S., 1989, A multi-channel system for use in biomagnetic diagnosis in neurology and cardiology: principle, method and initial results, *Electromedica*, 57:2.

Kajola, M., Ahlfors, S., Ehnholm, G.J., Hällström, J., Hämäläinen, M.S., Ilmoniemi, R.J., Kiviranta, M., Knuutila, J., Lounasmaa, O.V., Tesche, C.D., Vilkman, V., 1989, A 24-channel magnetometer for brain research, this volume.

Knuutila, J., Ahlfors, S., Ahonen, A., Hällström, J., Kajola, M., Lounasmaa, O.V., Vilkman, V., Tesche, C., 1987, A large-area low-noise seven-channel magnetometer for brain research, *Rev. Sci. Instrum.*, 58:2145.

Knuutila, J., Hämäläinen, M.S., 1989, On the spatial locating accuracy of multichannel magnetometers, this volume.

Plonsey, R., 1969, "Bioelectric Phenomena", McGraw-Hill, New York.

Shannon, C.E., Weaver, W., 1949, "The Mathematical Theory of Communication", The University of Illinois Press, Urbana.

A 24-CHANNEL PLANAR GRADIOMETER:

SYSTEM DESIGN AND ANALYSIS OF NEUROMAGNETIC DATA

Matti S. Hämäläinen

Low Temperature Laboratory
Helsinki University of Technology
02150 Espoo, Finland

INTRODUCTION

After the first neuromagnetic measurements with single-SQUID instruments in the early 1970's, multi-channel devices were built in several laboratories (for a review, see Ilmoniemi et al., 1989). However, the number of channels has been rather limited and multiple measurements at different dewar positions are generally needed for locating the neural current sources accurately. We are just getting ready a complete multichannel system for neuromagnetic studies. It consists of a 24-channel dc-SQUID gradiometer, signal detection electronics, signal preconditioning and measurement control electronics, data acquisition system, a probe position indicator (PPI), computer hardware, and software for measurement and analysis of data. This paper will first give an overview of our system and will then concentrate on features of the software which have been the main responsibility of the author.

GRADIOMETER AND ELECTRONICS

Our new instrument consists of 12 identical units, each incorporating two IBM dc SQUIDs (Tesche et al., 1985) and the associated wire-wound flux transformers. The planar gradiometers measure the two off-diagonal derivatives, $\partial B_z/dx$ and $\partial B_z/\partial y$, at 12 locations; B_z is the component of the magnetic field perpendicular to the curved bottom of the dewar, which is the same as used in our previous seven-channel instrument (Knuutila et al., 1987). The two orthogonal pickup coils were wound in a figure-of-eight configuration; the size of each unit is 30 by 30 mm^2. The array covers a spherical cap with a diameter of 125 mm.

The preamplifiers are mounted on top of the dewar, while the main SQUID electronics (Knuutila et al., 1987) is located in an rf-shielded cabinet outside our magnetically shielded room. The whole electronics is modular with 24 identical preamplifier detector-controller cards. The operating mode, the two available sensitivity ranges, and the autozero function of the electronics are computer controllable. The noise level of the instrument is in the range of 3 - 6 $\mathrm{fT/(cm\sqrt{Hz})}$. More details on the gradiometer and examples of the results obtained with can be found from another article in this volume (Kajola et al., 1989). The basic design principles and comparison with other feasible configurations are discussed by Knuutila et al. (1985) and by Knuutila and Hämäläinen (1989).

Advances in Biomagnetism
Edited by S.J. Williamson *et al.*
Plenum Press, New York

DATA ACQUISITION

The analog signals from the SQUID electronics are brought with shielded twisted-pair cables to the signal preconditioning electronics. The raw data are led, before digitizing, through a fourth-order low-pass Butterworth filter with a computer-selectable cut-off frequency and, optionally, through a second-order high-pass Bessel filter, fixed at 0.05 Hz. The lowpass filters are realized with switched-capacitor circuits, allowing a selection of the cut-off frequency by adjusting the filter clock frequencies. The filter rack also includes the stimulus output circuitry as well as three additional analog inputs directly connected to the A/D converter to be used for acquisition other signals of interest, e.g. stimulus waveforms.

The system also allows EEG measurements on up to 32 channels. Our commercial EEG amplifier unit contains the necessary bandpass filters whence the signal preconditioning electronics only consists of a differential-to-single-ended converter.

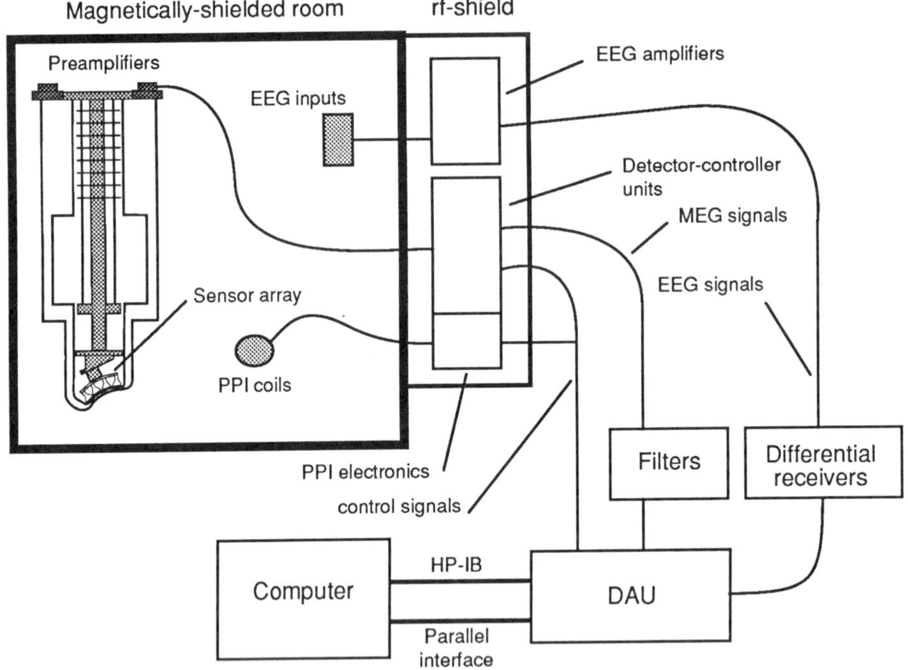

Fig. 1. Overview of the 24-channel MEG system including the EEG amplifiers and PPI.

The signals are then digitized with a HP 3852A data acquisition unit (DAU), equipped with two 48-channel FET multiplexers connected to high-speed voltmeters, together providing an aggregate sampling rate of 200 kHz which corresponds to 8.3 kHz per channel. Currently only one voltmeter is used in routine measurements. Digital output ports allow control of the SQUID electronics, low-pass filters, and of stimulus generation. The data acquisition unit is interfaced to the main computer via an IEEE-488 bus for control and program download and via dedicated parallel ports connected directly to voltmeters for data upload.

The filtered signals are also connected to an analog multiplexer which is used to select eight channels to be continuously monitored on a real-time display comprising a PC equipped with an AD-converter and a special data monitor card. An overview of the hardware is depicted in Fig. 1.

COMPUTERS

The main computer system consists of an HP 1000/A900 CPU with 3-Mbyte memory and a 576-Mbyte hard disk. Additional peripherals of the system include a graphics workstation, several terminals, a dedicated PC for fast on-line display of data, as well as printers and a plotter. The computer system is also connected to the university's local-area network (LAN).

The computer utilizes the HP-proprietary RTE-A (Real-Time-Executive) multitasking, multiuser operating system. The HP 1000 system provides excellent real-time capabilities, including a fast response to external interrupts (typical response time < 1 ms). Despite of its old-fashioned 16-bit architecture, the A900 has proved to be an ideal data-acquisition controller with a reasonable amount of computing power for analysis.

With increasing number of simultaneously measured channels the computer becomes very involved with data acquisition and on-line averaging: the measurement program uses more than 90% of the CPU time when 24 channels are acquired with an interstimulus interval (ISI) of 500 ms or less. Therefore, the off-line analysis programs are now being ported to a RISC-architecture HP 9000/835 UNIX workstation.

This new computer system has a 16-Mbyte main memory and a hard disk identical to that of the HP 1000 system. The workstation offers extended capabilities for data analysis through a high-performance 1024-by-1280-pixel resolution graphics display. In addition to the HP 1000 system, several UNIX-based workstations, Macintosh IIs, and IBM PCs will be later connected to the HP 835 system through LAN to provide additional graphics displays. On software level, this forthcoming new computer cluster will make use of standard interconnection tools: ARPA-Berkeley services for terminal connections and file transfer, the SUN Network File System (NFS) for file sharing, and the X-Window system for basic graphical user interface. The LAN also provides a possibility for convenient access to the Cray located on campus. Since this supercomputer also runs UNIX it provides an attractive option to off-load computationally exhaustive tasks from the local computer cluster.

REAL-TIME SOFTWARE

We have developed real-time measurement software for both evoked-response studies and for spontaneous activity measurements. Both transient and steady-state evoked responses can be processed with up to 40 channels. The data are, after rejection of artefacts, averaged on line and the evolution of the averages of up to 16 channels can be monitored during the measurement. In addition to the averages, the standard errors of the mean are routinely calculated to provide an estimate of the noise level during the measurement.

The software keeps in pace with the incoming data down to an ISI of 500 ms when 24 channels with 512 samples per epoch are acquired. If the ISI is further decreased or if the number of channels is increased, an intermediate file to hold the raw data records is automatically created. Therefore, it is possible to do on-line averaging even with short ISIs with the only drawback that averaging may eventually be somewhat out of phase, which implies waiting for the completition of the process after the data acquisition has actually stopped. If necessary, the individual epochs can be saved on disk for off-line analysis. This allows application of sophisticated signal analysis techniques and also makes it possible to view the individual epochs.

Six different stimuli can be delivered in a single transient response measurement under the control of a program residing in DAU. The TTL-level stimulus pulses can be used to trigger various kinds of stimulators. The data are grouped accordingly to produce separate averages for responses corresponding to each of the stimuli. The six averages are shown with separate colors on the average monitor. In addition to internally controlled stimuli, it is also possible to use an external trigger to indicate the time instant of the stimulus. In this case, however, only one type of stimulus can be employed in a single measurement.

In the steady-state paradigm, the determination of the stimulus repetition rate is done by software from a digitized trigger pulse prior to each stimulus. Two such trigger signals can be inspected to allow two stimuli with different repetition rates to be presented simultaneously.

All the acquisition parameters, such as the the sampling rate, the pre- and post-stimulus intervals, the ISIs between the stimuli, the sequence of stimuli delivered as well as the length of the stimulus pulses are completely user controllable. All the parameters can be saved in files making it easy to restore any previously used measurement setup.

In an MEG measurement it is of great importance to be able to determine the location of the dewar, in relation to the head, as accurately as possible. For this purpose we use a probe position indicator (PPI) comprising of small coils attached on the scalp. The coils are sequentially energized and their magnetic field is detected with the gradiometer. From these measurements the location and orientation of the dewar can be deduced. The achieved position accuracy is a few millimeters (for details, see Ahlfors and Ilmoniemi, 1989).

DATA ANALYSIS

The averaged responses are displayed and plotted off-line. Signal amplitudes at selected latencies can be determined interactively. Spatial features of the data may be viewed either as conventional isocontour plots or as 'arrow maps' (Cohen et al., 1976). The latter are constructed simply by rotating the measured two-dimensional gradient, at each sensor location, clockwise by 90 degrees:

$$\mathbf{v} = \frac{\partial B_z}{\partial y}\mathbf{e_x} - \frac{\partial B_z}{\partial x}\mathbf{e_y}\,. \tag{1}$$

The arrow maps are an useful visual tool, often giving a good hint about the location and orientation of the currents underlying the measured data.

The arrow maps can be considered as first-order approximations for minimum-norm current estimates (MNE, Hämäläinen and Ilmoniemi, 1984), which we have now introduced as a routine display. The MNE is defined as the current distribution which has the smallest norm among all square-integrable currents defined in a certain volume or surface G. Here the norm of a current distribution $\mathbf{J}$ is the usual L_2 norm:

$$\langle \mathbf{J},\mathbf{J} \rangle = \int_G \mathbf{J}\cdot\mathbf{J}\, dG\,. \tag{2}$$

It turns out that the MNE is a weighted sum of the lead fields, or sensitivity functions of the gradiometers used in the measurement. Being a linear combination of continuous vector fields, the MNE is continuous whereas the arrow maps are defined only at the discrete measurement points. Furthermore, by constructing the MNE on a surface at the approximate location of the real current distribution, it is more closely confined to the sites of activity than the 'raw' arrow maps. The estimates also provide a way for interpolation and extrapolation: the magnetic field that would be produced by the MNE can be used to construct an isocontour plot from the gradient measurements. An

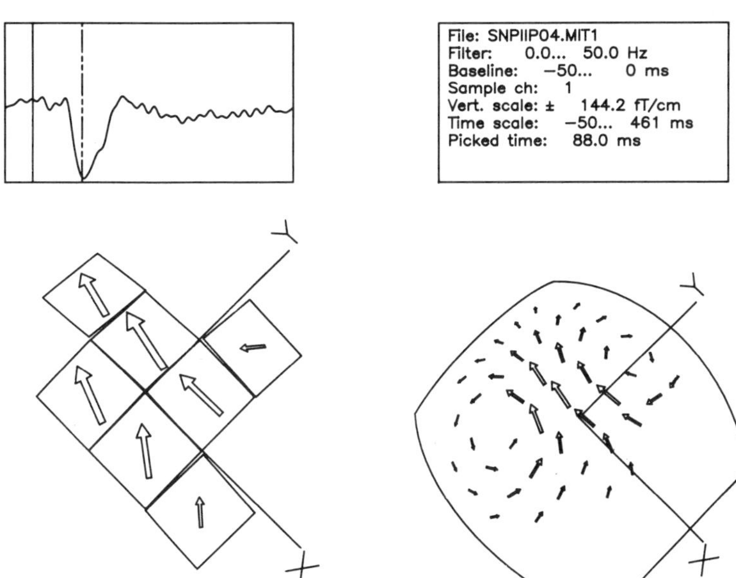

Fig. 2. An example of the output from the 'arrowmapper' program used to analyze the 24-channel MEG data. A sample auditory evoked response is shown in the upper left inset with the picked time instant (88 ms after stimulus) indicated by a dashed line. The upper right inset contains the information about the data being analyzed. The two lower insets show the arrow map computed from the 14-channel data at the picked time (left) and the corresponding minimum-norm current distribution estimate (right). The MNE has been constructed on a spherical cap 30 mm below the scalp.

example of an arrow map and a minimum norm estimate constructed from a measurement with 14 out of the 24 channels of our new gradiometer is shown in Fig. 2.

Further interpretation of the signals, in terms of currents flowing in the cortex, involves restrictive assumptions about the primary source and modeling of the surrounding conductor. We routinely use the current dipole model in a spherically symmetric conductor. As shown previously (Hämäläinen and Sarvas, 1989), a reasonable refinement to the sphere model is the homogeneous head model.

The calculation of the magnetic field with the homogeneous model involves two steps: (1) computation of the potential on the surface of the conductor and (2) integration of the magnetic field from the potential (Horacek, 1973). Dividing the conductor surface into n (typically from 300 to 500) triangles we find that the potential values $\mathbf{v} = (V_1 \ldots V_n)^T$ (superscript T denotes the matrix transpose) at the centers of the triangles are related to the corresponding potential values $\mathbf{v}^0 = (V_1^0 \ldots V_n^0)^T$ for an infinite homogeneous medium by

$$\mathbf{v}^0 = \mathbf{C}\mathbf{v}, \tag{3}$$

where $\mathbf{C}$ is an n-by-n matrix.

Our goal is to obtain the outputs of a particular set of gradiometers $\mathbf{b} = (b_1 \ldots b_m)^T$ We obtain $\mathbf{b}$ from

$$\mathbf{b} = \mathbf{M}\mathbf{v} + \mathbf{b}^0, \tag{4}$$

where $\mathbf{b}^0 = (b_1^0 \ldots b_m^0)^T$ are the values which would be measured if the conductor were infinite and $\mathbf{M}$ is an m-by-m matrix. Assuming that $\mathbf{C}$ can be inverted we obtain, combining Eqs. (3) and (4),

$$\mathbf{b} = \mathbf{T}\mathbf{v}^0 + \mathbf{b}^0 , \tag{5}$$

where $\mathbf{T} = \mathbf{M}\mathbf{C}^{-1}$. The last step requires that $\mathbf{C}^{-1}$ is explicitly known. Up to now, however, iterative techniques have been used to solve Eq. (3) for $\mathbf{v}$, which requires too much computation time to allow the application of the homogeneous model to on-line analysis. We recently found that $\mathbf{C}$ can actually be inverted using the singular-value decomposition allowing us to apply Eq. (5). Since $\mathbf{T}$ is an m-by-n matrix and m is typically much smaller than n ($m = 24$ for a single 24-channel measurement), computation of $\mathbf{b}$ via Eq. (5) is the simple task of performing n dot products of n-vectors and m additions. It turns out that the required computation time is only about twice the time for the sphere model.

ACKNOWLEDGEMENTS

The design and construction of the system has been a group effort of S. Ahlfors, A. Ahonen, J. Hällström, G. Ehnholm, R. Ilmoniemi, M. Kajola, J. Knuutila, M. Kiviranta, O.V. Lounasmaa, C. Tesche, and V. Vilkman. The project is financially supported by Finnish National Fund for Research and Development (SITRA).

REFERENCES

Ahlfors, S. and Ilmoniemi, R.J., 1989, Magnetometer position indicator for multichannel MEG, this volume.

Cohen, D. and Hosaka, H., 1976, Magnetic field produced by a current dipole, *J. Electrocardiology*, 9:409.

Horacek, B.M., 1973, Digital model for studies in magnetocardiography, *IEEE Trans. Magn.*, MAG-9:440.

Hämäläinen, M.S. and Ilmoniemi, R.J., 1984, Interpreting measured magnetic fields of the brain: estimates of current distributions, *Report TKK-F-A559*, Helsinki University of Technology.

Hämäläinen, M.S. and Sarvas, J., 1989, Realistic conductivity geometry model of the human head for interpretation of neuromagnetic data, *IEEE Trans. Biomed. Eng.*, BME-36:165.

Ilmoniemi, R., Knuutila, J., Ryhänen, T., and Seppä, H., 1989, Multi-SQUID devices and their applications, *Progr. Low Temp. Phys.*, 12, in press.

Kajola, M., Ahlfors, S., Ehnholm, G., Hällström, J., Hämäläinen, M.S., Ilmoniemi, R., Kiviranta, M., Knuutila, J., Lounasmaa, O.V., Tesche, C., and Vilkman, V., 1989, A 24-channel magnetometer for brain research, this volume.

Knuutila, J., Ahonen A.I., Hämäläinen, M.S., Ilmoniemi, R.J., and Kajola M.J., 1985, Design considerations for multichannel SQUID magnetometers, *in:* "SQUID'85 - Superconducting Quantum Interference Devices and their Applications", H.D. Hahlbohm and H. Lübbig, eds., Walter de Gruyter, Berlin.

Knuutila, J., Ahlfors, S., Ahonen, A., Hällström, J., Kajola, M., Lounasmaa, O.V., and Vilkman, V., 1987, Large-area low-noise seven-channel dc SQUID magnetometer for brain research, *Rev. Sci. Instrum.*, 58:2145.

Knuutila, J. and Hämäläinen M.S., 1989, On the spatial locating accuracy of multichannel magnetometers, this volume.

Tesche, C.D., Brown, K.H., Callegari, A.C., Chen, M.M., Greiner, J.H., Jones, H.C., Ketchen, M.B., Kim, K.K., Kleinsasser, A.W., Notarys, H.A., Proto, G., Wang, R.H., and Yogi, T., 1985, Practical dc SQUIDs with extremely low 1/f noise, *IEEE Trans. Magn.*, MAG-21:1032.

IMPROVED SQUID MAGNETOMETER
WITH AN EXTERNAL FEEDBACK CIRCUIT

Y. Igarashi, T. Goto, T. Hayashi, N. Fujimaki*,
K. Kawabe, T. Shimura, and H. Hayashi

Medical Electronics Laboratory, Exploratory Devices Laboratory*
FUJITSU LABORATORIES LTD.
1015 Kamikodanaka, Nakahara-ku, Kawasaki 221, Japan

INTRODUCTION

The large magnetic noise and weak magnetic signal level of the heart and brain in magnetic measurement require that a magnetometer have a wide dynamic range and be highly sensitive. The single-chip digital SQUID magnetometer proposed by Fujimaki (Fujimaki, 1988) featured an internal superconducting feedback circuit that made it compact (3.0 mm x 3.5 mm), but its dynamic range was limited by the volume of magnetic flux stored in the superconducting feedback loop.

We report here how we improved it to extend the dynamic range and verify its operation and sensitivity.

METHODS

The storage volume of the single-chip digital SQUID magnetometer can be increased by increasing internal feedback loop inductance to extend the dynamic range (covered by another group at this Conference). Here, we report on a wide-range magnetometer using external feedback.

Figure 1 shows the improved magnetometer, which consists of a pickup coil, SQUID sensor, amplifier, up/down counter, feedback circuit including a D/A converter, and AC-biased current source. The SQUID chip, which is about 2 x 10 mm, consists of a SQUID sensor made of two Josephson junctions, superconducting loop, input coil, and feedback coil. The pickup coil has the geometry of a second-order gradiometer 2.4 cm in diameter, has a 3.0-cm baseline, and is wound round a ceramic coil bobbin using NbTi wire. The amplitude of the AC-biased current is adjusted to the threshold current of the SQUID sensor to enable operation in pulse mode. A digital SQUID magnetometer proposed by Dr. Drung and his colleagues (Drung, 1986) produces only positive pulses, but our sensor produces positive or negative pulses based on the polarity of the magnetic flux in the SQUID loop. These pulses are amplified and counted up or down based on the polarity. The count is converted to a feedback current. When the feedback flux caused by the feedback current cancels the input flux in the SQUID loop, the SQUID sensor produces no pulse. At that time, the counter content represents the magnetic flux detected by the pickup coil. We use an 18-bit D/A converter to give the magnetometer a range of 100 dB (from 10 nT to 0.1 pT).

Fig. 2 shows the pickup coil and SQUID sensor immersed in liquid helium. The center cylinder is a SQUID sensor package covered by Nb metal and magnetically shielded.

Advances in Biomagnetism
Edited by S.J. Williamson *et al.*
Plenum Press, New York

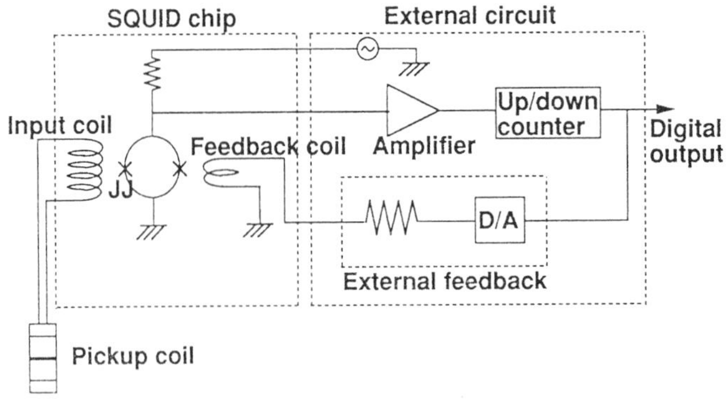

Fig. 1. Improved SQUID magnetometer

RESULTS

The faint alternate magnetic field generated with a 40-turn coil (2 cm in diameter) was measured in a magnetic shielded box placed in a RF-shielded room (Fig. 3). This coil was set 10 cm below the pickup coil cooled by liquid helium. The frequency f_B of the AC-biased current was 300 kHz. Fig. 4 shows the analog output for the alternate magnetic field. As shown by Fig. 4 (b), the noise level was about 10 pT. For a signal bandwidth of 100 Hz, this SQUID magnetometer's sensitivity was 0.3 pT / $\sqrt{Hz}$. The slew rate was 2.7 x 10^4 Φ_0 / s (in f_B = 300 kHz). The sensitivity was 2.3 x 10^{-5} Φ_0 / $\sqrt{Hz}$ for the flux in the SQUID sensor without a pickup coil.

Fig. 5 shows the results for different magnetic fields. The dynamic range was 65 dB and the magnetometer had good linearity.

DISCUSSION

The dynamic range, designed to be 100 dB. was actually 65 dB because the minimum sensitivity was still limited by the noise level. In our present magnetometer, we found that the external circuit and SQUID chip are readily disturbed by noise.

Improving of the external circuit and SQUID chip will improve sensitivity 20 to 30 dB on and enable measurement of the magnetocardiograms.

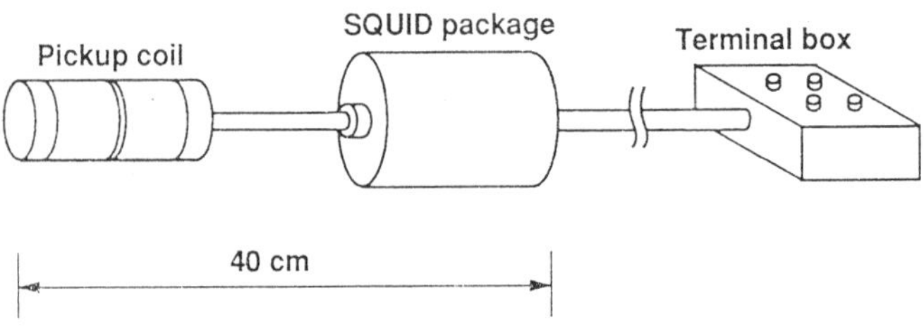

Fig.2. Pickup coil and SQUID package

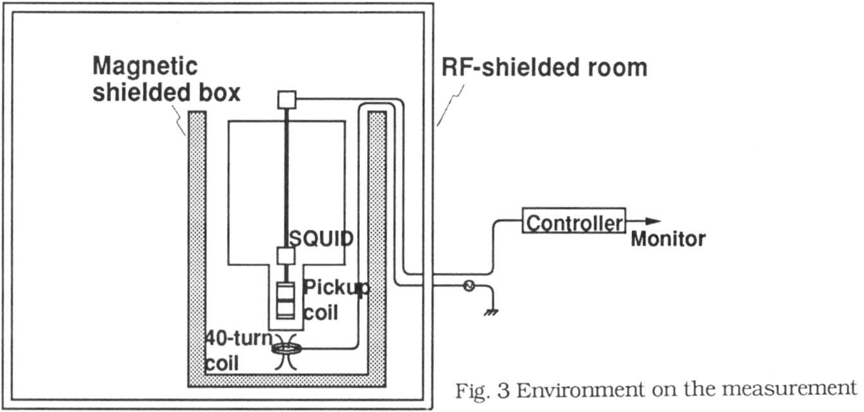

Fig. 3 Environment on the measurement

(a)

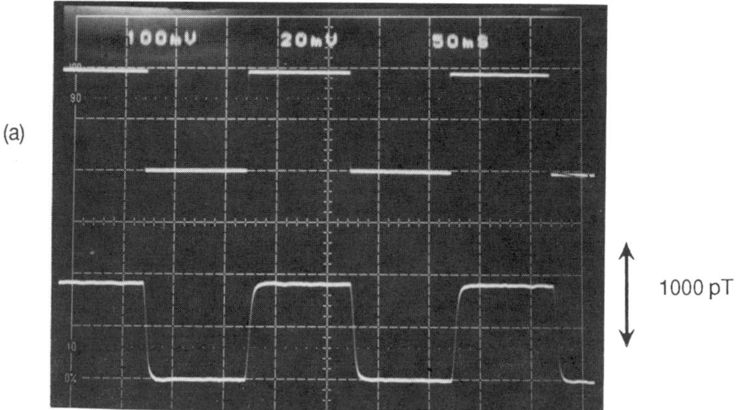

(b)

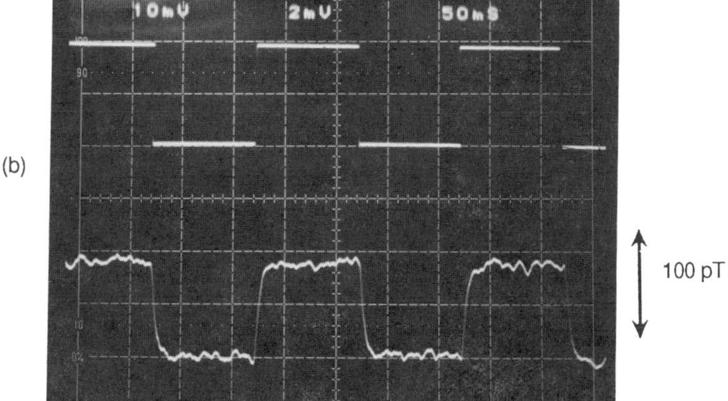

Fig. 4 Results; in (a) and (b), the upper lines show the signal input to the coil and lower lines show the output signal.
(a) Input magnetic field 1000 pT, freq. 5 Hz
(b) Input magnetic field 100 pT, freq. 5 Hz

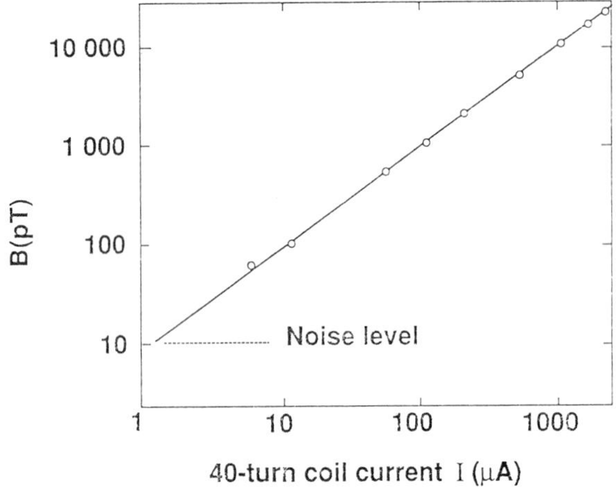

Fig. 5 Sensitivity and dynamic range

CONCLUSION

We confirmed that our external-feedback digital SQUID magnetometer has a sensitivity of 0.3 pT / $\sqrt{Hz}$ and dynamic range of 65 dB. The sensitivity was 2.3 x 10^{-5} Φ_0 / $\sqrt{Hz}$ for the flux in the SQUID sensor without a pickup coil.

The wide-range digital SQUID magnetometer promises to be a useful diagnostic tool in biomagnetic imaging.

REFERENCES

Drung, D. (1986). Digital feedback loops for d. c. SQUIDs. Cryogenics, 26, 623-627

Fujimaki, N., Tamura, H., Imamura, T., and Hasuo, S. (1988). A Single-Chip SQUID Magnetometer. IEEE Trans. Electron Devices, 35, 2412-2418

DESIGNING PLANAR GRADIOMETER ARRAYS : PRELIMINARY CONSIDERATIONS

A.C. Bruno and P. Costa Ribeiro

Departamento de Fisica, Pontificia Universidade Catolica
Caixa Postal 38071, Rio de Janeiro, 22453, RJ, Brasil

INTRODUCTION

A few years ago, when small scale multichannel systems (4 up to 7 channels) were built, a step forward was taken in biomagnetic measurements. The use of these systems shortened the time of measurement, allowing a more extensive source mapping and decreasing the risk of subject fatigue during the experiment. It is commonly said that the ultimate goal in this field is to build systems with a large number of detecting sensors, for instance 50 to 100 planar gradiometers. The purpose of this work is to begin a study on the design of these systems.

DESIGNING THE ARRAY

It will be discussed here some aspects of the array design: the array size and the number of gradiometers. The gradiometer coils' areas will be considered infinitely small because the analysis will be only on the sensor positioning. As the planar gradiometer is in linear shape, the study can be focused only on one array line, with the gradiometer orientation axis parallel to the array line. Finally it will be assumed that the source is under the center of the array.

As an example, the spatial properties of the most common model source used in biomagnetism, the current dipole, will be analysed. Fig. 1 shows different gradiometers outputs $B_z(x)$ of the magnetic field generated by a current dipole, at a $3\,cm$ depth and immersed in a semi-infinite conducting media. The dipole is oriented in the y direction. Curves a), b) and c) are the outputs for a magnetometer, first order ($2\,cm$ total length) and second order ($2\,cm$ total length) planar gradiometers respectively.

The array size, that in this case corresponds to the length (L) of the line of gradiometers, can be obtained considering the total signal energy by using the Parseval's Theorem (Antoniou A., 1979 and Bruno A.C. et al., 1986). The total energy of the signal is proportional to:

$$E \propto \int_{-\infty}^{\infty} \mid B_z(x) \mid^2 \; dx. \tag{1}$$

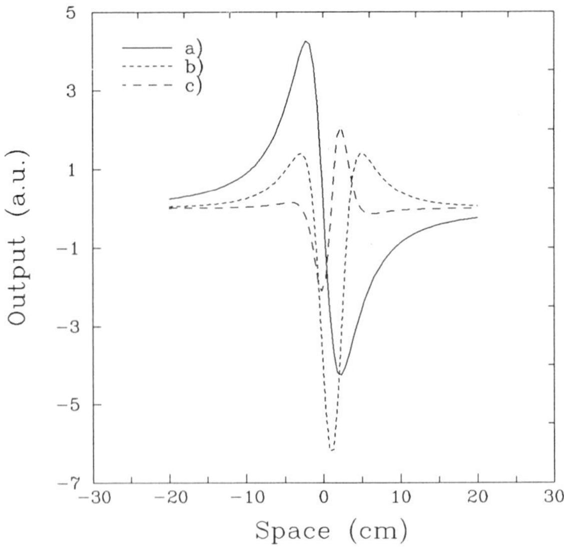

Fig. 1 B_z versus x for a magnetometer a), first order b) and second order c) planar gradiometers with 2 cm total length, detecting a current dipole at a distance of 3 cm below the gradiometer.

To be able to maintain nearly the total energy when measuring the signal, the limits L of integral (2) should be chosen in a way that 99% of the total energy is still present,

$$99\% \int_{-\infty}^{\infty} | B_z(x) |^2 \, dx = \int_{-L/2}^{L/2} | B_z(x) |^2 \, dx. \tag{2}$$

For the signals depicted in Fig. 1 the line lengths L that correspond to 99% of the total energy are 32 cm, 16 cm and 12 cm for the magnetometer, first and second order gradiometers respectively. For signals due to a deeper source of 7 cm, the values for L are 52 cm, 30 cm and 20 cm respectively. When building such array, one should consider the length that corresponds to the deeper source. The size of a planar gradiometer array can be smaller than the size of a magnetometer array because the output signal intensity decays more rapidly in the former. It also can be noticed that as the gradiometer order increases, the array size decreases.

On a first approach, a simple way to determine the array sampling period is to estimate the highest frequency component of the signal, investigating the smallest distance P between nearby peaks and valleys of the signal. This distance is related to the highest frequency component. The distance between a peak and a valley represents half of the period. Hence, the highest frequency is $F = 1/2P$. One may choose the array sampling frequency, obeying the Nyquist theorem, as $2.5F$ or, equivalently, the sampling period as $0.8P$. Inspecting Fig.1 one can see that the smallest distances between peaks and valleys are 4.5 cm, 3.7 cm and 2.5 cm for the magnetometer, first order and second order gradiometers respectively. Thus, the array sampling period should be 3.6 cm, 3.0 cm and 2.0 cm.

Another way to estimate the higher frequency component of the signal is to calculate its spatial Fourier transform and this has already been done for magnetometers (Romani et al., 1985). Fig. 2 shows spatial Fourier transforms of the output of a magnetometer, first and second order planar gradiometers due to a current dipole at a

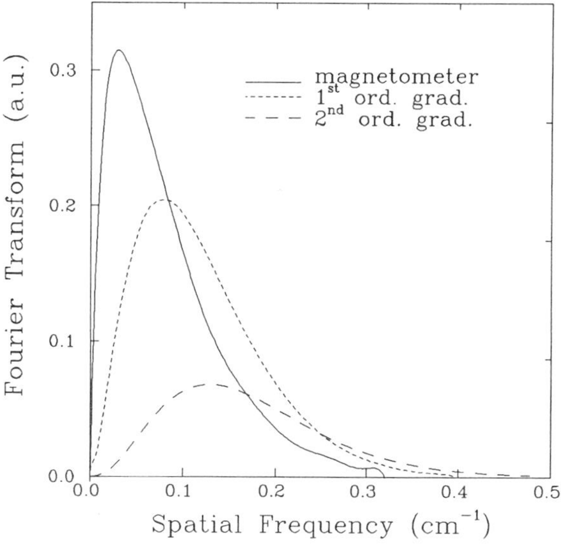

Fig. 2 Fourier Transforms $\mathcal{B}(k)$ for a current dipole at a $3\,cm$ depth detected by a magnetometer, first order and second order planar gradiometers.

$3\,cm$ depth.

By using the Parseval's theorem applied to the frequency domain:

$$E \propto \frac{1}{2\pi} \int_{-\infty}^{\infty} \mid \mathcal{B}(k) \mid^2 \, dk, \tag{3}$$

and calculating the following equation:

$$99\% \int_{-\infty}^{\infty} \mid \mathcal{B}(k) \mid^2 \, dk = \int_{-F}^{F} \mid \mathcal{B}(k) \mid^2 \, dk, \tag{4}$$

the magnetometer, first and second order planar gradiometers have the following values for the maximum frequency $F\,(cm^{-1})$: 0.16, 0.24 and 0.32 respectively. Applying the Nyquist theorem as $2.5F$, the sampling periods should be $2.5\,cm$, $1.7\,cm$ and $1.2\,cm$ for arrays of magnetometers, first and second order planar gradiometers respectively. By comparing to the values obtained in the first method, one should use these values since they are smaller. In this case a deeper source do not need to be considered since it will not generate higher frequency components.

Notice that since the gradiometer sensor has a $2\,cm$ length it will be difficult to build an array with first or second order planar gradiometers for detecting a $3\,cm$ depth source, since it will require a spacing less than $2\,cm$ between gradiometers. However, if one take into account the inner-outer dewar distance of about $1\,cm$ and the dewar-subject distance of about $0.5\,cm$, the minimum distance between gradiometer and source could increase to about $4.5\,cm$. In this case the distance between gradiometers should be $2.5\,cm$ for first order and $1.7\,cm$ for second order planar gradiometers. If the coil's area is taken into account, first order gradiometers could overlap again. However, taking into account the coil area leads to a spatial dependence varing more slowly in space and this will represent a smaller F and a larger distance between gradiometers. For first order planar gradiometers the array line should be $30\,cm$ long having 12 gradiometers with their centers separated by a 2.5 *cm* distance. It is worth noting that a deep source imposes a minimum limit to the array size and a shallow source imposes a maximum limit to the distance between gradiometers.

The correctness of this design is checked by using an algorithm to recover the gradiometer original input signal from the array output measurements (Bruno A.C. et al., 1989). In this test the dipole is at a 4.5 *cm* depth and it is detected by an array line of first order gradiometers as designed above. The result of the recovery algorithm at the gradiometer positions (circles) compared to the theoretical field values (continuous-line) can be seen in Fig. 3.

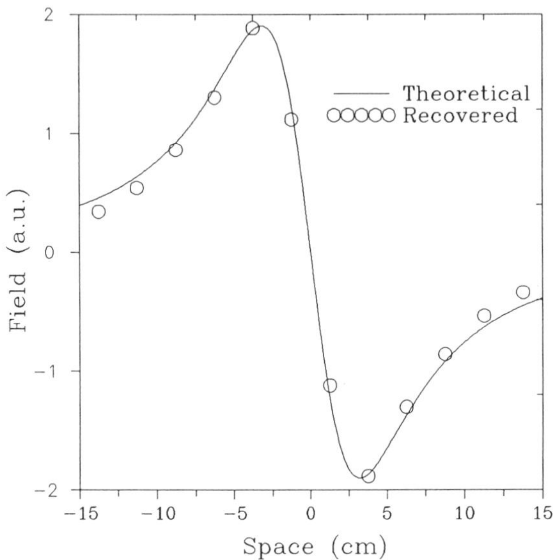

Fig. 3 Input signal recovered (circles) from the array line output measurements compared to the theoretical (continuous-line) dipole field. The array line has a 30 *cm* length and 12 first order gradiometers with a 2 *cm* baseline separeted by 2.5 *cm*.

ACKNOWLEDGEMENTS

This work has been partialy supported by FINEP, IBM of Brazil and CAPES.

REFERENCES

Antoniou, A., 1979, "Digital Filters: Analysis and Design," McGraw-Hill, New York.

Bruno, A.C., Costa Ribeiro, P., Weid, J.P., and Symko, O.G., 1986, Discrete spatial filtering with SQUID gradiometers in biomagnetism, J. Appl. Phys.,59 : 2584.

Bruno, A.C., and Costa Ribeiro, P., 1989, Spatial Deconvolution Algorithm for Superconducting Planar Gradiometer Arrays, IEEE Trans. Mags. 25 : 1216.

Romani, G.L., and Leoni, R., 1985, Localization of cerebral sources by neuromagnetic measurements, in: "Biomagnetism: Applicaton & Theory," H. Weinberg, G. Stroink, and T. Katila, eds., Pergamon Press, New York.

Pb-In WIRE BONDING FOR SUPERCONDUCTING CONNECTION BETWEEN THIN-FILM DC-SQUID AND PICKUP COIL

S.Kiryu, T.Ogashiwa*, K.Chinone**, N. Kasai, H.Kado,
N.Ishikawa***, M.Nakanishi and M.Koyanagi

Electrotechnical Laboratory, 1-1-4 Umezono, Tsukuba 305 Japan
*Tanaka Denshi Kogyo CO, 8-5-1 Shimorenjaku,
Mitaka, Tokyo 181 Japan
**Seiko Instrument Inc., 563 Takatșukasinden,
Matsudo 271, Japan
***SHIMIZU Corp.,3-4-17 Etchujima, Koto-ku, Tokyo 135, Japan

INTRODUCTION

During the last few years, integrated thin-film DC-SQUIDs have been introduced to biomagnetic measurements(Kado et al. 1987). Integrated thin-film DC-SQUIDs have many advantages such as low noise, tight coupling between SQUID and coils, and high reliability(Ketchen 1987). However, it is rather difficult to construct coil configurations for measuring diagonal gradient of the magnetic field by using thin-film coils except using multiple magnetometers. In such cases, the combination of a thin-film DC-SQUID and an external pickup coil is suitable. Usually, Nb wire is used for the pickup coil because of high reliability to mechanical stress. In order to connect the Nb pickup coil to the SQUID input coil, point contact connections made of Nb needles or the low temperature solder to the thin-film pads of the input coil are used. However, rather large contact pads of the input coil are necessary, and the reliability of the superconducting connection seems not to be enough. The reliable and compact superconducting connection between the thin film electrode of the input coil of the thin film DC-SQUID and the external pickup coil made of Nb wire is required.

Recently, a wire bonding technique using Pb-In alloy wire with the critical temperature of 6.9K has been developed(Ogashiwa et al. 1988). By using the Pb-In wire bonding, reliable superconducting connection between Nb pickup coil and the input coil of the thin-film SQUID without giving thermal and mechanical stress to the SQUID will be realized as follows: The Nb wire is mechanically connected to a superconducting plate, and the superconducting plate and the electrode of the SQUID input coil is connected with the Pb-In wire bonding.

In this paper, superconducting characteristics of the bonded part and the reliability of the bonded part against thermal cycle operations are reported. The practical second-order gradiometer with the superconducting connection by using Pb-In wire bonding is also described.

SUPERCONDUCTING CHARACTERISTICS OF BONDED PARTS WITH Pb-In WIRE

The mechanical strength of bonded part with Pb-In wire on bonding pads made of Nb thin film coated with Pb-In(1μm) has been investigated by Ogashiwa et al.(1989). The average tensile force was 0.05N and the force was not deteriorated in thermal cycle operations of 15 times.

As described in a following section, in our gradiometer, Pb-In wire was bonded to a thin-film bonding pad of the SQUID input coil and to a film coated with Au or PbIn, to Nb plate coated with Au and to Pb-In plate. In order to confirm the superconductivity of the bonded part, we measured the superconducting critical current of the bonded part using the following bonding pads: (1) Nb thin film (400nm) coated with Au (30nm), (2) Nb thin film coated with Pb-In (1μm) (3) Nb plate (100μm) coated with Au(30nm) and (4) Pb-In plate (100μm). In the experiment, 47μm-diameter Pb-In(12wt%In, 4wt%Au) wire of which critical temperature is 6.9k was used. The superconducting critical current was measured by four terminal measurement in the current range from -200mA to 200mA. In cases of (1), (2) and (4), in that current range, we could not detect voltage(< 1 μV). In the case(3), voltage was detect at above 2mA. Since the shielding current through the flux transformer composed of the input coil and the pickup coil is about several ten micro amperes for most biomagnetic measurements, the Pb-In bonding can be applied to the superconducting connection in the flux transformer.

We investigated reliability of the bonded part of the flux transformer against thermal cycle operation using the sample shown in Fig.1. The superconducting critical current* through the current path did not change after thermal cycle operations of 30 times.

* In the sample shown in Fig.1, the superconducting critical current was 36mA. the current might be limited in the thin-film input coil of the SQUID. When the bonding pads of the thin-film input coil in the sample were shorten by Pb-In wire, voltage could not be detected in the current range from -200mA to 200mA.

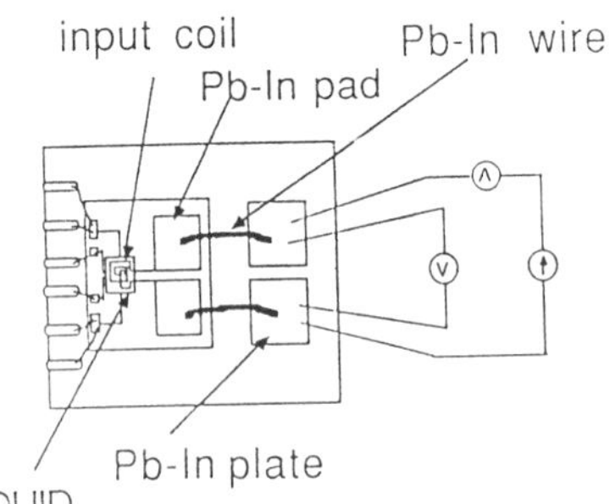

Fig.1 Configuration for measuring the effect of thermal cycle operation on the maximum superconducting current through Pb-In wire bonded connections and the input coil of the integrated planar-type SQUID in thermal cycle operation.

A SECOND-ORDER GRADIOMETER COMPOSED BY USING Pb-In WIRE BONDING

We fabricated a thin-film DC-SQUID integrated with an input coil and a modulation-feedback coil. The DC-SQUID was fabricated by the same process reported by Koyanagi(1989). The SQUID parameters are shown in Table 1. A second-order gradiometer was assembled with the SQUID and a wire wound pickup coil of 0.08mm-diameter Nb wire. Fig. 2 shows the schematic configuration of the SQUID and flux transformer which consists of a axial, second-order, symmetric gradiometer pickup coil and the input coil integrated on the SQUID chip. The diameter of the pickup coil is 15mm and the baseline is 50mm. The number of turns is 2(bottom), 4(center) and 2(top). The estimated inductance value of the pickup coil is 1.2μH. The bonding pad of the input coil and the superconducting plate(Nb plate coated with 30nm-thick Au or the Pb-In plate) was connected using Pb-In wire bonding. The pickup coil was connected to the superconducting plate using Nb arms as shown in Fig. 2. The Nb arms were used in order to replace the SQUID easily in the preliminary study.

To confirm the superconducting connection of the flux transformer, the frequency dependence of the gradiometer output was measured by applying the external magnetic field. The frequency dependence is shown in Fig. 3. If the connection had a resistance R, the gradiometer output would be

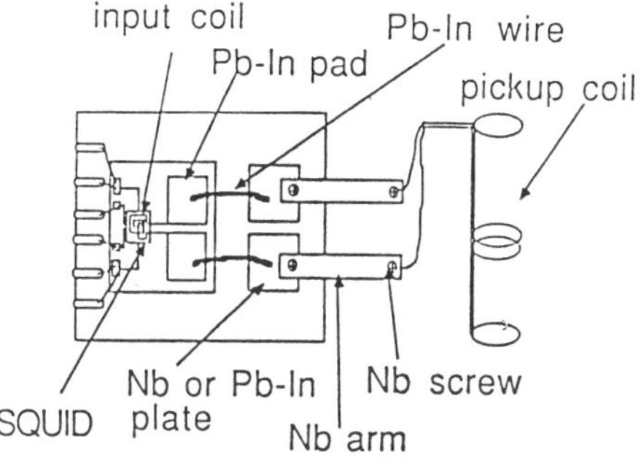

Fig.2 Configuration of the second-order gradiometer using Pb-In wire bonding.

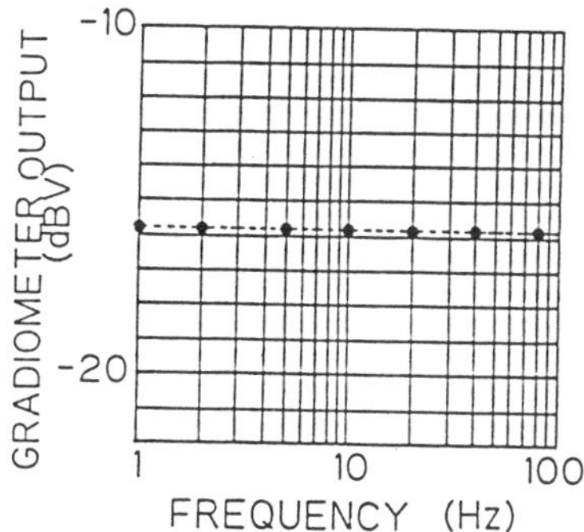

Fig.3 Frequency dependence of a gradiometer output measured by applying external magnetic field in the magnetically shielded room.

proportional to $1/\sqrt{1+(\omega_0/\omega)^2}$,where ω is an angular frequency, $\omega_0=R/(L_p+L_i)$, Lp is the inductance of the pickup coil and Li is the inductance of the input coil. The gradiometer output was constant over the measured frequency range from 1 to 100Hz. In the measurement, measurement error was less than 0.1dB. This result shows that the resistance of the flux transformer is less than several $\mu\Omega$.

In order to estimate the performance of the gradiometer, we measured the system noise and magnetocardiogram. the noise spectrum density of the gradiometer measured in a magnetically shielded room is shown in Fig. 4. It is assumed that the signal is detected with only the bottom coil of the pickup coil, The field sensitivity of the gradiometer was about 35 $fT/\sqrt{Hz}$ in the white-noise region. Using the gradiometer, magnetocardiogram was measured in a conventional electric shielded room. Fig. 5 shows an example of the magnetocardiogram. The signal was filtered to eliminate power line frequency component(50Hz) and was averaged over 64 times.

Table 1
SQUID Parameters

Critical current of one Josephson junction	$I_c=5\mu A$ *
Inductunce of SQUID loop	L = 78pH
Resistance	$R_{mn}=6\Omega$ *
Hysterisis parameter	$\beta_c=0.7$
Shielding parameter (when the input coil is open)	$\beta=0.4$
Input coil inductance	$L_i=0.7\mu H$
Modulation-feedback coil inductance	$L_m=0.9nH$
Coupling coefficient	k=0.97
Mutual inductance between SQUID and input coil	$M_i=7nH$
Mutual inductance between SQUID and modulation-feedback coil	Mm=200pH*

*values obtained experimentally

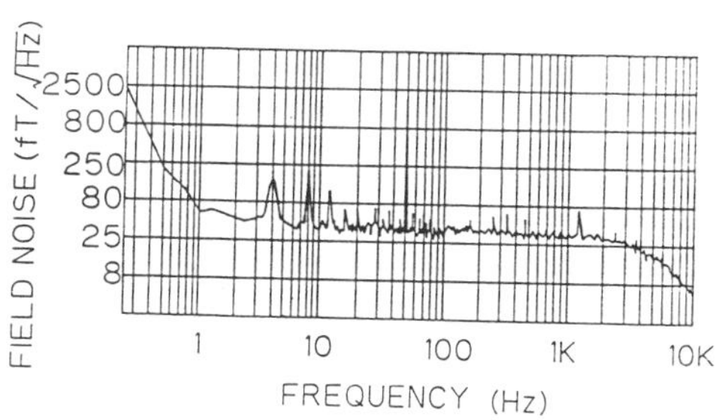

Fig.4 Spectrum density of the field noise of the gradiometer measured in the magnetically shielded room at a temperature of 4.2 k.

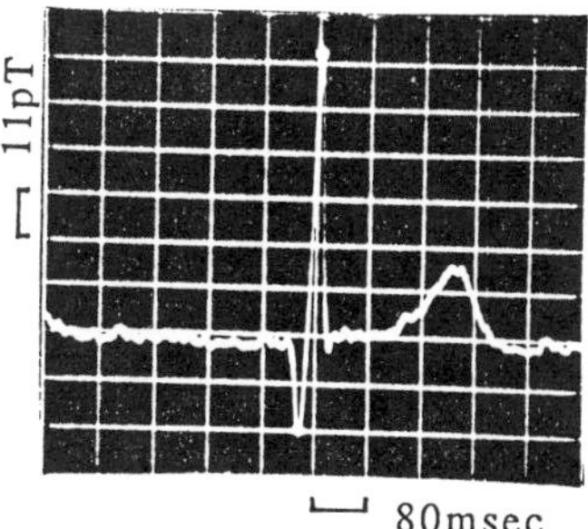

Fig.5 Example of the Magnetocardiogram was obtained in the ambient field. Signal was averaged over 64 times and the filter of the 50Hz power line frequency was used.

DISCUSSION

When a pickup coil made of Nb wire is mechanically connected to a superconducting metal plate, Nb plate is more reliable against mechanical stress than Pb-In plate. In our experiments, however, the superconducting critical current through the bonded part between the Nb plate coated with Au(30nm) and the Pb-In wire strongly depended on the surface condition of the Nb plate. In order to obtain enough performance for the flux transformer, careful preparation of Nb plate was required before evaporation of Au. On the other hand, in the case of Pb-In plate, the required performance could be easily obtained after cleaning with acetone.

The thermal compression bonding of Pb-Sn wire was used by Ketchen(1987) for superconducting connection between thin-film dc SQUID and the wire wound coil. However, the detailed comparison of our connection with that of Ketchen's was not carried out because we could not find the detailed report.

In our gradiometer, equivalent SQUID flux noise level estimated from Fig.4 was about $2 \times 10^{-5} \Phi_0/\sqrt{Hz}$. The noise would not be caused by the bonded connection because the above mentioned noise level corresponds to a resistance of several Ω in the flux transformer composed of the SQUID input coil and the pickup coil, however, the resistance of the bonded parts was less than several μΩ as mentioned in the previous section.

ACKNOWLEDGEMENT

The authors thank S. Takada and H. Miura for their encouragement throughout the work. S.K. thanks H.Nakagawa, I.Kurosawa and M.Aoyagi for their useful suggestions in the device fabrication process. T.O. thanks Research Development Corporation of Japan for useful suggestions. T.O would also like to thank Y.Fukui, N.Tadokoro and R.Utsumi of Tanaka Denshi Co., LTD. for their continuous encouragement.

REFERENCES

H.Kado et al.,1987,"Alpha Rhythm of Magnetoencephalogram Measured by 2-Channel DC-SQUID System",Proc. Biomagnetism'87,162:165.

M.B.Ketchen, 1987,"Integrated Thin-film dc SQUID Sensors", IEEE Trans. Magn., **MAG-23**, 1650:1657 .

M.Koyanagi et al., 1989, "An Integrated DC SQUID Gradiometer for Biomagnetic Application", IEEE Trans.Magn., **MAG-25**,1166:1169.

T.Ogashiwa et. al, 1988, "Superconductive Wire Bonding with $Pb_{84}In_{12}Au_4$ Wire", to be published on proc. Material Research Society International Meeting on Advanced Materials(May 30-June 3, 1988).

T.Ogashiwa et. al, 1989,to be submitted to Jpn. J. Appl. Phys.

A SINGLE-CHIP SQUID

N. Fujimaki, H. Tamura, H. Suzuki, T. Imamura,
S. Hasuo, and A. Shibatomi

Exploratory Devices Laboratory,
Fujitsu Laboratories Ltd.,
Morinosato-Wakamiya, Atsugi 243-01, Japan

INTRODUCTION

We have integrated a SQUID sensor and a superconducting feedback circuit on a single chip (Fujimaki, 1988). This aids in constructing multichannel SQUID systems, because it eliminates the need for massive feedback circuits outside the chip and the many electrical cables required to connect them to the SQUID sensors. In addition, since the output of our chip is a pulse sequence, it can be processed directly to obtain biomagnetic data. We improved the dynamic range and the sensitivity of the single-chip SQUID to bring it closer to practical applications.

CIRCUIT

Principle of operation

Figure 1 shows the circuit of the single-chip SQUID. The SQUID sensor is a two-junction interferometer. Unlike the dc SQUID, it is ac-biased and produces a positive or negative pulse with each positive or negative input flux. The superconducting feedback circuit consists of a superconducting loop and a write gate, which is a two-junction interferometer. When a positive or negative pulse arrives, the write gate adds a positive or negative flux quantum to the loop. The total flux stored in the loop represents the number of positive pulses minus the number of negative pulses and is fed back to the SQUID sensor to cancel the input flux. This feedback circuit works as an up/down counter. To determine the input flux, we count the output pulses, because the count represents the feedback flux with the same amplitude as the input flux.

Advances in Biomagnetism
Edited by S.J. Williamson *et al.*
Plenum Press, New York

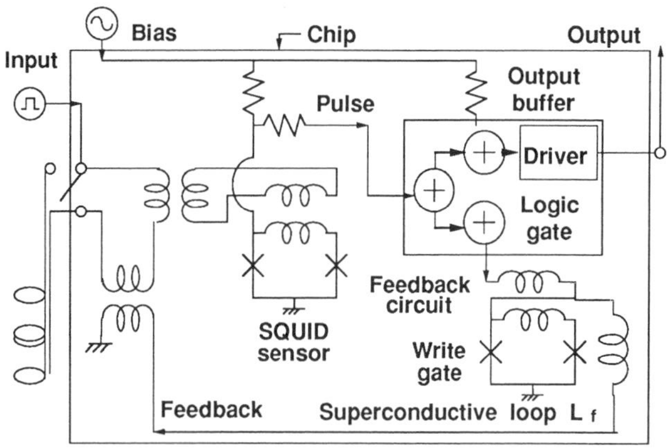

Fig. 1 Circuit integrated on a single chip.

Design improvements

The main improvements of this design over our previous one (Fujimaki, 1988) are:

(1) To increase dynamic range, we designed the superconducting loop inductance L_f to be 146 μH, which is much higher than the previous 20 nH. As a result, the capacity for storing flux quanta is increased from ±100 to $\pm 7 \times 10^5$.

(2) In our previous design, the output of the SQUID sensor was connected directly to the cables which transmit it to the counter operating at room temperature. In our new design, the added output buffer reduces the external noise coming through the output cable. It contains three Josephson logic gates (Fujimaki, 1989) and an output driver circuit (Suzuki, 1988) that produces a 9-mV pulse instead of the 1-mV sensor output.

Besides these improvements, the new chip does not use a pickup coil. In many biomagnetic applications, the pickup coil, made with Nb wire and called a gradiometer, is placed outside the chip. These pickup coils have a large inductance (around 1 μH). To match it to the SQUID's input inductance of 20 nH, we insert an intermediate transformer in the chip.

Design of the superconducting loop

Figure 2(a) shows the chip, which was fabricated using Nb/AlO_x/Nb junction, Mo resistor, and SiO_2 insulation (Imamura, 1987). The minimum line width is 2.5 μm, and the chip is 9.4 x 5 mm. To decrease magnetic coupling between the superconducting loop and the SQUID sensor, the loop is divided into 32 alternatively wound coils (Fig. 2(b)), to cancel the magnetic flux at the SQUID sensor and other chips. The magnetic field decreases as r^{-8} where r is the distance from the center of the 32 coils. When the maximum number of flux quanta is stored in the loop, its magnetic field is about 6×10^{-16} T at r=2 cm, while each coil produces 10^{-12} T. The total inductance of the 32 coils was measured as 30 μH. This is quite a bit less than the design value of 146 μH. The reason for this discrepancy is the approximation error in design equations.

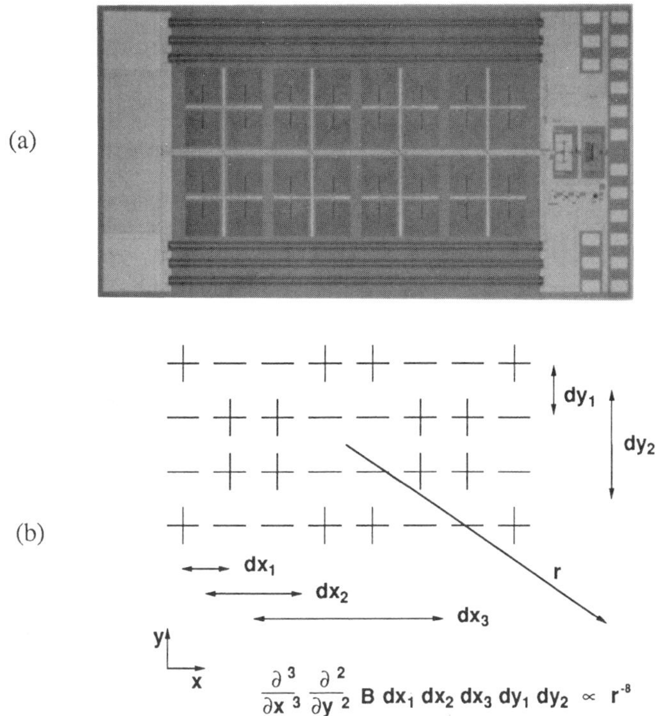

Fig. 2(a) The chip. (b) Polarities of the magnetic flux produced by the coils in the superconducting loop.

RESULTS

Figure 3 shows our results. We applied a 1 MHz ac-bias and a rectangular input pulse to obtain the pulse sequence of 9 mV. By counting this pulse sequence, we obtained the reconstructed waveform. The measured sensitivity was 1.4×10^{-5} $\Phi_0/Hz^{1/2}$ at frequencies above 1 Hz. The cut off frequency of the feedback loop was 18 Hz, which can be increased to 1.8 kHz by increasing the bias frequency to 100 MHz. The origin and characteristics of the noise require further study, but the measured sensitivity is nearly the same as the conventional dc SQUID (Knuutila, 1987).

With a large input, the loop stored flux quanta up to $\pm 2 \times 10^4$. This dynamic range is less than the design value of $\pm 7 \times 10^5$. This reduction is mainly due to the circulating current in the loop and the transformer which was caused by the flux trappings and the magnetic flux produced by the bias current and the output pulse. Thus, the dynamic range can be further improved by shielding the chip or by eliminating the circulating current in the loop.

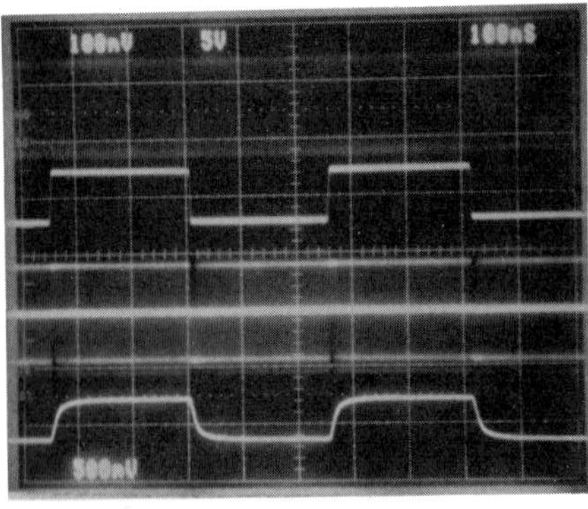

Fig. 3 Waveforms are from the top, the ac-bias, input pulse current, output pulse sequence, and reconstructed waveform. The horizontal axis is 0.1 s/div. The input pulse height corresponds to 0.11 Φ_0.

DISCUSSION

We have improved the performance of the single-chip SQUID. We obtained sensitivity nearly equal to the conventional dc SQUID. The dynamic range was $\pm 2 \times 10^4$, more than two orders of magnitude wider than the previous design. However, it can be further improved. The single-chip SQUID is a key element in constructing, for example, a 100-channel SQUID system.

REFERENCES

Imamura, T., Hoko, H., Ohara, S., Kotani, S., and Hasuo, S. (1987). Fabrication technology for Josephson integrated circuits with Nb/AlO_x/Nb junctions. In: Hara, K., Superconductivity Electronics. Prentice Hall & Ohmsha, Tokyo, pp. 22-33.

Fujimaki, N., Tamura, H., Imamura, T., and Hasuo, S. (1988). A single-chip SQUID magnetometer. IEEE Trans. Electron Devices, ED-35 ,pp. 2412-2418.

Fujimaki, N., Kotani, S., Imamura, T., and Hasuo, S. (1989). Josephson modified variable threshold logic gates for use in ultra-high-speed LSI. IEEE Trans. Electron Devices, ED-36, pp. 433-446.

Knuutila, J., Ahlfors, S., Ahonen, A., Hallsrtom, J., Kajola, M., Lounasmaa, O.V., and Vilkman, V. (1987). Large-area low-noise seven-channel dc SQUID magnetometer for brain research. Rev. Sci. Instrum. 58, pp. 2145-2156.

Suzuki, H., Inoue, A., Imamura, T., and Hasuo, S. (1988). A Josephson driver to interface Josephson junctions to semiconductor transistors. IEDM Technical Digest, pp. 290-293.

A MULTI-CHANNEL BIOMAGNETOMETER

C.N. Guy, A. Cayles, S. Walker, and K. Leedham-Green

Physics Department
Imperial College, London

INTRODUCTION

We have designed and constructed a seven channel biomagnetometer system at Imperial College using wirewound 2nd order gradiometers and RF squids working in an unscreened urban environment. The instrument was designed for and is currently in use in pilot clinical studies in MEG and MCG. The seven channels are arranged in a flat ,centred hexagonal array covering an area 135mm in diameter. After fine tuning the residual noise is measured to be 30-35 fT/√Hz in the frequency range 1-40Hz. At present five channels are fully operational,the remaining two channels are awaiting delivery of squid sensors.

The probe, housed in a vapour cooled fibre glass dewar, is supported in a gantry over a patient bed. Together these structures provide five degrees of relative movement between the probe and the patient. Location of the probe with respect to the patient's anatomy is achieved by a simple scheme in which the squids themselves are the detectors of a suitably patterned ac magnetic field whose source geometry is known accurately with respect to the anatomy.Analoque outputs from the squid channels are collected and analysed using an AT computer.

In the following sections we describe the main features of the system and illustrate its performance by means of examples.

LOW TEMPERATURE PROBE

Figure 1 shows the lower portion of the probe with five channels installed. Each channel consists of a coil barrel together with its associated squid. Both squid housing and coil barrel screw into the probe framework to allow easy maintenance and replacement. All the non_metallic parts are machined from linen based phenolic composite. Each coil barrel has four 0 BA screw threads cut into longitudinal internal holes and a surface vee-groove thread of 1.6 mm pitch. The former take the adjuster rods.The latter provides a very convenient method of accurate wire location at a given wire spacing that has been calculated to give a desired coil self-inductance. After winding and coating with low temperature epoxy resin the installed gradiometers typically are balanced to $2\text{-}3{:}10^4$ with respect to uniform applied fields.

The probe is housed in a flat bottom fibre glass dewar (CTF Inc.) whose neck diameter is 135mm. Without the gradiometer insert helium loss

Advances in Biomagnetism
Edited by S.J. Williamson *et al.*
Plenum Press, New York

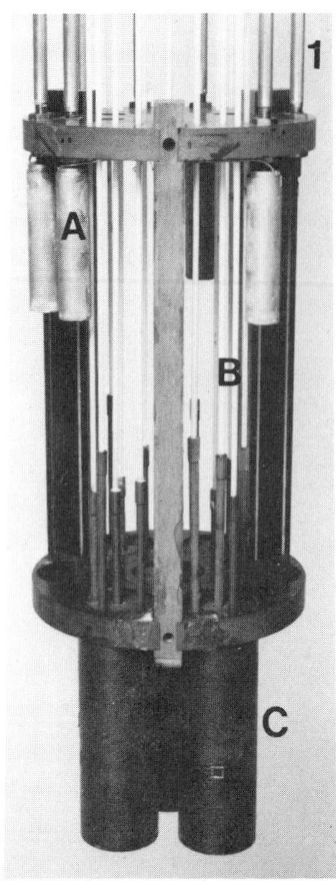

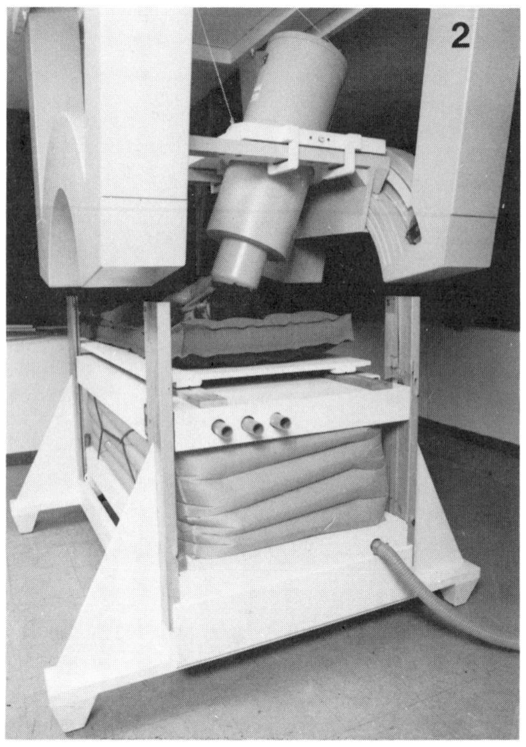

Figure 1. The lower part of the probe showing five installed gradiometer channels.A:Squid housing B: Adjuster rods C: Gradiometer coils.
Figure 2. The gantry and bed at installation.

is 2 l/day . The final complete probe has a loss of 3.5 l/day. The squids were manufactured by CCL. These devices have flux noise of less than $8.5*10^{-5}/\surd Hz$ and coupling efficiency (M/L) $8*10^{-3}$.

The details of our balancing procedure together with a detailed analysis are described elsewhere Guy et al (1989). Using 2.6 M square coils in situ we produce uniform fields in the Z and X directions and a uniform gradient in the Z direction. The coils are excited at 1.9Hz with a triangular waveform. The latter allows us to discriminate between true gradiometer imbalance with respect to the homogeneous test fields and quadrature signals that arise from eddy current sources within the dewar.The former gives rise to a triangular response whereas the latter give a square wave (α $\delta B/\delta t$). At the highest levels of balance we observe significant interactions between tabs in adjacent coils and a small degree of balance change with thermal cycling that is eliminated on all channels by tweaking the tab adjusters.

We estimate that about $10fT/\surd Hz$. of our residual noise arises directly from eddy current sources within the dewar. We have been able to localise these to an equivalent ring current at the top of the tail section of the dewar amounting to $8*10^{-9}$ Amps/nTHz. When this source is removed by rebuilding the vapour shields we anticipate being able to achieve a noise level of $21\text{-}23fT/\surd Hz$,the level achieved in our single channel prototype of the same design.

Calibration of the instrument is achieved using a low frequency ac current flowing in a horizontal straight wire of length 1.2 M, Grimes (1989). Movement of the wire in the horizontal plane beneath the probe allows simultaneous calibration of all channels and a fairly accurate estimate to be made of the wire to gradiometer distance (half distance between signal extrema).

GANTRY and BED

Figure 2 shows a photograph of the gantry /bed system at the time of installation. The dewar is held in gymbals on the ceiling mounted gantry which allows 4 degrees of freedom. The main arch allows $\pm$ 40^{0} of tip in the Z,Y plane with the dewar tip moving over a cylindrical surface of radius 0.11M. The gymbal mounting allows tipping in the X,Z plane about a centre 0.4M above the dewar tip. This mounting is on a carriage that allows a traverse of $\pm$ 0.3M in the X direction. Finally the dewar can be rotated about its own axis. This is particularly useful when balancing since it effectively removes the need for one helmholtz test coil in the X direction.The bed provides a platform that can be translated both horizontally and vertically. The latter movement is achieved using large low pressure airbags in combination with tensioned ropes running over a common capstan to ensure that the moving platform remains horizontal. The vertical range of movement is 0.6M and any position within this range can be achieved with an accuracy of 2mm. The ability to move the patient smoothly in the vertical direction allows us to use the XZ tip in combination with vertical and horizontal traveres to scan over the surface of a sphere whilst maintaining a radial probe orientation and a small dewar tip to body surface distance. Both gantry and bed are of an all wooden construction. The arms of the main gantry arch are hollow and contain dry sand to damp out inevitable mechanical resonances.

DATA ACQUISITION and ANALYSIS

Analogue outputs from the squids are passed via nominally identical signal conditioning cards to an 8 channel interface, Biodata Ltd, linked to an AT compatible microcomputer. Each card has selectable high and low pass filters and a 32 segment switched capacitor filter that removes 50 Hz (mains) and its first three harmonics. The computer/interface provides a sampling rate of 500Hz. and has a software circular buffer capable of storing 32 seconds of 8 channel data.

PROBE LOCATION

We have developed a very simple method in which a grid of wires carrying ac electrical currents is incorporated into closely fitting bonnets and chest patches that are worn by the patients. When each wire

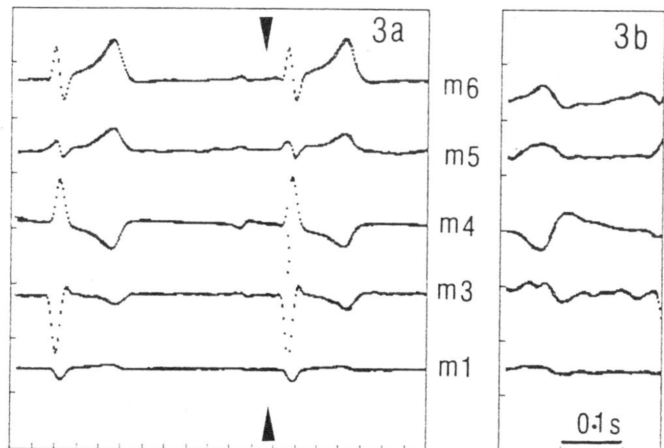

Figure 3(a). 5 channel MCG data from a normal male The arrow identifies the PQ interval chosen for 3b.(b) Enlargement of PQ interval showing ramp structure on M4,M6

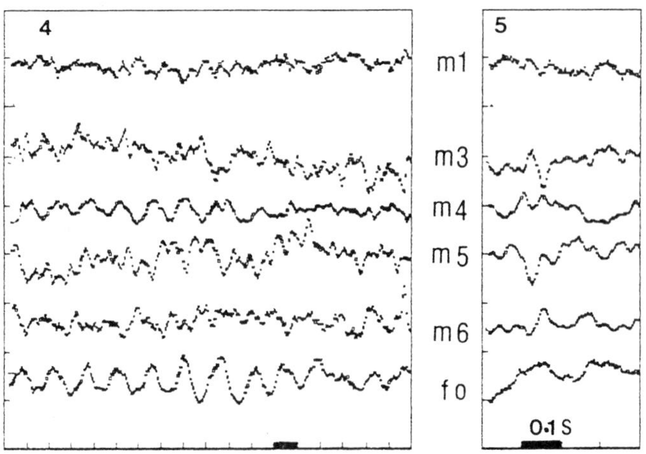

Figure 4. MEG and FO recordings from an epileptic patient. exhibiting diffuse quasi-periodic activity.
Figure 5. An isolated sharp wave recorded from the same patient.

in the grid is energised for a short time with a 20 Hz. sine wave a signal is produced in all of the squid channels and these signals are recorded in the normal way by the computer. A simple analysis shows that grid position of the centre of each channel is obtained by finding the point of signal phase reversal and position within a grid square is given to $\pm$ 1mm by interpolation using the signal strengths.
For flat grids we have shown that probe height and angle with respect to the grid plane are also obtained by signal processing, Guy et al (1989).

PERFORMANCE

Figure 3a shows some typical MCG data obtained from a normal male subject. Figure 3b shows an expanded version of the PQ interval taken at the arrowed point (figure 3a) showing the ramp structure that is probably, at this level of resolution, associated with P wave repolarisation, ten Voorde et al 1988. These traces show a clear phase reversal for one probe position.

Figure 4 shows data obtained from an epileptic patient on the five working squid channels together with one simultaneous Foramen Ovale electrical record. In this epoch the scalp EEG records showed the spatially diffuse quasi-periodic feature that is most visible on the foramen ovale and M4 channels in the figure. Figure 5 shows an interictal sharp wave recorded from the same patient. Although the signal to noise on the multichannel instrument is not yet as good as the single channel device this figure again demonstrates that the five

ACKNOWLEDGEMENTS
The authors thank the DHS and SERC for research grants and Mr. D. Bowerman for invaluable help in the design and construction of the bed/gantry.

REFERENCES

Biodata Ltd. Manchester ,UK
CCL, Cryogenic Consultants Ltd. ,London ,UK
CTF Inc. Vancouver Canada
Grimes D J (1989) Private communication
Guy C.N.,Cayless A.,Walker S.(1989) submit Phys. Med. Biol.
Guy C. N., Leedham Green K. (1989) In preparation
Ten Voorde B.J.,Peteres M.J.,Stroink G.,van der Wieken L.R. (1988) Med.and Biol. Eng. and Comp. March 1988

A NINE CHANNEL DC SQUID SYSTEM FOR BIOMAGNETISM

P. Carelli[*], C. Del Gratta[**], V. Foglietti, I. Modena[#], A. Pasquarelli, V. Pizzella, M. Pullano, G.L. Romani[##] and G. Torrioli

Istituto di Elettronica dello Stato Solido - CNR. Via Cineto Romano 42, 00156 Roma, ITALY
[*]Dipartimento di Energetica, Universita' de L'Aquila, L'Aquila, ITALY
[**]Supported by grant by CITEC S.p.A., Roma, ITALY
[#]Dipartimento di Fisica, II Universita' di Roma *"Tor Vergata"*, Roma, ITALY
[##]Istituto di Fisica Medica, Universita' *"G. D'Annunzio"*, Chieti, ITALY

INTRODUCTION

In the last few years several multi-channel systems for biomagnetic measurements have been developed. The first examples featured four-five sensors (Ilmoniemi et al., 1984; Romani, 1984; Williamson et al., 1984), whereas more recently a seven-channel system became commercially available, also in a configuration which endowes simultaneous investigation at 14 scalp sites with two twin systems (Biomagnetic Technologies Inc.). However several projects aimed to develop larger systems are being carried on in several countries both by groups involved in fundamental research and by industries. In general, these systems are designed to be used for neuromagnetic studies, even if efforts are being made also to setup large size cardiomagnetometers (Erne', personal communication). A common feature is that all systems are planned to work in shielded environments.

A 9-channel system for biomagnetic measurements has been developed in Italy in the frame of a national project on biomagnetic instrumentation and in collaboration with Elettronica S.p.A. In the present report we will present the features and performances of the superconducting detecting equipment, and the readout electronics.

INSTRUMENT DESCRIPTION

The basic idea was to set up a system able to perform both magnetocardiographic and neuromagnetic measurements in an unshielded environment. In order to achieve this double-purpose goal the nine gradiometers can be arranged *in situ* with their axes either parallely oriented or tilted in such a way to follow the orientation of the radii of a spherical surface. The minimum radius of curvature of this surface is 14 cm, corresponding to a radius of curvature of the outer surface of the dewar equal to about 12 cm. If the gradiometers are parallel, the system can be used to measure the normal component of the magnetic field in a plane (as is usually done in magnetocardiography) whereas if the gradiometers are opened downwards, so that the lower pick-up coils are positioned on the surface of a sphere, the system can be used to measure the radial component of the magnetic field around a sphere (as is done in neuromagnetic measurements). A schematic of the variable "umbrella"-like geometry for the gradiometer assembly is shown in Fig. 1. One gradiometer is located in the center and the other eight have their lower coils displaced in such a way to enclose a circle of radius 10.5 cm.

Gradiometers

The gradiometers are made of 80 μm niobium wire wound around a MACOR cylinder with a 7 cm baseline and 1.5 cm diameter; they are provided with three lead tabs and variable upper baseline for balancing. The 7 cm baseline have been chose to provide a better ability to investigate the heart and deep

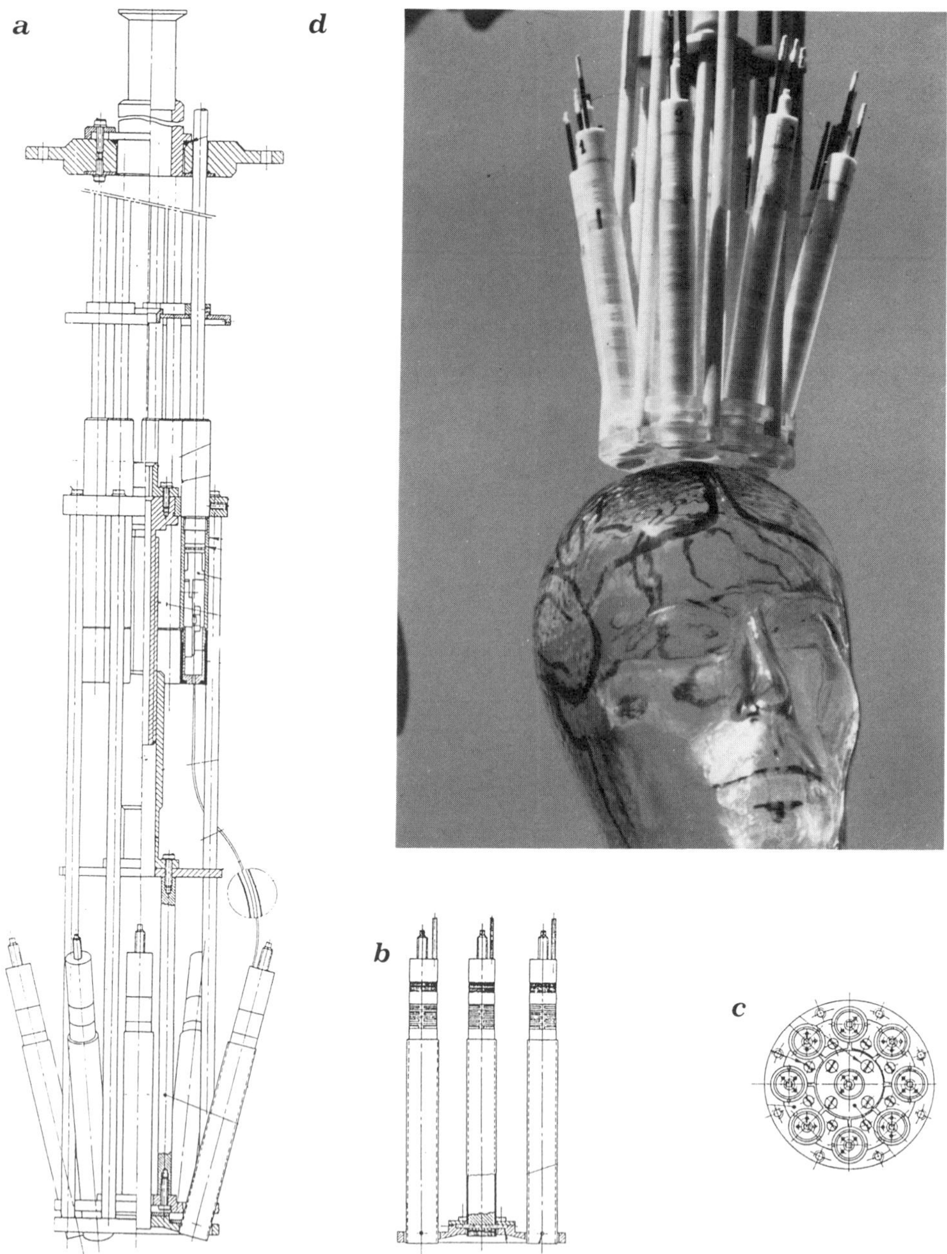

Fig. 1. a) Schematic illustration of the cryogenic insert of the nine-channel biomagnetic system. The variable orientation of the nine second-order gradiometers is shown in a) and b) respectively, whereas the relative position of the pick-up coils is depicted in c). When the system is used for cardiomagnetic measurements, as in b), the higher position of the central gradiometer with respect to the other eight must be taken into account for source localization. d) Close-up view of the gradiometer array as prepared for neuromagnetic measurements.

sources in the brain. The balancing mechanisms are similar to those already used in the previously developed four-channel system (Romani et al., 1985) but improved to fit a longer baseline and to ensure an enhanced "stability" with respect to thermal cycles. The gradiometers have been balanced singularly before assembling the system. Typical balancing factors range between 5×10^{-5} and 10^{-4} against spatially uniform fields, whereas gradient balancing factors range from 10^{-5} and 10^{-4}. After balancing, each gradiometer was carefully removed from the single channel assembly and put in the final position. During this procedure the balancing factors were found to be worsened no more than a factor of three.

SQUIDs and related electronics

The probe consists of nine steel pipes containing the connections from the SQUIDs to the room temperature electronics. Each gradiometer is coupled to a dc-SQUID by means of a flux-transformer. The dc-SQUIDs, microfabricated in our laboratory, are fully described elsewhere (Carelli et al., 1989); they have a multiloop geometry and an input coil patterned on the same lithographic process with a mutual inductance of 2×10^{-9} H (equal within the experimental error for the nine used device). The input coil of the dc-SQUID (1.5 μH) matches the inductance of the gradiometer. The transforming ratio between the flux coupled to each gradiometer and the flux sensed by each SQUID has been separately measured for each channel and its value (0.0021) is in good agreement with the expected value.

The SQUID package is made in a hybrid-like form. A fiberglass holder, with a double layer wiring of superconducting alloy, is the interface between the chip and the external wiring. All the connections to the SQUID, including the superconducting contacts with the gradiometer, are made by thermally bonding 50 μm Pb wire from the SQUID pads (the top layer of which is made of lead alloy) to the holder pads. The reliability of such a circuitry is 100%, at least for what concerns the tested devices. Included in the same package there are two coils used to send the external modulation signal and to close the feedback loop. The SQUID is connected to the biasing current and, through a 1.5 Ω resistor, to a helium temperature up-transformer (Wellstood et al., 1984) made of Cu wire wounded around a ferrite core (the transforming ratio is 6). This transformer is enclosed in a superconducting shield. A close-up view of the SQUID with its holder is shown in Fig. 2. A second room temperature transformer is used to feed the SQUID signal to the room temperature preamplifier. The total transforming ratio matches the low dynamic SQUID resistance to the preamplifier optimum resistance. Each dc-SQUID is coupled to a single channel electronics made of a "head" and a remote control unit. The head is made of a milled aluminium block containing the

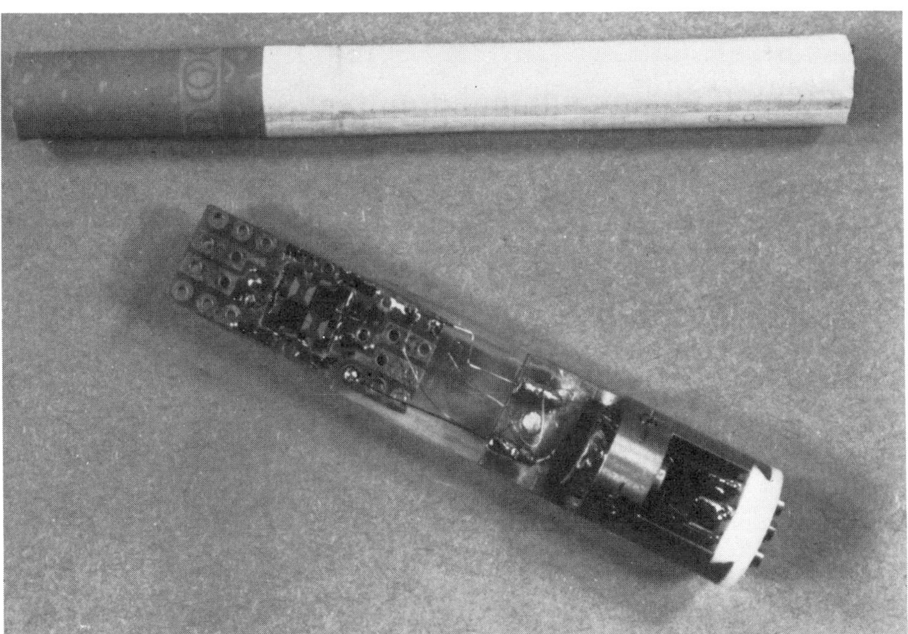

Fig. 2. Close-up view of the hybrid-like package. Note the fiberglass SQUID holder with the SQUID (left) and the first transformer inside the superconducting shield (right).

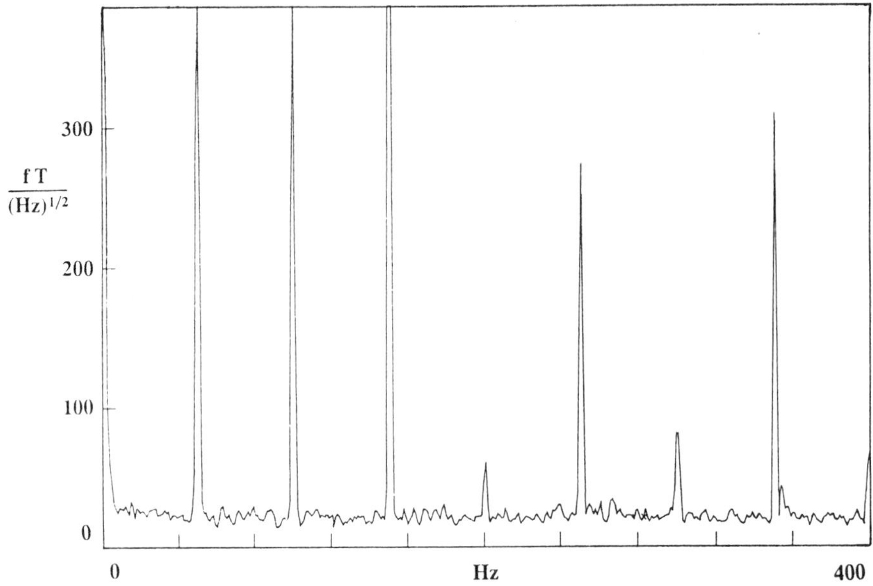

Fig. 3. Field noise spectral density of one of the nine channels under operating conditions.

preamplifier, the phase sensitive detector, and the modulation oscillator (500 KHz). Each of these units is in a different compartment. The remote control unit contains the SQUID current source, the amplitude modulation control, and other commands required to properly set the SQUID operation. The nine remote control units are inside an unique crate that also allows the separate use of each channel.

Performances and preliminary measurements

After being connected to the gradiometers, the white noise of the dc-SQUIDs spans between $3.5 \times 10^{-6}\ \phi_0/\surd\text{Hz}$ and $5 \times 10^{-6}\ \phi_0/\surd\text{Hz}$. Noise measurements are always performed in a phase-locked loop configuration. The corresponding field noise spectral density spans between 18 fT/$\surd$Hz and 25 fT/$\surd$Hz. The noise spectral density of one of the channels with "intermediate" performances is reported in Fig. 3. The white noise begins at frequencies larger than 2-3 Hz, when the SQUIDs are isolated. The same corner frequency is found for the devices in operating conditions only when the ambient is very quiet (such as the wooden hut at the Istituto di Elettronica dello Stato Solido) and particular care is taken to shield low frequency vibrations, by means of a specifically designed mount.

Experimental checks on both cardiomagnetic and neuromagnetic signals are in progress.

ACKNOWLEDGEMENTS

The authors thank all people who collaborated for the development and setup of the system. In particular, we mention S. Barbanera, W. Priore, and A. Piciccia for the design and construction of a cryogenic non-magnetic dewar of adequate dimensions, P. Maranci, and C. Grandi, for the development of the hardware to condition and acquire electric and magnetic signals, and M. Curti for adequate engineerization of the software for signal processing. We thank also to B. Polic, for supervision on the project from the ELETTRONICA S.p.A. side, and to A. Paoletti and P. De Gasperis for continuous help and encouragements. The whole project has been permitted by the support of MRST (Legge 46).

REFERENCES

Carelli, P., Foglietti, V., Leoni, R. and Pullano, M. (1989). Reliable low noise DC-SQUID. Proceedings of the ASC, San Francisco, August 1988, in press.

Romani, G.L., Leoni, R. and Salustri, C. (1985). Multichannel instrumentation for biomagnetism. In: Hahlbohm, H.D. and Lübbig, H., SQUID85: Superconducting Quantum Interference Devices and their Applications. Walter de Gruyter, Berlin-New York, pp. 918-932.

Wellstood, F., Heiden, C., Clarke, J. (1984). Integrated dc SQUID magnetometer with a high slew rate. Rev. Sci. Instrum., 55, 952-957.

DEVELOPMENT AND PERFORMANCE OF A MULTICHANNEL SYSTEM FOR STUDIES OF BIOMAGNETIC SIGNALS OF BRAIN AND HEART

S. Schneider, K. Abraham-Fuchs, G. Daalmans*, W. Folberth, H.E. Hoenig*, H. Reichenberger, G. Röhrlein, H. Seifert*, A. Wirth

Siemens Medical Engineering Group and Research Laboratory*, 8520 Erlangen, Federal Republic of Germany

INTRODUCTION

Biomagnetic systems operating with 4 to 7 channels have been described before [Ilmoniemi 1984, Williamson 1984, Romani 1985, Kajola 1987]. With noise levels of less than 20 fT/√Hz their performance was sufficient for various biomagnetic applications. So far the number of channels was insufficient for obtaining a complete set of magnetic signals. We have developed a biomagnetic system (KRENIKON) that is capable to collect complete coherent data sets under routine conditions.

METHOD

In order to reduce interfering noise a compact sensor design and a combination of first order gradiometers with a medium shielding were chosen. The multichannel sensor consists of a DC-SQUID-array integrated on four chips combined with a planar array of 31 first order gradiometers with an overall diameter of 20 cm. Each SQUID-chip contains 10 planar Ketchen-type DC-SQUIDs. The chip has been made in an all niobium technology [Daalmans 1980, 1989]. The SQUIDs are operated in the flux locked loop mode. The gradiometer array consists of axial first order gradiometers with a base line of 7 cm and a probing area of the pick up coil of about 6 cm^2 (Fig.1) [Hoenig 1989].The sensor is placed in a fiberglas epoxy dewar (HOXAN Corp.) with flat bottom mounted on a stable support. The support allows a vertical shift and an angular adjustment in two orthogonal directions.

The sensor system is operated inside a shielded room with two shields of soft magnetic material and one shield of aluminum (Vacuumschmelze). The shielding factor is more than 1000 for frequencies above 2 Hz. The data acquisition system includes a 12 bit ADC and a fast computer (μVAX 3600). The frequency band ranges from 0.016 Hz to 4 kHz.

Simultaneously with the biomagnetic measurements, ECG and EEG signals can be recorded as well as respiration, stimulation, and control signals. Patient position relative to the sensor is obtained from a plastic support connected to the couch. During MEG measurement the patient's head is fixed to this support by means of a silicon impression of the patient's upper teeth. The support also is used for positioning the patient during MR imaging.

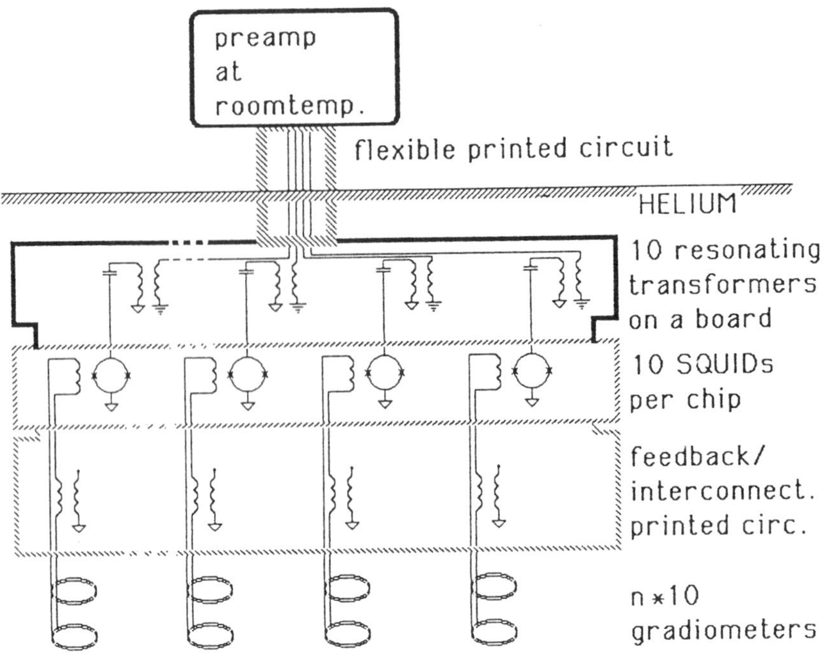

Fig. 1 Principle of the 31 channel DC-SQUID gradiometer array.

RESULTS

The noise performance of a SQUID with 300 h energy sensitivity corresponding to $3x10^{-6}$ $\phi_0/\sqrt{Hz}$ is given in Fig. 2. In the system SQUIDs with noise margins in between $2x10^{-6}$ $\phi_0/\sqrt{Hz}$ and $1x10^{-5}\phi_0/\sqrt{Hz}$ corresponding to values for the field resolution in between 0.8 and 4 $fT/\sqrt{Hz}$ are used. Due to other noise sources (dewar, electronics, shielded room) and under parallel operation of 31 channels in urban environment the overall system noise results to 10 $ft/\sqrt{Hz}$ - 20 $fT/\sqrt{Hz}$ at 5 Hz (Fig. 3).
The system was tested by localizing coils with a magnetic moment of 0.6 μAm^2. Up to a distance of 15 cm from the center of the pickup coil array these coils were localized within a sphere of 1.5 mm radius. Auditory evoked magnetic fields from volunteers were used to demonstrate the performance of the system. For stimulation we used tone bursts with frequencies 400 Hz, 800 Hz, 1600 Hz, and 3200 Hz and a repetition time of 4 s (risetime 15 ms, duration 500 ms, 60 dB HL /Hoke 1989). With 100 stimuli the total measurement time was 7 minutes. In extension of earlier findings [Hari 1980, Romani 1982 and Pantev 1988] frequency dependent locations of sources were found as function of frequency and visualized in 3D MR images in the auditory cortex (Fig. 4). During the N100 peak dipole positions (time resolution 2.5 ms) following an U-shaped path around the auditory fissure were found, which are shifted to deeper regions with increasing frequency (Fig. 5).

CONCLUSION

Tests on volunteers and clinical work on patients with focal epilepsy [Stefan 1988, 1989] and WPW syndrome [Weikl 1989, Abraham-Fuchs 1989] have shown, that with the new multichannel system coherent signals of high quality are recorded at any time of the day - including the untriggered acquisition of fieldmaps from spontaneous events.

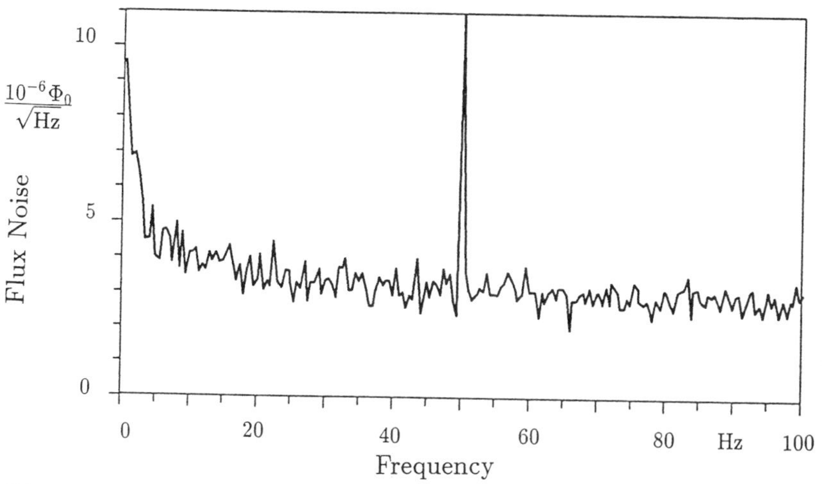

Fig. 2. Flux noise of a single SQUID in flux locked loop operation.

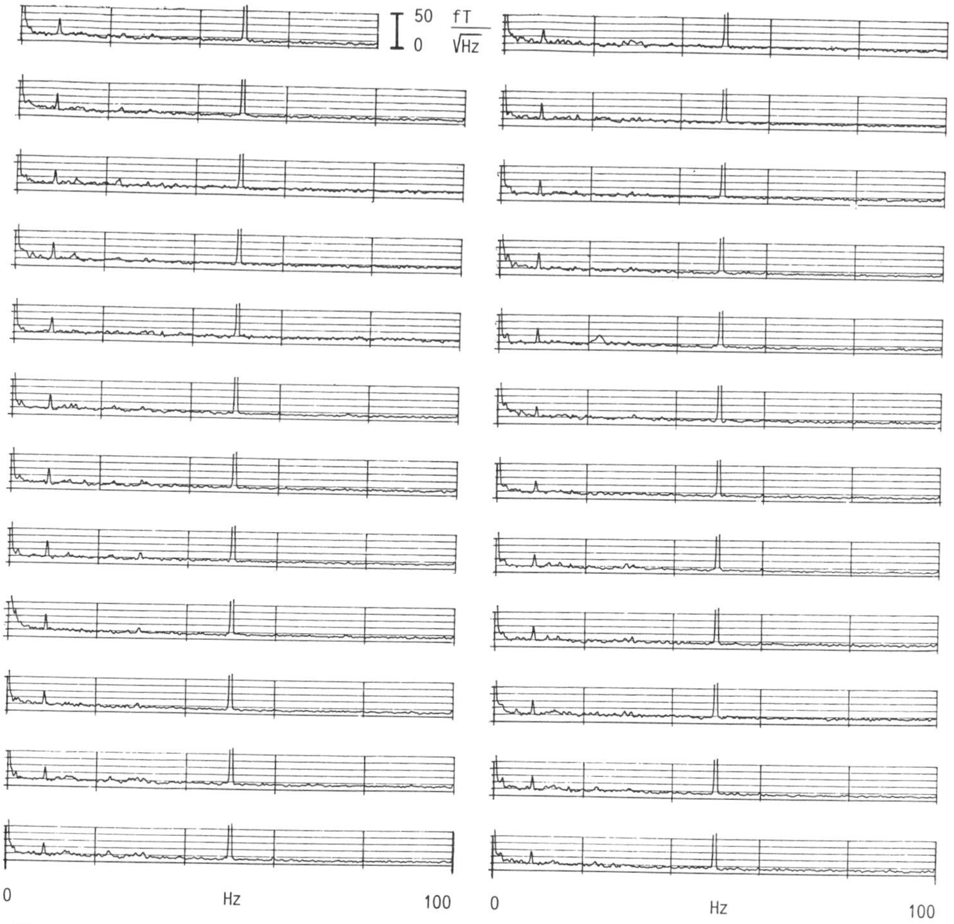

50 $\frac{fT}{\sqrt{Hz}}$ 0

0 Hz 100 0 Hz 100

Fig. 3 Noise spectra of 24 representative channels; parallel operation under regular urban noise conditions. (0-100 Hz; 0-5 ft/$\sqrt{Hz}$; res. = 0.24 Hz; Hanning window).

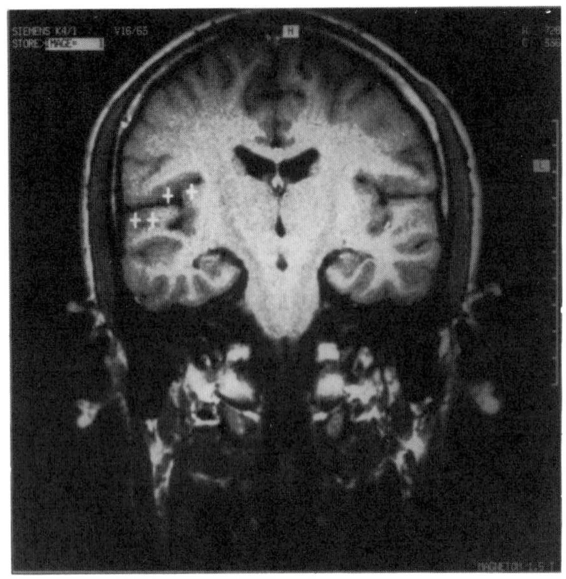

Fig.4 MR image (coronar slice), with center of dipolar activity for each frequency marked with a cross.

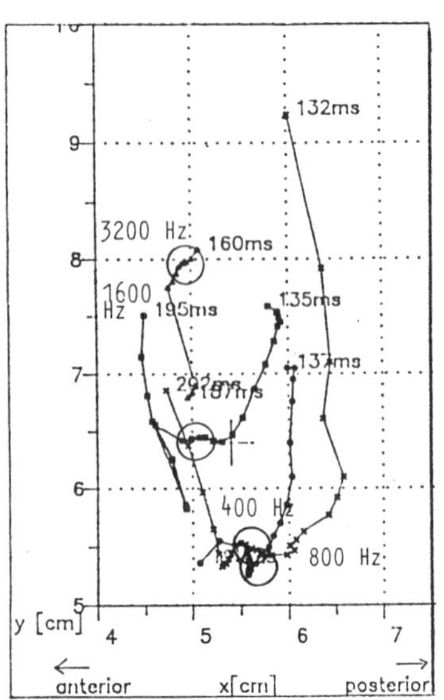

Fig.5 Dipole paths, sagittal projection during N100, for 4 stimulation frequencies.

From signal evaluation in combination with 3D MR imaging dipolar sources of electrical activity can be localized with a precision of a few millimeters. This for the first time allows clinical research of biomagnetism under routine conditions and also may provide a basis for improved modelling.

REFERENCES

Abraham-Fuchs et al., this conference.

Daalmans, G.M. (1980), SQUID '80, Edit. Hahlbohm,H.D., Lübbig,H., de Gruyter, Berlin, 399 - 415.

Daalmans, G.M. et al. (1989), Proc. Intern. Supercond. Elektr. Conf., ISEC'89, Tokyo, June 12-13 (1989).

Hari, R. et al. (1980), Exp. Brain Res. 40, 237 - 240.

Hoenig, H.E. et al. (1989), Cryogenics.

Hoke, M. et al. (1989), Hearing Res. 37, 281-286.

Ilmoniemi, R.J. et al. (1984), EEG clin.Neurophysiol. 58, 467-473.

Kajola, M. et al. Biomagnetism 87, Tokyo 1987, Edit. Atsumi, K.et al., Tokyo Denki University Press.

Pantev, C. et al. (1988), EEG clin. Neurophys. 69, 160 -170.

Romani, G.L. et al. (1982), Exp. Brain Res. 47, 381 - 393.

Romani, G.L. et al. (1985), SQUID '85 , Edit. Hahlbohm,H.D., Lübbig,H., de Gruyter, Berlin, 919-932.

Stefan, H. et al. (1988), contrib. (abstract) U7, Dt. EEG-Ges., 33 ann. conf., Hamburg, Sept. 29 - Oct.1.

Stefan, H. et al. (1989), this conference.

Weikl, A. et al. (1989) contrib. (abstract), Deutsche Ges.Innere Medizin, 95 Meeting, Wiesbaden, Apr. 2.-4.

Williamson, S.J. et al.(1984) Proc. 10th Int. Cryo Eng. Conf., Edit. Colland, H., Butterworth, Guildford, 339-348.

A 24-CHANNEL MAGNETOMETER FOR BRAIN RESEARCH

M. Kajola, S. Ahlfors, G.J. Ehnholm*, J. Hällström, M.S. Hämäläinen, R.J. Ilmoniemi, M. Kiviranta, J. Knuutila, O.V. Lounasmaa, C.D. Tesche**, and V. Vilkman

Low Temperature Laboratory, Helsinki University of Technology, 02150 Espoo, Finland
*Instrumentarium Imaging Ltd, Teollisuuskatu 27, 00510 Helsinki, Finland
**IBM Thomas J. Watson Research Center, Yorktown Heights, New York 10598, USA

INTRODUCTION

This paper describes the hardware of the 24-channel SQUID magnetometer being completed in the Low Temperature Laboratory. The overall system, including computer hardware and software, is discussed elsewhere (Hämäläinen 1989). The instrument will be used in a magnetically shielded room for brain research. We hope that this apparatus will enable us to locate current sources underlying evoked magnetic fields without moving the dewar.

MECHANICAL STRUCTURE

The device is kept at 4 K in a fiberglass dewar having a slanted spherical cap. The dewar was designed for this instrument and manufactured by CTF Inc., Canada. The structure of the device is shown in Fig. 1. The construction of the insert allows easy expansion to a 32 channel system by adding four sensor units of two SQUIDs each. Electronics in the insert has been divided into four identical groups of 8 channels, three of which are actually in use. The preamplifiers, located in 4 detachable aluminium boxes on top of the dewar, are connected to the SQUIDs via twisted pairs of leads inside shield tubes, which are separate for bias, modulation, and signal wires.

COIL CONFIGURATION

The pickup coil array consists of 12 sensor units, each measuring orthogonal tangential derivatives $\partial B_Z/\partial x$ and $\partial B_Z/\partial y$ of the radial field component. These units can be manufactured either using integrated planar sensors or conventional wire-wound coils. Although our integrated prototype sensors showed excellent sensitivity and tolerance to external disturbances (Knuutila et al., 1987b), we chose wire-wound coils for the present gradiometers because of technical difficulties encountered in fabricating reliable thin film structures in large quantities. Wire-wound coils also allow the use of other SQUID chips as well. In our instrument we employ dc SQUIDs provided by IBM (Tesche et al. 1985).

Advances in Biomagnetism
Edited by S.J. Williamson *et al.*
Plenum Press, New York

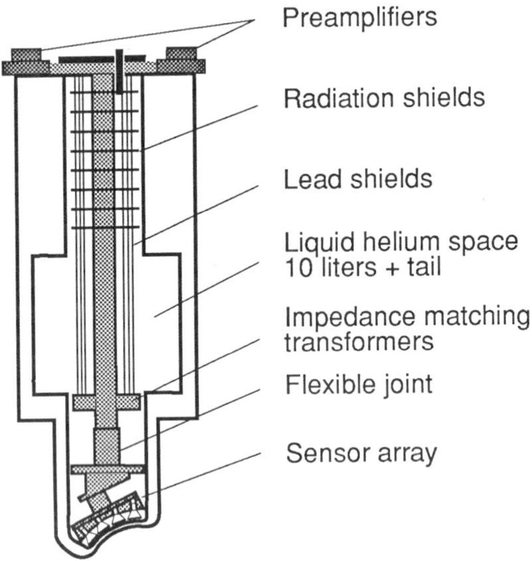

Figure 1. Schematic view of the dewar and insert.

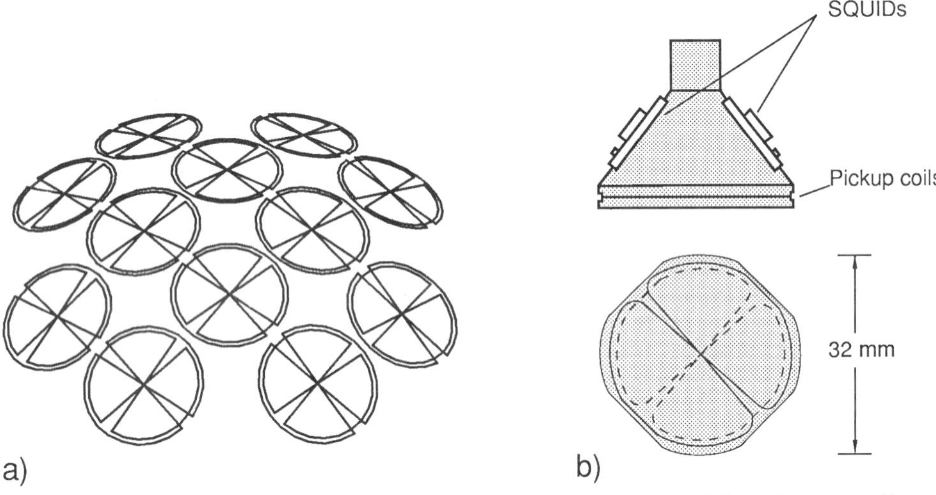

Figure 2. a) The 24-coil array. b) A two-channel sensor unit. The pick-up coils are connected to the signal coils of the two SQUIDs, mounted on the top of the conical ceramic glass coil former; the SQUIDs are in a fiberglass package and have no superconducting shielding.

The advantage of a planar coil configuration is its small size without sacrificing too much of the source locating accuracy. This enables us to use a dewar of reasonable size and to slant the bottom of the dewar for more flexible positioning. The locating capability of the device and the amount of information gained in measurements have been compared with several radial gradiometer coil configurations, and found adequate for practical work (Knuutila et al., 1985; Knuutila and Hämäläinen, 1989; Kemppainen and Ilmoniemi, 1989).

The two-SQUID units are placed on the spherical bottom of the dewar; the radius of curvature is 125 mm and the coils cover an area with a diameter of 125 mm. Each unit consists of two Nb wire-wound figure-of-eight gradiometer coils and the SQUIDs they are connected to. The area of each gradiometer loop is 3.7 cm^2 and the effective base length is 1.3 cm. The placement of the units and their structure is shown in Fig. 2. The gradient noise level is about 3-5 $fT/(cm\sqrt{Hz})$, using the IBM dc SQUIDs. The balance against homogeneous fields is better than 3%. The coupling between the orthogonal coils in a single unit is about 2% and between adjacent units less than 1%.

ELECTRONICS AND SIGNAL MONITORING

The electronics is a slightly modified version of that used in our seven channel system (Knuutila et al. 1987a). For each SQUID there is an impedance matching transformer in liquid helium, a preamplifier on top of the dewar, and a single eurocard detector-controller unit outside the magnetically shielded room in an rf-shielded cabinet. The 90-kHz flux modulation frequency is common and in phase for all channels. The SQUIDs can be operated either in an open loop or in a flux-locked loop mode, and the flux-voltage characteristics can be monitored for adjustment of the bias current. The operating mode, the output gain, and resetting of the feedback integrator can be controlled remotely by a computer. The main difference to the seven-channel system is the balancing of all lines between the SQUIDs and preamplifiers and between the preamplifiers and controllers. The structure of the impedance matching transformers is simplified. The real-time signal on 8 selectable channels can be monitored and the on-line averaged responses of 16 channels can be displayed during the measurements.

PRELIMINARY RESULTS

Tests have been made with 24 IBM dc SQUIDs out of which 21 worked satisfactorily with noise levels between 3 and 7 $fT/(cm\sqrt{Hz})$. Results from an auditory evoked field measurement are presented in Fig. 3. The dewar was placed above the right auditory cortex and the stimuli were tone pips, 50 ms long, delivered to the left ear. It should be noted that with this planar gradiometer the largest signal is obtained from the channel which is directly above the source and which measures the derivative perpendicular to the equivalent dipole.

ACKNOWLEDGMENTS

The project was financially supported by the Finnish National Fund for Research and Development (SITRA).

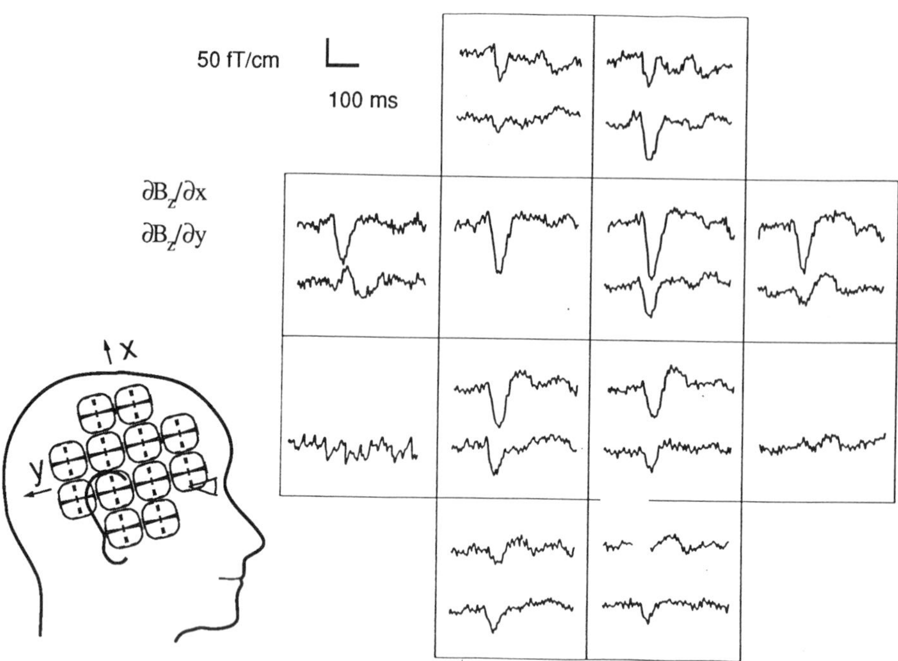

Figure 3. Responses to 50-ms tone pips of a 1000-Hz sine wave, delivered with an interstimulus interval of 3 s. Tones were given to the left ear and the recording was made on the right hemisphere. Traces are averages of 100 responses with a passband of 0.05 - 100 Hz. Both time sequences in each pair were measured over the same location, the upper traces represent the derivative $\partial B_Z/\partial x$ and the lower ones $\partial B_Z/\partial y$.

REFERENCES

Hämäläinen, M.S., 1989, A 24-channel planar gradiometer: system design and analysis of neuromagnetic data, this volume.

Kemppainen, P.K., and Ilmoniemi, R.J., 1989, Channel capacity of multichannel magnetometers, this volume.

Knuutila, J., Ahonen, A.I., Hämäläinen, M.S., Ilmoniemi, R.J., Kajola, M.J., Design considerations for multichannel SQUID magnetometers, 1985, *in:* SQUID'85, Superconducting Quantum Interference Devices and Their Applications, H.D. Hahlbohm and H. Lübbig, eds; Walter de Gruyter, Berlin, p. 939.

Knuutila, J., Ahlfors, S., Ahonen, A., Hällström, J., Kajola, M., Lounasmaa, O.V., Vilkman, V., and Tesche, C.D., 1987a, A large-area low-noise seven-channel dc SQUID magnetometer for brain research, *Rev. Sci. Instrum.*, 58: 2145

Knuutila, J., Kajola, M., Mutikainen, R., Salmi, J., 1987b, Integrated planar DC-SQUID magnetometers for multichannel neuromagnetic measurements, *in:* Extended Abstracts of the 1987 International Superconductivity Conference, Tokyo, p. 261.

Knuutila, J., Hämäläinen, M.S., 1989, On the spatial locating accuracy of multichannel magnetometers, this volume.

Tesche, C.D., Brown, K.H., Callegari, A.C., Chen, M.M., Greiner, J.H., Jones, H.C., Ketchen, M.B., Kim, K.K., Kleinsasser, A.W., Notarys, H.A., Proto, G., Wang, R.H., and Yogi, T., 1985, Practical dc SQUIDs with extremely low 1/*f* noise, *IEEE Trans. Magn.*, MAG-21: 1032.

MICROSQUID: A CLOSE-SPACED FOUR CHANNEL MAGNETOMETER

D.S. Buchanan, D.B. Crum, D. Cox[†], and J.P. Wikswo[‡]

Biomagnetic Technologies Inc.
San Diego, CA 92121, U.S.A.
[†]Quantum Design, Inc.
San Diego, CA 92121, U.S.A.
[‡]Vanderbilt University
Nashville, TN 37235, U.S.A.

INTRODUCTION

Typical SQUID-based magnetometers are currently constructed with 15 to 25 mm diameter coils that are spaced back from the room temperature measurement surface 12 to 20 mm. Both of these dimensions limit the spatial resolution of these systems. To understand the fundamental determinants of magnetic fields produced by bioelectric activity, better spatial resolution is needed (Wikswo, 1988). To address this need we have developed a close-spaced, four-channel magnetometer having 3mm diameter first-order assymetric gradiometer pick-up coils spaced on a 4.4mm grid and residing <1.5 mm from the measurement surface which is at room temperature: μSQUID™.

DEVICE

Fig. 1 shows a cross-section of the lower section of the μSQUID™. To achieve the close spacing several departures from more usual design practices were required. First the coils were mounted in the vacuum space of the dewar. This removed the inner wall of the dewar from between the coils and room temperature and it also facilitated the design of an actuator mechanism which allowed adjustment of the spacing between the pick-up coils and room temperature. Second, the rf shield which normally surrounds the coils was also absent again to reduce the material between the coils and the outside. Third, the section of the 77K thermal shield was eliminated from in front of the coils for the same reason. This left only the 4K shield, some super-insulation and the outer wall of the dewar between the coils and the outside allowing a closest spacing of 1.3 mm. At this spacing the loss of liquid helium becomes quite high, about 3.2 Lit./day. The adjustment of the coil spacing was included to allow the coils to be backed away from the measurement surface to reduce boil-off when not in use. Backing the coils away to 4mm reduces the boil-off to 1.8 Lit./day. Fig. 2 shows the boil-off as a function of coil spacing. The spacing was adjustable from the outside of the Dewar by means of screw adjustment on the bottom of the dewar. When at their closest spacing 0.1 mm of movement up or down would repeatedly drive the coils either normal or superconducting. The time for this transition to take place was approximately 20 seconds and was easily determined by

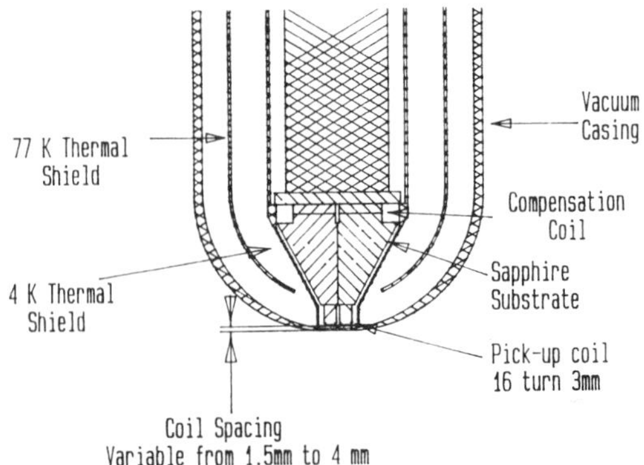

Fig. 1. Cross-section of tail of Dewar

observing the transfer function of the SQUIDs. Adjustment to closest spacing was done by slowly lowering the coils toward room temperature until they went normal and then backing off a small fraction of a turn on the adjustment screw.

To eliminate the effects of a 1.2% crosstalk between coils, external feedback was used. The system used standard Biomagnetic Technologies Inc. dc SQUIDS. If the system had operated at the SQUID noise level of $15\mu\phi_0/\sqrt{Hz}$ the system noise would have been approximately 55 ft/$\sqrt{Hz}$ equivalent. The final system noise was 90-100 ft/$\sqrt{Hz}$. We believe there are three possible sources of this noise which will be looked at in future devices: inadequate shielding of the transmission lines, insufficient cooling of the SQUIDs and possible noise coupling into the external feedback transformer. These sources were not pursued on the current system because of design difficulties which made the system difficult to modify.

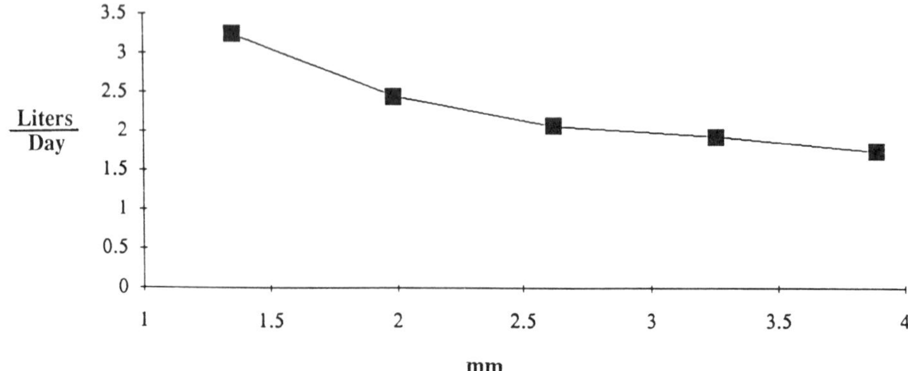

Fig. 2. Boiloff of the device in liters per day versus the coil spacing.

A number of preliminary measurement were made with this instrument (Wikswo 1989). We would like to present here measurements made on a wire phantom. The phantom was constructed of 70 wires of 0.28 mm diameter placed immediately side by side. The phantom was placed under the system and in contact with the vacuum casing so that the wires were approximately parallel to the axis connecting coils 3 and 4. Each wire was energized in turn with a 5 Hz, 20 μA peak-to-peak sine wave. The response of the magnetometer was then integrated over one half period of the sine wave. The resulting spatial transfer function is shown in Fig. 3.

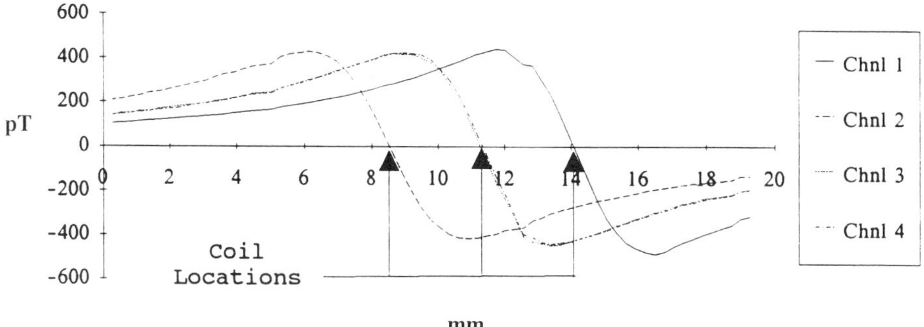

Fig. 3. Magnetometer response to a 20 μA peak-to-peak excitation current in a straight wire versus position. Response is integrated over 1/2 cycle of 5 Hz sine wave.

From Fig. 3 we derive a spatial sensitivity for the system for a 6.3 μ A current (the integral of a half cycle of a 10 μA sine wave) of 3.2×10^{-10} T/mm. Given a system noise of 90 ft/√Hz, a 1 Hz bandwidth, and a desired signal-to-noise ratio of 10 we calculate that this system would localize a straight line source to 2.5 μm. While this result might be misleading for a more generalized inverse of an unknown current source it is valid for localizing a source such as a power trace of an IC circuit.

ACKNOWLEDGEMENTS

This work supported in part by the Office of Naval Research, the National Institutes of Health, the Air Force Office of Scientific Research and Vanderbilt University.

REFERENCES

Wikswo, J. P., (1988). High-Resolution measurements of biomagnetic fields. Advances in Cryogenic Engineering, 33:107.

Wikswo, J. P. Friedman, R. N., Kilroy, A. W., van Egeraat, J. M., and Buchanan, D. S. (1989) Preliminary Measurements with MicroSQUID, This Proceedings.

PRELIMINARY MEASUREMENTS WITH MICROSQUID

John P. Wikswo[1], Richard N. Friedman[1], Anthony W. Kilroy[2], Jan M. van Egeraat[1], and D. Scott Buchanan[3]

[1]Department of Physics and Astronomy, Vanderbilt University, Nashville, TN 37235, U.S.A.
[2]Department of Neurology, Vanderbilt University Medical School
[3]Biomagnetic Technologies, Inc., San Diego, CA 92121, U.S.A.

INTRODUCTION

It is well known that for optimum sensitivity, the diameter of the pickup coil for a SQUID biomagnetometer should be no less than the source-to-coil spacing, and that this distance is the primary determinant of the spatial resolution of the magnetometer (Roth _et al_., 1989). As a result, SQUID systems with conventional Dewars _typically_ have spatial resolutions of 10 to 20 mm when resolution is measured in terms of the ability either to image a current distribution (Roth _et al_., 1989) or to resolve two closely-spaced dipolar current sources (Tan _et al_., 1989). While 1 to 2 cm resolution is adequate for many studies on _humans_, experiments on _in vitro_ preparations such as isolated nerves and muscles and slices of _brain and cardiac_ tissue would benefit from 1 to 2 mm resolution. Because the fields from these sources fall off as $1/r^2$ to $1/r^3$, it can be advantageous to trade absolute magnetometer sensitivity for decreased coil-to-source spacing (Roth _et al_. 1989; Wikswo, 1988). We describe measurements made with a 4-channel _SQUID_ gradiometer whose 3 mm diameter pickup coils are located 1.4 mm from the outer surface of the Dewar (Buchanan, _et al_., 1989).

METHODS

The SQUID system was operated in a magnetically shielded room, with a measurement bandwidth of 0.1 Hz to 6 kHz. Simultaneous electric and magnetic data were recorded with a microcomputer-based data acquisition system and, where appropriate, signal averaging was used to reduce noise. The four SQUID coils are located at the vertices of a square 4.4 mm on a side. In cases where the desired signals had opposite signs in pairs of SQUID channels, the signals could be subtracted to reduce both stimulus artifact and noise.

RESULTS

Figure 1a shows two simultaneously-recorded magnetoneurograms (MNGs) from compound action currents (CACs) conducted orthodromically by sensory components of the human median nerve, recorded at the wrist following a 1.0 ms, 11 mA stimulus applied to the index and middle fingers. Because the nerve was located beneath a point midway between the two pickup coils, the nerve-related components of the two signals had opposite signs, so that their difference in (b) exhibits reduced artifact. The electrically-recorded compound action potential (CAP) is given in (c). Figure 2 shows the slightly stronger magnetic fields from an isolated frog sciatic nerve.

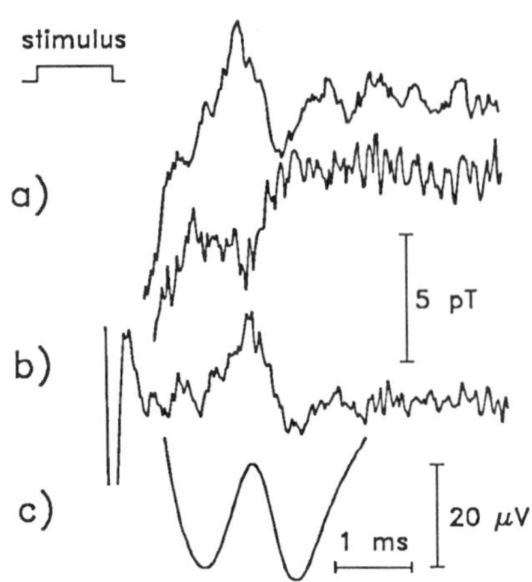

Fig. 1. a) The 2-channel MNG from sensory fibers in the human median nerve at the wrist. b) The difference of the two MNG signals. c) The CAP. (400 averages)

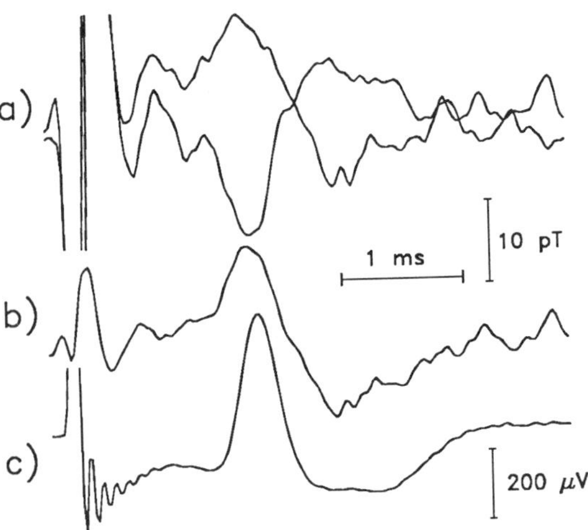

Fig. 2. a) The 2-channel MNG from an isolated frog sciatic nerve. b) The difference of the two MNG signals. c) The CAP. (64 averages)

The 4-channel magnetomyogram (MMG) of the human abductor pollicis brevis of the thumb was measured following stimulation (100 μs, 6 mA) of the median nerve at the wrist (Fig. 3). The similarities and differences between pairs of channels are determined by the relationships between the pickup coil geometry and the geometry of the muscle fibers, the location of the motor-endplate zone, and the direction of propagation along the fibers.

Figure 4 shows four simultaneous recordings of the voluntarily-activated MMG of the same muscle. It is clear that synchronous events were detected in all four channels, but with varying amplitudes and phases. Spikes from individual motor units can be resolved easily with an expanded time base, as shown by the six representative events in Fig. 5. Each of the four superimposed traces represents a single SQUID channel. Panels (a) and (b) show similar events (marked by an arrow), for which channel 2 (dashed) is positive but the other three channels are negative. Panel (c) shows a biphasic pulse for which all four channels have the same sign. Panel (d) has channel 2 negative and the other three positive, panel (e) has all positive, while panel (f) shows a spike with all channels negative. Events of each type could be found readily in the full record, demonstrating repeated firing of certain motor units. This suggests that the high-resolution MMG might be used to localize active motor units and determine their net action current, providing a new technique for quantitative assessment of motor unit behavior without the use of needle electrodes.

Simultaneously-recorded electric and magnetic compound action signals from an isolated frog gastrocnemius muscle are shown in Fig. 6. The muscle and sciatic nerve were dissected, removed from the frog, and immersed in saline. The nerve was stimulated by a 20 μs, 0.7 mA pulse once a second. The CAP was recorded differentially using a pair of Ag wires beneath the muscle. Panels (b) and (c) were from SQUID channels positioned above the axis of the muscle, while (a) and (d) were from SQUIDs on opposite sides of that line. The sign reversal between (a) and (d) is consistent with longitudinal action currents propagating parallel to the muscle axis, with the asymmetry probably due to error in positioning the magnetometer. The (b) and (c) traces are not as strongly biphasic as are the other two channels, and have a smaller amplitude. Their amplitude would have been expected to be zero if the action currents had been solely axial, if the muscle had been axially symmetric, and if the two pickup coils were directly above the axis. Detailed scans of the magnetic field will be required to understand its spatial variation and to determine whether or not we can detect the circumferential action currents reported by MacHattie and Pengelly.[5]

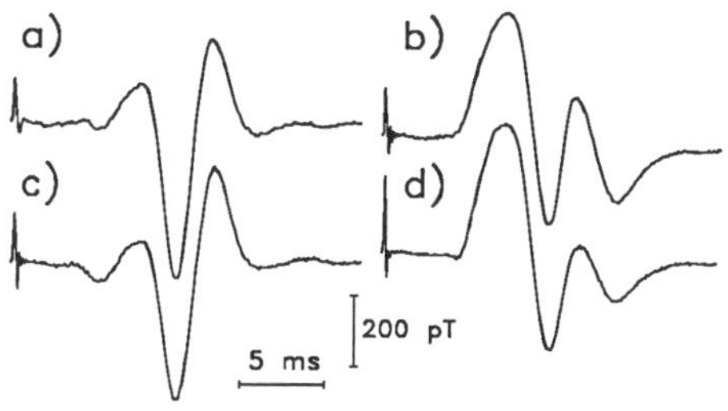

Fig. 3. A 4-channel evoked MMG of the human abductor pollicis brevis muscle in the hand. (16 averages)

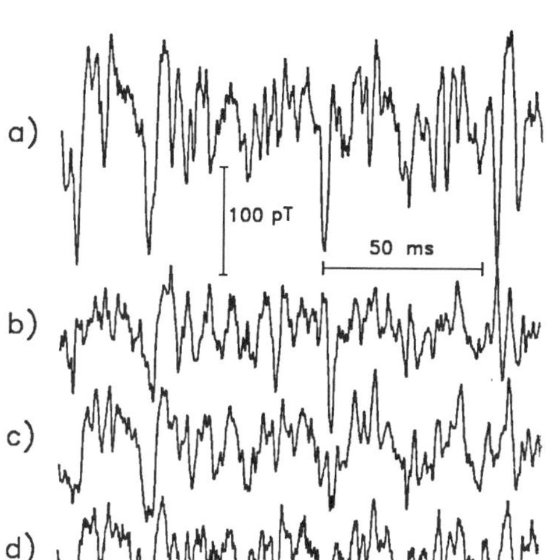

Fig. 4. A short sample of the voluntarily-activated, 4-channel MMG from the abductor pollicis brevis muscle.

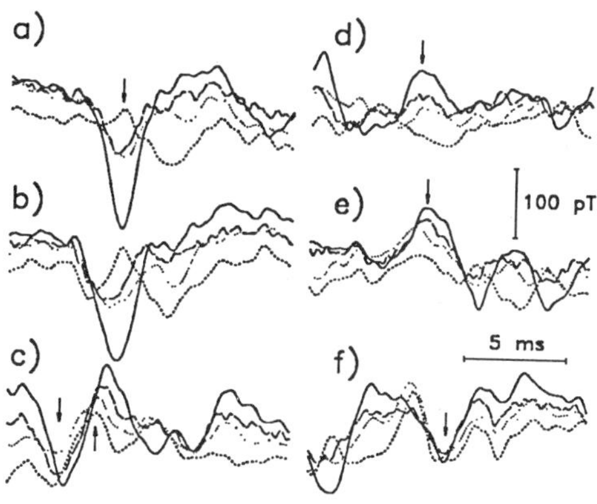

Fig. 5. Superimposed, 4-channel MMG spikes from the experiment in Fig.4.

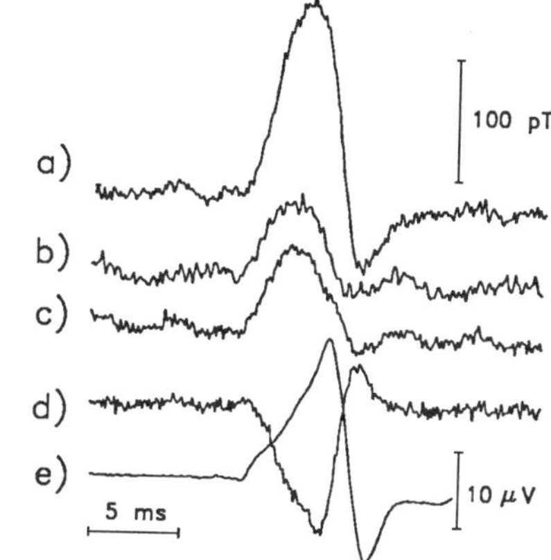

Fig. 6. (a-d) A 4-channel evoked MMG from an isolated frog gastrocnemius muscle. (e) The CAP. (8 averages).

Figure 7 shows three magnetocardiogram (MCG) signals and one electrocardiogram (ECG) signal recorded simultaneously from an exposed, in situ frog heart. From left to right, the peaks are produced by the activity of the atria, the ventricle, the sinus venosus, and the atria again. Note that, even for magnetometer channels separated by only 4.4 mm, there are distinct differences in the amplitude, shape, and sign of each peak.

While the absolute sensitivity of this SQUID system is lower than that reported for more conventional biomagnetometers, the outputs of the four independent channels can be combined to partially cancel the internal, uncorrelated system noise. When the source is so close to the coils that the desired signal has the opposite sign in pairs of coils, pairs of signals can be subtracted; when the source is so far away that the signals in all four coils are identical, the signals can be added. Other weightings can create lead systems optimized for specific sources and models. The human MCG in Fig. 8 is an example of the output of the SQUID system when the outputs of all four channels are averaged to reduce the noise by a factor of two.

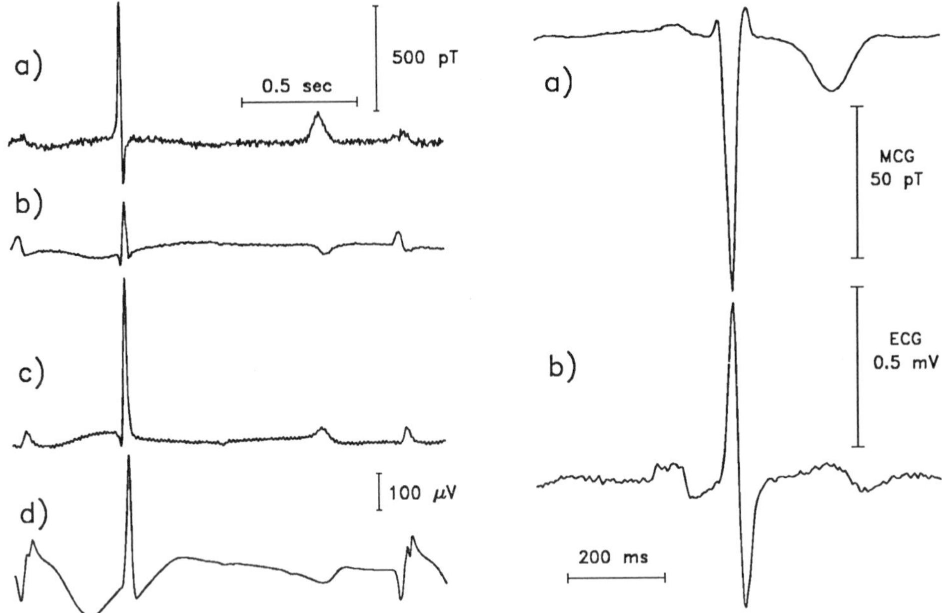

Fig. 7. (a-c) Frog MCG and (d) ECG. (32 averages, 100 Hz low pass filter).

Fig. 8. a) Human MCG at the xiphoid. b) Lead II ECG (30 averages)

DISCUSSION

The significant differences that we observe in waveform shape between SQUID pickup coils separated by only 4.4 mm suggest a wealth of information in the spatial variation of biomagnetic fields within 2 mm of electrically active tissue. While the 90-100 fT/√Hz noise in this system is larger than in conventional SQUID magnetometers, the increased resolution and the reduced coil-to-source spacing more than compensate. The availability of multiple SQUID channels gives the instrument the capability to perform real-time spatial filtering that is optimized for the particular source being studied, while at the same time improving the signal-to-noise ratio.

ACKNOWLEDGEMENT

Supported by the Office of Naval Research, the National Institutes of Health, the Air Force Office of Scientific Research, and Vanderbilt University. We are grateful to Ken Squires for encouragement and suggestions.

REFERENCES

Buchanan, D. S., Crum, D. B., Cox, D., and Wikswo, J.P. Jr., 1989, MICRO-SQUID: A close-spaced magnetometer, These proceedings.

MacHattie D. B., and Pengelly, L. D., 1988, Physiological and measurement factors affecting the magnetomyogram, Biomagnetism '87, K. Atsumi, M. Kotani, S. Ueno, T. Katila, and S. Williamson, Eds., Tokyo Denki Univ.Pr.

Roth, B. J., Sepulveda, N. G., and Wikswo, J. P., Jr., 1989, Using a magnetometer to image a two-dimensional current distribution, J. Appl. Phys., 65: 361-372.

Tan, S., Roth, B. J., and Wikswo, J. P., Jr., 1989, The magnetic field of cortical current sources: The application of a spatial filtering model to the forward and inverse problems, Submitted for publication.

Wikswo, J. P., Jr., 1988, High-resolution measurements of biomagnetic fields, Advances in Cryogenic Engineering, 33: 107-116.

SEQUENTIAL SPATIALLY DISTRIBUTED ACTIVITY OF THE HUMAN BRAIN DETECTED MAGNETICALLY BY CryoSQUIDS

G.A. Klemic, D.S. Buchanan,* Y.M. Cycowicz, and S.J. Williamson

Neuromagnetism Laboratory
Departments of Psychology and Physics and Center for Neural Science
4 Washington Place, New York University, New York, NY 10003
*Biomagnetic Technologies inc., San Diego, CA 92121, U.S.A

INTRODUCTION

Conventional SQUID-based magnetic sensors use a large reservoir of liquid helium (~10 liters) to maintain a low-temperature environment for the superconducting components. These systems waste helium, require refilling approximately every three days and may only be tipped up to 45 degrees from the vertical, constraining neuromagnetic measurements. Special dewars with canted tail surfaces and detection coils have been designed to overcome this problem, but still do not allow a full range of positions (Knuutila, et al, 1987). The recent development of a system called "CryoSQUID" based on helium gas refrigeration for cooling SQUID sensors elminates these limitations (Buchanan, Paulson, and Williamson, 1988). CryoSQUID has a completely closed system so it conserves helium and thus needs only a small reservoir of liquid (30 cm^3) and can be oriented in any direction, including upside down.

Two such single-channel CryoSQUIDs have been installed in a magnetically shielded room at New York University (Fig. 1). We report here the application of this system in two studies of spatially distributed neuronal activity in the human brain. These applications exploit the advantages of being able to orient the sensors in any direction. The first study monitors activity of auditory cortex in both hemispheres simultaneously, and the second is a study of sequential activity in a task involving a person's motor response following a visual stimulus.

Cooling of the SQUID sensor in each dewar is achieved by a three-stage cryocooler configuration in which a two-stage Gifford-McMahon (GM) cycle establishes a stage at 15 K and a Joule-Thomson (JT) cycle maintains the final stage at 4 K for the SQUID and detection coil (Buchanan, Paulson, Klemic, and Williamson, 1989). This avoids mechanical vibrations of the kind that may be introduced by a mechanical linkage as used for a Sterling cycle cryocooler (Zimmerman and Radebaugh, 1978). Valve motors controlling cryocooler operations are mounted outside the shielded room. Residual vibrations from the movement of the displacer in the GM cooler introduce magnetic noise. But since it is time-locked to the motion, a simple computer can be used to register a template and subtract this from the data in real time, removing all detectable noise of refrigerator origin. Both the GM and JT cycles operate from a common feed pressure of 2.3 MPa provided by a commercial compressor. The return at 0.6 MPa from the GM cooler is fed directly to this compressor, but the lower level return of 0.1 MPa from the JT cooler is first enhanced to 0.6 MPa by a second compressor. Cooling from room temperature is achieved after 20 hours simply by starting the compressors. One important feature of this device is provision for a reservoir where the JT stage stores liquid helium. The high specific heat of this liquid, compared to the much lower specific heat of solid structural materials provides a stable temperature for the SQUID, which is mounted outside the reservoir but in good thermal contact with it. The reservoir is important for

Advances in Biomagnetism
Edited by S.J. Williamson *et al.*
Plenum Press, New York

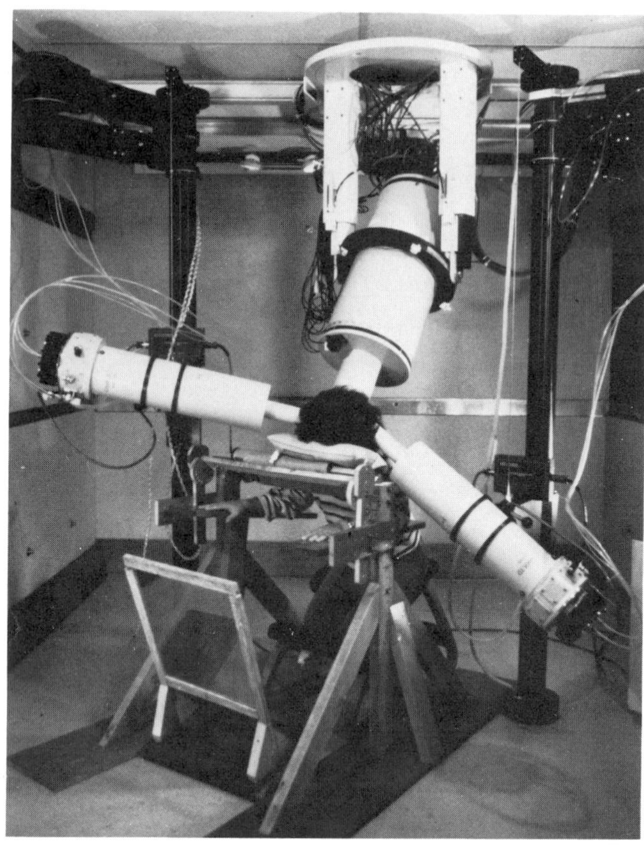

Fig. 1. Two CryoSQUIDs (small dewars on the left and right) shown here with a conventional five-sensor system (larger dewar supported from the ceiling) are positioned near a subject in a magnetically shielded room. Each CryoSQUID is supported by an individual tripod gantry permitting horizontal and vertical adjustment as well as positioning in any orientation. Flexible tubing provides high-pressure helium supply and low-pressure return for the refrigerators. Black fins at the top of the dewars are essential to dissipate heat convectively during the initial cool-down, but attain a temperature of only a few degrees above room temperature in operation.

another reason as well. Movement of the displacer of the GM stage and gas in the tubing produces acoustic noise which has proven impossible to eliminate. When this noise must be eliminated the system can be operated in an "intermittent" mode in which the GM cycle is shut down and the JT flow is reduced, with the residual evaporation of helium in the reservoir providing steady cooling. If neuromagnetic studies are carried out over a period of 2 - 3 minutes, followed by a similar time of renewed refrigeration the procedure can be extended for several hours. The whole operation is computer controlled. In the "one-shot" mode there is 20 minutes of operation before all the helium is evaporated. This system has most recently been in continuous operation for two months without failure, other than stoppages due to human error.

CONTRA AND IPSILATERAL DIFFERENCES IN RESPONSE

There are well-known functional differences between right and left hemispheres in humans. These are even evident in timing differences for certain processes. In the first experiment we compared simultaneous measurements of neuronal activity of auditory cortex in response to a short tone burst. One field extremum is generally found 2 - 4 cm anterior to the ear and about 3 - 5 cm above the line joining the ear canal to the corner of the eye. The other extremum is posterior to the ear and about 8 cm above that line. The field at both posterior extrema may be measured simultaneously with a conventional two dewar system. However experience has revealed strong alpha activity in occipital and parietal regions of the scalp, which introduces unwanted noise. Therefore there is considerable advantage in being able to monitor activity at the anterior extrema instead. This requires both sensors to be horizontal, or if the head is tipped to one side, one sensor can be pointed downward but the other must then be tipped upward to measure the normal component of the field.

The subject was presented monaurally with a 1000 Hz tone of 30 ms duration at 40 dB above threshold with an interstimulus interval of 2 s. CryoSQUIDs were positioned about 5 cm above and 3 cm forward of the ear canals, and operated in intermittent mode. Trials of 75 repetitions each

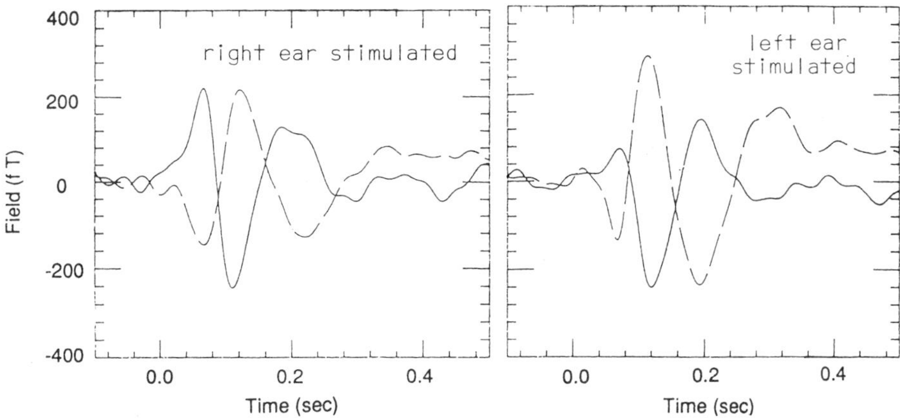

Fig. 2. Average of 150 responses to auditory stimuli. In each plot the dashed line represents field measured over the right hemisphere, and the solid line represents field measured over left hemisphere, as described in text.

were performed for stimuli presented in each ear. The results are shown in Fig. 2. Strong response components at about 70 ms ("P50m") and 120 ms ("N100m") were observed, with opposite polarities over the two hemispheres, as expected. In both cases the contralateral responses preceded the ipsilateral response: for N100m by about 6 ms for left ear stimulation and by 12 ms for right ear stimulation. Differences of comparable magnitudes for N100m have been reported for scalp potential measurements (Majkowski, Bochenek, Bochenek, Knapik-Fijalkowska, and Kopec, 1971). The latency differences for P50m are comparable for left ear stimulation, about 6ms, but not for right ear stimulation (3 ms) This may be compared with a similar difference of 7 - 8 ms that has been found for steady-state magnetic measurements of a response having an apparent latency of about 50 ms (Romani, Williamson, Kaufman, and Brenner, 1982). Such difference may well be explained by fewer synapses in contralateral projections.

SEQUENTIAL RESPONSES IN SENSORY-MOTOR PERFORMANCE

In the second experiment, the subject was instructed to view a screen and when a spot of light appeared to press a button with his left index finger. The visual stimulus was a circle of 0.5 deg diameter presented in the lower-right visual field, of 400 ms duration and 1.2 s interstimulus interval. One CryoSQUID was positioned over the left occipital scalp to record activity of visual cortex, (about 3 cm above and 2 cm to left of inion) and the other was placed over the right Rolandic fissure (19 cm back from the nasion, measured along the midline, and 10 cm above ear canal) because previous studies have shown that a field extrema from both motor and somatosensory areas in the fissure can be detected there (Okada, Williamson, and Kaufman, 1982).

Results shown in Fig. 3a depict the signals when 75 epochs are averaged with respect to onset of the visual stimulus. The two CryoSQUID outputs reveal that activity is first observed over occipital scalp, with a latency of about 110 ms, and this is followed about 50 ms later by a strong field over Rolandic fissure. Subsequently contact is made by the reaction time button, and about 75 ms later another strong field is observed over Rolandic fissure.

The time relation between these components and the subject's reaction time can be determined another way by averaging the same data with the moment of button contact as the time reference. Fig. 3b shows that the first field peak over the Rolandic fissure for the realigned average occurs 74 ms prior to the button press, and the subsequent peak occurs 86 ms following button press. These intervals are consistent with the indentification of the first being associated with neuronal activity of motor cortex and the second with activity of somatosensory cortex, the latter reflecting efferent input from proprioceptors involved in muscle flexation, perhaps with contributions from pressure on the finger tip from the button. We note also that the delay between peak activity in visual cortex and motor cortex is 51 ms. This means that the time interval between peak activity in visual cortex and reaction is 125 ms, in good agreement with the value of 115 ms

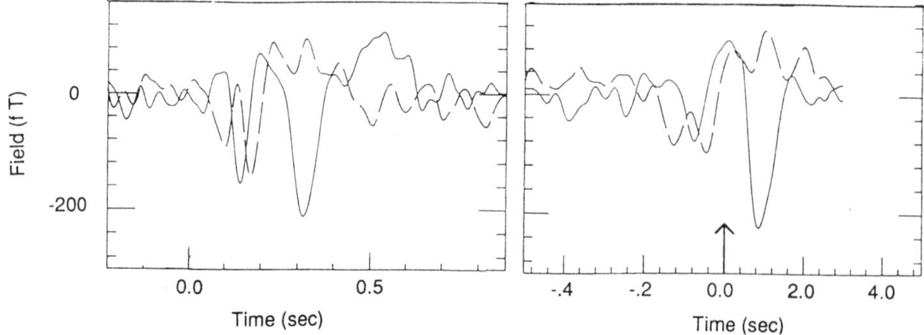

Fig. 3. (a) Observed fields in the two CryoSQUIDs for 75 responses averaged with onset of the visual stimulus as the time origin. (b) The same data when averaged with the button press as the time origin. In each plot, dashed lines represent field measured over occipital region and solid lines represent field measured over Rolandic fissure, as described in text.

obtained for the same subject using steady-state responses to determine the latency of visual cortex response (Williamson, Kaufman, and Brenner, 1978).

It is interesting to note that in the realigned average the amplitude of the motor peak is diminished relative to the average with respect to stimulus presentation, while all other peaks are about the same. This could indicate that response time jitter is related to a variability between first motor response and button press.

ACKNOWLEDGEMENTS

We thank Carlo Salustri for helpful advice. This work was supported in part by Air Force Office of Scientific Research contracts AFOSR-84-0313, F49620-85-K-0004, and F49620-86-C-0131.

REFERENCES

Buchanan, D.S., Paulson, D., and Williamson, S.J. (1987). Instrumentation for clinical applications of neuromagnetism. In: Fast, R.W., Ed., *Advances in Cryogenic Engineering* Vol. 33, Plenum Press, New York, pp. 97 - 106.

Buchanan, D.S., Paulson, D.N., Klemic, G.A., and Williamson, S.J. (1989). Development of a Hybrid Gifford-McMahon Joule-Thomson Based Neuromagnetometer: CryoSQUID, in press.

Knuutila, J., Ahlfors, S., Ahonen, A., Hallstrom, J., Kajola, M., Lounasmaa, O.V., Vilkman, V., Tesche, C. (1987). A Large-Area Low-Noise Seven-Channel DC SQUID Magnetometer for Brain Research. Helsinki Univ. fo Tech. Low Temp. Laboratory Report TKK-F-A613.

Majkowski, J., Bochenek, Z., Bochenek, W., Knapik-Fijalkowska, D., Kopec, J. (1971). Latency of averaged evoked potentials to contralateral and ipsilateral auditory stimulation in normal subjects. *Brain Research*, 25, 416-419.

Okada, Y.C., Williamson, S.J., and Kaufman, L. (1982). Magnetic field of the human sensorimotor cortex. *Intern. J. Neuroscience* 17, 33-38.

Romani, G.L., Williamson, S.J., Kaufman, L., and Brenner, D. (1982). Characterization of the human auditory cortex by the neuromagnetic method. *Exp. Brain Res.* 47, 381-393.

Williamson, S.J., Kaufman, L., and Brenner, D. (1978). Latency of the neuromagnetic response of the human visual cortex. *Vision Res.* 18, 107-110.

Zimmerman, J.E., and Radebaugh, R. (1978). Operation of a very low-power cryocooler. In: *Applications of Closed Cycle Cryocoolers to Small Superconducting Devices*, Zimmerman, J.E., and Flynn, T.M., Eds., NBS Special Publication No. 508, pp. 59-65.

THE LANL GRADIOMETER ORIENTATION DEVICE

D. B. van Hulsteyn, L. McGavran, L. Heller, J. George, P. Medvick and E. Flynn

Neuromagnetism Laboratory, Los Alamos National Laboratory
Los Alamos, New Mexico 87545

Introduction

A fundamental problem for neuromagnetic recording techniques is to determine the position and orientation of the sensors with respect to a subject's head. Until these parameters can be accurately characterized the ability to localize neuromagnetic signal sources precisely will be limited. At Los Alamos we are developing an inexpensive system designed to provide this essential information in a manner compatible with neuroscience experiments. Our approach is to place three sets of three mutually orthogonal magnetic loop dipole transmitters at salient points on the head surface. These can be activated sequentially to produce signals that are detected by each gradiometer. A program has been written to determine the positions of each transmitter cluster in the dewar reference frame. Because the locations of three points can also be determined in the head-centered coordinate system[1], it is possible to determine the translation and rotation transforms relating the gradiometer and the head coordinate systems.

Although similar principles are employed in a commercially available unit (the Probe Position Indicator, BTi), there are substantial and functionally significant differences in implementation. The BTi system uses an active magnetic transmitter which is attached to the neuromagnetic dewar. Room temperature pick-up coils are attached to the head surface or embedded in a wand which can be used to locate anatomical reference locations. In our unit the pick-up coils are the superconductor gradiometer sensors themselves. This approach allows us to toggle between localization procedures and conventional MEG operation without seriously disturbing the neuromagnetic detectors. It also eliminates the potential errors associated with inaccurate knowledge of the relative position of the internal gradiometers and an external system component. Knowing the positions *and the orientations* of each sensor will eliminate the need for prior knowledge or assumptions regarding a subject's head shape or the orientation of an equivalent current dipole source. The only disadvantage we anticipate is that the small angular separation between the individual gradiometers presents a moderately difficult computational geometry. This geometric complication increases the solution time, although preliminary results indicate that times of 3-5 seconds should be realistic on the computer used in our laboratory.

Advances in Biomagnetism
Edited by S.J. Williamson *et al.*
Plenum Press, New York

Methods

The major efforts in developing this unit have been to fabricate the hardware and develop software to solve the magnetic inverse problem. The hardware components consist of the three sets of loop dipoles, a multiplexing circuit to drive the dipoles in any specified order, a test stand for balancing the dipole magnetic moments and a head-stand for calibrating the software and isolating sources of error.

The dipoles are fabricated using 1 cm cubes of delrin as the forms. Three orthogonal slits, each .010" (.25 mm) in width, are cut in the faces of the cube to a depth of 4 mm. This provides a 2 mm cubical surface centered inside the delrin form; loop dipoles are then produced by wrapping 25 turns of #40 gauge wire to produce three orthogonal loops. The narrow slits (.25 mm) help assure that the dipoles are essentially perpendicular. The dipole leads are soldered to pairs of quick connect leads to allow the cubes to be installed and removed from the headband. The sockets are connected to the current driver via coaxial cables.

The current driver consists of a low impedance sinusoidal voltage and a multiplexing circuit containing nine latching reed relays. Each relay is connected to one of the dipoles through a ten ohm potentiometer. Upon command from a manually triggered pulse or a signal from the computer, a particular relay is closed while the others remain open; this directs the sinusoidal signal to the corresponding coil as long as the relay is closed. A subsequent trigger pulse opens this relay and closes the next one in the sequence.

In order to ensure that all the magnetic dipole moments are equal in strength, we adjust for geometric errors by noting that the moment is given by

$$M = NIA \ , \tag{1}$$

where M is the moment, N the number of windings, I the current and A the area of the loop. Variations in N and A can be compensated for by adjusting I; this is accomplished by varying the resistance of the 10 ohm potentiometers. In order to place the cubes in the correct orientation and positions for electrical balancing, we have assembled a simple test stand with three sets of sockets. This allows the cubes to be positioned so that X," Y", and Z" dipoles are alternatively aligned in the vertical direction corresponding to the calibration axis.

The final piece of hardware in the system is the calibration head-stand, which consists of a head mock-up installed in a gimballed mount. This permits rotation about three different axes and also makes it possible to translate the head in the X-Y plane. This system allows us to place the head at any desired point relative to the dewar and to rotate it in any specified direction. When the headband with the dipole clusters connected is placed on the head mock-up and the dipoles are activated, this head-stand will allow us to compare the calculated gradiometer positions and orientations with the prescribed values. This will test the software as well as other aspects of the system design and fabrication.

Results

In this presentation the major thrust will be to describe our approach for obtaining the second order gradiometer coordinates and orientations relative to a subject's head-centered axes. The seven sensor array used at Los Alaamos consists of a central gradiometer whose Z-axis is essentially the same as the dewar axis. The remaining six gradiometers are equally spaced about the Z-axis and inclined at an angle of 10°; the centers of the bottom coils are 2 cm from the dewar axis. The axes of all seven gradiometers, therefore, intersect at a point 11.4 cm below the bottom coils of the array. The X-axis is along a line that connects the center of the middle gradiometer (gradiometer #1) with the axis of gradiometer #7.

The head Y'-axis is defined by the periauricula adjacent to the ear canals; the X'-axis, which is perpendicular to the Y'-axis, points outward through the plane containing the nasion. The Z'-axis is orthogonal to the X'-Y' plane and points vertically through the top of the skull. Finally, each dipole triplet is defined by a set of X''_i, Y''_i, Z''_i axes which specify the directions of the magnetic dipole moments $\mathbf{M}''_{ij}$. The indices i = 1,2,3 and j = 1,2,3 indicate the number of the triplet and the number of the dipole in that triplet, respectively. Thus, for example, $\mathbf{M}''_{13}$ is the Z''_1-oriented dipole at position #1.

We consider set #i whose coordinates, relative to the dewar frame, are given by (X_i, Y_i, Z_i). By sequentially pulsing the three dipoles and measuring the fields sensed by the gradiometers, we can evaluate (X_i, Y_i, Z_i) and, if desired, the orientatations of the (X''_i, Y''_i, Z''_i) axes relative to the dewar frame. The matrix that rotates the dipole axes to the dewar coordinates is designated by $[\mathbf{A}_i]$. This allows us to relate the dipole set $[\mathbf{M}''_i]$ in its own frame to its representation $[\mathbf{M}_i]$ inthe dewar frame via the expression

$$[\mathbf{M}_i] = [\mathbf{A}_i]^t \, [\mathbf{M}''_i] = M \, [\, \mathbf{A}_i]^t \, . \tag{2}$$

Here, $[\mathbf{A}_i]^t$ is the transpose of $[\mathbf{A}_i]$. In the remainder of this discussion the subscript 'i' will be suppressed for simplicity, although it must be remembered that we are dealing with a specific triplet. The fact that M appears as a constant on the right hand side of eq (2) is a result of our having balanced the dipole strengths.

Using an observation made by Erne et. al.[2], the magnetic field sensed by gradiometer #k is given by

$$B_{kj} = \mathbf{S}_k \cdot \mathbf{M}_j \tag{3}$$

where $\mathbf{S}_k$ contains only geometric terms. Eq (3) provides the value of the magnetic field sensed by gradiometer #k due to dipole #j. This expression is applicable to single pick-up coils as well as to first and second order gradiometers, although the explicit form of the vector will be different. Viewing eq (3) as a 7x3 matrix (a result of seven gradiometers and three dipoles in a set) we can write

$$[\mathbf{B}] = [\mathbf{S}] \, [\mathbf{M}]^t \tag{4}$$

which, when combined with eq (2), yields

$$[\mathbf{B}] = M \, [\mathbf{S}] \, [\mathbf{A}] \tag{5}$$

If we now multiply eq (5) by its transpose we obtain

$$[\mathbf{B}] \, [\mathbf{B}]^t = M^2 \, [\mathbf{S}] \, [\mathbf{S}]^t \; ; \tag{6}$$

this matrix equation is independent of the dipoles' orientations by virtue of the fact that $[\mathbf{A}] \, [\mathbf{A}]^t = [\mathbf{1}]$. As an example, we consider the on-diagonal elements for gradiometer #2, which give us

$$M^2 \{ (S_{2x})^2 + (S_{2y})^2 + (S_{2z})^2 \} = \{ (B_{21})^2 + (B_{22})^2 + (B_{23})^2 \} \tag{7}$$

Because this equation contains only three unknowns (X, Y, Z), we can use it in conjunction with another pair to solve for the dipoles' coordinates. The terms on the right-hand side of eq (7) are the data; B_{21} for example is the field sensed by gradiometer #2 when dipole #1 is pulsed. The left-hand side represents the sum of the squares of the components of the geometric vector $\mathbf{S}_2$. What we have in eq (7) is a surface generated by adding the contributions from any set of three orthogonal dipoles *that does not depend upon the specific orientation of the dipole frame.*

When using idealized data containing no noise or measurement errors, the solution time for remote dipoles appears to increase somewhat with distance, although the resolution is not affected. A rigorous attempt to quantify the relationship between solution time and dipole distance will be made in the near future. In the mean time we are in the process of including the case where the gradiometer sensitivity is varied by 10% to determine the effect on spatial and angular resolution. We are also conducting calibration experiments using a specially designed dipole holder to test the accuracy of the theory.

The next step in determining the location and rotation of the dewar with respect to the head is to repeat the theoretical analysis for the other two dipole cluster positions. This establishes three points in the dewar reference coordinates; these same points can be specified in the head coordinates. With three points established in both the head and the dewar coordinates, the translation and rotation that relate the two frames are uniquely defined. In the present format, the solution time using an HP 825 is of order 30 seconds. We are investigating the use of a simple approximation as a method for obtaining a good set of starting values. This will avoid the systematic sampling of the solution space now employed and thus reduce the solution time by an order of magnitude.

Discussion

The rationale for fabricating this unit was to build an inexpensive device that could talk directly to the gradiometers and thus alleviate the need for an additional set of components. One difficulty we have encountered is that seven slightly inclined, second order gradiometers present a geometrically complicated problem. The time required to solve for the coordinates is significantly greater than if our dewar contained a set of orthogonal pick-up loops. A primary advantage promised by this system is that, because the pick-up coils are the gradiometer loops of the neuromagnetometer, it is not necessary to calibrate the position of an external system component with respect to the nominal positions of the gradiometers. Furthermore, it will be possible to determine these parameters without seriously affecting MEG data collection. By calculating the location *and* the orientation of each gradiometer directly, it will no longer be necessary to make assumptions about the orientations of brain electrical sources or about a subject's head shape.

Acknowledgement

This work is supported by the U. S. Department of Energy

References

J. S. George, P. S. Jackson, D. Ranken and E. R. Flynn, Three-Dimension Volumetric Reconstruction for Neuromagnetic Source Localization, this volume (1989).

S. N. Erne, L. Narici, V. Pizzella and G. L. Romani, The Positioning Problem in Biomagnetic Measurements: A Solution for Arrays of Superconducting Sensors, IEEE Trans. Magn. (USA) 23:1319, (1987.

MAGNETOMETER POSITION INDICATOR FOR MULTICHANNEL MEG

Seppo Ahlfors and Risto J. Ilmoniemi

Low Temperature Laboratory
Helsinki University of Technology
02150 Espoo, Finland

INTRODUCTION

We have constructed a system for the automatic determination of the relative position and orientation of a multichannel MEG magnetometer and the head. With this system and some fixed points as reference, the current sources in the brain can be related to the anatomy of the head. We first describe the principles of our method, and then examine the accuracy of our system.

METHODS

Small reference coils are placed on the head and the magnetic field generated by them is measured by means of a SQUID magnetometer using at least 3 channels. From the signals, the relative position of the coils and the magnetometer is calculated. In addition to standard MEG equipment, only the coils, a current generator, and computer software are required. The idea has been presented independently by Knuutila et al., 1985 and by Erné et al., 1987. In the latter paper, simulations, which assume a signal-to-noise ratio of 10^4, suggest an accuracy better than 1 mm. In practice, however, signal-to-noise ratios much better than 10^2 are not significant, because constructional uncertainties and inaccuracies in magnetometer calibration act as additional sources of error. To make the method independent of the orientations of the coils, and to improve the convergence of the calculations, we introduce sets of three nominally orthogonal transmitter coils at one position.

Our 5-mm-diameter coil sets are mounted on EEG electrodes (Ilmoniemi and Ahlfors, 1988). This allows automatic determination of the electrode positions, simplifying the future combination of MEG and EEG. Current is fed to each coil separately and the magnetic field is measured with a 7-channel magnetometer (Knuutila et al., 1987). Since the distance from a current loop to the magnetometer is always long, compared to the loop diameter, the loop can be approximated by a magnetic dipole.

The field generated by a dipole $\mathbf{m}_j$ $(j = 1,2,3)$ and detected by channel $i = 1,..,7$ of the magnetometer is $b_{ij} = \mathbf{m}_j^T \mathbf{R}_i \mathbf{e}_i$, where the 3×3 -matrix $\mathbf{R}_i$ depends only on the position $\mathbf{r}$ of the dipole and on the geometry of the flux transformer; $\mathbf{e}_i$ is a unit vector in the direction of the sensitivity axis of channel i; T indicates transpose. If the flux through each first-order gradiometer coil is approximated by the difference of the field strengths at the center of the pickup coil ($\mathbf{r}_i^p$, see Fig. 1) and the compensation coil ($\mathbf{r}_i^c$),

Advances in Biomagnetism
Edited by S.J. Williamson *et al.*
Plenum Press, New York

then

$$\mathbf{R}_i = \frac{\mu_0}{4\pi}\left(\frac{3(\mathbf{r}_i^p - \mathbf{r})(\mathbf{r}_i^p - \mathbf{r})^T}{|\mathbf{r}_i^p - \mathbf{r}|^5} - \frac{\mathbf{I}}{|\mathbf{r}_i^p - \mathbf{r}|^3} - \frac{3(\mathbf{r}_i^c - \mathbf{r})(\mathbf{r}_i^c - \mathbf{r})^T}{|\mathbf{r}_i^c - \mathbf{r}|^5} + \frac{\mathbf{I}}{|\mathbf{r}_i^c - \mathbf{r}|^3}\right).$$

We group the signals to vectors $\mathbf{b}_i = (b_{i1}, b_{i2}, b_{i3})^T = \mathbf{M}^T\mathbf{R}_i\mathbf{e}_i$, where the matrix $\mathbf{M} = (\mathbf{m}_1, \mathbf{m}_2, \mathbf{m}_3)$ has the dipole moment vectors as columns. If the $\mathbf{m}_j$ are linearly independent, $\mathbf{M}^{-1}$ exists. The seven numbers $\mathbf{b}_i^T\mathbf{M}^{-1}(\mathbf{M}^{-1})^T\mathbf{b}_i$ are invariant during rotations of the coil set; from them, the position $\mathbf{r}$ of the coil set in the magnetometer coordinate system can be obtained by nonlinear least-squares fitting.

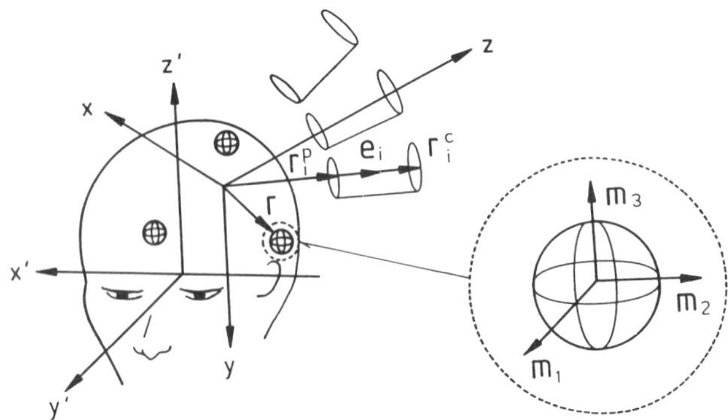

Fig. 1. Three three-coil sets, each approximated by three magnetic dipoles, attached on the head. First, the positions of the coil sets are determined both in the magnetometer (x, y, z) and the head (x', y', z') coordinate systems. Then, the position and orientation of the flux transformer array are calculated in the head coordinate system.

In our head coordinate system (Fig. 1), the x'-axis goes from the center of the left auditory canal to the right; the y'-axis intersects the x'-axis perpendicularly and passes through the nasion; the z'-axis points up. The magnetometer coordinate system is fixed to the flux transformer coils. The positions of the coil sets are determined (i) with a 3-dimensional digitizer in the head coordinate system and (ii) magnetically in the magnetometer coordinate system. Finally, with coordinate transformations, the position and orientation of the magnetometer in the head coordinate system is obtained.

RESULTS

The error in the calculated position of one coil set increases with the distance of the coils from the magnetometer. Small deviations in measured signals lead to large errors in positions when the coil set is far compared to the distance between the outermost pickup coils (72 mm in our magnetometer). At 80-mm distance, the standard deviation of the position of one coil set was measured to be about 3 mm; at longer distances, the performance deteriorates rapidly. Also, the accuracy with which the geometry of the coils and of the magnetometer are known is critical for proper positioning. Simulated

Table 1. Standard deviation $s(\mathbf{r})$ of the position of one coil set in a simulation in which the coil and magnetometer geometries were assumed inaccurately known.

parameter	*variation*	$s(\mathbf{r})$ [mm]
Magnetic moment, amplitude	1 %	0.2
Magnetic moment, direction	1°	0.1
Pickup coil position, tangential	0.5 mm	0.5
Pickup coil position, radial	0.5 mm	0.7
Magnetometer calibration	1 %	0.7

measurements from 100 different coil set positions, covering a normal MEG measurement area, were calculated varying different geometric factors, one at the time. The positions of the coil set were then deduced using the original parameter values without variation. The root-mean-square differences $s(\mathbf{r})$ of the positions are shown in Table 1. For example, 1-% error in one calibration coefficient causes an error of about 1 mm in the coil set position.

The error in the position of the magnetometer with respect to the head is not the same as the errors in the position of individual coils. When these are attached to the head 100 mm apart from each other, the estimated averaged error in the magnetometer position is about 3 mm. A series of test measurements, in which the coils were fixed to a head model, confirmed this estimate. The calculated positions could be reproduced with millimeter precision, which indicates that the error is not due to measurement noise.

The main objective of MEG is to determine the source current distribution $\mathbf{J}^p(\mathbf{r}')$ in the brain. Figure 2 illustrates how $\mathbf{J}^p(\mathbf{r}')$ is obtained, and how it can be related to the results of other brain imaging methods, like CT, MRI, and PET. Errors to $\mathbf{J}^p(\mathbf{r}')$ accumulate from different sources: the definition of the fixed points may be inaccurate; the mechanical digitizer and the magnetic locating system introduce errors; the subject may move his head during the measurement; MEG signals are noisy; the conductivity geometry model (e.g., a spherical head) and source current model (e.g., a current dipole) may be inadequate.

DISCUSSION

It seems that millimeter precision in the determination of magnetometer locations is reachable with our method. However, to succeed, calibration techniques must be improved. The true accuracy in the 7-channel magnetometer position achieved in our experiments so far was about 3 mm. The error is expected to diminish when devices with more channels become available. With our system we are able to locate neural current distributions with respect to chosen fixed points outside the head. Thus, it is also possible to relate MEG source locations with anatomical and functional features obtained by other imaging methods.

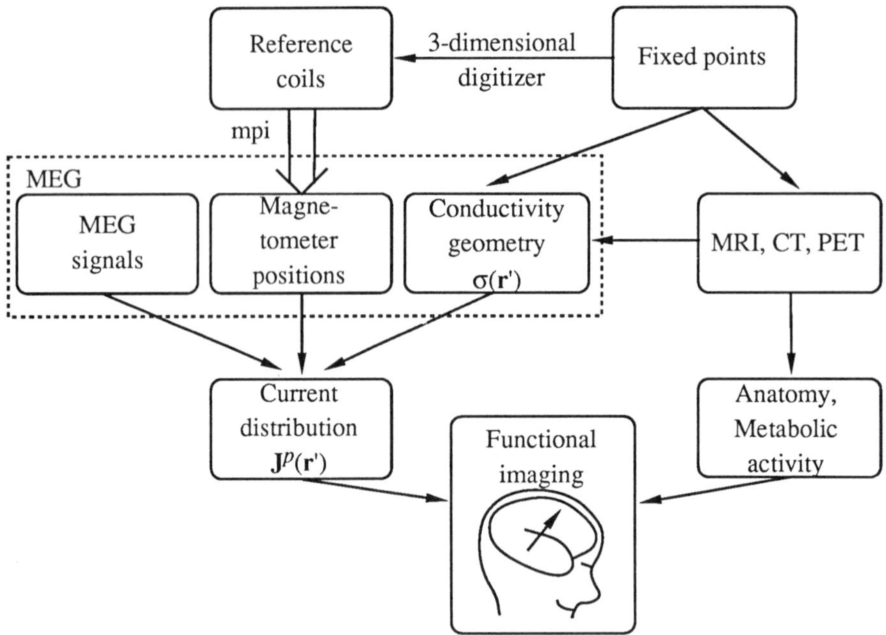

Fig. 2. Relations between the current distribution determined by MEG and the features obtained by other brain imaging methods. With the help of the reference coils, the magnetometer position indicator (mpi) gives the location and orientation of the magnetometer with respect to the fixed points.

ACKNOWLEDGMENTS

We thank Olli V. Lounasmaa for support and criticism, M. Hämäläinen for computer programs, M. Kajola for constructing the electronics, P. Kemppainen for making the coils, J. Hällström, J. Knuutila, and V. Vilkman for technical assistance.

REFERENCES

Erné, S. N., Narici, L., Pizzella, V., and Romani, G. L., 1987, The positioning problem in biomagnetic measurements: a solution for arrays of superconducting sensors, *IEEE Trans. Magn.*, MAG-23:1319.

Ilmoniemi, R. J. and Ahlfors, S., 1988, Finnish patent application, No. 884187, Sept 12, 1988.

Knuutila, J., Ahlfors, S., Ahonen, A., Hällström, J., Kajola, M., Lounasmaa, O. V., Vilkman, V., and Tesche, C., 1987, Large-area low-noise seven-channel dc SQUID magnetometer for brain research, *Rev. Sci. Instrum.*, 58:2145.

Knuutila, J., Ahonen, A. I., Hämäläinen, M. S., Ilmoniemi, R. J., and Kajola, M. J., 1985, Design considerations for multichannel SQUID magnetometers, *in* "SQUID 85 - Superconducting Quantum Interference Devices and their Applications", H. Hahlbohm and H. Lübbig, eds., Walter de Gruyter, Berlin.

SUBJECT AND GRADIOMETER POSITIONING FOR MEG RECORDING: A PRELIMINARY REPORT

P. Teale, J. E. Zimmerman, J. Edrich, S. Linnville, and M. Reite

Department of Psychiatry
University of Colorado Health Sciences Center
Denver, CO 80262, USA

INTRODUCTION

The estimation of neuromagnetic source location is facilitated by knowing where the magnetic sensing coils are located in space with reference to the center (or other reference point) of the head. The use of various grid systems referenced to the surface of the scalp, while not unreasonable for points near the center of the grid, is far from optimal for outlying sites. In addition, it is difficult to accurately determine the orientation of the sensing coils with respect to the intracranial space. While they may be normal to the local scalp surface, their position relative to the center of the total volume is unknown. In the case where a mapping session is interrupted or it is desirable to repeat measurements, the ability to return to the same location reliably is an obvious necessity. Another consideration is the ability to transfer an estimated source location obtained from MEG measurements to an alternate reference frame, e.g., a set of MRI or CAT scans.

We report here the design and construction of a gradiometer mounting system with automatic position encoding, and a subject chair which allows for the precise centering of the head, or intracranial space, using a laser crosshair alignment system, which insures that all measurements are accompanied by accurate coordinates of the coil positions in space with reference to the head.

METHODS

Figure 1 presents a schematic diagram of our dewar carriage and encoding system. The dewar (A) is encased in a teflon sleeve (B), to which is attached on one side a brass rack gear (C), and, on the other, an aluminum guide bar (D). This assembly is mounted in a square acrylic carriage block (E) between four pairs of nylon rollers (F). A pinion gear attached to a hand wheel (G) engages the rack and allows for the adjustment of radial position A spring loaded rubber drive wheel (H) contacts the guide bar and drives a ten turn, .2% linearity potentiometer connected to a five volt DC reference. The wiper arm is connected to an A/D converter channel in the data acquisition computer. The carriage block is sandwiched between two vertical acrylic panels (J), each having 1/4 circle milled slots in which nylon rollers (I) travel. This allows for a declination (theta) adjustment from 5 to 70 degrees off vertical. Another drive wheel-pot assembly (K) is located in one of the slots, and is connected to a second A/D channel. The acrylic sides share a common top panel of aluminum (L) through which a 5" hollow column is inserted. A collar at the bottom of the column (M) has a concentric V-groove in which 200 bronze balls are located allowing the entire assembly to rotate. This provides a phi adjustment of 360^0. The column is attached to the ceiling of our shielded room and a third drive wheel-pot unit (N) runs on the collar. The center for the gradiometer spherical coordinate system is the focal point for three cross-hair laser projectors[1], one mounted on a side wall, one on the back wall and one mounted inside the center of the support column. These are energized through fiber optic cables with an externally located laser. The projector housings are made of stainless steel and are sufficiently remote from the gradiometer so as to contribute no measurable increase in noise.

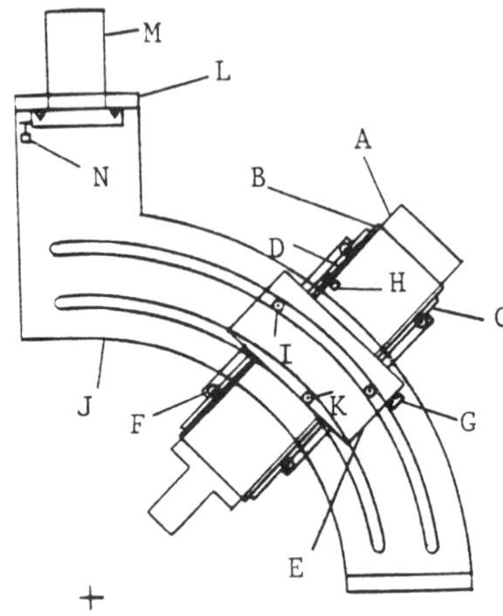

Figure 1 The gradiometer support mechanism

With the projectors and the center of the gradiometer system fixed, it is necessary to bring the subject's head into appropriate alignment. A wooden chair (see Fig. 2) is suspended in a frame such that it may be rotated from side to side up to 30 deg. off vertical in a fashion similar to a baby's cradle. The axis of rotation is co-linear with the x-axis of the gradiometer coordinate system and a fourth drive wheel-pot (A) is mounted to measure this rotation. The frame has four grooved wheels (B) which ride on two horizontal rails (C) allowing for back and forth positioning. On each side of the chair a lever arm pivots in such a way as to force the front of the chair upwards at the same time that a low-stretch cable (D), winding around a hand turned axle (E), is lifting the rear, thus raising or lowering the subject. A head support and

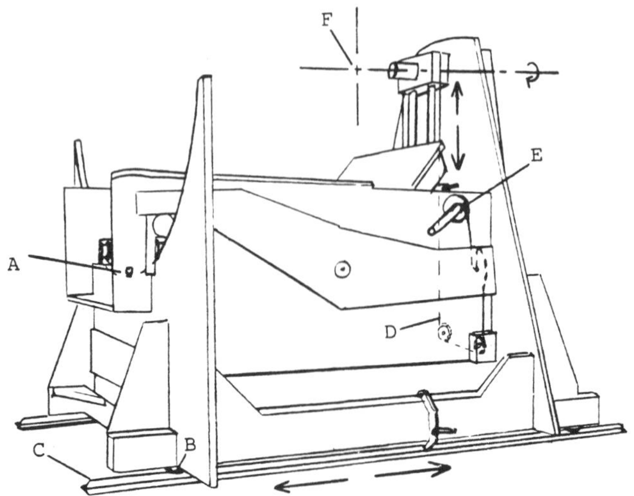

Figure 2 The subject chair

restrainer mechanism (not shown) rotates about the main chair shaft, and is fitted with a single removable arm located on the side opposite that being recorded from. This chair and head support system permits the center point of the head (F) to be located concentric with the origin of the gradiometer coordinate system, using the laser crosshairs for alignment.

RESULTS AND DISCUSSION

The apparatus is employed as follows: a subject is seated in the chair, a latex swim cap placed on the head and three lines inscribed (mid-sagittal nasion-inion line, mid-coronal vertex-tragus line, and horizontal nasion-inion line); the chair is then moved front to back and up or down until these lines (or lines referenced to these, if a different center, e.g. center of intracranial space based upon MR imaging, is desired) intersect the cross-hair projections; the chair is then rotated such that the declination range of the gradiometer is sufficient to cover the desired measurement region. The position information is read from the pots just prior to the start of data acquisition and the coordinates stored with the resulting waveform.

A three dimensional reconstruction of the brain using MRI scans is shown in Figure 3. The three orthoganal semi-circles surrounding the volume, represent the three inscribed lines (or arcs) described above, identified by taping rubber tubing filled with petroleum jelly to the subjects head just prior to the start of scanning. The intersection of the planes containing these arcs is the origin of the MEG coordinate system. Using the MRI information it is then possible to generate appropriate volume shapes, referenced to this system, to be used in solving the inverse problem, e.g., the method described by Hamalainen and Sarvas[2]. This is the modelling approach we expect to use in the near future.

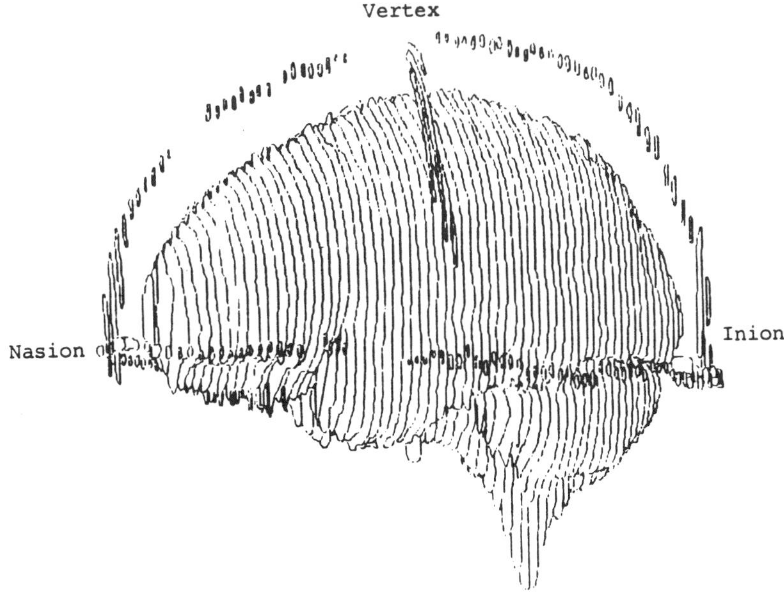

Figure 3

Our experience to date suggests that each coordinate can be known with an accuracy of approximately 1%, depending on how carefully the initial setup is done. The primary limitations being, the accuracy with which the reference lines are drawn, and the possible movement of the subject's head after alignment. The BTI Probe Position Indicator[3] is perhaps a more elegant method of associating spatial coordinates with field measurements, but it would appear to suffer from these same limitations at a considerably higher cost. This mechanism greatly enhances repeatability and should, in the future, significantly reduce the error bounds of localization estimates.

ACKNOWLEDGEMENT

This research was supported by USPHS Grants No. RR03259, MH41396, and MH46335.

RERERENCES

1 Gammex Model 30C002 fiber optic generator, model 30A115 fiber optic cables, and model 34A122 (MRI) output head. Gammex, Inc. Milwaukee Regional Medical Center, 9722 W. Watertown Plank Rd., Milwaukee, Wisconsin 53226.

2 Hamalainen, M.S. and Sarvas, J., (1987). Feasibility of the homogeneous head model in the interpretation of neuromagnetic fields. Physics in Medicine and Biology. 32, 91-97.

3 BTI model PPI Biomagnetic Technologies, Inc 4174 Sorrento Valley Blvd., San Diego, Calif. 92121.

THE POSITIONING OF MAGNETOMETER PICKUP COIL IN DEWAR BY ARTIFICIAL SIGNAL SOURCE

M.Higuchi, K.Chinone**, N.Ishikawa***,H.Kado*, N.Kasai*, M.Nakanishi*, M.Koyanagi* and Y.Ishibashi

Tsukuba University, 1 Ten-nohdai, Tsukuba 305 Japan
*Electrotechnical Laboratory, 1-1-4 Umezono,Tsukuba 305 Japan
Seiko Instruments Inc., * SHIMIZU Corp.

INTRODUCTION

It is necessary to determine precisely the position of a SQUID sensor for estimating the location of biomagnetic source. Usually in biomagnetic measurement, the sensor is moved near the points which are plotted on the subject. This operation is usually carried out by eye. For more precise positioning, the following two methods have been used. One is the method that the positions of the both the subject and the dewar in which SQUID is installed are determined by reading scales patched on a gantry and a bed. The other is that the relative position of the dewar to the subject is determined by using receivers on the subject and a transmitter mounted on the dewar[1]. In these methods, the position of the dewar is measured and the position of the sensor is estimated from the structure of the dewar and the SQUID holder. However the SQUID sensor position in liquid helium cannot be determined precisely because the strains of the dewar and the SQUID holder caused at low temperature are unknown. It is required that the relative position of the subject to the SQUID sensor is determined directly.

We propose a method to determine directly the position of the SQUID magnetometer pickup coil in liquid helium. In this method, the unknown SQUID position is estimated from known magnetic fields by using a least squeare method. The position is presented using a coodinate system defined by the artificial signal sources.

It is required to determine the relative position of the subject to the SQUID sensor precisely. We can know the relative position as follows. Another artificial signal source is located on the fixed point of the subject (for example nasion, inion, ear lobe). The SQUID sensor detects the magnetic field at several points. The relative position of the signal source to the SQUID sensor is estimated by the same method above mentioned. Erne et al. proposed a similar positioning method[2]. But the coodinate system is defined by an array of the SQUID sesors.

In this paper, we describe the analytical method to determine the position of the SQUID sensor by using artificial signal sources and the experiment.

ANALYTICAL METHOD

Magnetic field generated by the signal coil at the position of the pickup coil $\mathbf{r}_s$ is described as following;

$$\mathbf{B}(a,j,\mathbf{r}_c,\mathbf{n}_c,\mathbf{r}_s)$$

where a, j, $\mathbf{r}_c$ and $\mathbf{n}_c$ are a radius of the signal coil , current intensity fed to the coil, the position of the coil, normal vector of the coil as shown in Fig.1. The output of SQUID V_s is proportional to inner product between magnetic field and normal vector of the pickup coil $\mathbf{n}_s$,

$$V_s = G\mathbf{B} \bullet \mathbf{n}_s$$

where G is a transfer rate of SQUID system.

The following evaluation function L is adopted, to carry out the least square estimation of the unknown parameters $\mathbf{r}_s$ and $\mathbf{n}_s$.

Fig.1. Magnetic field generated by a one-turn coil.

$$L(\mathbf{r}_s,\mathbf{n}_s) = \Sigma(V_m - V_s)^2$$
$$= \Sigma(V_m - G\mathbf{B}(\mathbf{r}_c,\mathbf{n}_c,\mathbf{r}_s) \bullet \mathbf{n}_s)^2$$

where V_m is the value of SQUID output obtained experimentally and summation is over every magnetical field from all artifical source coils. The position $\mathbf{r}_s$ and direction $\mathbf{n}_s$ of a pickup coil are estimated so that the function can be made to minimize by using the Hooke-Jeeves method[3].

EXPERIMENT

Apparatus

Fig. 2 shows our experimental system. The vector magnetometer has been developed at Electrotechnical Laboratory[4]. It consists of 3 integrated SQUID magnetometers of which pickup coils are located perpendicularly to each other to detect 3 orthogonal components of the magnetic field. As an artificial signal source,we have used a coil of which radius is 2.0cm. To define the coordinate system, 4 sets of 3 orthogonal and unipositional signal coils were located at each corner of 50.0cm x 55.0cm square on a plate as shown in Fig. 3. So total number of coils as signal sources is 12. The plate could be moved to x-direction and y-direction, but the position of the vector magnetometer was fixed. Using the measured value of the magnetic fields generated by 12 signal coils, the position and direction of the pickup coil were estimated by the procedure mentioned above.

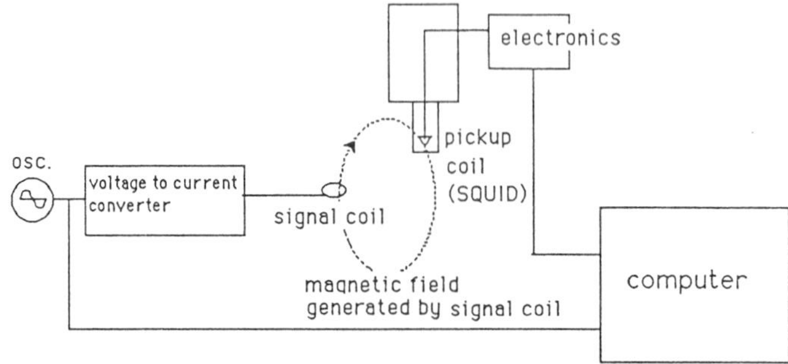

Fig.2. Block diagram of the positioning system with using artificial signal coil. The magnetic field was generated by a known current fed the signal coil. The field was measured by the SQUID magnetometer. Both the output of the SQUID and the reference signal of the current are collected to the computer system.

Results

We could estimate the SQUID position in our experimental system. There is a pickup coil in liquid helium, therefore the true values of the position and direction of the pickup coil could not be known. The position and direction of the pickup coil which is estimated from our experimental system could not be compared with the true values. We calculated the change of the SQUID position when the dewar was moved in the x-direction by 5.0cm. The result is indicated in Table 1. The mechanical accuracy of the moving system was smaller than 0.1cm. The results agreed with the moving distance within 0.1cm.

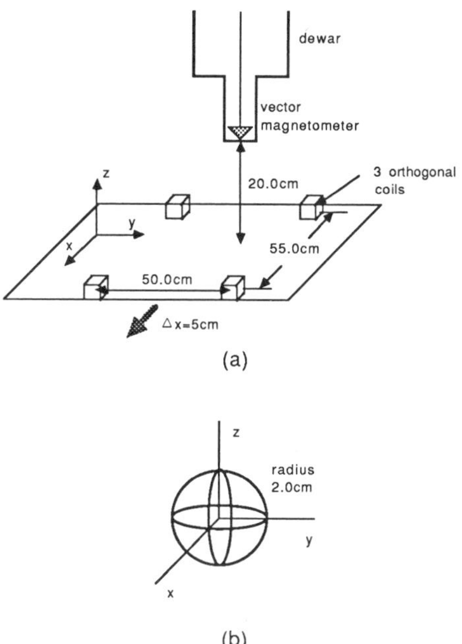

Fig.3. (a) Arrangement of the dewar and the signal coils. The SQUID magnetometer is located at the bottom of the dewar.
(b) 3 orthogonal and unipositional coils. 4 sets of these coils are placed on a plate to define the coordinate system.

Discussion

We suppose 3 main causes for the error of the estimated SQUID position. They are <u>(1) the error of the positions of the signal coils</u>, <u>(2)the error of the direction of the signal coils</u> and <u>(3)the error due to the noise in the detection</u>. We simulated the effects of the 3 causes on the estimated values.

At first, we examined the effect of the positional error of the signal coil to the estimated SQUID position. The SQUID position was estimated adding the error which obeys a Gaussian distribution to the position of the signal coil. The simulation was carried out 50 times. The mean and standard deviations of the estimated values are shown in Table 2. For example, when the standard deviation of the error of the signal coil position is 0.5cm, x-coordinate value of the estimated SQUID position scatters with a standard deviation 0.34cm (see the row which "d" is 0.5 in Table 2).

Table 1. The differences of the estimated values when the position of the SQUID changes 5.0cm in the x-direction .
The "Δx","Δy" and "Δz" columns give the difference of the position. The "Δθ" column indicates the difference of the direction of the pickup coil.

Δx(cm)	Δy(cm)	Δz(cm)	Δθ (degree)
5.10	-0.02	0.01	0.25

At second, we examined the effect of the dirctional error of the signal coil. In the same manner as above method, the SQUID position was estimated adding the directional error to the direction of the siganl coil. For example, when the standard deviation of the directional error is 2.0 degree, x-coordinate value of the estimated SQUID position scatters with a standard deviation 0.18cm (see the row which "a" is 2.0 in Table 3).

At third, we examined the effect of the effect of the system noise. The SQUID position was estimated adding pseudorandam numbers to the data produced by the siganl coils. In this table.it is defined that N is a ratio of the system noise to the maximum siganl of all siganls produced by the 12 signal coils. For example, when N is 0.05, x-coordinate of the estimated SQUID position scatters with standard deviation 0.42cm (see the row which "N" is 0.05 in Table 4).

To obtain the 0.1 cm accuracy of the estimated position in our experimental system, it requires that accuracy of the signal coil position is better than 0.1cm, accuracy of the direction of the signal coil is better than 1.0 degree and signal to noise ratio is better than 100.

d	x(cm)	y(cm)	z(cm)	Δθ (degree)
0.1	25.02 (0.07)	25.01 (0.07)	29.99 (0.07)	0.18 (0.08)
0.2	25.03 (0.13)	25.02 (0.15)	29.99 (0.14)	0.37 (0.15)
0.5	25.07 (0.34)	25.03 (0.36)	29.96 (0.33)	0.92 (0.40)
1.0	25.12 (0.68)	25.07 (0.72)	29.93 (0.65)	1.83 (0.81)

Table 2. Results of the simulation with the position error of the signal coil. The "d" column gives the standard deviation of the position error which obeys a Gaussian distribution with zero mean. The "x", "y"and "z" columns indicated the average of 50 simulations. The true values of them are x=25,y=25,z=30. The values in parentheses are standard deviation.

Table 3. Results of the simulation with the direction error of signal coil. The "a" column gives the standard deviation of the directional error.

a	x(cm)	y(cm)	z(cm)	Δθ (degree)
0.5	25.01 (0.05)	24.98 (0.04)	29.98 (0.07)	0.20 (0.10)
1.0	25.01 (0.09)	24.97 (0.09)	29.95 (0.14)	0.40 (0.18)
2.0	25.03 (0.18)	24.95 (0.17)	29.89 (0.28)	0.79 (0.35)
5.0	25.06 (0.47)	24.86 (0.43)	29.75 (0.69)	1.98 (0.88)

Table 4 Results of the simulation with noise. The "N" column gives the standard deviation of the Gaussian noise as a ratio to the maximum siganl of all signals produced by the 12 signal coils.

N	x(cm)	y(cm)	z(cm)	Δθ (degree)
0.01	25.01 (0.09)	25.02 (0.09)	29.98 (0.11)	0.29 (0.19)
0.02	25.01 (0.17)	25.05 (0.17)	29.97 (0.21)	0.59 (0.35)
0.05	25.02 (0.42)	25.11 (0.42)	29.90 (0.54)	1.47 (0.86)
0.10	25.01 (0.83)	25.21 (0.85)	29.82 (1.07)	2.94 (1.73)

CONCLUSION

We proposed a method to determine the position of the SQUID magnetometer pickup coil in dewar using artificial signal source. We could estimate the position of the SQUID in our experimental system. We estimated the accuracy of this method by simulation.

REFERENCE

1. T.Yamamoto, S.J.Williamson, L.Kaufman, C.Nicholson, and R.Llinas; "Magnetic Localization of neuronal Activity in The Human Brain", Proc. Natl. Acad. Sci. USA, Vol.85, 8732(1988)
2. S.N. Erne, L. Narici, V.Pizzella and G.L. Romani; "The Positioning Problem in Biomagnetic Measurements: A Solution for Arrays of Superconducting Sensors", IEEE Trans. Mag. **MAG-23**, No.2, 1319(1987)
3. R.Hooke and T.A.Jeeves, "Direct Search Solution of Numerical and Statistical Problems", J. Assoc. Comput. Mach., 8, 212(1961)
4. M.Nakanishi, N.Kasai, H.Kado and M.Koyanagi;"DC-SQUID Magnetometer system for Detecting Vector Value of Magnetic Field", IEEE Trans. Mag. **MAG-25**, No.2, 1162(1989)

NEUROMAGNETOMETER® CALIBRATION USING AN ARRAY OF SMALL COILS

D.S. Buchanan and D.N. Paulson

Biomagnetic Technologies Inc.
San Diego, CA 92121

INTRODUCTION

We have developed a technique for the *in-situ* calibration of multi-channel Neuromagnetometers using a small single turn excitation coil placed in a number of locations in close proximity to the sensors of the Neuromagnetometer. Previous methods of calibration have included the use of large coil arrangements to generate a known field pattern (Ribeiro et al. 1988), the use of a dipole at large distance or the use of a single small coil placed outside the dewar tail. Each of these methods suffers from various drawbacks, both practical and fundamental. The use of large coils requires both having sufficient space for the coils (the coils are 1-2 m on a side) and the removal of the neuromagnetometer from its normal location, such as in a magnetically shielded room, to place it in the coils in order to re-calibrate. Using large coils does not allow easy re-calibration of the instruments and it requires precise knowledge of the field balance of the sensors. Using a distant dipole requires having large magnetically clean space (2-3 m in size) for the measurements and in our experience also is not repeatable at the 10% level, probably due to the distortion of the dipole field by the building etc. The single small coil placed outside the dewar worked well if the dewar spacing is very accurately known. This usually requires the ability to x-ray the dewar to determine the spacing. By using an array of accurately constructed and accurately placed coils we have determined the position, orientation and gain of the sensors in the frame of the calibration coil array assuming only knowledge of the internal geometry of the sensors (i.e. how they are machined and wound). The effect of thermal shrinkage of the coil forms is less than 0.5% and should have less than a 1% effect on the absolute sensitivities and minimal effect on the relative sensitivities.

ARRAY

A 1.0 cm diameter single turn coil is consecutively placed in a plane approximately 4 cm below the sensor array at 16 locations on a 4 cm by 4 cm grid. The exact position and orientation of the excitation coil array relative to the sensors is not critical because they are free parameters in the fitting routine. A sampling distribution in a plane perpendicular to the axis of the sensor as opposed to one along the axis of the sensors is used because of the higher spatial frequency of the

Advances in Biomagnetism
Edited by S.J. Williamson *et al.*
Plenum Press, New York

coupling function when moving perpendicular to the sensor axis. The excitation coil crosses at least two zero crossings in this coupling function for each sensor. This increases the sensitivity of the fitting routines to the positions of the sensors.

The diameter of the excitation coil is known to 0.005 cm and its location in both x, y, and z in the calibration array frame to 0.005 cm. The excitation coils is driven with a 20 or 200 micro-amp 100 Hz current (the current is changed according to the coupling between the excitation coil and the sensors to prevent overloading of the amplifiers). The output of the sensors and their associated amplifiers along with the current is measured and integrated over a 5 second period for each of the 16 positions resulting in 16 data points for each sensor. The data is acquired in parallel for the sensors and serially for each of the 16 excitation coil positions. The gain, position and orientation of each sensor is then determined from the data. Each sensor is fit independently.

Each sensor can be characterized by six free parameters: gain, three translation coordinates and two angles. A non-linear least-squares fit is made to the data for each sensor to determine these parameters. The coupling between the excitation coil and the sensor is calculated by summing the mutual inductances between the excitation coil and each turn of the sensor. The mutual inductance is calculated using formulae from Grover (1946).

RESULTS

Determination of the absolute accuracy of the measurement of the gains is difficult but it is also not as important as the relative accuracy of the gains between sensors. It is the relative gain accuracy which determines the accuracy of localization of a source. The absolute gain enters only as a scaling factor. We have checked the accuracy of the gain measurements in three ways. First, we have repeated the measurement several times in succession on a number of systems without moving the array in-between measurements. This was done to look at the scatter in the measurements due to signal to noise. The result for three sets of these type of measurements is shown in Fig. 1. Second, we have repeated the measurements on two systems while lowering the excitation array away from the sensor array. This was done to reveal any systematics such as inaccuracies in the placement of the excitation coil. If the coil was not being accurately placed there would have been a systematic dependence of the results on the distance from the sensor array. The results for this are shown in Fig. 2. Third we have compared the gain results to those obtained from calibrations made on two first order systems using a set of Helmholtz coils which apply a known gradient to the coils. The first system consisted of seven 2 cm diameter 8 cm baseline coils. The difference between the Helmholtz and array averaged over the seven channels was 2.7% while error from channel to channel after normalizing to the average to remove systematic errors was between -1.3% to 0.6%. The second system was a set of four asymmetric 3 cm baseline first order gradiometer with 16 turns in the 3 mm diameter primary coil and a single turn compensation coil. The difference between the sensitivities measured with the Helmholtz coils and those measured with the array averaged over the four channels was 3.5% while error from channel to channel after normalizing to the average to remove systematic errors was between -1.5% to 1.5%.

The quality of the fit can be expressed as the maximum error between calculated and measured data which is typically less than 0.5% when scaled to the largest measured data point. This statistic is used because it has been found to be a very sensitive indicator of bad data points. If this statistic is much greater than 1.5% it usually indicates that a noise burst or other similar problem has occurred.

In addition to gain, the calibration procedure measures the position and orientation of the sensors. The angle between sensor coils, theta, was measured using X-rays for two seven channel systems and then compared to the results of the calibration. Agreement was better than ±1 degree. An independent measurement of the other orientation angle, phi. the rotation of the coil about the z axis, was not done. Similar comparisons for translational parameters shown an accuracy of ±0.5 mm.

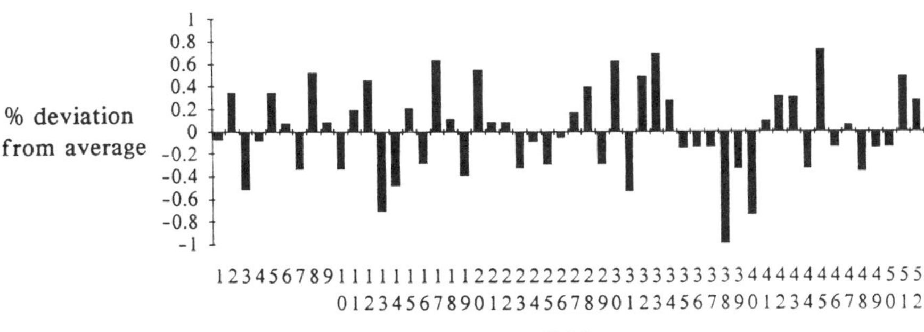

Fig. 1. Repeatability of gains of one five channel and two seven channel magnetometers. Shown is the percent deviation from the average of individual measurements on each channel. There are two sets of measurements on the five channel systems for a total of 52 sensors which have been measured. The array apparatus is not removed between measurements so that this indicates the signal to noise of the measurement.

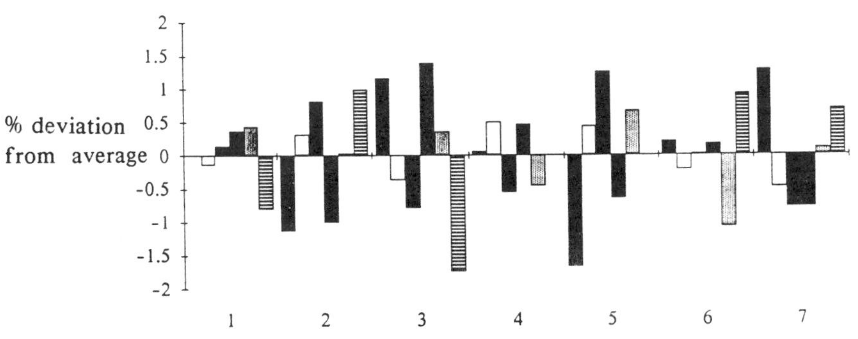

Fig. 2. Relative gains of two seven channel magnetometers from repeated measurements with the calibration array placed at different locations approximately 2, 4 and 6 cm below the Dewar tail. The gains of each probe are normalized to the average for a given probe in order to remove absolute gain offsets that occur from run to run. The absolute gain changes are of order 0.5%. Plotted is the percent difference between each measurement and the average for a given channel. Measurements were done at each of three different distances from each of two different seven channel probes.

This calibration procedure has several other advantages. First it can be done in a relatively short period of time. The collection of the data from setup to finish can be done in less than 1/2 hour. The data analysis for a seven channel second-order gradiometer system takes about 30 minutes for a HP350 computer system. This time can easily be reduced to 5 minutes if the coils are approximated by a 1-2-1 coil configuration instead of the 3-6-3 configuration used, the number of computations going approximately as the number of loops squared. The approximation does not seriously alter the results but the computation time has yet to be a problem in the field. The second advantage of this technique is that the system is calibrated on the gain settings that will be used to take neuromagnetic measurements thereby eliminating any gain variations present in the amplifiers.

CONCLUSION

We have developed a relatively fast, easy to use and accurate method for the in-situ calibration of multi-channel Neuromagnetometers. The system provides gain and position calibration as well and is easily adaptable to all manner of array configurations differing in arrangement, size and type of gradiometer. The technique measures relative gain to ±1.5% which is sufficient for most currently used source localization procedures, i.e. equivalent dipole localization (Buchanan 1989). It also measures sensor location to ±0.5 mm and sensor orientation, theta, to ±1 degree.

ACKNOWLEDGEMENTS

This work was supported in part by NINCDS Grant # 2R44 NS 24098 under the SBIR program. We would like to thank Sam Williamson and Risto Ilmoniemi for all their helpful input and discussions.

REFERENCES

Ribeiro, P.C., Williamson, S.J., and Kaufman L. (1988). SQUID Arrays for Simultaneous Magnetic Measurements: Calibration and Source Localization Performance. IEEE Trans. Biomed. Eng. 35n7:551.

Grover, F.W. (1946) in: "Inductance Calculations: Working Formulas and Tables" Dover Publications, Inc., New York, pp193-208.

Buchanan, D.S. (1989), Impact of Different Noise Sources on Dipole Localization In The Spherical Model: A Simulation, This proceedings.

SPATIAL FOURIER TECHNIQUE FOR CALIBRATING GRADIOMETERS

A.C. Bruno, C.S. Dolce, S.D. Soares and P. Costa Ribeiro

Departamento de Fisica, Pontificia Universidade Catolica
Caixa Postal 38071, Rio de Janeiro, 22453, RJ, Brasil

INTRODUCTION

One of the main features of the biomagnetic technique is the possibility to identify and locate sources of bioelectric activity with an uncertainty of a few millimeters. The use of multichannel systems not only eases this procedure shortening the time of the measurement session but also enables simultaneous measurement at different points in space, making possible the observation of non periodic phenomena. However, a multichannel system can introduce an important source of error in the localization result, if the calibration factor (field/voltage) of each channel is not measured with an extreme accuracy (Costa Ribeiro et al, 1988). The prospect of using planar gradiometers in biomagnetism imposes further difficulties to adapt the calibration procedures normaly used for axial gradiometers. In this work we propose a very general calibration method valid for all kinds of gradiometers and arrays. It is based on a spatial Fourier technique and in the fact that the gradiometer performs discrete spatial filtering.

THE GRADIOMETER AS A DISCRETE DEVICE

The gradiometer samples in space the magnetic field generated by both signal and noise sources at the discrete locations corresponding to the position of each coil. The sampled field is weighted by the value of the respective coil area and the output is the addition and subtraction of the weighted fields. Being a discrete device, the gradiometer has its spatial transfer function analogous to its time domain correspondent, the *moving average* filter. The transfer function $H(k)$ can be expressed as in the following equation:

$$H(k) = \sum_{i=1}^{N+1} A_i e^{-jki\lambda_s}, \tag{1}$$

where, N is the gradiometer order, A_i are the areas of the coils, k is the spatial frequency and λ the sampling period or baseline.

Advances in Biomagnetism
Edited by S.J. Williamson *et al.*
Plenum Press, New York

TRANSFER FUNCTION AND CALIBRATION

An experimental procedure has been designed to measure the spatial transfer function and this has been applied to different axial gradiometers (Bruno et al, 1988). It consists in moving a calibration coil along the gradiometer axis, calculating the theoretical input and recording the measured output values for the successive coil positions. The gradiometer input is defined as the theoretical flux that is induced in the first gradiometer coil (*pick-up coil*) and the output is the measured voltage values. Prior to taking the Fourier transforms of both series, the output voltages were converted into flux by using a conventional calibration procedure. The transfer function is the result of the division of the output by the input transforms. However, we have realized that this procedure could be used to determine the calibration factor itself, since the output is a voltage readout v_{out} and the input is the theoretical flux ϕ_{in} calculated in Weber.

From these previous experiments, it has been found that the unbalance effect alters the low frequency portion of the transfer function spectrum. Data quantitating this effect can be found elsewhere (Bruno et al, 1988). Also, it has been found that inaccuracies due to positioning the calibration coil modify the high frequency part of the transfer function spectrum. Thus, the calibration factor should be withdrawn, from the comparison between the experimental and theoretical transfer functions avoiding these two frequency extremes.

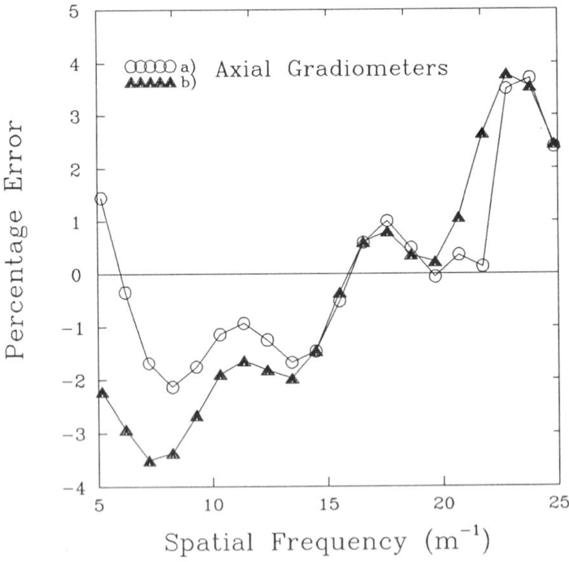

Fig. 1 Percentage error between theoretical and experimental transfer functions against the spatial frequency. Curves *a)* and *b)* correspond to axial 2nd order gradiometers with 1.5 cm diameter coils and 5 cm baselines.

Experimental transfer functions were evaluated in the frequency range between 0 and 30 m^{-1} (Knuutila et al, 1987). Curves *a)* and *b)* in Fig. 1 show the percentage difference between theoretical and experimental transfer functions for two axial 2nd order SQUID gradiometers in two different experiments. Gradiometer *a)* has a 5 cm baseline and 1.5 cm diameter coils. Gradiometer *b)* has a 5 cm baseline and 1.5 cm diameter coils. The calibration coil has a 32 cm diameter and was slipped axially over the dewar in steps of about 2 cm to an approximately equal distance of 10 baselines above and below the gradiometer. About 50 points were measured in both experiments and a spline routine was used before the Fourier process. Fitting the experimental transfer function by the theoretical one in the entire range i.e. 0.5 - 30 m^{-1} gives calibration factors of $2.158 \cdot 10^{-8}$ *Tesla/Volt (T/V)* with a standard deviation of about 22% for *a*) and $2.249 \cdot 10^{-8}$ T/V with a standard deviation of about 7% for *b*). The difference between the standard deviations of *a*) and *b*) is because only gradiometer *b*) is balanced. Fitting in the 5 - 25 m^{-1} range gives calibration factors of $2.295 \cdot 10^{-8}$ T/V with a standard deviation of 1.6% for *a*) and $2.301 \cdot 10^{-8}$ T/V with a standard deviation of 2.2%. Fitting in the 10 - 20 m^{-1} range gives calibration factors of $2.309 \cdot 10^{-8}$ T/V with a standard deviation of 0.9% for *a*) and $2.308 \cdot 10^{-8}$ T/V with a standard deviation of 1.1% for *b*).

The errors for different frequencies oscillate around zero having an average of about 10^{-5}%. Although the worst error of the two experiments reaches 3.7% the parameter that we should be concerned about is the average error. Notice that the calibration factor found in the 5 - 25 m^{-1} range differs from the one found in the 10 - 20 m^{-1} range about 0.5%. Even if the 0.5 - 30 m^{-1} range is used, the calibration factor differs from the ones in the middle frequency range about 5%. Standard deviations of few percents attest the reliability of the method.

Moreover, we have also realized that this procedure could be extremely useful for calibrating planar gradiometers, since this method does not depend on the gradiometer geometry. In this case it will be possible to have them calibrated in field units instead of the usual gradient units which do not seem to be adequate for clinical use.

For this purpose, a wound-wire first order planar gradiometer was built with a 2 cm baseline and 1 cm diameter coils. Fig. 2 displays the theoretical (dashed-line) and experimental (continuous-line) transfer functions. This transfer function was obtained by displacing the planar gradiometer along a line over a calibration coil of 80 cm diameter at a distance of 15 cm from its plane. It was taken about 100 measurements with a 1 cm interval. The calibration coil was excited by a sinusoidal current. The gradiometer was wound with copper wire and its output was detected with a PAR 124-A lock-in amplifier.

Then, Fourier transforms of the input and output sequences were computed and the division of the output by the input transforms was performed. The calibration factor could be chosen by fitting the experimental transfer function by the theoretical one, on an interval between 5 and 25 m^{-1}. The theoretical transfer function was obtained by using Eq. (1) and the gradiometer parameters. It was checked that for frequencies in this range, the error oscillates around zero with a maximum amplitude of 2% . The average error was 0.5% and the standard deviation was 1%. Similar results can be obtained for an interval between 10 and 20 m^{-1}.

For planar gradiometer calibration or for array of axial gradiometers, where the gradiometers lie off the calibration coil axis, the theoretical input should be calculated by using the following expression :

$$B_z(x,y,z) = \frac{\mu_0}{4\pi} I \int_0^{2\pi} \frac{a\,(a - y\sin\theta - x\cos\theta)}{\left[x^2 + y^2 + z^2 + a^2 - 2a\,(x\,cos\theta + y\,sin\theta)\right]^{\frac{3}{2}}}\,d\theta$$

where I is the calibration coil current and a is the calibration coil radius.

It is worth noting that for both planar and axial gradiometers we can have as much as 70% of the points in the experimental transfer functions coincident with

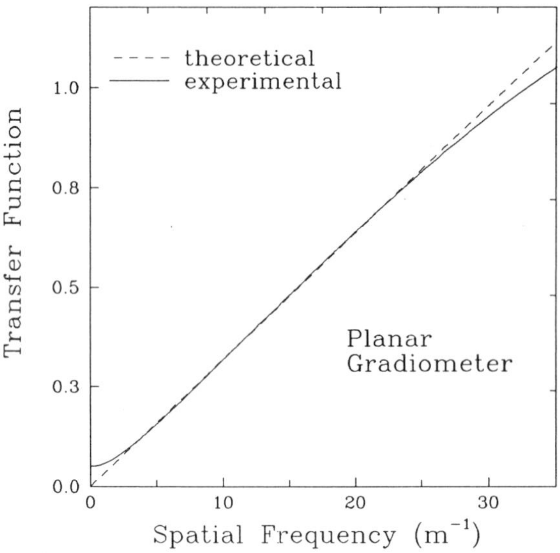

Fig. 2 Theoretical (dashed-line) and experimental (continuous-line) transfer functions of a planar first order gradiometer with 2 *cm* baseline and 1 *cm* diameter coils

the theoretical ones but for a small error. An advantage of this technique, besides its simplicity, is that in the frequency domain it is possible to graphically visualize, in the low frequency range, the unbalance effect, which is the main source of errors when using large calibration coils. Also, imprecisions in positioning the calibration coil, which is the major source of errors when using small calibration coils, appears only in the high frequency range. Due to this fact the fitting should be done in the middle frequency range. The choice of middle frequency range is a tradeoff between the standard deviation and the reliability of the result. Finally it should be emphasized that when using a conventional method for calibrating gradiometer arrays with a large number of detecting sensors, the amount of work is the same as in the procedure above, since the calibration coil has to be displaced near each gradiometer.

ACKNOWLEDGEMENTS

We gratefully acknowledge P.J.E. Hübscher for his help in computing work. This work has been partialy supported by FINEP, IBM of Brazil and CAPES.

REFERENCES

Bruno, A.C., Paulsen, C.C., Symko, O., and Costa Ribeiro, P., 1988, Measurements of gradiometers' spatial Transfer Function, in : "Biomagnetism'87," K. Atsumi, M. Kotani, S. Ueno, T. Katila and S.J. Williamson, eds., Tokyo Denki University Press, Tokyo.

Costa Ribeiro, P., Williamson, S.J., and Kaufman, L., 1988, SQUID arrays for simultaneous magnetic measurements: Calibration and source localizations performance, IEEE Trans. Biomed. Eng., 35 : 551.

Knuutila, J., Ahlfors, S., Ahonen, A., Hallstron, J., Kajola, M., Lounasmaa, O.V., Vilkman, V., and Tesche, C., 1987, A Large-Area Low Noise Seven-Channel DC SQUID Magnetometer for Brain Research, Rev. Sci. Instrum., 58 : 2145.

ON THE SPATIAL LOCATING ACCURACY

OF MULTICHANNEL MAGNETOMETERS

Jukka Knuutila and Matti S. Hämäläinen

Low Temperature Laboratory
Helsinki University of Technology
02150 Espoo, Finland

INTRODUCTION

Several projects are currently aiming at neuromagnetic devices with more than 20 SQUIDs. In addition to the sensor array design, the possible advantages of replacing the commonly used axial gradiometers by off-diagonal gradiometers have been discussed (Knuutila et al., 1985; Erné and Romani, 1985; Carelli and Leoni, 1986; Hari and Ilmoniemi, 1986; Bruno et al., 1989). The purpose of this study is to investigate how the spatial locating accuracy of a current dipole in the brain is affected by the pickup coil type, the shape of the dewar tail, the sensor distance from the head, and by the distribution and number of gradiometers.

METHODS

To compare the ability of different gradiometer configurations in locating cortical sources, we have calculated the 95-% confidence limits of an equivalent current dipole (Sarvas, 1987). A radius of curvature of 110 mm was assumed for the spherically symmetric head, and the confidence limits were calculated as a function of the position of a 10-nAm tangential dipole. A noise of 10 fT/$\sqrt{\text{Hz}}$, realizable with state-of-the-art dc SQUIDs, was used for the field differences measured by all the gradiometers. The true locating accuracies can be found by scaling the data with the actual noise levels. All results correspond to a bandwidth of 100 Hz and to 100 averages. The dewar was assumed to be at a fixed position.

We compared the 24-channel planar gradiometer (24M) built in our laboratory (Kajola et al., 1989; Hämäläinen et al., 1989) with several axial gradiometer arrays. The 24M measures the tangential derivatives $\partial B_z/\partial x$ and $\partial B_z/\partial y$ of the radial magnetic field component B_z at 12 points separated by 30 mm, on a spherical cap. The radius of curvature and the diameter of the cap are both 125 mm (Fig. 1a); the insulating gap at the dewar bottom is 15 mm and the pickup coil area is 3.7 cm^2. One of the axial configurations studied is a 25-channel device (25M) on a similar dewar bottom surface and with roughly the same total area as the 24M (Fig. 1b); the channel separations are 21 mm (along the circles) and 28 mm (between inner and outer circles). In addition, we calculated the confidence limits for a 31-channel gradiometer (31M, Fig. 1c) on a 200-mm-diameter flat dewar bottom with an insulating gap of 25 mm. Such an instrument has been announced to become commercially available (Siemens Corp.; Gudden et al., 1989). For the 31M, dewar tails with flat and curved bottoms and with insulating gaps of 25 and 15 mm were also studied. Finally, the 33-channel configuration of Fig. 1d (33M) was investigated to see the effect of elongated geometry; the insulating gap and the radius of curvature are similar to that of 24M and 25M. The channel separations for 31M and 33M are 30 mm for both; the pickup coil areas of 25M and 33M are 3.1 cm^2 and that of 31M is 7.1 cm^2. The base lengths for the off-diagonal and axial gradiometers are 13 and 60 mm, respectively.

Advances in Biomagnetism
Edited by S.J. Williamson *et al.*
Plenum Press, New York

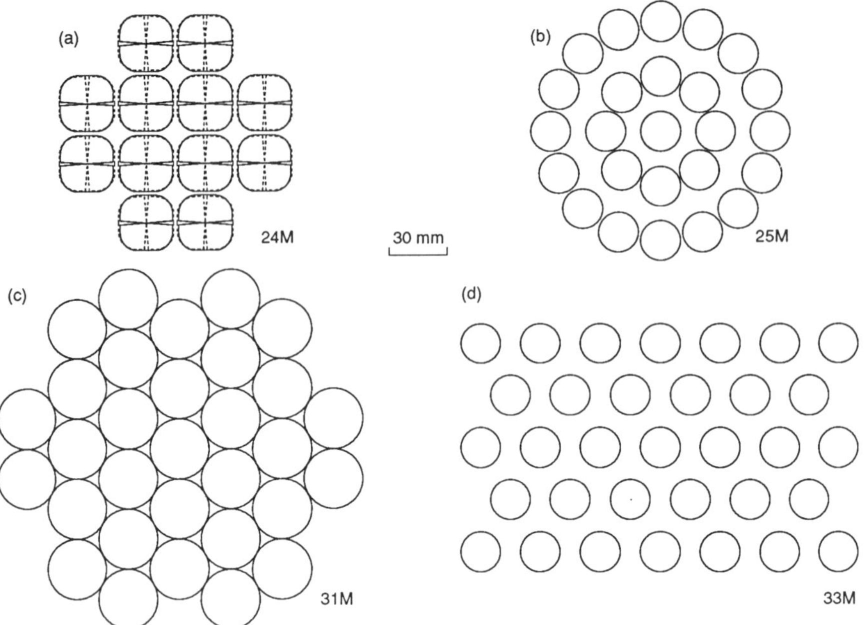

Fig. 1. The coil configurations studied in this work. Azimuthal equidistant projection is used for the arrays located on a spherical surface in (a), (b) and (d); (a) utilizes planar and (b)–(d) axial gradiometers. For more details, see text.

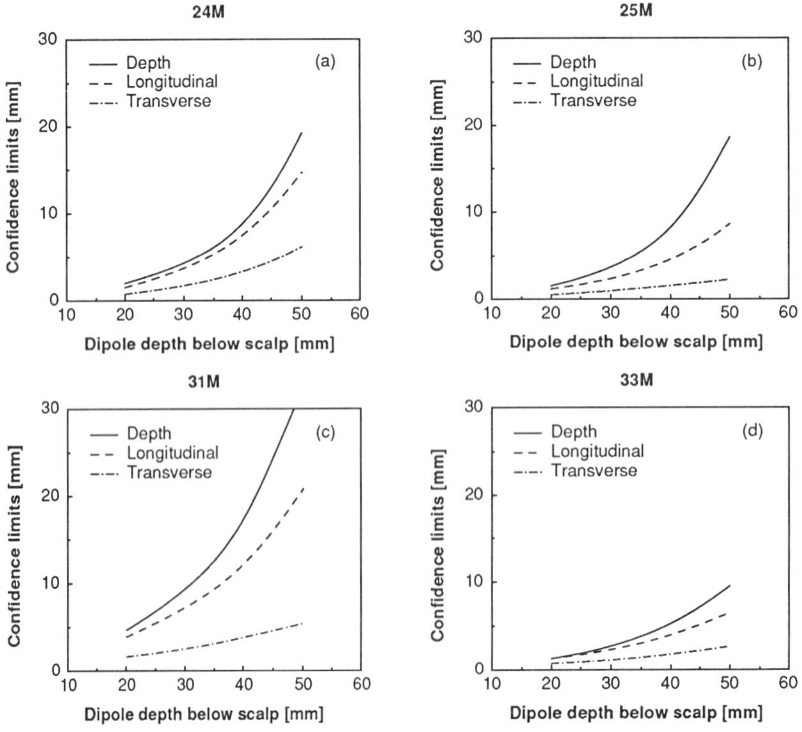

Fig. 2. Confidence limits as a function of dipole depth. The source is located at an angle 5° off the symmetry axis. Equal noise, 10 fT/√Hz, was assumed in all cases.

RESULTS

The spatial locating accuracy did not depend significantly on the location or the orientation of the source in the tangential θ and φ directions as long as the dipole was kept under the gradiometers, except for the less symmetric 33M. Dipoles oriented along the longer side of the 33M array resulted in depth errors 20–30 % larger than for perpendicularly oriented dipoles; in the latter case the field extrema fit better under the active area. The two dipole orientations had about the same confidence limits in the longitudinal and in the transverse directions.

Figure 2 illustrates the locating accuracy as a function of dipole depth below the scalp. The relative performances of the configurations depend on the dipole position and on the direction in which the confidence limit is considered. The locating error of the axial 25M is about 20–40 % smaller than that of the planar 24M. The difference is largest in the tangential directions and for the deepest sources. The 31-channel configuration with 25-mm dewar gap and flat bottom was found to be worse than the 24M by a factor of 1.5–2. The elongated configuration of the 33M was better than the approximately circular 24M by a factor of 1.4–2.2.

The poor performance of the 31M is attributable to the flatness of the bottom and the large insulating gap. In Fig. 3 we show the effect of reducing the gap from 25 to 15 mm and placing the magnetometers on a spherical surface with a radius of curvature of 135 or 125 mm. With a flat 15-mm gap the 31M would show comparable performance to the 24M, whereas the confidence limits of the curved-bottom 31M, with 15-mm gap, are slightly better than for the 25M device. A reduction of the dewar gap from 25 to 15 mm improves the locating accuracy by a factor of 1.5–2. With a curved dewar bottom the improvement is 30–40 %.

Comparison of the 25M with the curved thin-bottom 31M and 33M configurations shows that the effect of additional channels on the locating accuracy of a single dipole is an enhanced depth resolution, especially for the deepest sources. This is due to the increased area of the magnetometers, which covers better the more widely spread field pattern of the deep dipoles. When comparing the 31M and 33M it is seen that an elongated sensor array gives 10–30 % better depth resolution if the dipole is oriented along the shorter side of the array.

DISCUSSION

A good spatial locating accuracy is obtained with our 24-channel device using only a single measurement site. With the reported noise levels of 3–5 fT/(cm·$\sqrt{\text{Hz}}$) (Kajola et al., 1989) the true confidence limits are only one-half of those given in Fig. 2a. The fact that an axial configuration with roughly the same area and number of channels is somewhat better than the

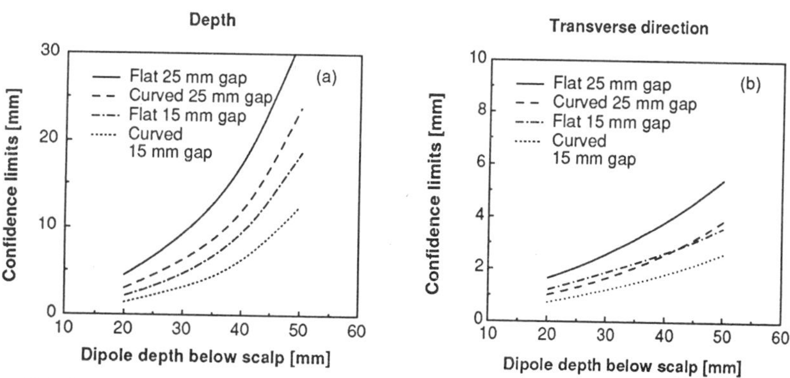

Fig. 3. The locating errors for depth (a) and transverse directions (b) for the 31M configuration (see Fig. 1) with different dewar bottoms. The other conditions are identical to those in Fig. 2.

24M is outweighed by the more compact size of the planar sensors; this was one of the main gradiometers would result in a substantially bulkier dewar.

The effect of a large distance from the sensors to the head, either because of a large gap at the dewar bottom or because of a flat bottom, is significant but not as prominent as that of the noise. Low-noise sensors are therefore the key to good accuracy. However, the instrumental noise, which may be as low as 5 fT/√Hz, is not the only contribution: the background activity of the subject's brain is significant as well (Knuutila and Hämäläinen, 1988). Therefore, the results presented here may not be valid as such in real measurements; especially, the sensitivities of planar and axial gradiometers to the background activity can be different.

Although these calculations suggest that the gain obtained by increasing the number of channels and the active area is relatively modest, a large area is convenient because exact positioning of the dewar above the source is not required. However, the price of large coverage is a very massive dewar. It must also be noted that the figure-of-merit used in this work is limited to a specific current-source model; its advantage is the close connection to present-day MEG practice. For comparison of multichannel magnetometers, a more universal measure of comparison, based on the information-theoretical channel capacity, has been proposed (Kemppainen and Ilmoniemi, 1989).

ACKNOWLEDGMENTS

This project was financially supported by the Finnish National Fund for Research and Development (SITRA). We acknowledge Riitta Hari for suggesting the 33M and thank Matti Kajola, Pia Kemppainen, and Olli V. Lounasmaa for their comments on the manuscript.

REFERENCES

Bruno, A.C., Pizzella, V., Torrioli, G., and Romani, G.L., 1989, Experimental localization ability of planar gradiometer systems for biomagnetic measurements, *IEEE Trans. Magn.,* MAG-25:1170.

Carelli, P. and Leoni, R., 1986, Localization of biological sources with arrays of superconducting gradiometers, *J. Appl. Phys.,* 59:645.

Erné, S.N. and Romani, G.L, 1985, Performances of higher order planar gradiometers for biomagnetic source localization, *in:* "SQUID'85, Superconducting Quantum Interference Devices and their Applications", H.D. Hahlbohm and H. Lübbig, eds., Walter de Gruyter, Berlin, p. 951.

Gudden, F., Hoenig, E., Reichenberger, H., Schittenhelm, R., Schneider, S., 1989, A multichannel system for use in biomagnetic diagnosis in neurology and cardiology: principle, method and initial results, *Electromedica,* 57:2.

Hari, R. and Ilmoniemi, R.J., 1986, Cerebral magnetic fields, *CRC Critical Reviews in Biomed. Eng.*, 14:93.

Hämäläinen, M.S., 1989, A 24-channel planar gradiometer: system design and analysis of neuromagnetic data, this volume.

Kajola, M., Ahlfors, S., Ehnholm, G.J., Hällström, J., Hämäläinen, M.S., Ilmoniemi, R.J., Kiviranta, M., Knuutila, J., Lounasmaa, O.V., Tesche, C.D., and Vilkman, V., 1989, A 24-channel magnetometer for brain research, this volume.

Kemppainen, P.K. and Ilmoniemi, R.J., 1989, Channel capacity of multichannel magnetometers, this volume.

Knuutila, J., Ahonen, A.I., Hämäläinen, M.S., Ilmoniemi, R.J., and Kajola, M.J., 1985, Design considerations for multichannel SQUID magnetometers, *in:* "SQUID'85, Superconducting Quantum Interference Devices and their Applications", H.D. Hahlbohm and H. Lübbig, eds., Walter de Gruyter, Berlin, p. 939.

Knuutila, J. and Hämäläinen, M.S., 1988, Characterization of brain noise using a high-sensitivity 7-channel magnetometer, *in:* "Biomagnetism '87", K. Atsumi, M. Kotani, S. Ueno, T. Katila, and S.J. Williamson, eds., Tokyo Denki University Press, Tokyo, p. 186.

Sarvas, J., 1987, Basic mathematical and electromagnetic concepts of the biomagnetic inverse problem, *Phys. Med. Biol.,* 32:11.

Siemens Ag, Bereich Medizinische Technik, D-8520 Erlangen, Federal Republic of Germany.

EXPERIMENTAL ACCURACY OF LOCALIZATION OF CURRENT DIPOLES IN A SPHERICAL PHANTOM

D. N. Paulson and D. S. Buchanan

Biomagnetic Technologies, Inc.
San Diego, CA 92121

INTRODUCTION

We have measured the accuracy of the BTi Neuromagnetometer® system in localizing current dipoles embedded in a spherical conductor. Several papers have been written on the accuracy of source localization possible in various phantom sources (Yamamoto et al.(1989) and Barth et al.(1986)). We have measured the performance possible with the existing BTi system and have measured some of the sources of error and the resulting inaccuracies in source localization.

METHODS

A hollow spherical plastic phantom (radius = 10 cm) was constructed with 5 separate tangential current dipoles located at nominal positions of 5 to 9 cm along the vertical radius of the sphere. The phantom was filled with 0.9% by weight saline solution. The dipoles had a nominal length of 4 mm.

The current dipoles were constructed by bending the ends of a tightly twisted pair of wires 90 degrees from the twisted pair and in opposite directions to each other thereby forming a "T". Five of these dipoles were then embedded into a 4 mm diameter cylindrical plastic rod so that only the ends of the wire were exposed. Electrodes were constructed of Pt(0.1 and 0.5 mm diameter), PtIr (0.13 mm diameter), sintered AgCl(2 mm diameter), and Cu both bare and Au plated (0.1 and 1.3 mm diameter). The impedance of these electrodes to the bath varied from 1 kΩ to 10 MegΩ and by factors of 2 to over 100 over the current range of .1 to 200 μA for a 5 Hz current sine pulse. These variations are illustrated in Figure 1. With time, the copper, copper-Au, and the sintered AgCl appeared to react with the saline solution yielding a higher impedance. The larger diameter Pt seemed to be most stable with time and gave impedances from 20-200 kΩ. All electrodes had nonlinear characteristics starting at about a few tenths of a Volt. The chemistry gave nonrepeatable currents (variations of 20%) at low duty cycles (1-2 sec) for a fixed amplitude voltage input. This was reduced to less than 1% by using a constant current driver. The output current pulse was symmetric with this driver.

The accuracy of the localization of a current dipole using a magnetometer detector system is a function of a number of factors including: 1) the relative locations of the coordinate system of the phantom, the BTi Source Positioning Indicator (SPI) transmitter, and the individual detector coils, 2) relative calibration gain errors between detectors , and 3) the detected magnetic field signal to noise ratio. The accuracy of the SPI was measured in the magnetically shielded room (MSR) in which the magnetic measurements were taken. Errors in the sensitivity have also been measured for this system (Buchanan and Paulson(1989)).

Advances in Biomagnetism
Edited by S.J. Williamson *et al.*
Plenum Press, New York

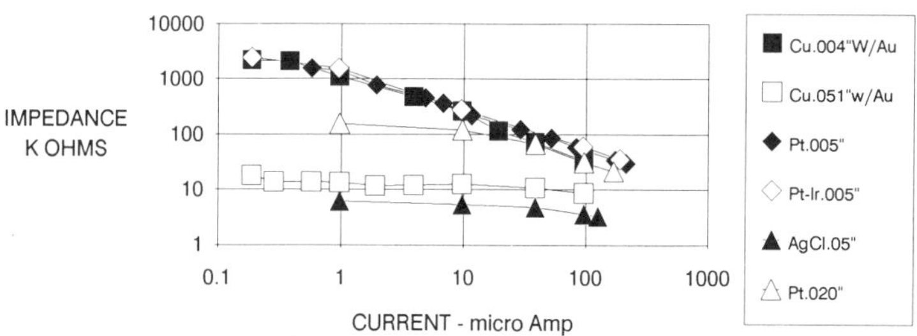

Fig. 1. Impedance of electrodes in saline solution versus applied current at 5 Hz.

The positions of the dipole electrodes relative to the head frame coordinates (defined by lead tabs placed at equivalent RPA, LPA, Nasion positions) were measured with two orthogonal X-rays. This method was compared with SPI and X-ray values (SPI for locations of top and bottom of the dipole rod and X-rays for depth along the rod) along with geometrically measured values, and differences were less than 2 mm. The current dipoles were then measured with the BTi Neuromagnetometer® system. The dipole sources used had dipole strengths of 5 to 1000 nA-m (about 1 to 200 μA sources), measurements averaged 64 trials using a single cycle 5 Hz sine wave current source. The dipole was oriented along the RPA/LPA (Y) axis.

The accuracy of relative position determined via the BTi SPI was within 1.5 mm for translational differences over the measurement volume (hemisphere of 48 cm radius below the transmitters). The standard deviation of relative positions in the MSR with the SPI system was < 1 mm over the measurement volume (0.6 m from the walls of the room). The measurement of the head shape location (4 points) was within ± 1 mm with a standard deviation of < 1 mm. The relative locations of the 4 reference points on the phantom as measured by the SPI in the MSR was repeatable to better than ± 1.5 mm with a standard deviation of < 0.8 mm in x ,y, and z.

Several different spherical containers were measured along with varying all the following parameters: dipole materials, 7-channel systems, shielded rooms, current amplitude levels, SPI systems, receiver locations, probe positions and sensitivity calibrations.

RESULTS

A set of measurements for locating a dipole were taken using a two sensor (two 7 channel probes) system from 7 basic positions of sensors relative to the phantom. These positions are shown in Figure 2. These positions were: 4 with both sensors tilted at 30° from vertical; 2 using one sensor tilted 15° along the dipole maximum (phantom rotated once), and one using one sensor directly over the top. This is equivalent to 11 single sensor placements. The equivalent set was repeated interchanging the sensor used at each location and the dipole locations reported by the software were compared. For adequate signal to noise there was no difference for results of either separate or combined (22 single sensor placements) data sets.

The location of the dipoles as measured by X-ray were compared with the value reported by the BTi software. Some results are shown in Figure 3 below. The magnitude of the error is the square root of the sum of the squares of errors in x, y, and z. Dipole location error was shown to be a function of field and positional noise. For adequate signal to noise ratio the dipole location is shown to be accurate to < 0.3 cm and the direction correct to < ± 3° relative to the X axis in the XY plane. The dipole amplitude reported by software varies by about 10 % but was 1.9 times greater in amplitude than the amplitude calculated by multiplying the current applied times the dipole physical length. The source localization results did not show an improvement in location accuracy for higher values of dipole strength. This indicates that the SPI positioning error will limit system accuracy even for large signal to noise ratios. For small dipole strengths (5 nA-m) the accuracy for 64 averages was better than 6 mm near the surface (first 4 dipoles) but only 1.5 cm at the deepest source. The sensitivity of the detection coils used by the software (Tesla/Volt) was also changed by about 10 % randomly relative to the other channels in a sensor and an effect < 0.3 cm in location was seen for the higher strength dipoles. However, there was a change in the dipole amplitude for this sensitivity change. The latency point (the point in time the localization was done) was varied over the waveform from about .25 to full amplitude applied current. The only effect seen for this variation in time was for low amplitude signals for which signal to noise became degraded. The analysis shown was for a latency of .25 sec.

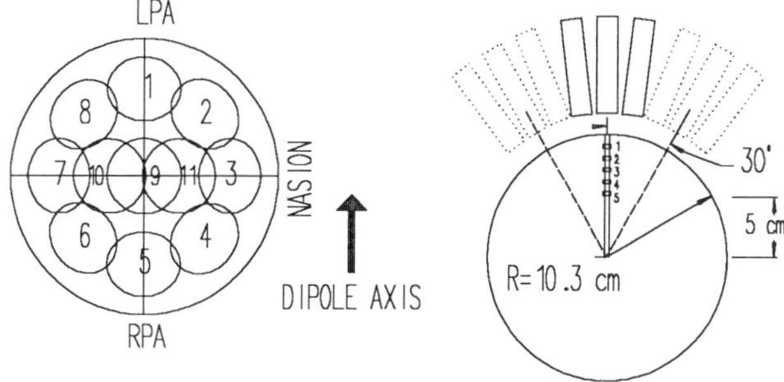

Fig. 2. Sensor positions used for dipole localization. The left figure is the view from the top (Z axis). The right hand figure shows the relative angles above the spherical phantom and the dipole locations from a side view (Y-Z plane).

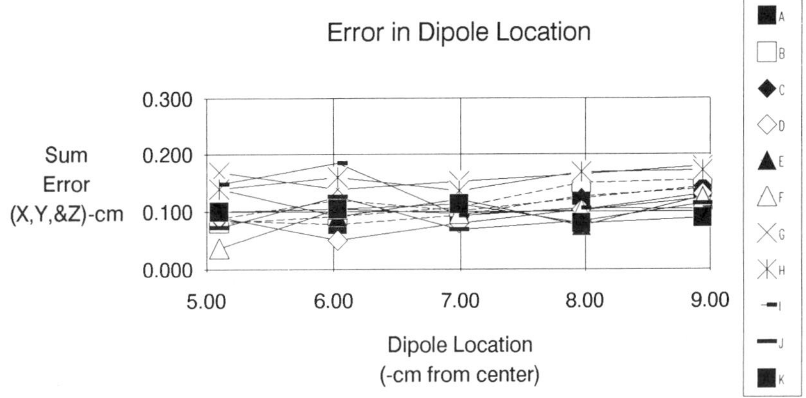

Fig. 3. Magnitude of error in dipole location versus distance from center of phantom sphere. The first three data sets are at 500 nA-m and the remainder are at 50 nA-m.

If the dipole location is determined from subsets of the 22 total data positions, the results indicate that if the dipole axis is known, a minimum of about 2 sensor measurement locations (14 detector coil positions) are needed (at a separation of about 15° from the dipole probe axis) for localization to better than 1 cm. For dipole strengths of 100-1000 nA-m and 64 trial averages localization to better than 4 mm was possible for a single two sensor placement (14 data points) with a relative 30° separation. Note that these readings were simultaneous.

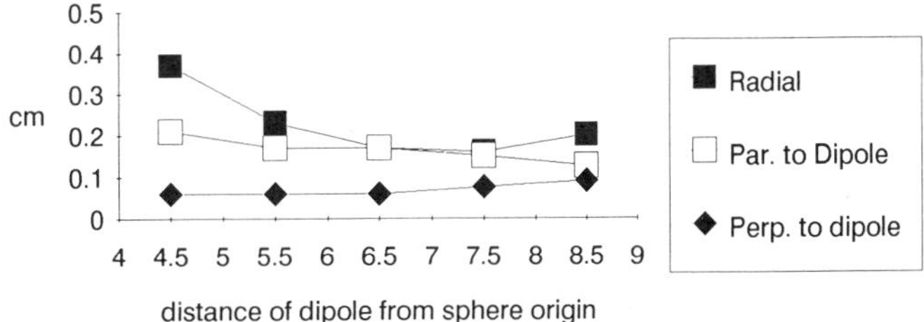

Fig. 4. Calculated localization error as a function of dipole depth. A seven channel sensor source is placed at seven locations to give 49 measurement points. Calculation is for a 50 nA-m source, field noise of 25 fT, sensor positioning error of 1.5 mm, sensor angular positioning error of 2 degrees and relative gain error of 1.5%.

The current dipole field was also calculated analytically for similar measurement locations. The size of the various noise sources was estimated and the forward calculation perturbed accordingly. The BTi software routines were then used for source location. The results are shown in Figure 4. Note that the values shown are standard deviations. This clearly shows that an error with a standard deviation of 2 mm can cause a final magnitude error of 2 mm for an electrode location of 5 cm to 9 cm.

SUMMARY

The accuracy in determining the location and magnitude of an artificial dipole in a spherical plastic phantom filled with saline was experimentally determined to be < 0.3 cm and the direction correct to < ± 3° in the XY plane with a repeatability of 10 % in dipole magnitude using the BTi Neuromagnetometer system. The degree of localization for this artificial source was shown to be mainly a function of the positional noise in the SPI positioning system.

ACKNOWLEDGEMENTS

The work was supported in part by NIH grant # NS24098-03.

REFERENCES

Barth, D. S., Sutherling, W. , and Broffman, J. (1986). Magnetic localization of a dipolar current source implanted in a sphere and a human cranium. Electroencephalogr Clin Neurophysiol, 63:260-273.

Buchanan, D. S. and Paulson, D. N. (1989). Neuromagnometer calibration using an array of small coils, 7th International Biomagnetism Conference.

Ribeiro, C. R., Williamson, S. J., and Kaufman, L. (1988). Squid arrays for simultaneous magnetic measurements: Calibration and source localization performance, IEEE Transactions on Biomedical Engineering, vol 35,#7,551-560.

Yamamoto, T., Williamson, S.J., Kaufman, L., Nicholson, C., and Linas, R. (1988). Magnetic localization of neuronal activity in the human brain. Proceedings of the National Acadamy of Sciences, 85:8732-8736.

ENVIRONMENTAL NOISE CANCELLATION

FOR BIOMAGNETIC MEASUREMENTS

Stephen E. Robinson

Technology Department
Biomagnetic Technologies, Inc.
San Diego, CA 92121

INTRODUCTION

An efficient algorithm has been developed for reducing the environmental magnetic noise (EMN) content of digitally recorded biomagnetic data. The EMN recorded by an indifferent reference sensor is subtracted from that of a biomagnetic sensor in an *a posteriori* fashion after measuring the amount of signal common to both sensors. This procedure contrasts with our previous efforts on adaptive recursive attenuation of magnetic noise using analog electronic noise cancellation (ENC) hardware (Williamson, *et al*, 1987).

BACKGROUND

Environmental magnetic noise cancellation should be regarded as distinctly different from gradiometer balance. Gradiometer balance refers only to the rejection of uniform field components and (for 2nd and higher-order gradiometers) the lower-order gradient terms. By contrast, magnetic noise cancellation refers to the attenuation of all signals measured simultaneously by the both the biomagnetometer and reference sensors, of which the imbalance components may be only part.

Since the magnitude of the EMN gradient components are expected to decline with increasing gradient order, the traditional approach to biomagnetic instrument design has been to construct higher-order shorter-baseline gradiometers with improved balancing with respect to the rejection of all uniform field and lower-order gradients. This path has led to an increase in the complexity of the biomagnetometer and a corresponding degradation in its overall sensitivity and SQUID noise level. This study demonstrates that sensitivity can be improved without a severe penalty of noise degradation by designing low-order gradiometers used together with reference sensors and noise cancellation processing.

ANALYTIC METHODS

An unprocessed signal is postulated to be the linear superposition of the desired signal and the unwanted noise. To eliminate the noise, one needs an independent measure of the interfering signal -- a reference signal. The superposition of signal and noise are resolved by subtraction of the reference signals, scaled by an appropriate weighting coefficient, from the unprocessed signal (Widrow and Stearns, 1985).

Let us assume that the reference channels measure only the EMN. Given a discrete time-series recording of signals detected simultaneously by an array of M reference channels and N biomagnetic sensor channels, the reference signal content and therefore the EMN present in the biomagnetic sensor signals can be measured statistically. Let $R_i(t)$ be the ith reference sensor time-series, and $S_j(t)$ be the jth biomagnetic sensor time-series. The signals

Advances in Biomagnetism
Edited by S.J. Williamson *et al.*
Plenum Press, New York

in common to any biomagnetic sensor and any reference channel may be estimated from the principal-axis matrix of the sensor-reference scattergram -- each element of which is given by:

$$W_{ij} = \begin{Bmatrix} -d_{ij} + \sqrt{d_{ij}^2 + 1} & \text{if } \sum r_i s_j \geq 0 \\ -d_{ij} - \sqrt{d_{ij}^2 + 1} & \text{if } \sum r_i s_j < 0 \end{Bmatrix}, \qquad \text{where} \qquad d_{ij} = \frac{\sum s_j^2 - \sum r_i^2}{2\sum s_j r_i}$$

and the sums-of-squares and products are the conventional statistical quantities:

$$\sum r_i s_j = \sum_{t=1}^{T} (R_i - R_{it})(\overline{S}_j - S_{it}), \qquad \sum r_i^2 = \sum_{t=1}^{T} (\overline{R}_i - R_{it})^2, \qquad \text{and} \qquad \sum s_j^2 = \sum_{t=1}^{T} (\overline{S}_j - S_{jt})^2$$

If the reference detector signals are both linearly independent and orthogonal to one another then the minimum EMN discrete time-series $S'_j(t)$ for each biomagnetic sensor is exactly:

$$S'_j(t) = S_j(t) - \sum_{i=1}^{M} W_{ij} R_i(t) \qquad j = 1 \cdots N$$

In practice, however, the reference signals are rarely orthogonal. To be so, a particular EMN signal would have to appear in only one of the reference sensors. Because of this, it is necessary to characterize the interdependence of signals from the reference sensors, using linear regression. We obtain the matrix of slopes for the signals of each reference sensor regressed onto that of every other reference sensor, of which each element is given by:

$$U_{ik} = \frac{\sum r_i r_k}{\sum r_k^2} \qquad i = 1 \cdots M, \quad k = 1 \cdots M$$

Inverting the reference regression matrix U results in the coefficients necessary to orthogonalize the compensation coefficients W. The noise-reduced time series then becomes:

$$S'_j(t) = S_j(t) - \sum_{i=1}^{N} \left(R_i(t) \sum_{k=1}^{N} W_{kj} U_{ik}^{-1} \right) \qquad j = 1 \cdots N$$

We now must consider minimizing the noise (primarily SQUID noise) added to $S'_j(t)$ by the reference sensor signal $R_i(t)$. If the ith reference sensor is assumed to be a gradiometer of the same geometry as the biomagnetic sensors, their sensitivities relative to the environmental and SQUID noise will be equal. Since random noise sums vectorially, adding a single gradient reference sensor having equal sensitivity to the biomagnetic sensors will increase the random noise content of $S'_j(t)$ by $\sqrt{2}$. This noise penalty was noted during the evaluation of the analog ENC method.

Since the EMN spectrum is rarely white, the reference signals can be band-limited. By passing only the interfering frequencies, the total random noise added by the reference sensors is reduced. The correct phase relationship between the reference and sensor channels is maintained by filtering the reference signals with a zero phase-shift digital filter. For frequency-dependent noise minimization, an independent set of weighting and orthogonalization coefficients may be computed for references in each spectral band.

EXPERIMENTAL METHODS

A moving permanent magnet was used to generate environmental magnetic noise outside a magnetically shielded room. Magnetic signals were recorded from a seven-channel 1st-order gradiometer sensor (baseline 5.0 cm). This multi-channel sensor was equipped with three field-reference magnetometers. A single channel 1st-order gradiometer in a separate dewar was used as a gradient reference. Several minutes of continuous data was acquired simultaneously from all channels in an analog bandwidth of DC to 50 Hz using a 12-bit analog to digital converter at a sample rate of 150 Hz. The digitally recorded signals were processed using the adaptive noise-reduction algorithm, which was coded for execution on an HP9000/350 computer. Noise-reduction was applied first using only the three magnetometer channels as references, next adding the separate 1st-order gradiometer as a reference, and lastly using one of the seven 1st-order gradiometer channels as a fourth reference. A noise reduction bandpass of DC to 1 Hz was selected.

RESULTS

The unprocessed response of one of the 1st-order gradiometer sensors to the EMN is shown in Figure 1. Environmental noise reduction performance for this sensor when using the three field reference magnetometer channels, alone, was on the order of 12 dB (Figure 2). Addition of the external 1st-order gradient reference channel, G_z, improved noise reduction to better than 40 dB in the DC to 1 Hz range (Figure 3).

The weighting coefficients, indicating the amount of each reference signal used for cancellation were examined for each of the trials. When one of the gradient references was included, the field reference weights, and therefore the contribution of the field reference channels to the noise reduction, was greatly reduced. On the average, better than 87 percent of the compensation was associated with the gradient reference, the field reference channels accounting for only 13 percent of the noise attenuation.

Noise weighting coefficients were found to be strongly dependent upon the location of the sensors within the magnetically shielded room. A set of noise reduction coefficients computed for one sensor position proved ineffective in reducing noise when the sensors were rotated or translated. Noise reduction was maximum when the external 1st-order gradient sensor was adjacent (25 cm) to and directed on the same axis as the biomagnetic sensors. Noise reduction dropped to 28 dB (average) when the gradient sensor was 1 meter away.

DISCUSSION

The adaptive noise-reduction algorithm tested was effective at reducing low-frequency artificial environmental magnetic noise detected by 1st-order gradiometer sensors. The relative weights computed for the field and gradient reference sensors demonstrate that, for environmental magnetic noise from a source external to the magnetically shielded room, the field reference terms are relatively unimportant when compared with the 1st-order gradient response term of the sensors. This hypothesis is strengthened further by the observation that the EMN signal was nearly identical in all seven biomagnetic sensors, prior to noise reduction (Figure 4). Had the EMN response been attributable to the residual field imbalance response of the detection coils, one would not have expected high coherence among all sensors. In addition, the gradients of the EMN could not be completely reconstructed by simply scaling the field components, even for the relatively simple artificial interference source used.

ACKNOWLEDGEMENTS

The author is grateful for the helpful suggestions and encouragement of D. Crum. This research was supported in part by NINCDS SBIR award 2 R44 NS24484.

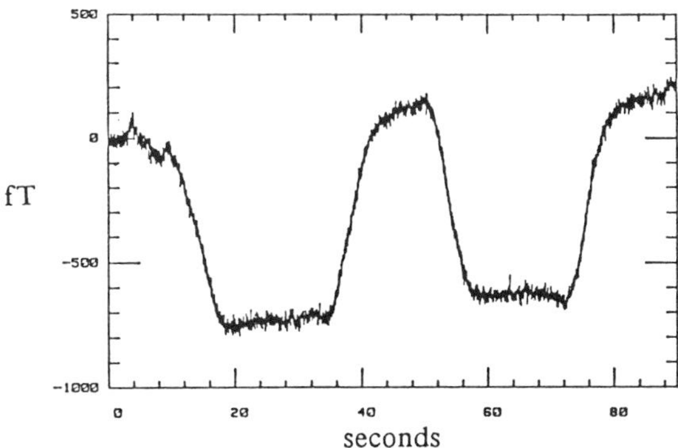

Figure 1. Environmental magnetic noise detected by 1st-order gradiometer, before noise-reduction processing.

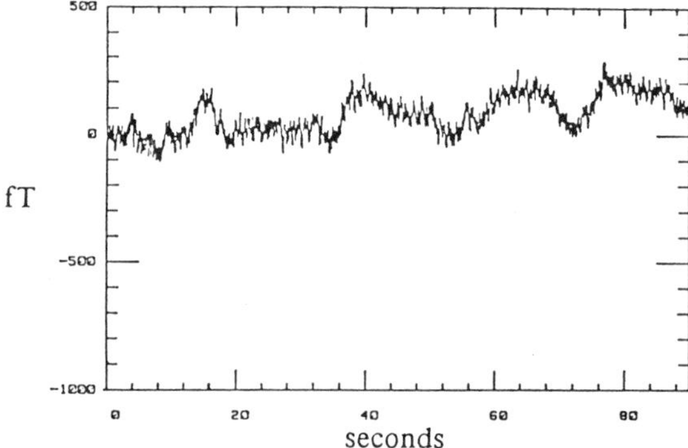

Figure 2. Residual environmental magnetic noise, after noise reduction using three orthogonal magnetometer reference signals. The data processed was the same as shown in Figure 1. The information present in the three reference channels was not sufficient for complete noise cancellation.

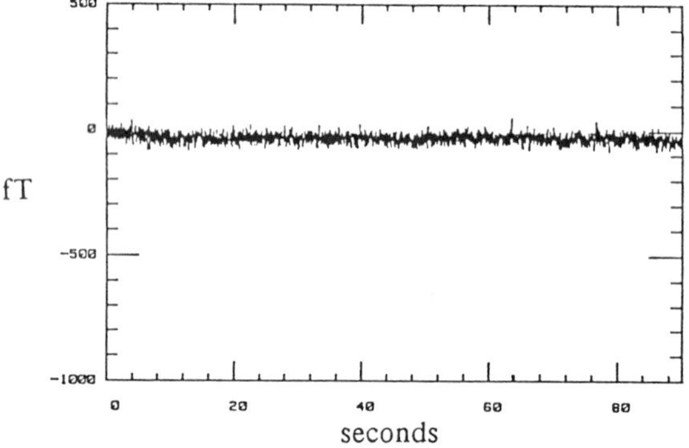

Figure 3. Residual environmental magnetic noise, after noise reduction using 1st-order gradiometer reference (G_z) plus three orthogonal magnetometer reference signals. The data processed was the same as shown in Figure 1. The EMN has been reduced to a level comparable with the SQUID noise.

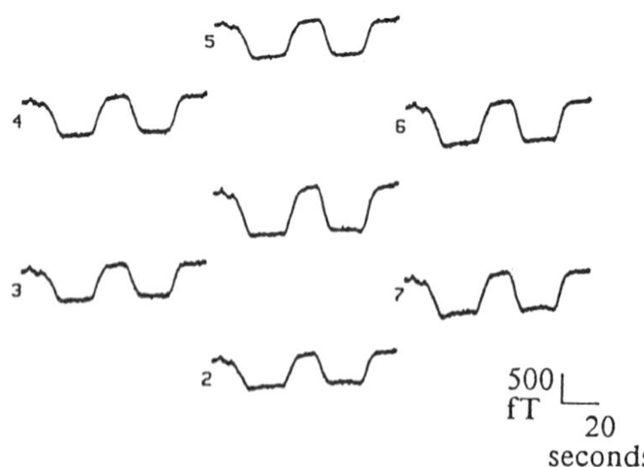

Figure 4. Environmental magnetic noise seen simultaneously by an array of seven 1st-order gradiometers. The similarity between channels suggests that the gradiometers are detecting the gradient components of the EMN. If this noise were due to gradiometer imbalance, the amplitudes and polarity of these signals would be random.

REFERENCES

Widrow, B. and Stearns, S.D. (1985). "Adaptive Signal Processing". Prentice-Hall, Inc.

Williamson, S.J., Robinson, S.E., and Kaufman L. (1987). Methods and instrumentation for biomagnetism. In: Atsumi, K., Kotani, M., Ueno, S., Katila, T, and Williamson S.J. (Eds.) "Biomagnetism, '87". Tokyo Denki University Press, pp. 18-25.

ELECTRONIC NOISE SUPPRESSION IN MULTICHANNEL NEUROMAGNETIC SYSTEM

A. Matlashov, Yu. Zhuravlev, A. Lipovich, A. Alexandrov, E. Mazaev, V. Slobodchikov, O. Wazhiewski

Institute of Radioengineering and Electronics
USSR Academy of Sciences
Moscow, USSR

INTRODUCTION

Usually when measuring biomagnetic signals without shielding second-order gradiometers are used. Satisfactory field registration requires the homogeneous field reduction factor to be more than 10^5 and the homogeneous gradient reduction factor about 10^3. Fine mechanical balancing which permits to overcome this problem becomes more complicated as the number of signal channels increases. Another possibility is an electronic suppression of low frequency ambient noise. Its efficiency for multichannel neuromagnetometer was first demonstrated by Williamson et al. [1]. Multichannel sensors contain three or more additional detection coils designed to monitor noise in the ambient magnetic field [2]. By suitable scaling the output of these reference channels and subtracting them from the output of each main signal channel, much of the magnetic noise can be canceled out [3]. The earnest problem is to choose correctly the method of calculating the scaling factors.

Design of neuromagnetic SQUID-based multichannel system with electronic noise suppression is described below. Operation of system units is controlled by personal computer. The neuromagnetic multichannel system includes sensor probe, automatic electronic noise suppression units, analog filter units and 8 or 16-channel digital control unit. We consider several algorithms to calculate the scaling factors.

SENSING SYSTEM

The array of detection (signal) coils is mounted on a probe suspended within a fiberglass dewar of 7.6 liter capacity. Inner diameter of the flat tail bottom is 60 mm. The array consists of one central coil aligned along the dewar's axis and six equally spaced surrounding coils. The distance between the centers of adjacent coils is 20 mm. The gradiometer axes are parallel to each other. Each signal coil has the geometry of a second-order gradiometer with a 7.5-mm radius and 50-mm baseline. Shielded superconducting leads connect each signal coil to the thin-film spiral input coil of the integrated dc-SQUID.

The SQUID with impedance matching transformer is placed within a 9-mm diameter and 70-mm length superconducting shield. The size can be diminished by using an additional dc-SQUID preamplifier [4]. The shields are positioned 20-cm above the tail bottom. The input coils and the SQUIDs were made separately and pressed to each other. The SQUID has intrinsic energy resolution of $5\cdot10^{-31}$ J/Hz above 0.2 Hz. Input inductance is 0.6 μH. The intrinsic noise level of the signal channel is about $8\cdot10^{-15}$ T/√Hz.

Ambient magnetic noise is registered by a vector magnetometer. It consists of three planar thin-film dc-SQUIDs without input coils placed at the sides of a small cube holder. Impedance matching transformers are placed at the room temperature. The cube holder is fixed 5 cm above the upper wind of the central gradiometer. The intrinsic noise level of the reference channels is less than 0.3 pT/√Hz in 10-kHz band. The vector magnetometer has stable parameters and requires no adjustment after temperature recycling.

ELECTRONIC SYSTEM

The signal channel gradiometer electronics contains separate analog and digital boards. The first provides current-gate feedback mode operation to reduce channel cross-talk. The analog part is controlled by the digital one. Four discrete and three continuous parameters can be adjusted simultaneously for up to 16 signal channels. Sequential code controlling the digital boards is formed by personal computer. The computer also forms test signals to provide an automatic adjustment. Compact electronic units for each signal channel are placed on the cryostat top. Each module dimensions are 160×80×35 mm. The block diagram of the whole system is shown in Fig.1.

The wide-band voltages in the seven signal and three reference channels pass through the suppression units and then through digitally-controlled analog bandpass filters with 48 db/octave rolloff and through comb filters to reduce the pickup of noise at the power line frequency and its harmonics.

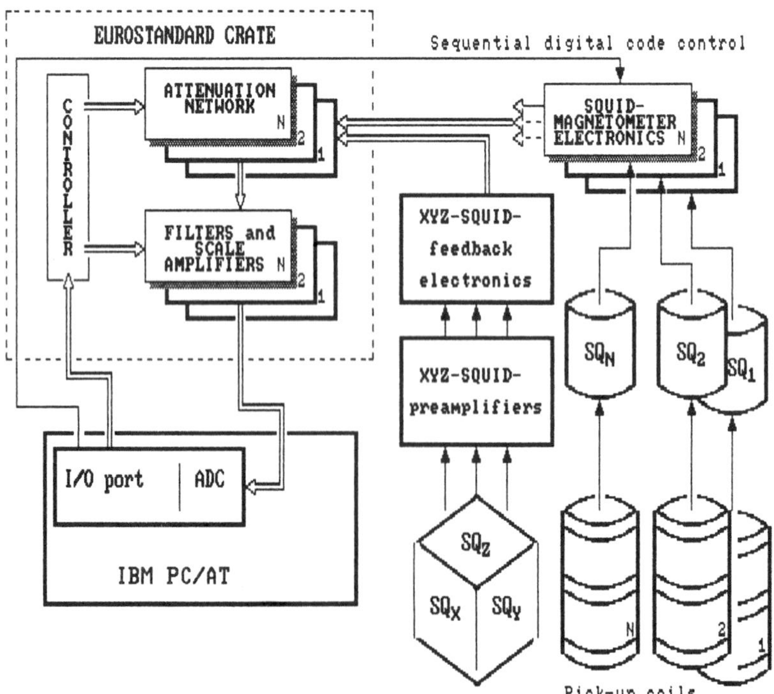

Fig. 1. Block diagram of the multichannel neuromagnetic system.

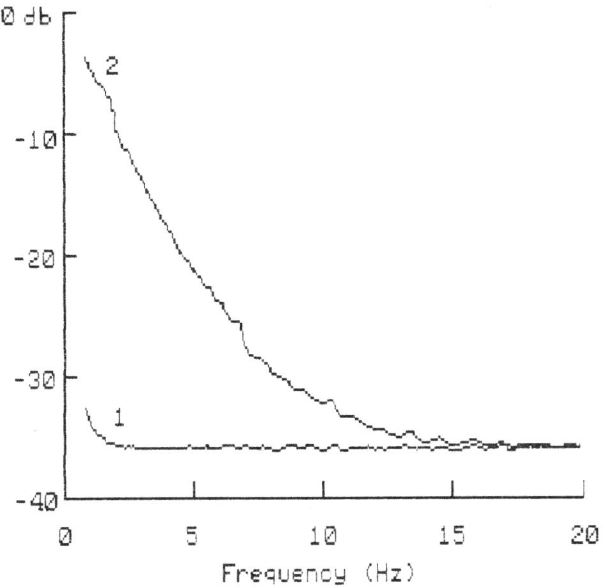

Fig. 2. Noise spectra for a signal channel with (1) and without (2) electronic noise suppression. The white noise level is 20 fT/$\sqrt{Hz}$.

Scaling factors are set by 12-bit digital code and filter cutoff frequencies by 8-bit digital code. Analog signal is converted to digital form with 14-bit resolution. Digital control is performed by IBM PC/AT computer.

PERFORMANCE AND RESULTS

Three signal channel modification of the neuromagnetic system was examined in a laboratory environment. Fig. 2 shows the averaged noise spectra for a signal channel with and without noise suppression. The white noise level is about 20 fT/$\sqrt{Hz}$. Its main source is the second spatial derivative of urban magnetic noise. The initial homogeneous field and homogeneous gradient reduction factors of each gradiometer are about 10^3. The homogeneous field reduction factors increase after electronic balancing by factor of 100 or more. One should note that the electronic noise suppression decreases signal output dynamic range from 120 dB to 70-80 dB. However in other respects this method is equivalent to the fine mechanical balancing method at least in the frequency band below 10 Hz.

To study the efficiency of the electronic suppression we also used mechanically balanced second-order gradiometer probe. The initial homogeneous field balance was set in the range 10^3 - $5 \cdot 10^5$. To obtain the optimum suppression scaling factors the cryogenic probe was placed at the common center of two Helmholtz coils for the transverse field and three-coil set for the axial field [5]. Manually-controlled electronic balancing was performed in 0.5-Hz sinusoidal uniform field [1]. The homogeneous field reduction factor obtained exceeded 10^5 independently of its initial value.

When using computer algorithms to calculate the scaling factors it's possible to exclude the unwieldy uniform field coils. To investigate the efficiency of different algorithms we compared the results in manually- and computer-controlled cases and estimated their stability and convergence rate.

We failed to obtain any satisfactory result by adaptive filtering. The correlation analysis of the signal and reference output data for short noise samples [3] yielded good efficiency. However the scaling factors were not the same for different noise samples and did not coincide with the uniform field results.

The important feature of the algorithm is the minimization criterion. We minimized the averaged absolute values of the suppression unit outputs instead of using standard least-mean-square error criterion. The best results were obtained by using sequential sorting over uniform grid in three-dimensional space of scaling factors followed by coordinate descent algorithm. At the first stage the absolute minimum point neighbourhood was found then this point was determined accurately. The optimum grid step which reduces computation time while retaining algorithm efficiency was determined experimentally. The results obtained by this procedure were the same as for the uniform field balancing technique. The complete computation time on the IBM PC/AT compatible computer (with math coprocessor) was about 10 minutes.

REFERENCES

1. S. J. Williamson, M. Pellizzone, Y. Okada, L. Kaufman, D. B. Crum and J. R. Marsden, Five channel SQUID installation for unshielded neuromagnetic measurements, in: "Biomagnetism: Applications and Theory," H. Weinberg, G. Stroink, T. Katila, eds., Pergamon Press, New York (1985).
2. New Biomagnetic Instruments From SHE. S.H.E. Corporation, San Diego, California (1984).
3. Magnetoencephalography. A New Window on the Brain. Biomagnetic Technologies Inc., San Diego, California (1987).
4. V. P. Koshelets, A. N. Matlashov, I. L. Serpuchenko, L. V. Filippenko and Yu. E. Zhuravlev, DC-SQUID preamplifier for DC-SQUID magnetometer, Appl. Supercond. Conf., California, rep.EH-14 (1988).
5. R. Merritt, C. Purcel and G. Stroink, Uniform magnetic field produced by three, four and five square coils, Rev. Sci. Instrum., 54: 879-882 (1983).

THERMAL NOISE OF A BIOMAGNETIC MEASUREMENT DEWAR

J. Nenonen, T. Katila and J. Montonen

Laboratory of Biomedical Engineering, Department of Technical Physics, Helsinki University of Technology, SF-02150 Espoo, Finland

INTRODUCTION

In our previous reports, we studied the effect of thermal magnetic noise arising from electrically conducing materials on the sensitivity of biomagnetic measurements. Such good conductor materials are commonly used for shielding purposes in the close vicinity of the sensing coil of the SQUID. The noise due to conducting plates was considered theoretically and experimentally by Varpula and Poutanen 1984, experimentally by Maniewski et al 1985, and both experimentally and computationally by Nenonen and Katila 1988. In the latter report, also the thermal magnetic noise arising from the walls of a magnetically shielded room was calculated. In some cases this noise may even be the limiting factor of the sensitivity. In addition, it was pointed out that small size mumetal shields, often used for checking the instrumental noise level, also contribute to external magnetic noise.

In most cases, however, the current limiting factor of the sensitivity in high-resolution biomagnetic measurements is the thermal noise caused by the measurement dewar. In this study, we report calculations of the magnitude and the spatial correlation of the thermal noise arising from electrically conducting thermal and radiation shields situated in the bottom and walls of a cryogenic dewar. The effect of different coil configurations on noise is considered. As an application to high-resolution biomagnetic measurements, we calculated the signal-to-noise ratio when measuring the magnetic field arising from an electric dipole source beneath the radiation shields.

NOISE CALCULATIONS

Thermal magnetic noise field, due to fluctuations of the conduction electrons in a volume conductor, was calculated with a model developed by Varpula and Poutanen. The volume conductor was assumed to be divided into infinitesimal subvolumes (van der Ziel 1970) and a noise current dipole, modeling thermal agitation of conduction electrons, was assigned into each subvolume. Assuming that the dipoles were non-correlated, the noise field of the volume conductor was obtained by summing up the

Advances in Biomagnetism
Edited by S.J. Williamson *et al.*
Plenum Press, New York

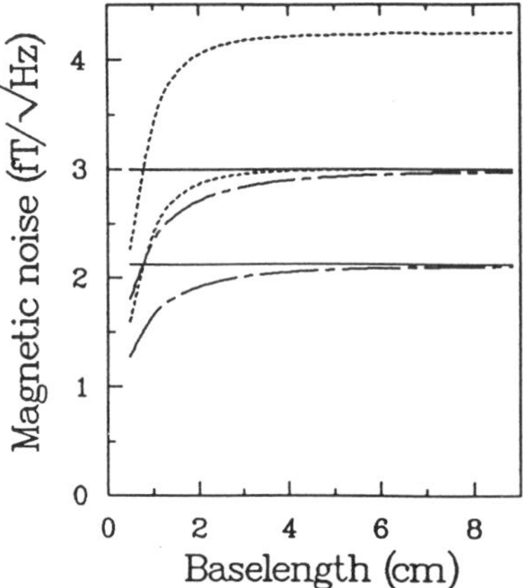

Fig. 1. Thermal noise arising from thin, infinite conducting foils. Solid curves: magnetometer, broken curves: axial gradiometer, dashed curves: planar gradiometer. The lower curves are calculated for a single infinite 25 nm thick aluminium slab at 250 K, and the upper curves for two infinite slabs at temperatures 225 and 265 K. (The temperatures are approximately the equilibrium temperatures for one and two floating radiation shields between walls at temperatures of 30 K and 293 K.)

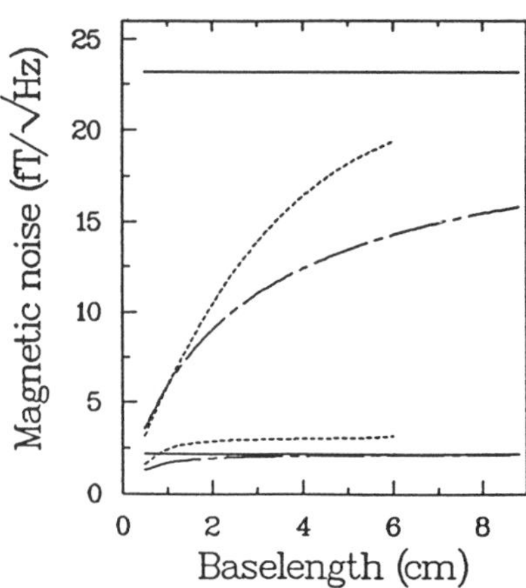

Fig. 2. Thermal noise calculated inside a rectangular enclosure of $8 \times 8 \times 80$ cm^3 for different coil configurations. Solid lines: magnetometer, broken lines: axial gradiometer, dashed lines: planar gradiometer. In the case of the three lowermost curves, the enclosure walls are 25 nm thick Al-foils at the temperature of 250 K. In the case of three uppermost curves, a 15 μm thick Al-foil at the temperature 293 K was added outside the dewar. The sensing coil was at a distance z=0.5 cm from the bottom of the enclosure, at a distance z=1.5 cm from the thicker foil, and x=y=4 cm from the walls.

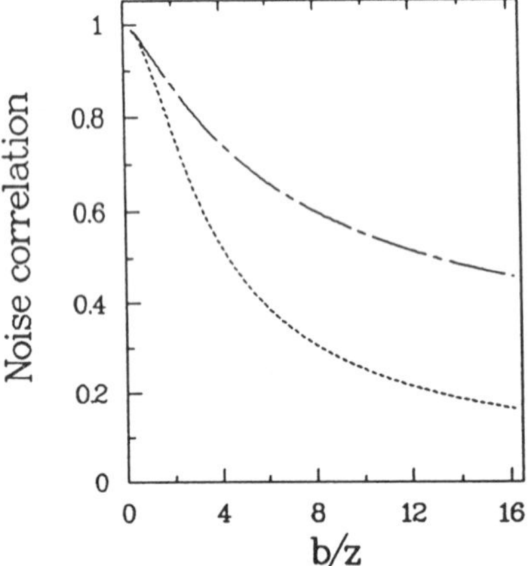

Fig. 3. The spatial correlation coefficient γ of the z-component of the thermal noise above a thin conducting slab. The parameter b is the distance between the observation points and z the distance to the surface of the slab. Broken curve: axial gradiometer, dashed curve: planar gradiometer.

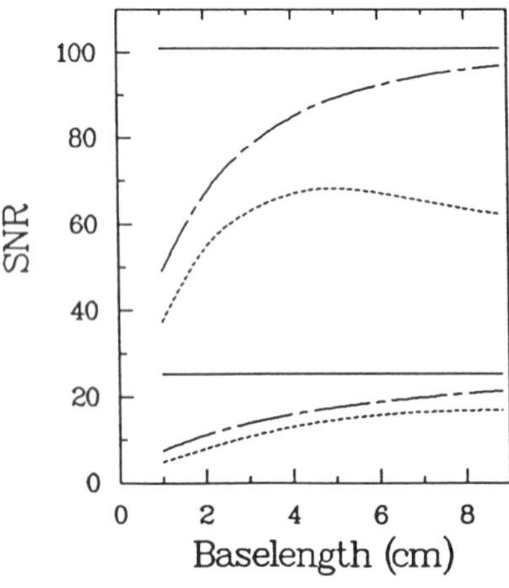

Fig. 4. The signal-to-noise ratio for a magnetic field of a current dipole at a distance of 4 cm (three uppermost curves) and 8 cm (three lowermost curves) from the pickup coil. Solid lines: magnetometer, broken lines: axial gradiometer, dashed lines: planar gradiometer. A 25 nm thick Al-foil at temperature of 250 K was at z=0.5 cm from the sensing coil.

contributions of all dipoles. Varpula and Poutanen (1984) measured and calculated the noise arising from different conducting slabs. Nenonen and Katila (1988) extended the calculations to soft magnetic materials and to layers of two different conductor plates. The main parameters determining the magnitude of the noise level are the electric conductivity, the magnetic permeability and the thickness of the plates. The slab calculations can be utilized to estimate the thermal magnetic noise inside a shielded rectangular enclosure.

In our one-channel test dewar, the radiation shields consist of layers with 25 nm thin semireflecting aluminium deposit on the surface of a mylar foil. To estimate the noise contribution of the radiation shields, we measured the electric conductivity of the foil at temperatures between 15 and 293 K at 1 K steps. The conductivity behaved almost linearly with temperature. The highest measured value was $\sigma = 3.2 \times 10^7 \frac{1}{\Omega \mathrm{m}}$ at a temperature T = 15 K and the measured conductivity at the room temperature was $\sigma = 1.9 \times 10^7 \frac{1}{\Omega \mathrm{m}}$.

Next we calculated the noise above a radiation shield, modeled by a thin infinite conducting slab, as sensed by magnetometers or axial or planar gradiometers. The finite area of the sensing coils was not taken into account. Using the calculated equilibrium temperature for one foil (250 K) between two walls at temperatures T = 30 K and T = 293 K, we calculated the noise of the main sensing coil at a distance z=5 mm from the foil. The calculations were repeated for two 25 nm aluminium layers at their respective equilibrium temperatures. The calculated noise spectra where white up to several MHz. The calculations match a practical measurement situation where the sensitivity of a first order gradiometer system with a baseline of 8 cm is ≥ 3 fT/$\sqrt{\mathrm{Hz}}$. The calculated noise curves are shown in Fig. 1.

As a first approximation to the noise contribution due to the radiation shields in the dewar walls, we calculated the noise inside a rectangular enclosure of 8×8×80 cm^3. The main sensing coil was at a distance of z=0.5 cm from the bottom and x=y=4 cm from the walls. The same calculation was repeated with a 15 μm thick aluminium foil, used as an rf-radiation shield and situated rectangularly outside the dewar, assuming the slabs are not in contact with each other. The calculations show that the main noise component sensed by the pickup coil(s) arises from the radiation shields at the bottom of the dewar. The results are presented in Fig. 2.

In addition to the magnitude of thermal noise we also calculated the correlation coefficient γ of the rms value of the z-component $B_{n,z}$ of the noise field above a conducting slab: $\gamma^2 = |B^{ij}_{n,z}|^2/|B^i_{n,z}||B^j_{n,z}|$, where i and j refer to two locations at a distance b from each other, either horizontally or vertically, the main sensing coil being at a distance z from the surface of the slab. The results, calculated as a function of b/z, are shown in Fig. 3.

Finally, as an application to high-resolution measurements, we calculated signal to noise ratios when the primary field source was a current dipole $p_x = p_y = 0.1$ μAm at a distance of z = 4 cm and z = 8 cm from the main sensing coil. The radiation shield was at a distance of 0.5 cm from the coil. The results for different coil configurations are depicted in Fig. 4.

DISCUSSION

The results clearly show that the sensitivity in high-resolution biomagnetic measurements is limited by thermal noise due to electrically conducting radiation shields in the dewar even if the measurements are carried out inside a magnetically shielded room. Assuming the slabs do not contact each other, it was shown that the shields at the bottom of the dewar have a clearly more significant effect on the thermal noise than the shields positioned at the sides of the dewar. Our calculations were performed for one or two very thin aluminium foils. In practice, however, the number of the layers is bigger. Calculation of the temperature distribution for several floating radiation shields results in approximately 80 % of the layers lying at a temperature higher than 200 K. According to our measurements, the conductivity of the shields is only a slowly varying function of temperature and computer simulations show that at frequencies of interest in biomagnetic measurements ($\leq$ 300 Hz) the thermal noise contributions of the shields sum up quadratically. On this basis it was calculated that e.g. ten 25 nm thick uniform aluminium layers at the bottom of the dewar lead to a thermal noise level of about 6.5 fT/$\sqrt{\text{Hz}}$ at a distance of 0.5 cm from the foils.

For planar gradiometers, the noise level due to uniform conducting slabs is higher by a factor of about $\sqrt{2}$ as compared to axial gradiometers with the same baselength ($\geq$ 1 cm). Planar sensing coils with small diameter are usually positioned as close to the dewar bottom as possible. Unfortunately, this increases thermal noise level due to the radiation shields. Axial gradiometers with larger coils can, on the contrary, be positioned further away from the noisy shields without losing the sensitivity to the field source and in addition the compensation coil locating even further away still diminishes the noise in this case.

By minimizing the number of the radiation shield layers we were able to increase the sensitivity of our one-channel DC-SQUID gradiometer from the level of 5 to $\sim$ 3 fT/$\sqrt{\text{Hz}}$. A further reduction of the noise level is possible by dividing the radiation shields into small pieces insulated from each other. For example, when a $100 \times 100 \times 0.5$ mm^3 Al-plate was cut into strips of 5×100 mm^2 the measured noise level dropped about 90 %. As a conclusion, dewar noise is an important problem and should not be neglected when optimizing the sensitivity of the biomagnetic measurement system.

REFERENCES

Maniewski, R., Derka, I., Katila, T., Ryhänen, T., and Seppänen, M. (1985), DC-SQUID system for high-resolution biomagnetic measurements, Med. & Biol. Eng. & Comput. 23(S2), pp. 1485-1486.

Nenonen, J., and Katila, T. (1988). Thermal noise in a magnetically shielded room, in: Atsumi, K., Kotani, M., Ueno, S., Katila, T., and Williamson, S., Proc. of the 6th Internat. Conf. on Biomagn., Tokyo Denki Univ. Press, pp. 426-429.

Van der Ziel, A. (1970), "Noise: Sources, Characterization, Measurement", 1st ed. Prentice-Hall, Englewood Cliffs, N.J., Chap. 5.1b.

Varpula, T., and Poutanen, T. (1984), Magnetic field fluctuations arising from thermal motion of electric charge in conductors, J. Appl. Phys. 55, pp. 4015-4021.

NOISE CANCELLATION IN BIOMAGNETOMETERS

J. Vrba, J. McCubbin, S. Lee, A. A. Fife, and M. B. Burbank

CTF Systems Inc.
Port Coquitlam, B.C.
Canada, V3C 1M9

INTRODUCTION

Noise cancellation in a system with a large number of biomagnetic sensors has been analysed, and three different noise cancellation techniques identified: gradiometer common mode balancing, formation of higher order gradiometers and adaptive subtraction of noise between various sensing channels. Examples of environmental noise cancellation by both common mode balancing and adaptive subtraction will be illustrated. Common mode balancing is more applicable to higher order gradiometers operated in magnetically harsh environments, while adaptive subtraction is most useful for similarly aligned 1st order gradiometers operated within a shielded room.

NOISE CANCELLATION METHODS

Biomagnetometer systems are usually equipped with reference sensors and numerous sensing channels of the same order. For these systems, two of the techniques mentioned in the introduction are independent of the character of the applied fields: **common mode balancing** and **formation of higher order gradiometers**. In situations where these two methods cannot be used, the **adaptive subtraction technique** becomes applicable (e.g. where there is an incomplete set of reference sensors available for balancing or where there are no gradiometers with identical orientation available for higher gradiometer formation). The selection of the most suitable noise cancellation technique thus depends on the gradiometer order, level of common mode balance and availability of reference sensors.

Throughout the paper, the following notation will be used: lower case quantities (b, g_1, g_2, or b_i, g_{ij}, g_{ijk}, ...) will refer to sensor outputs and the upper case quantities ($\mathbf{B}$, G_1, G_2, ..., or B_i, G_{ij}, G_{ijk}, ...) will refer to vector or tensor fields (the tensor components are defined as $G_{ij} = \partial B_i/\partial x_j$, or $G_{ijk} = \partial B_i/\partial x_j \partial x_k$). Coordinates x_1 and x_2 are in horizontal plane and x_3 is vertical, pointing up.

Gradiometer common mode balancing is understood to represent the removal of lower order terms from a higher order gradiometer signal output. For example, the general form of balancing for a 3rd order gradiometer is given by (Fife et al, 1984):

$$s = g_3 - \mathbf{C_B} \cdot \mathbf{b} - \mathbf{C_{G1}} \cdot \mathbf{g_1} - \mathbf{C_{G2}} \cdot \mathbf{g_2} \qquad (1)$$

where $\mathbf{b}$, $\mathbf{g_1}$, $\mathbf{g_2}$, and g_3 are direct outputs from magnetometers, 1st, 2nd, and 3rd order gradiometers, respectively, s is the balanced gradiometer output, and $\mathbf{C_B}$, $\mathbf{C_{G1}}$, $\mathbf{C_{G2}}$ are the common mode vectors (with 3, 5, and 7 components respectively). It is assumed in equation (1) that $\mathbf{b}$, $\mathbf{g_1}$, and $\mathbf{g_2}$ represent a complete set of reference sensors. The balancing coefficients are then independent of the character of the applied fields and are constant in time. Common mode signals result from various manufacturing errors and degrade the spatial discrimination of gradiometers. Balancing restores the spatial rejection close to the level of the intrinsic gradient response of perfect gradiometers.

Formation of higher order gradiometers involves the subtraction of signals from two identically oriented gradient sensors at different locations. For example, if the outputs of two identically oriented 1st order gradiometers located at points $\mathbf{x}$ and $(\mathbf{x} + \mathbf{d_2})$ are subtracted, a 2nd order gradiometer is formed with output g_2:

$$g_2 = g_1(\mathbf{x}) - \xi \cdot g_1(\mathbf{x} + \mathbf{d_2}) \qquad (2)$$

where the subtraction coefficients ξ compensate for the differences in gradiometer gains and are independent of applied fields and time. Higher order gradiometers have the benefit of improved noise rejection due to increased spatial discrimination. The drawback of the method is that the noise of the individual sensors is added in rms fashion (eg for identical sensors and $\xi = 1$ the noise increases by a factor of $\sqrt{2}$).

Adaptive subtraction is understood to consist of the determination and subsequent subtraction of common terms in the outputs of several sensing channels. Adaptive subtraction among N balanced sensor outputs, s_j, j = 1 ... N, can be described as follows:

$$\tilde{s}_k = s_k - \sum_{j=1,\, j \neq k}^{N} \xi_{kj} \cdot s_j \qquad (3)$$

where ξ_{kj} are the subtraction coefficients for minimizing the common terms among outputs s_j. They depend on the character of the applied fields and are therefore time dependent.

NOISE CANCELLATION EXAMPLES

Noise cancellation techniques have been investigated for a multi-channel biomagnetometer system, using software simulation which included the effects of sensor imperfections, noise, crosstalk, and environmental noise contributions. For present purposes, the techniques of gradiometer balancing and adaptive subtraction will be illustrated. It will be assumed that field common mode balancing is well understood and that the field common mode signals have been balanced out.

The noise cancellation examples were simulated using moving magnetic dipoles as noise sources. To reduce the complexity of presentation the dipole motions were constrained to horizontal x_1 - x_2 plane and dipoles were oriented either vertically ($\parallel x_3$) or horizontally ($\parallel x_2$). Two dipoles were moved along straight paths parallel to x_1 axis with distances of closest approach to the reference gradiometers of 2 m and 15 m and velocities of 2 m/sec and 4 m/sec, respectively. The near dipole was moved first, generating signal peak at $\approx$ 5 sec, the motion of the more distant dipole was delayed and it generated signal peak at $\approx$ 20 sec. The simulations were performed with SQUID sensor noise bandwidth of 1 Hz.

Common mode balancing is illustrated using a 3rd order gradiometer equipped with a complete set of field and 1st gradient reference sensors. The noise source dipole is vertical, for which only G_{13} and G_{23} components are non-zero. The field balanced 1st and 3rd gradiometer outputs are shown in Figs.1.a, b, and c. The presence of component G_{13} in the 3rd gradiometer output is indicated by asymmetry and a slight shift of the 3rd gradiometer peaks from the g_{23} peaks (Fig.1.c). The 1st gradients G_{13} and G_{23} are linearly independent and both are required to cancel the 1st gradient common mode signal of the 3rd gradiometer. The 3rd gradiometer outputs after balancing by only g_{13} or g_{23} are shown in Figs.1.d and 1.e. Obviously, balancing by only one of the 1st gradient components is insufficient. The 3rd gradiometer output after complete 1st gradient balancing is shown in Fig.1.f. This balanced 3rd gradiometer exhibits strong spatial discrimination, the peak due to the more distant dipole being greatly attenuated, while that due to the near dipole is quite strong.

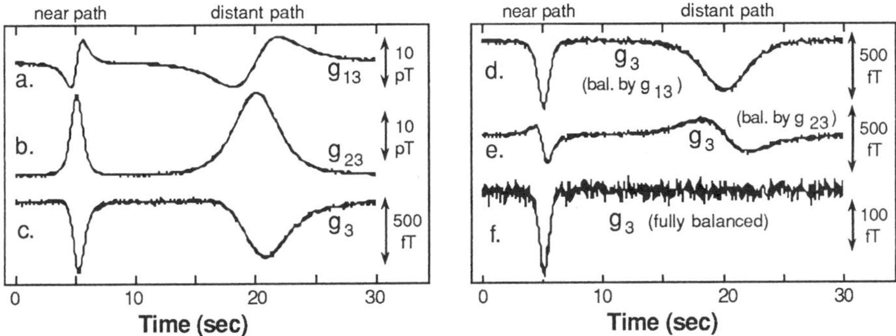

Fig.1. **1st gradient balancing of a 3rd order gradiometer.** a, b, c - g_{13}, g_{23}, and g_3 before 1st gradient balancing; d - g_3 balanced by g_{13} only; e - g_3 balanced by g_{23} only; f - g_3 fully balanced by g_{13} and g_{23}. BW = 1 Hz.

Adaptive subtraction is illustrated for a system of two slightly inclined 1st gradiometers ($\psi = 15°$ inclination). Gradiometers are located a short distance apart, exact position is not important. Assuming gradiometer baselines of $\mathbf{d_1} = d\cdot(0,0,1)$ and $\mathbf{d_2} = d\cdot(\sin\psi,0,\cos\psi)$ and gradiometer coil orientations of $\mathbf{p_1} = \mathbf{d_1}/d$ and $\mathbf{p_2} = \mathbf{d_2}/d$, the balanced 1st order gradiometer outputs, s_1 and s_2, are:

$$s_1 = (\mathbf{p_1}\, G\, \mathbf{d_1}) = d\cdot G_{33} \tag{4.a}$$

$$s_2 = (\mathbf{p_2}\, G\, \mathbf{d_2}) = d\cdot\left\{G_{33}\cdot\left(1 - \sin^2\psi\right) + G_{11}\cdot\sin^2\psi + G_{13}\cdot\sin 2\psi\right\} \tag{4.b}$$

Selecting the adaptive subtraction coefficient as $\xi_{21} = d\cdot\left(1 - \sin^2\psi\right)$, the adaptively subtracted signal is given by:

$$\tilde{s}_2 = s_2 - \xi_{21}\cdot s_1 = d\cdot\left(G_{11}\cdot\sin^2\psi + G_{13}\cdot\sin 2\psi\right) \tag{5}$$

With $\psi = 0$, the adaptive subtraction is perfect ($\tilde{s}_2 = 0$), and the procedure corresponds to the formation of a 2nd order gradiometer, G_{33i}, where i depends on the direction of the displacement between the two 1st order gradiometers. With $\psi \neq 0$, the success of adaptive subtraction depends on the character of the applied signals. With G_{33} dominant and G_{11} and G_{13} small, adaptive subtraction is successful. If the opposite is true, adaptive subtraction fails.

Based on the above rules, configurations for successful and unsuccessful adaptive subtractions are designed. Sensors used are three field balanced, axial, 1st gradiometers with tilts and azimuth orientations $(\psi,\varphi) = (0°,0°)$, $(15°,0°)$, $(15°,60°)$ and baselines of 5 cm. All gradiometers are located on the surface of 10 cm radius sphere with center at location (0,0,-18) cm. For successful adaptive subtraction, the two dipole are oriented in the direction of the x_2-axis, such that the components $G_{13} = G_{23} = 0$, and G_{11}, G_{22}, and G_{33} are large. The 1st gradient outputs and adaptively subtracted signals are shown in Fig.2.a. In this situation, the outputs of the 1st gradient sensors are very similar and adaptive subtraction is successful. For unsuccessful adaptive subtraction, the dipoles are oriented vertically, such that only G_{13} and G_{23} are non-zero. The 1st gradiometer outputs for this situation are shown in Fig.2.b. Adaptive subtraction is not possible, since the sensor outputs are linearly independent.

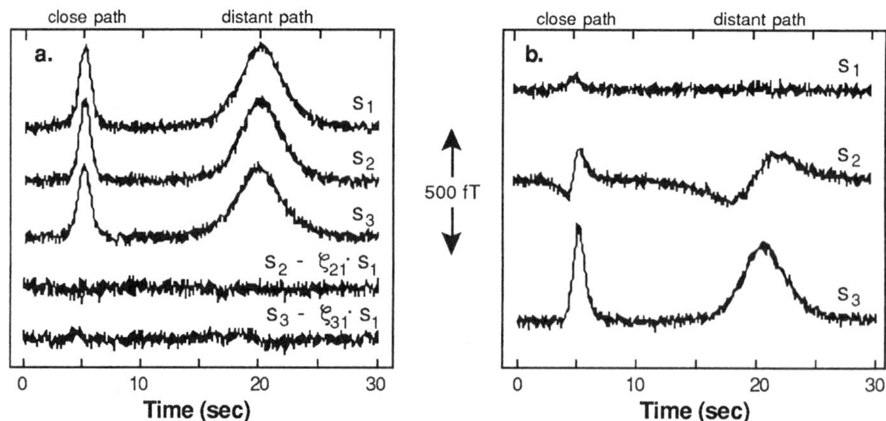

Fig.2: **Adaptive subtraction between 1st gradient channels.** a - successful (dipole ‖ x_2) and b - unsuccessful (dipole ‖ x_3) adaptive subtractions. BW = 1 Hz.

DISCUSSION

The results of this study indicate that field and 1st gradient common mode balancing are most effective for higher order gradiometers and must be performed with a full set of linearly independent, lower order, reference channels. Well balanced, higher order gradiometers exhibit strong spatial filtering and attenuate distant sources by many orders of magnitude. For 1st and well balanced 2nd and 3rd gradiometers, operated in their intrinsic gradient response regimes, further noise rejection can be achieved through adaptive subtraction of the common terms in the outputs of similarly aligned channels. The responses of similar gradiometers to distant noise sources will exhibit a large degree of linear dependency and in many situations, the noise can be reduced by adaptive subtraction between them. However, the adaptive subtraction may not be universally successful.

The findings of this work are being integrated into a multi-channel system (up to 60 channels) currently under development.

ACKNOWLEDGEMENTS

This work was supported in part by the Departments of National Defence, Supply and Services, and the Transport Development Center, Canada.

REFERENCES

Fife, A. A., Vrba, J., McCubbin, J., Weinberg, H., and Brickett, P., 1984, Biogradiometer Design for Noisy Environment, in: "BIOMAGNETISM: Applications & Theory," Proceedings of the Fifth World Conference on Biomagnetism, Vancouver, Canada, H. Weinberg, G. Stroink, T. Katila, eds., Pergamon Press, New York, page 41.

THREE-DIMENSIONAL VOLUMETRIC RECONSTRUCTION FOR NEUROMAGNETIC SOURCE LOCALIZATION

J. S. George, P. S. Jackson, D.M. Ranken, and E.R. Flynn

Neuromagnetism Laboratory, MS-M882
Los Alamos National Laboratory, Los Alamos, NM 87545

INTRODUCTION

Neuromagnetic measurements in conjunction with appropriate mathematical models permit the localization of centers of activity in the human brain. For large evoked response components, Monte Carlo error analyses suggest that location uncertainty due to measurement noise may be as low as 1 mm. However, in order to achieve and exploit this degree of accuracy in source localization it is necessary to improve procedures for documenting the location of sensors with respect to the head, and for locating anatomical sources which account for observed fields.

To satisfy these perceived needs, we have developed systems for modeling and displaying the three dimensional structure of the head and brain. The first system is a video-based device for rapidly digitizing the head surface. A shaded rendering of the head can be generated using software or hardware subsystems, and pseudocolor maps of observed evoked response fields can be painted on the head surface model. A second system allows neuromagnetic sources to be located on magnetic resonance images (MRIs). The system reconciles MRI and neuromagnetic coordinate systems and converts between them, selects appropriate images from series of sagittal, axial and coronal slices, and displays calculated sources in orthographic projection. A third system allows the production and manipulation of a 3-D volumetric model of brain structure from detailed anatomical data provided by MRI. This system will eventually be used to drive source modeling procedures utilizing accurate head geometry and anatomically constrained source configurations.

SYSTEMS

The head surface digitizer produces a plane of light which is oriented to pass through the vertical axis of the head. The bright contour arising from the intersection of the light plane with the head surface is viewed with a video camera rotated 30-45° off of the light source axis. The entire assembly is rotated around the subject's head, driven by a tightly coupled stepping motor. Superthreshold pixels along each scan line are analyzed to determine the peak of the distribution. The calculated horizontal offset from the center of rotation on the video screen is converted into the radius measure in a cylindrical coordinate system. The angular measure is calculated from the position reported by the stepping motor controller for each image location. Cylindrical coordinates are converted directly into cartesian coordinates which are used for analysis and graphic displays.

We have employed two different systems for producing the plane of light. A small laser directed at a rapidly rotating mirror produces a scanned beam which approximates a plane of light. Secondary mirrors above and below the rotating mirror can be used to help avoid

Advances in Biomagnetism
Edited by S.J. Williamson *et al.*
Plenum Press, New York

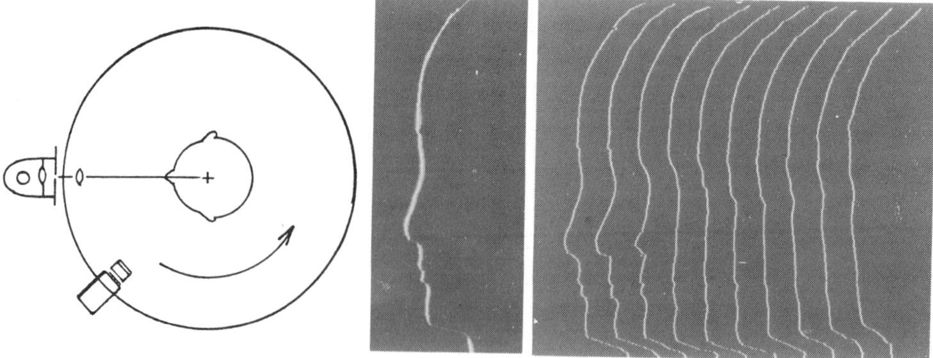

Figure 1. Operation of the head surface digitizer. **Left Panel:** Schematic diagram of system geometry. **Center panel:** A pattern of superthreshold pixels stored as an intermediate output of the system. **Right panel:** Calculated contours for a selected subset of radial slices. A horizontal offset between slices has been introduced for clarity.

shadowing on the top of the head, and under the chin. We currently use a system employing a linear halogen source which is focused using a reflector lamp housing and cylindrical lens onto a vertical slit. The image of the slit is collimated with a second cylindrical lens placed at the lens focal length.

The video camera is an NTSC compatible miniature CCD. In the prototype system, video signals are digitized using an IBM-PC/AT resident framegrabber (FG-100 or VS-100, Imaging Technology Inc.). These boards are also used for the generation of visual stimuli or displays of data. Video threshold levels are set and adjusted using input lookup tables. Because of the binary thresholding, the host computer can access data from a single bit plane for 8 pixels in parallel. This strategy significantly reduces data processing and storage requirements so that a single video frame can typically be processed in .5 to 1 sec, allowing a head scan to be completed in 2- 5 minutes depending on desired resolution. We are currently implementing the system on a CAMAC-resident digitizer (AC-100, Data Design Corporation). This system has a threshold storage mode implemented in hardware; only the x and y coordinates and intensity values of superthreshold pixels are stored in frame memory. This system will allow individual images to be processed in realtime (i.e. 30 frames per second) so that scans can be completed in 10-20 seconds, greatly alleviating the problem of mechanically stabilizing the subject during the digitization process. By preserving analog intensity data, the system will allow thresholds to be relaxed without increasing the ambiguity of the location of the peak of the surface contour.

The subject typically wears a swimming cap during the digitization process. For neuromagnetic experiments, markings on the cap provide a rough guide for placement of the dewar containing the sensor array. During digitization, the cap compresses the hair so that the digitized surface more closely approximates scalp contours. The use of a cap simplifies signal processing in other ways. Hair is a highly scattering medium so that video thresholds that are optimal for other surfaces may not produce a contour on hair. This problem could be resolved by differential imaging or adaptive thresholding, however both techniques would increase the complexity of signal processing during data acquisition. Simply lowering the threshold produces larger data files and can introduce ambiguities, but may prove workable with the new hardware configuration.

Shadowing or obstruction of the bright contour by prominent features on the head such as the nose or ears is typically a problem in a few slices in a complete scan. For graphical purposes this can be resolved by simple editing procedures or by reference to symmetry. The hardware solution employs two video cameras, one on either side of the plane of light. This approach is simple to implement on the Imaging Technology framegrabbers which have multiple, software selectible video inputs. An alternative strategy is to use a birfucated fiber optic image guide to mechanically combine images collected at two locations for input into a single video camera. This system more efficiently utilizes the camera's field of view and avoids additional data acquisition overhead, but is a more expensive solution.

We have developed simple algorithms for graphically rendering the head models as line drawings or as shaded surface images. Such images are typically displayed in 16 grey levels, stored in 4 bits of frame memory. The remaining bits can be used to contain a pseudocolor map prepared by interpolation of measured neuromagnetic field amplitudes as a spatial projection for one point in time. This map can be transparently painted on the head model by use of appropriate output lookup tables. A sequence of such images may be captured on video tape using a triggerable time lapse video recorder, or using a video animation controller in conjunction with an sVHS editing recorder.

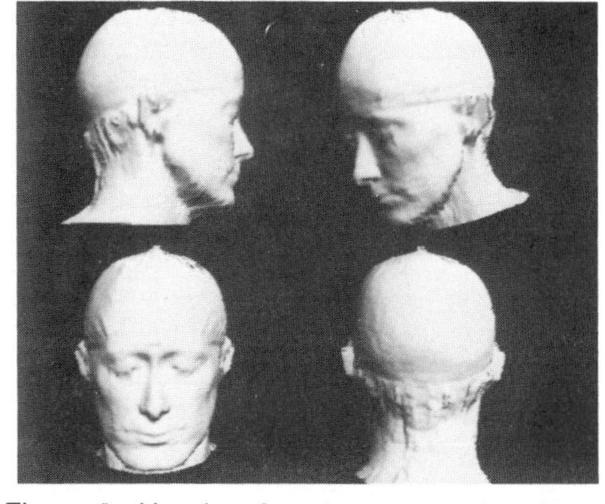

Figure 2. Head surface images produced by high performance 3-D graphics hardware in an IBM PC/AT.

In addition to the software systems we have developed, we have recently implemented this application on IBM compatible 3-D graphics hardware from Matrox, which dramatically improves system performance for interactive use. Using either system, the head model can be rotated mathematically and viewed from any angle. Small features can be captured; resolution <1mm can be achieved. A primary application of the system will be to document the location of reference transmitters (1 cm cubes) used to localize the neuromagnetic sensor array with respect to the head (Van Hulsteyn et al, this volume). The head surface model might also be used to define head geometry for modeling procedures when MRI data is not available.

Magnetic Resonance Imaging provides high quality anatomical images of the soft tissue of the brain. By choosing appropriate data acquisition timing parameters, it is possible to precisely define the skull cavity, or to resolve grey and white matter within cortex. MRI provides a powerful noninvasive tool for structural definition of the brain, complementing the functional measure provided by neuromagnetic techniques.

We typically work with image data downloaded directly from electronic media, however it is possible to use images digitized from film. Work to date has employed data collected on a Diasonics low-field imaging system. 12 or 16 bit data provided by this system is first compressed to 8 bits per pixel. In order to more efficiently use memory, image data can be further compressed to 4 bits (16 grey levels). If contrast enhancement or other adaptive mapping strategies are employed during this step, resulting images are adequate for anatomical descrimination. This storage strategy allows a representation of the original image data to be stored within a single byte voxel element while allowing one of 16 anatomical tags to be associated with the voxel. A display of image data or a pseudocolor representation of the categorical tags can be readily produced by simple manipulation of output lookup tables-- the "palettes" linking data values with displayed colors.

The MRI coordinate system must be reconciled with the head centered coordinate system employed for neuromagnetic measurements. This has been achieved by identifying anatomical reference features in MRI scans or by attaching oil-containing capsules to the head at designated reference locations to provide fiducial marks for registration of coordinate systems. Human stereotaxic frames compatible with MRI are commercially available, and may be useful for critical applications. Given a set of common reference locations in both coordinate systems, it is easy to transform the coordinates of a neural source into the corresponding location in voxel space so that the anatomical structure responsible for the signal can be identified. We have developed algorithms which select the appropriate MRI slices, calculate pixel coordinates, and display calculated neuromagnetic sources in three views. An example of such a display is included in a separate paper (George, Aine, Medvick and Flynn, this volume).

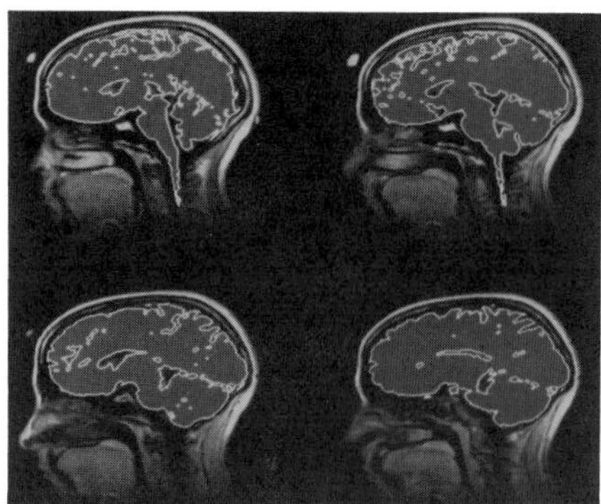

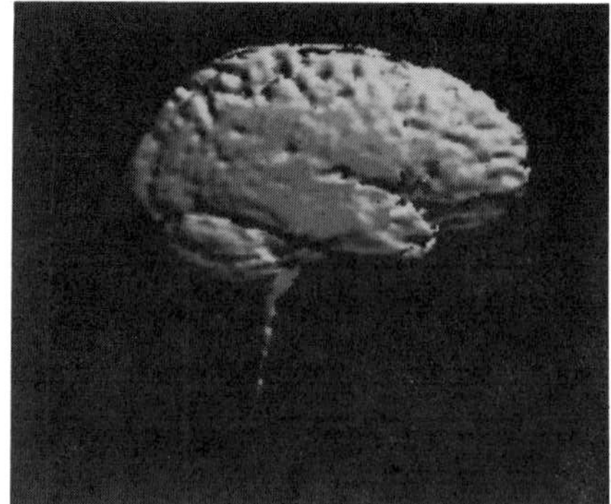

Figure 3. Anatomical modeling system. **Left panel:** Image processing of a series of MRI slices. Brain volume and surfaces have been identified using semiautomated procedures. **Right panel:** A shaded rendering of the brain volume produced by ray-tracing software in the context of the 3-D volumetric model.

The 3-D anatomical modeling system embodies two key design decisions. First, we employ a voxel space representation; every data element describes a small volume in cartesian space. This approach is very memory intensive, but offers a number of advantages for our application. It also provides a useful database management tool for MRI data collected using full volume acquisition techniques instead of as a series of discrete slices. A second primary feature is the integration of image analysis and editing features for structure tagging, edge detection,etc. This allows us to build a semi- automatic interactive system, avoiding the manual tracing of structures employed by many systems.

The basic structure of the model is a voxel space with variable resolution. A plane in the voxel space corresponds to a slice in the MRI dataset. Resolution within a plane is typically 256x256 corresponding to the resolution of a single MRI image. The thickness of a plane is set equal to the slice interval for a tomographic series. A typical contiguous volumetric series consists of 32 slices at 4.5 mm intervals. Voxel elements are tagged using flood routines; a seed point and tag value identifying a structure are specified by the user, and the system tags all contiguous points satisfying some criteria, e.g. all pixels falling within a specified range of intensity values. We have developed algorithms that extend the usual 2-D flood throughout the volumetric data structure. For 3-D rendering of an anatomical unit, the system can interrogate the data structure to identify all voxels on the surface of a designated structure. Surface shaded 3-D orthographic projections can be calculated from any viewing angle, using software or high performance hardware systems.

In the future, the use of a volumetric model should facilitate other analytical procedures. Our group as well as others are developing numerical models of neuromagnetic sources which account for such features as extended source geometries and volume conduction currents. Finite element analyses are a particularly powerful approach for handling such calculations and are well suited for volumetric modeling. We expect that an explicit knowledge of cortical geometry will be of significant benefit for current-dipole model fitting. For example, it might be possible to fit arbitrary patterns of source activation if sources are constrained to lie on the cortical surface. Our system can also simplify the development of two-dimensional maps of the cortical surface compatible with data provided by other experimental techniques.

ACKNOWLEDGEMENTS

This work was supported by the U.S. Army Research Institute, the Department of Energy contract W-7405-ENG-36 and the VA/LANL/UNM Magnetoencephalography Program. The assistance and cooperation of William Orrison , M.D., of the Dept of Radiology, University of New Mexico Medical Center is gratefully acknowledged.

AN INTEGRATED STIMULUS GENERATION AND DATA ACQUISITION SYSTEM FOR THE INVESTIGATION OF AUDITORY EVOKED MAGNETIC FIELDS

B. Ross, B. Lütkenhöner, M. Hoke, C. Pantev

Institute of Experimental Audiology
University of Münster, Münster
Federal Republic of Germany

INTRODUCTION

For the investigation of biomagnetic activity evoked by sensory stimuli (event related fields) usally two independent systems are used: a stimulus generator and a data acquisition system, consisting of SQUID sensor and electronics, analog-to-digital converter (ADC), and data acquisition computer. In general, the data acquisition process has to be interrupted if any stimulation or recording parameter is to be changed. This fact places considerable restrictions on the design of experimental procedures. For example, a complete randomization of stimuli is not feasible. Besides that, intermediate results as obtained by on-line analysis of the experimental data collected so far cannot be used for automatically controlling the further progress of the experiment. To avoid such restrictions, we have developed, for studies of the auditory system, an integrated stimulus generation and data acquisition system, which supports in a very flexible way almost any kind of experimental design.

HARDWARE CONFIGURATION

Fig.1 schematically shows the hardware components and their interaction. A home-made two-channel signal generator, consisting of function generators, noise sources, attenuators, switches for mixing different signals, and power amplifiers for driving a pair of headphones, allows to generate arbitrary monotic, diotic or dichotic acoustic signals. The generator is connected, via a serial interface (RS232), with the data acquisition computer, which serves to control all functions of the generator, to program the generator, and to set specified stimulus parameters. The generator is triggered by a TTL signal transmitted via a standard printer interface which is available in each computer system. The data acquisition computer, which is a VME-bus system equipped with a Motorola 68020 CPU and a 68881 floating-point coprocessor, has been built up using commercially available boards so that no special hardware developments were required. The ADC (12 bit resolution) contains 128 kBytes of on-board memory which can be used as a buffer with programmable length (between 4 words and 64 kwords). To allow independent read and write operations, the buffer is subdivided into two equal parts: While digitized data from the ADC are written into one part of the buffer, data stored in the other part are read out by the computer. If the part into which data are written is full, an interrupt signal is generated, and the roles of the two parts of the memory are interchanged. Fast switching from one part to the other ensures a continous data acquisition even at sampling rates as high as 200 kHz. The acquired data are stored on a 250 MByte disk. A graphic controller connected to the VME-bus allows fast generation and updating of the graphic output (1024*1024 pixels) displaying the results of on-line analysis.

SOFTWARE CONFIGURATION

Except for some special subroutines written in assembly language, all subroutines are written in FORTRAN 77 (F77). The disadvantage that F77 programs are uncapable of responding to unexpected external events is overcome by a special feature of the real-time operating system (VERSADOS): the asynchronous service queue (ASQ). The ASQ (in other operating systems a similar structure is represented by the "mailbox") is a data structure which receives messages from all interrupt sources of the system (Fig.2) and allows control of the course of the program. One major interrupt source is the ADC. Other interrupts are related to the generation of stimuli and the analysis of the biomagnetic data. Such interrupts may be elicited either software-controlled or hardware-controlled by a programmable timer. Using F77 subroutine calls, the timer on the CPU-board can be programmed to generate an interrupt once at a specified time, at a specified time after a certain event, or periodically with a given time interval. Whenever an interrupt occurs, the CPU executes an interrupt service routine (ISR) sending a message to the ASQ without interacting directly with the concurrently running F77 program.

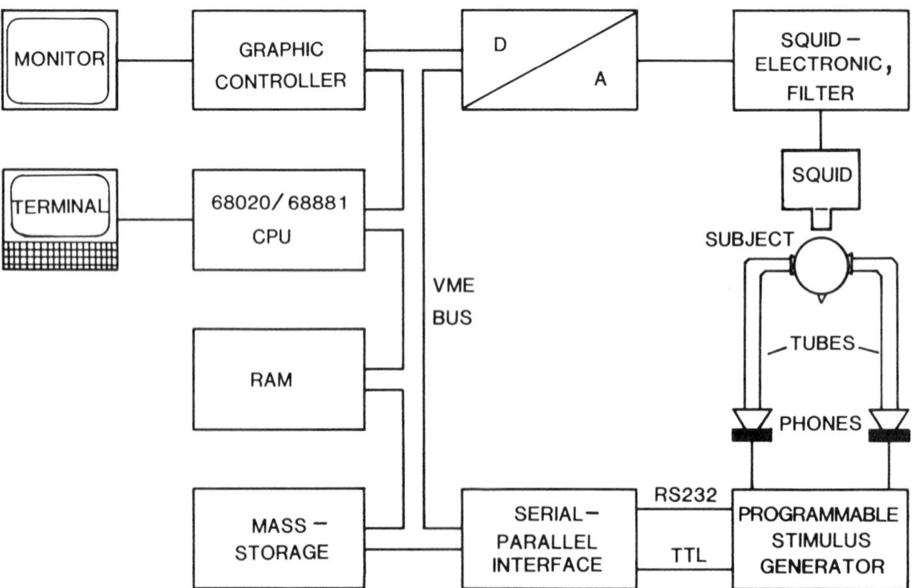

Fig.1. Hardware configuration of the integrated stimulus generation and data acquisition system.

The time required for the execution of one ISR, which typically consists of five lines of assembler source code, is of the order of 10 microseconds. In addition, the user may cause an interrupt by sending a message to the ASQ via keyboard input.

The F77 program interacts with the ASQ as follows: Whenever the execution of a specified task by a F77 program is terminated, the contents of the ASQ are checked. If the ASQ is empty, the program enters a wait state and remains in this state until the next event occurs. If there is only one message, the corresponding task will be executed. If there are more messages than one, the task with the highest priority will be executed. To overcome the restriction that the execution time of a task must be shorter than the minimal response time required for any other ASQ service, a long task has to be subdivided into several short subtasks so that the ASQ can be inspected between two subtasks, and a higher-priority task can be executed in between, if necessary. In this way it is achieved that a program with inherently serial nature controls several parallel processes.

A schematic timing diagram is shown in Fig.3. In response to the periodically occuring ADC interrupts (which have the highest priority), a subroutine reads the data from the ADC buffer and writes them into a software-realized cyclic buffer set up in the random access memory (RAM). The data are written to a disk file as soon as the data accumulated in the cyclic buffer suffice to fill one record. All parameters of the experimental setup, their modifications, the times of modifications, and the times of occurrence of external events are continously written into the file.

The change of stimulus parameters is controlled either automatically by a sophisticated software or interactively by the user. A signal for triggering the stimulus generator is elicited if the time since the last stimulus exceeds a predefined limit. This trigger may be suppressed (or postponed for a specified interval) if e.g. the biomagnetic signal is disturbed. After each stimulus presentation a software-realized on-line analyser (e.g. averager) is activated and the result of the respective analysis is updated. Separate analysers are provided for each channel and each stimulus condition.

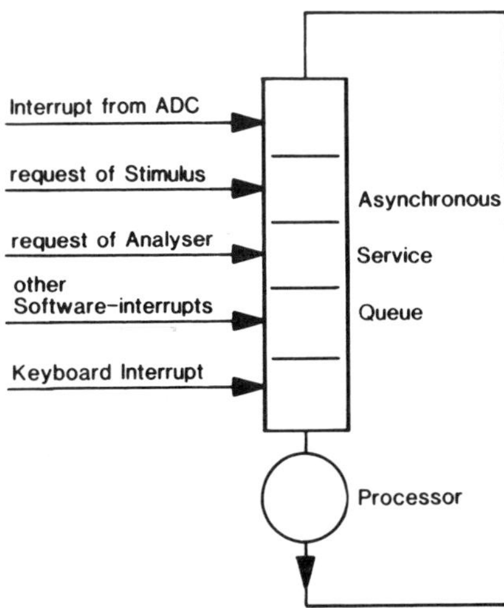

Fig.2. By means of an asynchronous service queue it is achieved that a single processor controls several parallel processes.

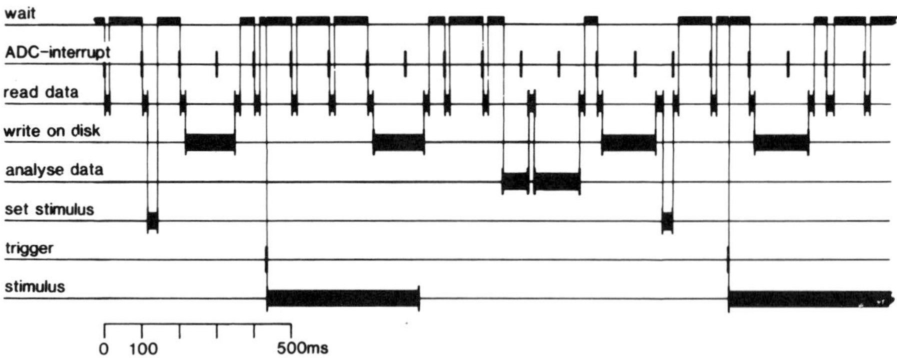

Fig.3. Timing diagram exemplifying how the processor switches between the different tasks.

DISCUSSION

The integrated stimulus generation and data acquisition system described above represents an extremely flexible and powerful tool for a great variety of biomagnetic (and bioelectric) investigations. For example, a quasi-simultaneous investigation of the influence of different stimulus parameters on the location of an equivalent current dipole in the auditory cortex can be easily done. Moreover, random presentation of different stimuli allows to shorten the interstimulus interval since adaptation and habituation effects will be diminished so that the overall investigation time can be considerably reduced. Furthermore, if such a paradigm is used to compare the effect of different stimulus parameters (e.g. functional organization of the auditory cortex), a randomization of stimulation and data collection will spread the influence of variations in the subject's state of vigilance or of inhomogeneities of the superimposed MEG over the responses collected in all stimulus conditions, so that even minute differences in the results, which otherwise would remain undiscovered, can be detected. Finally, an automatic change of the stimulus parameters without interrupting the data acquisition process considerably reduces the time required for an experimental session.

STUDY ON A DESIGN METHOD OF MAGNETICALLY SHIELDED ROOM USING MODELS

Keita. Yamazaki Kenichi Unno and Kazuo Seino*

Technical Research Laboratory, Takenaka. Corp.
*Metal Division Electro Materials Group, Tokin. Corp.
5-14, 2-Chome, Koto-ku, Tokyo, 107 Japan
*7-1, 6-Chome, Koriyama, Sendai City, 982 Japan

Purpose

Three 1/10 scale models were constructed and used in tests to estimate at the design stage the effectiveness of magnetically shielded rooms. In order to confirm the accuracy of the tests on a permalloy model, the results of these tests were compared with measurements taken from the completed room.

Method

The shielding factor of direct current magnetic field can be evaluated by next equation[1].

$$S = Ho/Hi = 1 + K \cdot (\mu \cdot t)/r$$

where K: form factor (cubes K=0.4)
μ: permeability of the material
t: thickness of the material
r: radius of the shielded room

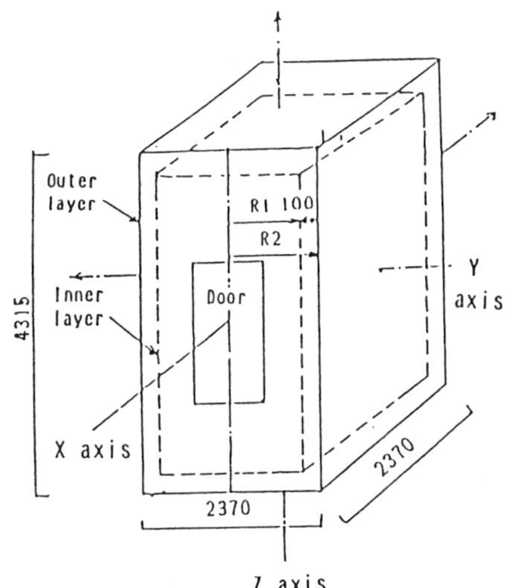

Fig. 1 Outline of magnetically shielded room

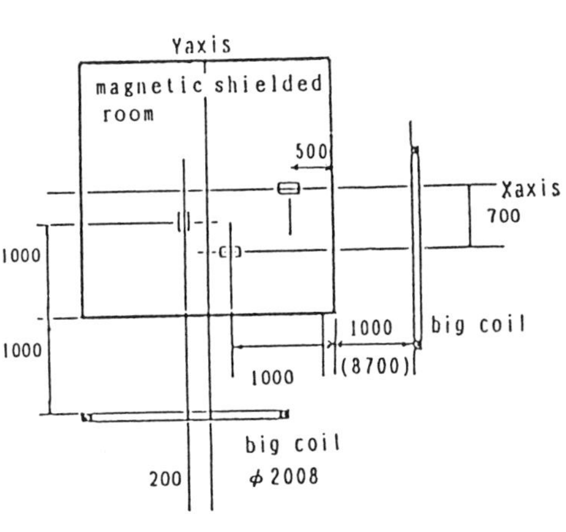

Fig. 2 Measuring method of fluctu-ation magnetic flux density in the room

Advances in Biomagnetism
Edited by S.J. Williamson *et al.*
Plenum Press, New York

For double layer shielded room:

$$S=Ho/Hi=1+S1+S2+S1 \cdot S2 \cdot (1-R1^2/R2^2) \quad (2)$$

where S1:shielding factor of inner layer(calculated by eq.(1))
S2:shielding factor of outer layer(calculated by eq.(1))
R1:radius of inner layer
R2:radius of outer layer

The thickness of the materials used in the models was 1/10 that of the actual thickness shown in Fig. 1 in accordance with equation (1) and (2) .One model was made of 2.0mm electromagnetic pure iron, one was made of 0.6mm silicon steel plate, and one was made of 0.2mm permalloy. In order to compare the magnetic shielding effect in the models, the internal magnetic field variation was measured by changing a magnetic field of direct current and 50Hz alternating current through the use of a helmholtz coil from outside.

In order to compare the magnetic shielding effect of the model with that of the actual room, both of which were made of permalloy, magnetic field variations in the room were measured. This is shown in Fig. 2. In these measurements, a magnetic field density majored in advance in an unshielded environment was given to a probe of a magnetometer in the rooms by using a coil having two meters in diameter, which was located one meter away from the walls of the actual magnetic shielded room. Magnetometer used in experiment is 428B CLIP-ON DC Millianmeter made by YHP.

Result

The external magnetic field density was varied from 5×10^{-7}T to 10^{-4}T both by a direct current and an alternating current of 50Hz, and was added to the models. Fig. 3 shows the magnetic shielding effect of the models to the direct current. The magnetic shielding factors were 50 or more for permalloy, 2-5 for electromagnetic pure iron and 5-20 for silicon steel plate. It was found that there was a tendency for the shielding effect of electromagnetic pure iron and silicon steel plate to increase when the magnetic field rose to 10^{-5}T or more.

The magnetic shielding effect of silicon steel plate and permalloy to alternating current magnetic field of 50Hz were almost the same as that to direct current field. However, shielding effect of electromagnetic pure iron improved in low magnetic fields of 10^{-5}T or less compered to the effect in a direct current magnetic field.

The shielding effect of the model and the actual permalloy magnetically shielded room against varying magnetic fields added from outside had almost same effect about direct current. Magnetic flux density was not perceived in actual room by magnetometer when an alternating current magnetic field of 50HZ was applied.

Discussion

In Table 1 (A) was obtained by calculating with shielding factor to direct current of three models majored in measurement using equations (1) and (2).The initial permeabilities (B) of electromagnetic pure iron and silicon steel plate is almost within the range of (A). (A) of permalloy has 1/6-1/4 on the X and Y axes, and 1/3-1/2 on the Z axis of the initial permeability of (B). These results were due to the differences in composition shown in Fig.6. The small models made of silicon steel plate and electromagnetic pure iron are composed of six steel plates; four plates for the walls,and one plate each for the ceiling and the floor. On the other hand,the permalloy model uses eighteen plates in the walls, nine plates in the ceiling and nine plates in the floor. The model of permalloy has the most and longest gaps of the three models. Therefore it is significant to decrease a length of gaps between members of plates. Since in permalloy model and silicon steel model the plates are jointed by plastic tape, there is no possibility to decrease initial permeabilities of materials when they are built.

The differences in the shielding effect between the actual rooms and the models against alternating current magnetic field of 50HZ arise from the aluminum which covers the exterior surfaces of the actual room.

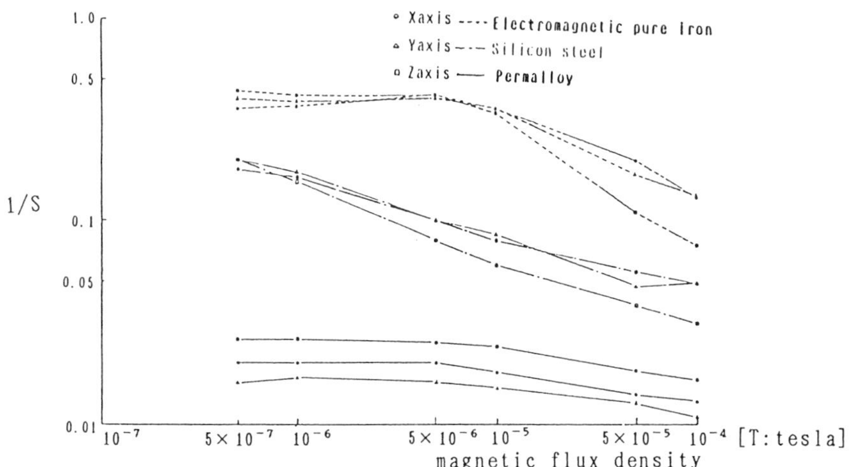

Fig. 3 Magnetic shielding effect to DC in three models

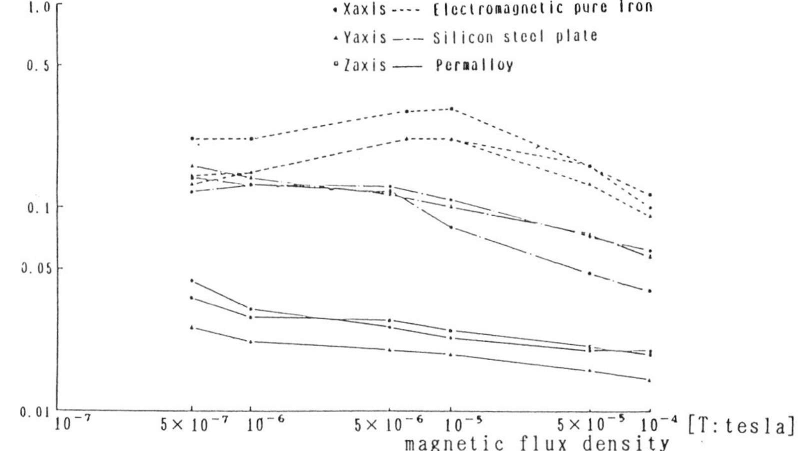

Fig. 4 Magnetic shielding effect to AC 50HZ in three models

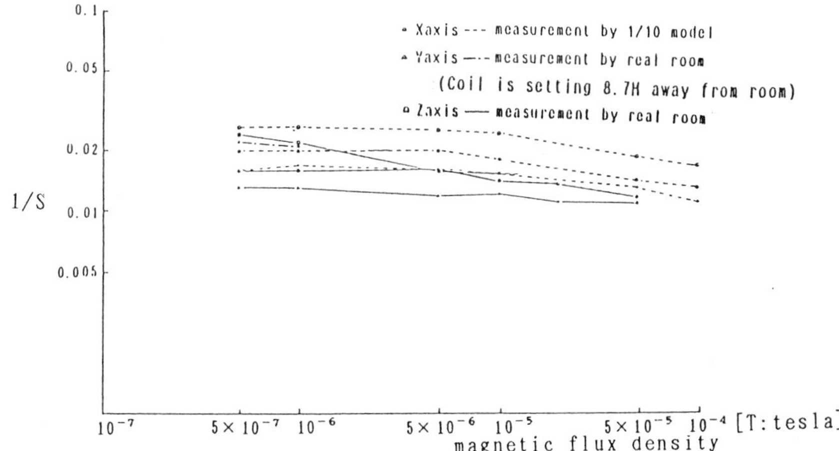

Fig. 5 Comparison of the magnetic shielding effect to DC between 1/10 scale model and real room

Tab. 1 Comparison between pearmiability obtained by eq. (1) and eq. (2) from measurement and initial permeability of material of models

material	(A) Permeability obta- -ined by measurement	(B) Initial perme- -ability of material
Permalloy	X, Yaxis 14000～20000 Zaxis 27000～36000	80000
Electromagnetic pure iron	X, Yaxis 100～300 Zaxis 120～900	300
Silicon steel iron	X, Yaxis 600～2400 Zaxis 1500～7800	1000

Conclusions

The measurement of shielding effect in 1/10 scale models is effective for design of magnetically shielded rooms in direct current magnetic fields on the following condition. Thickness and size of scale model are calculated by equations (1) and (2), and the models should be constructed with the same number of structual members utilized in actual room. According to the measured values of scale models, shielding effects of highly permeable materials such as permalloy are influenced by both the length of the gaps between materials, and the degree of adhesion between materials.

References

(1) VAIO O. KELHA: Design, Construction, and Performance, of a Large-Volume Magnetic Shield. IEEE Trans. Magn. Vol. MAG-18, No. 1 JAN 1982

(2) A. MAGER: The Berlin Magnetically Shielded Room (BMSR), Section A: Design And Construction. 1981 Walter de Gruyer & Co., Berlin. New York Biomagnetism

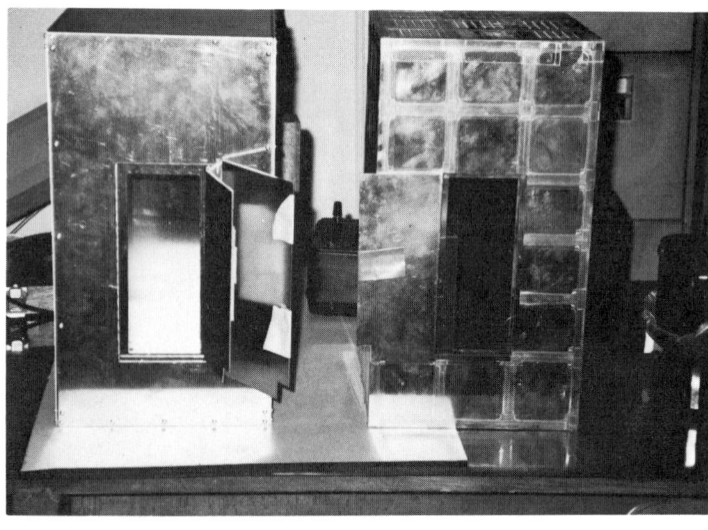

Fig. 6 Models of magnetically shielded room
left: model of electro-magnetic pure iron
right: model of permalloy

PREPARATION OF HIGH-T_c SUPERCONDUCTING MAGNETIC SHIELDS BY A LOW PRESSURE PLASMA SPRAYING

K.Tachikawa, O.Tsukamoto*, Y.Shimbo**, K.Niki***, M.Ono**, M.Kabasawa** and S.Kosuge**
Department of Materials Science, Tokai University, Hiratsuka, Kanagawa 259-12, Japan. *Division of Electrical and Computer Engineering, Yokohama National University Yokohama 240, Japan **Steel Research Center, ***Electronics Research Center, NKK Corporation, Kawasaki-ku, Kawasaki 210, Japan

INTRODUCTION

A perfect magnetic shielding can be achieved by superconductors, because the magnetic flux can not penetrate into superconductors at magnetic field of less than their lower critical magnetic field ;H_{c1}, (Meissner effect). Thus, the superconducting magnetic shields are much advantageous for biomagnetic and other applications whereby an absolute minimum of magnetic background noise is required. However, metallic superconductors such as Nb or Nb-Ti require a cooling by liquid helium. Meanwhile, the high-T_c oxide superconductors developed recently have critical temperature (T_c) over liquid nitrogen temperature. For example, $YBa_2Cu_3O_{7-x}$[1)] has T_c of 90K. Therefore, oxide superconductors enable the operation of the sperconducting shields at more practically favorable liquid nitrogen temperature. We have developed a low pressure plasma spraying technique for the deposition of $YBa_2Cu_3O_{7-x}$ superconductor thick film[2)]. This technique facilitates the deposition of dense $YBa_2Cu_3O_{7-x}$ films on the substrate with complicated shapes and large areas at a high deposition rate. Thus, a low pressure plasma spraying has a great advantage to fabricate magnetic shields with thick films of oxide superconductor. However, single phase $YBa_2Cu_3O_{7-x}$ film is difficult to obtain by the plasma spraying[3)], because $YBa_2Cu_3O_{7-x}$ decomposes into other phases such as Y_2BaCuO_5 and $BaCuO_2$ during melting[4)]. Therefore, we have developed a melt-reaction method to avoid the formation of the second phases. By this method, a plasma sprayed Y-Ba-Cu oxide layer is converted into a dense and uniform $YBa_2Cu_3O_{7-x}$ layer, which increases critical current density (J_c) and improves the magnetic shielding property of the films. In this study, we prepared a magnetic shielding tube with Y-Ba-Cu-oxide film by the low pressure plasma spraying and the melt-reaction method. And we evaluated the magnetic shielding performance of the tubes.

Advances in Biomagnetism
Edited by S.J. Williamson *et al.*
Plenum Press, New York

EXPERIMENTAL PROCEDURE

Fig.1 shows the schematic drawing of present low pressure plasma spraying. The powders were injected into the plasma jet, then melted and blasted onto the substrate to form the film. Spraying was carried out in a chamber under 60 torr O_2. The feedstock powder were prepared by the solid state reaction method. Mixed powder of Y_2O_3, $BaCO_3$ and CuO with nominal composition of Y:Ba:Cu=3:3:4 (powder I) and Y:Ba:Cu:=1:13:26 (powder II) were calcined at 950℃ and pulverlized. Powder I, which is composed of mixture of $YBa_2Cu_3O_{7-x}$ and Y_2BaCuO_5, melts above 1000℃. And, powder II, which is composed of mixture of CuO, $BaCuO_2$ and $YBa_2Cu_3O_{7-x}$, melts at about 930℃. Powders with particle size ranging 26-44μm were used for spraying. The tube-shaped magnetic shields were prepared by the melt-reaction method (see fig 2.). Layer I was formed with powder I on the outer surface of Ni plated Cu tubes (18mm in diameter and 140mm in length). Then, layer II was overlaid on layer I with powder II. The thickness of layer I and layer II were 150μm and 50μm respectively. The tubes were annealed in oxygen at 950℃ for 30 minutes, where layer II melted. The molten oxide diffuses into the layer I as a flux which enhances grain growth of $YBa_2Cu_3O_{7-x}$ in the layer I. The excess flux reacts with Y_2BaCuO_5 to form $YBa_2Cu_3O_{7-x}$[5]. These reactions yield a dense uniform $YBa_2Cu_3O_{7-x}$ layer. Magnetic shielding property was evaluated by applying AC magnetic field in the axial direction of the tube. Fig.3 showes the experimental apparatus. The tube was immersed in liquid nitrogen and placed in a coil applying magnetic field, and a pick-up coil placed in the center of the tube detected magnetic flux passing within the tube. Measurements were made at a range of alternating current amplitude up to 1.0A and at freqencies between 30Hz and 300Hz.

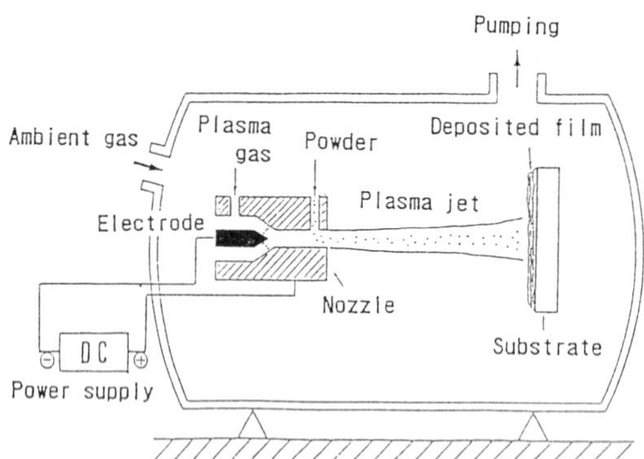

Fig.1 Schematic drawing of low pressure plasma spraying apparatus.

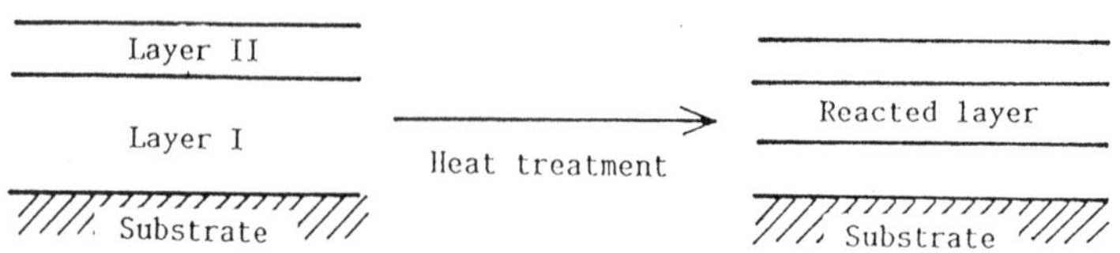

Fig.2 Schematic diagram of melt-reaction method.

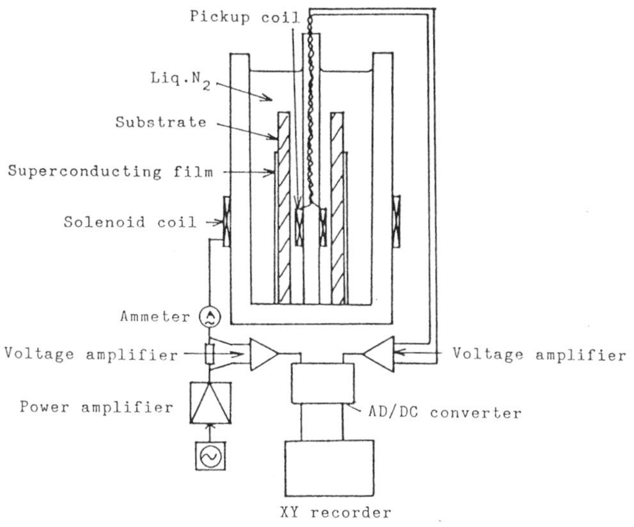

Fig.3 Schematic drowing of the apparatus used for shielding measurement.

RESULTS AND DISCUSSION

The microstructure of the oxide layer on the tube after annealing was studied by an optical microscope, SEM, and EDX analysis. Layer I and layer II reacted each other, and as a result, a dense and uniform layer with thickness of about 50μm grew between layer I and layer II. Fig.4 shows a SEM image of the reacted layer. It consists of large rectangular grains about 20μm long and 5μm wide. EDX analysis revealed that the reacted layer mainly consisted of $YBa_2Cu_3O_{7-x}$ and contained a small amount of Y_2BaCuO_5 and CuO grains. The critical current density of the superconducting layer was measured by a four probe method at liquid nitrogen temperature of 77K, and exceeded 1000A/cm^2. This value is much higher than those of ordinary plasma sprayed films due to the densification and uniformity of the films. Fig.5 shows the relations between the exciting solenoid current (30Hz) and the magnetic flux density in the superconducting tube. In the figure the result without tube is also shown. The present result revealed that the plasma sprayed Y-Ba-Cu oxide tube can shield magnetic fields up to 3.8×10^{-4}T at 77K. However, magnetic shielding property at biomagnetic levels has not been measured, because the sensitivity of the magnetic sensor used in this experiment was not so high. The preparation for measuring its property by use of highly sensitive sensors, such as SQUID sensors is under way.

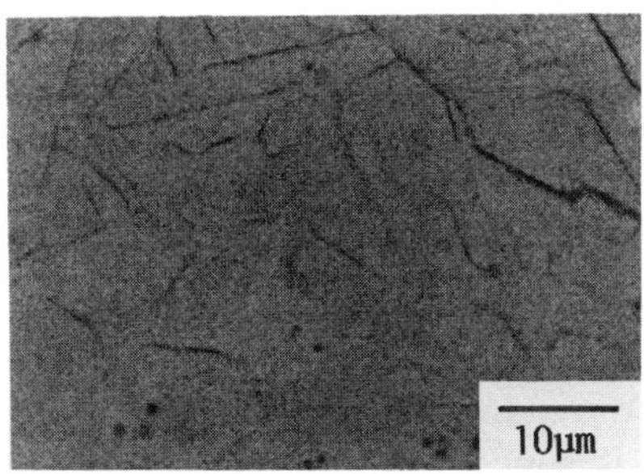

Fig.4 SEM image of a cross-section of the reaction layer.

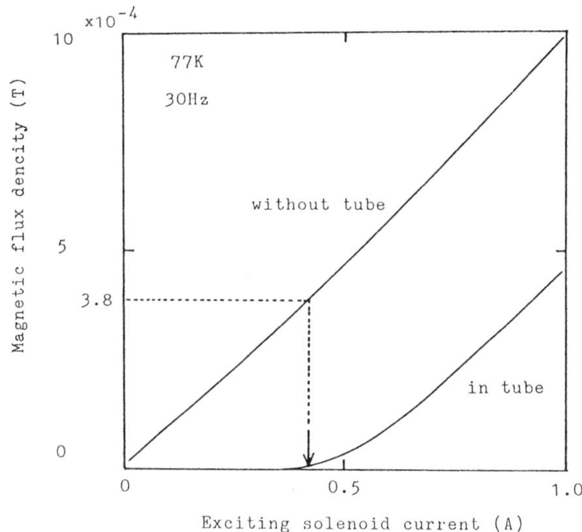

Fig.5 Relation between exciting current of the solenoid outside of the tube and magnetic flux density in the superconducting tube.

CONCLUSIONS

We prepared a superconducting oxide shield by a low pressure plasma spraying, and improved the performance of the shield by densifing the film with a melt-reaction method. We confirmed that the shield is effective for magnetic shielding at a certain level. So, we are planning to prepare the sheilds of more practical scale equipped with cooling systems, and examine the magnetic shielding properties of them at the biomagnetic level using SQUID sensors to evaluate the feasibility of the superconducting shield for biomagnetic measurements.

REFERENCES

1. M. K. Wu, J. R. Ashburn, C. J. Torng, P. H. Hor, R. L. Meng, L. Gao, Z. J. Huang, Y. Q. Wang and C. W. Chu, Superconductivity at 93K in a New Mixed-Phase Y-Ba-Cu-O Compound System at Ambient Pressure. Physical Review Letters. 58; 908 (1987).
2. K. Tachikawa, I. Watanabe, S. Kosuge, M. Kabasawa, T. Suzuki, Y. Matsuda and Y.Shimbo, High-Tc Superconducting Films of Y-Ba-Cu Oxides Prepared by Low-pressure Plasma Spraying. Applied Physics Letters. 52; 1011 (1988).
3. K. Tachikawa, M. Ono, Y. Shimbo, T. Suzuki, M. Kabasawa and S. Kosuge, Preparation of High-Tc Superconducting Thick Films and Power Conducting Tubes by a Low-Pressure Plasma Spraying. IEEE Transactions on Magnetics. 25; 2029, (1989).
4. R. S. Roth, K. L. Davis and J. R. Dennis, Phase Equilibria and Crystal Chemistry in the System BaYCuO. Advanced Ceramic Materials. 2; 303 (1987).
5. N. Sadakata, M. Sugimoto, O. Kohno and K. Tachikawa. IEEE Transactions on Magnetics. 25; 2180 (1989).

AUTHOR INDEX

Abraham-Fuchs, K. 279, 369, 669
Ahlfors, S. 673, 693
Aine, C.J. 193, 197, 229, 543
Aizawa, Y. 489
Albrecht, G. 349
Alexandrov, A.A. 725
Al-Sewaidan, H. 481, 485
Armstrong, R.A. 315
Arthur, D.L. 113, 229
Awano, N. 425

Bachmann, K. 369
Backonja, M. 185
Badeau, A.F. 551
Baffa, O. 185, 513
Bak, C.K. 93, 295
Barkley, G.L. 323, 327
Balish, M. 269
Barth, D.S. 161, 291, 299, 339
Basar, E. 93
Bauer, J. 279
Baumann, S. 101, 105
Baumgartner, C. 161, 291, 299, 339
Biscay, R. 615
Blankenship, M.H. 217
Blott, B.H. 481
Bodis-Wollner, I. 193
Bolton, J.P.R. 587, 591
Brenner, D. 189
Brockmeier, K. 421, 453
Bruno, A.C. 389, 649, 709
Buchanan, D.C. 539, 677, 681, 685, 705, 717
Burbank, M.B. 733
Burghoff, M. 349
Busch, C. 221, 233

Cappell, J. 165
Cappelli, A. 361, 365, 441
Carelli, P. 665
Cayless, A. 661
Chan, C.Y. 331
Cheyne, D. 177
Chinone, K. 253, 425, 653, 701
Chiyotani, K. 489
Clarke, C.J.S. 587, 591
Cleeland, C. 185
Cohen, D. 611
Comani, S. 505
Costa Monteiro, E. 389
Costa Ribeiro, P. 389, 649, 709
Cox, D. 677
Crowley, C.W. 603
Crum, D.B. 677
Cuffin, B.N. 611
Curio, G. 133
Cycowicz, Y.M. 241, 685

Daalmans, G. 669
Dallas, W.J. 571
Darcey, T.M. 291
Davies, S. 481, 485
Deecke, L. 177
Del Gratta, C. 287, 505, 665
De Luca, C. 361, 365, 441
De Munck, J.C. 595
DeRego, P.J. 551
Di, S. 299, 339
Di Luzio, S. 505
do Carmo, S.J. 389
Dolce, C.S. 709
Ducla-Soares, E. 533
Durand, D. 583
Durin, G.F. 393

Edelsack, E.A. 73
Edrich, J. 697
Ehnholm, G.J. 673
Eich, E. 501
Eisenberg, H.M. 105
Engle, D.J. 141
Engelhardt, R. 497, 501
Erné, S.N. 133, 287, 303, 421, 453, 559

Feistel, H. 279
Feldman, H. 319
Fenici, R.R. 361, 365, 409, 441
Ferguson, A.S. 583
Ferris, S.H. 311
Fife, A.A. 733
Fischer, R. 497, 501
Flynn, E.R. 113, 193, 197, 225, 229, 543, 689, 737
Foglietti, V. 81, 665
Folberth, W. 669
Fonseca Costa, A. 389
Forsman, M. 477
Freake, S.M. 509
Friedman, R.N. 137, 681
Fujiki, M. 529
Fujimaki, N. 645, 657
Fujino, K. 373, 417, 457
Furuie, S.S. 445, 607

Gallagher, W.J. 81
Gardner-Medwin, A.R. 323
Gardner, M.J. 433, 437
Gehr, P. 473
George, J.S. 193, 197, 229, 689, 737
Gießler, F. 349
Glanzer, M. 241
Godik, E.E. 353
Goldstein, L. 555
Gonnelli, R.S. 393
Gonzalez, S.L. 615
Gorbach, A.M. 623, 283
Gordon, E. 153
Goto, T. 645
Grave de Peralta, R. 615
Grebenkin, A.P. 245
Greenblatt, R.E. 603
Grognard, R.J-M. 149, 153
Grummich, P. 307
Gulyaev, Yu.V. 353
Gupta, A. 81
Gurtovoy, K.G. 245, 249
Guy, C.N. 661

Haberkorn, W. 349
Hällström, J. 673
Hämäläinen, M.S. 97, 125, 169, 639, 673, 713
Hamaya, T. 521
Haneishi, H. 575
Harding, G.F.A. 315
Hari, R. 87, 97, 117, 121, 169
Harumi, K. 397
Hasegawa, T. 173
Hashimoto, K. 489
Hashimoto, T. 397
Hasuo, S. 657
Hasson, R. 591
Hatanaka, K. 265
Hayashi, T. 645
Hayashi, H. 645
Heinrich, H.C. 497, 501
Heller, L. 547, 689
Henry, W.P. 137
Higuchi, M. 253, 425, 579, 701
Hillyard, S. 113
Hoenig, H.E. 669
Högstedt, P. 477
Hoke, M. 319, 563, 627, 741
Horikoshi, K. 521
Hosaka, H. 173
Howland, E. 185
Hu, P. 493
Huang, J.-C. 335
Huiskamp, G. 343
Huk, W.J. 279

Igarashi, Y. 645
Ilmoniemi, R.J. 257, 635, 673, 693
Imamura, T. 657
Im Hof, V. 473
Inlow, M. 217
Ioannides, A.A. 587, 591
Iori, G. 261
Iramina, K. 619
Ishibashi, Y. 701
Ishikawa, N. 653, 701

Jackson, P.S. 737
Janday, B.S. 315, 509
Jandt, K.D. 571
Jazbinšek, V. 517, 559
Jerčinović, A. 517
Jimenez, J.C. 615
Joseph, J. 185

Kabasawa, M. 749
Kado, H. 253, 265, 425, 579, 653, 701
Kafer, C.J. 357
Kajola, M. 169, 249, 673
Kariyone, S. 425
Kasai, N. 253, 425, 653, 701
Kashiwaya, S. 579
Katayama, M. 373, 417, 457
Katila, T. 19, 377, 381, 385, 729
Kaufman, L. 213, 237, 241, 209
Kaukoranta, E. 125
Kawabe, K. 645
Kemppainen, P.K. 635
Kessler, M. 501
Khalil, I. 603
Kholodov, Yu.A. 283, 623
Kida, K. 173
Kilroy, A.W. 137, 681
Kim, K.W. 141
Kiryu, S. 653

Kiviranta, M. 673
Klauser, M. 473
Klemic, G.A. 209, 685
Kluger, A. 311
Knuutila, J. 673, 713
Koch, R. 81
Konyshev, V.A. 283, 623
Koren, G. 81
Kosuge, S. 749
Koyanagi, M. 253, 653, 701
Kotani, M. 173, 489
Krauskopf, J. 209
Kristeva, R. 177
Križaj, D. 517
Kullmann, W.H. 571
Kumpf, W. 319
Kuriki, S. 109, 129, 181

Laibowitz, R.B. 81
Lamothe, R. 357, 437
Lang, W. 177
Lant, J. 433
Lebech, J. 93, 295
Lee, S. 733
Lee, W.Y. 81
Leedham-Green, K.E. 661
Lefèbre, Ch. ... 303
Lehnertz, K. 319, 563, 627
Leiniö, M. 377, 381, 385
Lemagne, J. 615
Lewine, J.D. 229
Lewis, G.W. 217
Lewis, P.S. 543
Li, L. 493
Lim, C.L. 153
Lindinger, G. 177
Linnville, S. 697
Lipovich, A.Y. 353, 725
Llinás, R.R. 311, 165
Lopes Côrrea, S. 513
Lopez, L. 331
Lounasmaa, O.V. 209, 673
Lu, S.T. 117
Luber, B. 213
Lütkenhöner, B. 319, 563, 627, 741
Lužnik, J. 517

Mäkijärvi, M. 377, 381, 385
Mäkiniemi, K. 377, 381, 385
Malmivuo, J. 449
Maniewski, R. 611
Maragey, R.A. 283, 623
Mashima, S. 397
Masselli, M. 361, 365, 441
Matlashov, A.N. 353, 725
Matsuda, T. 529
Matsunaga, T. 525
Mazaev, E.S. 725
McCubbin, J. 733
McGavran, L. 689
Medvick, P.A. 193, 197, 543, 689
Melillo, G. 361, 365, 409, 441
Melo, C.P. 445, 607
Mikkelsen, K.B. 93, 295
Milek, M.A. 137
Miura, H. 579
Mizutani, Y. 181
Modena, I. 261, 665
Montague, T.J. 429
Montonen, J. 377, 381, 385, 729
Moran, J.E. 323, 327
Mori, H. 373, 403, 417, 457, 373
Moshage, W. 369
Murase, M. 109, 129

Näätänen, R. 125
Nagel-Leiby, S. 323
Naitoh, P. 217
Nakamura, N. 525
Nakanishi, M. 253, 425, 653, 701
Nakasato, N. 265
Nakaya, Y. 373, 403, 417, 457
Narici, L. 157, 261
Naurzakov, S.P. 245
Nemoto, I. 469
Nenonen, J. 377, 381, 385, 729
Neubauer, U. 279
Ni, C. 481
Nicholson, C. 331, 335
Nielsen, P. 501
Niessen, R. 631
Niki, K. 749
Nishiyama, G. 397
Nomura, M. 373, 403, 417, 457
Nousiainen, J. 449
Nowak, H. 349

Oakley, M.T. 225, 229
Obletter, G. 505
Ogashiwa, T. 653
Ogura, K. 469
Oh, B. 81
Ohwada, K. 425
Ohyama, N. 575
Oja, O.S. 449
Okada, Y.C. 273, 331, 335
Okano, K. 181
Oliver, C. 233
Ono, M. 749
Oostendorp, T.F. 343
Orr, C. 221, 233
Ozhogin, V.I. 245

Pääkkö, P. 485
Palfreyman, N.M. 567
Pantev, C. 319, 563, 627, 741
Papanicolaou, A. 101, 105, 221, 233

Parente Ribeiro, E. 389
Pascual, R.D. 615
Pasquarelli, A. 665
Paulson, D.N. 497, 705, 717
Pelá, C.A. 513
Peresson, M. 287
Pirnat, J. 517
Pizzella, V. 157, 287, 665
Potenti, F. 185
Pullano, M. 665
Purcell, C. 429, 611

Rankin, D.M. 737
Rassi, D. 481, 485
Regan, D. 201, 205
Regan, M.P. 201, 205
Rehm, K. 571
Reichenberger, H. 669
Reite, M. 555, 697
Rennie, C. 153
Ribary, U. 165, 311
Ricci, G.B. 287
Rif, J. 121
Robinson, S.E. 599, 721
Roeder, S.W. 225, 229
Roenager, J. 295
Rogers, R. 101, 105
Röhrlein, G. 369, 669
Romani, G.L. 33, 157, 287, 261, 505, 665
Rosettani, E. 393
Ross, E. 741
Rossini, P.M. 157, 261

Sabers, A. 295
Sack, G. 307
Saermark, K. 93, 295
Sakauchi, Y. 425
Salustri, C. 237
Sams, M. 117, 125
Sandforth, J. 133
Sanmartino, A. 393
Sato, S. 269
Saydjari, C. 101, 105
Scheer, J. 133
Scherg, M. 97
Scheuler, W. 303
Schittenhelm, R. 369
Schlitt, H.A. 571
Schmidt, A. 113
Schmitz, L. 421, 453
Schneider, S. 279, 307, 369, 669
Schueler, P. 307
Schulman, T. 381
Schwartz, B.J. 237
Sclabassi, R.J. 141
Seagar, A.D. 149, 153
Seifert, H. 669
Seino, K. 745
Seki, K. 265
Sekihara, K. 575
Shabanov, S.Yu. 245
Shibatomi, A. 657
Shimbo, Y. 749
Shimizu, K. 397
Shimura, T. 645
Siltanen, P. 377, 381, 385
Simkins, R.T. 323, 327
Singh, K.D. 567
Sirota, S. 445, 607
Slaven, A. 315
Slobodchikov, V. 725
Sloggett, G.J. 153
Smith, W.E. 571
Soares, S.D. 709
Spekreijse, H. 595
Stefan, H. 279
Stehr, R. 133, 303
Stroink, G. 47, 357, 429, 433, 437
Suk, J. 165, 189, 311
Sullivan, G. 225
Supek, S. 193
Sutherling, W.W. 161, 291, 299, 339
Suzuki, H. 657
Suzuki, S. 145
Swithenby, S.J. 57, 509, 567

Tachinardi, U. 445, 607
Tachikawa, K. 749
Taikina-aho, O. 485
Takata, T. 489
Takeuchi, A. 373, 417, 457
Takeuchi, F. 109, 129
Tamura, H. 657
Tannus, A. 513
Tatsumi, H. 489
Teale, P. 555, 697
Tepley, N. 323, 327
Tesche, C.D. 673
Thomas, I.M. 509
Tiihonen, J. 121, 169
Timbrell, V. 485
Tominaga, M. 489
Torrioli, G. 261, 287, 665
Trahms, L. 133, 303, 421, 453, 559
Traversa, R. 157, 261
Travis, D. 209
Trejo, L.J. 217
Trontelj, Z. 517, 559
Tsukamoto, O. 749
Tsunakawa, H. 397

Uchikawa, Y. 173
Ueno, S. 145, 529, 619
Unno, K. 745

Valberg, P. 461
Valdes, P.A. 615
Valenčič, V. 517
van der Wal, A.J. 631
van Egeraat, J.M. 137, 681
van Hulsteyn, D.B. 689
van Oosterom, A. 343
Vardy, D. 433, 437
Verkhlutov, V.M. 283, 623
Vieth, J. 307
Vijn, P.C.M. 595
Vilkman, V. 673
Vodovnik, L. 517
Voskamp, J.H. 631
Vrba, J. 733
Vvedensky, V.L. 245, 249

Wakai, R. 185
Waki, H. 469
Walker, S.R. 661
Wang, J.-Z. 257
Watanabe, K. 373, 417, 457
Wazhiewski, O. 725
Wedemeyer, J. 303
Weikl, A. 369
Welch, K.M.A. 323, 327
Wijesinghe, R.S. 137
Wikswo, J.P. 1, 137, 681, 677
Williamson, S.J. 209, 213, 237, 241, 257, 685
Wilson, G.F. 221, 233
Wirth, A. 369, 669

Xiang, K. 493

Yamazaki, K. 745
Yamamoto, H. 173
Yamomoto, T. 165
Yoshimoto, T. 265
Yiannikas, C. 153
Yu, B. 493
Yunokuchi, K. 611

Zaner, K.S. 461
Zhuravlev, Yu.E. 353, 725
Zimmerman, J.E. 67, 697

SUBJECT INDEX

Accessory pathway (*see* Magnetoencephalography)
Action current (*see* Action potential, Magneto-neurography)
Action field (*see also* Action current, Action potential)
compound
correlation with potential, 141
measurement technique, 141
median nerve, 137
sciatic nerve, 141
thumb, 682
of isolated axon
of motor neuron, 11
origin, 11, 36
pattern, 13
relationship to potential, 12
of sciatic nerve, 141
Action potential (*see also* Action field, Magneto-neurography)
cellular processes, 10
compound
correlations with field, 144
measurement technique, 142
current dipole model, 13
of motor neuron, 11
depolarization, 11, 34
extracellular potential, 10
intracellular potential, 10
propagation, 10
relationship to magnetic field, 12, 13
repolarization, 13, 34
After discharge
following periodic stimulation
somatosensory, 40
visual, 40
Alpha rhythm, magnetic studies (*see also* Magneto-encephalography)
coherence, 253
first measurements
with inductance coil, 77
with a SQUID system, 78
pattern across scalp, 254, 284
phase distribution, 249
compared with potential, 246, 265
sources
alphon, 257
from relative covariance, 40
spindles, 257, 265
spiral waves, 284
Alpha rhythm (continued)
sleep, 265
suppression
during mental imagery, 237
during silent rhyming, 241
Alphon, 257
Alzheimer's disease
auditory evoked response, 311
neuropathology, 315
visual evoked response, 316
Analysis of variance, 390
Angina pectoris, 420
Annealing (*see* Inverse problem)
ANOVA (*see* Analysis of variance)
Arrhythmia (*see* Magnetocardiography)
Arrow maps, 642
Artifact identification, 225, 308, 327
Asbestos miners
lung asbestos contamination,
correlation with ash, 486
correlation with occupation, 486
correlation with magnetite, 487
asbestosis, 485
Atria (*see* Heart, Magnetocardiography)
Attentional effects
evoked response (*see* specific modality of evoked response)
spontaneous activity (*see* Alpha rhythm)
Auditory processing
dichotic rectifier, 203
Auditory evoked field
amplitopic representation, 40
effect of
attention, 109, 113
deviant stimuli, 88, 125 (*see also* mismatch)
interstimulus interval, 88, 109
masking, 121
mismatch, 117, 121, 126, 635
oddball stimulus, 90
omitted stimulus, 76
paired tones, 88, 121
simultaneous visual stimulation, 221
lateralized stimulation, 105, 686
periodicity pitch, 117
ratio of component amplitudes
N100 versus P200, 320
selective averaging, 93

Auditory evoked field (continued)
sources
activation path, 105
comparison with MRI, 102, 672
in frontal cortex, 90
long latency responses, 101, 105, 113, 118, 123, 125, 130, 601, 672, 677
middle latency responses, 97
mismatch field response, 117, 121, 126
Nd component, 113
P300, 229
replicability of sources, 101, 672
steady-state responses, 89
stimulus generation system, 741
steady-state response, 311
as sum of middle latency responses, 89
in Alzheimer's disease, 311
tinnitus, objective evidence for, 319
tonotopic representations, 39, 99, 672
Auditory evoked potential
sources
middle latency responses, 99
Nd component, 113
P300, 229
Aura, of migraine, 327
Axon (*see also* Action field, Action current, Action potential)
action potential, 7
current pattern, 13, 34
current dipole model, 34

B field (*see* Magnetic field)
Bacteria (*see* Biogenic ferrimagnetism, Magnetotactic bacteria)
Balancing (*see* Gradiometer)
Baseline (*see* Gradiometer)
Battery, biological, 6
BER (*see* specific modality for brainstem evoked response)
Bereitschaftsfeld (*see* Readiness field)
Beta rhythm,
suppression during mental imagery, 238
Bi-domain, 275
Biomagnetic field
abdomen (*see* Steady fields)
brain (*see* Magnetoencephalography)
eye (*see* Magneto-oculography, Magnetoretinography)
heart (*see* Magnetocardiography)
isolated tissue (*see In vitro* studies)
limbs (*see* Steady fields)
liver susceptibility (*see* Biosusceptibility)
lung (*see* Magnetopneumography)
nerve (*see* Magnetoneurography)
Biomagnetism
definition, *vii*
first measurement, 23
Biopsy, 503 (*see also* Biosusceptometry)
Biosusceptometry (*see also* Susceptibility)
leg, 505
liver (*see* Liver)
instrumentation, 497
methodology, 497, 501
susceptibility of body tissue, 505
thorax scan, 481, 505
field distribution, 482

Biosusceptometry (continued)
torso effects, 505
whole body scan, 507
Biot-Savart law, 5
discretized, 571
use of, 374, 575, 579
Body surface potential map, 50, 358, 433 (*see also* Electrocardiography)
Boltzmann probability statistics, 576
Brain disfunction (*see also* Alzheimer's disease, Epilepsy, Spreading cortical depression, Tinnitus)
ischemic lesions, 308
Brain shape
digitized surface from MRI, 699, 739
volumetric representations, 699, 739
Brain signals
evoked responses (*see* specific sensory modality)
spontaneous activity (*see* Electroencephalography, Magnetoencephalography)
stimulated activity (*see* Electromagnetic stimulation)
Brainstem evoked response (*see* specific modality)
Brownian motion, of particles in lung, 469
BSPM (*see* Body surface potential map)
Bundle branch activity (*see* Magnetocardiography)

Ca (*see* Calcium)
Calcium
transmembrane channel, 331
role in cardiac action potential, 13
role in evoked field, 331
Capacitance, 11
Cardiac field (*see* Magnetocardiography)
Cardiac pacing, 361
Cardiac potential (*see* Electrocardiography)
Cerebellum, of turtle
in vitro studies, 273, 331
Channel capacity
for multisensor systems, 635
Channels, transmembrane
blocking studies, 332
Charge dipole, 3
relationship to current dipole, 3
Charge multipole, 5, 7
Chip (*see* Circuit)
Chitons, 521
Chrominance stimulus (*see* Visually evoked response)
Circuit
integrated, 657, 669, 673
superconducting feedback, 657
Clearance, of lung particles (*see* Magnetopneumography)
Climbing fibers of cerebellum, 275
Cochlear prosthesis
neuromagnetic evaluation, 43
Coding (*see* Computer, Signal processing)
Cognitive processes (*see also* P300)
mental imagery, 237
silent rhyming, 241
Coherence length (*see* Superconductivity)
Coil (*see* Detection coil)
Color stimulus (*see* Visually evoked field)
Computer (*see also* Signal processing)
control of measurements, 631, 645
data
compression, 627
encoding procedure, 629

Computer (continued)
processing, 662, 669
system, 645, 742
Conductance, transmembrane
calcium channels, 331
sodium channels, 331
Conduction velocity (*see* Nerve)
Conduction system of heart (*see* Electrocardiography, Magnetocardiography)
Conductivity (*see* Electric conductivity)
Confidence limits (*see* Inverse problem)
Contribution maps, 346
cardiac, 346
Cooper, Leon
superconducting electron pairs, 20
Correlation (*see also* Covariance, Signal Processing)
for noise reduction
spatio-temporal, 279
temporal, 258
noise from random dipoles, 597
relative smoothness criterion, 421, 453
Cortex, as source of field
current source-density analysis, 339
Cortical Electroencephalography (*see also* Electroencephalography)
comparison with magnetoencephalography, 162
Counter, up/down, 645, 657
Covariance (*see also* Correlation, Signal Processing)
of random dipoles, 596
relative, for locating a source, 40, 297, 307
Critical current (*see* Superconductivity)
Cryocoolers
for low T_c SQUID, 685
for high T_c SQUID, 85
CryoSQUID, 685
Current dipole (*see also* Current monopole, Current multipole)
artificial, 717
automated localization, 369
deduced from field data (*see* Inverse problem)
definition, 3, 35
field pattern, 2, 4
in a half space, 49, 559
in a sphere, 533
localization (*see* Inverse problem)
moment, 3, 35
of intracellular current, 35
relationship to charge dipole, 3
random distribution
stochastic field, 595
stochastic potential, 595
Current, electric (*see* Electric current)
Current of injury (*see* Electric current)
Current monopole, 5
magnetic field
of conducting half space, 583
of conducting sphere, 584
model for neuronal source, 584
Current multipole (*see also* Current dipole)
deduced from field data (*see* Inverse problem)
expansion for field, 349
for cardiac activity, 17
quadrupole moments, 559
field for conducting half space, 559
vector potential, 559
source in WPW syndrome, 349
Current source (*see* Current monopole, Current dipole, Current multipole, Impressed current, Primary source, Secondary source)
Current source-density
analysis, 276
definition, 275
Cylindrical conductor model, of neuron
relation to neuromagnetic field, 340
Cytomagnetometry, 61, 473 (*see also* Magnetopneumography)
instrumentation, 463
twisting, 462
Cytoplasm viscoelastic studies, 462
Cytoskeleton (*see* Macrophage)

DC current, of the body (*see* Electric current)
DC field
epilepsy, 308
myocardial infarction, 52
spreading cortical depression, 323, 327
DC magnetoencephalogram, 323
DC SQUID (*see* SQUID)
Data processing (*see* Computer, Signal Processing)
Decay time
charge in electrolyte, 5
charge on cellular membrane, 11
Delta activity
during sleep, 265
wave, 374
Dendrites, cellular
activity (*see* Postsynaptic activity)
as source of field, 36
Depolarization, 34
cellular (*see* Action potential)
wavefront of heart, 15
Depression (*see* Spreading depression)
Depth electrode measurements (*see* Epilepsy)
Desynchronization
of alpha rhythm, 237, 241
of beta rhythm, 237
Detection coil (*see also* Gradiometer, Magnetometer, SQUID sensor)
asymmetric, 22
axial, 22
connection to SQUID, 21, 653
sensitivity pattern (*see* Lead field)
virtual, from lead field synthesis, 599
Dewar, 28, 29
radiation shields, 29
thermal magnetic noise, 729
Diabetes, and abnormal magnetocardiogram, 417
Diamagnetism, of the body, 57
Diastole
overload, 457
Diffusion of electric charge, 5
Digitized shape (*see* Brain shape, Head shape)
Dipole (*see* Charge dipole, Current dipole, Inverse Problem, Magnetic dipole)
Direct problem (*see also* Biot Savart law, Inverse problem)
projective method, 615
Dorsal horn, field source, 133

ECG (*see* Electrocardiography)
ECoG (*see* Electrocorticography)

EEG (*see* Electroencephalography)
EF (*see* specific modality of evoked field)
Egg magnetic field, 65, 509
  localization of source, 511
EKG (*see* Electrocardiography)
Electric conductivity, nonuniform
  effect on magnetic field, 5 (*see also* Secondary source)
  magnetic flux reversal, 620
Electric current (*see also* Current source)
  DC current, 57, 65
  embryonic development, 509
  induced, as source of noise, 662
  impressed, 13
    definition, 64, 273
  of injury
    cardiac, 398
    surgical incision, 517
  primary (*see* Primary source)
  reconstruction (*see* Inverse problem)
  secondary (*see* Secondary source)
  source of magnetic field (*see* Primary source, Secondary source)
  transmembrane, 9, 14
  volume
    contribution to magnetic field, 274 (*see also* Secondary source)
    effect on *in vitro* studies, 315, 393
    variational principle for, 547
Electric dipole (*see* Charge dipole)
Electric fish, Gymnotus Carapó
  magnetic field, 513
    determination of electric current, 515
Electric force vector, of heart, 48
Electric multipole (*see* Charge multipole)
Electrocardiography (*see also* Magnetocardiography)
  arrhythmia, 54, 366
    comparison with magnetic field, 54, 366
  atria
    flutter, 389
    repolarization, 358
    comparison with Magnetocardiography, 358
  body surface potential mapping, 48, 51, 429, 433
    complement to magnetocardiography, 348
  computation of signal, 343
    contribution map, 347
  conduction system
    accessory pathway, 366
    high-resolution recording, 378
    His spike, 378
    His-Purkinje system, 53, 377
    Kent bundle, 54, 366, 400
    WPW syndrome, 367, 400
  in vitro studies, 390, 393
  late potentials, 437
  leads
    Frank lead recordings, 419
    standard V_1 to V_6 leads, 344
  principles, 47
  QRS complex, 53, 401
    prolongation with ventricular tachycardia, 385
  spatial velocity, 419
  ST shift, 398
  T wave, 53, 401
Electrocardiography (continued)
  tachycardia
    late potentials, 54
    prolongation of QRS complex, 385
  torso effects, 344
  vector cardiography, 51
    unipositional leads, 449
  ventricles
    hypertrophies, 52, 397
    Romano-Ward syndrome, 423
Electrocatheter
  compatibility with MCG, 412
Electrocorticography (*see also* Epilepsy)
  for medial nerve stimulation, 291
Electrode placement
  10-20 system, 154
Electroencephalography (*see also* Epilepsy, Magnetoencephalography)
  spontaneous activity
    during sleep, 265
  template analysis, 287
Electromagnetic stimulation, 529
  stimulator, 529
Electromyography (*see also* Magnetomyography)
  response to electromagnetic stimulation, 529
EMG (*see* Electromyography)
Endogeneous field
    auditory studies, 113
Energy sensitivity (*see* SQUID)
Envelope curve, for QRS complex, 385
Enzymatic synthesis, 521
EP (*see* specific modality of evoked potential)
Epilepsy (*see also* Electroencephalography, Magnetoencephalography)
  activation states, 305
  DC shift, 308
  depth electrode studies, 291
  electroencephalography
    frontal lobe, 288, 291
    sharp potentials, 301
    temporal lobe, 280
  electrocorticography, 280, 291
  epidemiology, 269
  frequency spectra, 283
  frontal lobe, 291
  generalized, 289
  MRI relationship to source, 280
  multiple sources, 299
    polymorphic activity, 42
  propagation, 280
  source localization, 281, 292, 299
    delta bandwidth, 284
    pattern across scalp, 285
    theta bandwidth, 284
    relative covariance, 301
  spatio-temporal correlation, 279
  SPECT comparison, 280
  surgical confirmation, 294
  template analysis, 287
  temporal lobe, 279
  time records, 299, 664
EPSF (*see* specific modality of evoked field)
EPSP (*see* specific modality of evoked potential)
ERF (*see* specific modality of evoked field)
ERP (*see* specific modality of evoked potential)

Errors
  in source localization (*see* Inverse problem)
  in temporal mapping, 607
Estimation of a source (*see* Inverse problem)
Event related response (*see* specific modality)
Evoked field (*see* also specific modality)
  comparison with intracellular recordings, 331
  cross-modality interaction, 221
  definition, 34
  nonlinear response, 201
  selective averaging, 93
  steady-state response, 165, 311
  transient response (*see* specific modality)
Evoked potential (*see also* specific modality)
  definition, 34
  nonlinear response, 201
Expert system source analysis, 567 (*see also* Inverse problem)
Extracellular current (*see* Electric current)
Eye (*see* Magneto-oculography, Magnetoretinography)

F-actin
  magnetic determination of viscosity, 464
Face coil (*see* Detection coil)
Fast-Fourier transform
  zoom technique, 201, 205
Feedback circuit (*see* SQUID)
Ferrimagnetic particles (*see* Magnetopneumography)
  as tracers, 469, 473, 489
Ferritin in liver
  measurement of (*see* Biosusceptometer)
Fiber (*see* Nerve)
Fibrosis, of lung, 485
Field (*see* Magnetic field)
Finger (*see also* Somatosensory evoked field)
  movement-associated field, 181
Finite element analysis, 603, 623
Fish (*see* Electric fish)
Fluxgate (*see also* Magnetopneumography)
  gradiometer
    sensitivity, 477
  in lung studies, 469, 477, 490, 493
Flux-locked mode (*see* SQUID)
Flux quantum, 20
Flux transformer (*see* SQUID sensor)
Forward problem (*see* Biot-Savart law, Finite element analysis, Inverse problem)
  cardiac analysis, 343
Fourier composition,
  harmonics indicating nonlinearity, 201, 205
  spatial sampling, 649, 709
  zoom technique, 201
    auditory studies, 205
    visual studies, 207
Fourier descriptors, for 3D surface, 617
Frank leads (*see* Electrocardiography)
Frequency, spatial
  sampling procedure, 649, 709
frog, *in vitro* studies
  in situ heart, 683
  sciatic nerve, 681
  gastrocnemius muscle, 682

Gabor-Heisenberg uncertainty relation, 205
Gantry, for SQUID systems, 27, 697
Gifford-McMahon refrigerator, 685 (*see also* Cryocooler)
Ginzburg-Landau theory, 19
  superconductor order parameter, 20
Gradiometer (*see also* Detection coil, SQUID sensor)
  2-D configuration, 19
  asymmetric, 22
  axial, 22
  baseline
    effect on noise, 725
  calibration, 709
  common mode balancing, 721, 725, 733
  diameter
  inductance, 22
  order
    first, 22, 669
    second, 22, 645
    third, 22, 735
    zeroth (magnetometer), 22
  planar, 639, 649

Head,
  Fourier descriptors, 617
  models
    homogeneous head, 643, 537
    realistic, 38
    spherical, 37
  representation (*see* Phantom)
  shape (*see* Brain shape)
    characterization by MRI, 624
    digitized surface, 737
    obtained from TV image, 623
    spherical harmonic description, 149, 153
Heart
  anatomy, 48
  conduction system, 48
    His-Purkinje system, 13
  depolarization sequence, 48
  displacement in the body, 445
  double layer model, 343
  electric potential (*see* Electrocardiography)
  magnetic field (*see* Magnetocardiography)
  myocardium, 13
  torso model, 49
  ventricular overload, 457
Heart studies (*see* also Electrocardiography, Magnetocardiography)
  isolated heart, 389, 393
Heart vector, 48
Helmholtz, Hermann von
  non-uniqueness theorem for inverse problem, 16
Hematite, as magnetic tracer, 462
  in cytomagnetometry, 462
Hemochromatosis, 62 (*see also* Biosusceptibility)
Hemosiderin, in lung
  measurement of (*see* Biosusceptometry)
Hexadecapole (*see* Current multipole)
High-resolution MCG (*see* Magnetocardiography)
High-resolution spectrum (*see* Fourier spectrum, zoom)
High-temperature superconductor (*see* Superconductor)
Hippocampal formation,
  and endogeneous activity, 229
His-Purkinje system (*see also* Magnetocardiography)
  magnetic field, 13
Hodgkin-Huxley model, action potential, 10

Huffman, encoding for data, 629
Hyperventilation, 308

Image source, 336
Impressed current (*see* Electric Current)
In vitro studies
 cardiac tissue, 390, 393
 importance of secondary source, 335
 image source, 336
 instrumentation, 331
 high spatial resolution, 681
Induction coil,
 ferrite core, 513
 toroidal, 137
Industrial lung contaminants, 493
Infarction (*see* Magnetocardiography)
Information, from detection coil array, 635
Inhomogeneity (*see* Electric Conductivity)
Injury current (*see* Electric Current)
Intercalated disk, 13
Interferometer (*see* SQUID)
Integrated SQUID circuit (*see* SQUID)
Interstimulus interval
 effect on auditory evoked response, 109
Intracellular kinetics
 monitoring with magnetic tracers, 469
Intra-operative monitoring (*see* Magnetoneurography, Nerve)
Inverse problem – electric, for current dipole
 electrodes in the heart, 401
Inverse problem – electric, for other sources
 multiple dipoles, 401
Inverse problem – magnetic, for current dipole
 accuracy for multisensor system, 713
 definition, 16
 effects of conductivity
  inhomogeneities, 619
 estimating errors (*see also* Monte Carlo simulation)
 localization studies
  for pacing catheter, 362
  phantom, 535, 551, 611, 670, 717
  skull, 535
  subdural electrodes, 536
 non-uniqueness of solution, 16
 procedure, 38
 sources of error
  placement of center of model head, 535
  field noise, 39, 105, 539, 575, 717
  choice of measurement positions, 649
  sensor gain errors, 539
  sensor position errors, 39, 539, 717
  source variability, 39, 539
 test for a single source, 301
Inverse problem – magnetic, for other sources, 16
 effect of detection coil, 559
 examples of sources
  continuous current distribution, 579, 587, 591
  current monopole, 583
  multiple current dipoles, 98, 551, 567
  multipoles, 17
  opposing dipoles, 403
  parallel wires, 680
  partial temporal overlap, 97, 551
  two current dipoles, 97, 563
Inverse problem – magnetic (continued)
 influence of noise, 565
 linear estimation, 571
 localizing abnormalities, 607
 maximum entropy criterion, 587
 minimum norm procedure, 603
  for evoked field, 601
  for cardiac cycle, 601
 nonuniqueness of solution, 16
 simulated annealing procedure, 575
 source probability distribution, 587
  examples, 527, 590
 susceptibility distribution, 501
 three-dimensional source distribution, 592
 with potential and field data, 98
Iron overload, liver, 497
Ischemia of the brain, 307

Josephson, Brian
 AC effects, 23, 24
 DC effects, 20, 23
 junction, 22, 68
  current bias, 69
 oscillation, 26
  frequency, 68
Joule-Thomson
 refrigeration cycle, 85, 685
 refrigerator (*see* Cryocooler)

Karhuner-Loéve expansion, 358
KCl infusion
 initiation of spreading cortical depression, 329

Latency, of sensory response (*see* specific modality)
Latex spheres
 effect on lung clearance, 489
Lead field, magnetic
 applications
  electric sources, 603
  estimation of sensor channel capacity, 635
  spatial filter, 254
  synthesis of a virtual sensor, 599
 definition, 603, 635
Lesion, of brain
 effect on Magnetoencephalography, 619
Liver iron
 magnetic susceptibility (*see* Biosusceptometry)
  comparison with biopsy, 501
 model computation, 502
 noise effect on accuracy, 503
 instrumentation, 497
 overload, 503
 thorax mapping, 481
Localization of field sources (*see* Inverse problem, *see* specific modality of evoked field)
Locator loop
 for positioning detection coil, 497
Logic gate, for SQUID, 658
London, Fritz
 superconducting phase coherence, 67
Luminance stimulus (*see* Visual evoked response)
Lung
 anatomy, 58
 magnetic particles (*see* Magnetopneumography)
  post mortem studies, 485
 thorax mapping, 481

Macrophages
cytoskeleton dynamics (*see* Cytomagnetometry)
of lung, 465
magnetic studies, 469, 473 (*see also* Magneto-pneumography)
organelle motility, 473
Magnet, pulsed, 529
Magnetic biopsy (*see* Biosusceptometry)
Magnetic dipole (*see also* Magnetic multipoles)
definition, 3
of current loop, 3
field pattern of heart, 51
Magnetic field
of current dipole, 559
of current quadrupole, 559
of earth, 2
of loop of wire, 2
sources (*see also* Inverse problem)
current dipole in homogeneous conductor, 5
current element, 2
vector potential
of current dipole, 559
of current quadrupole, 559
Magnetic field sensor (*see* Fluxgate, Induction coil, SQUID sensor)
Magnetic flux (*see also* Magnetic field)
of current dipole, 559
of current quadrupole, 559
quantization law, 20, 67
Magnetic materials in the body, 20
Magnetic particles (*see also* Ferrimagnetism and Ferromagnetism)
synthesis, 521
Magnetic permeability (*see* Permeability)
Magnetic pole
north versus south, 3
Magnetic relaxation (*see* Magnetopneumography)
Magnetic resonance image
alignment with MEG recording coordinates, 669
comparison with neuronal activity (*see* Auditory evoked response, Visual evoked response)
Magnetic particles
probe of intracellular dynamics (*see* Cytomagnetometry)
tracers of lung retention (*see* Magnetopneumography)
Magnetic resonance image
3D reconstruction, 699
relation to coordinates of field recordings, 197
Magnetotactic bacteria, 265
Magnetic shielding (*see* Shielded room, Shielding)
Magnetic stimulation (*see* Electromagnetic stimulation)
Magnetic susceptibility
in vivo studies (*see* Biosusceptibility)
Magnetically shielded room (*see* Shielded room, Shielding)
Magnetite
in bacteria (*see* Magnetotactic bacteria)
magnetic tracer, 461
synthesis, 521
Magnetocardiography
arrhythmia, 54, 349, 353, 358, 369, 373, 381, 424, 441
source, 442
Magnetocardiography (continued)
atria
depolarization, 404
flutter, 389
overload, 404
repolarization, 354, 358
signals from right and left, 404
cardiomyopathy, 453
catheterization done simultaneously, 410
comparison with electrocardiography, 366
complemently aspects, 348
computation of signal, 343
contribution map, 346
conduction system
accessory pathway, 366, 374, 381
bundle branch block, 353, 457
delta wave, 370, 381
high-resolution studies, 409
His-Purkinje system, 53, 353, 358
His spike, 378
Kent bundle localization, 54, 365, 411
localization of activity, 353, 369, 380, 381
relative smoothness as measure of risk, 424
respiratory gating, 369
septal accessory pathways, 411
WPW syndrome, 349, 369, 373, 381, 407, 411
constitutional variables, 449
age and sex differences, 449
contribution map, 346
diabetes effect, 417
effect of cardiac motion, 445
endocardial mapping, 441
first recording
with induction coil, 73
with a SQUID sensor, 71, 77
frog, 683
fusion beat, 372
high resolution, 385
in vitro studies, 390
localization of pacing catheter, 361
measurement grid for sensor, 51, 403
myocardial infarction, 52, 429, 433
DC shift, 52
normal magnetocardiogram, 52
P wave, 48, 404
principles, 47
R wave, 48
relative smoothness
measure for disfunction, 455
QRS complex, 53
prolongation for ventricular tachycardia, 386
time-series recording, 655
torso effects, 50, 344, 407
ventricles (*see also* arrhythmia)
deduced current, 606
hypertrophies, 52
overload, 406, 457
repolarization, 404, 417, 429, 437
Romano-Ward syndrome, 421
source localization, 442
tachycardia, 54, 411, 413, 441
association with prolonged QRS interval, 385
ventricular late fields, 385, 437
relation to electrocardiogram, 385
T wave, 48, 53, 375, 422

Magnetocardiography (continued)
  endocardial mapping, 441
  trajectory plot, 433
  vector cardiography, 51, 425
Magnetoencephalography (*see also* Electroencephalography, Neuromagnetic Field, specific modality of sensory evoked field)
  abnormal activity (*see* Alzheimer's disease, Epilepsy, Ischemia, Migraine, Tinnitus)
  definition, 34
  DC record, 323
  evoked responses (*see* specific modality)
  first measurements, 78
  physiological basis, 273
  spontaneous activity
    alpha bandwidth, (*see* Alpha rhythm, Mu rhythm)
    beta bandwidth, 213
    delta bandwidth, 284 (*see also* Mu rhythm)
      during sleep, 265
    effect of mental activity, 214, 242
    relationship to potential, 265
    theta bandwidth, 284
Magnetometer (*see also* SQUID sensor)
  differential (*see* Gradiometer)
  optically pumped, 75
  simplest detection coil, 22
  vector, 702
Magnetomyography, 682
  definition, 12
  of skeletal muscle, 12
Magnetoneurography, 137 (*see also* Nerve)
  definition, 12
Magneto-oculography (*see also* Magnetoretinography)
  blink, 225
  eye movement, 225
  movement-related, 227
    lambda wave, 225
Magnetopneumography, 58 (*see also* Cytomagnetometry)
  clearance
    effect of occupational exposure, 493
    measures, 489, 493 (*see also* Macrophages)
  coercivity
    means of identifying material, 59
  contamination levels, 485
    correlation with ash, 486
    correlation with occupation, 486
  detection methods, 493
  in vivo, 481
  instrumentation for, 477, 493
  monitor for phagocytosis, 61
  post mortem studies, 485
    asbestos miners, 485
  preselection advantage, 488
  relaxation, 60, 478, 489
    measure of viscoelasticity, 461
    particles in lung, 469, 489, 493
  remanent moment, 59
  techniques, 58, 477, 481, 493
    thorax mapping, 481
  tissue sample, 485
  total lung burden, 60
  welding fumes, 60, 477
Magnetoretinography
  movement aspects (*see* Magneto-oculography)
  response to changing luminance, 225
Magnetotactic bacteria
  cultured, 521
  as immunosensor, 525
Migraine, 328 (*see also* Spreading cortical depression)
Mapping, localization of abnormalities, 607
MCG (*see* Magnetocardiography)
Median nerve
  electrical stimulation, 153, 161
MEG (*see* Magnetoencephalography)
Meissner, Hans
  magnetic flux expulsion by superconductor, 20
Membrane
  of cell, 8
    role in action potential, 10
Memory, 125
Mental processes
  imagery, 237
  rhyming, 241
Metabolic processes
  field of an egg, 511
Method of images (*see* Image source)
MicroSQUID, 677
  high spatial resolution, 681
Migraine
  spreading depression, 327
Minimum norm estimate, 642 (*see also* Inverse problem)
Mismatch field, 635 (*see also* Auditory evoked field)
  source compared with N100m, 126
MMG (*see* Magnetomyography)
MNG (*see* Magnetoneurography)
Models, of sources (*see* Inverse Problem)
MOG (*see* Magneto-oculography)
Monte Carlo simulation
  evaluation of precision
    in source parameters, 114, 151, 198, 544, 555, 566
    two-source discrimination, 544, 563
  linearization, for source fitting, 557
  maximum likelihood, 556
  measure for lack of fit, 557
Mössbauer spectra, 522
Motility (*see* Macrophage)
Motor cortex,
  activity, 177
  activation, 529
Motor field (*see* Sensorimotor field)
Motor neuron, 11
Motor potential, 183
Motor unit, of muscle
  magnetic field, 682
MNE (*see* Minimum norm estimate)
MPG (*see* Magnetopneumography)
MRG (*see* Magnetoretinography)
MRI (*see* Magnetic resonance image)
Mu rhythm (*see also* Magnetoencephalography)
  frequency spectrum, 171, 262
  pattern across scalp, 169, 262
  sources, 171, 261
  synchronized, 262
Multipole (*see* Charge multipole, Current multipole, Magnetic multipole)

Muscle field (*see also* Magnetocardiography, Magnetomyography)
skeletal, 181
Myocardium (*see* Heart)

Na (*see* Sodium)
Negative wave
in evoked response, 111
Nerve fiber (*see also* Action field, Action potential)
compound action field, 140, 145 (*see* Magneto-neurography)
deconvolution, 140
compound action potential, 141, 145
conduction speed, 138, 145
intraopertive monitoring, 137
peripheral nerve, 141, 682
Nerve stimulation (*see also* Somatosensory evoked field, Somatosensory evoked potential)
in vitro, 10
median nerve, 133, 153, 157, 161, 169, 261
tibial nerve, 173
Neuromagnetic field (*see also* Magnetoencephalography, specific modality of evoked response)
from *in vitro* source, 331, 335, 677
principles for investigations, 33
Neuron (*see also* Motor neuron)
pyramidal cells of cortex
current source-density analysis, 339
source of magnetic field, 12, 341
Noise, electric
of random dipoles, 595
Noise, magnetic (*see* also SQUID)
ambient field spectra, 31
cancellation procedure, 721, 725, 733
sources
brain, 597
conductors, 729
environment, 31
magnetic shield, 31
thermal, 31
random dipole models, 595
Nonlinear effects on a signal (*see* Fourier transform, zoom)

Octupole (*see* Current multipole)
Oddball paradigm, 121
Ohmic current, 5
Onnes, Kamerlingh,
discovery of superconductivity, 19
Operculum, frontal
site of evoked activity, 186
Optical magnetometer, 21
Overload (*see* Magnetocardiography, ventricular overload)

P300 (*see* Auditory evoked field, Visual evoked field)
Pacing (*see* Cardiac pacing)
Pain stimulation, 185
Parallel processor
for inverse problem, 591
Particles, as magnetic tracers, 461
Pb-In wire, for bonding, 653
PCA (*see* Principal component analysis)
Penicillin
induction of epileptic spikes, 339
Periodicity pitch
for auditory stimulus, 117
Peripheral nerve (*see* Nerve)
Permeability of free space, 2
Phagocytosis (*see* Magnetopneumography)
Phagosomes (*see* Macrophages)
Phantom, for assessment of measurement accuracy
source localization
skull, 717
spherical, 717
wire, 679
biosusceptometry
thorax, 482
leg, 506
Phase-locked loop (*see* SQUID, SQUID sensor)
Phase-sensitive detection, 27 (*see also* SQUID)
Phospholipid, 8
Pickup coil (*see* Detection coil, Gradiometer)
Plexus brachialis
magnetic field, 133
Poisson equation, 333
Position indicator (*see* SQUID sensing system)
Post mortem
lung studies, 485
Postsynaptic neuronal activity
current dipole model, 15, 34
relationship to magnetic field, 34, 36
Potassium ions
role in transmembrane potential, 9
Potential (*see* Action potential, Electric current, Transmembrane potential)
Power dissipation
by volume current, 548
Precentral gyrus
source of magnetic field, 178
Primary source
definition, 3
of a battery, 3
of the heart, 14
impressed component, 14
representation as current dipole, 3
Principal component analysis
for epileptic spikes, 300
for somatically evoked response, 162
Probe (*see also* SQUID sensor)
magnetic particles in the lung, 461
Processing (*see* Sensory processing, Signal processing)
Protein polymer viscoelasticity, 461
Pulsed field (*see* Electromagnetic stimulation)
Purkinje cells
cerebellum, 275
depolarization, 331
Purkinje system of heart, 13
magnetic activity (*see* Magnetocardiography)
Pyramidal cells, 36
source of magnetic field, 341

QRS (*see* Magnetocardiography)
Quadrupole moment, 559 (*see also* Charge multipole, Current multipole, Magnetic multipole)
Quantization of flux (*see* Magnetic flux)
Quasi-static regime,
definition, 6

R wave (*see* Magnetocardiography)
Rabbit
effect of surgical injury, 517
isolated heart, 393
spreading cortical depression, 323, 329
Radial current
magnetically silent, 17
Radiation shield
magnetic noise, 729
Rat, neuromagnetic studies, 339
Reaction time
for mental imagery, 237
for silent rhyming, 241
relationship to alpha suppression, 239, 243
Readiness field, 178
source location, 179
Reconstruction of current (*see* Inverse problem)
Rectification (*see* Sensory processing)
Readiness field (*see* Sensorimotor field)
Reference sensor (*see also* SQUID sensor)
to reduce field noise, 721, 725
Refrigerators (*see* Giffard-McMahon, Joule-Thomson)
Relaxation time, of charge distribution
in biological conductor, 5
Relaxation, magnetic (*see* Magnetopneumography)
Relative covariance (*see* Covariance)
Relative smoothness parameter, 421, 453
Remanent moment,
of industrial dusts, 493
of particles in lung, 485, 489, 493
Repolarization (*see also* Action potential, Wolf-Parkinson-White syndrome)
of cell membrane, 34
of myocardium, 373, 417, 437
Respiration gating
for cardiac study, 371
Resting potential
transmembrane, 8
RF SQUID (*see* SQUID)
Right-hand rule, for predicting field direction, 2
Rolandic fissure (*see also* Sensorimotor field, Somatosensory field)
somatosensory responses, 155, 161, 175

S wave (*see* Magnetocardiography)
Sampling theorem (*see* Fourier technique)
Scalp shape (*see* Head shape)
Sciatic nerve
action field, 141
Secondary source
as a dominant source, 335
definition, 5, 274
of the heart, 343
of the torso, 344
Sensing coil (*see* Detection coil)
Sensitivity (*see also* Fluxgate sensor, Inductance coil, SQUID sensor)
pattern for a coil (*see* Lead field theory)
Sensorimotor field (*see also* Somatosensory field)
finger, 686
readiness field, 178
somatotopic representation, 178
face, 178
finger, 178
foot, 178
Sensorimotor field (continued)
hand, 178
Sensory processing
classification of nonlinearities, 201
test for multistage models, 201
Shielded room, 28
performance, 29, 669, 745
Shielding, of magnetic fields
eddy current, 745
magnetic, 749
permeability effect, 746
high-T_c materials, 749
Signal processing, 641 (*see also* Correlation, Covariance)
averaging,
backward, 633
forward, 633
selective, 93
template trigger (*see* Template analysis)
data compression, 627
noise reduction (*see* Correlation)
by correlation measures
spatial, 255
spatio-temporal, 279
temporal, 258
respiration trigger, 369
Signal space, 189, 599
Silica
effect on lung clearance, 489
Silicosis, 493
Simplex algorithm, 563
Simulation
by computer (*see also* Monte Carlo simulation)
linear estimation of current source, 572
Singular value decomposition, 607
Skeletal muscle, 12
Sleep study
alpha rhythm, 265
Slew rate (*see* SQUID sensor)
SMA (*see* Supplementary motor area)
Smokers
lung studies (*see also* Macrophage, Magneto-pneumography)
assessment of phagocytosis, 473
Sodium
biological concentrations, 9
role in evoked field, 332
transmembrane channels, 12
Somatosensory evoked field (*see also* Mu rhythm, Sensorimotor field)
after discharge
synchronized, 41
dorsal horn generator, 134
latency,
in sensorimotor task, 687
lateralization, 165
signal space characterization, 189
somatotopic representation, 165
sources
activation path, 192
comparison with MRI, 166
long latency, 186
short latency, 134, 149, 153, 159, 170
steady-state response, 165
stimulation location
fingers, 166

Somatosensory evoked field (continued)
intracutaneous, 185
median nerve, 133, 153, 157, 161, 169, 261
pial surface,
tibial nerve, 173
Somatosensory evoked potential, 153
median nerve stimulation, 134, 153, 158, 161
Source, neuronal
electric localization (*see* Electrocardiography, Electroencephalography, Epilepsy, specific sensory modality for evoked response)
magnetic localization (*see* Epilepsy, Magnetocardiography, Epilepsy, Magnetoencephalography, specific sensory modality for evoked response)
models (*see* Inverse problem)
Source, of magnetic field (*see* Magnetic materials, Primary source, Secondary source)
Spatial discrimination (*see* Inverse problem)
Spatial filter
Backus-Gilbert theory, 254
lead field synthesis, 254
Spatial sampling by gradiometer, 649, 709
Spectral analysis (*see also* Fourier composition)
compressed spectrum, 296
Spherical harmonics
for field pattern, 153, 615
for head shape, 149, 153
for potential pattern, 615
Spherical model, of head, 37
field of current dipole, 37
Spike (*see* Epilepsy)
Spinal cord magnetic field, 133
Spindle
of alpha rhythm, 257
during sleep, 265
source localization, 257
Spiral wave propagation, 593
Spontaneous brain activity (*see also* Electroencephalography, Magnetoencephalography)
source models
alphons, 257
random dipoles, 595
Spreading cortical depression
evidence in human, 328
in rabbit, 323, 329
SQUID (*see also* SQUID sensor, SQUID sensing system)
dc bias, 26
high T_c material, 81
junctions
edge, 84
granular, 81
oxide, 23
thin-film Josephson, 25
magnetic hysteresis, 82, 85
phase sensitive detection, 27
principle of operation, 25
thin film superconductor, 25, 81, 667, 669
flux-locked mode, 661, 669, 675
history of development, 67, 69
interferometer, 69, 657
1/f noise, 84
magnetic hysteresis, 82
SQUID (continued)
rf bias, 24, 646, 657
history of, 67
phase sensitive detection, 27
point contact junction, 69
principle of operation, 23, 26
two-hole SQUID, 23, 71
sensitivity, energy, 83, 670
thermal cycling effects, 654
weak link hysteresis, 21
SQUID sensor (*see also* SQUID, SQUID sensing system)
calibration, 682, 705, 709
dc bias
dynamic range, 646, 658
field sensitivity, 19, 254, 646, 668
high T_c material, 84
dewar noise, 729
flux transformer, 21, 654
gradiometer
balance, 667, 675
detection coil (*see* Detection coil)
determing imbalance, 662
tangential, 245
magnetometer, 645
tangential, 245
vector, 425, 725
noise
spectra, 668, 671
thermal, 729
phase-locked loop, 70
refrigerated,
CryoSQUID, 685
rf bias
field sensitivity, 25
tank circuit, 25
sensitivity, field, 425, 662, 668, 670, 675
slew rate, 646
small size, 510
MicroSQUID, 677
SQUID sensing system (*see also* SQUID, SQUID sensor)
calibration, 662, 705, 709
chair for subject, 698
computer system (*see* Computer)
concept, 26
dewar, 673
gantry (*see* Gantry)
high spatial resolution, 681
illustration, 78
multisensor array, 157, 254, 349, 639, 657, 662, 665, 669, 673, 681, 725
information capacity, 637
source localizing accuracy, 713
noise, 19, 27, 29
spectra, 655
orientation indicator, 663, 689, 693, 705
position indicator, 30, 663, 671, 689, 693, 698, 705
reference sensors
noise cancellation, 721, 725
sensitivity, 30, 639, 646, 655, 670, 675
shielded room (*see* Shielded room)
single sensor
tangential magnetometer, 245
vector magnetometer, 425

Static approximation, for field, 6
Steady field (*see* DC field)
Steepest descent method, 577
Stimulation
  of brain (*see* Electromagnetic stimulation)
  of nerve (*see* Nerve stimulation)
Stochastic field
  random current dipoles, 595
Subdural electrode
  for evoked response, 162
Superconducting
  epitaxial film for SQUID, 81
  feedback circuit for SQUID, 657
  high T_c shield, 749
  transformer, 22
Superconductivity (*see also* Ginzburg-Landau, Josephson, London, Meissner)
  coherence length, 67
    of high T_c materials, 82
  critical current, 70
  critical temperature T_c
    new materials with high values, 19, 81
  definition, 20
  diamagnetism, 20
  energy gap, 23
  flux quantization, 20
  high T_c, 19, 81
  quantum state, 19
    phase, 20
  shielding current, 22
  tunneling, 74, 82
  weak link, 20, 23
  zero resistance, 19
Superinsulation, 27
Supplementary motor area
  magnetic field, 385
Surgical injury
  magnetic field, 517
Susceptibility, magnetic
  in vivo measurements (*see* Biosusceptometry)
  of body tissue, 505
Susceptometry, 499
Synapses, neural, 15
Syncytium, 13
Système International
  standard physical units
    for magnetic field, 2
Systole (*see also* Magnetocardiography)
  overload, 457

T wave (*see* Magnetocardiography)
Tachycardia (*see* Magnetocardiography)
Template analysis, 287
Temporal information
  in auditory stimulus, 117
Tesla, Nicola
  unit of magnetic flux density, 2
Thalamo-cortical activity, 314
Thalassemia, 62 (*see* Biosusceptometry)
Thenar muscle, 530
  point, 530
Thermal cycling
  of a SQUID, 654
Thermal magnetic noise, 729
  spatial correlation, 730
Theta rhythm (*see* Electroencephalography, Magnetoencephalography)
Thorax (*see also* Magnetocardiography, Magnetopneumography, Torso)
  magnetic field distribution, 482
  susceptibility model, 481
TIA (*see* Transitory ischemic attack)
Tibial nerve
  stimulation, 173
Theta activity (*see* Electroencephalography, Magnetoencephalography)
Tinnitus
  neuromagnetic evaluation, 43, 319
  remission, 320
Tonotopic representation (*see* Auditory evoked field)
Torso
  conductivity distribution, 345
  volume conduction model, 344
Trajectory plot (*see* Magnetocardiography)
Transfer function, spatial
  for gradiometer, 709
Transitory ischemic attack, 307
Transmembrane current (*see also* Action potential)
  components, 273
Transmembrane potential, 8 (*see also* Action potential)
  electric field, 9
  relation to evoked field, 331
  resting, 9
Turtle cerebellum
  in vitro studies, 275, 331
    importance of secondary sources, 277, 335

Unipositional lead system, 449

Variational principle
  for volume current, 547
VECG (*see* Vector electrocardiography)
Vector electrocardiography (*see* Electrocardiography, Magnetocardiography)
Vector potential, magnetic
  of current dipole, 559
  of current quadrupole, 559
VEF (*see* Visual evoked field)
Ventricles (*see* Heart, Magnetocardiography)
VEP (*see* Visual evoked potential)
Virtual magnetic sensor, 599
Viscoelasticity
  magnetic measurements of cytoplasm, 462
Viscosity, magnetic
  of particles, 469
Visual desynchronization
  of alpha rhythm, 237
Visual processing
  dichoptic rectifier, 203
Visual evoked field
  after discharge
    synchronized, 41
  alpha suppression
    during mental imagery, 237
    during silent rhyming, 241
  Alzheimer's disease, 315
  attentional effects, 213, 235
  chrominance stimulus, 209

Visual evoked field (continued)
latency,
relation to reaction time, 687
laterality, 221
luminance stimulus, 209
mental resource allocation, 233
P300 paradigm, 229
simultaneous auditory stimulation, 221
sources,
activation path, 198
comparison with MRI, 197
long latency response, 193, 198, 209, 213, 545
P300, 229
spiral wave propagation, 593
two-dipole model, 193
spatial attention effect, 213
variability across trials, 217
relationship to job performance, 219
Visual evoked potential
compared with field, 233
resource allocation, 233
sources,
P300, 229
VMCG (*see* Vector magnetocardiography)
Volume conductor
effect on field, 274 (*see also* Secondary source)
Volume current (*see* Electric current)
variational principle for pattern, 547
Voluntary movement (*see* Sensorimotor field)

Water bag
for biosusceptometry, 482
Wave function, 20 (*see also* Superconductivity)
Weak link, superconducting, 21, 70
Wire
bonding for detection coil, 653
magnetic field of, 2
Wolf-Parkinson-White syndrome (*see* Magnetocardiography)
magnetic studies,
accessory pathway, 369, 373

Zimmerman two-hole SQUID, 26, 71